PRINCIPLES *of* PHARMACOLOGY

The Pathophysiologic Basis of Drug Therapy

Second Edition

PRINCIPLES *of* PHARMACOLOGY

The Pathophysiologic Basis of Drug Therapy

Second Edition

David E. Golan, MD, PhD
Editor-in-Chief

Armen H. Tashjian, Jr., MD
Deputy Editor

Ehrin J. Armstrong, MD, MSc
April W. Armstrong, MD
Associate Editors

Wolters Kluwer | Lippincott Williams & Wilkins
Health
Philadelphia · Baltimore · New York · London
Buenos Aires · Hong Kong · Sydney · Tokyo

Acquisitions Editor: Donna Balado
Managing Editor: Stacey Sebring / Melissa Blaney
Marketing Manager: Emilie Linkins
Associate Production Manager: Kevin P. Johnson
Creative Director: Doug Smock
Artist: Rob Duckwall
Compositor: Maryland Composition
Printer: Quebecor World - Versailles

351 West Camden Street
Baltimore, MD 21201

530 Walnut Street
Philadelphia, PA 19106

Printed in the United States of America

First Edition, 2005

Library of Congress Cataloging-in-Publication Data

Library of Congress Cataloging-in-Publication Data

The pathophysiologic basis of drug therapy / [edited by] David E. Golan. —2nd ed.
p. ; cm.
Rev. ed. of: Principles of pharmacology. c2005.
Includes bibliographical references and index.
ISBN 978-0-7817-8355-2
1. Pharmacology. 2. Physiology, Pathological. I. Golan, David E. II. Principles of Pharmacology.
[DNLM: 1. Drug Therapy. 2. Pharmacology. QV 38 P297 2008]
RM301.P65 2008
615'.1—dc22

2006037708

The publishers have made every effort to trace the copyright holders for borrowed material. If they have inadvertently overlooked any, they will be pleased to make the necessary arrangements at the first opportunity.

To purchase additional copies of this book, call our customer service department at **(800) 638-3030** or fax orders to **(301) 223-2320.** International customers should call **(301) 223-2300.**

Visit Lippincott Williams & Wilkins on the Internet: http://www.LWW.com. Lippincott Williams & Wilkins customer service representatives are available from 8:30 am to 6:00 pm, EST.

07 08 09 10 11
1 2 3 4 5 6 7 8 9 10

To my loving parents, Irene Soble Golan and the late Harold Philip Golan, who set a shining example from day one. To my wife and life-partner, Laura Carolyn Green. To my children, Liza and Sarah Green-Golan, who are all that any father could ask for. To my mentor and scientific soul-mate, the late Will Veatch. To my colleagues, students, and patients, from whom I am constantly learning.

David E. Golan

To my teachers, students, fellows, and colleagues who have enlivened my mind and who have created for me the excitement of analyzing data, interpreting and challenging what is thought to be known, and exchanging ideas in such a constructively critical environment. Throughout my academic life, the interest and understanding of my wife, three daughters, parents, and sisters have been indispensable. Thanks be to all.

Armen H. Tashjian, Jr.

To my parents, Douglas Johnson and Carole Peet, who always supported me down any path. To my fellow students and residents, for making this collaborative process possible. And, of course, to my wife April Armstrong, who is a constant source of creativity and energy. May we work on many more life projects together.

Ehrin J. Armstrong

To my husband, Ehrin Armstrong: you are the inspiration and joy in my life. To my grandmother Xiaochun, mother Susan, and sister Amy; your love and encouragement are a constant source of support. And to the rest of the editorial board, for tireless work and companionship: you are like family to me.

April W. Armstrong

CONTENTS

FOREWORD

Almost every practicing physician prescribes drugs; most write many prescriptions every day. The learning of pharmacology, the science that deals with the action and use of drugs, is among the most important steps in becoming a physician. Rather than reflexly ordering a medication to treat a specific symptom or disease, modern therapeutics requires an understanding of the underlying mechanism of action of a pharmacologic agent, how it influences and is influenced by the disease for which it is prescribed and its capacity for causing both beneficial and harmful clinical effects.

Medical textbooks play a vital role in the education of students, residents, fellows, practicing physicians, and paramedical professionals. The large majority are written for anyone who will read—or preferably buy—them. As a consequence, they often provide a little for everyone but not enough for anyone. The sparsity of medical texts designed specifically for students leads faculty to spend countless hours preparing and duplicating voluminous lecture notes, and providing students with custom-designed "camels" (a camel is a cow created by a committee). Occasionally, these lecture notes are collated and published but these products have not been widely adopted. *Principles of Pharmacology: The Pathophysiologic Basis of Drug Therapy*, a collaborative project of Harvard Medical Faculty and Students, represents a refreshing and innovative departure in the preparation of a medical text. The close collaboration between students and faculty experts, under the leadership of two distinguished scientist-educators, Drs. David E. Golan and Armen H. Tashjian, Jr., has resulted in this fine introductory text *specifically* designed to meet the needs of medical, dental, and pharmacy students. The superb illustrations greatly enhance the text and help to make complex concepts readily comprehensible.

Pharmacology is uniquely positioned among the biomedical sciences. It depends on and contributes to genetics, biochemistry, cell biology, organ physiology and clinical medicine. Similarly, pharmacology occurs at a critical juncture in the medical curriculum, after completion of most of the basic science courses but before intense clinical experiences have begun. At this vital point in their education, most students are anxious to begin to apply their knowledge of science to clinical medicine. The clinical vignettes and questions at the opening of every chapter demonstrate the critical importance of understanding pharmacologic principles to the solution of important clinical problems.

In my Foreword to the first edition of this book I predicted "...with confidence that *Principles of Pharmacology: The Pathophysiologic Basis of Drug Therapy* will play a vital role in the teaching and learning of pharmacology." I was not mistaken. Medical and dental students are extremely discerning and vote with their dollars. The first edition was accepted widely and has already been translated into four languages. Much is learned by editors and authors in the preparation of the first edition of any textbook. Almost universally the second edition of a text is superior to the first. This is certainly the case with *Principles of Pharmacology: The Pathophysiologic Basis of Drug Therapy*. Readers will find the numerous new drug summary tables helpful and the many new illustrations especially illuminating.

Drs. Golan and Tashjian and their colleagues—both students and faculty—have made a significant and unique contribution in preparing this important book. Future generations of teachers and students, and ultimately the patients they serve, will be indebted to them for this important contribution.

Eugene Braunwald, M.D.
Distinguished Hersey Professor of Medicine
Harvard Medical School
Boston, Massachusetts

PREFACE

The editors are grateful for the constructive suggestions we have received from students, readers, and reviewers of the first edition of *Principles of Pharmacology: The Pathophysiologic Basis of Drug Therapy*. In response to these suggestions, and in light of the many important changes that have taken place across the landscape of pharmacology and therapeutics over the past several years, we have made a number of significant improvements in this second edition of the textbook. We hope and expect that the following additions will aid students and faculty in the learning and teaching of pharmacology:

- Addition of a *new chapter* on the principles and mechanisms of drug toxicity
- Reorganization of the 9-chapter section on principles of chemotherapy — this section has been completely reorganized according to therapeutic target, including two chapters on the principles of antimicrobial and antineoplastic pharmacology, two chapters on the pharmacology of bacterial infections, one chapter each on the pharmacology of fungal, parasitic, and viral infections, and two chapters on the pharmacology of cancer, with the addition of a *new chapter* on the pharmacology of signal transduction in cancer
- Addition of a 3-chapter section on drug discovery, development, and regulation — this new section describes the "life cycle" of a drug from the identification of its potential target through phase IV postmarketing surveillance, with the addition of a *new chapter* on the systematic detection of adverse events in marketed drugs
- Creation of a comprehensive set of 37 *drug summary tables* that group drugs and drug classes according to their mechanism of action and that list clinical applications, serious and common adverse effects, contraindications, and therapeutic considerations (including important drug interactions) for each drug
- Comprehensive updating of all chapters, including new drugs approved through 2006
- Comprehensive updating of all figures and tables, including 100 new or substantially modified figures — as in the first edition of the textbook, all the figures have been produced by the same artist for uniformity of style and presentation
- Comprehensive updating of state-of-the-art chapters at the *frontiers of pharmacology*, including pharmacogenomics, protein-based therapies, and drug delivery modalities

In addition, we have recruited a panel of new chapter authors who have added tremendous strength and depth to the existing panel of authors, and the second edition of the textbook has been edited even more carefully than the first edition for clarity of content and style and for uniformity of presentation.

Last but certainly not least, the second edition of *Principles of Pharmacology* is accompanied by the expertly prepared case-based *Principles of Pharmacology Workbook*, by Susan Farrell, MD, which reviews all of the important concepts in pharmacology and the majority of the important drug classes in a question-and-answer format that is conducive to course and board exam review.

David E. Golan, MD, PhD
Armen H. Tashjian, Jr., MD
Ehrin J. Armstrong, MD, MSc
April W. Armstrong, MD

PREFACE TO THE FIRST EDITION

This book represents a new approach to the teaching of a first or second year medical school pharmacology course. The book, titled *Principles of Pharmacology: The Pathophysiologic Basis of Drug Therapy,* departs from standard pharmacology textbooks in several ways. *Principles of Pharmacology* provides an understanding of drug action in the framework of human physiology, biochemistry, and pathophysiology. Each section of the book presents the pharmacology of a particular physiologic or biochemical system, such as the cardiovascular system or the inflammation cascade. Chapters within each section present the pharmacology of a particular aspect of that system, such as vascular tone or eicosanoids. Each chapter presents a clinical vignette illustrating the relevance of the system under consideration; then discusses the biochemistry, physiology, and pathophysiology of the system; and finally presents the drugs and drug classes that activate or inhibit the system by interacting with specific molecular and cellular targets. In this scheme, the therapeutic and adverse actions of drugs are understood in the framework of the drug's mechanism of action. The physiology, biochemistry, and pathophysiology are illustrated using clear and concise figures, and the pharmacology is depicted by displaying the targets in the system on which various drugs and drug classes act. Material from the clinical vignette is referenced at appropriate points in the discussion of the system. Contemporary directions in molecular and human pharmacology are introduced in chapters on modern methods of drug discovery and drug delivery and in a chapter on pharmacogenomics.

This approach has several advantages. We anticipate that students will use the text not only to learn pharmacology, but also to review essential aspects of physiology, biochemistry, and pathophysiology. Students will learn pharmacology in a conceptual framework that fosters mechanism-based learning rather than rote memorization, and that allows for ready incorporation of new drugs and drug classes into the student's fund of knowledge. Finally, students will learn pharmacology in a format that integrates the actions of drugs from the level of an individual molecular target to the level of the human patient.

The writing and editing of this textbook have employed a close collaboration among Harvard Medical School students and faculty in all aspects of book production, from student-faculty co-authorship of individual chapters to student-faculty editing of the final manuscript. In all, 43 HMS students and 39 HMS faculty have collaborated on the writing of the book's 52 chapters. This development plan has blended the enthusiasm and perspective of student authors with the experience and expertise of faculty authors, to provide a comprehensive and consistent presentation of modern, mechanism-based pharmacology.

David E. Golan, MD, PhD
Armen H. Tashjian, Jr., MD
Ehrin J. Armstrong, MD, MSc
Joshua M. Galanter, MD
April W. Armstrong, MD
Ramy A. Arnaout, MD, DPhil
Harris S. Rose, MD
FOUNDING EDITORS

ACKNOWLEDGMENTS

The editors are very grateful for support and assistance from a number of individuals. Valuable feedback on the first edition of *Principles of Pharmacology* was provided by scores of student and faculty readers and reviewers from around the world. Salahadin Abdi, Rami Burstein, Carl Rosow, and Joachim Scholz provided valuable comments on the draft of Chapter 16. Shreya Kangovi and Gia Landry kindly provided initial drafts of the case in Chapter 39 and the discussion in the chapter related to the case. Laura Green and Sarah Armstrong provided much-appreciated editorial assistance at critical stages in the preparation of the final manuscript.

Rob Duckwall devoted tremendous energy, enthusiasm, and creativity to the art generation and revision process. We are most fortunate to be working closely with an artist of such talent and vision.

Stuart Ferguson was a superb executive assistant to the authors and editors in every aspect of this project. We benefited tremendously from his dedication, determination, organization, and good humor throughout the planning, preparation, writing, and editing of this edition.

Liz Allison was superb as our advisor, mentor, guide, cheerleader, and friend throughout this project.

We are very grateful to David Filman for his expertise and patience in rendering the cover images. Radhakrishnan Rathnachalam was also very helpful in the early stage of the cover design.

We are especially grateful to Sue Farrell for her dedication and generosity in preparing the expert case-based workbook that accompanies this edition.

We are also most grateful to the editors and production managers at LWW, especially Betty Sun, Donna Balado, Stacey Sebring, and Melissa Blaney, for their unwavering support and encouragement.

David Golan would like to thank the many individuals whose support and understanding allowed him to maintain a teaching, research, and clinical presence while working on this project. Members of the Golan laboratory, Ed Harlow and the faculty and staff in the Department of Biological Chemistry and Molecular Pharmacology at Harvard Medical School, and the faculty and staff in the Hematology Division at Brigham and Women's Hospital and the Dana-Farber Cancer Institute were especially supportive and gracious throughout. Laura, Liza, and Sarah were constant sources of support and rejuvenation.

Armen Tashjian thanks Carol for her enthusiastic encouragement and tolerance for time spent throughout the highs and lows of this project. Julie Larrabee helped me navigate the electronic literature in ways I could never have done alone.

Ehrin Armstrong would like to thank the Massachusetts General Hospital Internal Medicine program and especially Hasan Bazari for providing research time during the hectic years of residency. Bigelow and Ellison were also always by his side during the editing and never complained despite the long hours.

April Armstrong would like to thank the faculty and residents of the Harvard Dermatology Residency program. Drs. Martin Mihm, Charles Taylor, Joseph Kvedar, and Harley Haynes have been mentors and a constant source of support throughout the process.

Credit lines identifying the original source of a figure or table borrowed or adapted from copyrighted material, and acknowledging the use of non-copyrighted material, are gathered together in a list at the end of the book. We thank all of these sources for permission to use this material.

CONTRIBUTORS

Ryan Lloyd Albritton, MD
Resident Physician
Diagnostic Radiology Resident
Department of Radiology
UCSF Medical Center
University of California, San Francisco
San Francisco, CA

Seth L. Alper, MD, PhD
Professor of Medicine, Harvard Medical School
Associate Physician, Department of Medicine
Beth Israel Deaconess Medical Center
Boston, MA

April W. Armstrong, MD
Clinical Fellow
Harvard Combined Dermatology Program, Harvard
Medical School
Department of Dermatology, Massachusetts General
Hospital
Boston, MA

Ehrin J. Armstrong, MD, MSc
Clinical Fellow
Department of Medicine
Massachusetts General Hospital
Boston, MA

Sarah R. Armstrong, MS, DABT
Senior Scientist
Cambridge Environmental Inc.
Cambridge, MA

Ramy A. Arnaout, DPhil, MD
Clinical Fellow in Pathology
Department of Pathology
Brigham and Women's Hospital
Boston, MA
Program for Evolutionary Dynamics
Harvard University
Cambridge, MA

Alireza Atri, MD, PhD
Instructor in Neurology
Harvard Medical School
Assistant in Neurology
Department of Neurology
Massachusetts General Hospital
Boston, MA

Jerry Avorn, MD
Professor of Medicine, Harvard Medical School
Senior Physician and Chief, Division of
Pharmacoepidemiology and Pharmacoeconomics
Brigham and Women's Hospital
Boston, MA

David A. Barbie, MD
Chief Resident in Internal Medicine
Department of Medicine
Massachusetts General Hospital
Instructor in Medicine
Harvard Medical School
Boston, MA

Robert L. Barbieri, MD
Kate Macy Ladd Professor of Obstetrics, Gynecology and
Reproductive Biology
Department of Obstetrics, Gynecology and Reproductive
Biology
Harvard Medical School
Chairman
Department of Obstetrics and Gynecology
Brigham and Women's Hospital
Boston, MA

Mallar Bhattacharya, MD, MSc
Senior Resident
Department of Medicine
Johns Hopkins Hospital
Johns Hopkins University
Baltimore, MD

Christopher W. Cairo, Ph.D.
Assistant Professor
Department of Chemistry
University of Alberta
Edmonton, AB Canada

Michael S. Chang, MD
Department of Orthopaedic Surgery
University of Iowa Hospitals and Clinics
Iowa City, IA

William W. Chin, MD
Vice President
Discovery Research and Clinical Investigation
Eli Lilly & Company
Volunteer Professor of Medicine
Department of Medicine
Indiana University School of Medicine
Indianapolis, IN

Deborah Yeh Chong, MD
Ophthalmology Resident
Kellogg Eye Center
University of Michigan
Ann Arbor, MI

Janet Chou, MD
Clinical Fellow
Department of Pediatrics, Harvard Medical School
Resident
Department of Pediatric Medicine, Children's Hospital
Boston
Boston, MA

Vinh Quoc Chung, MD, MPharmSci, MTh
Dermatology Resident
Department of Dermatology
Emory University
Atlanta, GA

Jay Hwan Chyung, MD, PhD
Consultant
Boston Consulting Group
Boston, MA

David E. Clapham, MD, PhD
Aldo R. Castañeda Professor of Cardiovascular Research
Director of Cardiovascular Research
Professor of Pediatrics, Children's Hospital Boston
Professor of Neurobiology, Harvard Medical School
Boston, MA

Donald M. Coen, PhD
Professor of Biological Chemistry and Molecular
Pharmacology
Harvard Medical School
Boston, MA

David E. Cohen, MD, PhD
Associate Professor, Harvard Medical School
Director of Hepatology
Department of Medicine, Brigham and Women's Hospital
Boston, MA

John P. Dekker, PhD
MD-PhD Student
Department of Neurobiology
Harvard Medical School
Boston, MA

George D. Demetri, MD
Associate Professor of Medicine, Harvard Medical School
Director, Center for Sarcoma and Bone Oncology
Department of Medical Oncology
Dana-Farber Cancer Institute
Boston, MA

Robert G. Dluhy, MD
Professor of Medicine, Harvard Medical School
Senior Physician
Department of Medicine
Brigham and Women's Hospital
Boston, MA

David M. Dudzinski, MD, JD
Clinical Fellow in Internal Medicine
Department of Medicine
Harvard Medical School
Massachusetts General Hospital
Boston, MA

Stuart A. Forman, MD, PhD
Associate Professor of Anaesthesiology
Department of Anaesthesiology, Harvard Medical School
Associate Anesthetist
Department of Anesthesia & Critical Care
Massachusetts General Hospital
Boston, MA

David A. Frank, MD, PhD
Assistant Professor of Medicine, Harvard Medical School
Assistant Professor, Department of Medical Oncology
Dana-Farber Cancer Institute
Boston, MA

Joshua M. Galanter, MD
Fellow
Pulmonary and Critical Care Medicine
University of California, San Francisco
San Francisco, CA

David E. Golan, MD, PhD
Professor of Biological Chemistry and Molecular
Pharmacology, Professor of Medicine, Harvard Medical
School
Scholar and Founding Member, The Academy at Harvard
Medical School
Physician, Hematology Division, Brigham and Women's
Hospital and Dana-Farber Cancer Institute
Department of Biological Chemistry and Molecular
Pharmacology, Department of Medicine
Harvard Medical School
Boston, MA

Laura C. Green, PhD, DABT
Senior Scientist and President
Cambridge Environmental Inc.
Cambridge, MA
Lecturer
Biological Engineering Division
Massachusetts Institute of Technology
Cambridge, MA

Edmund A. Griffin, Jr., MD, PhD
Resident Physician
Department of Psychiatry
Columbia University
New York State Psychiatric Institute
New York, NY

Robert S. Griffin, PhD
MD-PhD Program
Harvard Medical School
Boston, MA

F. Peter Guengerich, PhD
Professor
Department of Biochemistry
Vanderbilt University School of Medicine
Nashville, TN

Heidi Harbison, MD
Emergency Medicine Resident
Brigham and Women's Hospital
Boston, MA

David C. Hooper, MD
Associate Professor of Medicine, Harvard Medical School
Associate Chief
Division of Infectious Diseases
Massachusetts General Hospital
Boston, MA

Louise Ivers, MD, MPH, DTM&H
Instructor in Medicine, Department of Medicine
Harvard Medical School
Associate Physician
Department of Medicine
Brigham and Women's Hospital
Boston, MA

Anne G. Kasmar, MD, MSc
Research Fellow
Combined MGH-BWH Program in Infectious Diseases
Harvard Medical School
Fellow
Department of Infectious Diseases
Massachusetts General Hospital
Boston, MA

Lloyd B. Klickstein, MD, PhD
Translational Medicine Head
Musculoskeletal Diseases
Novartis Institutes for Biomedical Research
Cambridge, MA
Associate Physician
Division of Rheumatology, Immunology & Allergy
Brigham and Women's Hospital
Boston, MA

Joseph C. Kvedar, MD
Associate Professor
Department of Dermatology
Harvard Medical School
Vice Chairman & Residency Program Director
Department of Dermatology
Massachusetts General Hospital
Boston, MA

John C. LaMattina, MD
Surgical Resident
Department of Surgery
Massachusetts General Hospital
Boston, MA

Robert S. Langer, ScD
Institute Professor
Department of Chemical Engineering
Massachusetts Institute of Technology
Cambridge, MA

Stephen C. Lazarus, MD
Professor of Medicine
Department of Pulmonary & Critical Care Medicine
University of California, San Francisco
San Francisco, CA

Benjamin Leader, MD, PhD
Senior Resident Physician
Department of Emergency Medicine
Brown University Medical School
Rhode Island Hospital
Providence, RI

David C. Lewis, MD
Donald G. Millar Distinguished Professor of Alcohol and Addiction Studies
Community Health and Medicine
Center for Alcohol & Addiction Studies
Brown University
Providence, RI

Allen Shuyuan Liu, MD
Surgical Resident
Department of Surgery
Brigham and Women's Hospital
Boston, MA

Eng H. Lo, PhD
Professor, Radiology and Neurology
Harvard Medical School
Director, Neuroprotection Research Laboratory
Departments of Neurology and Radiology
Massachusetts General Hospital
Boston, MA

Daniel H. Lowenstein, MD
Professor of Neurology
Director, UCSF Epilepsy Center
Department of Neurology
University of California, San Francisco
San Francisco, CA

Thomas Michel, MD, PhD
Professor of Medicine (Biochemistry), Harvard Medical School
Senior Physician, Cardiovascular Division, Brigham and Women's Hospital
Boston, MA

Keith W. Miller, MA, DPhil
Edward Mallinckrodt Professor of Pharmacology
Department of Biological Chemistry and Molecular
Pharmacology
Harvard Medical School
Pharmacologist
Department of Anesthesia and Critical Care
Massachusetts General Hospital
Boston, MA

Joshua D. Moss, MD
Fellow
Cardiovascular Division
Hospital of the University of Pennsylvania
Philadelphia, PA

Martin G. Myers, Jr., MD, PhD
Associate Professor of Medicine
Division of Metabolism, Endocrinology and Diabetes
University of Michigan Medical School
Ann Arbor, MI

Mireya Nadal-Vicens, MD, PhD
Resident Tutor in Medicine
Mather House
Harvard University
Cambridge, MA
Child and Adolescent Psychiatry Fellow
Department of Child and Adolescent Psychiatry
Massachusetts General Hospital
Boston, MA

Dalia Shoretz Nagel, MD
Resident
Department of Ophthalmology
The Mount Sinai School of Medicine
New York, NY

Thomas P. Rocco, MD
Associate Professor of Medicine, Harvard Medical School
Cardiovascular Division, Brigham and Women's Hospital
Boston, MA
Associate Chief, Cardiology Section, VA Boston
Healthcare System
West Roxbury, MA

Harris S. Rose, MD
Resident
Department of Orthopaedic Surgery
University of Texas Health Science Center - Houston
Houston, TX

Edward T. Ryan, MD
Assistant Professor of Medicine, Harvard Medical School
Director, Tropical and Geographic Medicine Center,
Division of Infectious Diseases, Massachusetts General
Hospital
Boston, MA

Marvin Ryou, MD
Clinical & Research Fellow
Division of Gastroenterology
Brigham and Women's Hospital
Boston, MA

Joshua M. Schulman
Harvard Medical School
Boston, MA

Charles N. Serhan, PhD
Simon Gelman Professor of Anesthesia (Biological
Chemistry and Molecular Pharmacology), Harvard
Medical School
Director, Center for Experimental Therapeutics and
Reperfusion Injury
Department of Anesthesiology, Perioperative and Pain
Medicine
Brigham and Women's Hospital
Boston, MA

Helen M. Shields, MD
Associate Professor, Harvard Medical School
Physician, Department of Medicine
Beth Israel Deaconess Medical Center
Boston, MA

Steven E. Shoelson, MD, PhD
Professor, Department of Medicine, Harvard Medical
School
Associate Director, Research Division, Joslin Diabetes
Center
Boston, MA

Aimee D. Shu, MD
Clinical Fellow
Division of Endocrinology
Department of Medicine
Columbia University Medical Center
New York, NY

Josef B. Simon, MD
Resident
Orthopedic Surgery
Harvard Medical School
Massachusetts General Hospital
Boston, MA

David G. Standaert, MD, PhD
Professor
Department of Neurology
University of Alabama at Birmingham
Birmingham, AL

Gary R. Strichartz, PhD
Professor of Anaesthesia, Harvard Medical School
Director, Pain Research Center
Department of Anesthesiology, Perioperative and Pain
Medicine
Brigham and Women's Hospital
Boston, MA

Robert M. Swift, MD, PhD
Professor
Department of Psychiatry & Human Behavior
Center for Alcohol & Addiction Studies
Brown University
Associate Chief of Staff for Research
Providence Veterans Administration Medical Center
Providence, RI

Cullen Taniguchi, MD, PhD
Postdoctoral Fellow
Molecular and Cellular Physiology
Joslin Diabetes Center
Harvard Medical School
Boston, MA

Armen H. Tashjian, Jr., MD
Professor of Biological Chemistry and Molecular
Pharmacology, *emeritus*
Harvard Medical School
Professor of Toxicology, *emeritus*
Harvard School of Public Health
Department of Genetics and Complex Diseases
Harvard School of Public Health
Boston, MA

Charles Russell Taylor, MD
Associate Professor
Department of Dermatology
Harvard Medical School
Director of Phototherapy; Staff Dermatologist
Department of Dermatology
Massachusetts General Hospital
Boston, MA

Timothy John Turner, PhD
Assistant Research Professor
Department of Neuroscience
Tufts University School of Medicine
Boston, MA

*Michael Tsan Ty, MD, MS
Clinical Fellow in Neurology
Massachusetts General Hospital/Brigham and Women's
Hospital Neurology Program
Boston, MA
*deceased

John L. Vahle, DVM, PhD
Senior Research Advisor
Pathology and Toxicology
Lilly Research Laboratories
Greenfield, IN

Andrew J. Wagner, MD, PhD
Instructor in Medicine
Harvard Medical School
Department of Medical Oncology
Dana-Farber Cancer Institute
Boston, MA

Liewei Wang, MD, PhD
Assistant Professor
Department of Molecular Pharmacology and Experimental
Therapeutics
Mayo Clinic College of Medicine
Associate Consultant
Department of Molecular Pharmacology and Experimental
Therapeutics
Mayo Clinic
Rochester, MN

Richard M. Weinshilboum, MD
Professor
Department of Molecular Pharmacology and Experimental
Therapeutics
Mayo Clinic College of Medicine
Consultant
Department of Molecular Pharmacology and Experimental
Therapeutics
Mayo Clinic
Rochester, MN

*Ariel Weissmann, MD, MPH
Resident in Internal Medicine
Boston Medical Center
Boston, MA
*deceased

Freddie M. Williams, MD
Fellow
Cardiovascular Division
University of Virginia
Charlottesville, VA

Clifford J. Woolf, MD, PhD
Richard J. Kitz Professor of Anesthesia Research, Harvard
Medical School
Director, Neural Plasticity Research Group, Department of
Anesthesia and Critical Care
Massachusetts General Hospital
Boston, MA

Jacob Wouden, MD
Clinical Fellow
Department of Radiology
Harvard Medical School
Resident
Department of Radiology
Brigham and Women's Hospital
Boston, MA

Robert W. Yeh, MD, MBA, MSc
Cardiology Fellow
Cardiology Division
Department of Medicine
University of California, San Francisco
San Francisco, CA

Fundamental Principles of Pharmacology

1

Drug-Receptor Interactions

Christopher W. Cairo, Josef B. Simon, and David E. Golan

INTRODUCTION

Why is it that one drug affects cardiac function and another alters water and ion balance in the kidney? Why does **ciprofloxacin** effectively kill bacteria, but rarely harms a patient? These questions can be answered by first examining the interaction between a drug and its specific molecular target and then considering the role of that action in a broader physiologic context. This chapter focuses on the molecular details of drug–receptor interactions, emphasizing the variety of receptors and their molecular mechanisms. This discussion provides a conceptual basis for the action of the many drugs and drug classes discussed in this book. It also serves as a background for Chapter 2, Pharmacodynamics, which discusses the quantitative relationships between drug–receptor interactions and pharmacologic effect.

Although drugs can theoretically bind to almost any three-dimensional target, most drugs achieve their desired (therapeutic) effects by interacting selectively with target molecules that play important roles in physiologic or pathophysiologic functioning. In many cases, selectivity of drug binding to receptors also determines the undesired (adverse)

effects of a drug. In general, **drugs** are molecules that interact with specific molecular components of an organism to cause biochemical and physiologic changes within that organism. Drug **receptors** are macromolecules that, upon binding to a drug, mediate those biochemical and physiologic changes.

Case

Intent on enjoying his newly found retirement, Mr. B has made a point of playing tennis as often as possible during the past year. For the past 3 months, however, he has noted increasing fatigue. Moreover, he is now unable to finish a meal, despite being an avid life-long eater. Worried and wondering what these nonspecific symptoms mean, Mr. B schedules an appointment with his doctor. On physical examination, the physician notes that Mr. B has an enlarged spleen, extending approximately 10 cm below the left costal margin; the physical exam is otherwise within normal limits. Blood tests show an increased total white blood cell count (70,000 cells/mm^3) with an absolute increase in neutrophils, band forms, metamyelocytes, and myelocytes, but no blast cells (undifferentiated precursor cells). Cytogenetic analysis of metaphase cells demonstrates that 90% of Mr. B's myeloid cells possess the Philadelphia chromosome (indicating a translocation between chromosomes 9 and 22), confirming the diagnosis of chronic myeloid leukemia. The physician initiates therapy with **imatinib**, a highly selective inhibitor of the BCR-Abl tyrosine kinase that is encoded by the Philadelphia chromosome. Over the next month, the cells containing the Philadelphia chromosome disappear completely from Mr. B's blood, and he begins to feel well enough to compete in a seniors' tennis tournament. Mr. B continues to take imatinib every day, and he has a completely normal blood count and no feelings of fatigue. He is not sure what the future will bring, but he is glad to have been given the chance to enjoy a healthy retirement.

QUESTIONS

■ **1.** How does the BCR-Abl receptor tyrosine kinase affect intracellular signaling pathways?
■ **2.** How does imatinib interrupt the activity of the BCR-Abl protein?
■ **3.** Unlike imatinib, most of the older therapies for chronic myeloid leukemia (such as interferon-α) had significant "flu-like" side effects. Why did these therapies cause significant adverse effects in most patients, whereas (as in this case) imatinib causes side effects in very few patients?
■ **4.** Why is imatinib a specific therapy for chronic myeloid leukemia? Is this specificity related to the lack of side effects associated with imatinib therapy?

CONFORMATION AND CHEMISTRY OF DRUGS AND RECEPTORS

Why does imatinib act specifically on the BCR-Abl receptor tyrosine kinase and not on other molecules? The answer to this question, and an understanding of why any drug binds to a particular receptor, can be found in the structure and chemical properties of the two molecules. This section discusses the basic determinants of receptor structure and the chemistry of drug–receptor binding. The discussion here focuses primarily on the interactions of drugs that are small organic molecules with target receptors that are mainly macromolecules (especially proteins), but many of these principles also apply to the interactions of protein-based therapeutics with their molecular targets (see Chapter 53, Protein-Based Therapies).

Because many human and microbial drug receptors are proteins, it is useful to review the four major levels of protein structure (Fig. 1-1). At the most basic level, proteins consist of long chains of amino acids, the sequences of which are determined by the sequences of the DNA that code for the proteins. A protein's amino acid sequence is referred to as its **primary structure.** Once a long chain of amino acids has been synthesized on a ribosome, many of the amino acids begin to interact with nearby amino acids in the polypeptide

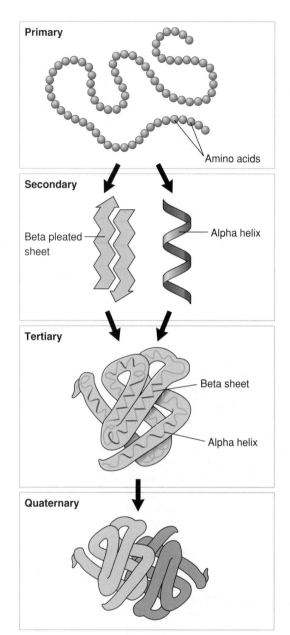

Figure 1-1. Levels of protein structure. Protein structure can be divided into four levels of complexity, referred to as *primary, secondary, tertiary*, and *quaternary* structure. Primary structure is determined by the sequence of amino acids that make up the polypeptide chain. Secondary structure is determined by the interaction of positively charged hydrogen atoms with negatively charged oxygen atoms on carbons from the same polypeptide chain. These interactions result in a number of characteristic secondary patterns of protein conformation, including the α helix and β pleated sheet. Tertiary structure is determined by the interactions of amino acids that are relatively far apart on the protein backbone. These interactions, which include ionic bonds and covalent disulfide linkages (among others), give proteins their characteristic three-dimensional structure. Quaternary structure is determined by the binding interactions among two or more independent protein subunits.

chain. These interactions result in the **secondary structure** of the protein, forming well-defined conformations such as the α helix, β pleated sheet, and β barrel. As a result of their highly organized shape, these structures often pack tightly with one another, further defining the overall shape of the protein. **Tertiary structure** results from the interaction of amino acids more distal to one another along a single amino acid chain. These interactions include ionic bond formation and the covalent linkage of sulfur atoms to form intramolecular disulfide bridges. Finally, polypeptides may oligomerize to form more complex structures. The conformation that results from the interaction of separate polypeptides is referred to as the **quaternary structure.**

Different portions of a protein's structure generally have different affinities for water, and this feature has an additional effect on the protein's shape. Because both the extracellular and intracellular environments are composed primarily of water, **hydrophobic** protein segments are often drawn to the inside of the protein or shielded from water by insertion into lipid bilayer membranes. Conversely, **hydrophilic** protein segments are often located on a protein's exterior surface. After all of this twisting and turning is completed, each protein has a unique shape that determines its function, location in the body, relationship to cellular membranes, and binding interactions with drugs and other macromolecules.

The site on the receptor at which the drug binds is called its **binding site.** Each drug-binding site has unique chemical characteristics that are determined by the specific properties of the amino acids that make up the site. The three-dimensional structure, shape, and reactivity of the site, and the inherent structure, shape, and reactivity of the drug, determine the orientation of the drug with respect to the receptor and govern how tightly these molecules bind to one another. Drug–receptor binding is the result of multiple chemical interactions between the two molecules, some of which are fairly weak (such as van der Waals forces) and some of which are extremely strong (such as covalent bonding). The sum total of these interactions provides the specificity of the overall drug–receptor inter-

action. The favorability of a drug–receptor interaction is referred to as the **affinity** of the drug for its binding site on the receptor. This concept is discussed in more detail in Chapter 2. The chemistry of the local environment in which these interactions occur—such as the hydrophobicity, hydrophilicity, and pK_a of amino acids near the binding site—may also affect the affinity of the drug–receptor interaction. The primary forces that contribute to drug–receptor affinity are described below and in Table 1-1.

van der Waals forces, resulting from the induced polarity on a molecule caused by the shifting of its electron density, provide a weak attractive force for drugs and their receptors. This induced polarity is a ubiquitous component of all molecular interactions. **Hydrogen bonding,** mediated by the interaction between positively polarized atoms (such as hydrogen attached to nitrogen or oxygen) and negatively polarized atoms (such as oxygen, nitrogen, or sulfur), results in bonds of significant strength. Hydrogen bonds give β pleated sheets and α helices their structure. **Ionic interactions,** which occur between atoms with opposite charges, are stronger than hydrogen bonds but less strong than covalent bonds. **Covalent bonding** results from the sharing of a pair of electrons between two atoms on different molecules. Covalent interactions are so strong that, in most cases, they are essentially irreversible. Table 1-1 indicates the mechanism of interaction and relative strength of each of these types of bonds. As noted above, the environment in which drugs and receptors interact also affects the favorability of binding. The **hydrophobic effect** refers to the mechanism by which the unique properties of the ubiquitous solvent water cause the interaction of a hydrophobic molecule with a hydrophobic binding site to be enhanced.

Rarely is drug–receptor binding caused by a single type of interaction; rather, it is a combination of these binding interactions that provides drugs and receptors with the forces necessary to form a stable drug–receptor complex. In general, multiple weak forces comprise the majority of drug–receptor interactions: a typical drug–receptor interaction may consist of 10 or more van der Waals interactions and a few hydrogen bonds; ionic interactions and covalent

TABLE 1-1	Relative Strength of Bonds between Receptors and Drugs		
BOND TYPE	**MECHANISM**	**BOND STRENGTH**
van der Waals	Shifting electron density in areas of a molecule, or in a molecule as a whole, results in the generation of transient positive or negative charges. These areas interact with transient areas of opposite charge on another molecule.	+
Hydrogen	Hydrogen atoms bound to nitrogen or oxygen become more positively polarized, allowing them to bond to more negatively polarized atoms such as oxygen, nitrogen, or sulfur.	+ +
Ionic	Atoms with an excess of electrons (imparting an overall negative charge on the atom) are attracted to atoms with a deficiency of electrons (imparting an overall positive charge on the atom).	+ + +
Covalent	Two bonding atoms share electrons.	+ + + +

bonding are much less common. For example, imatinib forms many van der Waals interactions and hydrogen bonds with the ATP-binding site of the BCR-Abl tyrosine kinase. The sum total of these forces creates a strong (high affinity) interaction between this drug and its receptor (Fig. 1-2).

Although relatively rare, covalent interactions between a drug and its receptor are a special case. The formation of a covalent bond is often essentially irreversible, and in such cases the drug and receptor form an inactive complex. To regain activity, the cell must synthesize a new receptor molecule to replace the inactivated protein; and the drug molecule, which is also part of the inactive complex, is not available to inhibit other receptor molecules. Drugs that modify their target receptors (often enzymes) through this mechanism are sometimes called **suicide substrates**.

The molecular structure of a drug dictates the physical and chemical properties that contribute to its specific binding to the receptor. Important factors include hydrophobicity, ionization state (**pK$_a$**), conformation, and stereochemistry of the drug molecule. All of these factors combine to determine the complementarity of the drug to the binding site. Receptor binding pockets are highly specific, and small changes in the drug can have a large effect on the affinity of the drug–receptor interaction. For example, the **stereochemistry** of the drug has a great impact on the strength of the binding interaction. **Warfarin** is synthesized and administered as a racemic mixture (a mixture containing 50% of the right-handed molecule and 50% of the left-handed molecule); however, the S enantiomer is four times more potent than the R because of a stronger interaction of the S form with its binding site on vitamin K epoxide reductase. Stereochemistry can also affect toxicity in cases where one enantiomer of a drug causes the desired therapeutic effect and the other enantiomer causes an undesired toxic effect, perhaps due to an interaction with a second receptor or to metabolism to a toxic species. Although it is sometimes difficult for pharmaceutical companies to synthesize and purify individual enantiomers on a large scale, a number of currently marketed drugs are produced as individual enantiomers in cases where one enantiomer has higher efficacy and/or lower toxicity than its mirror image.

IMPACT OF DRUG BINDING ON THE RECEPTOR

How does drug binding produce a biochemical and/or physiologic change in the organism? In the case of receptors with enzymatic activity, the binding site of the drug is often the **active site** at which an enzymatic transformation is catalyzed. Therefore, the catalytic activity of the enzyme is inhibited by drugs that prevent substrate binding to the site or that covalently modify the site. In cases where the binding site is not the active site of the enzyme, drugs can cause a change by preventing the binding of endogenous ligands to their receptor binding pockets. In many drug–receptor interactions, however, the binding of a drug to its receptor results in a change in the conformation of the receptor. Altering the shape of the receptor can affect its function, including enhancing the affinity of the drug for the receptor. Such an interaction is often referred to as **induced fit**, because the receptor's conformation changes so as to improve the quality of the binding interaction.

The principle of induced fit suggests that drug–receptor binding can have profound effects on the conformation of the receptor. By inducing conformational changes in the re-

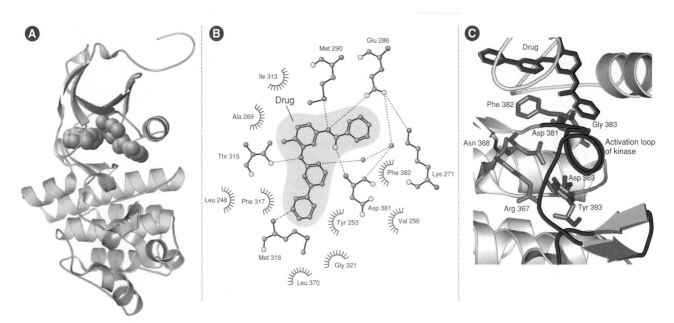

Figure 1-2. Structural basis of specific enzyme inhibition: imatinib interaction with the BCR-Abl kinase. A. The kinase portion of the BCR-Abl tyrosine kinase is shown in a ribbon format (*gray*). An analogue of imatinib, a specific inhibitor of the BCR-Abl tyrosine kinase, is shown as a space-filling model (*blue*). **B.** Detailed diagram of the intermolecular interactions between the drug (*shaded in blue*) and amino acid residues in the BCR-Abl protein. Hydrogen bonds are indicated by dashed lines, while van der Waals interactions (indicated by halos around the amino acid name and its position in the protein sequence) are shown for nine amino acids with hydrophobic side chains. **C.** The interaction of the drug (*blue*) with the BCR-Abl protein (*gray*) inhibits phosphorylation of a critical activation loop (*blue-highlighted ribbon format*), thus preventing catalytic activity.

ceptor, many drugs not only improve the quality of the binding interaction but also alter the action of the receptor. The change in shape induced by the drug is sometimes identical to that caused by the binding of an endogenous ligand. For example, exogenously administered **insulin** analogues all stimulate the insulin receptor to the same extent, despite their slightly different amino acid sequences. In other cases, drug binding alters the shape of the receptor so as to make it more or less functional than normal. For example, imatinib binding to the BCR-Abl tyrosine kinase causes the protein to assume an enzymatically inactive conformation, thus inhibiting the kinase activity of the receptor.

Another way to describe the induced fit principle is to consider that many receptors exist in multiple conformational states—such as inactive (or closed), active (or open), and desensitized (or inactivated)—and that the binding of a drug to the receptor stabilizes one or more of these conformations. Quantitative models that incorporate these concepts of drug–receptor interactions are discussed in Chapter 2.

MEMBRANE EFFECTS ON DRUG–RECEPTOR INTERACTIONS

The structure of the receptor determines not only its binding affinities for drugs and endogenous ligands, but also where the protein lies in relationship to cellular boundaries such as the plasma membrane. Proteins that have large hydrophobic domains are able to reside in the plasma membrane because of the membrane's high lipid content. Many receptors that span the plasma membrane have lipophilic domains that sit in the membrane and hydrophilic domains that reside in the intracellular and extracellular spaces. Other drug receptors, including a number of transcription regulators (also called **transcription factors**), have only hydrophilic domains and can reside in the cytoplasm, nucleus, or both.

Just as the structure of the receptor determines its location in relationship to the plasma membrane, *the structure of a drug affects its ability to gain access to the receptor.* For example, drugs that are highly water-soluble are often less able to pass through the plasma membrane and bind to target molecules in the cytoplasm. In contrast, certain hydrophilic drugs that are able to pass through transmembrane channels or use other transport mechanisms can gain ready access to cytoplasmic receptors. Drugs that are highly lipophilic, such as many steroid hormones, are able to pass through the hydrophobic lipid environment of the plasma membrane without special channels or transporters, and thereby gain access to intracellular targets.

The ability of drugs to alter receptor shape enables drug binding to receptors on the cell surface to affect functions inside cells. Many cell surface protein receptors have extracellular domains that are linked to intracellular effector molecules through receptor domains that span the plasma membrane. In some cases, changing the shape of the extracellular domain can alter the conformation of the membrane-spanning and/or intracellular domains of the receptor, resulting in a change in receptor function. In other cases, drugs can crosslink the extracellular domains of two receptor molecules, forming a dimeric receptor complex that activates effector molecules inside the cell.

All of these factors—drug and receptor structure, the chemical forces influencing drug–receptor interaction, drug solubility in water and in the plasma membrane, and the function of the receptor in its cellular environment—confer significant **specificity** on the interactions between drugs and their target receptors. This book discusses numerous examples of drugs that can gain access and bind to receptors in such a way as to induce a conformational change in the receptor, and thereby to produce a biochemical or physiologic effect. This principle suggests that, armed with the knowledge of the structure of a receptor, one could theoretically design a drug that interrupts receptor activity. In fact, much investigation is currently underway to enhance the efficacy and reduce the toxicity of drugs by altering their structure so that they bind more selectively to their targets. This process, referred to as **rational drug design,** has enabled the development of protease inhibitors that have profoundly affected the course of HIV disease as well as antineoplastic agents such as imatinib. This approach to drug design is discussed in greater detail in Chapter 48, Drug Discovery and Preclinical Development.

MOLECULAR AND CELLULAR DETERMINANTS OF DRUG SELECTIVITY

The ideal drug would interact only with a molecular target that causes the desired therapeutic effect but not with molecular targets that cause unwanted adverse effects. Although no such drug has yet been discovered (i.e., all drugs currently in clinical use have the potential to cause adverse effects as well as therapeutic effects), pharmacologists can take advantage of several determinants of drug **selectivity** in an attempt to reach this goal. Selectivity of drug action can be conferred by at least two classes of mechanisms, including (1) the cell-type specificity of receptor subtypes, and (2) the cell-type specificity of receptor-effector coupling.

Although many potential receptors for drugs are widely distributed among diverse cell types, some receptors are more limited in their distribution. Systemic administration of drugs that interact with such localized receptors can result in a highly selective therapeutic effect. For example, drugs that target ubiquitous processes such as DNA synthesis are likely to cause significant toxic side effects; this is the case with many currently available chemotherapeutics for the treatment of cancer. Other drugs that target cell-type restricted processes such as acid generation in the stomach may have fewer adverse effects. Imatinib is an extremely selective drug because the BCR-Abl protein is not expressed in normal (noncancerous) cells. In general, *the more restricted the cell-type distribution of the receptor targeted by a particular drug, the more selective the drug is likely to be.*

Similarly, even though many different cell types may express the same molecular target for a drug, the effect of that drug may differ in the various cell types because of differential receptor–effector coupling mechanisms or differential requirements for the drug target in the various cell types. For example, although voltage-gated calcium channels are ubiquitously expressed in the heart, cardiac pacemaker cells are relatively more sensitive to the effects of calcium channel blocking agents than are cardiac ventricular muscle cells. This differential effect is attributable to the

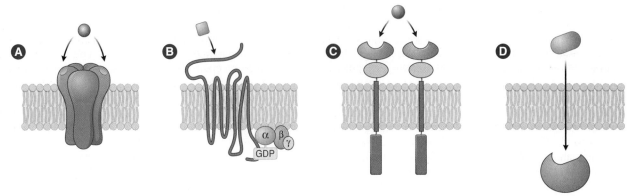

Figure 1-3. Four major types of interactions between drugs and receptors. Most drug–receptor interactions can be divided into four groups. **A.** Drugs can bind to ion channels spanning the plasma membrane, causing an alteration in the channel's conductance. **B.** Heptahelical receptors spanning the plasma membrane are functionally coupled to intracellular G proteins. Drugs can influence the actions of these receptors by binding to the extracellular surface or transmembrane region of the receptor. **C.** Drugs can bind to the extracellular domain of a transmembrane receptor and cause a change in signaling within the cell by activating or inhibiting an enzymatic intracellular domain (rectangular box) of the same receptor molecule. **D.** Drugs can diffuse through the plasma membrane and bind to cytoplasmic or nuclear receptors. This is often the pathway used by lipophilic drugs (e.g., drugs that bind to steroid hormone receptors). Alternatively, drugs can inhibit enzymes in the extracellular space without the need to cross the plasma membrane (*not shown*).

fact that action potential propagation depends mainly on the action of calcium channels in cardiac pacemaker cells, whereas sodium channels are more important than calcium channels in the action potentials of ventricular muscle cells. In general, *the more the receptor–effector coupling mechanisms differ among the various cell types that express a particular molecular target for a drug, the more selective the drug is likely to be.*

MAJOR TYPES OF DRUG RECEPTORS

Given the great diversity of drug molecules, it might seem likely that the interactions between drugs and their molecular targets would be equally diverse. This is only partly true. In fact, *most of the currently understood drug–receptor interactions can be classified into six major groups.* These groups comprise the interactions between drugs and (1) transmembrane ion channels, (2) transmembrane receptors coupled to

intracellular G proteins, (3) transmembrane receptors with enzymatic cytosolic domains, (4) intracellular receptors, including enzymes, transcription regulators, and structural proteins, (5) extracellular enzymes, and (6) cell surface adhesion receptors (Fig. 1-3). Table 1-2 provides a summary of each major interaction type.

Knowing whether and to what extent a drug activates or inhibits its target provides valuable information about the interaction. Although **pharmacodynamics** (the effects of drugs on the human body) is covered in detail in the next chapter, it is useful to state briefly the major pharmacodynamic relationships between drugs and their targets before examining the molecular mechanisms of drug–receptor interactions. *Agonists are molecules that, upon binding to their targets, cause a change in the activity of those targets.* **Full agonists** bind to and activate their targets to the maximal extent possible. For example, acetylcholine binds to the nicotinic acetylcholine receptor and induces a conformational change in the receptor-associated ion channel from a nonconducting to a fully conducting state. **Partial agonists** produce a submaximal response upon binding to their targets.

TABLE 1-2	Six Major Types of Drug-Receptor Interactions	

RECEPTOR TYPE	SITE OF DRUG-RECEPTOR INTERACTION	SITE OF RESULTANT ACTION
Transmembrane ion channel	Extracellular, intrachannel, or intracellular	Cytoplasm
Transmembrane linked to intracellular G protein	Extracellular or intramembrane	Cytoplasm
Transmembrane with enzymatic cytosolic domain	Extracellular	Cytoplasm
Intracellular	Cytoplasm or nucleus	Cytoplasm or nucleus
Extracellular enzyme	Extracellular	Extracellular
Adhesion	Extracellular	Extracellular

Inverse agonists cause constitutively active targets to become inactive. *Antagonists inhibit the ability of their targets to be activated (or inactivated) by physiologic or pharmacologic agonists.* Drugs that directly block the binding site of a physiologic agonist are called **competitive antagonists**; drugs that bind to other sites on the target molecule, and thereby prevent the conformational change required for receptor activation (or inactivation), may be either **noncompetitive** or **uncompetitive antagonists** (see Chapter 2). As the mechanism of each drug–receptor interaction is outlined in the next several sections, it will be useful to consider at a structural level how these different pharmacodynamic effects could be produced.

TRANSMEMBRANE ION CHANNELS

Many cellular functions require the passage of ions and other hydrophilic molecules across the plasma membrane. Specialized transmembrane channels regulate these processes. The functions of **ion channels** are diverse, including fundamental roles in neurotransmission, cardiac conduction, muscle contraction, and secretion. Because of this, drugs targeting ion channels can have a significant impact on major body functions.

Three major mechanisms are used to regulate the activity of transmembrane ion channels. In some channels, the conductance is controlled by ligand binding to the channel. In other channels, the conductance is regulated by changes in voltage across the plasma membrane. In still other channels, the conductance is controlled by ligand binding to plasma membrane receptors that are linked to the channel in some way. The first group of channels is referred to as **ligand-gated,** the second as **voltage-gated,** and the third as **second messenger-regulated.** Table 1-3 summarizes the mechanism of activation and function of each channel type.

Channels are generally highly selective for the ions they conduct. For example, action potential propagation in neurons of the central and peripheral nervous systems occurs as a result of the synchronous stimulation of voltage-gated ion channels that permit the selective passage of Na^+ ions into the cell. When the membrane potential in such a neuron becomes sufficiently positive, the voltage-gated Na^+ channels open, allowing a large influx of extracellular sodium ions that further depolarize the cell. The role of ion-selective channels in action potential generation and propagation is discussed in Chapter 6, Principles of Cellular Excitability and Electrochemical Transmission.

Most ion channels share some structural similarity, regardless of their ion selectivity, the magnitude of their conductance, or their mechanisms of activation (gating) or inactivation. Ion channels tend to be tube-like macromolecules consisting of a number of protein subunits that pass through the plasma membrane. The **ligand-binding domain** can be extracellular, within the channel, or intracellular, while the domain that interacts with other receptors or modulators is most often intracellular. The structure of the nicotinic acetylcholine (ACh) receptor has been determined to 4.6 Å resolution, providing an example of the structure of an important ligand-gated ion channel. This receptor consists of five subunits, each of which crosses the plasma membrane (Fig. 1-4). Two of the subunits have been designated α; each contains a single extracellular binding site for ACh. In the free (nonliganded) state of the receptor, the channel is occluded by amino acid side chains and does not allow the passage of ions. Binding of two molecules of acetylcholine to the receptor induces a conformational change that opens the channel and allows ion conductance.

Although the nicotinic ACh receptor appears to assume only two states, open or closed, many ion channels are able to assume other states as well. For example, some ion channels are able to become **refractory** or **inactivated.** In this state, the channel's permeability cannot be altered for a certain period of time, known as the channel's refractory period. The voltage-gated sodium channel undergoes a cycle of activation, channel opening, channel closing, and channel inactivation. During the inactivation (refractory) period, the channel cannot be reactivated for a number of milliseconds, even if the membrane potential returns to a voltage that normally stimulates the channel to open. Some drugs bind with different affinities to different states of the same ion channel. This **state-dependent binding** is important in the mechanism of action of some local anesthetic and antiarrhythmic drugs, as discussed in Chapters 10 (Local Anesthetic Pharmacology) and 18 (Pharmacology of Cardiac Rhythm), respectively.

Two important classes of drugs that act by altering the conductance of ion channels are the local anesthetics and the benzodiazepines. Local anesthetics block the conductance of sodium ions through voltage-gated sodium channels in neurons that transmit pain information from the periphery to the central nervous system, thereby preventing action potential propagation and, hence, pain perception (nociception). Benzodiazepines also act on the nervous system, but by a different mechanism. These drugs inhibit neurotransmission in the central nervous system by potentiating the

TABLE 1-3 **Three Major Types of Transmembrane Ion Channels**

CHANNEL TYPE	MECHANISM OF ACTIVATION	FUNCTION
Ligand-gated	Binding of ligand to channel	Altered ion conductance
Voltage-gated	Change in transmembrane voltage gradient	Altered ion conductance
Second messenger-regulated	Binding of ligand to transmembrane receptor with G protein-coupled cytosolic domain, leading to second messenger generation	Second messenger regulates ion conductance of channel

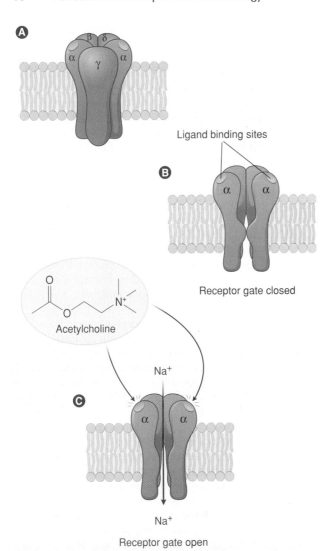

Figure 1-4. Ligand-gated nicotinic acetylcholine receptor. A. The plasma membrane acetylcholine (ACh) receptor is composed of five subunits—two α subunits, a β subunit, a γ subunit, and a δ subunit. **B.** The γ subunit has been removed to show an internal schematic view of the receptor, demonstrating that it forms a transmembrane channel. In the absence of ACh, the receptor gate is closed, and cations (most importantly, sodium ions [Na^+]) are unable to traverse the channel. **C.** When ACh is bound to both α subunits, the channel opens, and sodium can pass down its concentration gradient into the cell.

ability of the neurotransmitter gamma-aminobutyric acid (**GABA**) to increase the conductance of chloride ions across neuronal membranes, thereby driving the membrane potential farther away from its threshold for activation.

TRANSMEMBRANE G PROTEIN-COUPLED RECEPTORS

G protein-coupled receptors are the most abundant class of receptors in the human body. These receptors are exposed at the extracellular surface of the cell membrane, traverse the membrane, and possess intracellular regions that activate a unique class of signaling molecules called **G proteins.**

(G proteins are so named because they bind the guanine nucleotides GTP and GDP.) G protein-coupled signaling mechanisms are involved in many important processes, including vision, olfaction, and neurotransmission.

G protein-coupled receptors all have seven transmembrane regions within a single polypeptide chain. Each transmembrane region consists of a single α helix, and the α helices are arranged in a characteristic structural motif that is similar in all members of this receptor class. The extracellular domain of this class of proteins usually contains the ligand-binding region, although some G protein-coupled receptors bind ligands within the transmembrane domain of the receptor. In the resting (unstimulated) state, the cytoplasmic domain of the receptor is noncovalently linked to a G protein that consists of α and $\beta\gamma$ subunits. Upon activation, the α subunit exchanges GDP for GTP. The α-GTP subunit then dissociates from the $\beta\gamma$ subunit, and the α or $\beta\gamma$ subunit diffuses along the inner leaflet of the plasma membrane to interact with a number of different effectors. These effectors include adenylyl cyclase, phospholipase C, various ion channels, and other classes of proteins. Signals mediated by G proteins are usually terminated by the hydrolysis of GTP to GDP, which is catalyzed by the inherent GTPase activity of the α subunit (Fig. 1-5).

One major role of the G proteins is to activate the production of **second messengers**; that is, signaling molecules that convey the input provided by the first messenger—usually an endogenous ligand or an exogenous drug—to cytoplasmic effectors (Fig. 1-6). The activation of cyclases such as adenylyl cyclase, which catalyzes the production of the second messenger cyclic adenosine-3',5'-monophosphate (cAMP), and guanylyl cyclase, which catalyzes the production of cyclic guanosine-3',5'-monophosphate (cGMP), constitutes the most common pathway linked to G proteins. In addition, G proteins can activate the enzyme phospholipase C (PLC) which, among other functions, plays a key role in regulating the concentration of intracellular calcium. Upon activation by a G protein, PLC cleaves the membrane phospholipid phosphatidylinositol-4,5-bisphosphate (PIP_2) to the second messengers diacylglycerol (DAG) and inositol-1,4,5-trisphosphate (IP_3). IP_3 triggers the release of Ca^{2+} from intracellular stores, thereby dramatically increasing the cytosolic Ca^{2+} concentration and activating downstream molecular and cellular events. DAG activates protein kinase C, which then mediates other molecular and cellular events including smooth muscle contraction and transmembrane ion transport. All of these events are dynamically regulated, so that the different steps in the pathways are activated and inactivated with characteristic kinetics.

A large number of Gα protein isoforms have now been identified, each of which has unique effects on its targets. A few of these G proteins include G-stimulatory (G$_s$), G-inhibitory (G$_i$), G$_q$, G$_o$, and G$_{12/13}$. Examples of the effects of these isoforms are shown in Table 1-4. The differential functioning of these G proteins, some of which may couple in different ways to the same receptor in different cell types, is likely to be important for the potential selectivity of future drugs. The $\beta\gamma$ subunits of G proteins can also act as second messenger molecules, although their actions are not as thoroughly characterized.

One important class in the G protein-coupled receptor family is the β-adrenergic receptor group. The most thor-

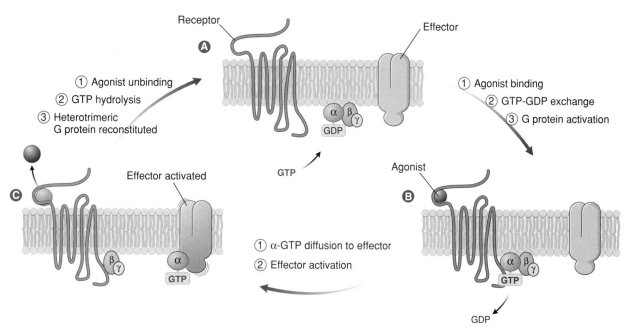

Figure 1-5. Receptor-mediated activation of a G protein and the resultant effector interaction. A. In the resting state, the α and $\beta\gamma$ subunits of a G protein are associated with one another, and GDP is bound to the α subunit. **B.** Binding of an extracellular ligand (agonist) to a G protein-coupled receptor causes the exchange of GTP for GDP on the α subunit. **C.** The $\beta\gamma$ subunit dissociates from the α subunit, which diffuses to interact with effector proteins. Interaction of the GTP-associated α subunit with an effector activates the effector. In some cases (*not shown*), the $\beta\gamma$ subunit can also activate effector proteins. Depending on the receptor subtype and the specific $G\alpha$ isoform, $G\alpha$ can also inhibit the activity of an effector molecule. The α subunit possesses intrinsic GTPase activity, which leads to hydrolysis of GTP to GDP. This leads to reassociation of the α subunit with the $\beta\gamma$ subunit and the cycle can begin again.

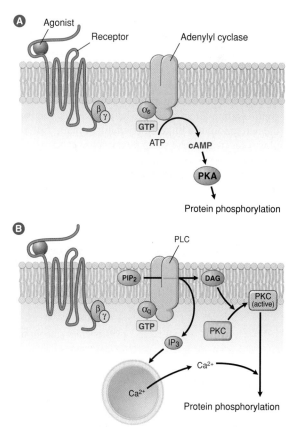

Figure 1-6. Activation of adenylyl cyclase (AC) and phospholipase C (PLC) by G proteins. G proteins can interact with several different types of effector molecules. The subtype of $G\alpha$ protein that is activated often determines which effector the G protein will activate. Two of the most common $G\alpha$ subunits are $G\alpha_s$ and $G\alpha_q$, which stimulate adenylyl cyclase and phospholipase C, respectively. **A.** When stimulated by $G\alpha_s$, adenylyl cyclase converts ATP to cyclic AMP (cAMP). cAMP then activates protein kinase A (PKA), which phosphorylates a number of specific cytosolic proteins. **B.** When stimulated by $G\alpha_q$, phospholipase C (PLC) cleaves the membrane phospholipid phosphatidylinositol-4,5-bisphosphate (PIP$_2$) into diacylglycerol (DAG) and inositol-1,4,5-trisphosphate (IP$_3$). DAG diffuses in the membrane to activate protein kinase C (PKC), which then phosphorylates specific cellular proteins. IP$_3$ stimulates release of Ca^{2+} from the endoplasmic reticulum into the cytosol. Calcium release also stimulates protein phosphorylation events that lead to changes in protein activation. Although not shown, the $\beta\gamma$ subunits of G proteins can also affect certain cellular signal transduction cascades.

TABLE 1-4 **The Major G Proteins and Examples of Their Actions**

G PROTEIN	ACTIONS
G-stimulatory (G_s)	Activates Ca^{2+} channels, activates adenylyl cyclase
G-inhibitory (G_i)	Activates K^+ channels, inhibits adenylyl cyclase
G_o	Inhibits Ca^{2+} channels
G_q	Activates phospholipase C
$G_{12/13}$	Diverse ion transporter interactions

oughly studied of these receptors have been designated β_1, β_2, and β_3. As discussed in more detail in Chapter 9, Adrenergic Pharmacology, β_1 receptors play a role in controlling heart rate; β_2 receptors are involved in the relaxation of smooth muscle; and β_3 receptors play a role in the mobilization of energy by fat cells. Each of these receptors is stimulated by the binding of endogenous catecholamines, such as **epinephrine** and **norepinephrine**, to the extracellular domain of the receptor. **Epinephrine** binding induces a conformational change in the receptor, activating G proteins associated with the cytoplasmic domain of the receptor. The activated (GTP-bound) form of the G protein activates adenylyl cyclase, resulting in increased intracellular cAMP levels and downstream cellular effects. Table 1-5 indicates some of the diverse tissue localizations and actions of the β-adrenergic receptors.

TRANSMEMBRANE RECEPTORS WITH ENZYMATIC CYTOSOLIC DOMAINS

The third major class of cellular drug targets consists of transmembrane receptors that transduce an extracellular ligand-binding interaction into an intracellular action through the activation of a linked enzymatic domain. Such receptors play roles in a diverse set of physiologic processes, including cell metabolism, growth, and differentiation. Receptors that have an intracellular enzymatic domain can be grouped into

five major classes based on their cytoplasmic mechanism of action (Fig. 1-7). All of these receptors are single–membrane-spanning proteins, in contrast to the seven–membrane-spanning motif present in G protein-coupled receptors. Many receptors with enzymatic cytosolic domains form dimers or multisubunit complexes to transduce their signals.

Many of the receptors with enzymatic cytosolic domains modify proteins by adding or removing phosphate groups to or from specific amino acid residues. *Phosphorylation is a ubiquitous mechanism of protein signaling.* The large negative charge of phosphate groups can dramatically alter the three-dimensional structure of a protein and thereby change that protein's activity. In addition, phosphorylation is easily reversible, thus allowing this signaling mechanism to act specifically in time and space.

Receptor Tyrosine Kinases

The largest group of transmembrane receptors with enzymatic cytosolic domains is the receptor tyrosine kinase family. These receptors transduce signals from many hormones and growth factors by phosphorylating tyrosine residues on the cytoplasmic tail of the receptor. This leads to recruitment and subsequent tyrosine phosphorylation of a number of cytosolic signaling molecules.

The insulin receptor is a well-characterized receptor tyrosine kinase. This receptor consists of two extracellular α subunits that are covalently linked to two membrane-spanning β subunits. Binding of insulin to the α subunits results in a change in conformation of the adjacent β subunits, causing the β subunits to move closer to one another on the intracellular side of the membrane. The proximity of the two β subunits promotes a transphosphorylation reaction, in which one β subunit phosphorylates the other ("autophosphorylation"). The phosphorylated tyrosine residues then act to recruit other cytosolic proteins, known as insulin receptor substrate (IRS) proteins. Type 2 diabetes mellitus may, in some cases, be associated with defects in post-insulin receptor signaling; thus, understanding the insulin receptor signaling pathways is relevant for the potential design of rational therapeutics. The mechanism of insulin receptor signaling is discussed in more detail in Chapter 29, Pharmacology of the Endocrine Pancreas.

Recognizing that receptor tyrosine kinases play an im-

TABLE 1-5 **Tissue Localization and Action of β-Adrenergic Receptors**

RECEPTOR	TISSUE LOCALIZATION	ACTION
β_1	SA node of heart	Increases heart rate
	Cardiac muscle	Increases contractility
	Adipose tissue	Increases lipolysis
β_2	Bronchial smooth muscle	Dilates bronchioles
	Gastrointestinal smooth muscle	Constricts sphincters and relaxes gut wall
	Uterus	Relaxes uterine wall
	Bladder	Relaxes bladder
	Liver	Increases gluconeogenesis and glycolysis
	Pancreas	Increases insulin release
β_3	Adipose tissue	Increases lipolysis

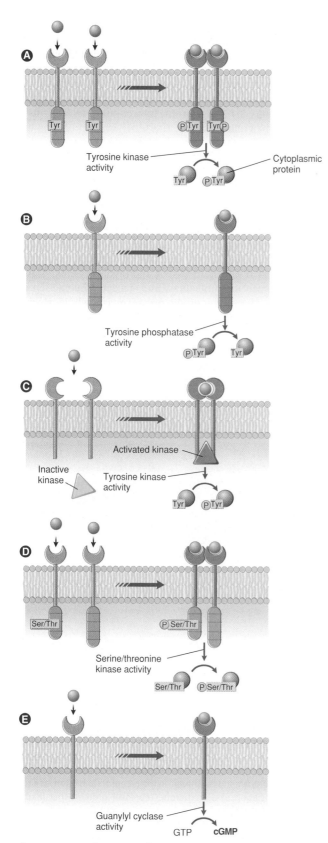

portant role in cellular growth and differentiation, it is not surprising that "gain-of-function" mutations in these receptors (i.e., mutations that cause *ligand-independent* activity of these molecules) can lead to uncontrolled cell growth and cancer. Recall from the introductory case that chronic myeloid leukemia is associated with the Philadelphia chromosome, which results from a reciprocal translocation between the long arms of chromosomes 9 and 22. The mutant chromosome codes for a constitutively active receptor tyrosine kinase referred to as the BCR-Abl protein (BCR and Abl are short for "break-point cluster region" and "Abelson," respectively, the two chromosomal regions that undergo translocation with high frequency in this form of leukemia). The constitutive activity of this kinase results in phosphorylation of a number of cytosolic proteins, leading to dysregulated myeloid cell growth and chronic myeloid leukemia. Imatinib inhibits BCR-Abl activity by neutralizing its ability to phosphorylate substrates; this is the first example of a drug targeted specifically to receptor tyrosine kinases, and its success is leading to the development of a number of drugs that act by similar mechanisms.

Receptor Tyrosine Phosphatases

Just as receptor tyrosine kinases phosphorylate the tyrosine residues of cytoplasmic proteins, receptor tyrosine phosphatases remove phosphate groups from specific tyrosine residues. In some cases, this may be an example of receptor convergence (discussed later), where the differential effects of two receptor types can negate one another. However, receptor tyrosine phosphatases possess novel signaling mechanisms as well. Many receptor tyrosine phosphatases are found in immune cells, where they regulate cell activation. These receptors are discussed further in Chapter 44, Pharmacology of Immunosuppression.

Tyrosine Kinase-Associated Receptors

Tyrosine kinase-associated receptors constitute a diverse family of proteins that, although lacking inherent catalytic activity, recruit active cytosolic signaling proteins in a li-

Figure 1-7. Major types of transmembrane receptors with enzymatic cytosolic domains. There are five major categories of transmembrane receptors with enzymatic cytosolic domains. **A.** The largest group is comprised of receptor tyrosine kinases. After ligand-induced activation, these receptors dimerize and transphosphorylate tyrosine residues in the receptor and, often, on target cytosolic pro-

teins. Examples of receptor tyrosine kinases include the insulin receptor and the BCR-Abl protein. **B.** Some receptors can act as tyrosine phosphatases. These receptors dephosphorylate tyrosine residues either on other transmembrane receptors or on cytosolic proteins. Many cells of the immune system have receptor tyrosine phosphatases. **C.** Some tyrosine kinase-associated receptors lack a definitive enzymatic domain, but binding of ligand to the receptor triggers activation of receptor-associated protein kinases (termed **nonreceptor tyrosine kinases**) that then phosphorylate tyrosine residues on certain cytosolic proteins. **D.** Receptor serine/threonine kinases phosphorylate serine and threonine residues on certain target cytosolic proteins. Members of the TGF-β superfamily of receptors are in this category. **E.** Receptor guanylyl cyclases contain a cytosolic domain that catalyzes the formation of cGMP from GTP. The receptor for B-type natriuretic peptide is one of the receptor guanylyl cyclases that has been well characterized.

gand-dependent manner. These cytosolic proteins are also called (somewhat confusingly) **nonreceptor tyrosine kinases.** Ligand activation of cell surface tyrosine kinase-associated receptors causes the receptors to cluster together. This clustering event recruits cytoplasmic proteins that are then activated to phosphorylate other proteins on tyrosine residues. Thus, the downstream effect is much like that of receptor tyrosine kinases, except that tyrosine kinase-associated receptors rely on a nonreceptor kinase to phosphorylate target proteins. Important examples of tyrosine kinase-associated receptors include cytokine receptors and a number of other receptors in the immune system. These receptors are discussed in detail in Chapter 44.

Receptor Serine/Threonine Kinases

These receptors, which are all members of the transforming growth factor β (TGF-β) receptor superfamily, are important mediators of cell growth and differentiation that have been implicated in cancer progression and metastasis. They act by phosphorylating serine and threonine residues on cytoplasmic target proteins. No pharmacologic agents currently exist that target serine/threonine kinases, although such drugs are under development.

Receptor Guanylyl Cyclases

Recall that the activation of G protein-coupled receptors may cause Gα subunits to alter the activity of adenylyl and guanylyl cyclases. Receptor guanylyl cyclases have no intermediate G protein. Instead, ligand binding stimulates intrinsic receptor guanylyl cyclase activity, in which GTP is converted to cGMP. This is the smallest family of transmembrane receptors. B-type natriuretic peptide, a hormone secreted by the ventricles in response to volume overload, acts via a receptor guanylyl cyclase. A recombinant version of the native peptide ligand, **nesiritide,** is approved for treatment of decompensated heart failure, as discussed in Chapter 20, Pharmacology of Volume Regulation.

INTRACELLULAR RECEPTORS

Enzymes are a common cytosolic target, and many drugs that target intracellular enzymes produce their effect by altering the enzyme's production of critical signaling or metabolic molecules. Vitamin K epoxide reductase, a cytosolic enzyme involved in the post-translational modification of glutamate residues in certain coagulation factors, is the target of the anticoagulant drug **warfarin.** Many lipophilic inhibitors of cytosolic **signal transduction molecules** are under development, including drugs that target mediators of apoptosis (programmed cell death) or inflammation.

The transcription regulatory factors are important cytosolic receptors that are targeted by lipophilic drugs. All proteins in the body are encoded by DNA. The transcription of DNA into RNA and the translation of RNA into protein are controlled by a diverse set of molecules. Transcription of many genes is regulated, in part, by the interaction between lipid-soluble signaling molecules and tran-

scription regulatory factors. Because of the fundamental role played by control of transcription in many biological processes, **transcription regulators** (also called **transcription factors**) are the targets of some important drugs. **Steroid hormones** are a class of lipophilic drugs that can diffuse readily through the plasma membrane and achieve their actions by binding to transcription factors in the cytoplasm or nucleus (Fig. 1-8).

Just as the shape of a transcription factor governs to which drugs it will bind, the shape also determines where on the genome the transcription factor will attach, and which coactivator or corepressor molecules will bind to it. By activating or inhibiting transcription, thereby altering the intracellular or extracellular concentrations of specific gene products, drugs that target transcription factors can have a profound impact on cellular function. The cellular responses to such drugs, and the effects that result from this cellular response in tissues and organ systems, provide links between the molecular drug–receptor interaction and the effects of the drug on the organism as a whole. Because gene transcription is a relatively slow (minutes to hours)

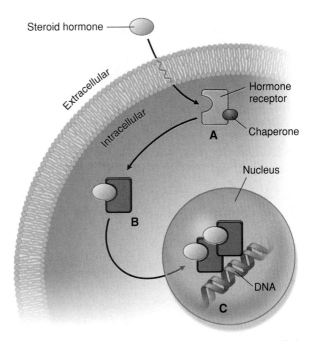

Figure 1-8. Lipophilic molecule binding to an intracellular transcription factor. A. Small lipophilic molecules can diffuse through the plasma membrane and bind to intracellular transcription factors. In this example, steroid hormone binding to a cytosolic hormone receptor is shown, although some receptors of this class may be located in the nucleus before ligand binding. **B.** Ligand binding triggers a conformational change in the receptor (and often, as shown here, dissociation of a chaperone repressor protein) that leads to transport of the ligand–receptor complex into the nucleus. In the nucleus, the ligand–receptor complex typically dimerizes. In the example shown, the active form of the receptor is a homodimer (two identical receptors binding to one another), but heterodimers (such as the thyroid hormone receptor and the retinoid X receptor) may also form. **C.** The dimerized ligand–receptor complex binds to DNA, and may then recruit coactivators or corepressors (*not shown*). These complexes alter the rate of gene transcription, leading to a change (either up or down) in cellular protein expression.

and long-lasting process, drugs that target transcription factors often require a longer period of time for the onset of action to take place, and have longer-lasting effects, than do drugs that alter more transient processes such as ion conduction (seconds to minutes).

Not all drugs with cytosolic targets act on transcription factors. **Structural proteins,** such as tubulin, are important targets for antineoplastic drugs that are able to diffuse through the plasma membrane of the cancer cell. For example, the antimitotic vinca alkaloids bind to tubulin monomers and prevent the polymerization of this molecule into microtubules. This inhibition of microtubule formation arrests the affected cells in metaphase. Other drugs bind directly to RNA or ribosomes; such drugs are important agents in antimicrobial and antineoplastic chemotherapy.

EXTRACELLULAR ENZYMES

Many important drug receptors are enzymes with active sites located outside the plasma membrane. The environment outside of cells consists of a milieu of proteins and signaling molecules. While many of these proteins serve a structural role, others are used to communicate information between cells. Therefore, enzymes that modify the molecules mediating these important signals can influence physiologic processes such as vasoconstriction and neurotransmission. One example of this class of receptor is **angiotensin converting enzyme** (ACE), which converts angiotensin I to the potent vasoconstrictor angiotensin II. **ACE inhibitors** are drugs that inhibit this enzymatic conversion and thereby lower blood pressure (among other effects; see Chapter 20). Another example is **acetylcholinesterase,** which degrades acetylcholine after this neurotransmitter is released from cholinergic neurons. **Acetylcholinesterase inhibitors** significantly enhance neurotransmission at cholinergic synapses by preventing neurotransmitter degradation at these sites (see Chapter 8, Cholinergic Pharmacology).

CELL SURFACE ADHESION RECEPTORS

Cells are often required to interact directly with other cells in order to perform specific functions or to communicate information. Some important functions requiring cell–cell adhesive interactions are the formation of tissues and the migration of immune cells to a site of inflammation. A region of contact between two cells is termed an **adhesion,** and cell–cell adhesive interactions are mediated by pairs of **adhesion receptors** on the surfaces of the individual cells. In many cases, a number of such receptor–counter-receptor pairs combine to secure a firm adhesion, and intracellular regulators control the activity of the adhesion receptors by changing their affinity or by controlling their expression and localization on the cell surface. Several adhesion receptors involved in the inflammatory response are attractive targets for selective inhibitors. Inhibitors of a specific class of adhesion receptors, known as **integrins,** have entered the clinic in recent years, and these drugs are being studied in the treatment of a range of conditions including inflammation, multiple sclerosis, and cancer (see Chapter 44).

PROCESSING OF SIGNALS RESULTING FROM DRUG–RECEPTOR INTERACTIONS

Many cells in the body are continuously bombarded with multiple inputs, some stimulatory and some inhibitory. How do cells integrate these signals to produce a coherent response? G proteins and other second messengers appear to provide important points of integration. As noted above, relatively few second messengers have been identified, and it is unlikely that many more remain to be discovered. Thus, second messengers are an attractive candidate mechanism for providing cells with a set of common points upon which numerous outside stimuli could converge to generate a coordinated cellular effect (Fig. 1-9).

Ion concentrations provide another point of integration for cellular effects because the cellular concentration of a particular ion is the result of the integrated activity of *multiple* ionic currents that both enhance and diminish the concentration of the ion within the cell. For example, the contractile state of a smooth muscle cell is a function of the intracellular calcium ion concentration, which is determined by several different Ca^{2+} conductances. These conductances include calcium ion leaks into the cell and calcium currents into and out of the cytoplasm through specialized channels in the plasma membrane and smooth endoplasmic reticulum.

Because the magnitude of cellular response is often considerably greater than the magnitude of the stimulus that caused the response, cells appear to have the ability to amplify the effects of receptor binding. G proteins provide an excellent example of signal amplification. Ligand binding to a G protein-coupled receptor serves to activate a single G protein molecule. This G protein molecule can then bind to and activate many effector molecules, such as adenylyl cyclase, which can then generate an even greater number of second messenger molecules (in this example, cAMP). Another example of signal amplification is ''trigger Ca^{2+},'' in which a small influx of Ca^{2+} through voltage-gated Ca^{2+} channels in the plasma membrane ''triggers'' the release of larger amounts of Ca^{2+} into the cytoplasm from intracellular stores.

CELLULAR REGULATION OF DRUG–RECEPTOR INTERACTIONS

Drug-induced activation or inhibition of a receptor often has a lasting impact on the receptor's subsequent responsiveness to drug binding. Mechanisms that mediate such effects are important because they prevent overstimulation that could lead to cellular damage or adversely affect the organism as a whole. Many drugs show diminishing effects over time; this phenomenon is called **tachyphylaxis.** In pharmacologic terms, the receptor and the cell become **desensitized** to the action of the drug. Mechanisms of desensitization can be

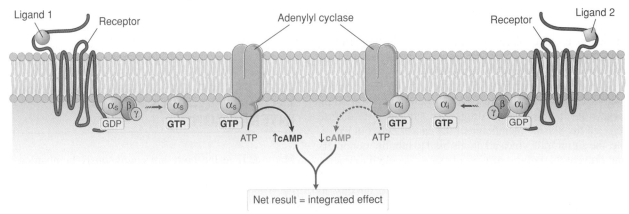

Figure 1-9. **Signaling convergence of two receptors.** A limited number of mechanisms are used to transduce intracellular signal cascades. In some cases, this allows for convergence, where two different receptors have opposite effects that tend to negate one another in the cell. In a simple example, two different G protein-coupled receptors could be stimulated by different ligands. The receptor shown on the left is coupled to $G\alpha_s$, a G protein that stimulates adenylyl cyclase to catalyze the formation of cAMP. The receptor shown on the right is coupled to $G\alpha_i$, a G protein that inhibits adenylyl cyclase. When both of these receptors are activated simultaneously, they can attenuate or even neutralize each other, as shown. Sometimes, signaling through a pathway may alternate as the two receptors are sequentially activated.

divided into two types: **homologous,** in which the effects of agonists at only one type of receptor are diminished; and **heterologous,** in which the effects of agonists at two or more types of receptors are coordinately diminished. Heterologous desensitization is thought to be caused by drug-induced alteration in a common point of convergence in the mechanisms

of action of the involved receptors, such as a shared effector molecule.

Many receptors exhibit desensitization. For example, the cellular response to repeated stimulation of β-adrenergic receptors by epinephrine diminishes steadily over time (Fig. 1-10). β-adrenergic receptor desensitization is mediated by

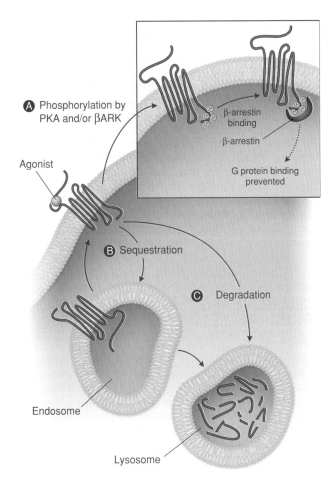

Figure 1-10. **β-Adrenergic receptor regulation.** Agonist-bound β-adrenergic receptors activate G proteins, which then stimulate adenylyl cyclase activity. **A.** Repeated or persistent stimulation of the receptor by agonist results in phosphorylation of amino acids at the C-terminus of the receptor by protein kinase A (PKA) and/or β-adrenergic receptor kinase (βARK). β-Arrestin then binds to the phosphorylated domain of the receptor and blocks G_s binding, thereby decreasing adenylyl cyclase (effector) activity. **B.** Binding of β-arrestin also leads to receptor sequestration into endosomal compartments, effectively neutralizing β-adrenergic receptor signaling activity. The receptor can then be recycled and reinserted into the plasma membrane. **C.** Prolonged receptor occupation by agonist can lead to receptor down-regulation and eventual receptor degradation. Cells can also reduce the number of surface receptors by inhibiting the transcription or translation of the gene coding for the receptor *(not shown)*.

TABLE 1-6	Mechanisms of Receptor Regulation
MECHANISM	**DEFINITION**
Tachyphylaxis	Repeated administration of the same dose of a drug results in a reduced effect of the drug over time
Desensitization	Decreased ability of a receptor to respond to stimulation by a drug or ligand
Homologous	Decreased response at a single type of receptor
Heterologous	Decreased response at two or more types of receptor
Inactivation	Loss of ability of a receptor to respond to stimulation by a drug or ligand
Refractory	After a receptor is stimulated, a period of time is required before the next drug-receptor interaction can produce an effect
Down-regulation	Repeated or persistent drug-receptor interaction results in removal of the receptor from sites where subsequent drug-receptor interactions could take place

epinephrine-induced phosphorylation of the cytoplasmic tail of the receptor. This phosphorylation promotes the binding of β-arrestin to the receptor; in turn, β-arrestin inhibits the receptor's ability to stimulate the G protein G_s. With lower levels of activated G_s present, adenylyl cyclase produces less cAMP. In this manner, repeated cycles of ligand–receptor binding result in smaller and smaller cellular effects. Other molecular mechanisms have even more profound effects, completely turning off the receptor to stimulation by ligand. The latter phenomenon, referred to as **inactivation,** may also result from phosphorylation of the receptor; in this case, the phosphorylation completely blocks the signaling activity of the receptor or causes removal of the receptor from the cell surface.

Another mechanism that can affect the cellular response caused by drug–receptor binding is called **refractoriness.** Receptors that assume a refractory state following activation require a period of time to pass before they can be stimulated again. As noted above, voltage-gated sodium channels, which mediate the firing of neuronal action potentials, are subject to refractory periods. Following channel opening induced by membrane depolarization, the voltage-gated sodium channel spontaneously closes, and cannot be reopened for some period of time (called the **refractory period**). This inherent property of the channel determines the maximum rate at which neurons can be stimulated and transmit information.

The effect of drug–receptor binding can also be influenced by drug-induced changes in the number of receptors on or in a cell. One example of a molecular mechanism by which receptor number can be altered is called **down-regulation.** In this phenomenon, prolonged receptor stimulation by ligand induces the cell to endocytose and sequester receptors in endocytic vesicles. This sequestration prevents the receptors from coming into contact with ligands, resulting in cellular desensitization. When the stimulus that caused the receptor sequestration subsides, the receptors can be recycled to the cell surface and thereby rendered

functional again (Fig. 1-10). Cells also have the ability to alter the level of synthesis of receptors and thereby to regulate the number of receptors available for drug binding. Receptor sequestration and alteration in receptor synthesis occur on a longer time scale than does phosphorylation, and have longer-lasting effects as well. Table 1-6 provides a summary of the mechanisms by which the effects of drug–receptor interactions can be regulated.

DRUGS THAT DO NOT FIT THE DRUG–RECEPTOR MODEL

Although many drugs interact with one of the basic receptor types outlined above, others act by nonreceptor-mediated mechanisms. Two examples are the osmotic diuretics and the antacids.

Diuretics control fluid balance in the body by altering the relative levels of water and ion absorption and secretion in the kidney. Many of these drugs act on ion channels. One class of diuretics, however, alters water and ion balance not by binding to ion channels or G protein-coupled receptors, but by changing the osmolarity in the nephron directly. The sugar **mannitol** is secreted into the lumen of the nephron and increases the osmolarity of the urine to such a degree that water is drawn from the peritubular blood into the lumen. This fluid shift serves to increase the volume of urine while decreasing the blood volume.

Another class of drugs that does not fit the drug–receptor model is the antacids, which are used to treat gastroesophageal reflux disease and peptic ulcer disease. Unlike antiulcer agents that bind to receptors involved in the physiologic generation of gastric acid, antacids act nonspecifically by absorbing or chemically neutralizing stomach acid. Examples of these agents include bases such as $NaHCO_3$ and $Mg(OH)_2$.

Conclusion and Future Directions

Although the molecular details of drug–receptor interactions vary widely among drugs of different classes and receptors of different types, the six fundamental mechanisms of action described in this chapter serve as paradigms of the principles of pharmacodynamics. The ability to classify drugs based on their mechanisms of action makes it possible to simplify the study of pharmacology, because the molecular mechanism of action of a drug can usually be linked to its cellular, tissue, organ, and system levels of action. In turn, how a given drug mediates its particular therapeutic effects and its unwanted or adverse effects in a particular patient becomes easier to understand. The major aim of modern drug development is to identify drugs that are highly selective by tailoring drug molecules to unique targets responsible for disease. As knowledge of drug development and the genetic and pathophysiologic basis of disease progresses, physicians and scientists will learn to combine the *molecular* specificity of a drug with the *genetic* and *pathophysiologic* specificity of the drug target to provide more and more selective therapies.

Suggested Reading

Alexander SP, Mathie A, Peters JA. Guide to receptors and channels. 2nd ed. *Br J Pharmacol* 2006;147(Suppl 3):S1–S168. (*Brief overview of molecular targets for drugs, organized by types of receptors.*)

Berg JM, Tymoczko JL, Stryer L. *Biochemistry.* 6th ed. New York: WH Freeman and Company; 2006. (*Contains structural information on receptors, especially G proteins.*)

Krause DS, Van Etten RA. Tyrosine kinases as targets for cancer therapy. *N Engl J Med* 2005;353:172–187. (*Discusses the dysregulation of protein tyrosine kinases in cancer and the targeting of these molecules by drugs such as imatinib.*)

Perez DM, Karnik SS. Multiple signaling states of G protein-coupled receptors. *Pharmacol Rev* 2005;57:147–161. (*Discusses the many roles played by G proteins in cell signaling.*)

Pratt WB, Taylor P, eds. *Principles of drug action: the basis of pharmacology.* 3rd ed. New York: Churchill Livingstone; 1990. (*Contains a detailed discussion of drug–receptor interactions.*)

Savage DG, Antman KH. Imatinib mesylate—a new targeted therapy. *N Engl J Med* 2002;346:683–693. (*Summarizes the pathophysiologic basis of chronic myeloid leukemia and reviews the mechanistic basis of imatinib specificity.*)

2

Pharmacodynamics

Harris S. Rose and David E. Golan

INTRODUCTION

Pharmacodynamics is the term used to describe the effects of a drug on the body. These effects are typically described in quantitative terms. The previous chapter considered the molecular interactions by which pharmacologic agents exert their effects. The integration of these molecular actions into an effect on the organism as a whole is the subject addressed in this chapter. It is important to describe the effects of a drug quantitatively in order to determine appropriate dose ranges for patients, as well as to compare the potency, efficacy, and safety of one drug to that of another.

Case

Admiral X is a 66-year-old retired submarine captain with a 70 pack/year smoking history (two packs a day for 35 years) and a family history of coronary artery disease. Although he usually ignores the advice of his physicians, he does take the pravastatin prescribed to reduce his cholesterol level and aspirin to reduce his risk of coronary artery occlusion.

One day, while working in his wood shop, Admiral X begins to feel tightness in his chest. The feeling rapidly becomes painful, and the pain begins to radiate down his left arm. He calls 911, and an ambulance transports him to the local emergency room. After evaluation, it is determined that Admiral X is having an anterior myocardial infarction. Because the hospital has no cardiac catheterization laboratory and Admiral X has no specific contraindications to thrombolytic therapy (such as uncontrolled hypertension, history of stroke, or recent surgery), the physician initiates therapy with both a thrombolytic agent, tissue-type plasminogen activator (tPA), and an anticoagulant, heparin. Improper dosing of both of these drugs can have dire consequences (hemorrhage and death) because of their low therapeutic indices, so Admiral X is closely monitored, and the pharmacologic effect of the heparin is measured periodically by testing the partial thromboplastin time (PTT). Admiral X's symptoms resolve over the next several hours, although he remains in the hospital for monitoring. He is discharged after 4 days in the hospital; his discharge medications include pravastatin, aspirin, atenolol, lisinopril, and clopidogrel for secondary prevention of myocardial infarction.

QUESTIONS

■ **1.** How does the molecular interaction of a drug with its receptor determine the potency and efficacy of the drug?

2. What properties of certain drugs, such as aspirin, allow them to be taken without monitoring of plasma drug levels, whereas other drugs, such as heparin, require such monitoring?

3. Why does the fact that a drug has a low therapeutic index mean that the physician must use greater care in its administration?

DRUG–RECEPTOR BINDING

The study of pharmacodynamics is based on the concept of drug–receptor binding. When either a drug or an endogenous ligand (such as a hormone or neurotransmitter) binds to its receptor, a response may result from that binding interaction. When a sufficient number of receptors are bound (or "occupied") on or in a cell, the cumulative effect of receptor "occupancy" may become apparent in that cell. At some point, all of the receptors may be occupied, and a maximal response may be observed (an exception is the case of spare receptors; see below). When the response occurs in many cells, the effect can be seen at the level of the organ or even the patient. But this all starts with the binding of drug or ligand to a receptor (for the purpose of discussion, "drug" and "ligand" will be used interchangeably for the remainder of this chapter). A model that accurately describes the binding of drug to receptor would therefore be useful in predicting the effect of the drug at the molecular, cellular, tissue (organ), and organism (patient) levels. This section describes one such model.

Consider the simplest case, in which the receptor is either free (unoccupied) or reversibly bound to drug (occupied). We can describe this case as follows:

$$L + R \underset{k_{off}}{\overset{k_{on}}{\rightleftarrows}} LR \qquad \text{Equation 2-1}$$

where L is ligand (drug), R is free receptor, and LR is bound drug–receptor complex. At equilibrium, the fraction of receptors in each state is dependent on the dissociation constant, K_d, where $K_d = k_{off}/k_{on}$. K_d is an intrinsic property of any given drug–receptor pair. Although K_d varies with temperature, the temperature of the human body is relatively constant, and it can therefore be assumed that K_d is a constant for each drug–receptor combination.

According to the law of mass action, the relationship between free and bound receptor can be described as follows:

$$K_d = \frac{[L][R]}{[LR]}, \text{ rearranged to } [LR] = \frac{[L][R]}{K_d} \qquad \text{Equation 2-2}$$

where $[L]$ is free ligand concentration, $[R]$ is free receptor concentration, and $[LR]$ is ligand–receptor complex concentration. Because K_d is a constant, some important properties of the drug–receptor interaction can be deduced from this equation. First, as ligand concentration is increased, the concentration of bound receptors increases. Second, and not so obvious, is that as free receptor concentration is increased (as it may, for example, in disease states or upon repea-

ted exposure to a drug), bound receptor concentration also increases. Therefore, *an increase in the effect of a drug can result from an increase in the concentration of either the ligand or the receptor.*

The remainder of the discussion in this chapter, however, assumes that the total concentration of receptors is a constant, so that $[LR] + [R] = [R_o]$. This allows Equation 2-2 to be arranged as follows:

$$[R_o] = [R] + [LR] = [R] + \frac{[L][R]}{K_d}$$

$$= [R]\left(1 + \frac{[L]}{K_d}\right) \qquad \text{Equation 2-3}$$

Solving for $[R]$ and substituting Equation 2-3 into Equation 2-2 yields:

$$[LR] = \frac{[R_o][L]}{[L] + K_d}, \text{ rearranged to}$$

$$\frac{[LR]}{[R_o]} = \frac{[L]}{[L] + K_d} \qquad \text{Equation 2-4}$$

Note that the left side of this equation, $[LR]/[R_o]$, represents the fraction of all available receptors that are bound to ligand.

Figure 2-1 shows two plots of Equation 2-4 for the binding of two hypothetic drugs to the same receptor. These plots are known as **drug–receptor binding curves.** Figure 2-1A shows a linear plot, and Figure 2-1B shows the same plot on a semilogarithmic scale. Because drug responses occur over a wide range of doses (concentrations), the semilog plot is often used to display drug–receptor binding data. The two drug–receptor interactions are characterized by different values of K_d; in this case, $K_{dA} < K_{dB}$.

Notice from Figure 2-1 that maximum drug–receptor binding occurs when $[LR]$ is equal to $[R_o]$, or $[LR]/[R_o] = 1$. Also notice that, according to Equation 2-4, when $[L] = K_d$, then $[LR]/[R_o] = K_d/2K_d = 1/2$. Thus, K_d can be defined as the concentration of ligand at which 50% of the available receptors are occupied.

DOSE–RESPONSE RELATIONSHIPS

The pharmacodynamics of a drug can be quantified by the relationship between the dose (concentration) of the drug and the organism's (patient's) response to that drug. One might intuitively expect the dose–response relationship to be related closely to the drug–receptor binding relationship, and this turns out to be the case for many drug–receptor combinations. Thus, a useful assumption at this stage of discussion is that *the response to a drug is proportional to the concentration of receptors that are bound (occupied) by the drug.* This assumption can be quantified by the following relationship:

$$\frac{\text{response}}{\text{max response}} = \frac{[DR]}{[R_o]} = \frac{[D]}{[D] + K_d} \qquad \text{Equation 2-5}$$

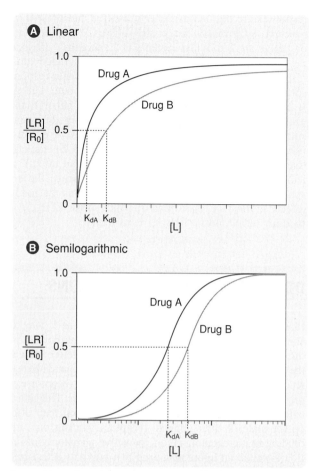

whereas quantal relationships show the effect of various doses of a drug on a population of individuals.

GRADED DOSE–RESPONSE RELATIONSHIPS

Figure 2-2 shows graded dose–response curves for two hypothetical drugs that elicit the same biological response. The curves are presented on both linear and semilog scales. The curves are similar in shape to those in Figure 2-1, consistent with the assumption that response is proportional to receptor occupancy.

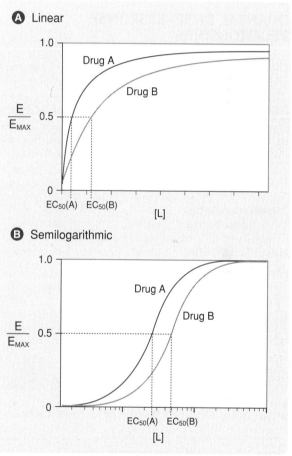

Figure 2-1. Ligand–receptor binding curves. A. Linear graphs of drug–receptor binding for two drugs with different values of K_d. **B.** Semilogarithmic graphs of the same drug–receptor binding. K_d is the equilibrium dissociation constant for a given drug–receptor interaction—a lower K_d indicates a *tighter* drug–receptor interaction (higher affinity). Because of this relationship, Drug A, which has the lower K_d, will bind a higher proportion of total receptors than Drug B at any given drug concentration. Notice that K_d corresponds to the ligand concentration [L] at which 50% of the receptors are bound (occupied) by ligand. [L] is the concentration of free (unbound) ligand (drug), [LR] is the concentration of ligand–receptor complexes, and R_o is the total concentration of occupied and unoccupied receptors. Thus,

$$\frac{[LR]}{[R_o]}$$

is the *fractional occupancy* of receptors, or the fraction of total receptors that are occupied (bound) by ligand.

where $[D]$ is the concentration of free drug, $[DR]$ is the concentration of drug–receptor complex, $[R_o]$ is the concentration of total receptors, and K_d is the equilibrium dissociation constant for the drug–receptor interaction. (Note that the right side of Equation 2-5 is equivalent to Equation 2-4, with $[D]$ substituted for $[L]$.) The generalizability of this assumption is examined below.

There are two major types of dose–response relationships—graded and quantal. The difference between the two methods is that graded dose–response relationships describe the effect of various doses of a drug on an individual,

Figure 2-2. Graded dose–response curves. Graded dose–response curves demonstrate the effect of a drug as a function of its concentration. **A.** Linear graphs of graded dose–response curves for two drugs. **B.** Semilogarithmic graphs of the same dose–response curves. Note the close resemblance to Figure 2-1: the fraction of occupied receptors [LR]/[R_o] has been replaced by the fractional effect E/E_{max}, where E is a quantifiable response to a drug (for example, an increase in blood pressure). EC_{50} is the potency of the drug, or the concentration at which the drug elicits 50% of its maximal effect. In the figure, Drug A is more potent than Drug B because it elicits a half-maximal effect at a lower concentration than Drug B. Drugs A and B exhibit the same efficacy (the maximal response to the drug). Note that potency and efficacy are not intrinsically related—a drug can be extremely potent but have little efficacy, and vice versa. [L] is drug concentration, E is effect, E_{max} is efficacy, and EC_{50} is potency.

Two important parameters—potency and efficacy—can be deduced from the graded dose–response curve. The **potency (EC$_{50}$)** of a drug is *the concentration at which the drug elicits 50% of its maximal response.* The **efficacy (E$_{max}$)** is *the maximal response produced by the drug.* In accordance with the assumption stated above, efficacy can be thought of as the state at which receptor-mediated signaling is maximal and, therefore, additional drug will produce no additional response. This usually occurs when all the receptors are occupied by the drug. Some drugs, however, are capable of eliciting a maximal response when fewer than 100% of the drug's receptors are occupied; the remaining receptors can be called **spare receptors.** This concept is discussed further in the text that follows. Note again that the graded dose–response curve of Figure 2-2 bears a close resemblance to the drug–receptor binding curve of Figure 2-1, with EC_{50} replacing K_d and E_{max} replacing R_o.

QUANTAL DOSE–RESPONSE RELATIONSHIPS

The quantal dose–response relationship plots the fraction of the population that responds to a given dose of drug as a function of the drug dose. Quantal dose–response relationships describe the concentrations of a drug that produce a given effect in a population. Figure 2-3 shows an example of quantal dose–response curves. Because of differences in biological response among individuals, the effects of a drug are seen over a range of doses. The

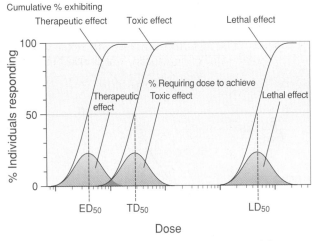

Figure 2-3. Quantal dose–response curves. Quantal dose–response curves demonstrate the average effect of a drug, as a function of its concentration, in a population of individuals. Individuals are typically observed for the presence or absence of a response (for example, sleep or no sleep), and this result is then used to plot the percentage of individuals who respond to each dose of drug. Quantal dose–response relationships are useful for predicting the effects of a drug when it is administered to a population of individuals, and for determining population-based toxic doses and lethal doses. These doses are called the *ED$_{50}$* (dose at which 50% of subjects exhibit a therapeutic response to a drug), *TD$_{50}$* (dose at which 50% of subjects experience a toxic response), and *LD$_{50}$* (dose at which 50% of subjects die). Note that *ED$_{50}$* is the dose at which 50% of subjects respond to a drug, while *EC$_{50}$* (as described in the previous figure) is the dose at which a drug elicits a half-maximal effect in an individual subject.

responses are defined as either present or not present (i.e., *quantal,* not *graded*). Endpoints such as ''sleep/no sleep'' or ''alive at 12 months/not alive at 12 months'' are examples of quantal responses; in contrast, graded dose–response relationships are generated using scalar responses such as change in blood pressure or heart rate. The goal is to generalize a result to a population, rather than to examine the graded effect of different drug doses on a single individual. Types of responses that can be examined using the quantal dose–response relationship include effectiveness (therapeutic effect), toxicity (adverse effect), and lethality (lethal effect). The doses that produce these responses in 50% of a population are known as the **median effective dose (ED$_{50}$), median toxic dose (TD$_{50}$),** and **median lethal dose (LD$_{50}$),** respectively.

DRUG–RECEPTOR INTERACTIONS

Many receptors for drugs can be modeled as having two conformational states that are in reversible equilibrium with one another. These two states are called the **active state** and the **inactive state.** Many drugs function as ligands for such receptors and affect the probability that the receptor exists preferentially in one conformation or the other. The pharmacologic properties of drugs are often based on their effects on the state of their cognate receptors. A drug that, upon binding to its receptor, favors the active receptor conformation is called an **agonist;** a drug that prevents activation of the receptor by agonist is referred to as an **antagonist.** Some drugs do not fit neatly into this simple definition of agonist and antagonist; these include **partial agonists** and **inverse agonists.** The following sections describe these pharmacologic classifications in more detail.

AGONISTS

An agonist is a molecule that binds to a receptor and stabilizes the receptor in a particular conformation (usually, the active conformation). When bound by an agonist, a typical receptor is more likely to be in its active conformation than its inactive conformation. Depending on the receptor, agonists may be drugs or endogenous ligands. A useful model for understanding the relationship between agonist binding and receptor activation is shown in Equation 2-6:

$$D + R \rightleftarrows D + R^*$$
$$\text{⇕} \qquad \text{⇕}$$
$$DR \rightleftarrows DR^*$$

Equation 2-6

where D and R are unbound (free) drug and receptor concentrations, respectively, DR is the concentration of the agonist–receptor complex, and R^* indicates the active conformation of the receptor. For most receptors and agonists, R^* and DR are unstable species that exist only briefly and are quantitatively insignificant compared to R and DR^*. Therefore, in most cases, Equation 2-6 simplifies to

$$D + R \rightleftarrows DR^*$$

Equation 2-7

Note that Equation 2-7 is identical to Equation 2-1, which was used for the analysis of drug–receptor binding. This suggests that, for most receptors, agonist binding is proportional to receptor activation. Some receptors, however, do have limited stability in the R^* and/or DR conformations; in these cases, Equation 2-6 must be revisited (see below).

Equation 2-6 can also be used to illustrate quantitatively the concepts of potency and efficacy. Recall that potency is the agonist concentration required to elicit a half-maximal effect, and efficacy is the maximal effect of the agonist. Assuming that a receptor is not active unless bound to a drug (i.e., R^* is insignificant compared to DR^*), Equation 2-8 provides a quantitative description of potency and efficacy:

$$D + R \underset{k_{off}}{\overset{k_{on}}{\rightleftarrows}} \underset{\text{Potency}}{DR} \underset{k_{\beta}}{\overset{k_{\alpha}}{\rightleftarrows}} \underset{\text{Efficacy}}{DR^*} \qquad \text{Equation 2-8}$$

Here, k_{α} is the rate constant for receptor activation and k_{β} is the rate constant for receptor deactivation. This equation demonstrates the relationship between potency ($K_d = k_{off}/k_{on}$) and agonist binding ($D + R \rightleftarrows DR$), as well as the relationship between efficacy (k_{α}/k_{β}) and the conformational change required for activation of the receptor ($DR \rightleftarrows DR^*$). These relationships are intuitive when we consider that more potent drugs are those that have a higher affinity for their receptors (lower K_d), and more efficacious drugs are those that cause a higher proportion of receptors to be activated.

ANTAGONISTS

An antagonist is a molecule that inhibits the action of an agonist but has no effect in the absence of the agonist.

Figure 2-4 shows one approach to classifying the various types of antagonists. Antagonists can be divided into receptor and nonreceptor antagonists. A **receptor antagonist** binds to either the active site (agonist binding site) or an allosteric site on a receptor. Binding of antagonist to the active site prevents the binding of agonist to the receptor, whereas binding of antagonist to an allosteric site either alters the K_d for agonist binding or prevents the conformational change required for receptor activation. Receptor antagonists can also be divided into **reversible** and **irreversible antagonists;** that is, antagonists that bind to their receptors reversibly and those that bind irreversibly. Figure 2-5 illustrates the general effects of these antagonist types on agonist binding; more detail is provided in the following sections.

A **nonreceptor antagonist** does not bind to the receptor for agonist, but it nonetheless inhibits the ability of an agonist to initiate a response. At the molecular level, this inhibition can occur by inhibiting the agonist directly (e.g., using antibodies), by inhibiting a downstream molecule in the activation pathway, or by activating a pathway that opposes the action of the agonist. Nonreceptor antagonists can be divided into chemical antagonists and physiologic antagonists. **Chemical antagonists** inactivate an agonist before it has the opportunity to act (e.g., by chemical neutralization); **physiologic antagonists** cause a physiologic effect opposite to that induced by the agonist.

The following section discusses competitive receptor antagonists and noncompetitive receptor antagonists. Nonreceptor antagonists are also examined briefly.

Competitive Receptor Antagonists

*A **competitive antagonist** binds reversibly to the active site of a receptor.* Unlike an agonist, which also binds to the

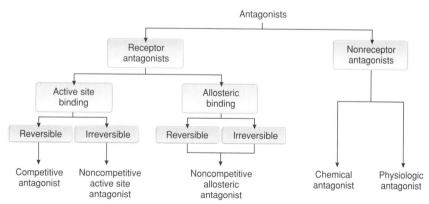

Figure 2-4. Antagonist classification. Antagonists can be categorized based on whether they bind to a site on the receptor for agonist (receptor antagonists) or interrupt agonist–receptor signaling by other means (nonreceptor antagonists). Receptor antagonists can bind either to the agonist (active) site or to an allosteric site on the receptor; in either case, they do not affect basal receptor activity (i.e., the activity of the receptor in the absence of agonist). Agonist (active) site receptor antagonists prevent the agonist from binding to the receptor. If the antagonist competes with the ligand for agonist site binding, it is termed a **competitive antagonist**; high concentrations of agonist are able to overcome competitive antagonism. Noncompetitive agonist site antagonists bind covalently or with very high affinity to the agonist site, so that even high concentrations of agonist are unable to activate the receptor. Allosteric receptor antagonists bind to the receptor at a site other than the agonist site. They do not compete directly with agonist for receptor binding, but rather alter the K_d for agonist binding or inhibit the receptor from responding to agonist binding. High concentrations of agonist are generally unable to reverse the effect of an allosteric antagonist. Nonreceptor antagonists fall into two categories. Chemical antagonists sequester agonist and thus prevent the agonist from interacting with the receptor. Physiologic antagonists induce a physiologic response opposite to that of an agonist, but by a molecular mechanism that does not involve the receptor for agonist.

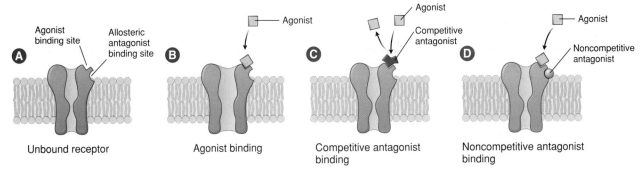

Figure 2-5. Types of receptor antagonists. A schematic illustrating the differences between agonist (active) site and allosteric antagonists. **A.** The unbound inactive receptor. **B.** The receptor activated by agonist. Note the conformational change induced in the receptor by agonist binding, for example, the opening of a transmembrane ion channel. **C.** Agonist site antagonists bind to the receptor's agonist site but do not activate the receptor; these agents block agonist binding to the receptor. **D.** Allosteric antagonists bind to an allosteric site (different from the agonist site) and thereby prevent receptor activation, even if the agonist is bound to the receptor.

active site of the receptor, a competitive antagonist does not stabilize the conformation required for receptor activation. Therefore, the antagonist blocks an agonist from binding to its receptor, while maintaining the receptor in the inactive conformation. Equation 2-9 is a modification of Equation 2-7 that incorporates the effect of a competitive antagonist (A).

$$AR \rightleftarrows A + D + R \rightleftarrows DR* \qquad \text{Equation 2-9}$$

In this equation, a fraction of the free receptor molecules (R) are unable to form a drug (agonist)–receptor complex ($DR*$), because receptor binding to antagonist results in the formation of an antagonist–receptor complex (AR) instead. In effect, the formation of the AR complex sets up a second equilibrium reaction that competes with the equilibrium for agonist–receptor binding. Note that AR is incapable of undergoing a conformational change to the active ($R*$) state of the receptor.

Quantitative analysis yields the following equation for agonist (D) binding to receptor in the presence of a competitive antagonist (A):

$$\frac{[DR]}{[R_o]} = \frac{[D]}{[D] + K_d\left(1 + \dfrac{[A]}{K_A}\right)} \qquad \text{Equation 2-10}$$

Equation 2-10 is similar to Equation 2-4, except that the effective K_d has been increased by a factor of $(1 + [A]/K_A)$, where K_A is the dissociation constant for binding of the antagonist to the receptor (i.e., $K_A = [A][R]/[AR]$). Because an increase in K_d is equivalent to a decrease in potency, *the presence of a competitive antagonist (A) reduces the potency of an agonist (D) by a factor of (1 + [A]/K_A)*. Although the potency of an agonist decreases as the concentration of competitive antagonist increases, the efficacy of the agonist is unaffected. This occurs because the agonist concentration [D] can be increased to counteract ("out-compete") the antagonist, thereby "washing out" or reversing the effect of the antagonist. Figure 2-6A shows the effect of a competitive antagonist on the agonist dose–response relationship. Note that the competitive antagonist has the effect of shifting the agonist dose–response

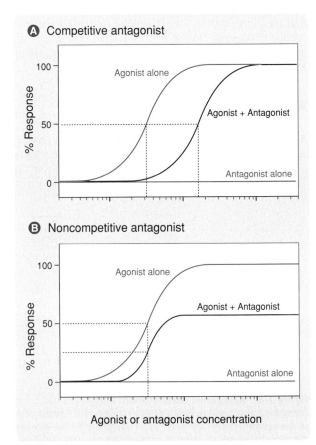

Figure 2-6. Antagonist effects on the agonist dose–response relationship. Competitive and noncompetitive antagonists have different effects on potency (the concentration of agonist that causes a half-maximal response) and efficacy (the maximal response to an agonist). **A.** A competitive antagonist reduces the potency of an agonist, without affecting agonist efficacy. **B.** A noncompetitive antagonist reduces the efficacy of an agonist. As shown here, most allosteric noncompetitive antagonists do not affect agonist potency.

curve to the right, causing a decrease in agonist potency while maintaining agonist efficacy.

Pravastatin, the drug used in the case at the beginning of this chapter to lower the Admiral's cholesterol, is an example of a competitive antagonist. Pravastatin is a member of the HMG CoA reductase inhibitor (statin) class of lipid-lowering drugs. HMG CoA reductase is an enzyme that catalyzes the reduction of HMG CoA, which is the rate-limiting step in cholesterol biosynthesis. The similarity between the chemical structures of statins and HMG CoA allows the statin molecule to bind to the active site of HMG CoA reductase, and thereby to prevent HMG CoA from binding. Inhibition of HMG CoA reductase decreases endogenous cholesterol synthesis and thereby lowers the patient's cholesterol levels. This inhibition is reversible because no covalent bonds are formed between the statin and the enzyme. For a more detailed discussion of pravastatin and other HMG CoA reductase inhibitors, see Chapter 23, Pharmacology of Cholesterol and Lipoprotein Metabolism.

Noncompetitive Receptor Antagonists

Noncompetitive antagonists can bind to either the active site or an allosteric site of a receptor (Fig. 2-4). A noncompetitive antagonist that binds to the active site of a receptor can bind either covalently or with very high affinity; in either case, the binding is effectively irreversible. Because an irreversibly bound active site antagonist cannot be ''outcompeted,'' even at high agonist concentrations, such an antagonist exhibits noncompetitive antagonism.

A noncompetitive allosteric antagonist acts by preventing the receptor from being activated, even when the agonist is bound to the active site. An allosteric antagonist exhibits noncompetitive antagonism regardless of the reversibility of its binding, because such an antagonist acts not by competing with agonist for binding to the active site, but rather by preventing receptor activation. The reversibility of antagonist binding is nonetheless important, because the effect of an irreversible antagonist does not diminish when the free (unbound) drug is eliminated from the body, whereas the effect of a reversible antagonist can be ''washed out'' over time as it dissociates from the receptor (see Equation 2-9).

A receptor that is bound by a noncompetitive antagonist can no longer respond to the binding of an agonist. Therefore, the maximal response (efficacy) of the agonist is reduced. A characteristic difference between competitive and noncompetitive antagonists is that *competitive antagonists reduce agonist potency, whereas noncompetitive antagonists reduce agonist efficacy*. This difference can be explained by considering that a competitive antagonist continuously competes for receptor binding, effectively reducing the receptor's affinity for agonist without limiting the number of available receptors. In contrast, a noncompetitive antagonist removes functional receptors from the system, thereby limiting the number of available receptors. Figures 2-6A and 2-6B compare the effects of competitive and noncompetitive antagonists on the agonist dose–response relationship.

Aspirin is one example of a noncompetitive antagonist. This agent irreversibly acetylates cyclo-oxygenase, the enzyme responsible for generating thromboxane A_2 in platelets. In the absence of thromboxane A_2 generation, platelet aggregation is inhibited. Because the inhibition is irreversible, and platelets are not capable of synthesizing new cyclo-oxygenase molecules, the effects of a single dose of aspirin last for 7 to 10 days (the time required for the bone marrow to generate new platelets), even though the free drug is cleared from the body much more rapidly.

Nonreceptor Antagonists

Nonreceptor antagonists can be divided into chemical antagonists and physiologic antagonists. A **chemical antagonist** inactivates the agonist of interest by modifying or sequestering it, so that the agonist is no longer capable of binding to and activating the receptor. **Protamine** is an example of a chemical antagonist; this basic protein binds stoichiometrically to the heparin class of anticoagulants and thereby inactivates these agents (see Chapter 22, Pharmacology of Hemostasis and Thrombosis). Because of this chemical antagonism, protamine can be used to terminate the effects of heparin rapidly.

A **physiologic antagonist** most commonly activates or blocks a receptor that mediates a response physiologically opposite to that of the receptor for agonist. For example, in the treatment of hyperthyroidism, **β-adrenergic antagonists** are used as physiologic antagonists to counteract the tachycardic effect of endogenous thyroid hormone. Although thyroid hormone does not produce its tachycardic effect via β-adrenergic stimulation, blocking β-adrenergic stimulation can nonetheless relieve the tachycardia caused by hyperthyroidism (see Chapter 9, Adrenergic Pharmacology, and Chapter 26, Pharmacology of the Thyroid Gland).

PARTIAL AGONISTS

A *partial agonist is a molecule that binds to a receptor at its active site but produces only a partial response, even when all of the receptors are occupied (bound) by the agonist.* Figure 2-7 shows a family of dose–response curves for several full and partial agonists. Each agonist acts by binding to the same site on the muscarinic acetylcholine (ACh) receptor. Note that butyl trimethylammonium (TMA) is not only more potent than longer-chain derivatives at stimulating muscle contraction, but also more efficacious than some of the derivatives (e.g., the heptyl and octyl forms) at producing a greater maximum response. For this reason, butyl TMA is a *full agonist* at the muscarinic ACh receptor, whereas the octyl derivative is a *partial agonist* at this receptor.

Because partial agonists and full agonists bind to the same site on a receptor, a partial agonist can reduce the response produced by a full agonist. In this way, the partial agonist can act as a competitive antagonist. For this reason, partial agonists are sometimes called ''partial antagonists'' or even ''mixed agonist-antagonists.''

It is interesting to consider how an agonist could produce a less-than-maximal response if a receptor can exist in only the active or the inactive state. This is an area of current investigation, for which several hypotheses have

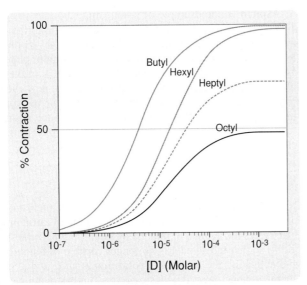

Figure 2-7. Full and partial agonist dose–response curves. There are many instances in which drugs that all act at the agonist site on the same receptor produce different maximal effects. For example, various alkyl derivatives of trimethylammonium all stimulate muscarinic acetylcholine (ACh) receptors to cause muscle contraction in the gut, but they produce different maximal responses, even when all receptors are occupied. In the figure, the butyl and hexyl trimethylammonium derivatives are full agonists—although they have different potencies, they are both capable of eliciting a maximal response. Agonists that produce only a partial response, such as the heptyl and octyl derivatives, are called **partial agonists.** Note that the dose–response curves of partial agonists plateau at values less than those of full agonists. ACh acts as a full agonist in this system (*not shown*).

been proposed. Recall that Equation 2-6 was simplified to Equation 2-7 based on the assumption that R and DR^* are much more stable than R^* and DR. But what would happen if a drug (call it a partial agonist) could stabilize DR as well as DR^*? In that case, addition of the partial agonist would result in stabilization of some receptors in the DR form and some receptors in the DR^* form. At full receptor occupancy, some receptors would be in the active state and some in the inactive state, and the efficacy of the drug would be reduced compared to that of a full agonist (which stabilizes only DR^*). In this formulation, a pure antagonist binds preferentially to the inactive state of the receptor, a full agonist binds preferentially to the active state of the receptor, and a partial agonist binds with comparable affinity to both the active and inactive states of the receptor.

A second hypothesis for the action of partial agonists is that a receptor may have multiple DR^* conformations, each with a different intrinsic activity. Depending on the particular conformations of the receptor that are bound by the agonist, a fraction of the maximum possible effect may be observed even when a partial agonist is bound to 100% of the receptors. This may be the case with the so-called **selective estrogen receptor modulators (SERMs)** such as **raloxifene** and **tamoxifen** (see Chapter 28, Pharmacology of Reproduction). Raloxifene acts as a partial agonist at estrogen receptors in bone and an antagonist at estrogen receptors in breast. The crystal structure of raloxi-

fene bound to estrogen receptor, when compared to that of estrogen bound to estrogen receptor, reveals that the side chain of raloxifene inhibits an α helix of the estrogen receptor from aligning in the active site (see inside front cover). This may result in inhibition of some downstream effects of the estrogen receptor, while maintaining other effects. At a physiologic level, this would be observed as partial agonist activity in bone.

Another example of a partial agonist is **pindolol**, a drug often classified as a β-adrenergic antagonist (see Chapter 9). In actuality, however, pindolol demonstrates partial agonist properties, and this drug may be of clinical value because of the intermediate response that it produces. Although resting heart rate and blood pressure are not reduced as much by pindolol as by other pure β-adrenergic antagonists, pindolol does inhibit the potentially dangerous heart rate and blood pressure increases that would otherwise occur with sympathetic stimulation (e.g., with exercise) in patients with cardiovascular disease.

INVERSE AGONISTS

The action of inverse agonists can be understood by considering Equation 2-6 again. As noted above, in some cases, receptors can have inherent stability in the R^* state. In these cases, there is intrinsic activity (''tone'') of the receptor system, even in the absence of an endogenous ligand or an exogenously administered agonist. *An **inverse agonist** acts by abrogating this intrinsic (constitutive) activity of the free (unoccupied) receptor.* Inverse agonists may function by binding to and stabilizing the receptor in the DR (inactive) form. This has the effect of deactivating receptors that had existed in the R^* form in the absence of drug. The physiologic importance of receptors that have inherent stability in the R^* state is currently under investigation, and receptors with mutations that render them constitutively active (e.g., BCR-Abl and EGFR tyrosine kinases) are becoming attractive targets for inverse agonist approaches in cancer chemotherapy (see Chapter 38, Pharmacology of Cancer: Signal Transduction).

Consider the similarities and differences between the actions of inverse agonists and competitive antagonists. Both types of drug act to reduce the activity of a receptor. In the presence of a full agonist, both competitive antagonists and inverse agonists act to reduce agonist potency. Recall, however, that a competitive antagonist has no effect in the absence of agonist, whereas an inverse agonist deactivates receptors that are constitutively active in the absence of agonist. Using Equations 2-6 through 2-9 as models, these concepts can be summarized by stating that *full agonists stabilize DR^*, partial agonists stabilize both DR and DR^* (or alternate forms of DR^*), inverse agonists stabilize DR, and competitive antagonists ''stabilize'' R (or AR) by preventing full, partial, and inverse agonists from binding to the receptor.*

SPARE RECEPTORS

Recall that the initial discussion of drug–receptor binding assumed that 100% receptor occupancy is required for an

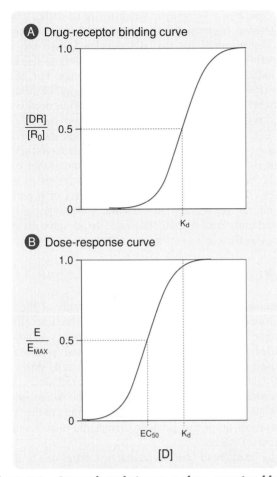

A Drug–receptor binding curve

B Dose–response curve

$\dfrac{[DR]}{[R_0]}$

$\dfrac{E}{E_{MAX}}$

[D]

At least two molecular mechanisms are thought to be responsible for the spare receptor phenomenon. First, the receptor could remain activated after the agonist departs, allowing one agonist molecule to activate several receptors. Second, the cell signaling pathways described in Chapter 1 could allow for significant amplification of a relatively small signal, and activation of only a few receptors could be sufficient to produce a maximal response. The latter is true, for example, with many G protein-coupled receptors; activation of a single $G\alpha_s$ molecule can stimulate adenylyl cyclase to catalyze the formation of dozens of molecules of cAMP.

The presence of spare receptors alters the effect of a noncompetitive antagonist on the system. At low antagonist concentrations, the noncompetitive antagonist binds receptors that are not required to produce a maximal response; therefore, the efficacy of the agonist is not decreased. The potency of the agonist is affected, however, because potency is proportional to the fraction of available receptors that must be occupied to produce a 50% response. A noncompetitive antagonist reduces the number of available receptors, thereby increasing the fraction of receptors that must be bound at any agonist concentration to produce the same response. At high antagonist concentrations, the noncompetitive antagonist binds not only the ''spare'' receptors but also receptors that are required to produce a maximal response, and the efficacy as well as the potency of the agonist is decreased. Figure 2-9 illustrates this concept.

Figure 2-8. Comparison between a drug–receptor binding curve and a dose–response curve in the presence of spare receptors. In the absence of spare receptors, there often exists a close correlation between a drug–receptor binding curve and a dose–response curve—the binding of additional drug to the receptor causes an incremental increase in response, and EC_{50} is approximately equal to K_d. In situations with spare receptors, however, a half-maximal response is elicited when less than half of all receptors are occupied (the term *spare* implies that occupation of every receptor with drug is not necessary to elicit a full response). **A.** Drug–receptor binding curve. **B.** Dose–response curve for the same drug, in the presence of spare receptors. Note that the maximal response occurs at a lower agonist concentration than does maximal binding, and $EC_{50} < K_d$. These two relationships confirm the presence of spare receptors. *D* is drug, *R* is receptor, and $[DR]/[R_o]$ is fractional receptor occupancy. *E* is response (effect), E_{max} is maximal response (efficacy), and E/E_{max} is fractional response. EC_{50} is potency, and K_d is the equilibrium dissociation constant for drug–receptor binding.

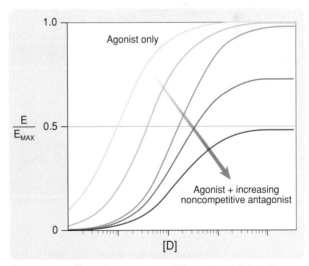

$\dfrac{E}{E_{MAX}}$

Agonist only

Agonist + increasing noncompetitive antagonist

[D]

Figure 2-9. Effect of a noncompetitive antagonist on the agonist dose–response curve in the presence of spare receptors. In a system without spare receptors, a noncompetitive antagonist causes efficacy to decrease at all concentrations of the antagonist (see Figure 2-6B). In a system with spare receptors, however, potency is decreased but efficacy is unaffected at low concentrations of the antagonist, because a sufficient number of unoccupied receptors is available to generate a maximal response. As increasing concentrations of antagonist bind noncompetitively to more and more receptors, the antagonist eventually occupies all of the ''spare'' receptors, and efficacy is also reduced.

agonist to exert its maximal effect. Now, consider the possibility that a maximal response could be achieved with less than 100% receptor occupancy. Figure 2-8 shows an example of a drug–receptor binding curve and a dose–response curve that illustrate this situation. In this example, a maximal effect is achieved at a lower dose of agonist than that required for receptor saturation, that is, the EC_{50} is less than the K_d for this system. This type of discrepancy between the drug–receptor binding curve and the dose–response curve signifies the presence of **spare receptors**.

CONCEPTS IN THERAPEUTICS

THERAPEUTIC INDEX AND THERAPEUTIC WINDOW

The **therapeutic window** is the range of doses (concentrations) of a drug that elicits a therapeutic response, without unacceptable adverse effects (toxicity), in a population of patients. For drugs that have a small therapeutic window, plasma drug levels must be monitored closely to maintain effective dosing without exceeding the level that could produce toxicity. The next chapter discusses some of the techniques used in clinical therapeutics to maintain plasma concentrations of drugs within the therapeutic window.

The therapeutic window can be quantified by the **therapeutic index (TI)** (sometimes called the **therapeutic ratio**), commonly defined as

$$\text{Therapeutic Index (TI)} = \frac{TD_{50}}{ED_{50}} \qquad \text{Equation 2-11}$$

where TD_{50} is the dose of drug that causes a toxic response in 50% of the population, and ED_{50} is the dose of drug that is therapeutically effective in 50% of the population. The TI provides a single number that quantifies the relative safety margin of a drug in a population of people. A large TI represents a large (or "wide") therapeutic window (for example, a thousand-fold difference between the therapeutic and toxic doses), and a small TI represents a small (or "narrow") therapeutic window (for example, a twofold difference between the therapeutic and toxic doses).

The potential for toxicity associated with the use of heparin and tPA in the case at the beginning of this chapter is indicated by the low TIs of these drugs. For example, the dose of heparin that can cause major bleeding in a patient is often less than twice the dose needed for a therapeutic effect; heparin can therefore be defined as having a therapeutic index of less than two. For this reason, patients treated with heparin must have their PTT, a marker of the coagulation cascade, monitored every 8 to 12 hours. Aspirin's high TI is indicative of its relative safety. Note that the pharmacologic effect of heparin was monitored periodically in the case, whereas aspirin could be administered without the need to monitor its plasma drug level.

Conclusion and Future Directions

Pharmacodynamics is the quantitative study of the effects of drugs on the body. Several tools have been developed to compare the efficacy and potency of drugs, including the graded and quantal dose–response relationships. The former is used to examine the effects of various drug doses on an individual, whereas the latter is used to examine the effects of various drug doses on a population. The therapeutic window and therapeutic index are used to compare the concentrations of drugs that produce therapeutic effects and toxic (adverse) effects.

In the study of pharmacodynamics, drugs can be divided

TABLE 2-1 **Summary of Agonist and Antagonist Action**

CLASSES OF AGONISTS	
AGONIST CLASS	**ACTION**
Full agonist	Activates receptor with maximal efficacy
Partial agonist	Activates receptor but not with maximal efficacy
Inverse agonist	Inactivates constitutively active receptor

CLASSES OF ANTAGONISTS			
ANTAGONIST CLASS	**EFFECTS ON AGONIST POTENCY**	**EFFECTS ON AGONIST EFFICACY**	**ACTION**
Competitive antagonist	Yes	No	Binds reversibly to active site of receptor; competes with agonist binding to this site
Noncompetitive active site antagonist	No	Yes	Binds irreversibly to active site of receptor; prevents agonist binding to this site
Noncompetitive allosteric antagonist	No	Yes	Binds reversibly or irreversibly to site other than active site of receptor; alters K_d for agonist binding or prevents conformational change required for receptor activation by agonist

into two broad classes—agonists and antagonists. Most agonists cause a receptor to maintain its conformation in the active state, whereas antagonists prevent activation of the receptor by agonists. Antagonists are further divided according to the molecular location of their effect (i.e., receptor or nonreceptor), the site at which they bind to the receptor (i.e., active site or allosteric site), and the mode of their binding to the receptor (i.e., reversible or irreversible). Table 2-1 provides a summary of the various types of agonists and antagonists presented in this chapter.

The information presented in this chapter is used repeatedly throughout this book and throughout one's career as a health professional. Whenever drugs are compared according to potency or efficacy, or the appropriate dose of a drug for a specific patient must be determined, a working knowledge of pharmacodynamics is essential.

Suggested Reading

Berg JM, Tymoczko JL, Stryer L. *Biochemistry.* 6th ed. New York: WH Freeman and Company; 2006. (*Discusses the structural basis for protein–protein interactions.*)

Leff P. The two-state model of receptor activation. *Trends Pharmacol Sci* 1995;16:89–97. (*Provides the theoretic grounding for Equation 2-6; discusses quantitative treatment of drug–receptor interactions.*)

Pratt WB, Taylor P, eds. *Principles of drug action: the basis of pharmacology.* 3rd ed. New York: Churchill Livingstone; 1990. (*Contains an in-depth discussion of pharmacodynamics.*)

3

Pharmacokinetics

John C. LaMattina and David E. Golan

INTRODUCTION

Even the most promising of pharmacologic therapies will fail in clinical trials if the drug is unable to reach its target organ at a concentration sufficient to have a therapeutic effect. Many of the characteristics that render the human body resistant to harm by foreign invaders and toxic substances also limit the ability of modern drugs to combat pathologic processes within the patient. An appreciation of the many factors that affect a drug's ability to act within a patient, and the dynamic nature of these factors over time, are vitally important to the clinical practice of medicine.

All drugs must meet certain minimal requirements to achieve clinical effectiveness. A successful drug must be able to cross the physiologic barriers that exist to limit the access of foreign substances to the body. Drug **absorption** may occur by a number of mechanisms that are designed either to exploit or to breach these barriers. After absorption, the drug uses **distribution** systems within the body, such as the blood and lymphatic vessels, to reach its target organ in an appropriate concentration. The drug's ability to access its target is also limited by several processes within the patient. These processes fall broadly into two categories: **metabolism,** in which the body inactivates the drug through enzymatic degradation (primarily in the liver), and **excretion,** in which the drug is eliminated from the body (primarily by the kidneys and liver, and in the feces). This chapter presents a broad overview of the pharmacokinetic processes of absorption, distribution, metabolism, and excretion (often abbreviated as **ADME**; Fig. 3-1), with a conceptual emphasis on basic principles that, when applied to an unfamiliar situation, should enable the student or physician to understand the pharmacokinetic basis of drug therapy.

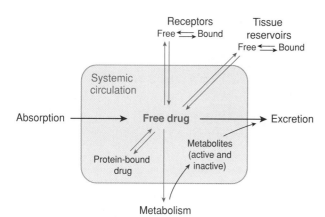

Figure 3-1. Drug absorption, distribution, metabolism, and excretion (ADME). The basic principles of pharmacokinetics affect the amount of free drug that ultimately reaches the target site. To elicit an effect on its target, a drug must be absorbed and then distributed to its target before being metabolized and excreted. At all times, free drug in the systemic circulation is in equilibrium with tissue reservoirs, plasma proteins, and the target site (which usually consists of receptors); only the fraction of drug that successfully binds to specific receptors will have a pharmacologic effect. Note that metabolism of drug can result in both inactive and active metabolites; active metabolites may also be able to exert a pharmacologic effect, either on the target receptors or sometimes on other receptors.

■ Case

Mr. W is a 66-year-old technology consultant who makes frequent trips abroad as part of his job in the telecommunications industry. His only medical problem is chronic atrial fibrillation and his only chronic medication is **warfarin**. Mr. W flies to Turkey for a consulting job. On the last night of the trip, he attends a large dinner featuring shish kebabs and other foods he does not often eat. The next day, he develops profuse, watery, foul-smelling diarrhea. A physician makes a diagnosis of traveler's diarrhea and prescribes a 7-day course of **trimethoprim-sulfamethoxazole**.

Mr. W feels entirely well 2 days into the course of antibiotics, and 4 days later (while still taking his antibiotics), he entertains some clients at another lavish dinner. Mr. W and his guests become intoxicated at the dinner, and Mr. W stumbles and falls on the curb as he is leaving the restaurant. The next day, Mr. W has a markedly swollen right knee that requires evaluation in a local emergency room. Physical examination and imaging studies are consistent with a moderate-sized hemarthrosis of the right knee, and laboratory studies show a markedly elevated international normalized ratio (INR), which is a standardized measure of prothrombin time and, in this clinical setting, a surrogate marker for plasma warfarin level. The emergency physician advises Mr. W that his warfarin level is in the supratherapeutic (toxic) range, and that this effect is likely due to adverse drug–drug interactions involving his warfarin, his antibiotics, and his recent **alcohol** intoxication.

QUESTIONS

■ **1.** How does a patient with well-established therapeutic levels of a chronic medication suddenly develop clinical manifestations of drug toxicity?

■ **2.** Could this situation have been avoided? If so, how?

PHYSIOLOGIC BARRIERS

A drug must overcome physical, chemical, and biological barriers to reach its molecular and cellular sites of action. The epithelial lining of the gastrointestinal tract and other mucous membranes is one sort of barrier; additional barriers are encountered after the drug enters the blood and lymphatics. Most drugs must distribute from the blood into local tissues, a process that may be impeded by structures such as the blood–brain barrier. Typically, drugs leave the intravascular compartment at the level of the postcapillary venules, where there are larger gaps between the endothelial cells through which the drug can pass. Drug distribution occurs mainly through passive diffusion, the rate of which is affected by local ionic and cellular conditions. This section describes the major physical, chemical, and biological barriers presented by the body and the properties of drugs that favor or disfavor the drugs' ability to overcome these barriers.

BIOLOGICAL MEMBRANES

All human cells are limited by a lipid bilayer membrane. The membrane contains a hydrophobic lipid core and presents a hydrophilic surface to the aqueous extracellular and intracellular environments. The major lipid components of biological membranes are amphiphilic molecules, including phospholipids, cholesterol, and other minor species. The hydrophilic phosphate-containing head groups of phospholipids and the polar hydroxyl groups of cholesterol are exposed at the outer and inner membrane surfaces, while the hydrophobic tails of the lipids face the interior of the membrane. In addition to lipid components, biological membranes contain many different proteins. Some of these proteins are exposed only at the extracellular or intracellular membrane surface; others (called **transmembrane proteins**) penetrate through the lipid bilayer and are exposed at both membrane surfaces. This design has important implications for drug therapy. For a drug either to affect intracellular targets or to pass through a cell, it must be able to cross at least one, and usually several, biological membranes.

Traversing the Membrane

The hydrophobic core of a biological membrane presents the major barrier to drug transport. Small nonpolar molecules, such as steroid hormones, are able to diffuse easily through membranes. Many therapeutic drugs are sufficiently large and polar, however, as to render this an ineffective mechanism of transport across the membrane. Some transmembrane proteins in the **human solute linked carrier (SLC)** superfamily—which includes 43 families of proteins such as the **organic anion transporter (OAT)** and **organic cation transporter (OCT)** families—allow passage of polar drugs and molecules across the membrane. Some members of this superfamily are specialized transmembrane carrier proteins that are specific for the drug and related endogenous molecules; upon binding of the drug to the extracellular surface of the protein, the protein undergoes a conformational change that may be energy-independent (called **facilitated diffusion**) or require the input of energy (called **active transport**). This conformational change allows the bound drug access to the interior of the cell, where the drug molecule is released from the protein. Alternatively, some drugs bind to specific cell surface receptors and trigger a process called **endocytosis**, in which the cell membrane involutes around the molecule to form a closed cavity or vesicle from which the drug is subsequently released into the interior of the cell.

Membrane Diffusion

In the absence of other factors, a drug will enter a cell until the intracellular and extracellular concentrations of the drug are equal. The rate of diffusion depends on the concentration gradient of the drug across the membrane and on the thickness, area, and permeability of the membrane. Fick's law of diffusion states that the net drug flux across the membrane is

$$\text{Flux} = \frac{(C2 - C1) \times (\text{Area} \times \text{Permeability})}{\text{Thickness}_{\text{membrane}}} \quad \text{Equation 3-1}$$

where $C1$ and $C2$ are the intracellular and extracellular concentrations of the drug, respectively. This definition applies to an ideal situation where there is an absence of complicating factors such as ionic, pH, and charge gradients across the membrane. In vivo, however, these additional factors affect the tendency of a drug to enter cells. For example, a higher concentration of drug outside the cell would ordinarily tend to favor net drug entry into the cell, but if both the cell interior and the drug are negatively charged, then net drug entry into the cell may be impeded. A positively charged drug would show the opposite electrical tendency, and entry into the cell would be favored.

Net diffusion of acidic and basic drugs across lipid bilayer membranes may also be affected by a charge-based phenomenon known as **pH trapping**. The extent of drug trapping on one side of the membrane is determined by the drug's acid dissociation constant (pK_a) and by the pH gradient across the membrane. For weakly acidic drugs, such as phenobarbital and aspirin, the protonated form of the drug that predominates in the highly acidic environment of the stomach is electrically neutral. This uncharged form of the drug is more likely to pass through the lipid bilayers of the gastric mucosa, speeding the drug's absorption (Fig. 3-2). The weakly acidic drug is then deprotonated to its electrically charged form in the more basic environment of the plasma, and this form is less likely to diffuse back across the gastric mucosa. Together, these equilibria effectively trap the drug within the plasma.

In quantitative terms, the pK_a of a drug represents the pH value at which one-half of the drug is present in its ionic form. The Henderson-Hasselbalch Equation describes the

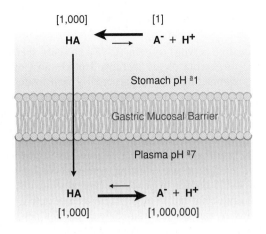

Figure 3-2. pH trapping across lipid bilayers. In the example shown, consider a hypothetical drug with $pK_a = 4$. Although this drug is a weak acid, in the highly acidic environment of the stomach, it is largely protonated. If the stomach pH is approximately 1, then for every 1,001 molecules of drug, 1,000 molecules are protonated (and neutral) and only 1 is deprotonated (and negatively charged). The protonated, neutral form of the drug is able to diffuse across the gastric mucosal barrier into the blood. Because the blood plasma has a pH of approximately 7 (it is actually 7.4), and the drug has a pKa of 4, the vast majority of drug now exists in the deprotonated (negatively charged) form: for every 1,001 molecules of drug, only 1 molecule is protonated (and neutral), while 1,000 molecules are deprotonated (and negatively charged). The negatively charged form of the drug is no longer able to diffuse across the lipid bilayers of the gastric mucosa, and the drug is effectively trapped in the plasma.

relationship between the pK_a of an acidic or basic drug A and the pH of the biological medium containing the drug:

$$pK_a = \text{pH} + \log \frac{[HA]}{[A^-]} \quad \text{Equation 3-2}$$

where HA is the protonated form of drug A. For example, consider the hypothetical case of a weakly acidic drug with a pK_a of 4. In the stomach, which has a pH of approximately 1, Equation 3-2 becomes

$$pK_{a_{drug}} = \text{pH}_{stomach} + \log \frac{[HA]}{[A^-]},$$

which simplifies to:

$$3 = \log \frac{[HA]}{[A^-]},$$

and finally:

$$1,000 = \frac{[HA]}{[A^-]}.$$

Therefore, in the stomach, the protonated form of the drug exists in 1,000 times the concentration of the deprotonated form, and 99.9% of the drug is in the neutral form. A similar calculation for the plasma, in which the pH is approximately 7 (plasma pH is actually 7.4), demonstrates that the situation is reversed, with 99.9% of the drug in the deprotonated form (see Fig. 3-2).

CENTRAL NERVOUS SYSTEM

The central nervous system (CNS) presents special challenges to pharmacologic therapy. Unlike most other anatomic regions, the CNS is particularly well insulated from foreign substances. The **blood–brain barrier** uses specialized tight junctions to prevent the passive diffusion of most drugs from the systemic to the cerebral circulation. Therefore, drugs designed to act in the CNS must either be sufficiently small and hydrophobic to traverse biological membranes easily or use existing transport proteins in the blood–brain barrier to penetrate central structures. Hydrophilic drugs that fail to target facilitated or active transport proteins in the blood–brain barrier cannot penetrate the CNS. The blood–brain barrier can be bypassed using intrathecal drug infusion, in which drugs are delivered directly into the cerebrospinal fluid (CSF). Although this approach can be used to treat infectious or carcinomatous meningitis, the intrathecal route is impractical for drugs that must be taken regularly by the patient.

ABSORPTION

The human body presents formidable obstacles to microorganisms that would seek to invade it. The integument, with its keratinized outer layer and the defensins found within its epithelium, presents an inhospitable surface for invasion. The mucous membranes, while presenting a more feasible penetration point, are also replete with nonspecific defense mechanisms, including mucociliary clearance in the trachea, lysozyme secretion from lacrimal ducts, acid in the stomach, and base in the duodenum. These nonspecific mechanisms must also be overcome by any drug, or the amount of the drug available to the target organ, referred to as the drug's **bioavailability** (also known as the fraction absorbed), will never be sufficiently high for the drug to be efficacious. The route by which the drug is administered, the chemical form of the drug, and a number of patient-specific factors—such as gastrointestinal and hepatic transporters and enzymes—combine to determine the drug's bioavailability.

Bioavailability is defined quantitatively as follows:

$$\text{Bioavailability} = \frac{\text{Quantity of drug reaching systemic circulation}}{\text{Quantity of drug administered}} \qquad \text{Equation 3-3}$$

This definition of bioavailability is based on the important fact that *most drugs reach their molecular and cellular sites of action directly from the systemic circulation.* Intravenously administered drugs are injected directly into the systemic circulation; for these drugs, the quantity administered is equivalent to the amount reaching the systemic circulation, and the bioavailability is, by definition, 1.0. In contrast, incomplete gastrointestinal absorption and "first-pass" hepatic metabolism (see below) typically cause the bioavail-

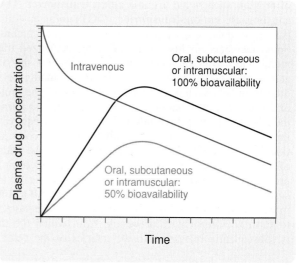

Figure 3-3. Bioavailability after administration of a single dose of drug. An intravenously administered drug is immediately available in the circulation. The drug is then distributed to other body compartments (see Fig. 3-7) and eliminated by first-order kinetics (see Fig. 3-6). In contrast, other routes of administration (e.g., oral, subcutaneous, and intramuscular) demonstrate slower entry of drug into the blood. In addition, other routes of administration must take into account bioavailability—for example, many orally administered drugs are incompletely absorbed or undergo first-pass metabolism in the liver. If a drug has 100% bioavailability, the total amount of drug reaching the systemic circulation will be the same for all routes of drug administration, but non-intravenous routes will require a longer period of time to reach a maximal concentration of drug in the plasma. If the bioavailability of an oral, subcutaneous, or intramuscular dosage form is less than 100%, then the dose of the drug would have to be increased in order for the total amount of drug reaching the systemic circulation to be the same as that of an intravenous dose. Note that the total amount of drug reaching the systemic circulation can be quantified by integrating the **area under the curve** (**AUC**) of the plasma drug concentration versus time plot.

ability of an orally administered drug to be less than 1.0 (Fig. 3-3).

ADMINISTRATION ROUTES AND RATIONALE

Each new drug is designed and tested in a dosage form that is administered by a specific route. Routes of administration are chosen to enable the drug to penetrate barriers presented by the body, often taking advantage of transport molecules and other mechanisms that permit the drug to enter body tissues. This section discusses the advantages and disadvantages of drug administration by enteral (oral), parenteral, mucous membrane, and transdermal routes (Table 3-1).

Enteral

Enteral drug administration, or the administration of a drug by mouth, is the simplest of drug routes. The enteral route of administration exploits existing weaknesses in human barrier defenses, but it exposes the drug to harsh acidic (stomach) and basic (duodenum) environments that could limit

TABLE 3-1	Routes of Drug Administration	
ROUTE	**ADVANTAGES**	**DISADVANTAGES**
Enteral (e.g., aspirin)	Simple, inexpensive, convenient, painless, no infection	Drug exposed to harsh GI environments and first-pass metabolism, requires GI absorption, slow delivery to site of pharmacologic action
Parenteral (e.g., morphine)	Rapid delivery to site of pharmacologic action, high bioavailability, not subject to first-pass metabolism or harsh GI environments	Irreversible, infection, pain, fear, skilled personnel required
Mucous membrane (e.g., beclomethasone)	Rapid delivery to site of pharmacologic action, not subject to first-pass metabolism or harsh GI environments, often painless, simple, convenient, low infection, direct delivery to affected tissues (e.g., lung) possible	Few drugs available to administer via this route
Transdermal (e.g., nicotine)	Simple, convenient, painless, excellent for continuous or prolonged administration, not subject to first-pass metabolism or harsh GI environments	Requires highly lipophilic drug, slow delivery to site of pharmacologic action, may be irritating

GI, gastrointestinal.

its absorption. This route provides many advantages for the patient: oral drugs are easily and conveniently self-administered, and these dosage forms are less likely than other methods to introduce systemic infection as a complication of treatment.

An orally administered drug must be stable during its absorption across the gastrointestinal tract epithelium. Gastrointestinal epithelial cell junctions make paracellular transport across an intact epithelium difficult. Instead, ingested substances (such as drugs) must usually traverse the cell membrane at both apical and basal surfaces before entering the blood. The efficiency of this process is determined by drug size and hydrophobicity, and sometimes by the presence of carriers through which the drug may enter and/or exit the cell. *In general, hydrophobic and neutral drugs cross cell membranes more efficiently than do hydrophilic or charged drugs, unless the membrane contains a carrier molecule that facilitates the passage of hydrophilic substances.*

Upon traversing the gastrointestinal epithelium, drugs are carried by the portal system to the liver before entering the systemic circulation. While the portal circulation serves to protect the body from the systemic effects of ingested toxins by delivering these substances to the liver for detoxification, this system may complicate drug delivery. All orally administered drugs are subjected to **first-pass metabolism** in the liver. In this process, liver enzymes may inactivate a fraction of the ingested drug. Any drug that exhibits significant first-pass metabolism must be administered in a quantity sufficient to ensure that an effective concentration of active drug exits the liver into the systemic circulation, from which it can reach the target organ. Nonenteral routes of drug administration are not subjected to first-pass liver metabolism.

Parenteral

Parenteral drug administration, in which a drug is introduced directly across the body's barrier defenses into the systemic circulation or some other tissue space, immediately overcomes barriers that can limit the effectiveness of orally administered drugs. Drugs can be administered parenterally into vascularized tissue or injected directly into the blood or cerebrospinal fluid (Table 3-2). Tissue administration results in a rate of onset of drug action that differs among the various body tissues, depending on the rate of blood flow to the tissue. Subcutaneous (SC) administration of drug into poorly vascularized adipose tissue results in a slower onset of action than does injection into well-vascularized intramuscular (IM) spaces. Drugs that are soluble only in oil-based solutions are often administered intramuscularly. Direct introduction of drug into the venous [intravenous (IV)] or arterial [intra-arterial (IA)] circulation, or into the cerebrospinal fluid [intrathecal (IT)], results in the drug reaching its target organ the fastest. Intravenous injection is not typically limited in the amount of drug that can be delivered, as subcutaneous and intramuscular injections may be. Continuous intravenous infusions also have the advantage of controlled drug delivery, so that the dose of drug delivered can be adjusted at any time.

Although the physical properties of certain drugs (e.g., size and hydrophobicity) may necessitate a particular route of drug administration, the clinician will often have a choice among several different routes. Parenteral administration may be associated with several potential disadvantages, including an increased risk of infection and the requirement for administration by a health care professional. The rate of onset of parenterally administered drugs is often rapid, potentially resulting in increased toxicity when such drugs are administered too rapidly or in incorrect doses. These disadvantages must be weighed against the advantages of parenteral administration (such as speed of onset and control of the delivered dose) and the urgency of the indication for pharmacologic therapy.

TABLE 3-2	Routes of Parenteral Drug Administration	
PARENTERAL ROUTE	**ADVANTAGES**	**DISADVANTAGES**
Subcutaneous (e.g., Xylocaine)	Slow onset, may be used to administer oil-based drugs	Slow onset, small volumes
Intramuscular (e.g., haloperidol)	Intermediate onset, may be used to administer oil-based drugs	Can affect lab tests (creatine kinase), intramuscular hemorrhage, painful
Intravenous (e.g., morphine)	Rapid onset, controlled drug delivery	Peak-related drug toxicity
Intrathecal (e.g., methotrexate)	Bypasses blood-brain barrier	Infection, highly skilled personnel required

Mucous Membrane

Administration of drugs across mucous membranes can potentially provide rapid absorption, low incidence of infection, convenience of administration, and avoidance of harsh gastrointestinal environments and first-pass metabolism. Sublingual, ocular, pulmonary, nasal, rectal, urinary, and reproductive tract epithelia have all been used to deliver drugs in the form of liquid drops, rapidly dissolving tablets, aerosols, and suppositories (among other dosage forms). The mucous membranes are highly vascular, permitting the drug to enter the systemic circulation rapidly and to reach its target organ with minimal delay. Drugs may also be administered directly into the target organ, resulting in virtually instantaneous onset of action. This is advantageous in critical conditions such as acute asthma, where drugs such as β-adrenergic agonists are administered via aerosol directly into the airways.

Transdermal

A limited set of drugs has sufficiently high lipophilicity that passive diffusion across the skin provides a viable route of administration. Transcutaneously administered drugs are absorbed from the skin and subcutaneous tissues directly into the blood. This route of administration is ideal for a drug that must be slowly and continuously administered over extended periods. There is no associated risk of infection, and drug administration is simple and convenient. The success of transdermal nicotine, estrogen, and scopolamine patches demonstrates the potential utility of this route of administration (see Chapter 54, Drug Delivery Modalities, for more details on transdermal drug delivery).

LOCAL FACTORS AFFECTING ABSORPTION

The rate and extent of absorption of a drug are affected by several factors that are specific to the treatment situation. In general, a higher and/or more rapidly administered dose results in a greater increase in local drug concentration (Fig. 3-4). This increases the tendency for the drug to diffuse across membranes or into the blood, which then causes the local drug concentration to decrease. Thus, factors that increase the rate of distribution of the drug away from the site

of administration decrease the likelihood that the concentration of the drug will reach equilibrium across biological membranes. Regional blood flow has the greatest effect in this regard; in a highly perfused region, drug molecules crossing into that compartment are rapidly removed. This effect maintains the drug concentration at a low level in the compartment, allowing the driving force for entry of new

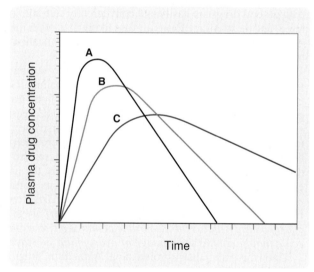

Figure 3-4. Effect of rate of absorption on peak plasma concentration of drug and on duration of drug action. The duration of action and peak plasma concentration of a drug can be affected markedly by the drug's absorption rate. In this example, three drugs with identical bioavailability, volume of distribution, and clearance are administered in identical doses. The drugs demonstrate different rates of absorption—drug A is absorbed quickly, drug C is absorbed slowly, and drug B's absorption rate is between those of drugs A and C. Drug A reaches the highest peak plasma concentration, since all of the drug is absorbed before significant elimination can take place. Drug C is absorbed slowly and never achieves a high plasma concentration, but it persists in the plasma for longer than drugs A or B because absorption continues during the elimination phase. It should be noted that the hypothetical drugs A, B, and C could all be the same drug administered by three different routes. For example, curve A could represent intravenous glucocorticoid administration, curve B could be a depot intramuscular injection, and curve C could be an ultraslow-release subcutaneous formulation of the same drug.

TABLE 3-3	Drug Distribution to Different Body Compartments

COMPARTMENT	EXAMPLES
Total body water	Small water-soluble molecules (e.g., ethanol)
Extracellular water	Larger water-soluble molecules (e.g., mannitol)
Blood plasma	Highly plasma protein-bound molecules, very large molecules, highly charged molecules (e.g., heparin)
Fat	Highly lipid-soluble molecules (e.g., diazepam)
Bone and teeth	Certain ions (e.g., fluoride, strontium)

drug molecules into the compartment to remain high (see Equation 3-1). For example, volatile general anesthetics are administered via inhalation. The lungs are highly perfused, and the anesthetic is removed rapidly from the lungs into the circulation. Because blood flows through the lung rapidly, an increased concentration of anesthetic does not develop in the local circulation, and there is little diffusional force to oppose the entry of anesthetic into the blood. Therefore, many volatile anesthetics enter the blood compartment readily until this compartment begins to become saturated with drug (see Chapter 15, General Anesthetic Pharmacology, for more details). A similar trend is seen in patients of greater body mass, who have both an increased surface area across which diffusion can occur and a larger tissue volume into which the drug can distribute. Both of these factors increase the tendency for a drug to be absorbed by the patient. The absorption of some orally administered drugs is affected by the presence or absence of food in the lumen of the gastrointestinal tract at the time of drug administration.

DISTRIBUTION

Although absorption of a drug is a prerequisite for establishing adequate plasma drug levels, the drug must also reach its target organ(s) in therapeutic concentrations to have the desired effect on a pathophysiologic process. Drug distribution is achieved primarily through the circulatory system; a minor component is contributed by the lymphatic system. Once a drug has been absorbed into the systemic circulation, it is then capable of reaching any target organ (with the possible exception of sanctuary compartments such as the brain and testes). The concentration of drug in the plasma is often used to define and monitor therapeutic drug levels, because the amount of drug that is actually taken up by the target organ is difficult to measure. In some cases, the plasma concentration of a drug may represent a relatively poor measure of the actual tissue concentration. In most cases, however, the effect of the drug in the target tissue correlates well with the plasma drug concentration.

Organs and tissues vary widely in their capacity to take up different drugs and in the proportion of systemic blood flow that these tissues receive. The forces governing the distribution of a drug among the various tissues and compartments (Table 3-3) greatly affect the concentration of the drug in the plasma. Blood flow also varies markedly among the different organ systems, with the liver, kidneys, and brain (CNS) receiving the highest flow (Table 3-4). These kinetic factors determine the amount of drug that must be administered to achieve the desired concentration of drug within the vascular compartment. The ability of nonvascular tissues and plasma proteins to take up and/or bind the drug adds complexity to dosing regimens and must also be accounted for in order to achieve therapeutic drug levels.

VOLUME OF DISTRIBUTION

The **volume of distribution** of a drug (V_d) represents the fluid volume that would be required to contain the total amount of absorbed drug in the body at a uniform concentration equivalent to that in the plasma at steady state:

$$V_d = \frac{\text{Dose}}{[\text{Drug}]_{\text{plasma}}}$$

Equation 3-4

TABLE 3-4	Total and Weight-Normalized Tissue Blood Flow in an Adult

ORGAN PERFUSED	BLOOD FLOW (mL/min)	ORGAN MASS (kg)	NORMALIZED BLOOD FLOW (mL/min/kg)
Liver	1,700	2.5	680
Kidneys	1,000	0.3	3,333
Brain	800	1.3	615
Heart	250	0.3	833
Fat	250	10.0	25
Other (muscle, etc.)	1,400	55.6	25
Total	5,400	70.0	—

The extent to which a drug is taken up by the body as a whole is greater when the drug is highly distributed among body tissues. Thus, the volume of distribution is relatively low for drugs that are retained primarily within the vascular compartment and relatively high for drugs that are highly distributed into muscle, adipose, and other nonvascular compartments. In fact, for very highly distributed drugs, the volume of distribution is often much greater than the volume of total body water, reflecting the low concentration of drug in the vascular compartment at steady state. A number of drugs have very large volumes of distribution; examples include amiodarone (4,620 liters [L] for a 70-kg person), amitriptyline (1,050 L), amlodipine (1,120 L), azithromycin (2,170 L), chloroquine (9,240 L), chlorpromazine (1,470 L), digoxin (645 L), fluoxetine (2,450 L), gefitinib (1,400 L), haloperidol (1,260 L), itraconazole (980 L), ivermectin (700 L), olanzapine (1,150 L), and triamterene (940 L), among others. These numerical examples demonstrate that V_d is an extrapolated volume based on the concentration of drug in the plasma, rather than a physical volume. This concept is quantified in Equation 3-4.

The capacity of the blood and the various body organs and tissues to take up and retain a drug depends on both the volume (mass) of the tissue and the density of specific and nonspecific binding sites for the drug within that tissue. A drug that is taken up in large quantities by body tissues such as adipose and muscle will be largely removed from the circulation at steady state. In most cases, these tissues must be saturated before plasma levels of such drugs can increase sufficiently to affect the drug's target organ. Thus, for drugs of equal potency, a drug that is more highly distributed among body tissues generally requires a higher initial dose to establish a therapeutic plasma concentration than does a drug that is less highly distributed.

Plasma Protein Binding

The capacity of muscle and adipose tissue to bind a drug increases the tendency of the drug to diffuse from the blood into nonvascular compartments, but this tendency can be counteracted to some extent by plasma protein binding of the drug. Albumin is the most abundant plasma protein (its concentration is about 4 g/dL) and is the protein that is most responsible for drug binding. Many drugs bind with low affinity to albumin through both hydrophobic and electrostatic forces. Plasma protein binding tends to reduce the availability of a drug for diffusion or transport into the drug's target organ because, in general, only the free or unbound form of the drug is capable of diffusion across membranes (Fig. 3-5). Plasma protein binding may also reduce the transport of drugs into nonvascular compartments such as adipose tissue and muscle. Because a highly protein-bound drug tends to remain within the vasculature, such a drug often has a relatively low volume of distribution (typically, 7 to 8 L for a 70-kg person).

Theoretically, plasma protein binding could be important as a mechanism for some drug–drug interactions. Coadministration of two or more drugs, each of which is highly bound to plasma protein, could result in a higher-than-expected plasma concentration of the free form of either or both drugs. This would occur because the coadministered drugs compete for the same binding sites on

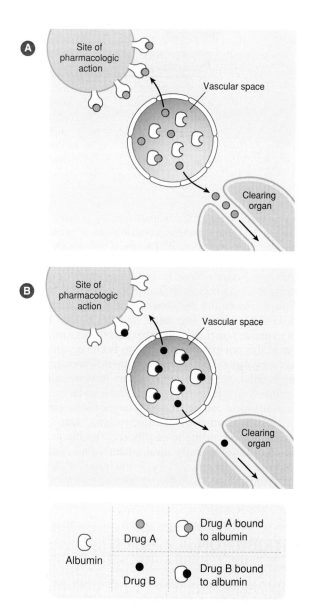

Figure 3-5. Protein binding and drug trapping. A drug that is bound to albumin or other plasma proteins cannot diffuse from the vascular space into surrounding tissues. **A.** Drugs that do not bind plasma proteins appreciably (shown here as Drug A) diffuse readily into tissues. This results in both a high level of binding to the site of pharmacologic action (usually receptors) and a high rate of elimination (represented by flux through a clearing organ). Examples of such drugs include acetaminophen, acyclovir, nicotine, and ranitidine. **B.** In contrast, for drugs that exhibit high levels of binding to plasma proteins (shown here as Drug B), a higher total drug concentration is required to ensure an adequate concentration of free (unbound) drug in the circulation. Otherwise, only a small fraction of the drug can diffuse into the extravascular space and only a small percentage of the receptors are occupied. Examples of such drugs include amiodarone, fluoxetine, naproxen, and warfarin. *It should be emphasized that plasma protein binding is only one of many variables that determine drug distribution.* Drug molecule size, lipophilicity, and rate of metabolism are other important parameters that must be taken into account when considering the pharmacokinetics of a particular drug.

plasma proteins. The increased free drug concentration could have the potential to cause increased therapeutic and/or toxic effects of the drug. In such cases, one could imagine that the dosing regimen of one or both of the drugs would need to be adjusted so as to bring the free drug concentration back into the therapeutic range. In practice, however, it has been difficult to demonstrate clinically significant drug–drug interactions caused by competition between the binding of two drugs to plasma proteins. This somewhat surprising result may be attributable to the increased clearance of the free drugs as they are displaced from their plasma protein binding sites (see below).

MODELING THE KINETICS AND THERMODYNAMICS OF DRUG DISTRIBUTION

Most drugs are distributed rapidly from the systemic circulation (intravascular compartment) to other compartments in the body. This **distribution phase** results in a sharp decrease in the plasma drug concentration shortly after intravenous administration of a drug bolus. Even after the drug equilibrates among its tissue reservoirs, the plasma drug concentration continues to decline because of drug elimination from the body. The rate of decline of plasma drug concentration during the elimination phase is slower than that during the distribution phase, because during the elimination phase the "reservoir" of drug in the tissues can diffuse back into the blood to replace the drug that has been eliminated (Figs. 3-6 and 3-7).

The tendency for a drug to be taken up by adipose and muscle tissue during the distribution phase results in a set of dynamic equilibria among drug concentrations in the various body compartments. As shown in Figure 3-8, the rapid decline of plasma drug concentration after administration of an intravenous bolus of drug can be approximated more accurately by using a four-compartment model consisting of the blood and vessel-rich, muscle-rich, and adipose-rich tissues. The vessel-rich group is the first extravascular compartment in which the concentration of drug increases, because the high blood flow received by this group *kinetically* favors drug entry into this compartment. However, the muscle-rich group and fat group often have a higher *capacity* for taking up drug than the vessel-rich group. Because the fat group often has the highest capacity to take up drug and the lowest blood flow, the fat group can take up a greater amount of drug than the other groups, but at a slower rate.

The capacity of a compartment for drug and the rate of blood flow to the compartment also affect the rate at which drugs exit from that compartment. Drugs tend to exit first from the vessel-rich group, followed by the muscle group and then the fat group. Most drugs are taken up to greater or lesser extents by all of these tissues, creating a complex and dynamic pattern of changing blood concentrations over time that is specific for each drug. This pattern may also be patient-specific, depending on factors such as the size, age, and fitness level of the patient. For example, an older patient typically has less skeletal muscle mass than does a younger patient, decreasing the contribution of muscle uptake to changes in the plasma concentration of drug. An opposite effect may be seen in an elite athlete, who would be expected to have both greater muscle mass and greater proportional muscle blood flow. As a third example, an obese person would be expected to exhibit greater capacity for drug uptake into adipose tissue.

METABOLISM

A number of organs are capable of metabolizing drugs to some extent, using enzymatic reactions that are elucidated further in Chapter 4, Drug Metabolism. Thus, the kidneys, gastrointestinal tract, lungs, skin, and other organs all contribute to systemic drug metabolism. However, the liver contains the greatest diversity and quantity of metabolic enzymes, and the majority of drug metabolism occurs there. The ability of the liver to modify drugs depends on the amount of drug that enters the hepatocytes. Highly lipophilic drugs can generally enter cells (including liver cells) more readily. As a result, the liver preferentially metabolizes hydrophobic drugs. However, the liver contains a multitude of transporters in the SLC superfamily that allow entry of some hydrophilic drugs into hepatocytes as well. Hepatic enzymes are able to chemically modify a variety of substituents on drug molecules, thereby either rendering the drugs inactive or facilitating their elimination. These modifications are collectively referred to as **biotransformation.** Biotransformation reactions are classified into two types, termed **oxidation/reduction reactions** and **conjugation/hydrolysis reactions**. (Although biotransformation reactions are often called **Phase I** and **Phase II** reactions, in this book we use

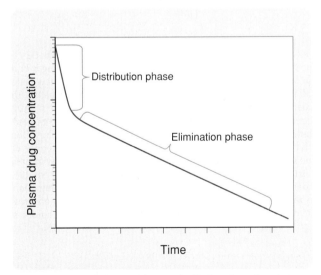

Figure 3-6. Drug distribution and elimination after intravenous administration. Immediately after intravenous administration of a drug, the plasma drug concentration declines rapidly as the drug distributes from the vascular compartment to other body compartments. This rapid decline is followed by a slower decline as the drug is metabolized and excreted from the body. Both drug distribution and elimination display first-order kinetics, as demonstrated by linear kinetics on a semilogarithmic plot.

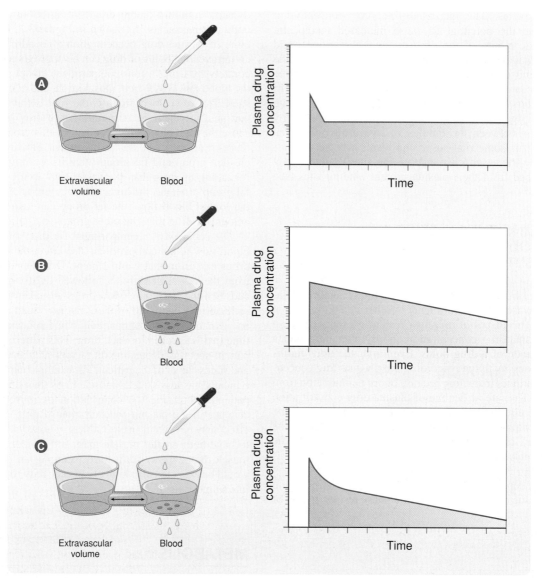

Figure 3-7. Schematic model of drug distribution and elimination. A two-compartment pharmacokinetic model can be used to describe drug distribution and elimination after administration of a single intravenous dose. The drug concentration rises rapidly as the drug is added to the first compartment. **A.** In the absence of elimination, the initial rise in drug concentration is followed by a rapid decline to a new plateau as the drug equilibrates (distributes) between the two compartments. **B.** If the distribution of the drug is confined to the blood volume, then the plasma drug concentration declines more slowly as the drug is eliminated from the body. In both cases, as the concentration of drug in the plasma decreases, the forces driving **(A)** drug distribution and **(B)** elimination decrease, and the absolute amount of drug distributed or eliminated per unit time decreases. Therefore, the kinetics of both distribution and elimination appear as straight lines on a semilogarithmic plot; this is the definition of *first-order kinetics*. Note that the half-time for drug elimination is generally longer than the half-time for drug distribution. **C.** When drug distribution and elimination are occurring simultaneously, the decline of plasma drug concentration with time is represented by the sum of the two processes. Note that the curve in **(C)** is the sum of the two first-order processes shown in **(A)** and **(B)**. In the schematics on the left of the figure, the volume in the "Blood" compartment represents plasma drug concentration, the volume in the "Extravascular volume" compartment represents tissue drug concentration, the dropper above the "Blood" compartment represents absorption of drug into the systemic circulation, and the drops below the "Blood" compartment represent elimination of drug by metabolism and excretion.

the more precise terms *oxidation/reduction* and *conjugation/hydrolysis;* see Chapter 4.)

OXIDATION/REDUCTION REACTIONS

Oxidation/reduction reactions modify the chemical structure of a drug through oxidation or reduction. The liver has en-

zymes that facilitate each of these reactions. The most common pathway, the microsomal **cytochrome P450 system**, mediates a large number of oxidative reactions. One common oxidative reaction involves the addition of a hydroxyl group to the drug. It should also be noted that some drugs are administered in inactive **(prodrug)** form, so that they can be altered metabolically by oxidation/reduction reactions to the active (drug) form in the liver. This prodrug strategy can

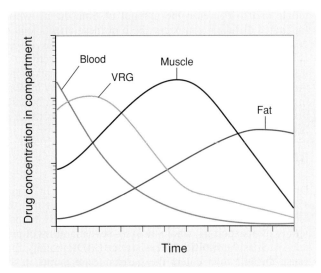

Figure 3-8. Four-compartment model of drug distribution. After administration of an intravenous bolus, the drug is delivered to various tissues via the systemic circulation. Drug concentration is initially highest in the vascular compartment (blood), but the blood concentration subsequently falls rapidly as the drug is distributed to the different tissue compartments. The most vessel-rich tissues (i.e., the tissues that are supplied by the highest fraction of the cardiac output) are generally the first to accumulate drug. However, the tissue compartments also vary in their capacity for taking up drug. Because the mass of the muscle group is larger than that of the vessel-rich group (VRG), the muscle group has a larger uptake capacity. But because the muscles are less well perfused than the vessel-rich group, this effect is manifested only after the drug has begun to distribute to the VRG. The most poorly perfused group is the fat group, but this group has the highest capacity to accumulate drug. The peak level of drug in the fat group is not as high as that in the muscle-rich group, because a significant amount of drug has been eliminated by metabolism or excretion before the fat group begins to accumulate drug. After the administration of drug has been completed, the reverse pattern is seen—the drug leaves first from the vessel-rich group and then from the muscle and fat groups, respectively.

be used to facilitate oral bioavailability, decrease gastrointestinal toxicity, and/or prolong the elimination half-life of a drug.

CONJUGATION/HYDROLYSIS REACTIONS

Conjugation/hydrolysis reactions hydrolyze a drug or conjugate a drug to a large, polar molecule in order to inactivate the drug or, more commonly, to enhance the drug's solubility and excretion in the urine or bile. Occasionally, hydrolysis or conjugation can result in the metabolic activation of prodrugs. The most commonly added groups include glucuronate, sulfate, glutathione, and acetate.

As described in more detail in the next chapter, the effects of oxidation/reduction and conjugation/hydrolysis reactions on a particular drug also depend on the presence of other drugs that are being taken concomitantly by the patient. Certain classes of drugs, such as barbiturates, are powerful inducers of enzymes that mediate oxidation/reduction reactions; other drugs are capable of inhibiting these enzymes. An understanding of these **drug–drug interactions** is an essential prerequisite to the appropriate dosing of drug combinations.

Physicians and researchers have begun to elucidate the important role of genetic differences among individuals in the various transporters and enzymes responsible for drug absorption, distribution, excretion, and especially metabolism. For example, an individual's complement of cytochrome P450 enzymes in the liver determines the rate and extent to which that individual can metabolize numerous therapeutic agents. This topic is discussed in detail in Chapter 52, Pharmacogenomics.

EXCRETION

Oxidation/reduction and conjugation/hydrolysis reactions enhance the hydrophilicity of a hydrophobic drug and its metabolites, enabling such drugs to be excreted along a final common pathway with drugs that are intrinsically hydrophilic. Most drugs and drug metabolites are eliminated from the body through renal and biliary excretion. Renal excretion provides the most common mechanism of drug excretion; this form of excretion relies on the hydrophilic character of a drug or metabolite. Only a relatively small number of drugs are excreted primarily in the bile. Many orally administered drugs are incompletely absorbed from the upper gastrointestinal tract, and residual drug is eliminated by fecal excretion. Otherwise, drugs can be excreted in minor quantities through respiratory and dermal routes.

RENAL EXCRETION

Renal blood flow comprises about 25% of total systemic blood flow, ensuring that the kidneys are continuously exposed to any drug found in the blood. The rate of drug elimination through the kidneys depends on the balance of drug filtration, secretion, and reabsorption rates (Fig. 3-9). The afferent arteriole introduces both free (unbound) drug and plasma protein-bound drug into the glomerulus. Typically, however, only the free drug form is filtered into the renal tubule. Therefore, renal blood flow, glomerular filtration rate, and drug binding to plasma protein all affect the amount of drug that enters the tubule at the glomerulus. Enhancing blood flow, increasing glomerular filtration rate, and decreasing plasma protein binding all cause a drug to be excreted more rapidly. Renal excretion plays a role in the clearance of many drugs; vancomycin, atenolol, and ampicillin are three among many examples of drugs for which the kidneys provide the primary route of excretion. *Drugs such as these can accumulate to toxic levels in patients with compromised renal function and in elderly patients (who often manifest some degree of renal compromise).*

Urinary drug concentration rises in the proximal tubule because of passive diffusion of uncharged drug molecules, facilitated diffusion of charged or uncharged molecules, and active secretion of anionic and cationic molecules from the blood into the urinary space. The secretory mechanisms are generally not specific for the drugs; rather, drug secretion takes advantage of molecular similarities between the drug and naturally occurring substances such as organic anions (transported by OAT family proteins) and cations (trans-

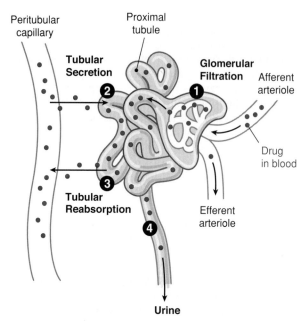

Figure 3-9. Drug filtration, secretion, and reabsorption in the kidney. Drugs may be (1) filtered at the renal glomerulus, (2) secreted into the proximal tubule, (3) reabsorbed from the tubular lumen and transported back into the blood, and (4) excreted in the urine. The relative balance of filtration, secretion, and reabsorption rates determines the kinetics of drug elimination by the kidney. Enhancing blood flow, increasing glomerular filtration rate, and decreasing plasma protein binding all cause a drug to be excreted more rapidly, because all these changes result in increased filtration of drug at the glomerulus. Some drugs, such as penicillin, are actively secreted into the proximal tubule. Although reabsorption can decrease the elimination rate of a drug, many drugs exhibit pH trapping in the distal tubule and are therefore efficiently excreted in the urine. For drugs that are dependent on the kidney for elimination, compromised renal function can result in higher plasma drug concentrations, and the dose and frequency of drug administration must be altered accordingly.

ported by OCT family proteins). Penicillin is an example of a drug that is eliminated largely by active transport in the proximal tubule. The extent of plasma protein binding appears to have a relatively small effect on drug secretion into the proximal tubule, because the highly efficient transporters that mediate active tubular secretion rapidly remove free (unbound) drug from the peritubular capillaries and thereby alter the equilibrium between free and protein-bound drug at these sites.

The urinary concentration of drug may fall as the drug is reabsorbed in the proximal and distal tubules. Reabsorption is limited primarily by **pH trapping**, as described above. The renal tubular fluid is typically acidic in and beyond the proximal tubule, which tends to favor trapping of the ionic form of weak bases. Because this region of the tubule contains transporter proteins that are different from those in preceding segments of the nephron, ionic drug forms resist facilitated diffusional reabsorption, and their excretion is thereby enhanced. Drug reabsorption in the tubule can be enhanced or inhibited by chemical adjustment of the urinary pH. Changing the rate of urine flow through the tubules can also modify the rate of drug reabsorption. An increased rate of urine output tends to dilute the drug concentration in the

tubule and to decrease the amount of time during which facilitated diffusion can occur; both of these effects tend to decrease drug reabsorption. For example, aspirin is a weak acid that is excreted by the kidney. Aspirin overdose is treated by administering sodium bicarbonate to alkalinize the urine (and thus trap aspirin in the tubule) and by increasing the urine flow rate (and thus dilute the tubular concentration of the drug). Both of these clinical maneuvers result in faster elimination of the drug.

BILIARY EXCRETION

Drug reabsorption also plays an important role in biliary excretion. Some drugs are secreted from the liver into the bile by members of the **ATP binding cassette** (**ABC**) superfamily of transporters, which includes seven families of proteins such as the **multidrug resistance** (**MDR**) family. Because the bile duct enters the gastrointestinal tract in the duodenum, such drugs must pass through the length of the small and large intestine before being eliminated. In many cases, these drugs undergo **enterohepatic circulation**, in which they are reabsorbed in the small intestine and subsequently retained in the portal and then the systemic circulation. Drugs such as steroid hormones, digoxin, and some cancer chemotherapeutic agents are largely excreted in the bile.

CLINICAL APPLICATIONS OF PHARMACOKINETICS

The dynamic interactions among drug absorption, distribution, metabolism, and excretion determine the plasma concentration of a drug and dictate the ability of the drug to reach its target organ in an effective concentration. Often, the desired duration of drug therapy exceeds that achievable by a single dose, and multiple doses are needed to provide a relatively constant plasma concentration of drug within the limits of efficacy and toxicity. The results of clinical trials of drugs under development, as well as clinical experience using FDA-approved drugs, suggest target plasma levels for a drug in the average patient. However, pharmacokinetic and other differences among patients (such as disease status and pharmacogenomic profile) must also be considered in designing a dosing regimen for a drug or drug combination in the individual patient.

CLEARANCE

The clearance of a drug is the pharmacokinetic parameter that most significantly limits the time course of action of the drug at its molecular, cellular, and organ targets. Clearance can be conceptualized in two complementary ways. First, it is defined as the rate of elimination of the drug from the body relative to the concentration of the drug in plasma. Alternatively, clearance is the rate at which plasma would have to be cleared of the drug to account for the observed kinetics of change of the total amount of drug in the body, assuming that all the drug in the body is present at the same concentration as that in the plasma. Therefore, clearance is expressed in units of volume/time, as follows:

$$\text{Clearance} = \frac{\text{Metabolism} + \text{Excretion}}{[\text{Drug}]_{\text{plasma}}} \qquad \text{Equation 3-5}$$

where metabolism and excretion are expressed as rates (amount/time).

Although metabolism and excretion are distinct physiologic processes, the pharmacologic endpoint is equivalent—a reduction in circulating levels of active drug. As such, metabolism and excretion are often referred to collectively as **clearance** mechanisms, and the principles of clearance can be applied to both:

$$\text{Clearance}_{\text{total}} = \text{Clearance}_{\text{renal}} + \text{Clearance}_{\text{hepatic}}$$
$$+ \text{Clearance}_{\text{Other}} \qquad \text{Equation 3-6}$$

Metabolism and Excretion Kinetics

The rate of drug metabolism and excretion by an organ is limited by the rate of blood flow to that organ. The majority of drugs demonstrate **first-order kinetics** when used in standard therapeutic doses; that is, the amount of drug that is metabolized or excreted in a given unit of time is directly proportional to the concentration of drug in the systemic circulation at that time. Because the clearance mechanisms for most drugs are not saturated under ordinary circumstances, increases in plasma drug concentration are matched by increases in the rate of drug metabolism and excretion (see Equation 3-5). The first-order elimination rate (where elimination includes both metabolism and excretion) follows Michaelis–Menten kinetics:

$$E = \frac{V_{\text{max}} \times C}{K_m + C} \qquad \text{Equation 3-7}$$

where V_{max} is the maximum rate of drug elimination, K_m is the drug concentration at which the rate of elimination is $\frac{1}{2} V_{\text{max}}$, C is the concentration of drug in the plasma, and E is the elimination rate (Fig. 3-10). Because elimination is usually a first-order process, a semilogarithmic plot of plasma drug concentration versus time typically shows a straight line during the elimination phase (see Fig. 3-6).

A small number of drugs (e.g., phenytoin) and recreational substances (e.g., ethanol) demonstrate **saturation kinetics,** in which the clearance mechanisms become saturated at or near the therapeutic concentration of the drug. Once saturation occurs, the clearance rate fails to increase with increasing plasma drug concentrations. Instead, the clearance rate remains constant (a characteristic of **zero-order** rather than first-order kinetics) despite increasing plasma drug levels. This can result in dangerously elevated plasma concentrations of the drug that can cause toxic (or even lethal) effects.

The extent to which an organ contributes to drug clearance is quantified by its **extraction ratio,** which compares the drug levels in plasma immediately before entering and just after exiting the organ:

$$\text{Extraction} = \frac{C_{\text{in}} - C_{\text{out}}}{C_{\text{in}}} \qquad \text{Equation 3-8}$$

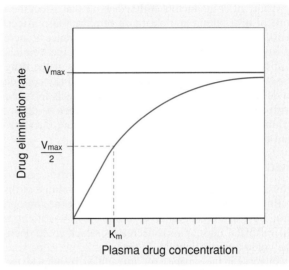

Figure 3-10. Michaelis–Menten kinetics. Drug elimination typically follows Michaelis–Menten (first-order) kinetics. The rate of drug elimination increases as the plasma drug concentration increases, until the elimination mechanisms become saturated and reach a maximal elimination rate (V_{max}) at high plasma concentrations. K_m (the Michaelis-Menten constant) is the drug concentration at which the drug elimination rate is $1/2$ V_{max}.

where C = concentration. An organ that contributes significantly to drug clearance is expected to have a higher extraction ratio (closer to 1) than does an organ that does not participate significantly in drug clearance (closer to zero). For example, the liver extraction ratio is high for drugs that have significant first-pass metabolism, and the brain extraction ratio is high for intravenous barbiturates that are used for rapid induction of general anesthesia (see Chapter 15).

HALF-LIFE

By decreasing the concentration of active drug in the blood, drug metabolism and excretion shorten the time during which a drug is capable of acting on a target organ. The **elimination half-life** of a drug is defined as *the amount of time over which the drug concentration in the plasma decreases to one-half of its original value.* Knowledge of a drug's elimination half-life allows the clinician to estimate the frequency of dosing required to maintain the plasma concentration of the drug in the therapeutic range (see below). There are many potentially confounding factors in any clinical situation, and it is useful to consider here the simplest of cases. Because most drugs are eliminated by first-order kinetics, the body can often be modeled as a single compartment with a volume that is equivalent to the volume of distribution. In this model, the elimination half-life ($t_{1/2}$) depends only on the volume of distribution and clearance of the drug:

$$t_{1/2} = \frac{0.693 \times V_d}{\text{Clearance}} \qquad \text{Equation 3-9}$$

where V_d is the volume of distribution and 0.693 is an approximation of ln 2.

Thus, all of the factors outlined above that affect the volume of distribution and clearance of a drug also affect the half-life of the drug. A decrease in drug clearance or increase in volume of distribution tends to prolong the elimination half-life, and thereby to enhance the effect of the drug on the target organ. The half-life must be carefully considered in designing any dosing regimen, as the effects from a drug with a long half-life may last for a number of days. For example, the half-life of chloroquine is more than 1 week and that of amiodarone is almost 1 month.

Factors Altering Half-Life

Physiologic and pathologic changes in the volume of distribution must be considered when determining the appropriate drug dose and dosing interval (Table 3-5). As patients age, their skeletal muscle mass decreases, which could decrease the volume of distribution. In contrast, an obese person has an increase in the capacity for drug uptake by adipose tissue, and a drug that distributes into fat may need to be given in a higher dose in order to reach therapeutic plasma drug levels. As a third example, if drug dosage is based on body weight but the fat group does not take up the drug, then potentially toxic drug levels could be reached in an obese individual. Finally, some drugs may partition preferentially into pathologic fluid spaces such as ascites or a pleural effusion, causing long-term toxicity if the drug dosage is not adjusted accordingly.

Physiologic and pathologic processes may also affect drug clearance. For example, the cytochrome P450 enzymes responsible for drug metabolism in the liver can be induced, increasing the rate of drug inactivation, or inhibited, decreasing the rate of drug inactivation. Specific P450 enzymes are induced by some drugs (such as carbamazepine, phenytoin, prednisone, and rifampin) and inhibited by others (such as cimetidine, ciprofloxacin, diltiazem, and fluoxetine); see

TABLE 3-5   **Factors Affecting Drug Half-Life**

FACTOR AFFECTING HALF-LIFE	MOST COMMON EFFECT ON HALF-LIFE
Effects on Volume of Distribution	
Aging (decreased muscle mass → decreased distribution)	Decreased
Obesity (increased adipose mass → increased distribution)	Increased
Pathologic fluid (increased distribution)	Increased
Effects on Clearance	
Cytochrome P450 induction (increased metabolism)	Decreased
Cytochrome P450 inhibition (decreased metabolism)	Increased
Cardiac failure (decreased clearance)	Increased
Hepatic failure (decreased clearance)	Increased
Renal failure (decreased clearance)	Increased

Table 4-3 for an extensive list of inducers and inhibitors of specific enzymes. Organ failure is another critical factor in determining appropriate drug regimens. Hepatic failure may both alter liver enzyme function and decrease biliary excretion. Decreased cardiac output reduces the amount of blood that reaches clearance organs. Renal failure decreases drug excretion because of decreased drug filtration and secretion into the renal tubules (see Box 3-1). In summary, *hepatic, cardiac, and renal failure can each lead to a decreased ability to inactivate or eliminate a drug, and thereby increase the elimination half-life of the drug.*

THERAPEUTIC DOSING AND FREQUENCY

The basic principles of pharmacokinetics—absorption, distribution, metabolism, and excretion—each influence the design of an optimal dosing regimen for a drug. Absorption determines the potential route(s) of administration and helps to determine optimal drug dose. A highly absorbed drug—as evidenced by a high bioavailability—generally requires a lower dose than does a poorly absorbed drug. (It is important to note, however, that the most important determinant of drug dose is the **potency** of the drug; see Chapter 2.) In contrast, a highly distributed drug—as evidenced by a high volume of distribution—necessitates higher drug dosing. The elimination rate of a drug influences its half-life and thereby determines the frequency of dosing required to maintain therapeutic plasma drug levels.

In general, *therapeutic dosing of a drug seeks to maintain the peak (highest) plasma drug concentration below the toxic concentration, and the trough (lowest) drug concentration above the minimally effective level* (Fig. 3-11). This can be accomplished most efficiently using continuous drug delivery by intravenous (continuous infusion), subcutaneous (continuous pump or implant), oral (sustained-release tablet), and other routes of administration, as described in more detail in Chapter 54, Drug Delivery Modalities. In many cases, however, the dosing regimen must also consider patient convenience. Frequent small doses (usually oral) can be administered to achieve minimal variation in steady-state plasma drug concentration, but this strategy subjects the patient to the inconvenience of frequent drug administration. Less frequent dosing requires the use of higher doses and leads to greater fluctuations in peak and trough drug levels; this type of regimen is more convenient for the patient but also more likely to cause problems due to excessive (toxic) or insufficient (subtherapeutic) drug levels (Fig. 3-12).

Optimal dosing regimens typically maintain the steady-state plasma drug concentration within the therapeutic window for that drug. Because steady state is reached when the rate of drug input is equal to its output, the steady-state drug concentration is affected by drug bioavailability, clearance, dose, and dosing interval (the frequency of administration):

$$C_{\text{steady state}} = \frac{\text{Bioavailability} \times \text{Dose}}{\text{Interval}_{\text{dosing}} \times \text{Clearance}} \qquad \text{Equation 3-10}$$

where C is the plasma concentration of the drug.

Immediately following the initiation of drug therapy, the rate of drug entry into the body (k_{in}) is much greater than the elimination rate (k_{out}); therefore, the drug concentration

BOX 3-1. Application to Therapeutic Decision-Making: Drug Use in Chronic Kidney Disease
by Vivian Gonzalez Lefebre and Robert H. Rubin

Many drugs are excreted by the kidneys, and the decreased creatinine clearance that accompanies chronic kidney disease often necessitates dosage adjustment or use of a different drug. Consider the following scenario.

Mr. R is a 59-year-old man with diabetes mellitus, hypertension, and chronic kidney disease (creatinine clearance, <10 mL/min). He has required hemodialysis for 5 years. One night he is admitted to the hospital with fever and hypotension. The presumed source of infection is the central venous catheter used for hemodialysis. Blood cultures are obtained from both the catheter and a peripheral site. The Gram stain of the catheter tip is remarkable for gram-positive cocci, and empiric treatment is started with vancomycin and gentamicin. The culture eventually identifies methicillin-resistant *Staphylococcus aureus* (MRSA).

Kidney disease can lead to many physiologic changes that affect the pharmacokinetics of a drug. For example, in patients with edema, pleural effusion, or ascites, there may be an increase in the volume of distribution of highly water-soluble or protein-bound drugs. *The most concerning pharmacologic consequence of renal insufficiency is its effect on drug clearance.* Plasma concentrations of drugs that have narrow therapeutic indices and are predominantly cleared by the kidneys, such as gentamicin and methotrexate, may reach sustained toxic levels if administered at standard doses to a patient with renal failure. Therefore, the doses of these drugs must be reduced in proportion to the extent of renal compromise. Renal function is most commonly measured by creatinine clearance. Use of the plasma creatinine level to establish the presence of normal renal status can be misleading, however, because the plasma creatinine may fall within the normal range in elderly or debilitated patients with mild-to-moderate renal failure as a result of diminished muscle mass. Assuming that such patients have normal renal function can cause serious overdoses and toxic drug accumulation.

Renal insufficiency may also alter the pharmacodynamics of some drugs. Potassium salts, potassium-sparing diuretics, nonsteroidal anti-inflammatory drugs (NSAIDs), and ACE inhibitors are more likely to cause hyperkalemia in patients with renal dysfunction. Thiazide diuretics tend to be ineffective in a patient whose glomerular filtration rate is less than 30 mL/min, because these drugs must be secreted by the kidney to act at the luminal membrane of the renal tubules. Refer to Chapter 20, Pharmacology of Volume Regulation, for a review of the physiology and pharmacology of diuretics.

How does Mr. R's chronic kidney disease affect the choice and dosing of a safe and effective antibiotic regimen for his infection? Infectious complications are a source of substantial morbidity and a common cause of death among dialysis patients. Gram-positive organisms, including *S. aureus,* are responsible for most catheter-related infections. Because septicemia is a therapeutic emergency, empiric treatment should not be delayed while waiting for culture results. Therapy can be modified subsequently, once the culture and sensitivity results are known. In this case, empiric treatment consists of vancomycin and gentamicin for broad-spectrum coverage of Gram-positive and Gram-negative organisms. Gentamicin, an aminoglycoside, is often used to treat infections caused by Gram-negative bacilli. It is eliminated by the kidney and effectively removed by hemodialysis and hence is usually administered immediately after a hemodialysis session. In the case of Mr. R, gentamicin would be discontinued once the cultures reveal MRSA. The tricyclic glycopeptide vancomycin is the antibiotic of choice for MRSA infections. Vancomycin is cleared by the kidneys but, unlike the small molecule gentamicin, is not removed by conventional hemodialysis. In individuals with normal kidney function, the dosing interval for vancomycin is 12 hours. In severe kidney disease, as in this case, therapeutic levels of the drug may persist for 7 days following a single intravenous dose, allowing convenient outpatient treatment once the patient has become hemodynamically stable.

in the blood increases. As the plasma drug concentration increases, the rate of elimination also increases, because this rate is proportional to the plasma drug concentration. Steady state is reached when the two rates (k_{in} and k_{out}) are equal. Because k_{in} is a constant, *the approach to steady state is governed by k_{out}, the composite rate for all drug clearance mechanisms.* (k_{out} can also be called k_e, the composite rate for drug elimination.) In most dosing regimens, drug levels accumulate following each successive dose, and the steady state is reached only when the amount of drug entering the system is equal to the amount being removed from the system (see Fig. 3-11). Clinically, this principle must be remembered when the dosing regimen is altered, because at least four to five elimination half-lives must pass before the new steady state is reached.

The steady-state plasma concentration can also be altered by the addition of another drug to a patient's treatment regimen. In the case of Mr. W, the addition of the drug trimethoprim-sulfamethoxazole inhibited the metabolism of warfarin, decreasing the clearance rate of the latter drug and causing its steady-state concentration to reach supratherapeutic levels. This effect was exacerbated by Mr. W's acute intoxication with ethanol, which also inhibited warfarin metabolism. Assuming that Mr. W's weight is approximately 70 kg, he is taking 5 mg of warfarin every 24 hours, and the bioavailability of warfarin is 0.93, then his initial steady-state plasma warfarin concentration can be calculated as follows:

$$C_{steady\ state} = \frac{0.93 \times 5\ mg}{24\ h \times 0.192\ L/h} = 1.01\ mg/L$$

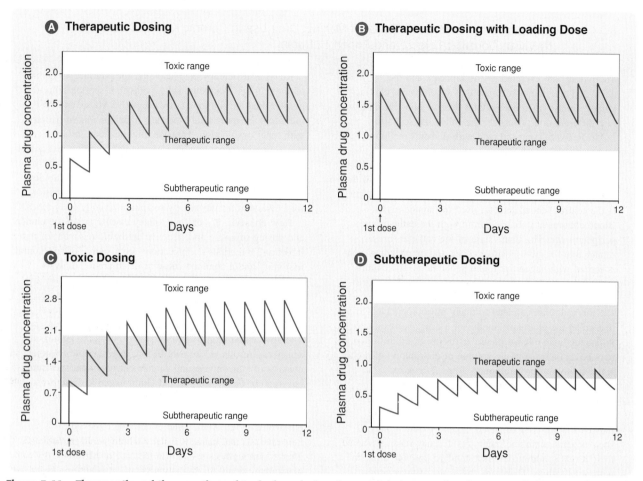

Figure 3-11. Therapeutic, subtherapeutic, and toxic drug dosing. From a clinical perspective, drug concentrations in plasma can be divided into subtherapeutic, therapeutic, and toxic ranges. The goal of most drug-dosing regimens is to maintain the drug at concentrations within the therapeutic range (referred to as the "therapeutic window"). **A.** The first several doses of a drug are typically subtherapeutic as the drug equilibrates to its steady-state concentration (approximately four elimination half-lives are required to achieve steady state). Appropriate drug dosing and dosing frequency result in steady-state drug levels that are therapeutic, and the maximal and minimal concentrations of the drug remain within the therapeutic window. **B.** If the initial (loading) dose is larger than the maintenance dose, the drug reaches therapeutic concentrations more rapidly. The magnitude of the loading dose is determined by the volume of distribution of the drug. **C.** Excessive maintenance doses or dosing frequency result in drug accumulation and toxicity. **D.** Insufficient maintenance doses or dosing frequency result in subtherapeutic steady-state drug concentrations. In all four panels, the drug is administered once daily, distributed very rapidly to the various body compartments, and eliminated with first-order kinetics.

where the clearance value of 0.192 L/hour is determined from the half-life and volume of distribution of the drug (see Equations 3-9 and 3-10). When his warfarin clearance was decreased by the addition of trimethoprim-sulfamethoxazole and ethanol, the steady-state plasma concentration of warfarin increased to toxic levels.

Loading Dose

After administration of a drug by any route, the plasma concentration of the drug initially increases. Distribution of drug from the vascular (blood) compartment to body tissues then causes the plasma drug concentration to decrease. The rate and extent of this decrease are significant for drugs with high volumes of distribution. If the administered dose of drug fails to take account of this volume of distribution, instead accounting only for the blood volume, then therapeutic drug levels will not be reached promptly. Initial (loading)

doses of drug are often administered in order to compensate for drug distribution into the tissues. Such doses may be much higher than would be required if the drug were retained in the intravascular compartment. Loading doses may be used to achieve therapeutic levels of drug (i.e., levels at the desired steady-state concentration) with only one or two doses of drug:

$$\text{Dose}_{\text{loading}} = V_d \times C_{\text{steady state}} \qquad \text{Equation 3-11}$$

where V_d is the volume of distribution and C is the desired steady-state plasma concentration of the drug.

In the absence of a loading dose, four to five elimination half-lives are required for a drug to reach equilibrium between tissue distribution and plasma concentration of the drug. Use of a loading dose circumvents this process by providing a sufficient amount of drug to attain an appropriate (therapeutic) drug concentration in the blood and tissues

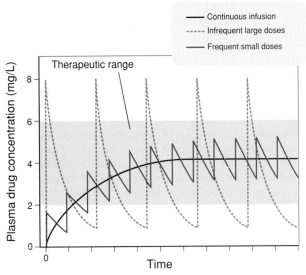

Figure 3-12. Fluctuations in steady-state drug concentration depend on dosing frequency. The same average steady-state plasma drug concentration can be achieved using a variety of different drug doses and dosing intervals. In the example shown, the same total amount of a drug is administered by three different dosing regimens: continuous infusion; frequent small doses; and infrequent large doses. The smooth curve represents the effect of a continuous infusion of drug. Discontinuous dosing results in fluctuations above and below the continuous-infusion curve. Note that all three dosing regimens have the same time-averaged plasma drug concentration at steady state (4 mg/L), but the discontinuous regimens result in peaks and troughs above and below the target drug concentration. If these peaks and troughs fall above or below the boundaries of the therapeutic window (as in the infrequent large-dose regimen), then clinical outcome can be adversely affected. For this reason, frequent small-dose regimens are generally more efficacious and better tolerated than infrequent large-dose regimens. However, this concern must be balanced against the convenience of (and improved patient compliance with) less frequent (e.g., once daily) dosing regimens.

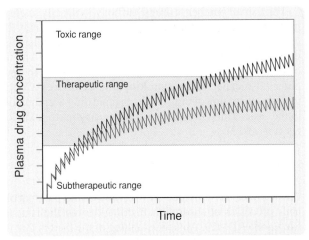

Figure 3-13. Saturation kinetics and drug toxicity. Drug elimination typically follows first-order Michaelis–Menten kinetics, increasing as the plasma drug concentration increases. At optimal dosing, the steady-state plasma drug concentration remains within the therapeutic window (*bottom curve*). However, excessive drug dosing may saturate the body's capacity to eliminate the drug, for example, by overwhelming the hepatic cytochrome P450 enzyme system. In this case, the elimination rate of the drug does not increase with increasing plasma drug concentration (i.e., elimination follows zero-order rather than first-order kinetics). Continued administration of the drug results in drug accumulation, and the plasma drug concentration may reach toxic levels *(top curve)*.

maintenance dose rate would provide a drug input greater than the drug clearance, and the drug could accumulate to toxic levels within the tissues. In Mr. W, the calculated maintenance dose for warfarin is

$$\text{Dose}_{\text{maintenance}} = 0.192 \text{ L/h} \times 1.01 \text{ mg/L}$$

$$= 0.194 \text{ mg/h} = 4.65 \text{ mg/day}$$

The appropriate maintenance dose for Mr. W is therefore 4.65 mg/day. Because warfarin is only 93% bioavailable, Mr. W should take 5 mg/day to maintain an adequate steady-state plasma concentration. (Note also that, because warfarin has a low therapeutic index and toxic levels of the drug can lead to potentially fatal hemorrhage, the biological activity of warfarin should be monitored carefully by periodic measurement of the INR.)

after only one or two doses of drug. For example, lidocaine has a volume of distribution of 77 L in a 70-kg person. Assuming that a steady-state plasma concentration of 3.5 mg/L is needed to control ventricular arrhythmias, the appropriate loading dose of lidocaine in this person can be calculated as

$$\text{Dose}_{\text{loading}} = 77 \text{ L} \times 3.5 \text{ mg/L} = 269.5 \text{ mg}$$

Maintenance Dose

Once the steady-state plasma drug concentration is achieved, and equilibrium is established between the drug concentrations in the tissues and the plasma, subsequent doses need to replace only the amount of drug that is lost through metabolism and excretion. The maintenance dose rate of a drug is dependent on the drug clearance, according to the principle that *rate in = rate out at steady state*:

$$\text{Dose}_{\text{maintenance}} = \text{Clearance} \times C_{\text{steady state}} \qquad \text{Equation 3-12}$$

Administration of a dose rate greater than the calculated

TABLE 3-6	Summary of Key Pharmacokinetic Relationships

Initial concentration	$=$	$\dfrac{\text{Loading dose}}{\text{Volume of distribution}}$
Steady-state concentration	$=$	$\dfrac{\text{Fraction absorbed} \times \text{Maintenance dose}}{\text{Dosing interval} \times \text{Clearance}}$
Elimination half-life	$=$	$\dfrac{0.693 \times \text{Volume of distribution}}{\text{Clearance}}$

For a small number of drugs, the body's capacity to eliminate the drug (e.g., through hepatic metabolism) may become saturated at therapeutic or only slightly supratherapeutic plasma drug concentrations. In these cases, the kinetics of drug elimination may change from first-order to zero-order (also called **saturation kinetics**; see above). Continued administration of drug results in rapid drug accumulation in the plasma, and drug concentrations may reach toxic levels (Fig. 3-13).

Conclusion and Future Directions

This chapter has provided an overview of the pharmacokinetic processes of absorption, distribution, metabolism, and excretion (ADME). An understanding of the factors that determine a drug's ability to act in an individual patient, and the changing nature of these factors over time, is vitally important to the safe and efficacious use of drug therapy. The *key equations governing the relationships among dosing, clearance, and plasma drug concentration* (Table 3-6) are important to consider when making therapeutic decisions about drug regimens.

At present, the clinical applicability of pharmacokinetics is mainly based on drug effects that have been observed in a population of individuals. There are nearly infinite major and minor variations among individuals, however, and these variations influence the effects of drug therapy. For example, clear differences in pharmacokinetics are present among persons of different ages, genders, body mass, fitness levels, ethnicities, genomic makeup, and disease states. For some drugs, advances in therapeutic drug monitoring have enabled the real-time determination of plasma drug concentrations. A more extraordinary revolution in pharmacokinetics is offered by **pharmacogenomics**. Future drug therapy may involve the administration of drugs that have been engineered specifically for the patient who is receiving them. Knowledge of a patient's genomic makeup could enable drug therapies to exploit strengths and compensate for weaknesses in a host of patient-specific variables. This topic is discussed in Chapter 52.

Suggested Reading

Godin DV. Pharmacokinetics: disposition and metabolism of drugs. In: Munson PL, ed. *Principles of pharmacology.* New York: Chapman & Hall; 1995. (*A solid introductory text, this chapter illustrates the various aspects of pharmacokinetics with many examples of specific drugs.*)

Pratt WB, Taylor P, eds. *Principles of drug action: the basis of pharmacology.* 3rd ed. New York: Churchill Livingstone; 1990, Chapters 3 and 4. (*This text provides a comprehensive treatment of pharmacokinetics and pharmacokinetic principles.*)

4

Drug Metabolism

Cullen Taniguchi and F. Peter Guengerich

INTRODUCTION

Our tissues are exposed on a daily basis to **xenobiotics**—foreign substances that are not naturally found in the body. Most drugs are xenobiotics that are used to modulate bodily functions for therapeutic ends. Drugs and other environmental chemicals that enter the body are modified by a vast array of enzymes. The biologic transformations performed by these enzymes can alter the compound to render it beneficial, harmful, or simply ineffective. The processes by which biochemical reactions alter drugs within the body are collectively called **drug metabolism** or **drug biotransformation.**

The previous chapter introduced the importance of renal clearance in the pharmacokinetics of drugs. Although the biochemical reactions that alter drugs to renally excretable forms are an essential part of drug metabolism, drug metabolism encompasses more than this one function. Drug biotransformation can alter drugs in four important ways:

- An *active drug* may be converted to an *inactive drug.*
- An *active drug* may be converted to an *active* or *toxic metabolite.*
- An *inactive prodrug* may be converted to an *active drug.*
- An *unexcretable drug* may be converted to an *excretable metabolite* (e.g., to enhance renal or biliary clearance).

This chapter presents the major processes of drug metabolism. Following the case is an overview of the sites of drug metabolism, focusing principally on the liver. The two major types of biotransformation are then discussed; these are often termed **phase I** and **phase II reactions,** although the terminology is imprecise and it incorrectly implies a temporal order of the reactions. (In addition, "**phase III**" is sometimes used to describe the process of drug transport, which is even more confusing.) In this chapter we use "oxidation/reduction" and "conjugation/hydrolysis" to describe these processes more accurately. The chapter concludes with a discussion of the factors that can lead to differences in drug metabolism among individuals.

Case

Ms. B is a 32-year-old Caucasian woman who complains of sore throat and difficulty swallowing for the past 5 days. Physical examination reveals creamy white lesions on the tongue that are identified as oral thrush, a fungal infection. Her history includes sexual activity with multiple partners, inconsistent use of condoms, and continuous use of oral contraceptives for the past 14 years. The presentation suggests a diagnosis of HIV-1 infection, which is confirmed by polymerase chain reaction (PCR) analysis. Ms. B has a low

CD4 T-cell count, and is immediately started on a standard anti-HIV regimen that includes the protease inhibitor saquinavir. Her oral thrush resolves with a topical antifungal agent. Despite aggressive therapy, her CD4 cell count continues to decrease, and she presents to her physician several months later with fatigue and a persistent cough. Further investigation leads to a diagnosis of tuberculosis.

QUESTIONS

■ **1.** What factors should a physician consider in devising a drug regimen to treat both Ms. B's acute tuberculosis and her underlying HIV disease?

■ **2.** One of the first-line drugs in the treatment of tuberculosis is rifampin, which decreases the effectiveness of HIV protease inhibitors. What is the mechanism for this drug-drug interaction?

■ **3.** Isoniazid is another drug commonly used in the treatment of tuberculosis. Why does Ms. B's ethnic background give her physician reason for concern when considering the use of this drug?

SITES OF DRUG METABOLISM

The liver is the main organ of drug metabolism. This fact figures prominently in the phenomenon known as the **first-pass effect.** Orally administered drugs are often absorbed unchanged in the gastrointestinal (GI) tract and transported directly to the liver via the portal circulation (Fig. 4-1). In this manner, the liver has the opportunity to metabolize drugs before they reach the systemic circulation and, therefore, before they reach their target organs. The first-pass effect must be taken into account when designing dosing regimens because, if hepatic metabolism is extensive, the amount of drug that reaches the target tissue is much less than the amount (dose) that is administered orally (see Chapter 3, Pharmacokinetics). Certain drugs are inactivated so efficiently upon their first pass through the liver that they cannot be administered orally and must be given parenterally. One such drug is the antiarrhythmic lidocaine, which has a bioavailability of only 3% when taken orally.

Although the liver is quantitatively the most important organ in metabolizing drugs, every tissue in the body is capable of drug metabolism to some degree. Particularly active sites include the skin, the lungs, the gastrointestinal tract, and the kidneys. The gastrointestinal tract deserves special mention because this organ, like the liver, can contribute to the first-pass effect by metabolizing orally administered drugs before they reach the systemic circulation.

PATHWAYS OF DRUG METABOLISM

Drugs and other xenobiotics undergo biotransformation before excretion from the body. Many pharmaceuticals are li-

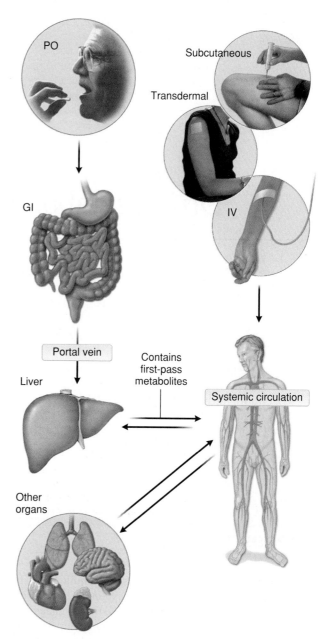

Figure 4-1. Portal circulation and the first-pass effect. Drugs administered by mouth (*per os,* or PO) are absorbed in the GI tract and then delivered, via the portal vein, to the liver. This pathway allows the liver to metabolize drugs before they reach the systemic circulation, a process responsible for the **first-pass effect.** In contrast, drugs that are administered intravenously (IV), transdermally, or subcutaneously enter the systemic circulation directly and can reach their target organs before hepatic modification. The first-pass effect has important implications for bioavailability; the oral formulation of a drug that undergoes extensive first-pass metabolism must be administered in a much larger dose than the equivalent IV formulation of the same drug.

pophilic, which enables the drug to pass across cell membranes, such as those of the intestinal mucosa or of the target tissue. Unfortunately, the same chemical property that enhances bioavailability of drugs may also make renal excretion difficult, since clearance by the kidney requires that these drugs be made more hydrophilic so that they can dissolve in the aqueous urine. Thus, biotransformation reactions often enhance the hydrophilicity of compounds to render them more susceptible to renal excretion.

Biotransformation reactions are classically divided into two main types: oxidation/reduction (phase I) and conjugation/hydrolysis (phase II). Oxidation reactions typically transform the drug into more hydrophilic metabolites by adding or exposing polar functional groups such as hydroxyl (-OH), thiol (-SH), or amine (-NH₂) groups (Table 4-1). Such metabolites are often pharmacologically inactive and, without further modification, may be excreted. Some products of oxidation and reduction reactions, however, require further modifications prior to excretion. Conjugation (phase II) reactions modify compounds through attachment of hydrophilic groups, such as glucuronic acid, to create more polar conjugates (Table 4-2). It is important to note that these conjugation reactions occur independently of the oxidation/reduction reactions, and the enzymes involved in oxidation/reduction and conjugation/hydrolysis reactions often compete for substrates.

OXIDATION/REDUCTION REACTIONS

Oxidation reactions involve membrane-associated enzymes expressed within the endoplasmic reticulum (ER) of hepatocytes and, to a lesser extent, of cells in other tissues. The enzymes that catalyze these phase I reactions are typically oxidases; the majority of these enzymes are **heme protein mono-oxygenases** of the **cytochrome P450** class. P450 enzymes (sometimes abbreviated CYP) are also known as microsomal mixed-function oxidases and are involved in the metabolism of approximately 75% of all drugs used today. (The term P450 refers to the 450-nm absorption peak characteristic of these heme proteins when they bind carbon monoxide.)

The net result of a cytochrome P450-dependent oxidation reaction is

$$Drug + O_2 + NADPH + H^+ \longrightarrow$$

$$Drug\text{-}OH + H_2O + NADP^+ \qquad \text{Equation 4-1}$$

The reaction proceeds when the drug binds to the oxidized (Fe^{3+}) cytochrome P450 to form a complex, which is then reduced in two sequential oxidation/reduction steps as outlined in Figure 4-2A. Nicotinamide adenine dinucleotide phosphate (NADPH) donates the electrons in both of these steps via a flavoprotein reductase. In the first step, the donated electron reduces the cytochrome P450-drug complex. In the second step, the electron reduces molecular oxygen to form an activated oxygen-cytochrome P450-drug complex. Finally, as the complex becomes more active through rearrangement, the reactive oxygen atom is transferred to the drug, resulting in the formation of the oxidized drug product and recycling oxidized cytochrome P450 in the process. The mechanism of these reactions is illustrated in Figure 4-2B.

Most liver cytochrome P450 oxidases exhibit broad substrate specificity (Table 4-1). This is due in part to the activated oxygen of the complex, which is a powerful oxidizing agent that can react with a variety of substrates. The names of the cytochrome P450 enzymes are sometimes designated by ''P450'' followed by the number of the P450 enzyme

family, capital letter of the subfamily, and an additional number to identify the specific enzyme (e.g., P450 3A4). Many of the P450 enzymes have partially overlapping specificities that together allow the liver to recognize and metabolize a wide array of xenobiotics.

Together, P450-mediated reactions account for more than 95% of oxidative biotransformations. Other pathways may also oxidize lipophilic molecules. A pertinent example of a non-P450 oxidative pathway is the **alcohol dehydrogenase** pathway that oxidizes alcohols to their aldehyde derivatives as part of the overall process of excretion. These enzymes are the basis for the toxicity of methanol. Methanol is oxidized by alcohol dehydrogenase to formaldehyde, which does considerable damage to some tissues. The optic nerve is particularly sensitive to formaldehyde, and methanol toxicity can cause blindness.

Another important non-P450 enzyme is **monoamine oxidase** (**MAO**). This enzyme is responsible for the oxidation of amine-containing endogenous compounds such as catecholamines and tyramine (see Chapter 9, Adrenergic Pharmacology) and some xenobiotics, including drugs.

CONJUGATION/HYDROLYSIS REACTIONS

Conjugation and hydrolysis reactions provide a second set of mechanisms for modifying compounds for excretion (Fig. 4-3). Although hydrolysis of ester- and amide-containing drugs is sometimes included among the phase I reactions (in the older terminology), the biochemistry of hydrolysis is more closely related to conjugation than to oxidation/reduction. Substrates for these reactions include both metabolites of oxidation reactions (e.g., epoxides) and compounds that already contain chemical groups appropriate for conjugation, such as hydroxyl (-OH), amine (-NH₂), or carboxyl (-COOH) moieties. These substrates are coupled by transfer enzymes to endogenous metabolites (e.g., glucuronic acid and its derivatives, sulfuric acid, acetic acid, amino acids, and the tripeptide glutathione) in reactions that often involve high-energy intermediates (Table 4-2). The conjugation and hydrolysis enzymes are located in both the cytosol and the endoplasmic reticulum of hepatocytes (and other tissues). In most cases, the conjugation process makes the drug more polar. Virtually all of the conjugated products are pharmacologically inactive, with some important exceptions (e.g., morphine glucuronide).

Some conjugation reactions are important clinically in the case of neonates, who have not yet fully developed the capacity to carry out this set of reactions. UDP-glucuronyl transferase (UDPGT) is responsible for conjugating bilirubin in the liver and facilitating its excretion. The developmental deficiency of this enzyme at birth puts infants at risk for neonatal jaundice, which results from increased serum levels of unconjugated bilirubin. Neonatal jaundice is a problem because neonates have not only underdeveloped activity of this enzyme but also an undeveloped blood–brain barrier. Unconjugated bilirubin is water-insoluble and very lipophilic; it binds easily to the unprotected neonate brain and is capable of causing significant damage to the central nervous system. This pathologic condition is known as bilirubin encephalopathy or **kernicterus**. Prophylactic treatments for kernicterus include: (1) phototherapy with 450-nm light,

text continues on page 55

TABLE 4-1 **Oxidation and Reduction Reactions**

REACTION CLASS	STRUCTURAL FORMULA	REPRESENTATIVE DRUGS
I. Cytochrome P450-Dependent Oxidations		
1. Aliphatic Hydroxylation		Barbiturates Digitoxin Cyclosporine
2. Aromatic Hydroxylation		Propranolol Phenytoin
3. N-Dealkylation		Methamphetamine Lidocaine
4. O-Dealkylation		Codeine
5. S-Oxidation		Phenothiazine Cimetidine
6. N-Oxidation		Quinidine
7. Desulfuration		Thiopental
8. Epoxide Formation		Carbamazepine
II. Cytochrome P450-Independent Oxidations		
1. Alcohol Dehydrogenation/Aldehyde Dehydrogenation		Ethanol Pyridoxine
2. Oxidative Deamination		Histamine Norepinephrine
3. Decarboxylation		Levodopa
III. Reductions		
1. Nitro Reduction		Nitrofurantoin Chloramphenicol
2. Dehalogenation		Halothane Chloramphenicol
3. Carbonyl Reduction		Methadone Naloxone

TABLE 4-2 Hydrolysis and Conjugation Reactions

REACTION CLASS	STRUCTURAL FORMULA	REPRESENTATIVE DRUGS

I. Hydrolysis

1. Ester Hydrolysis

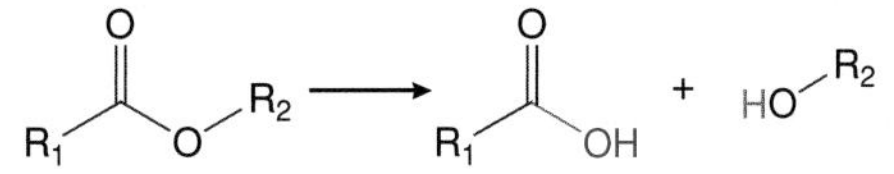

Procaine
Aspirin
Succinylcholine

2. Amide Hydrolysis

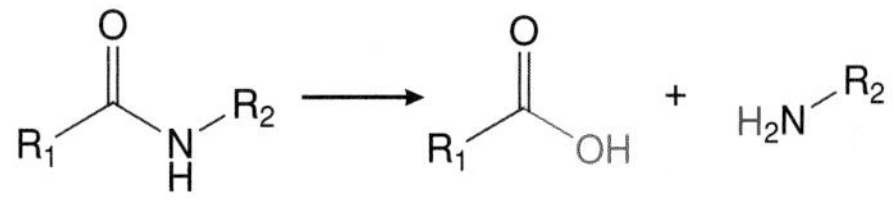

Procainamide
Lidocaine
Indomethacin

3. Epoxide Hydrolysis

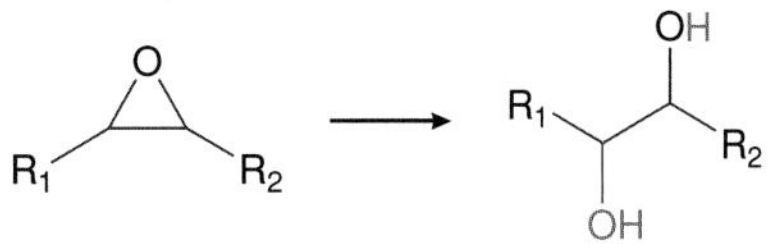

Carbamazepine (epoxide metabolite)

II. Conjugation

1. Glucuronidation

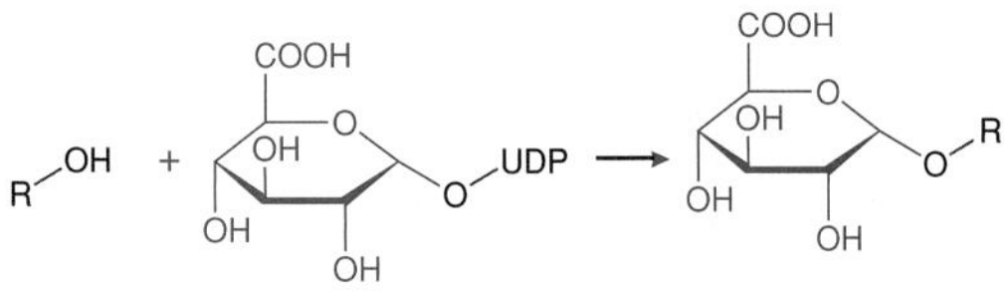

Diazepam
Digoxin
Ezetimibe

2. Acetylation

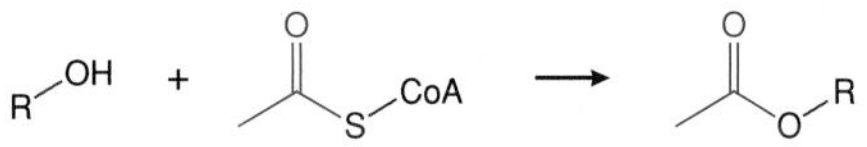

Isoniazid
Sulfonamides

3. Glycine Conjugation

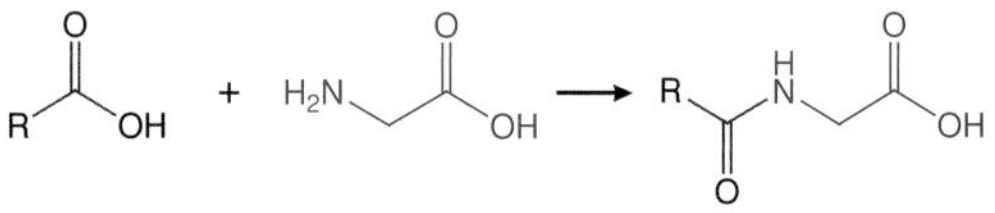

Salicylic acid

4. Sulfate Conjugation

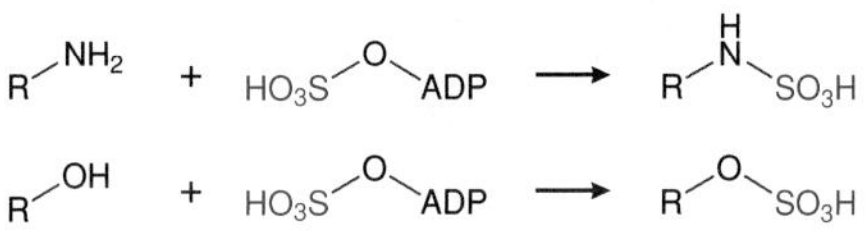

Estrone
Methyldopa

5. Glutathione Conjugation (and processing to mercapturic acids)

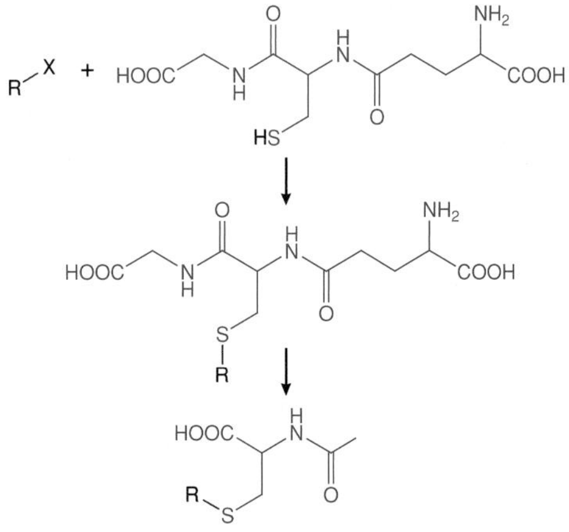

Ethacrynic acid
Dichloroacetic acid
Acetaminophen (metabolite)
Chlorambucil

6. N-Methylation

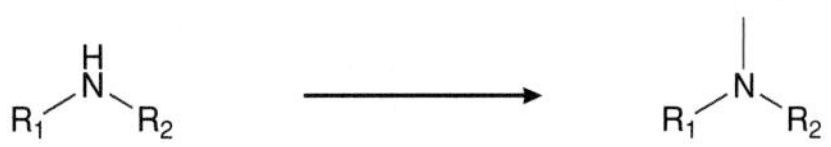

Methadone
Norepinephrine

7. O-Methylation

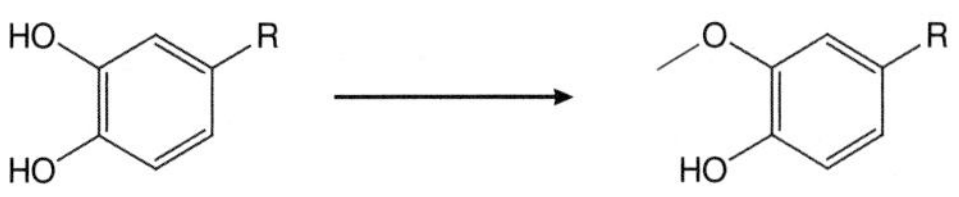

Catecholamines

8. S-methylation

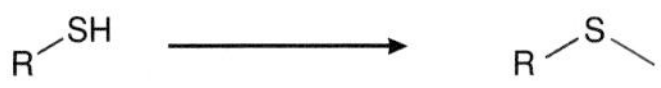

Thiopurines

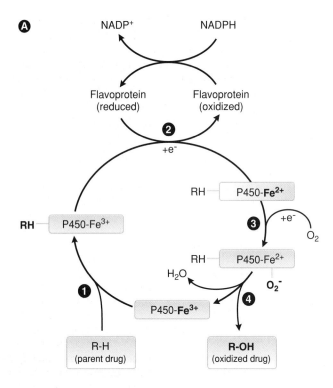

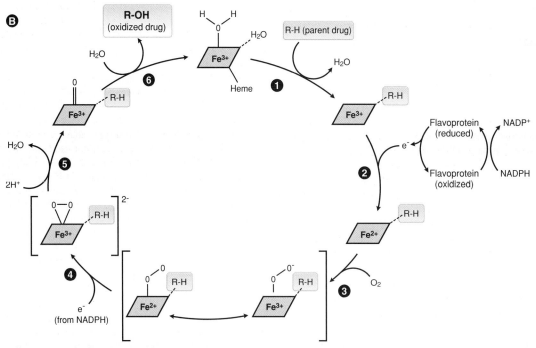

Figure 4-2. Cytochrome P450-mediated drug oxidation. Many drug metabolism reactions involve a system of hepatic P450 microsomal enzymes that catalyze the oxidation of drugs. **A.** An overview of the reaction involves a set of oxidation/reduction steps in which an iron moiety in the P450 enzyme acts as an electron carrier to transfer electrons from NADPH to molecular oxygen. The reduced oxygen is then transferred to the drug, resulting in an additional -OH group on the now-oxidized drug (for this reason, P450 enzymes are sometimes referred to colloquially as "oxygen guns" or even "nature's blowtorch"). The addition of the -OH group results in increased drug hydrophilicity and an increased rate of drug excretion. **B.** The detailed mechanism of the P450 reaction can be divided into six steps: (1) drug complexes with oxidized cytochrome P450; (2) NADPH donates an electron to the flavoprotein reductase, which reduces the P450-drug complex; (3 and 4) oxygen joins the complex, and NADPH donates another electron, creating the activated oxygen–P450-substrate complex; (5) iron is oxidized, with the loss of water; and (6) the oxidized drug product is formed. There are multiple P450 enzymes; each has a somewhat different specificity for substrates (such as drugs). Five of the human P450s (1A2, 2C9, 2C19, 2D6, and 3A4) account for approximately 95% of the oxidative metabolism of drugs.

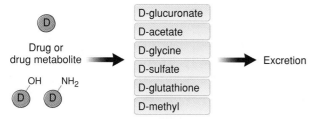

Figure 4-3. Conjugation reactions. In these reactions, a drug (represented by D) or drug metabolite (represented by D-OH and D-NH₂) is conjugated to an endogenous moiety. Glucuronic acid, a sugar, is the most common group that is conjugated to drugs, but conjugations of acetate, glycine, sulfate, glutathione, and methyl groups are also common. The addition of one of these moieties makes the resulting drug metabolite more hydrophilic and often enhances drug excretion. (Methylation, an important exception, does not increase drug hydrophilicity.) Transport mechanisms also play a major role in the elimination of drugs and their metabolites.

which converts bilirubin to an isomer that is more rapidly excreted, and (2) administration of the barbiturate phenobarbital, which induces UDPGT and thereby reduces serum levels of unconjugated bilirubin.

It is important to note that conjugation and hydrolysis reactions do not necessarily constitute the last step of biotransformation. Since the conjugation of these highly polar moieties occurs intracellularly, they often require active transport across cellular membranes to be excreted. (Active transport of the parent drug can also occur.) Moreover, some conjugation products may be subjected to further metabolism.

DRUG TRANSPORT

Although many drugs are sufficiently lipophilic to passively cross cell membranes, it is now appreciated that many drugs need to be actively transported into cells. This fact has significant consequences for oral bioavailability (transport into enterocytes or active excretion into the intestinal lumen), hepatic metabolism (transport into hepatocytes for enzymatic metabolism and for excretion into bile), and renal clearance (transport into proximal tubular cells and excretion into the tubular lumen). Several important molecules mediate these processes. The **multidrug resistance protein 1 (MDR1)**, or **P-glycoprotein**, which is a member of the ABC family of efflux transporters, actively transports compounds back into the intestinal lumen. This process limits the oral bioavailability of several important drugs, including digoxin and HIV-1 protease inhibitors. The metabolism of drugs from the portal circulation (i.e., the first-pass effect) often requires the transport of compounds into hepatocytes via the **organic anion transporting polypeptide (OATP)** and the **organic cation transporter (OCT)** family of proteins. These transporters are particularly relevant for the metabolism of several 3-hydroxy-3-methylglutaryl-coenzyme A (HMG-CoA) reductase inhibitors (statins), which are used in the treatment of hypercholesterolemia. For example, metabolism of the HMG-CoA reductase inhibitor pravastatin is dependent on the transporter OATP1B1, which transports the drug into hepatocytes. Drug uptake into hepatocytes via OATP1B1 is thought to be the rate-limiting step in the clearance of pravastatin. The uptake of pravastatin on its first

pass through the liver also provides a potential advantage by keeping the drug out of the systemic circulation, from which it could be taken up by muscle cells and thereby cause toxic effects such as rhabdomyolysis. The **organic anion transporter (OAT)** family of transporters is responsible for renal secretion of many clinically important anionic drugs, such as β-lactam antibiotics, nonsteroidal anti-inflammatory drugs (NSAIDs), and antiviral nucleoside analogs.

INDUCTION AND INHIBITION

The use of phenobarbital to prevent neonatal jaundice demonstrates that drug metabolism can be influenced by the expression levels of drug metabolizing enzymes. Although some P450 enzymes are constitutively active, others can be **induced** or **inhibited** by different compounds. Induction or inhibition can be incidental (a side effect of a drug) or deliberate (the desired effect of therapy).

The primary mechanism of P450 enzyme induction is an increase in the expression of the enzyme through increased transcription, increased translation, or decreased degradation. P450 enzyme induction typically occurs via increased transcription. Drugs, environmental pollutants, industrial chemicals, or even foodstuffs can enter hepatocytes and bind to several different xenobiotic receptors, including the pregnane X receptor (PXR), constitutively active/androstane receptor (CAR), or aryl hydrocarbon receptor (AhR) (Fig. 4-4). Xenobiotic receptors function in a manner similar to nuclear hormone receptors; binding of a xenobiotic compound activates the receptor, allowing it to translocate to the nucleus and bind to the promoters of various biotransformation enzymes.

There are multiple consequences of P450 enzyme induction. *First*, a drug can increase its own metabolism. For example, carbamazepine, an antiepileptic drug, not only induces P450 3A4 but also is metabolized by P450 3A4. Hence, carbamazepine hastens its own metabolism by inducing P450 3A4. *Second*, a drug can increase the metabolism of a coadministered drug. For example, P450 3A4 is responsible for metabolizing more than 50% of all clinically prescribed drugs. Should such a drug be coadministered with carbamazepine, its metabolism would also be increased. This situation can be problematic, because the increased P450 3A4 activity can reduce drug concentrations below their therapeutic levels if standard doses of the drugs are administered. In Ms. B's case, the administration of rifampin in conjunction with her HIV therapy could be detrimental, because rifampin induces P450 3A4 and thereby increases the metabolism of protease inhibitors such as saquinavir. *Third*, induction of P450s or some of the other biotransformation enzymes can result in the production of toxic levels of reactive drug metabolites, resulting in tissue damage or other side effects.

Just as certain compounds can induce P450 enzymes, other compounds can inhibit these enzymes. *An important consequence of enzyme inhibition is the decreased metabolism of drugs that are metabolized by the inhibited enzyme.* Such inhibition can both allow drug levels to reach toxic concentrations and prolong the presence of active drug in the body.

Enzyme inhibition can be achieved in several different ways (Fig. 4-4). For example, ketoconazole, a widely used antifungal drug, has a nitrogen moiety that binds to the heme

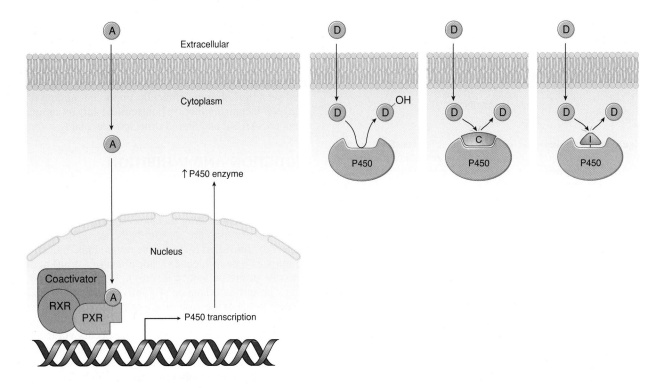

Figure 4-4. Conceptualization of P450 induction and inhibition. Drugs can both induce the expression and inhibit the activity of P450 enzymes. Some drugs can induce the synthesis of P450 enzymes (*left panel*). In this example, drug A activates the pregnane X receptor (PXR), which heterodimerizes with the retinoid X receptor (RXR) to form a complex with coactivators and initiate transcription of the P450 enzyme. Induction can also occur via the constitutively active/androstane receptor (CAR) or the aryl hydrocarbon receptor (AhR) (*not shown*). Drug D enters the cell and is hydroxylated by a P450 enzyme (*right panel*). The P450 enzyme can be inhibited by a second drug acting as a competitive inhibitor (drug C) or an irreversible inhibitor (drug I). The mechanism by which a drug inhibits P450 enzymes is not necessarily predictable from the drug's chemical structure; the mechanism can only be determined experimentally. In addition, metabolites of drugs A, C, and I can play a role in enzyme induction and inhibition (*not shown*).

iron in the active site of P450 enzymes; this binding prevents the metabolism of coadministered drugs by competitive inhibition. An example of irreversible inhibition is secobarbital, a barbiturate, which alkylates and permanently inactivates the P450 complex. On occasion, the inhibition of P450 enzymes can be used to therapeutic advantage: for example, the protease inhibitor lopinavir cannot achieve therapeutic levels as a single agent because of extensive first-pass metabolism, but coadministration of lopinavir with the P450 3A4 inhibitor ritonavir (also a protease inhibitor) allows lopinavir to reach therapeutic concentrations.

Drug transporters can also be induced or inhibited by other drugs. For example, the macrolide antibiotics can inhibit MDR1, and this inhibition can lead to increased serum levels of drugs, such as digoxin, that are excreted by MDR1. MDR1 is also transcriptionally regulated by PXR. Consequently, drugs that induce up-regulation of P450 enzymes via the PXR pathway (e.g., P450 3A4) concomitantly increase transcription of the MDR1 drug transporter.

A detailed list of compounds that can inhibit or induce the common P450 enzymes can be found in Table 4-3.

ACTIVE AND TOXIC METABOLITES

Knowing the routes by which therapeutic agents are metabolized can affect the choice of drug to prescribe in a particular clinical situation. This is true both when the metabolite is active, in which case the administered agent may be acting as a **prodrug,** and when the agent has **toxic metabolites** (see Chapter 5, Drug Toxicity).

Prodrugs are inactive compounds that are metabolized by the body into their active, therapeutic forms. One example of a prodrug is the selective estrogen receptor antagonist **tamoxifen;** this drug has little activity until it is hydroxylated to become 4-hydroxytamoxifen, a metabolite that is 30- to 100-fold more active than the parent compound. Another example is the angiotensin II receptor antagonist **losartan;** the potency of this drug is increased 10-fold upon oxidation of its alcohol group to a carboxylic acid by P450 2C9.

The strategy of selective prodrug activation can be used for therapeutic benefit in cancer chemotherapy. One example of this strategy is the use of **mitomycin C,** a naturally occurring compound that is activated to a powerful DNA alkylating agent after it is *reduced* by several enzymes including a cytochrome P450 *reductase.* Mitomycin C selectively kills hypoxic cancer cells in the core of solid tumors because: (1) these cells have increased levels of the cytochrome P450 reductase that activates mitomycin C; and (2) reoxidation of the drug is inhibited under hypoxic conditions.

Other examples of toxic metabolites, including the important case of **acetaminophen,** are discussed in Chapter 5.

P450 ENZYME	SUBSTRATES	INHIBITORS	INDUCERS
P450 3A4	**Anti-HIV agents** Indinavir Nelfinavir Ritonavir Saquinavir **Benzodiazepines** Alprazolam Midazolam Triazolam **Calcium channel blockers** Diltiazem Felodipine Nifedipine Verapamil **Immunosuppressants** Cyclosporine Tacrolimus **Macrolide antibiotics** Clarithromycin Erythromycin **Statins** Atorvastatin Lovastatin **Others** Loratadine Losartan Quinidine Sildenafil	**Antifungal agents (azoles)** Itraconazole Ketoconazole **Anti-HIV agents** Delavirdine Indinavir Ritonavir Saquinavir **Calcium channel blockers** Diltiazem Verapamil **Macrolide antibiotics** Clarithromycin Erythromycin Troleandomycin (not azithromycin) **Others** Cimetidine Grapefruit juice Mifepristone Nefazodone Norfloxacin	**Antiepileptics** Carbamazepine Oxcarbazepine Phenobarbital Phenytoin **Anti-HIV agents** Efavirenz Nevirapine **Rifamycins** Rifabutin Rifampin Rifapentine **Others** St. John's wort
P450 2D6	**5-HT reuptake inhibitors** Fluoxetine Paroxetine **Antiarrhythmic agents** Flecainide Mexiletine Propafenone **Antidepressants** Amitriptyline Clomipramine Desipramine Imipramine Nortriptyline **Antipsychotics** Haloperidol Perphenazine Risperidone Venlafaxine **Beta-antagonists** Alprenolol Bufuralol Carvedilol Metoprolol Penbutolol Propranolol Timolol	**5-HT reuptake inhibitors** Fluoxetine Paroxetine **Antiarrhythmic agents** Amiodarone Quinidine **Antidepressants** Clomipramine **Antipsychotics** Haloperidol	None identified

(continued)

TABLE 4-3	Some Pharmacologic Substrates, Inducers, and Inhibitors of Cytochrome P450 Enzymes *(Continued)*		
P450 ENZYME	**SUBSTRATES**	**INHIBITORS**	**INDUCERS**
	Opioids Codeine Dextromethorphan		
P450 2C19	**Antidepressants** Clomipramine Imipramine **Proton pump inhibitors** Lansoprazole Omeprazole Pantoprazole **Others** Propranolol R-warfarin	**Proton pump inhibitors** Omeprazole **Others** Fluoxetine Ritonavir Sertraline	Norethindrone Prednisone Rifampin

P450 2C9	**Angiotensin II receptor
	  antagonists**
	Irbesartan
	Losartan
	
	**Nonsteroidal anti-inflammatory
	  drugs (NSAIDs)**
	Ibuprofen
	Suprofen
	
	Others
	S-warfarin
	Tamoxifen
		Antifungal agents (azoles)
		Fluconazole
		Miconazole
		
		Others
		Amiodarone
		Phenylbutazone
			Rifampin
			Secobarbital

P450 2E1	**General anesthetics** Enflurane Halothane Isoflurane Methoxyflurane Sevoflurane **Others** Acetaminophen Ethanol	Disulfiram	Ethanol Isoniazid
P450 1A2	**Antidepressants** Amitriptyline Clomipramine Clozapine Imipramine **Others** R-warfarin Tacrine	**Quinolones** Ciprofloxacin Enoxacin Norfloxacin Ofloxacin **Others** Fluvoxamine	Char-grilled meat Cruciferous vegetables Insulin Omeprazole Phenobarbital Rifampin Tobacco

INDIVIDUAL FACTORS AFFECTING DRUG METABOLISM

For a number of reasons, the rates of biotransformation reactions may vary greatly from one person to another. The most important of these factors are discussed below.

PHARMACOGENOMICS

The effects of genetic variability on drug metabolism are an important part of the new science of pharmacogenomics (see Chapter 52, Pharmacogenomics). Certain populations exhibit polymorphisms or mutations in one or more enzymes of drug metabolism, changing the rate of some of these reactions and eliminating others altogether. These pharmacogenetic differences must be taken into account in therapeutic decision-making and drug dosing.

For example, 1 in every 2,000 Caucasians carries a genetic alteration in the plasma enzyme cholinesterase, which metabolizes the muscle relaxant succinylcholine (among other functions). This altered form of the enzyme has an approximately 1,000-fold reduced affinity for succinylcholine, resulting in slowed elimination and prolonged circulation of the active drug. Should a sufficiently high plasma concentration of succinylcholine be reached, respiratory paralysis and death can occur unless the patient is supported with artificial respiration until the drug is cleared.

A similar situation can occur with isoniazid, one of the drugs considered for treatment of Ms. B's tuberculosis. Genetic variability, in the form of a widespread autosomal recessive trait that results in decreased synthesis of an enzyme, causes the metabolism of this drug to be slowed in certain subsets of the U.S. population. The enzyme at issue is *N*-acetyltransferase, which inactivates isoniazid by an acetylation (conjugation) reaction. The ''slow acetylator'' phenotype is expressed by 45% of whites and blacks in the U.S. and by some Europeans living in high northern latitudes. The ''fast acetylator'' phenotype is found in more than 90% of Asians and in Inuits in the U.S. Blood levels of isoniazid are elevated four- to six-fold in slow acetylators relative to fast acetylators. Moreover, because the free drug acts as an inhibitor of P450 enzymes, slow acetylators are more susceptible to adverse drug interactions. If Ms. B expresses the slow acetylator phenotype, and her dose of isoniazid is not decreased accordingly, then the addition of isoniazid to her drug regimen could potentially have a toxic effect.

RACE AND ETHNICITY

Some genetic aspects of race and/or ethnicity affect drug metabolism. In particular, differences in drug action among races/ethnicities have been attributed to polymorphisms in specific genes. For example, P450 2D6 is functionally inactive in 8% of Caucasian individuals, but in only 1% of Asians. Moreover, African Americans have a high frequency of a P450 2D6 allele that encodes an enzyme of reduced activity. These observations are clinically relevant, in that P450 2D6 is responsible for the oxidative metabolism of about 20% of drugs—including many beta-antagonists and tricyclic antidepressants—and for the conversion of codeine to morphine.

In some cases, a polymorphism in the target gene is the basis for racial differences in drug action. The activity of the enzyme vitamin K epoxide reductase (VKORC1), which is the target of the anticoagulant warfarin, is affected by single nucleotide polymorphisms (SNPs) that render an individual either more or less sensitive to warfarin and that dictate administration of lower or higher doses of the drug, respectively. In one study, Asian-American populations were found to be enriched in haplotypes (inherited combinations of individual base/SNP differences) associated with increased sensitivity to warfarin, while African-American populations exhibited haplotypes associated with increased resistance to warfarin. Perhaps the most prominent example of a race-based therapeutic is the combination of fixed-dose isosorbide dinitrate and hydralazine (also known as BiDil).

This combination of vasodilators was reported to cause a 43% decrease in mortality in African Americans with heart failure. Although the biochemical basis of this effect is not known, these clinical data demonstrate that race may be a key consideration in choosing drug treatments and doses.

AGE AND GENDER

Drug metabolism can also differ among individuals as a result of age and gender differences. Many reactions of biotransformation are slowed in both young children and the elderly. At birth, neonates are capable of carrying out many but not all oxidative reactions; however, most of these drug-metabolizing enzyme systems mature gradually over the first 2 weeks of life and throughout childhood. Recall that neonatal jaundice results from a deficiency of the bilirubin-conjugating enzyme UDPGT. Another example of a conjugating enzyme deficiency that puts infants at risk for toxicity is the so-called **gray baby syndrome**. *Hemophilus influenza* infections in infants were once treated with the antibiotic chloramphenicol; excretion of this drug requires an oxidative transformation followed by a conjugation reaction. The oxidation metabolite of chloramphenicol is toxic; if this metabolite fails to undergo conjugation, it can build up in the plasma and may reach toxic concentrations. Toxic levels of the metabolite can cause neonates to experience shock and circulatory collapse, leading to the pallor and cyanosis that give the syndrome its name.

In the elderly, a general decrease in metabolic capacity is observed. As a result, particular care must be taken in prescribing drugs for the elderly. This decline in function has been attributed to age-related decreases in liver mass, hepatic enzyme activity, and hepatic blood flow.

There is some evidence for gender differences in drug metabolism, although the mechanisms are not well understood and data from experimental animals have not been particularly illuminating. Decreased oxidation of ethanol, estrogens, benzodiazepines, and salicylates has been reported anecdotally in women relative to men and may be related to androgenic hormone levels.

DIET AND ENVIRONMENT

Both diet and environment can alter drug metabolism by inducing or inhibiting enzymes of the P450 system. An interesting example is grapefruit juice. The psoralen derivatives and flavonoids in grapefruit juice inhibit both P450 3A4 and MDR1 in the small intestine. Inhibition of P450 3A4 significantly decreases the first-pass metabolism of coadministered drugs that are also metabolized by this enzyme, and inhibition of MDR1 significantly increases the absorption of coadministered drugs that are substrates for export (efflux) by this enzyme. The **grapefruit juice effect** is important when grapefruit juice is ingested together with drugs that are acted upon by these enzymes. Such drugs include some protease inhibitors, macrolide antibiotics, hydroxymethyl glutaryl CoA reductase inhibitors (statins), and calcium channel blockers. Saquinavir is one of the protease inhibitors that is both metabolized by P450 3A4 and exported by MDR1. In the case that opens this chapter, Ms. B should be alerted to the fact that the simultaneous ingestion of grapefruit juice and saquinavir could inadvertently lead to toxic serum levels of the protease inhibitor.

Because many endogenous substances used in the conjugation reactions are ultimately derived from the diet (and also require energy for the production of the appropriate cofactors), nutrition can affect drug metabolism by altering the pool of such substances available to the conjugating enzymes. Pollutant exposures can produce similarly dramatic effects on drug metabolism; one common example is the AhR-mediated P450 enzyme induction by polycyclic aromatic hydrocarbons in cigarette smoke.

METABOLIC DRUG INTERACTIONS

Drugs can potentially affect oral bioavailability, plasma protein binding, hepatic metabolism, and renal excretion of co-administered drugs. Among the categories of drug-drug interactions, the effects on biotransformation have special clinical importance. The concept of P450 enzyme induction and inhibition has already been introduced. A common clinical situation that must take this type of drug-drug interaction into consideration is the prescription of certain antibiotics to women who are already using hormonal contraception. For example, enzyme induction by the antibiotic rifampin causes estrogen-based hormonal contraception to be ineffective at standard doses because P450 3A4 is induced by rifampin and this is the main enzyme involved in the metabolism of the common estrogenic component 17α-ethynylestradiol. In this situation, other means of birth control should be recommended during the course of rifampin therapy. Ms. B should be made aware of this interaction if rifampin is added to her therapeutic regimen. The herbal supplement St. John's wort also induces P450 3A4, and thus has a similar effect on estrogen-based hormonal contraception. Another phenomenon associated with enzyme induction is **tolerance**, which can occur when a drug induces its own metabolism and thus reduces its efficacy over time (see the discussion of carbamazepine above and the discussion of tolerance in Chapter 17, Pharmacology of Drug Dependence and Addiction).

Because drugs are often prescribed in combination with other pharmaceuticals, careful attention should be paid to drugs that are metabolized by the same hepatic enzymes. The concomitant administration of two or more drugs that are metabolized by the same enzyme will generally result in higher serum levels of the drugs. The mechanisms of drug-drug interaction can involve competitive substrate inhibition, allosteric inhibition, or irreversible enzyme inactivation; in any case, drug levels can increase acutely, possibly leading to deleterious results. For example, erythromycin is metabolized by P450 3A4, but the resulting nitrosoalkane metabolite can form a complex with P450 3A4 and inhibit the enzyme. This inhibition can lead to potentially fatal drug-drug interactions. A notable example is the interaction between erythromycin and cisapride, a drug that stimulates GI tract motility. Toxic concentrations of cisapride can inhibit HERG potassium channels in the heart and thereby induce potentially fatal cardiac arrhythmias; for this reason, cisapride was withdrawn from the market in 2000. Before its withdrawal, cisapride was often well tolerated as a single agent. However, because cisapride is metabolized by P450 3A4, when the activity of P450 3A4 was compromised due to the concomitant administration of erythromycin or another inhibitor of P450 3A4, serum cisapride concentrations could increase to levels associated with arrhythmia induction. In other cases, drug interactions may be beneficial. For example, as noted above, the ingestion of methanol (a component of wood alcohol) can result in blindness or death because its metabolites (formaldehyde, an embalming agent, and formic acid, a component of ant venom) are highly toxic. One treatment for methanol poisoning is the administration of ethanol, which competes with methanol for oxidation by alcohol dehydrogenase (and, to a lesser extent, by P450 2D1). The resulting delay in oxidation allows the methanol to be cleared renally before its toxic byproducts can form in the liver.

DISEASES AFFECTING DRUG METABOLISM

Many disease states can affect the rate and extent of drug metabolism in the body. Because the liver is the main site of biotransformation, many liver diseases significantly compromise drug metabolism. Hepatitis, cirrhosis, cancer, hemochromatosis, and fatty infiltration of the liver each impair cytochrome P450s and other hepatic enzymes that are crucial to drug metabolism. As a result of this slowed metabolism, the levels of the active forms of many drugs may be significantly higher than intended and thereby cause toxic effects. Thus, the doses of many drugs may need to be lowered for individuals with hepatic disease.

Concomitant cardiac disease can also affect drug metabolism. The rate of metabolism of many drugs, such as the anti-arrhythmic lidocaine and the opioid morphine, is dependent on drug delivery to the liver via the bloodstream. Because blood flow is commonly compromised in cardiac disease, there must be heightened awareness of the potential for supra-therapeutic levels of drugs in patients with heart failure. In addition, some antihypertensive agents selectively reduce blood flow to the liver and, therefore, can increase the half-life of a drug such as lidocaine, leading to potentially toxic levels.

Thyroid hormone regulates the basal metabolic rate of the body, which, in turn, affects drug metabolism. Hyperthyroidism can increase the rate of metabolism of some drugs, whereas hypothyroidism can do the opposite. Other conditions, such as pulmonary disease, endocrine dysfunction, and diabetes, are also thought to affect drug metabolism, but the mechanisms for these effects are not yet completely understood.

■ *Conclusion and Future Directions*

This chapter has reviewed a number of issues relating to drug metabolism, including the sites of biotransformation, the transport and enzymatic metabolism of drugs at those sites, and individual factors that can affect those reactions. The case of Ms. B illustrates the clinical implications of drug metabolism, including the possible influences of ethnicity and drug-drug interactions on pharmacologic therapy. Understanding drug metabolism, and particularly the interaction of drugs within the body, allows the principles of biotransformation to be applied in the design and use of therapeutics. As pharmacogenomics and rational drug design lead pharmacology research into the future, increased understanding of biotransformation will also render the pharmacologic treatment of disease more individualized, efficacious, and safe. This topic is discussed in Chapter 52.

 Suggested Reading

Burchard EG, Ziv E, Coyle N, et al. The importance of race and ethnic background in biomedical research and practice. *N Engl J Med* 2003;348:1170–1175. (*Current understanding regarding ethnic variability in response to drug administration.*)

Fura A. Role of pharmacologically active metabolites in drug discovery and development. *Drug Discov Today* 2006;11:133–142. (*More detail on the role of active metabolites in drug activity.*)

Guengerich FP. Cytochrome P450s, drugs, and diseases. *Mol Interv* 2003;3:194–204. (*Review of the P450 system, its role in drug metabolism, and the effects of diseases on drug metabolism.*)

Ho RH, Kim RB. Transporters and drug therapy: implications for drug disposition and disease. *Clin Pharmacol Ther* 2005;78: 260–277. (*Review of the crucial role played by drug transporters in drug metabolism.*)

Wilkinson GR. Drug metabolism and variability among patients in drug response. *N Engl J Med* 2005;352:2211–2221. (*An excellent basic review of the P450 system and drug-drug interactions.*)

5

Drug Toxicity

Cullen M. Taniguchi, Sarah R. Armstrong, Laura C. Green, David E. Golan, and Armen H. Tashjian, Jr.

INTRODUCTION

Physicians prescribe drugs to prevent or treat disease. Those same drugs can be toxic to certain patients, however, because of genetic predisposition, nonselective action, or inappropriate use or administration of the drug. The United States Food and Drug Administration (FDA) spends a significant portion of its $1 trillion budget to ensure that new drugs are not overtly or unnecessarily dangerous. Moreover, pharmaceutical and biotechnology companies spend years and millions of dollars in clinical trials to understand the safety and inherent toxicity of their drugs. Potential drug candidates often fail because of unacceptable levels of toxicity in preclinical experiments or in clinical studies (see Chapter 48, Drug Discovery and Preclinical Development, and Chapter 49, Clinical Drug Evaluation and Regulatory Approval). Despite all of these efforts, even common over-the-counter drugs such as **acetaminophen** can be lethal (in this case, by causing fulminant hepatitis) if taken in supratherapeutic doses.

It must be recognized that no drug is entirely specific. All drugs have both primary intended effects and secondary unintended effects, the latter known as **side effects** or **ad-verse effects**. Although side effects can be neutral or even beneficial, side effects are typically undesirable. Adverse effects can range in severity from nuisance to life threatening. These effects make many patients unwilling to take drugs on a regular basis, and this lack of compliance represents a major practical limitation of pharmacotherapy.

Drug toxicology focuses on the harmful effects of drugs in the animal and human body. In virtually all respects, the pharmacologic principles discussed in the preceding chapters apply to the study of drug toxicity. Thus, just as drug-receptor interactions are fundamental to understanding the beneficial properties of a drug, so too are these interactions crucial in understanding the adverse effects of a drug. Although understanding the various toxicities of every drug is important, it can be an arduous and daunting task to learn and remember the myriad adverse drug effects. Thus, instead of repeating the general principles discussed in Chapters 1 through 4, or presenting extensive tables of information that can be found in many digital resources, this chapter focuses on the *common mechanisms* that underlie the toxic effects of drugs. Toxicities that derive from inappropriate activation or inhibition of the intended drug target (**on-target adverse effects**) or unintended targets (**off-target adverse effects**) begin the discussion. The phenotypic effects of these drug toxicities are then discussed at the physiologic, cellular, and molecular levels. A number of general principles and specific examples are also illustrated in the Workbook that accompanies this text (Farrell SE. *Principles of Pharmacology Workbook*. Baltimore: Lippincott Williams & Wilkins; 2007), and important drug-specific toxicities are also highlighted in the Drug Summary Tables at the ends of most chapters throughout this book. The toxicity of nondrug xenobiotics—such as carbon monoxide, lead, and pesticides—and the treatment of poisoning are discussed in Chapter 51, Poisoning by Drugs and Environmental Toxins.

■ Case

Ms. G is an 80-year-old piano teacher with progressively severe right leg pain over a period of 5 to 10 years. She has continued to teach in her studio but at the cost of increasing pain and fatigue. Imaging studies reveal severe osteoarthritis of the right hip. She is scheduled for elective replacement of the right hip with a prosthetic joint.

The total hip replacement is performed without immediate complications. During the first few days after the operation, Ms. G is given low-molecular-weight heparin and warfarin as prophylaxis against deep vein thrombosis. Six days after the operation, she develops excruciating pain in the area of the operation. Right lateral hip and buttock swelling is noted on physical examination. A complete blood count reveals significant blood loss (drop in hematocrit from 35% to 25%), and she is taken back to the operating room for evacuation of a large hematoma around the prosthetic joint. Although the hematoma does not appear to be grossly infected, cultures of the hematoma are positive for *Staphylococcus aureus*.

Because prosthetic joint infections are difficult to treat successfully without removal of the prosthesis, Ms. G is started on an aggressive 12-week course of combination antibiotics in which intravenous vancomycin and oral rifampin are administered for 2 weeks followed by oral ciprofloxacin and rifampin for 10 weeks. She tolerates the first 2 weeks of antibiotics without complications. However, 36 hours after switching her antibiotic from vancomycin to ciprofloxacin, she develops a high fever to 103°F and extreme weakness. Aspiration of the hip reveals only a scant amount of straw-colored (i.e., nonpurulent) fluid. Ms. G is therefore admitted to hospital for close observation.

Twelve hours after her admission, Ms. G develops an extensive maculopapular rash over her chest, back, and extremities. Her ciprofloxacin and rifampin are discontinued and vancomycin is restarted. Gradually, over the next 72 hours, her temperature returns to normal and her rash begins to fade. There is no growth in the culture of the right hip aspirate. Ms. G is continued on vancomycin as a single agent for the next 4 weeks without incident; rifampin is restarted, again without incident; and the 12-week antibiotic course is eventually completed using a combination of trimethoprim-sulfamethoxazole and rifampin.

Four months after her hip surgery, Ms. G is back to teaching her piano students and making slow but steady progress in her rehabilitation program.

QUESTIONS

■ 1. What was the rationale for coadministration of low-molecular-weight heparin and warfarin in the immediate postoperative period?

■ 2. Was there a cause-and-effect relationship between administration of the prophylactic anticoagulants and Ms. G's life-threatening bleeding complication?

■ 3. What was the rationale for administration of vancomycin and rifampin followed by ciprofloxacin and rifampin for treatment of the *S. aureus* infection?

■ 4. How likely was it that Ms. G's high fever, weakness, and skin rash represented a drug reaction to ciprofloxacin?

MECHANISMS OF DRUG TOXICITY

Whether a drug will do more harm than good in an individual patient depends on many factors, including the patient's age, genetic makeup and preexisting conditions, the dose of the drug administered, and other drugs the patient may be taking. For example, the very old or the very young may be more susceptible to the toxic effects of a drug because of age-dependent differences in pharmacokinetic profiles or in drug-metabolizing enzymes. As discussed in Chapter 4, Drug Metabolism, genetic factors can alter how a patient metabolizes or responds to a drug. Therefore, individual responses can also occur because of genetic differences in drug metabolism or receptor activity, as well as differences in the activities of repair mechanisms. Adverse drug reactions may be more likely in patients with preexisting conditions, such as liver or kidney dysfunction, depressed immune function, or pregnancy. The clinical determination of a drug's toxicity may not always be straightforward: as seen in the case of Ms. G, for example, a patient being treated with an antibiotic to combat an infection can develop a high fever, skin rash, and significant morbidity due either to recurrence of the infection or an adverse reaction to the antibiotic.

While a spectrum of adverse effects may be associated with the use of any drug or drug class, it is helpful to conceptualize the mechanisms of drug toxicity based on several general paradigms:

- "On-target" adverse effects, which are the result of the drug binding to its intended receptor, but at an inappropriate concentration, with suboptimal kinetics, or in the incorrect tissue (Fig. 5-1)
- "Off-target" adverse effects, which are caused by the drug binding to a target or receptor for which it was not intended (Fig. 5-1)
- Production of toxic metabolites (Figs. 5-1 and 5-2)
- Production of harmful immune responses (Fig. 5-2 and Table 5-1)
- Idiosyncratic responses

Each of these mechanisms is discussed below.

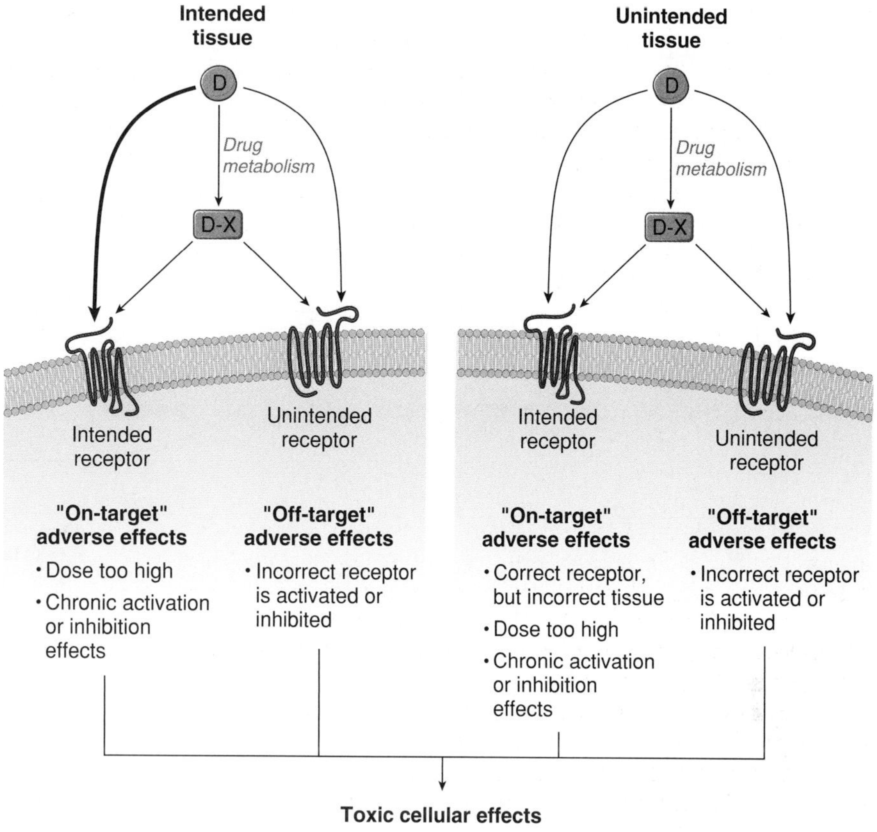

Figure 5-1. On-target and off-target adverse drug effects. Drug D is intended to modulate the function of a specific receptor (*Intended receptor*) in a particular tissue (*Intended tissue*). On-target adverse effects in the intended tissue could be caused by a supratherapeutic dose of the drug or by chronic activation or inhibition of the intended receptor by Drug D or its metabolite D–X. The same on-target effects could occur in a second tissue (*Unintended tissue*); in addition, the intended receptor could mediate an adverse effect because the drug is acting in a tissue for which it was not designed. Off-target effects occur when the drug and/or its metabolites modulate the function of a target (*Unintended receptor*) for which it was not intended.

ON-TARGET EFFECTS

An important concept in drug toxicity is that an adverse effect may be an exaggeration of the desired pharmacologic action due to alterations in exposure to the drug (see Fig. 5-1). This can occur by deliberate or accidental dosing error, by alterations in the pharmacokinetics of the drug (e.g., due to liver or kidney disease or to interactions with other drugs), or by changes in the pharmacodynamics of the drug-receptor interaction that alter the pharmacologic response (e.g., changes in receptor number). All such changes can lead to an increase in the effective concentration of the drug and thus to an increased biological response.

An important class of on-target adverse effects may occur because the drug, or one of its metabolites, interacts with the appropriate receptor but in the incorrect tissue. Many drug targets are expressed in more than one cell type or tissue. For example, the antihistamine **diphenhydramine hydrochloride** is an H_1 receptor antagonist used to reduce the unpleasant symptoms of histamine release in allergic conditions. Diphenhydramine also crosses the blood-brain barrier to antagonize H_1 receptors in the central nervous system, leading to somnolence. This adverse effect led to the design of second-generation H_1 receptor antagonists that do not cross the blood-brain barrier, and so do not induce drowsiness.

Sometimes on-target side effects unmask important and previously unknown functions of the biologic target. A prominent example of this phenomenon occurs with administration of hydroxymethylglutaryl coenzyme A (HMG CoA) reductase inhibitors (so-called *statins*), which are used

clinically to decrease cholesterol levels. The intended target tissue of these drugs is the liver, where they inhibit HMG CoA reductase, the rate-limiting enzyme of isoprenoid synthesis. A rare adverse effect of statin therapy is muscle toxicity, including rhabdomyolysis and myositis; this side effect is due to the physiologic role of HMG CoA reductase in regulating the posttranslational modification of several muscle proteins through a lipidation process called *geranyl-geranylation*.

OFF-TARGET EFFECTS

Off-target adverse effects occur when the drug interacts with unintended targets. Indeed, few drugs are so selective that they interact with only one molecular target. An example of an off-target effect is given by the antihistamine **terfenadine**, which also inhibits a cardiac potassium channel (hERG). The unintended inhibition of the ion channel unfortunately led to fatal cardiac arrhythmias in some patients, and terfenadine was withdrawn from the market for this reason. The active metabolite of terfenadine, **fexofenadine**, was later discovered to inhibit the hERG channel only weakly, and fexofenadine is now marketed as a safer antihistamine.

Enantiomers (mirror-image isomers) of a drug can also cause off-target effects. As described in Chapter 1, Drug-Receptor Interactions, drug receptors are often exquisitely sensitive to the three-dimensional arrangement of atoms in the drug molecule; therefore, receptors can distinguish between enantiomers of a drug. A tragic and well-known example of this phenomenon occurred with the administration of racemic thalidomide (mixture of [R] and [S]-enantiomers)

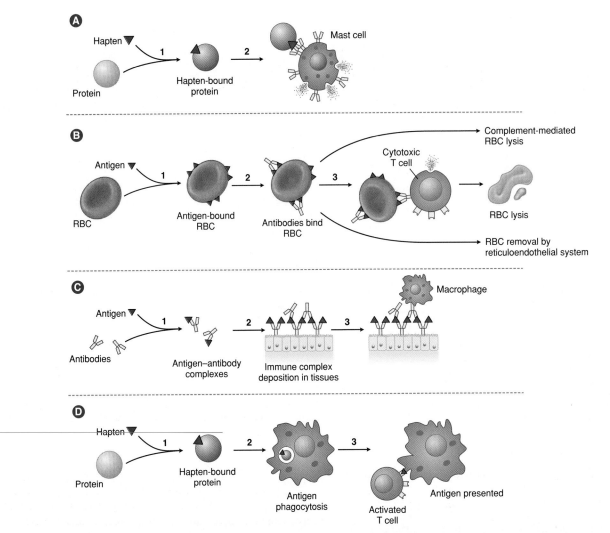

Figure 5-2. Mechanisms of hypersensitivity reactions. A. Type I hypersensitivity reactions occur when a hapten binds to a protein (1). The antigen crosslinks IgE antibodies on the surface of a mast cell, leading to mast cell degranulation (2). Mast cells release histamine and other inflammatory mediators. **B.** Type II hypersensitivity reactions occur when an antigen binds to the surface of a circulating blood cell, usually a red blood cell (RBC) (1). Antibodies to the antigen then bind the surface of the RBC (2), attracting cytotoxic T cells (3), which release mediators that lyse the RBC. Binding of antibody to RBCs can also directly stimulate complement-mediated RBC lysis and RBC removal by the reticuloendothelial system. **C.** Type III hypersensitivity reactions occur when antibodies bind to a soluble toxin, acting as an antigen (1). The antigen–antibody complexes are then deposited in the tissues (2), attracting macrophages (3) and starting a complement-mediated reaction sequence (*not shown*). **D.** Type IV hypersensitivity reactions occur when a hapten binds to a protein (1) and the hapten-bound protein is phagocytosed by a Langerhans cell (2). The Langerhans cell migrates to a regional lymph node, where it presents the antigen to a T cell, thereby activating the T cell (3).

in the 1960s as a treatment for morning sickness in pregnant women. While the (*R*)-enantiomer of thalidomide was an effective sedative, the (*S*)-enantiomer was a potent teratogen, which caused severe birth defects such as phocomelia in an estimated 10,000 newborns in 46 countries. These defects are now known to be linked to the anti-angiogenic properties of (*S*)-thalidomide. Notably, thalidomide was never approved for this indication in the United States because FDA pharmacologist Frances Kelsey believed that the initial toxicity testing results were inadequate.

The potential for pronounced pharmacologic differences between enantiomers has led the FDA to treat enantiomers of drugs as separate chemical entities. If a single enantiomeric preparation of a drug can be shown to have improved pharmacologic properties over a racemic version, then the puri-

fied enantiomer can be recognized as a new drug. For example, the racemic proton pump inhibitor **omeprazole** and its (*S*)-enantiomer **esomeprazole** (as in [*S*]-omeprazole) are marketed as separate drugs.

Another common off-target effect is the unintended activation of different receptor subtypes. For example, the β_1-adrenergic receptor is expressed in the heart, and its activation increases heart rate and myocardial contractility. Closely related β_2-adrenergic receptors are expressed primarily in smooth muscle cells in the airways and in the vasculature, and activation of β_2 receptors leads to smooth muscle relaxation and dilation of these tissues (see Chapter 9, Adrenergic Pharmacology). The clinical uses of β-adrenergic receptor antagonists (so-called *β-blockers*) are often targeted to the β_1 receptor to control heart rate and reduce

TABLE 5-1	Types of Hypersensitivity Reactions

CLASSIFICATION	PRIMARY TRIGGERS	PRIMARY MEDIATORS	EXAMPLES OF SIGNS AND SYMPTOMS	EXAMPLES OF DRUGS
Type I or immediate-type hypersensitivity (humoral)	Antigen-binding IgE on mast cells	Histamine and serotonin	Hives and urticaria, bronchoconstriction, hypotension, and shock	Penicillin
Type II or antibody-dependent cellular cytotoxicity (humoral)	IgG and complement-binding cell-bound antigen	Neutrophils, macrophages, and natural killer cells	Hemolysis	Cefotetan
Type III or immune-complex disease (humoral)	IgG and complement-binding soluble antigen	Neutrophils, macrophages, and natural killer cells; reactive oxygen species and chemokines	Cutaneous vasculitis	Mitomycin C
Type IV or delayed-type hypersensitivity (cell-mediated)	Antigen in association with major histocompatibility complex (MHC) protein on the surface of antigen-presenting cells	Cytotoxic T lymphocytes, macrophages, and cytokines	Macular rashes and organ failure	Sulfamethoxazole

The four types of hypersensitivity reactions and their triggers, mediators, and clinical manifestations are shown. Examples of drugs that cause each type of hypersensitivity reaction are also provided. (Adapted from Table 2, Bugelski PJ. Genetic aspects of immune-mediated adverse drug effects. *Nat Rev Drug Discov* 2005;59–69.)

myocardial oxygen demand in patients with angina or heart failure. However, some β_1 receptor antagonists are not entirely selective for the β_1 receptor and can also antagonize the β_2 receptor. β-Adrenergic receptor antagonists with nonselective effects are therefore contraindicated in patients with asthma, because these drugs could inadvertently cause airway constriction by antagonizing β_2 receptors.

Interestingly, the off-target effects of a drug can be explored by using genetically modified animals in which the intended target receptor is genetically deleted. If the mice lacking the intended target respond to the drug in some way, then the actions of the drug must be occurring via a target other than the intended target. Modern molecular biology techniques have also made possible tissue-specific deletion of the target receptor, making it easier to identify off-target effects and previously unknown on-target adverse effects.

PRODUCTION OF TOXIC METABOLITES

As described in Chapter 4, virtually all drug molecules are metabolized by the liver and/or other tissues. Sometimes metabolism produces a pharmacologically active metabolite, as with the angiotensin receptor antagonist **losartan** and the antihistamine **ebastine**, which are converted from inactive prodrugs to the active drugs **E3174** and **carebastine**, respectively.

In other cases, a drug metabolite can have an adverse effect. A clinically significant example is that of acetaminophen, a commonly used analgesic and antipyretic. In its therapeutic dose range, acetaminophen is metabolized predomi-

nantly by glucuronidation and sulfation, and these conjugated products account for approximately 95% of the total excreted metabolites. P450 enzymes oxidize a small percentage of acetaminophen to a reactive intermediate, **N-acetyl-benzoquinoneimine**, which is immediately conjugated to glutathione. However, when the level of acetaminophen exceeds the therapeutic range, the glucuronidation and sulfation pathways become saturated and the stores of glutathione in the liver become depleted. This results in excessive accumulation of *N*-acetyl-benzoquinoneimine, an electrophile that reacts with nucleophilic groups on proteins to produce covalent protein derivatives.

Although the biological mechanisms are still not well understood, some of these complexes between the drug metabolite and cellular proteins are highly toxic to the liver and, in the case of acetaminophen overdose, can cause fulminant hepatotoxicity and death. An antidote for acetaminophen overdose is **N-acetylcysteine**, which reacts directly with (and thereby detoxifies) the iminoquinone. Administered within 8 to 16 hours of an overdose of acetaminophen, *N*-acetylcysteine can be lifesaving. This example demonstrates the importance of **dose**, an axiom of toxicology. Although acetaminophen is used safely by millions of individuals every day, the same drug is responsible for roughly 50% of the cases of acute liver failure in the United States.

The toxicity of drug metabolites can only be determined empirically. This underscores the importance of extensive drug testing, both in preclinical experiments and in clinical trials. Despite such testing, some rare drug toxicities are discovered only when exposure occurs in a much larger population than that required for clinical trials. For example, **fluoroquinolones**, a class of broad-spectrum antibiotics derived from nalidixic acid, had minimal toxicities in preclinical studies and clinical trials. However, wider clinical exposure of these drugs led to reports of anaphylaxis, QTc-interval prolongation, and potential cardiotoxicity, resulting in the removal of two drugs of this class, **temafloxacin** and **grepafloxacin**, from the market. Use of another drug in this class, **trovafloxacin**, is significantly restricted due to liver toxicity. In comparison, **ciprofloxacin and levofloxacin** are generally well-tolerated fluoroquinolones and are frequently used for treatment of bacterial infections. As seen in the introductory case, however, even these agents can occasionally cause a severe drug hypersensitivity reaction.

HARMFUL IMMUNE RESPONSES

Drugs are xenobiotics that can be recognized by the immune system as foreign substances. Most small molecule drugs with a mass of less than 600 daltons are not direct immunogens, but act as **haptens**, where the drug binds (often covalently) to a protein in the body and is then capable of triggering an immune response. If a drug is sufficiently large (e.g., a therapeutic peptide or protein), it may directly activate the immune system. The two principal immune mechanisms by which drugs can produce damage are **hypersensitivity responses** (allergic responses) and **autoimmune reactions.**

The hypersensitivity responses are classically divided into four types, which are described further in Figure 5-2. Table 5-1 provides more detailed information about the mediators of hypersensitivity reactions and the clinical manifestations of the four types of hypersensitivity reactions. Prior exposure to a substance is required for each of the four types of hypersensitivity reactions.

A **type I** hypersensitivity response (**immediate hypersensitivity**) results from the production of IgE after exposure to an antigen. The antigen may be a foreign protein, such as the bacterially derived thrombolytic drug **streptokinase**, or it may be an endogenous protein modified by a **hapten** to become immunogenic. **Penicillin** fragments formed either in vivo or in the administered drug formulation can act as haptens and are responsible for such hypersensitivity reactions. Subsequent exposure to the antigen causes mast cells to degranulate, releasing inflammatory mediators such as histamine and leukotrienes that promote bronchoconstriction, vasodilatation, and inflammation. Manifested in the skin, a type I hypersensitivity response results in a **wheal-and-flare reaction.** In the upper respiratory tract, symptoms of "hay fever" such as conjunctivitis and rhinitis develop, while in the lower respiratory tract, asthmatic bronchoconstriction may occur (see Chapter 46, Integrative Inflammation Pharmacology: Asthma).

A **type II** hypersensitivity response (**antibody-dependent cytotoxic hypersensitivity**) results when a drug binds to cells, usually red blood cells, and is recognized by an antibody, usually IgG. The antibody triggers lysis of the cell by enabling complement fixation or by the action of cytotoxic T cells or phagocytosis by macrophages. Type II responses are rare adverse responses to several drugs, including penicillin and **quinidine**.

Type III hypersensitivity responses (**immune complex-mediated hypersensitivity**) occur when antibodies, usually IgG or IgM, are formed against soluble antigens. The antigen–antibody complexes are deposited in tissues such as kidneys, joints, and lung vascular endothelium (Table 5-1). These complexes cause damage by initiating an inflammatory response called **serum sickness**, in which leukocytes and complement are activated within the tissues. For example, type III hypersensitivity can be caused by the administration of **antivenins,** horse serum proteins obtained by inoculating a horse with the venom to be neutralized. Examples of other drugs that may pose a risk of serum sickness are **buproprion** and **cefaclor**.

A **type IV** hypersensitivity response (**delayed-type hypersensitivity**) results from the activation of T_H1 and cytotoxic T cells. It most commonly presents as **contact dermatitis** when a substance acts as a hapten and binds to host proteins. The first exposure does not normally produce a response; however, subsequent dermal exposures can activate Langerhans cells, which migrate to local lymph nodes and activate T cells. The T cells then return to the skin and initiate an immune response. Well-known type IV hypersensitivity responses include the reactions to poison ivy and the development of latex allergies. Repeated exposure to a drug that the immune system recognizes as foreign can trigger a massive immune response. This "cytokine storm" can lead to fever, hypotension should, and even organ failure. Thus, physicians should consider possible immune reactions to any drug treatment, even those that have appeared to be safe in broader populations. In the case at the beginning of the chapter, Ms. G had fever and rash that were likely caused by a T-cell mediated hypersensitivity reaction to ciprofloxacin. Once this was recognized and the ciprofloxacin was stopped, her complication resolved as well.

Autoimmunity results when the organism's immune system attacks its own cells (see Chapter 44, Pharmacology of Immunosuppression). Several drugs and a number of other chemicals can initiate autoimmune reactions. **Methyldopa** can cause hemolytic anemia by eliciting an autoimmune reaction against the Rhesus antigens (Rh factors). Several other drugs, such as **hydralazine, isoniazid,** and **procainamide,** can cause a lupus-like syndrome by inducing antibodies to myeloperoxidase (hydralazine and isoniazid) or DNA (procainamide).

IDIOSYNCRATIC TOXICITY

Idiosyncratic drug reactions are rare adverse effects for which no obvious mechanism is apparent. These idiosyncratic reactions are often thought to reflect unique individual genetic differences in the response to the drug molecule, possibly through variations in drug metabolism or immune response. As the classification denotes, idiosyncratic reactions are difficult to explain and often difficult to study in animal models, precisely because the genetic variation that may be causing the adverse response is not known. It is believed that the systematic study of patient variations in response to different drugs (pharmacogenomics) may help to elucidate the mechanisms that underlie idiosyncratic drug reactions.

CONTEXTS OF DRUG TOXICITY

DRUG OVERDOSE

The Swiss physician and chemist Paracelsus noted nearly 500 years ago that "all substances are poison; there is not which is not a poison. The right dose differentiates a poison and a remedy." In some cases, such as a suicide attempt, the overdose of a drug is intentional. However, many more cases of overdose occur accidentally in both the hospital and outpatient setting. Adverse drug events due to accidental dosing errors are estimated to affect nearly 775,000 people each year, with associated hospital costs of $1.5 to $5.5 billion annually. This significant cost to both the patient and the health care system has led to significant changes in prescribing and dosing practices in an attempt to avoid such adverse events.

DRUG-DRUG INTERACTIONS

As the population has aged and increasing numbers of patients have been prescribed multiple medications, the potential for drug-drug interactions has grown. Numerous adverse interactions have been identified, and the mechanisms often involve pharmacokinetic or pharmacodynamic effects. Drug-herb interactions are also an important subset of drug-drug interactions.

Pharmacokinetic Drug-Drug Interactions

Pharmacokinetic interactions between drugs arise if one drug changes the absorption, distribution, metabolism, or excretion of another drug, thereby altering the concentration of active drug in the body. These mechanisms are discussed more extensively in Chapter 4, but reviewed here for emphasis.

As discussed in Chapter 4, drugs can *inhibit* or *induce* hepatic P450 enzymes. If two drugs are metabolized by the same P450 enzyme, the competitive or irreversible inhibition of that P450 enzyme by one drug can lead to an *increase* in the plasma concentration of the second drug. On the other hand, the induction of a specific P450 enzyme by one drug can lead to a *decrease* in the plasma concentrations of other drugs that are metabolized by the same enzyme.

In addition to altering the activity of P450 enzymes, drugs can affect the transport of other drugs into and out of tissues. As discussed in Chapter 4, the multidrug resistance 1 (MDR1) efflux pump transports drugs into the intestinal lumen. A drug that inhibits MDR1 can lead to an increase in the plasma concentration of other drugs that are normally pumped out of the body by this mechanism. Other transporters, such as the organic anion transporting polypeptide 1 (OATP1), mediate the uptake of drugs into hepatocytes for metabolism and the transport of drugs across the tubular epithelium of the kidney for excretion; both of these mechanisms promote clearance of drug from the body. Interactions of a drug or one of its metabolites with these classes of transporters can lead to inappropriately high plasma concentrations of other drugs that are handled by the same transporter.

A pharmacokinetic interaction can sometimes be desirable. For example, because **penicillin** is cleared via tubular-secretion in the kidney, the elimination half-life of this drug can be increased if the drug is given concomitantly with **probenecid**, an inhibitor of renal tubular transport. A second example is provided by the combination of **imipenem**, a broad-spectrum antibiotic, and **cilastatin**, a selective inhibitor of a renal brush border dipeptidase (dehydropeptidase I). Because imipenem is rapidly inactivated by dehydropeptidase I, coadministration of imipenem with cilastatin is required to achieve therapeutic plasma concentrations of the antibiotic.

A drug that binds to plasma proteins, such as albumin, may displace a second drug from the same protein to increase its free plasma concentration and thereby increase its bioavailability to target and nontarget tissues. This effect can be enhanced in a situation where circulating albumin levels are low, such as liver failure or malnutrition (decreased albumin synthesis) or nephrotic syndrome (increased albumin excretion).

Pharmacodynamic Drug-Drug Interactions

Pharmacodynamic interactions arise when one drug changes the response of target or nontarget tissues to another drug. Toxic pharmacodynamic interactions can occur when two drugs activate complementary pathways, leading to an exaggerated biological effect. One example of such a drug interaction is provided by the coadministration of **sildenafil** (for erectile dysfunction) and **nitroglycerin** (for angina pectoris). Sildenafil inhibits phosphodiesterase type 5 (PDE5) and thus prolongs the action of cyclic GMP, and nitroglycerin stimulates guanylyl cyclase to increase cyclic GMP levels in vascular smooth muscle. Co-exposure to the two drugs increases cGMP to an even greater degree, increasing the risk of severe hypotension (see Chapter 21, Pharmacology of Vascular Tone).

A second example is the coadministration of antithrombotic drugs. After hip replacement surgery, patients are treated with prophylactic warfarin for a number of weeks to prevent the development of postoperative deep vein thrombosis. Because plasma warfarin concentrations may not reach a therapeutic level for several days, patients are sometimes coadministered low-molecular-weight heparin and warfarin during this time. As seen in the case of Ms. G, however, significant bleeding may result if the effects of the heparin and warfarin synergize to produce supratherapeutic levels of anticoagulation.

Drug-Herb Interactions

The safety and efficacy of a drug may also be altered by co-exposure with various non-pharmaceuticals, such as foods, beverages, and herbal and other dietary supplements. Many herbal products are complex mixtures of biologically active compounds, and their safety and effectiveness have rarely been tested in controlled studies. The wide use of unregulated herbal products among the public should lead clinicians to inquire about patient use of such products.

The literature contains a number of reports of therapeutic failure of drugs taken in conjunction with herbal products, and some reports of toxicity. For example, the herbal preparation **ginkgo biloba** (from the tree of the same name) inhibits platelet aggregation. Simultaneous use of ginkgo and

nonsteroidal anti-inflammatory drugs (NSAIDs), which also inhibit platelet aggregation, may increase the risk of bleeding. **Echinacea** products contain alkaloids that may deplete hepatic glutathione stores, increasing the risk of acetaminophen toxicity. In combination with **selective serotonin reuptake inhibitors**, **St. John's wort** may cause a mild serotonergic syndrome.

PATHOLOGY OF DRUG TOXICITY

As illustrated in Figure 5-3, drugs and their metabolites can interact with a diverse array of receptors to mediate adverse effects in vivo. Sometimes the parent, unmetabolized drug causes toxicity, but often a metabolite of the drug reacts with proteins, DNA, and oxidative defense molecules (such as glutathione) to cause cellular damage and other adverse reactions.

TEMPORAL ASPECTS OF TOXICITY

Drug toxicity can occur on many different time scales. **Acute toxicity** results from a single exposure to a drug, with adverse effects resulting in minutes to hours. Examples of acute toxicity are the massive hepatic necrosis that can occur after a single toxic dose of **acetaminophen** and exacerbations of acute bronchoconstriction in patients with **aspirin**-intolerant asthma. Many immune-mediated adverse effects occur within hours to days after administration of the drug.

Chronic toxicity, on the other hand, refers to an adverse effect of a drug that occurs over a prolonged period of time. Long-term treatment with dopamine receptor antagonists for schizophrenia can result in tardive dyskinesia, an unfortunate

on-target adverse effect that results from the critical role of dopamine as a neurotransmitter in the motor cortex (see Chapter 12, Pharmacology of Dopaminergic Neurotransmission).

Sometimes the toxicity of a drug is not revealed until it has been on the market for a number of years. For example, the insulin-sensitizing agent **troglitazone** was removed from the market only after it was noted that approximately 1 in 10,000 patients taking the drug died from acute liver failure.

Hormone replacement therapy for postmenopausal women is another important example of chronic toxicity. While the administration of estrogens significantly reduces several of the effects of menopause (e.g., hot flashes, vaginal atrophy, and skin thinning), continued activation of the estrogen receptor pathway can lead to endometrial cancer. As discussed below, prolonged exposure to certain drugs or their metabolites can lead to fibrosis, organ dysfunction, and birth defects as well as cancer.

CELLULAR TOXICITY: APOPTOSIS AND NECROSIS

Cells have mechanisms for damage repair, and toxic exposures that cause cellular dysfunction do not necessarily lead to cell death. One example of macromolecular damage repair is the reduction of oxidized thiol groups on proteins by **thioredoxin** and **glutaredoxin**. Denatured proteins can be refolded by molecular chaperones, such as heat shock proteins. DNA damage, such as adduct formation due to covalent binding of cancer cytotoxic drugs to double-stranded DNA or to specific nucleotides, can be reversed by DNA repair mechanisms. In some cases, chronic exposure to DNA-damaging drugs can overwhelm these repair mechanisms, leading to mutagenesis, carcinogenesis (see below), or cell death.

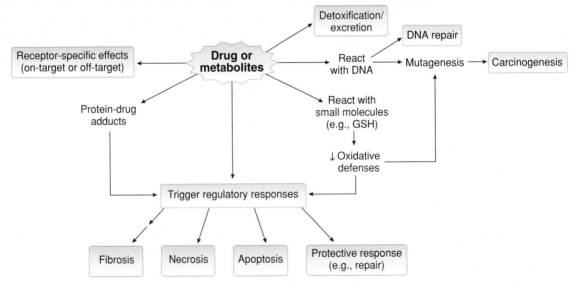

Figure 5-3. Mechanisms of drug toxicity. A drug or its metabolites or both interact with specific receptors to mediate on-target or off-target adverse effects. In addition, metabolites can be detoxified and excreted, or can react with a variety of macromolecules including DNA, small antioxidants such as glutathione (GSH), or cellular or plasma proteins. The formation of unrepaired or misrepaired DNA adducts is often mutagenic and may lead to cancer. The impairment of oxidative defenses can lead to inflammation and cell death (apoptosis or necrosis). The formation of drug-protein adducts can trigger immune responses that can damage cells and tissues (see Fig. 5-2). Regardless of the mechanism of damage, a gradation of acute responses from protective to apoptosis (programmed cell death) and necrosis can result, depending on the extent of damage and the temporal and dose relationships. Chronic inflammation and repair can also lead to tissue fibrosis.

Depending on the severity of the toxic insult, a cell may undergo **apoptosis** (programmed cell death). Apoptosis allows the cell to undergo ordered self-destruction by the coordinated activation of a number of dedicated proteins. Apoptosis can be beneficial when it is able to eliminate damaged cells. Inhibition of apoptosis is common in many cancer cells.

If the toxic insult is significant enough that ordered cell death cannot be accomplished, the cell undergoes **necrosis.** Necrosis is characterized by enzymatic digestion of cellular contents, denaturation of cellular proteins, and disruption of cellular membranes. While apoptotic cells undergo cell death with minimal inflammation and disruption of adjacent tissue, necrotic cells attract inflammatory cells and can damage nearby healthy cells.

ORGAN AND TISSUE TOXICITY

Fibrosis

The response to injury after cellular damage is largely determined by the regenerative capacity of the target organ. In organs that are capable of regeneration, such as the liver, repeated insults may be followed by regeneration. Over time, however, cellular injury can lead to excessive deposition of collagen and extracellular matrix proteins, causing **fibrosis.** Organ systems with limited or no regenerative function, such as cardiac and neuronal tissue, lose function as tissue is destroyed.

Chronic toxicity in the lungs can be manifested as both loss of function and fibrosis. Emphysematous changes are caused by the destruction of pulmonary **elastin** by neutrophil-derived **elastase.** Agents that elicit an inflammatory response, such as those found in cigarette smoke, can lead to **emphysema. Pulmonary fibrosis,** on the other hand, is caused by excessive and abnormal collagen deposition in the alveolar interstitium. The antiarrhythmic drug **amiodarone** and the chemotherapeutic agent **bleomycin** are known to cause pulmonary fibrosis; therefore, these drugs are contraindicated in patients with existing disease of the lung parenchyma.

Because of its central role in drug metabolism, the liver is particularly susceptible to toxic insult. Drugs or their metabolites can injure hepatocytes by disruption of calcium homeostasis (leading to cell membrane blebbing and cell lysis), canalicular injury, mitochondrial injury, and induction of apoptosis. Repeated exposure to toxic drug metabolites may cause drug-induced liver disease, a spectrum of clinical injuries that include inflammation (**hepatitis),** necrosis, fibrosis (in this case, **cirrhosis), cholestasis,** and **liver failure.** Nonalcoholic steatohepatitis (NASH) can also be an adverse drug effect; NASH may be caused, in part, by the release of cytokines after hepatocellular injury.

The kidney is also susceptible to toxic insult because it concentrates many xenobiotics for excretion. Nephrotoxicity may manifest as alterations in renal hemodynamics, tubular damage and obstruction, glomerular nephropathy, and interstitial nephritis. When a sufficient number of nephrons are lost, compensatory hemodynamic changes increase glomerular pressures, leading to glomerular sclerosis, further glomerular loss, diminished glomerular filtration rate, and progressive renal failure. Examples of drugs that can cause renal failure include certain antibiotics, NSAIDs, and angiotensin-converting enzyme inhibitors.

Carcinogenesis

Carcinogenesis occurs when a normal cell transforms to a neoplastic cell and the neoplastic cell undergoes clonal expansion. A **carcinogen** is a chemical, physical, or biologic insult that acts by causing DNA damage (mutations). Carcinogenesis is a complex process, involving multiple genetic changes, that usually takes place over years to decades in human beings.

The development of cancer requires sequential genetic changes (the first of which is termed **initiation**) and epigenetic changes (characterized as **promotion** and **progression**). **Initiators** act by damaging DNA, interfering with DNA replication, or interfering with DNA repair mechanisms. Most initiators are reactive species that covalently modify the structure of DNA, preventing accurate replication and, if unrepaired or misrepaired, leading to a mutation(s). If the mutation(s) affects a gene(s) that controls cell cycle regulation, neoplastic transformation may be initiated.

Carcinogenesis may involve mutations in at least two types of genes, **proto-oncogenes** and **tumor suppressor genes** (of which there are several dozen). **Proto-oncogenes** encode proteins that encourage cell cycle progression. **Tumor suppressor genes** often encode proteins responsible for inhibiting growth and cell cycle progression. Tumor suppressors can down-regulate important signaling pathways for growth, such as the phosphoinositide 3-kinase pathway, or they may directly suppress cell cycle progression. A mutation in a tumor suppressor gene thus encourages neoplastic growth by removing the normal inhibitory checks on cell growth.

An important on-target adverse effect of cytotoxic alkylating agents used in cancer chemotherapy (**chlorambucil, cyclophosphamide, melphalan, nitrogen mustards,** and **nitrosoureas**) is that they not only kill cancer cells but also damage normal blood cell progenitors. These agents are therefore toxic to bone marrow and can cause myelodysplasia and/or acute myeloid leukemia (AML). Indeed, 10% to 20% of cases of AML in the United States are secondary to treatment with such cancer drugs.

Tamoxifen, an estrogen receptor antagonist, is an effective treatment in patients with breast cancer. While tamoxifen is an antagonist of estrogen receptors in the breast, it acts as a *partial agonist* in other tissues that express the estrogen receptor, most notably the uterus. Therefore, an adverse effect of breast cancer treatment with tamoxifen can be the development of endometrial cancer. Newer estrogen receptor antagonists, such as **raloxifene,** do not stimulate uterine estrogen receptors and may therefore be safer drug choices for treatment or prevention of breast cancer.

Teratogenesis

Drugs given to pregnant women may have serious, unwanted effects on the health of the fetus. **Teratogenesis** is the induction of defects in the fetus, and a **teratogen** is a substance that can induce such defects. Exposure of the fetus to a teratogen necessarily involves maternal exposure. For this reason, the interaction between maternal tissues and the teratogenic drug is important to the severity of fetal exposure. In particular, the fetus's exposure to the agent is determined by maternal absorption, distribution, metabolism, and excretion of the drug, by the toxification of inert precursors to toxic metabolites in maternal tissues, and by the ability of the active teratogen to cross the placenta. These issues are further discussed in Box 5-1.

Because development of the fetus is precisely timed, the teratogenic effect of any substance is dependent on the developmental timing of the exposure. Thus, drugs that might have few adverse effects on the mother may cause substantial damage to the fetus. For example, **retinoic acid** (vitamin A) possesses significant on-target teratogenic toxicity. Retinoic acid activates nuclear retinoid receptors (RAR) and retinoid X receptors (RXRs) that regulate a number of key transcriptional events during development. In humans, **organogenesis** generally occurs between the 3rd and 8th weeks of gestation. It is during the period of organogenesis that teratogens have the most profound effect. Before the 3rd week, most toxic compounds result in death to the embryo and spontaneous abortion, whereas after organogenesis, teratogenic compounds may affect growth and functional maturation of organs but do not affect the basic developmental plan. Given the severity of birth defects that can occur, women who take RAR/RXR agonists such as **isotretinoin** for the treatment of acne must sign FDA-mandated informed consent forms to demonstrate that they are aware of the risk of serious drug-related birth defects.

Another example of an on-target teratogenic effect is *in utero* exposure of the fetus to ACE inhibitors. Although ACE inhibitors were previously not contraindicated in the first trimester of pregnancy, recent data indicate that fetal exposure during this period significantly increases the risks of cardiovascular and central nervous system malformations. ACE inhibitors can cause a group of conditions including oligohydramnios, intrauterine growth retardation, renal dysplasia, anuria, and renal failure, reflecting the importance of the angiotensin pathway on renal development and function.

▮ Conclusion and Future Directions

This chapter has presented a mechanism-based approach to understanding drug toxicity. Using these concepts, pharma-

---

BOX 5-1. Application to Therapeutic Decision-Making: Drugs in Pregnancy
by Vivian Gonzalez Lefebre and Robert H. Rubin

Pregnancy introduces several special considerations in therapeutic decision-making. These factors include the health of the woman as well as the delivery of a healthy baby; the altered pharmacokinetics and pharmacodynamics associated with pregnancy; and a lack of information regarding the effects of drugs on the developing fetus.

Most drugs are labeled with disclaimers regarding their use during pregnancy. This paucity of data makes it difficult to estimate the risk-benefit ratio for use of a drug in pregnancy. Physicians depend partly on animal studies and epidemiologic studies (which may be fraught with confounding factors) to establish the teratogenic potential of a drug. **Teratogenesis** refers to the structural or functional dysgenesis of developing organs; each tissue and organ of a fetus has a critical period during which its development may be disrupted by the administration of a teratogenic drug.

The FDA has established a system that classifies drugs on the basis of human and animal data, ranging from class A (safe) to class X (proven teratogenicity) drugs. For example, methyldopa has an excellent safety record in the treatment of hypertension during pregnancy; it is therefore considered a class A drug for use in pregnancy. In contrast, ACE inhibitors (another class of antihypertensives) are absolutely contraindicated during the second and third trimesters of pregnancy (class X) because of their association with fetal and neonatal renal dysfunction, including oligohydramnios, neonatal anuria, and renal failure. This classification system is helpful when a drug fits one of the two extremes; classifications in the middle, though, are often confusing and ambiguous. Therefore, the physician relies heavily on clinical judgment to decide whether a drug's potential benefits to the mother outweigh the risk to the fetus. Often, physicians err on the side of not treating.

The following issues should be addressed when prescribing a drug to a pregnant woman:

- the probability of placental transfer of the drug, given the drug's molecular weight, charge, hydrophobicity, and potential for carrier-mediated transport into or out of the placental circulation
- a physiologic explanation for how the drug could affect the fetus, e.g., through effects on organogenesis, organ development, organ function, or a delivery complication
- the risk to both fetus and mother associated with the underlying maternal illness for which the drug is being considered

When assessing the risk-benefit ratio for administering a drug, it should also be recognized that drugs that have teratogenic effects in animals when administered in high doses (e.g., aspirin) may not present a risk to humans when given in therapeutic doses. Other drugs, such as thalidomide and 13-cis-retinoic acid, are teratogenic in both animals and humans. Furthermore, it is important to remember that the population baseline risk of birth malformations is 3% to 5%. When appropriate, drugs that have proven effective for treating a patient's underlying condition should be continued, and experimenting with new drugs should be avoided. Finally, to minimize fetal risk, drugs should be prescribed at the lowest therapeutic dose, taking into account the normal metabolic and physiologic changes that occur during pregnancy (e.g., placental metabolism; increased water retention, renal filtration, heart rate, and plasma volume).

ceutical companies are investigating how to predict which patient populations will be most susceptible to an adverse drug reaction. One approach is to find correlations between individual single nucleotide polymorphisms (SNPs) and possible adverse reactions by comparing the SNPs of patients who have adverse reactions with those who do not. The identification of patients with genetic variants of the molecular target (and closely related targets) of a drug could also provide useful information about patients who might be more likely to experience adverse effects.

Certain pharmacokinetic drug-drug interactions may be better predicted with the advent of P450 chips that allow investigators to screen many compounds for the ability to inhibit specific P450 enzymes. Drug-related cellular toxicity is now being predicted by the ability of drugs to bind important antioxidants, such as glutathione, in large-scale preclinical drug screening. During clinical trials, plasma alanine aminotransferase (ALT) levels are measured to approximate the risk of hepatotoxicity that could occur in a broader population. An ALT reading three times greater than normal is considered to be predictive of impending liver damage. Vigilant postmarketing surveillance of a drug in a large population can also help to identify rare adverse drug reactions.

The therapeutic benefit of a drug must always be weighed against its toxic effects in the context of a patient's disease, treatment, and genetic makeup. The use of evolving biomarkers and genetic tests may help to identify patients at greatest risk for adverse drug reactions.

 Suggested Reading

Agranat I, Caner H, Caldwell J. Putting chirality to work: the strategy of chiral switches. *Nat Rev Drug Discov* 2002;1:753–768. (*An overview of enantiomeric-specific properties of drugs and the strategies of switching drugs from achiral to chiral preparations.*)

Bugelski PJ. Genetic aspects of immune-mediated adverse drug effects. *Nat Rev Drug Discov* 2005;4:59–69. (*Overview of immune-mediated adverse effects, including detailed mechanistic information.*)

Cooper WO, Hernandez-Diaz S, Arbogast PG, et al. Major congenital malformations after first-trimester exposure to ACE inhibitors. *N Engl J Med* 2006;354:2443–2451. (*Recent report of teratogenic effects of ACE inhibitors.*)

Knowles SR, Uetrecht J, Shear NH. Idiosyncratic drug reactions. *Lancet* 2000;356:1587–1591. (*Reviews mechanisms of idiosyncratic reactions, with focus on toxic metabolites.*)

Koop R. Combinatorial biomarkers: from early toxicology assays to patient population profiling. *Drug Discov Today* 2005;10:781–788. (*Use of biomarkers for preclinical and early clinical testing.*)

Liebler DC, Guengerich FP. Elucidating mechanisms of drug-induced toxicity. *Nat Rev Drug Discov* 2005;4:410–420. (*Introduces the concept of a mechanism-based approach to drug toxicity.*)

Navarro VJ, Senior JR. Drug-related hepatotoxicity. *N Engl J Med* 2006;354:731–739. (*Overview of pharmacogenomic approaches to understanding and predicting drug hepatotoxicity.*)

II

Principles of Neuropharmacology

IIA

Fundamental Principles of Neuropharmacology

6

Principles of Cellular Excitability and Electrochemical Transmission

John Dekker, Michael Ty, and Gary R. Strichartz

INTRODUCTION

Cellular communication is essential for the effective functioning of any complex multicellular organism. The major mode of intercellular communication is the transmission of chemical signals, such as neurotransmitters and hormones. In excitable tissues, such as nerves and muscles, rapid intracellular communication relies on the propagation of electrical signals—action potentials—along the plasma membrane of the cell. Both chemical and electrical transmission commonly involve the movement of ions across the plasma membrane that separates the cell from its environment or across the membranes of internal organelles such as the endoplasmic reticulum or mitochondria. Ionic movements can directly change the cytoplasmic concentration of ions, such as Ca^{2+}, that are key regulators of biochemical and physiologic processes such as phosphorylation, secretion, and contraction. Ionic movements also change the electrical potential across the membrane through which the ions flow, thus regulating various **voltage-dependent** functions, such as the opening of other ion channels. Some of these events are brief, with durations and actions of several milliseconds (0.001 sec). Others can take many seconds, with biochemical consequences that can persist for minutes or hours. Even gene expression can be regulated by changes in ion concentrations, resulting in long-term changes in cellular physiology, growth, differentiation, and other processes.

Many drugs modify chemical or electrical signaling to increase or decrease cellular excitability and electrochemical transmission. To appreciate how such drugs act, the present chapter explains the electrochemical foundations that underlie these phenomena. These general principles are applicable to many areas of pharmacology, including those discussed in Chapters 8 to 10 (Section IIB, Principles of Autonomic and Peripheral Nervous System Pharmacology), Chapters 11 to 17 (Section IIC, Principles of Central Nervous System Pharmacology), and Chapter 18, Pharmacology of Cardiac Rhythm.

Case

Karl is a 47-year-old man who works for the Virginia state government. He is traveling to Japan to meet with several CEOs to discuss the prospective openings of their companies' satellite offices in Roanoke. While visiting Yamaguchi, his hosts take him to dinner at an expensive restaurant where the specialty is fugu fish. Karl is impressed because he has heard that this special dish is not available in the United States and is an expensive delicacy in Japan.

Before the meal is over, Karl notes an unusual and delightful sensation of tingling and numbness in his mouth and around his lips. His hosts are pleased that he is experiencing the desired effect of fugu fish ingestion.

Karl is fascinated and somewhat fearful of the potential toxic effects of the fugu neurotoxin (tetrodotoxin) as they are described to him by his knowledgeable hosts. However, the Japanese assure him that the sushi chef at this fine restaurant is fully licensed to prepare fugu fish and is certified by the government. Still, back at his hotel, thoughts of the meal make him feel somewhat nauseated.

Karl is relieved when he awakens the next morning, feeling well and energized. He tests his muscles and his strength is as good as ever! However, he decides that he will politely forgo seafood for the rest of the trip and ask for Kobe beef instead.

QUESTIONS

■ **1.** What is the molecular mechanism of action of tetrodotoxin?

■ **2.** What is the effect of tetrodotoxin on the neuronal action potential?

CELLULAR EXCITABILITY

Excitability refers to the ability of a cell to generate and propagate electrical **action potentials**. Neuronal, cardiac, smooth muscle, skeletal muscle, and many endocrine cells have an excitable character. Action potentials may propagate over large distances, as in peripheral nerve axons that conduct over several meters, or they may stimulate activity in cells of much smaller size, such as the 30- to 50-μm-long interneurons that are contained within a single autonomic ganglion. The function of action potentials differs depending on the cells in which they occur. Propagating waves of action potentials carry encoded information with fidelity over long distances along axons. Within a small cell, action potentials excite the whole cell at once, causing an increase in intracellular ions (such as Ca^{2+}) followed by a rapid release of chemical transmitter molecules or hormones. These chemicals then travel to specific receptors, near or far from the releasing cell, to effect **chemical transmission**, which is discussed in the second part of this chapter.

Cellular excitability is fundamentally an electrical event. Therefore, an understanding of basic electricity is necessary to explain the biological processes of excitability and synaptic transmission. The following sections present basic principles of electricity as applied to two important cellular components—the plasma membrane and ion-selective channels.

OHM'S LAW

The magnitude of a current (I, measured in amperes) flowing between two points is determined by the potential difference (V, measured in volts) between those two points and the resistance to current flow (R, measured in Ohms):

$$I = V/R \qquad \text{Equation 6-1a}$$

For example, current may flow from the extracellular to the intracellular compartment in response to a potential difference (also known as a voltage difference) across the plasma membrane. Voltage can be thought of as a potential energy or as the propensity for charge to flow from one area to another. Resistance is the obstacle to this flow. Decreased resistance allows greater ion flow and therefore increased current (current has units of charge/time). When this relationship, known as Ohm's law, is applied to biological membranes such as the plasma membrane, the electrical resistance is often replaced by its reciprocal, the conductance (g, measured in reciprocal Ohms, or Siemens [S]):

$$I = gV \qquad \text{Equation 6-1b}$$

For simplicity, assume that all resistive elements in the cell membrane behave in an "ohmic way;" that is, their current-voltage (I-V) relationship is described by Equation 6-1b. In this case, the I-V relationship is linear, with a slope given by the conductance, g. Figure 6-1 represents the transmembrane current (I) measured at different transmembrane potentials (V) in a hypothetical cell. The slope of the I-V curve represents the conductance. From a conceptual perspective, current increases as voltage increases because a higher voltage results in a greater potential energy difference between the inside and outside of the cell, which in turn favors an increased rate of charge movement across the membrane.

The convention used in most texts and in this chapter is that the voltage across a membrane is expressed as the difference between the intracellular and extracellular potentials ($V_m = V_{in} - V_{out}$). For most normal cells, V is negative when the cell is at rest ($V_{in} < V_{out}$). The membrane is termed **hyperpolarized** when V is more negative than at rest, and it is described as **depolarized** when V is more positive than at rest. Current is conventionally defined with respect to the direction in which positive charge flows. Positive charge moving from inside to outside is called outward current and is represented graphically by positive values. Positive charge moving from outside to inside is called inward current and is represented graphically by negative values. Movement of negative charge is defined in the exact opposite way.

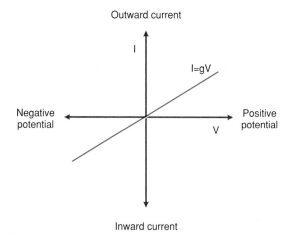

Figure 6-1. Ohm's law. Ohm's law states that there is a linear relationship between current (*I*) and voltage (*V*), and that the slope of the *I* versus *V* plot yields the conductance (*g*). By convention, outward current is the flow of positive charge from inside the cell to outside the cell. Transmembrane potential is defined by the difference in potential (voltage) between the inside and outside of the cell. For most cells, the resting potential inside the cell is negative relative to that outside the cell. Conductance, *g*, is the reciprocal of resistance.

ION CHANNELS

How does current actually flow across a cell membrane? Biological membranes are composed of a lipid bilayer in which some proteins are embedded and to which other proteins are attached (Fig. 6-2). Pure lipid membranes are virtually impermeable to most polar or charged substances. From an electrical perspective, the lipid bilayer acts as a capacitor by maintaining charge separation between the extracellular and intracellular ions. To allow the passage of ions that carry electrical current, ion channels or pores are embedded in the membrane. Most ion channels discriminate among the various types of ions, and most also remain closed until specific signals dictate their opening. From an electrical perspective, a set of ion channels is a variable conductor—it provides many individual conductances for ion flow between the extracellular and intracellular environments. The magnitude of the overall conductance depends on the fraction of channels in the open state and the conductance of the individual open channels.

CHANNEL SELECTIVITY, THE NERNST EQUATION, AND THE RESTING POTENTIAL

By itself, the hypothetical I-V relation in Figure 6-1 does not explain the electrical behavior of most real cells. If a cell behaved according to Equation 6-1, then the potential difference across the membrane would be zero in the absence of an externally applied current. Instead, most cells maintain

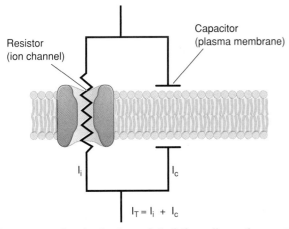

Figure 6-2. Electric circuit model of the cell membrane. The cell membrane can be modeled as a simple electric circuit containing a resistor and a capacitor. Ion-selective channels function as resistors (identical to conductors), through which ions can flow down their electrochemical gradient. The lipid bilayer acts as a capacitor by maintaining a separation of charges between the extracellular and intracellular spaces. This circuit (referred to as an *RC*, or *resistor-capacitor*, circuit) changes the timing between the flow of charges across the membrane (current) and changes in transmembrane potential (voltage), because the lipid bilayer, acting as a capacitor, stores some of the charge that passes across the membrane. Time is required to store this charge; therefore, the initial change in voltage associated with a step of current is slow. As the capacitor (lipid bilayer) fills with charges and the voltage change grows, more of the charge passes through the resistor, until a new steady state is reached and the current-voltage relationship becomes more linear. (I_c, capacitor current; I_i, ionic current; I_T, total current.)

a negative potential difference across their plasma membrane. This voltage difference is most pronounced in neuronal and cardiac ventricular cells, where a resting potential (the voltage difference across the membrane in the absence of external stimuli) of -60 to -80 mV can be recorded. The resting potential results from three factors: (1) an unequal distribution of positive and negative charges on each side of the plasma membrane; (2) a difference in permeability of the membrane to the various cations and anions; and (3) the action of active (energy-requiring) and passive pumps that help to maintain the ion gradients. The effects of these three interrelated factors can be explained best with an example.

Consider the case when there are only potassium ions (K^+) and protein-bound anions (A^-) inside the cell, and no other ions outside the cell (Fig. 6-3). If this cell membrane is permeable to potassium alone, then K^+ will flow outward, while A^- will remain inside. The K^+ flows outward because of a chemical gradient; that is, K^+ efflux is favored because the K^+ concentration inside the cell is greater than that outside the cell. Efflux of the anion, A^-, would also be favored by its **chemical gradient**, but the absence of transmembrane channels permeable to A^- prevents this anion from flowing across the membrane. (In other words, the membrane is impermeable to A^-.) Because of this selective permeability for K^+, every K^+ ion that exits the cell leaves one net negative charge (an A^- ion) on the inside of the cell and adds one net positive charge (a K^+ ion) on the outside of the cell. This separation of charges across the membrane creates a negative membrane potential.

If a negative membrane potential were not established as K^+ leaves the cell, then K^+ ions would continue to exit until the extracellular concentration of K^+ is equal to the intracellular concentration of K^+. However, the establishment of a voltage difference creates an **electrostatic force** that eventually prevents net K^+ efflux (Fig. 6-3B). Thus, the electrical gradient (V_m) and the chemical gradient "pull" the K^+ ions in opposite directions; the electric gradient favors an inward flow of K^+ ions, while the chemical gradient favors an outward flow of K^+ ions. These forces combine to create an **electrochemical gradient**, which is equal to the sum of the electrical gradient and the chemical gradient. *The transmembrane electrochemical gradient is the net driving force for ion movement through channels in biological membranes.*

As a result of the electrochemical gradient, the extracellular concentration of K^+ does not equilibrate with the intracellular concentration. Instead, an equilibrium is established in which the electrostatic force "pulling" K^+ back into the cell is balanced exactly by the chemical gradient favoring K^+ efflux. The potential at which this equilibrium occurs, for any permeant ion X, is a function of the charge of the ion (z), the temperature (T), and the intracellular and extracellular concentrations of the ion. This relationship is expressed as the **Nernst equation**:

$$V_x = V_{in} - V_{out} = \frac{RT}{zF} \ln \frac{[X]_{out}}{[X]_{in}} \qquad \text{Equation 6-2}$$

where V_x is the transmembrane potential that a membrane selectively permeable to ion X would reach at equilibrium (i.e., the **Nernst potential** for that ion), $V_{in} - V_{out}$ is the transmembrane voltage difference, RT/zF is a constant for a given temperature and charge (this number simplifies to 26.7 mV for a charge of $+1$ at a temperature of 37°C),

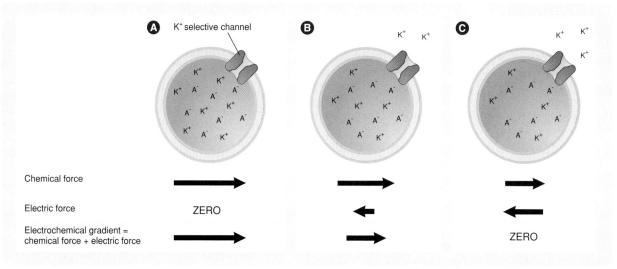

Figure 6-3. Electrochemical basis of the resting membrane potential. A. Consider a prototypical cell that initially contains equal concentrations of intracellular potassium ions (K^+) and impermeant anions (A^-). Assume further that ions can exit the cell only via a single K^+-selective channel. In this case, there is a strong chemical gradient for both K^+ and A^- to exit the cell, but there is no electrical force favoring ion flow because the electrical sum of the intracellular charges is zero. **B.** K^+ begins to exit the cell through the K^+-selective channel, but A^- remains inside the cell because it has no exit route. Therefore, the K^+ chemical gradient across the membrane becomes smaller. As K^+ exits the cell, the net negative charge from the A^- remaining inside the cell produces a negative membrane potential that exerts an electrical force disfavoring K^+ efflux. This force is opposite in direction to that of the chemical gradient; as a result, the total electrochemical gradient (the sum of the chemical force and the electrical force) is less than the chemical gradient alone. **C.** When the electrical gradient is equal and opposite to the chemical gradient, the system is in equilibrium and no net ion flow occurs. The voltage resulting from the separation of charges at equilibrium is referred to as the **Nernst potential.**

and $[X]_{out}$ and $[X]_{in}$ are the extracellular and intracellular concentrations, respectively, of ion X. The electrochemical driving force on ion X is equal to the difference between the actual membrane potential and the Nernst potential for that ion, $V_m - V_x$.

The third determinant of the resting membrane potential, that active and passive ion pumps maintain ion gradients across the membrane, governs the concentration of ions inside and outside the cell. Numerous pumps play an important physiologic role in maintaining ion gradients; these include the ATP-dependent Na^+/K^+ pump (which extrudes three Na^+ ions for every 2 K^+ ions that enter the cell) and the Na^+/Ca^{2+} exchanger (which extrudes one Ca^{2+} for every three Na^+ ions that enter the cell). The coordinated action of these pumps closely regulates the intracellular and extracellular concentrations of all biologically important cations and anions. By knowing the values of these ion concentrations, it is possible to calculate the Nernst potentials for these cations and anions at physiologic temperature and, hence,

the value of the transmembrane potential at which the net driving force for each ion vanishes (Table 6-1).

The differences between the extracellular and intracellular concentrations of the four major ions are attributable to variations in the extent of transport for each ion—mediated by pumps and exchangers in the plasma membrane—and to variations in membrane permeability—mediated by channels selective for each ionic species. The relative ionic permeabilities of the neuronal membrane at rest are $K^+ \gg Cl^- > Na^+ \gg Ca^{2+}$. Because K^+ is the most permeant ion under resting conditions, the resting membrane potential most closely approximates the Nernst potential for K^+ (about -90 mV). In reality, the weak permeability of other ionic species raises the resting membrane potential above that for K^+. Thus, although K^+ is the most permeant ion, the permeability of the other ions and the action of so-called "electrogenic" pumps (i.e., pumps that produce net movement of charge) also contribute to the overall resting potential. At the steady state that describes the true resting mem-

TABLE 6-1	Nernst Equilibrium Potentials for Major Ions			
ION	**EXTRACELLULAR CONCENTRATION**	**INTRACELLULAR CONCENTRATION**	**NERNST EQUATION FOR ION**	**NERNST POTENTIAL FOR ION**
Na^+	145 mM	15 mM	$26.7 \ln (145/15)$	$V_{Na^+} = +61$ mV
K^+	4 mM	140 mM	$26.7 \ln (4/140)$	$V_{K^+} = -95$ mV
Cl^-	122 mM	4.2 mM	$-26.7 \ln (122/4.2)$	$V_{Cl^-} = -90$ mV
Ca^{2+}	1.5 mM	$\approx 1 \times 10^{-5}$ mM	$26.7/2 \ln (1.5/1 \times 10^{-5})$	$V_{Ca^{2+}} = +159$ mV

The calculated values of the Nernst potential are typical of mammalian skeletal muscle. Many human cells have similar transmembrane ion gradients.

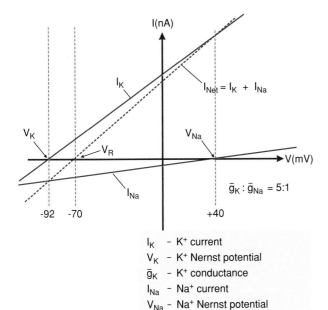

- I_K - K$^+$ current
- V_K - K$^+$ Nernst potential
- $\bar{g}_K$ - K$^+$ conductance
- I_{Na} - Na$^+$ current
- V_{Na} - Na$^+$ Nernst potential
- $\bar{g}_{Na}$ - Na$^+$ conductance
- V_R - Resting membrane potential
- I_{Net} - Net current

Figure 6-4. Relative contribution of K$^+$ and Na$^+$ to the resting membrane potential. The relative membrane permeabilities of K$^+$, Na$^+$, and other ions, and the Nernst (electrochemical equilibrium) potentials of these ions, together, determine the resting membrane potential. In the example shown, the conductance of K$^+$ is five times the conductance of Na$^+$ (shown by the slopes of the *I* versus *V* lines for I_K and I_{Na}, respectively). That is, the membrane is five times more permeable to K$^+$ than to Na$^+$. The K$^+$ current is described by I_K [$I_K = \bar{g}_K(V - V_K)$], while the Na$^+$ current is described by I_{Na} [$I_{Na} = \bar{g}_{Na}(V - V_{Na})$]. (In this example, $\bar{g}_K$ and $\bar{g}_{Na}$ are constant conductances over all voltages.) I_{Net}, the net membrane current, is the sum of these two currents ($I_{Net} = I_K + I_{Na}$). The "resting" membrane potential (V_R) is the value of V at which I_{Net} equals zero. In this example, note that V_R is close to, but greater than, V_K. This is because, although K$^+$ is the primary determinant of the resting potential, the minor Na$^+$ current depolarizes V_R to a value more positive than V_K.

brane potential (Fig. 6-4), V_m does not equal the Nernst potential for any of the individual ions, and each ionic species experiences a net electrochemical force. In other words, ($V_m - V_{ion}$) is nonzero, and small ion fluxes occur. The algebraic sum of these inward and outward currents is small and is balanced by currents from active, electrogenic pumps, so there is no *net* current across the resting membrane. It has been estimated that up to 25% of all cellular energy is expended in maintaining ion gradients across cellular membranes.

THE GOLDMAN EQUATION

The example shown in Figure 6-3 addresses a situation where only one ionic species flows across the plasma membrane. In reality, many cells possess a number of different ion-selective channels, all of which contribute to the overall resting membrane potential. When the resting potential is determined by two or more species of ions, the influence of each species is governed by its concentrations inside and outside the cell and by the permeability of the membrane to

that ion. Quantitatively, this relationship is expressed as the **Goldman-Hodgkin–Katz Equation**:

$$V_m = \frac{RT}{F} \ln \frac{P_K[K^+]_o + P_{Na}[Na^+]_o + P_{Cl}[Cl^-]_i}{P_K[K^+]_i + P_{Na}[Na^+]_i + P_{Cl}[Cl^-]_o} \quad \text{Equation 6-3}$$

where P_x is the membrane permeability of ion x. (P_x is expressed as a fraction, with a value of 1 indicating maximum permeability.) Essentially, this expression states that the higher the concentration of a particular ion and the greater its membrane permeability, the greater its role in determining the membrane potential. In the extreme case, when the permeability of one ion is exclusively dominant, the Goldman equation reverts to the Nernst equation for that ion. For example, if $P_K \gg P_{Cl}$, P_{Na}, the equation becomes

$$V_m = \frac{RT}{F} \ln \frac{[K^+]_o}{[K^+]_i}$$

Alternatively, if P_{Na} greatly exceeds P_K, P_{Cl}, then $V_m \sim V_{Na}$, and the membrane is strongly depolarized. This important concept links changes in ion channel permeability to changes in membrane potential. *Whenever an ion-selective channel opens, the membrane potential is driven toward the Nernst potential for that ion.* The relative contribution of a given channel to the overall membrane potential depends on the extent of ion flow through that channel (represented by the permeability). Time-dependent changes in the membrane permeabilities of Na$^+$ and K$^+$ (and, in cardiac cells, Ca^{2+}) account for the major distinguishing feature of electrically excitable tissues—the action potential.

THE ACTION POTENTIAL

According to Ohm's law, passage of a small amount of current across a cell membrane causes the voltage across the membrane to change, reaching a new steady-state value that is determined by the membrane's resistance (see above). The time course of this voltage change is determined by the product of the resistance r_m and the capacitance C_m of the membrane, with a rate constant equal to $[r_m \times C_m]^{-1}$. (The membrane's capacitance results from having an insulator, the hydrocarbon core of the phospholipids in the membrane, between two conductors, the ionic solutions on either side of the membrane [see Fig. 6-2]. Capacitors store charge at both surfaces and require time to change this charge.) If the stimulated potential change is less than the **threshold** value, then the membrane voltage changes smoothly and returns to its resting value when the current is turned off (Fig. 6-5A). On the other hand, if the membrane voltage changes positively by more than the threshold value, then a more dramatic event occurs: the membrane voltage rises rapidly to a value of approximately +50 mV and then drops to its resting value of approximately −80 mV (Fig. 6-5B). This "suprathreshold" event is known as the **action potential** (AP). An AP cannot be produced by even a large hyperpolarizing stimulus; in this case, the membrane voltage response remains continuous and scaled to the external current, depending only on the resting membrane's resistance and capacitance (Fig. 6-5C).

In most neurons, the balance between voltage-gated Na$^+$ and K$^+$ channels regulates the AP. (In some cardiac cells,

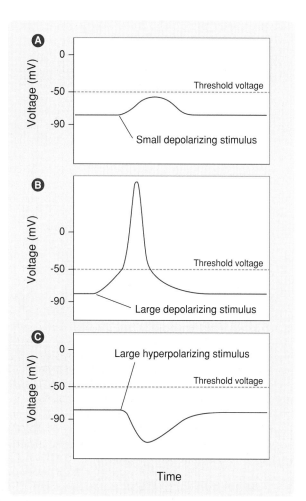

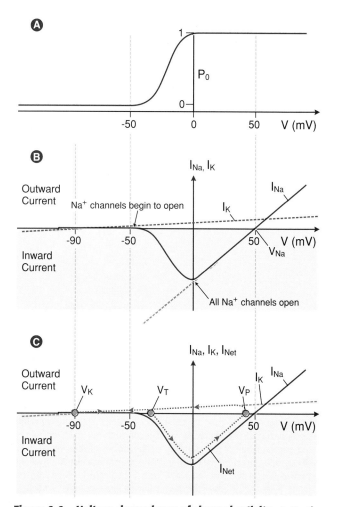

Figure 6-5. The action potential. A. In the example shown, a resting cell has a membrane potential of approximately −80 mV. If a small depolarizing stimulus is applied to the cell (for example, a stimulus that opens a few voltage-gated Ca^{2+} channels), the membrane slowly depolarizes in response to the influx of Ca^{2+} ions. Once the stimulus ends and the Ca^{2+} channels close, the membrane returns to its resting potential. The time course of the voltage change is determined by the membrane capacitance (see Fig. 6-2). **B.** If a larger depolarizing stimulus is applied to the cell, such that the membrane potential exceeds its "threshold" voltage, the membrane rapidly depolarizes to about +50 mV and then returns to its resting potential. This event is known as an **action potential**; its magnitude, time course, and shape are determined by voltage-gated Na^+ and K^+ channels that open in response to membrane depolarization. **C.** In comparison, application of a hyperpolarizing stimulus to a cell does not generate an action potential, regardless of the magnitude of hyperpolarization.

Figure 6-6. Voltage dependence of channel activity. A. P_o, the probability that an individual voltage-gated Na^+ channel will open, is a function of the membrane voltage (V). At voltages more negative than −50 mV, there is a very low probability that a voltage-gated sodium channel will open. At voltages more positive than −50 mV, this probability begins to increase and approaches 1 (i.e., a 100% chance of opening) at 0 mV. These probabilities are also generalizable to a population of voltage-gated Na^+ channels, so that virtually 100% of voltage-gated Na^+ channels in the membrane will open at 0 mV. **B.** The Na^+ current across a membrane (I_{Na}) is a function of the voltage-dependence of the Na^+ channels that carry the current. At voltages more negative than −50 mV, the Na^+ current is zero. As the voltage increases above −50 mV, Na^+ channels begin to open, and there is an increasingly inward (negative) Na^+ current. The maximum inward Na^+ flux is reached at 0 mV, when all the channels are open. As the voltage continues to increase above 0 mV, the Na^+ current is still inward, but decreasing, because inward flow of the positively charged Na^+ ions is opposed by the increasingly positive intracellular potential. The Na^+ current is zero at V_{Na} (the Nernst potential for Na^+) because, at this voltage, the electric and chemical gradients for Na^+ ion flow are balanced. At voltages more positive than V_{Na}, the Na^+ current is outward (positive). The dashed line indicates the relationship that would exist between Na^+ current and voltage if the open probability of the Na^+ channels were not voltage-dependent. The potassium current that flows through voltage-independent K^+ "leak channels" is shown by the broken line (I_K). **C.** The summation of plasma membrane Na^+ currents (I_{Na}) and K^+ currents (I_K) demonstrates three key transition points in the I-V graph (*denoted by blue circles*) at which the net current is zero. The first of these points occurs at a membrane potential of −90 mV, where $V = V_K$. At this voltage, a small increase in potential (i.e., a

voltage-gated Ca^{2+} channels are also involved in AP regulation; see Chapter 18.) Voltage-gated Na^+ channels conduct an inward current that depolarizes the cell at the beginning of the AP. Voltage-gated K^+ channels conduct an outward current that repolarizes the cell at the end of the AP, in preparation for the next excitatory event. Figure 6-6 shows the current-voltage (I-V) relationships for the voltage-gated Na^+ channel and the "resting" K^+ channel. The total Na^+ conductance of the membrane is the product of the conductance of a single open Na^+ channel, the total number of Na^+ channels, and the probability that an individual Na^+ channel is open, P_o. *Key to the excitability of the membrane* *is the voltage-dependence of P_o,* shown in Figure 6-6A. Rapid membrane depolarizations to -50 mV or above cause Na^+ channels to open, with a probability that increases to 1.0, the maximum value, at about zero millivolts. The open channel probability represents the fraction of all Na^+ channels that open in response to a single voltage step. For example, at very negative potentials (e.g., -85 mV) essentially no Na^+ channels are open; as the AP depolarizes the membrane through 0 mV most or all Na^+ channels open; and fast depolarizations to -25 mV open about half of the Na^+ channels.

Recall that ionic current is the product of the ionic conductance (g) and a potential difference. For ions, the potential difference is the same as the electrochemical driving force, $V_m - V_x$, where V_x is the Nernst potential for the specified ion. For example, for Na^+ current:

$$I_{Na} = g_{Na}(V_m - V_{Na})$$

or

$$I_{Na} = \bar{g}_{Na}P_o(V_m - V_{Na}) \qquad \text{Equation 6-4}$$

Here, $\bar{g}_{Na}$ is the Na^+ conductance of the membrane when all Na^+ channels are open, and P_o is, as above, the probability that any individual Na^+ channel is open. The graphic illustration of this equation is shown in Figure 6-6B, where the Na^+ current for a "fully activated" membrane is described by the straight line that passes with positive slope through V_{Na}. If there were no voltage-dependence to the Na^+ conductance (i.e., if g_{Na} were always equal to $\bar{g}_{Na}$), this line would extend throughout the negative voltage range, as shown by its dashed-line extrapolation. However, the voltage-dependence of P_o (Fig. 6-6A) causes the actual Na^+ conductance g_{Na} to be voltage-dependent, resulting in deviation of the real I_{Na} from this theoretical "fully activated" condition. Thus, increasing depolarizations from rest (caused, for example, by an applied stimulus) result in inward Na^+ currents that first become larger as more channels open and then become smaller as V_m approaches V_{Na} (Fig. 6-6B).

Potassium channels conduct outward currents that oppose the depolarizing actions of inward Na^+ currents. Although there are many types of K^+ channels with diverse "gating" properties, only two types need to be considered in order to appreciate the role of K^+ channels in excitability. These two K^+ channel types include the voltage-independent "leak" channels and the voltage-gated "delayed rectifier" channels. **Leak channels** are the K^+ channels that contribute to the resting membrane potential by remaining open throughout the negative range of membrane potentials. The K^+ current that flows through these channels is shown by the broken line in Figure 6-6B; for these channels, K^+ current is outward for all $V_m > V_K$.

The summation of I_{Na} and $I_{K(leak)}$ is represented by the dashed line in Figure 6-6C. Three important points on this line define three critical aspects of the AP. The net ionic current (I_{Net}) is zero at all three of these points. First, at rest, $V_m \approx V_K$. Under this condition, small membrane depolarizations caused by "external" influences result in net outward currents that repolarize the membrane back to rest when the external stimulus ends. Second, at $V_m = V_T$, the outward potassium currents are matched by inward sodium currents, and the net current is also zero. Under this condition, however, even a small further depolarization results in a net inward current that further depolarizes the membrane, which leads to a larger inward current and further membrane depolarization. This positive feedback loop constitutes the rising phase of the AP. Thus, the AP occurs in response to any rapid depolarization beyond V_T, which is defined as the **threshold potential**. Third, V_p is the potential at the peak of the AP. Once V_m reaches this maximum depolarization, the net current switches sign from inward to outward and, consequently, the membrane begins to be repolarized.

Voltage-gated (**delayed rectifier**) K^+ channels contribute to the rapid repolarization phase of the AP. Although membrane depolarization opens these channels, they open and close more slowly than do Na^+ channels in response to depolarization. Therefore, inward Na^+ current dominates the early (depolarization) phase of the AP, and outward K^+ current dominates the later (repolarization) phase (Fig. 6-7). This is why the AP is characterized by an initial rapid depolarization (caused by fast inward Na^+ current) followed by a prolonged repolarization (caused by slower and more sustained outward K^+ current).

The final feature determining membrane excitability is the limited duration of Na^+ channel opening in response to membrane depolarization. After opening in response to rapid membrane depolarization, Na^+ channels enter a closed state in which they are **inactivated** (i.e., prevented from subsequent opening). Recovery from inactivation occurs only when the membrane is repolarized, whereupon the Na^+ channels return to the closed, resting state from which they can open in response to a stimulus. This inactivation of Na^+ conductance, combined with the slowly decaying voltage-gated K^+ conductance, produces dynamic changes in membrane excitability. Following just one AP, fewer Na^+ channels are available to open (i.e., $\bar{g}_{Na}$ is temporarily smaller), more K^+ channels are open (i.e., g_K is larger), the corresponding ionic currents are changed, and *V_T is more positive than it was before the AP.* An excitable membrane is in its so-called **refractory state** during this period, which lasts from just after the AP until the conditions of fast g_{Na} inactivation and slow g_K activation have returned to their resting values. Slow depolarizing stimuli will fail to induce an AP, even when the membrane reaches the threshold potential defined by a rapid depolarizing stimulus, because of the accumulation of inactivated Na^+ channels during the slow depolarizing stimulus. The inactivation property of Na^+ channels is important in the concept of **use-dependent block**, as discussed in Chapter 10, Local Anesthetic Pharmacology, and Chapter 18, Pharmacology of Cardiac Rhythm.

---

small depolarization) results in an outward (positive) K^+ current that brings the membrane potential back toward V_K. The second point occurs at $V_{Threshold}$, the threshold voltage (V_T). At this voltage $I_{Na} = -I_K$; further depolarization results in the opening of more voltage-dependent Na^+ channels and a net negative (inward) current, which initiates the action potential. The third point occurs at V_{Peak}, the peak voltage (V_P). At this voltage, the transition occurs from a net negative current to a net positive (outward) current. As the Na^+ channels inactivate, the net positive current is dominated by I_K, and the membrane potential returns toward V_K (i.e., the membrane is repolarized).

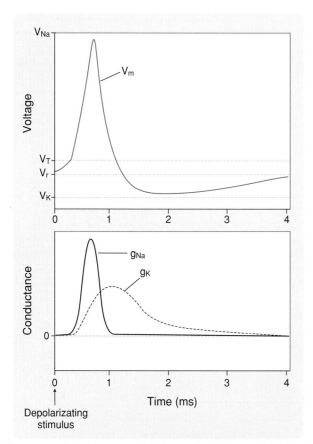

Figure 6-7. Time course of voltage-dependent Na⁺ and K⁺ conductances. During the course of an action potential, the transmembrane voltage (V_m) first increases rapidly from V_T toward V_{Na}, then decreases below V_T and more slowly approaches V_K. The shape and duration of the action potential can be explained by the differential time courses of the voltage-dependent Na⁺ and K⁺ currents. In response to a depolarizing stimulus, the Na⁺ conductance (g_{Na}) increases rapidly because of the rapid opening of voltage-gated Na⁺ channels, then decreases because of Na⁺ channel inactivation. The K⁺ conductance (g_K) increases concurrently with g_{Na} but takes a longer time to reach its maximum conductance because there is a slower rate constant for opening of voltage-dependent K⁺ channels. Eventually, g_K is greater than g_{Na}, and the membrane repolarizes. (V_{Na}, V_K, Nernst potentials for Na⁺ and K⁺, respectively; V_r, resting membrane potential; V_T, threshold potential for action potential firing.)

PHARMACOLOGY OF ION CHANNELS

Many drugs act directly on ion channels to produce changes in membrane excitability. For example, local anesthetics are injected locally at high concentrations to block Na⁺ channels in peripheral and spinal neurons; this Na⁺ channel block inhibits AP propagation and prevents sensory transmission (e.g., pain) by these nerves (see Chapter 10). At much lower concentrations, these and structurally similar antiarrhythmic drugs act systemically to suppress abnormal APs in the heart and to treat neuropathic pain and some forms of myotonia (see Chapter 18). Drugs that block K⁺ channels are used to treat certain types of cardiac arrhythmias, and may be used in the future to overcome nerve con-

duction deficits secondary to demyelinating conditions such as multiple sclerosis and spinal cord injury. Calcium channels are blocked directly by some drugs used in the treatment of hypertension; such drugs act by relaxing vascular smooth muscle and lowering systemic vascular resistance. Some heart conditions are also treated by selective blockers of cardiac Ca^{2+} channels (see Chapter 21, Pharmacology of Vascular Tone). Highly potent and selective blockers of a certain class of neuronal Ca^{2+} channel have been purified from the venom of a marine snail (*Conus* sp.) and administered into the spinal fluid to treat severe cases of neuropathic pain. Some toxins block ion channels and thereby inhibit AP propagation; **tetrodotoxin**, the fugu neurotoxin, blocks voltage-gated Na⁺ channels with high affinity and can cause fatal paralysis if ingested in sufficient amounts. Ion channels can also be modified by drugs indirectly, through pharmacologic modulation of the receptors that regulate the channels, as described below.

ELECTROCHEMICAL TRANSMISSION

Neurons communicate with one another and with other cell types through the regulated release of small molecules or peptides known as **neurotransmitters**. Neurotransmitters may be released into the circulation, from which they can act on distant organs, or they may diffuse only a short distance to act on juxtaposed target cells at a specialized connection called a **synapse**. Synaptic transmission thus integrates electrical signals (voltage changes in the plasma membrane of the presynaptic cell) with chemical signals (release of neurotransmitter by the presynaptic cell and subsequent binding of the transmitter to receptors in the membrane of the postsynaptic cell). For this reason, synaptic transmission is often referred to as **electrochemical transmission**.

The general sequence of processes essential for electrochemical transmission is as follows (Fig. 6-8):

1. Neurotransmitters are synthesized by cytoplasmic enzymes and stored in the neuron. Common neurotransmitters include acetylcholine, norepinephrine, γ-aminobutyric acid (GABA), glutamate, dopamine, and serotonin. Most neurons are specialized to release only one type of neurotransmitter, and this specialization is determined largely by the synthetic enzymes expressed in that neuron. After synthesis, neurotransmitters are actively transported from the cytoplasm into intracellular vesicles (often called **synaptic vesicles**) in which they reach high concentrations. Loading of these vesicles is accomplished by the coordinated activity of a number of vesicular membrane proteins. In most cases, an ATP-dependent transporter pumps protons from the cytoplasm into the vesicle, thereby creating a proton gradient across the vesicle membrane. The electrochemical energy in this proton gradient is used to provide specialized neurotransmitter transporters with the fuel for active transport of neurotransmitter molecules from the cytoplasm into the vesicle. Neurotransmitter-filled vesicles undergo a priming process and dock on the ''active zone'' of the plasma membrane of the presynaptic terminal, a cellular structure that is specialized for neurotransmitter release.

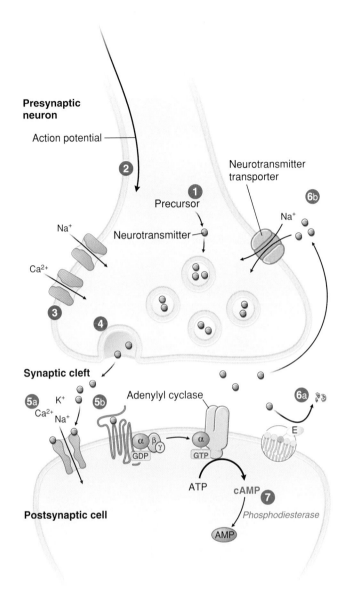

Figure 6-8. Steps in synaptic transmission. Synaptic transmission can be divided into a series of steps that couple electrical depolarization of the presynaptic neuron to chemical signaling between the presynaptic and postsynaptic cells. **1.** Neuron synthesizes neurotransmitter from precursor, and stores the transmitter in vesicles. **2.** An action potential traveling down the neuron depolarizes the presynaptic nerve terminal. **3.** Membrane depolarization activates voltage-dependent Ca^{2+} channels, allowing Ca^{2+} entry into the presynaptic nerve terminal. **4.** The increased cytosolic Ca^{2+} enables vesicle fusion with the plasma membrane of the presynaptic neuron, with subsequent release of neurotransmitter into the synaptic cleft. **5.** Neurotransmitter diffuses across the synaptic cleft and binds to one of two types of postsynaptic receptors. **5a.** Neurotransmitter binding to ionotropic receptors causes channel opening and changes the permeability of the postsynaptic membrane to ions. This may also result in a change in the postsynaptic membrane potential. **5b.** Neurotransmitter binding to metabotropic receptors on the postsynaptic cell activates intracellular signaling cascades; the example shows G protein activation leading to the formation of cAMP by adenylyl cyclase. In turn, such a signaling cascade can activate other ion-

selective channels. **6.** Signal termination is accomplished by removal of transmitter from the synaptic cleft. **6a.** Transmitter can be degraded by enzymes (*E*) in the synaptic cleft. **6b.** Alternatively, transmitter can be recycled into the presynaptic cell by reuptake transporters. **7.** Signal termination can also be accomplished by enzymes (such as phosphodiesterase) that degrade postsynaptic intracellular signaling molecules (such as cAMP).

2. When the threshold voltage is reached in the neuron, an AP is initiated and propagated along the axonal membrane to the presynaptic nerve terminal.

3. Depolarization of the nerve terminal membrane causes opening of voltage-dependent Ca^{2+} channels and influx of Ca^{2+} through these open channels into the presynaptic nerve terminal. In many neurons, this Ca^{2+} influx is regulated by P/Q-type (Ca_v 2.1) or N-type (Ca_v 2.2) Ca^{2+} channels.

4. In the presynaptic terminal, the rapid rise in cytosolic free Ca^{2+} concentration causes neurotransmitter-filled vesicles to fuse with specialized protein machinery in the presynaptic plasma membrane (see Synaptic Vesicle Regulation in the next section). After vesicle fusion, neurotransmitter is released into the synaptic cleft.

5. Released neurotransmitter diffuses across the synaptic cleft, where it can bind to two classes of receptors on the postsynaptic membrane:

   a. Binding of neurotransmitter to ligand-gated **ionotropic receptors** opens channels that permit ion flux across the postsynaptic membrane. Within milliseconds, this ion flux leads to **excitatory** or **inhibitory postsynaptic potentials**.

   b. Binding of neurotransmitter to **metabotropic receptors** (e.g., G protein-coupled receptors) causes activation of intracellular second messenger signaling cascades. These signaling events can also lead to changes in the postsynaptic potential, although their time course is slower (generally seconds to minutes).

   Some neurotransmitters may also bind to a third class of receptors on the *presynaptic* membrane. These receptors are called **autoreceptors** because they regulate neurotransmitter release.

6. Excitatory postsynaptic potentials (EPSPs) and inhibitory postsynaptic potentials (IPSPs) propagate passively (i.e., without generating an AP) along the membrane of the postsynaptic cell. A large number of EPSPs can summate to cause the postsynaptic membrane to exceed threshold voltage (V_T). If this occurs, an AP can be generated in the postsynaptic cell. (This process is not shown in Fig. 6-8.)

7. Stimulation of the postsynaptic cell is terminated by removal of the neurotransmitter, desensitization of the postsynaptic receptor, or a combination of both. Neurotransmitter removal occurs by two mechanisms:

   a. Degradation of the neurotransmitter by enzymes in the synaptic cleft.

   b. Uptake of the neurotransmitter by specific transporters into the presynaptic terminal (or by surrounding glial cells), which terminates synaptic action and allows the neurotransmitter to be recycled into synaptic vesicles in preparation for a new release event.

8. For G protein-coupled metabotropic receptors in the postsynaptic cell, termination of the response to a transmitter stimulus is also dependent on intracellular enzymes that inactivate second messengers (e.g., phosphodiesterases that convert cAMP to its inactive metabolite AMP).

The prototypic chemical synapse is that of the neuromuscular junction (see Fig. 8-4 for more detail). At this junction, terminal branches of the motor axon lie in a synaptic trough on the surface of the muscle cells. When the neuron fires, acetylcholine (ACh) is released from the motor neuron terminals. The released ACh diffuses across the **synaptic cleft** to bind to ligand-gated ionotropic receptors located on the postsynaptic muscle membrane. This binding of ACh to its receptors causes a transient increase in the probability of opening of receptor-associated ion channels. The channel pore is equally permeable to Na^+ and K^+, and these channels have a **reversal potential** (i.e., a potential at which there is no net current flowing through the channel) of approximately 0 mV (the average of the individual Na^+ and K^+ Nernst potentials). The net inward current passing through these open channels depolarizes the muscle cell membrane. Although this particular **end-plate potential** is sufficiently large to stimulate an AP in the muscle, its magnitude is unusual, because most neuronal excitatory postsynaptic potentials are of insufficient magnitude to stimulate an AP. Instead, several neuronal excitatory postsynaptic potentials must occur together, within a short time ($\sim$10 ms) and at closely spaced synapses, in order for the postsynaptic depolarization to reach the threshold value for firing of an AP.

The following discussion highlights points in the basic steps of neurotransmission that can be modified by pharmacologic agents.

SYNAPTIC VESICLE REGULATION

Nerve terminals contain two types of secretory vesicles: small, **clear-core synaptic vesicles** and large, **dense-core synaptic vesicles**. The clear-core vesicles store and secrete small organic neurotransmitters, such as acetylcholine, GABA, glycine, and glutamate. Dense-core vesicles are more likely to contain peptide or amine neurotransmitters. The larger dense-core vesicles are similar to the secretory granules of endocrine cells because their release is not limited to "active zones" on the presynaptic cell. Dense-core vesicle release is also more likely to follow a train of impulses (continuous or rhythmic stimulation) than a single AP. Hence, the smaller clear-core vesicles are involved in rapid chemical transmission, while the larger dense-core vesicles are implicated in slow, modulatory, or distant signaling.

Over the past several years, many of the proteins that control synaptic vesicle trafficking have been identified. **Synapsin** is an intrinsic membrane protein that binds both to synaptic vesicles and to actin. This protein links vesicles to the cytoplasmic actin matrix at nerve terminals. Because synapsin is a major substrate for protein kinases regulated by cAMP and Ca^{2+}/calmodulin, it is thought that these second messengers act in neurotransmitter release by controlling the availability of synaptic vesicles for Ca^{2+}-dependent exocytosis. **Synaptobrevin** is a small protein anchored to the vesicle membrane at its hydrophobic C-terminal region. It is one of several proteins, collectively called **SNAREs** (soluble N-ethylmaleimide-sensitive factor attachment protein re-

ceptors), which are essential for both Ca^{2+}-regulated and Ca^{2+}-independent vesicle exocytosis (Fig. 6-9). Certain neurotoxins, such as tetanus toxin and botulinum toxin (see Chapter 8), appear to act by selectively cleaving synaptobrevin and thereby inhibiting synaptic vesicle exocytosis. Synapsin, synaptobrevin, and other recently discovered proteins involved in neurotransmitter release may provide targets for pharmacologic control of synaptic transmission.

POSTSYNAPTIC RECEPTORS

A large number of neuropharmacologic drugs act on postsynaptic receptors. These integral membrane proteins fall into two classes: **ionotropic** and **metabotropic**.

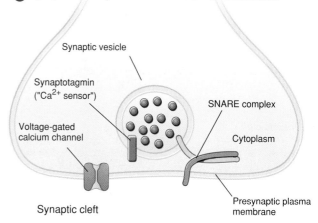

A Synaptic vesicle primed for release of neurotransmitter

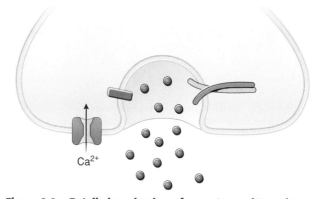

B Local Ca^{2+} transient triggers release of neurotransmitter into synaptic cleft

Figure 6-9. Detailed mechanism of neurotransmitter release. A. Synaptic vesicles are tethered close to the plasma membrane of the presynaptic neuron by several protein-protein interactions. The most important of these interactions involve SNARE (soluble N-ethylmaleimide-sensitive factor attachment protein receptor) proteins in the vesicle membrane and the plasma membrane. Voltage-gated Ca^{2+} channels are located in proximity to these SNARE complexes in the plasma membrane; this facilitates the sensing of Ca^{2+} entry by synaptotagmin in the vesicle membrane. **B.** Voltage-gated calcium channels open in response to an action potential, allowing entry of extracellular Ca^{2+} into the cell. The increase in intracellular Ca^{2+} triggers fusion of the vesicle membrane with the plasma membrane, releasing neurotransmitter molecules into the synaptic cleft.

Ionotropic receptors, such as nicotinic acetylcholine receptors and "A" type GABA receptors, are almost always composed of four to five subunits that oligomerize in the membrane to form a ligand-gated channel. Binding of one (or sometimes two) ligand molecules to the receptor leads to an allosteric conformational change that opens the channel pore. The subunits composing the same functional receptor often differ among different tissues and, as a consequence, the detailed molecular pharmacology of the receptors is tissue-dependent. For example, although acetylcholine is the endogenous transmitter for all nicotinic cholinergic receptors, a number of synthetic agonists (or antagonists) selectively activate (or inhibit) these receptors in skeletal muscle, autonomic ganglia, or the central nervous system (see Chapter 8).

Metabotropic receptors are similarly diverse. Although most are G protein-coupled receptors, the extracellular and cytoplasmic domains of these receptors differ significantly. These differences enable the development of agonists (or antagonists) that activate (or inhibit) specific subtypes of metabotropic receptors.

TRANSMITTER METABOLISM AND REUPTAKE

Altering the metabolism of the neurotransmitter provides an important mechanism for pharmacologic intervention at the synapse. The two major types of intervention involve inhibition of neurotransmitter degradation and antagonism of neurotransmitter reuptake. Acetylcholinesterase, the enzyme responsible for degrading acetylcholine, is an example of the first type of drug target. **Acetylcholinesterase inhibitors** are the mainstays of treatment for myasthenia gravis (see Chapter 8).

The transporters that facilitate neurotransmitter reuptake from the synaptic cleft into the presynaptic cell are of even greater importance. Because these reuptake transporters are crucial for the termination of synaptic transmission, their inhibition has profound effects. For example, the psychotropic effects of **cocaine** derive from this drug's ability to inhibit dopamine and norepinephrine reuptake in the brain, and the therapeutic benefit of antidepressants such as **fluoxe-** tine results from their inhibition of serotonin-selective reuptake (see Chapter 13, Pharmacology of Serotonergic and Central Adrenergic Neurotransmission). Because reuptake transporters tend to be substrate-specific, it is anticipated that new drugs can be designed to selectively target other specific transporter subtypes as well.

Conclusion and Future Directions

Cellular excitability is a crucial component of intercellular communication. The fundamental basis for cellular excitability lies in the electrochemical gradients that are established by ion pumps across the lipid bilayer of the plasma membrane. Ion-selective channels enable cellular membranes to regulate selectively the permeability of the membrane to different ionic species, allowing a change in membrane voltage to be coupled to a chemical stimulus or response. The action potential, a special type of stereotyped response found in excitable cells, is made possible by the voltage-dependent properties of Na^+ and K^+ channels.

The basic processes of electrochemical transmission provide the substrate for pharmacologic modulation of cellular excitation and communication, topics that are addressed in more detail throughout this book.

Suggested Reading

Conley EC, Brammer WJ. *The ion channel facts book, vol. IV: voltage-gated channels.* San Diego: Academic Press; 1996. (*Basic information on ion channels.*)

Hille B. *Ionic channels of excitable membranes.* 3rd ed. Sunderland, MA: Sinauer Associates; 2001. (*Clearly discusses the basis of cellular excitability and the biology of ion channels.*)

Nestler EJ, Hyman SE, Malenka RC. *Molecular neuropharmacology: a foundation for clinical neuroscience.* New York: McGraw-Hill/Appleton & Lange; 2001. (*An overview of neuropharmacology.*)

Rizzoli SO, Betz WJ. Synaptic vesicle pools. *Nat Rev Neurosci* 2005;6:57–69. (*Advances in synaptic vesicle biology.*)

Sudhof TC. The synaptic vesicle cycle. *Annu Rev Neurosci* 2004; 27:509–547. (*Review of mechanisms that regulate synaptic vesicle fusion and recycling.*)

7

Principles of Nervous System Physiology and Pharmacology

Joshua M. Galanter and Daniel H. Lowenstein

INTRODUCTION

The nervous system contains more than 10 billion neurons. Most neurons form thousands of synaptic connections, giving the nervous system complexity unlike that seen in any other organ system. Interactions among neuronal circuits mediate functions ranging from primitive reflexes to language, mood, and memory. To perform these functions, the individual neurons that comprise the nervous system must be organized into functional networks, which, in turn, are organized into larger anatomical units.

The previous chapter reviewed the physiology of individual neurons by describing electrical transmission within a neuron and chemical transmission from one neuron to another. This chapter discusses neuronal systems by examining two levels of organization. First, the gross anatomical organization of the nervous system is presented, to place in context the sites of action of pharmacologic agents that act on this system. Second, the major patterns of neuronal connectivity (so-called *neuronal tracts*) are presented, because knowledge of the ways in which neuronal cells are organized

to transmit, process, and modulate signals facilitates a deeper understanding of the actions of drugs on these tracts. This chapter also discusses the major types of neurotransmitters and the blood-brain barrier; these functional and metabolic concepts have important pharmacologic consequences for drugs that act on the nervous system.

Case

Martha P is a 66-year-old woman with a 4-year history of worsening Parkinson's disease, a neurological disorder resulting from the progressive degeneration of nigrostriatal neurons that use dopamine as a neurotransmitter. The disease causes a resting tremor, rigidity, difficulty initiating movement, and postural instability. While visiting her physician, Ms. P registers an unusual complaint: "It seems that my Sinemet doesn't work as well when I take it with meals." Ms. P explains that she has recently started on a new "low-carb" diet that has increased her protein intake at the expense of high-carbohydrate foods. Concerned, Ms. P asks, "Could my diet have anything to do with this?" Her physician explains that levodopa, a component of her Sinemet, helps replace a chemical in her brain that is produced in insufficient quantities because of the loss of certain neurons in her brain. Although many factors could lead to the decreased effectiveness of her medication, Ms. P's doctor confirms her suspicion that her high-protein diet could indeed be interfering with the medication's ability to reach her brain. He recommends that she moderate her protein intake, and, if necessary, take a higher dose of Sinemet after a high-protein meal. At her follow-up visit, Ms. P is happy to report that her medication is more effective now that she is eating less protein.

QUESTIONS

■ **1.** Where is the nigrostriatal tract located? How does the degeneration of a specific group of neurons result in specific symptoms such as those seen in Parkinson's disease?

■ **2.** Why is levodopa used in the treatment of Parkinson's disease, and what is the relationship of this compound to dopamine?

■ **3.** Why does protein consumption interfere with the action of levodopa?

NEUROANATOMY

The nervous system can be divided structurally and functionally into peripheral and central components. The **peripheral nervous system** includes all nerves traveling between the central nervous system and somatic and visceral sites. It is divided functionally into the **autonomic** (involuntary) **nervous system** and the **sensory and somatic** (voluntary) **nervous system**.

The **central nervous system (CNS)** includes the cerebrum, diencephalon, cerebellum, brainstem, and spinal cord. The CNS relays and processes signals received from the peripheral nervous system; the processing results in responses that are formulated and relayed back to the periphery. The CNS is responsible for important functions such as perception—including sensory, auditory, and visual processing—wakefulness, language, and consciousness.

ANATOMY OF THE PERIPHERAL NERVOUS SYSTEM

The autonomic nervous system regulates involuntary responses of smooth muscle and glandular tissue. For example, it controls vascular tone, heart rate and contractility, pupillary constriction, sweating, salivation, piloerection (''goose bumps''), uterine contraction, gastrointestinal (GI) motility, and bladder function. The autonomic nervous system is divided into the **sympathetic** nervous system, responsible for ''fight or flight'' responses, and the **parasympathetic** nervous system, responsible for ''rest and digest'' responses. The sensory and somatic peripheral nervous system carries sensory signals from the periphery to the CNS and motor signals from the CNS to striated muscle; these signals regulate voluntary movement (Fig. 7-1).

Autonomic Nervous System

Autonomic nerve fibers interact with their target organs by a two-neuron pathway. The first neuron originates in the brainstem or spinal cord and is termed a **preganglionic neuron**. The preganglionic neuron synapses outside the spinal cord with a **postganglionic neuron** that innervates the target organ. As discussed below, the anatomical location of these connections differs for neurons of the sympathetic and parasympathetic divisions of the autonomic nervous system.

Anatomy of the Sympathetic Nervous System

The sympathetic nervous system is also known as the **thoracolumbar system**, because its preganglionic fibers arise from the first thoracic segment to the second or third lumbar segment of the spinal cord (Fig. 7-2). Specifically, the preganglionic nerve cell bodies arise from the **intermediolateral** columns in the spinal cord. Preganglionic nerves exit the spinal cord at the ventral roots of each vertebral level and make synaptic connections with postganglionic neurons in sympathetic ganglia. Most sympathetic ganglia are located in the sympathetic chains, which consist of 25 pairs of interconnected ganglia that lie on either side of the vertebral column. The first three sympathetic ganglia, whose postganglionic fibers are carried with the cervical spinal nerves, are termed the **superior cervical ganglion, middle cervical ganglion,** and **inferior cervical ganglion.** The superior cervical ganglion innervates the pupil, salivary glands, and lacrimal glands, as well as blood vessels and sweat glands in the head and face (Fig. 7-2). Postganglionic neurons arising in the middle and inferior cervical ganglia, as well as the thoracic ganglia, innervate the heart and lungs. Fibers arising from the remaining paravertebral ganglia innervate sweat glands, pilomotor muscles, and blood vessels of skeletal muscle and skin throughout the body.

Postganglionic neurons that innervate the GI tract down to the sigmoid colon, including the liver and pancreas, arise from ganglia that are located anterior to the aorta, at the origins of the celiac, superior mesenteric, and inferior mesenteric blood vessels (Fig. 7-2). Hence, these ganglia, collectively known as **prevertebral ganglia**, are named the **celiac ganglion, superior mesenteric ganglion,** and **inferior mesenteric ganglion,** respectively. In contrast to the paravertebral ganglia, the prevertebral ganglia have long preganglionic fibers and short postganglionic fibers.

The **adrenal medulla** is contained within the adrenal glands that lie on the superior surface of the kidneys. The adrenal medulla contains postsynaptic neuroendocrine cells (Fig. 7-2). Unlike sympathetic postganglionic neurons, which synthesize and release norepinephrine, neuroendocrine cells of the adrenal medulla synthesize primarily epinephrine (85%) and release this neurotransmitter into the bloodstream rather than at synapses on a specific target organ (see Chapter 9, Adrenergic Pharmacology).

Many pharmacologic agents modulate sympathetic nervous system activity. As discussed in Chapter 9, the sympathetic nervous system has an organ-specific distribution of adrenergic receptor types. This organ-specific receptor

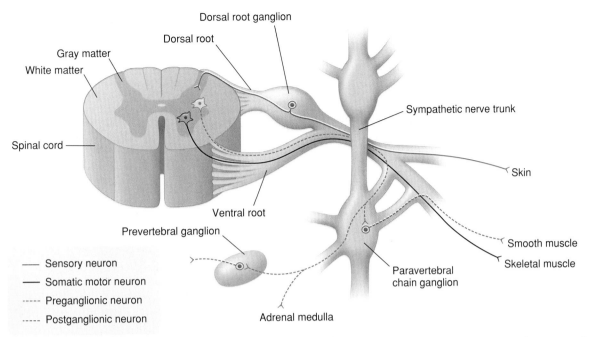

Figure 7-1. Organization of the peripheral nervous system. The peripheral nervous system contains sensory, somatic motor, and autonomic components. Sensory neurons (*solid blue line*) arise principally in the skin or joints, have cell bodies and nuclei in the dorsal root ganglia, and project onto neurons located in the dorsal horn of the spinal cord. Somatic motor neurons (*solid black line*) arise in the ventral horn of the spinal cord, exit through the ventral roots, and join fibers of sensory neurons to form spinal nerves, which then innervate skeletal muscle. The autonomic component of the peripheral nervous system consists of a two-nerve system; the two nerves are called *preganglionic* and *postganglionic* neurons, respectively. Sympathetic preganglionic neurons (*dashed gray line*) arise in the ventral horn of the thoracic and lumbar segments of the spinal cord and project onto postganglionic neurons in the paravertebral and prevertebral ganglia. Sympathetic postganglionic neurons (*dashed blue line*) innervate many organs, including smooth muscle. The adrenal medulla is also innervated by preganglionic neurons of the sympathetic nervous system (see Fig. 7-2). Parasympathetic preganglionic neurons (*not shown*) arise in nuclei in the brainstem and the sacral segments of the spinal cord and project onto postganglionic neurons in ganglia located near the innervated organs.

expression allows drugs to modulate sympathetic activity selectively. For example, certain sympathetic agonists, such as **albuterol,** can dilate bronchioles selectively, while certain sympathetic antagonists, such as **metoprolol,** can selectively decrease heart rate and contractility.

Anatomy of the Parasympathetic Nervous System

Nearly all of the parasympathetic ganglia lie in or near the organs they innervate. The preganglionic fibers of the parasympathetic nervous system arise in the brainstem or in sacral segments of the spinal cord; thus, the parasympathetic system is also called the **craniosacral system** (Fig. 7-2). In some cases, parasympathetic preganglionic neurons can travel almost one meter before synapsing with their postganglionic targets. Preganglionic nerve fibers of cranial nerve (CN) III, the **oculomotor nerve,** arise from a region of the midbrain termed the **Edinger-Westphal nucleus** and innervate the pupil, stimulating it to constrict. The medulla of the brain contains nuclei for parasympathetic nerve fibers in CNs VII, IX, and X. Parasympathetic fibers in the facial nerve (CN VII) stimulate salivary secretion by the submaxillary and sublingual glands as well as tear production by the lacrimal gland. Parasympathetic fibers in the ninth cranial nerve, the **glossopharyngeal nerve,** stimulate the parotid gland. The 10th cranial nerve, termed the **vagus nerve,** pro-

vides parasympathetic innervation to the major organs in the chest and abdomen, including the heart, tracheobronchial tree, kidneys, and GI system down to the proximal colon. Parasympathetic nerves originating in the sacral region of the spinal cord innervate the remainder of the colon, urinary bladder, and genitalia.

Many pharmacologic agents modulate parasympathetic nervous system activity. For example, **bethanechol** is a parasympathomimetic that promotes GI and urinary tract motility.

Antagonists of parasympathetic activity include **atropine**, a drug used locally to dilate the pupils or systematically to increase heart rate, and **ipratropium**, a drug used to dilate bronchioles. These agents and others are discussed in Chapter 8, Cholinergic Pharmacology.

Peripheral Motor and Sensory Nerves

Fibers of the somatic nervous system innervate their target striated muscles directly (Fig. 7-1). These neurons originate in the **ventral horns** of the spinal cord, and exit through the **ventral roots.** They join the **dorsal roots,** which carry sensory nerve fibers, to form the **spinal nerves.** Spinal nerves exit the vertebral column through the intervertebral foramina, after which they separate into peripheral nerves. Somatic components of the peripheral nerves innervate muscles directly. Muscles are innervated in a **myotomal distri-**

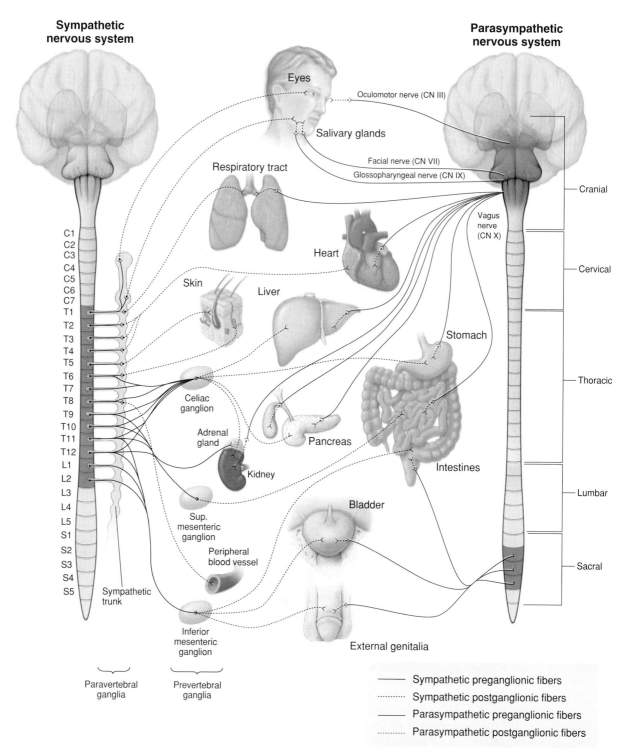

Figure 7-2. Patterns of sympathetic and parasympathetic innervation. Sympathetic preganglionic neurons arise in the thoracic and lumbar segments of the spinal cord. Sympathetic preganglionic neurons project onto postganglionic neurons in ganglia that lie close to the spinal cord, most notably the paravertebral ganglia, and in the prevertebral ganglia located near the aorta. Parasympathetic ganglia generally lie close to the organs they innervate. Thus, parasympathetic preganglionic neurons, which arise in nuclei in the brainstem and the sacral segments of the spinal cord, are generally long and project onto short postganglionic neurons.

bution. That is, neurons originating from a particular ventral root level of the spinal cord (e.g., C6) innervate specific muscles (e.g., flexor muscles of the forearm).

Sensory neurons have cell bodies in the **dorsal root ganglia.** The endings of sensory nerves lie in the skin and joints and enter the spinal cord through the **dorsal roots.** Neurons for vibration and position sense (proprioception) ascend through the **dorsal columns** in the spinal cord and synapse with secondary neurons in the lower medulla. Sensory neurons that carry sensations of pain, temperature, and touch synapse with secondary neurons in the **posterior horn** of the spinal cord. Sensory information is encoded in a **dermatomal distribution.** That is, neurons originating from a particular dorsal root level of the spinal cord (e.g., C6) carry sensory information corresponding to a particular area of the skin (e.g., the lateral aspects of the forearm and hand).

A number of pharmacologic agents modulate the activity of the somatic nervous system. For example, antagonists of neuromuscular junction activity, such as **pancuronium,** are used to induce paralysis during surgery. In contrast, drugs that increase neuromuscular junction activity, such as **edrophonium** and **neostigmine,** are used in the diagnosis and treatment of myasthenia gravis, an autoimmune disease characterized by decreased skeletal muscle stimulation at the neuromuscular junction. These agents and others are discussed in Chapter 8.

ANATOMY OF THE CENTRAL NERVOUS SYSTEM

The CNS is divided anatomically into seven major divisions, namely, the **cerebral hemispheres, diencephalon, cerebellum, midbrain, pons, medulla,** and **spinal cord** (Fig. 7-3). The midbrain, pons, and medulla are collectively known as the **brainstem** and together connect the spinal cord with the cerebrum, diencephalon, and cerebellum.

Cerebrum

The cerebral hemispheres constitute the largest division of the human brain. These structures contain several subdivisions, including the **cerebral cortex,** its underlying **white matter,** and the **basal ganglia** (Fig. 7-4). The cerebral hemispheres are divided into left and right sides that are connected by the **corpus callosum.** The cerebral cortex is responsible for high-level functions, including sensory perception, planning and ordering motor functions, cognitive functions, such as abstract reasoning, and language. The cortex is divided anatomically and functionally into the **frontal, temporal, parietal,** and **occipital** lobes (Fig. 7-4A). Subregions of the cortex have specific functions. For example, stimulation of part of the precentral gyrus, which lies in the frontal cortex, induces peripheral motor function (movement), and ablation of this structure inhibits movement. From a pharmacologic perspective, the cerebral cortex is a site of action of many drugs, sometimes as part of their intended mechanism of action and sometimes as a side effect. **Barbiturates** and **benzodiazepines** (see Chapter 11, Pharmacology of GABAergic and Glutamatergic Neurotransmission) are commonly prescribed hypnotics and sedatives that potentiate the action of inhibitory neurotransmit-

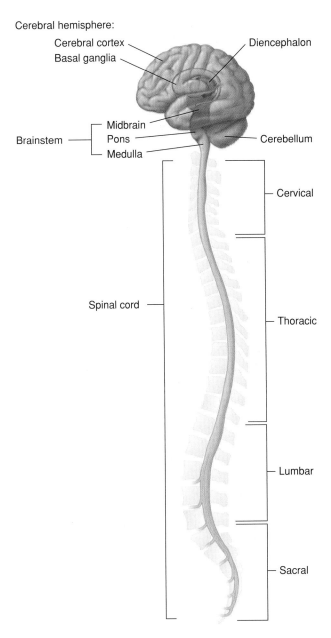

Figure 7-3. Anatomic organization of the central nervous system. The central nervous system is divided into seven major regions: the cerebral hemispheres, diencephalon (thalamus), cerebellum, midbrain, pons, medulla, and spinal cord. The cerebral hemispheres include the cerebral cortex, underlying white matter (*not shown*), and basal ganglia. The midbrain, pons, and medulla together make up the brainstem. The spinal cord is further divided into cervical, thoracic, lumbar, and sacral segments.

ters in the cortex. **General anesthetics** (see Chapter 15, General Anesthetic Pharmacology) are also thought to have effects on the cerebral cortex.

The cerebral white matter, which includes the corpus callosum (Fig. 7-4B), transmits signals between the cortex and other areas of the central nervous system and from one area of the cortex to another. The white matter consists primarily of myelinated axons that, as in other areas of the brain, have an associated vascular network of small arteries, veins, and

A

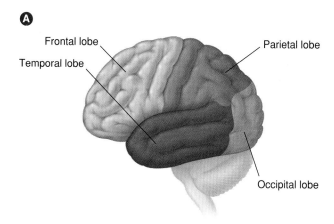

B

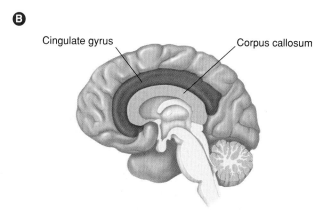

C

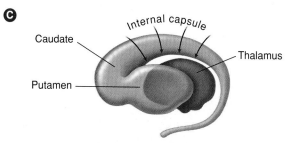

Figure 7-4.   Anatomy of the cerebral hemispheres. A. In this lateral view, the cerebral hemispheres are divided into four lobes—frontal, parietal, occipital, and temporal—which are structurally and functionally distinct from each other. **B.** A sagittal view of the cerebral hemispheres shows the corpus callosum and cingulate gyrus. The corpus callosum connects the left and right hemispheres and coordinates their actions. The cingulate gyrus is part of the limbic system; it lies immediately superior to the corpus callosum. **C.** The basal ganglia include the caudate and putamen, which are together known as the *striatum,* and the globus pallidus (medial to the putamen, *not shown*). The thalamus lies medial to the basal ganglia. Arrows indicate the trajectory of neurons in the internal capsule, a bundle of white matter that carries motor commands from the cortex to the spinal cord.

capillaries. It is around these small vessels that inflammatory cells collect in diseases such as multiple sclerosis, and it is the small arterioles that are especially affected by systemic hypertension.

The basal ganglia consist of three deep nuclei of gray matter (Fig. 7-4C), including the **caudate** and **putamen**—together known as the **striatum**—and the **globus pallidus**. In a general sense, these nuclei help initiate and

control cortical actions. These actions include not only intended movement, but also behavior and certain rudimentary aspects of cognition. Regions of the basal ganglia responsible for movement ensure that intended actions are carried out and irrelevant movements are inhibited. As seen in the case of Ms. P, Parkinson's disease is caused by degeneration of a dopaminergic pathway that arises in the **substantia nigra** in the midbrain (see below) and terminates in the striatum (hence its name, the **nigrostriatal tract** or pathway). This degeneration prevents the basal ganglia from properly initiating motor activity—resulting in decreased intended movement and an unintended tremor—and causes the decreased ("flat") affect characteristic of Parkinson's disease. **Levodopa,** a component of Ms. P's Sinemet medication, acts on the striatum to ameliorate these clinical manifestations of the disease (see Chapter 12, Pharmacology of Dopaminergic Neurotransmission).

A rim or "limbus" around the cortex has "older," more basic functions, and is loosely termed the **limbic system.** This system consists of the **cingulate gyrus** (Fig. 7-4B), the **hippocampal formation** (including the **hippocampus** and surrounding structures), and the **amygdala.** These structures are responsible for emotion, social behavior, autonomic control, the perception of pain, and memory. For example, the memory loss associated with Alzheimer's disease is caused by degeneration of the hippocampal formation. Only a few drugs that specifically affect the limbic system are currently available, although many agents affecting this region of the brain are in development. It should be noted that many drugs of abuse (see Chapter 17, Pharmacology of Drug Dependence and Addiction) stimulate the brain reward pathway, which includes the **nucleus accumbens** and its projections to the limbic system.

Diencephalon

The diencephalon is divided into the **thalamus** and **hypothalamus.** The thalamus, which has several distinct nuclei, is located medially in the brain and inferior to the cerebral cortex. Some thalamic nuclei link sensory pathways from the periphery to the cerebral cortex. Other nuclei act as connections between the basal ganglia and the cortex. The thalamus is not a simple signal relay; rather, it filters and modulates sensory information, in part dictating which signals reach conscious awareness.

The hypothalamus lies ventral to the thalamus. It controls the autonomic nervous system, the pituitary gland, and essential behaviors such as hunger and thermoregulation. Descending pathways from the medial hypothalamus regulate autonomic preganglionic neurons in the medulla and spinal cord. It is generally believed that the antihypertensive effect of **clonidine** is mediated by its action at receptors on brainstem neurons controlled by the hypothalamus (see Chapter 9). Other neurons originating in the medial hypothalamus secrete hormones either directly into the systemic circulation (e.g., **vasopressin** from axon terminals in the posterior pituitary gland) or into a portal system that, in turn, controls hormone secretion by the anterior pituitary gland (see Chapter 25, Pharmacology of the Hypothalamus and Pituitary Gland). The hypothalamus also initiates complex behaviors in response to hunger, extremes in temperature, thirst, and time of day.

Cerebellum

The cerebellum lies inferior to the posterior end of the cerebrum and dorsally to the brainstem. It has three functionally distinct regions: the central **cerebellar vermis,** the lateral **cerebellar hemispheres,** and the small **flocculonodular lobe** (Fig. 7-5). The cerebellum has a relatively well-defined pattern of neural connections, receiving inputs from a wide variety of sources and sending output primarily to the motor areas of the cerebral cortex via the thalamus. The cerebellum coordinates voluntary movement in space and time, maintains balance, controls eye movement, and has roles in motor learning (for example, hand-eye coordination) and certain cognitive functions such as the timing of repetitive events and language. Few drugs are designed primarily to affect the cerebellum. However, several agents, notably alcohol and certain antiepileptic drugs, are toxic to the cerebellum. These agents especially affect the vermis, which controls balance.

Brainstem

The midbrain, pons, and medulla are collectively known as the **brainstem.** The brainstem connects the spinal cord to the thalamus and cerebral cortex. It is arranged with the midbrain superior, the medulla inferior, and the pons bridging the midbrain and medulla (Fig. 7-3). White matter pathways interconnecting the spinal cord, cerebellum, thalamus, basal ganglia, and cerebral cortex course through this small region of the brain. In addition, the brainstem gives rise to most of the **cranial nerves.** Some of these nerves are conduits for sensation from the head and face, including hearing, balance, and taste. The cranial nerves also control the motor output to the skeletal muscles of mastication, facial expression, swallowing, and eye movement. The brainstem also regulates parasympathetic output to the salivary glands and the iris.

The medulla contains several control centers that are essential for life, including centers that direct the output of the autonomic nuclei, pacemakers that regulate heart rate and breathing, and centers that control reflex actions such as coughing and vomiting. Several relay structures in the pons also play a role (in conjunction with the midbrain) in regulating vital functions such as respiration. The base of the pons contains white matter tracts connecting the cerebral cortex and the cerebellum. Neurons in the **periaqueductal gray,** especially in the midbrain, send descending projections to the spinal cord that modulate pain perception (see Chapter 16, Pharmacology of Analgesia).

Clusters of diffusely projecting neurons lie throughout the brainstem, hypothalamus, and the surrounding base of the brain. These nuclei, which include the **locus ceruleus, raphé nucleus,** and several others, comprise the **reticular activating system,** which is responsible for consciousness. Many widely prescribed and illicit drugs influence one or more of these nuclei.

Spinal Cord

The spinal cord is the most caudal division of the central nervous system. It runs from the base of the brainstem (medulla) at the level of the first cervical vertebra down to the first lumbar vertebra. Like the cerebrum, the spinal cord is organized into white matter tracts and regions of gray matter. The white matter tracts connect the periphery and spinal cord to more rostral divisions of the CNS, while the gray matter forms the nuclear columns that lie in an H pattern in the center of the spinal cord (Fig. 7-6).

Neurons in the spinal cord can be defined by their spatial location relative to the gray matter H. These neurons include sensory neurons located in the dorsal horns of the H, motor neurons located in the ventral horns of the H, and spinal

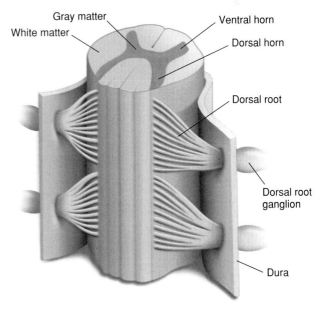

Figure 7-6. Anatomy of the spinal cord. The spinal cord has an H-shaped wedge of gray matter that includes the dorsal and ventral horns. The dorsal horn is responsible for sensory relays to the brain, and the ventral horn is responsible for motor relays to skeletal muscle. The white matter carries signals to and from more rostral divisions of the CNS.

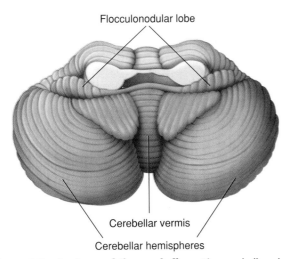

Figure 7-5. Anatomy of the cerebellum. The cerebellum is divided into the cerebellar hemispheres (laterally), the vermis (medially), and the small flocculonodular node. The area immediately above the flocculonodular lobe in this drawing is a cross section of the cerebellar peduncles.

interneurons. The sensory neurons relay information from the periphery to more rostral divisions of the CNS, whereas the motor neurons relay commands arising in the central motor areas of the cortex and brainstem to peripheral muscles. Interneurons connect sensory and motor neurons and are responsible for mediating reflexes, such as the deep tendon reflexes, by coordinating the action of opposing muscle groups. Because the spinal cord carries sensory signals—including sensations of pain—to the central nervous system, it is an important target for analgesic drugs such as opioids (see Chapter 16).

CELLULAR ORGANIZATION OF THE NERVOUS SYSTEM

Cellular organization in the autonomic and peripheral nervous system involves a limited number of neurons that make few connections. For example, somatic and sensory information is carried directly between the spinal cord and the periphery. Autonomic nerves are slightly more complex, in that the signal must undergo synaptic transmission between a preganglionic and a postganglionic neuron. In both cases, however, few ancillary neuronal connections are made, and little or no modification of information occurs.

In contrast, cellular organization in the central nervous system is far more complex. Information is not simply relayed from one area to another; instead, central neurons receive signals from numerous sources and distribute their own axons widely. Some neurons synapse with hundreds of thousands of other neurons. Moreover, not every synaptic connection is excitatory (i.e., designed to depolarize the postsynaptic neuron). Some connections are inhibitory (i.e., designed to hyperpolarize the postsynaptic neuron). Other neurons projecting onto a target neuron can modulate the relative excitability of the cell, affecting the response of the

postsynaptic neuron to other signals. The complexity generated by this variability is needed to carry out the many intricate processes performed by the brain.

Although the CNS possesses immense complexity at the level of neuronal connectivity, three major motifs are used to organize neurons into functional units in the nervous system: the **long tract neuronal systems, local circuits,** and **single-source divergent systems** (Fig. 7-7). The peripheral nervous system is organized exclusively as a long tract system, while the central nervous system uses all three motifs.

Long Tract Neuronal Organization

Long tract neuronal organization involves neural pathways that connect distant areas of the nervous system to one another (Fig. 7-7A). It is the organization used by the peripheral nervous system, and it is important for the transmission of signals from one region to another within the central nervous system.

In the peripheral nervous system, signals are transmitted with little modification. Sensory neurons respond to stimuli such as touch, temperature, pressure, vibration, and noxious chemicals, and, if the initial membrane depolarization is strong enough, transmit an action potential directly to the spinal cord. There, sensory neurons synapse directly with somatic motor neurons, forming reflex arcs, and with ascending spinal neurons that transmit the information to higher levels. Motor neurons carry information directly from the spinal cord out through the ventral roots, and project directly on the motor end plates of the muscles they innervate. The long axon tracts of the peripheral sensory and motor neurons are bundled together and travel as peripheral nerves.

As described above, preganglionic neurons of the autonomic nervous system form synaptic connections with postganglionic neurons at ganglia that are located prevertebrally,

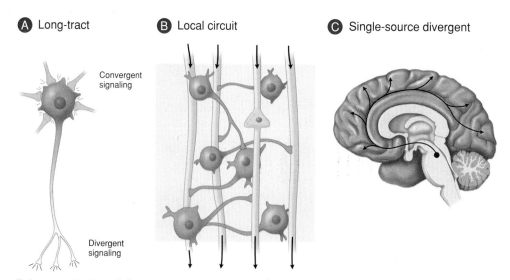

A Long-tract **B** Local circuit **C** Single-source divergent

Convergent signaling

Divergent signaling

Figure 7-7. Cellular organization of the central nervous system. The CNS has three main organizational motifs. **A.** Long-tract neurons act as relays between the periphery and higher sites in the CNS. Long-tract neurons receive signals from many different neurons (convergent signaling) and synapse with many downstream neurons (divergent signaling). **B.** Local circuit neurons show a complicated structural motif, arranged in layers, which includes both excitatory and inhibitory neurons. These circuits are used to process information. **C.** Single-source divergent neurons typically originate in a nucleus in the brainstem and have axonal terminals that innervate thousands of neurons, usually in the cerebral cortex.

paravertebrally, or near the innervated visceral organs. One preganglionic neuron typically makes synaptic connections with up to several thousand postganglionic neurons, an organization that is termed **divergent signaling**. Although divergent signaling does result in some processing and modification of information, the autonomic nervous system does not generally modify neural signals appreciably.

In contrast to neurons in the peripheral pathways, neurons in long tract systems of the central nervous system not only relay but also integrate and modify signals. CNS long tract neurons display divergent signaling like autonomic neurons, but also receive synaptic connections from many upstream neurons (**convergent signaling**). The CNS uses both excitatory and inhibitory neurotransmitters to localize a signal, a strategy that is known as **center-surround signaling**. For example, sensory perception in the CNS can precisely localize a signal by activating cortical neurons that map to one area of the body and inhibiting neurons that map to surrounding areas of the body.

Local Circuit Neuronal Organization

Local circuit neurons *maintain connectivity primarily within the immediate area.* These neurons are generally responsible for *modulating* signal transmission (Fig. 7-7B). For example, neurons in the cerebral cortex are organized in layers, usually six in number. While information flows into one layer and out of a different layer through long tract connections, links between the layers process the signals and interpret the inputs. Local synaptic connections can be both excitatory and inhibitory, ensuring that only certain patterns of inputs are passed along. For example, information originating in the lateral geniculate neurons enters the primary visual cortex through a long tract connection called the **optic tract.** In an area of the cortex designed to perceive lines, the outgoing neurons will be excited only if the incoming neurons fire in a particular pattern, in this case designating a line in a particular orientation. The outgoing signal might then serve as the input to another area of the brain that recognizes shapes. If this area receives an appropriate pattern of lines from the appropriate sources, it might recognize a particular object, such as the grid on a tic-tac-toe board.

Single-Source Divergent Neuronal Organization

Nuclei in the brainstem, hypothalamus, and basal forebrain follow **single-source divergent circuit organization** (Fig. 7-7C), in which *neurons originating in one nucleus innervate many target cells.* Because single-source divergent neuronal organization involves the action of signals on a wide variety of neurons, it is also commonly referred to as a **diffuse system of organization.** Instead of stimulating their targets directly, divergent neurons typically exert a modulatory influence by using neurotransmitters—generally, biogenic amines (see below)—that act on G protein-coupled receptors. These receptors alter the resting potential and ion channel conductance of the neuronal membranes in which they are embedded, thereby altering the ease of depolarization of these neurons. Neurons constituting single-source divergent circuits do not generally have myelin sheaths, because their modulatory influences vary over the course of minutes or hours rather than fractions of a second. In addition, their axons are highly branched, enabling synaptic connections with a large number of target neurons.

The principal single-source divergent neuronal systems are summarized in Table 7-1. They include pigmented dopaminergic neurons that originate in the **substantia nigra,** widely innervate the striatum, and are responsible for regulating the activity of neurons that control intended actions (Fig. 7-8A). Specifically, neurons in the nigrostriatal tract excite downstream pathways that initiate movement and inhibit pathways that suppress movement. The nigrostriatal tract degenerates in Parkinson's disease, which is why Ms. P displayed a paucity of movement. Other dopaminergic neurons medial to the substantia nigra project to the prefrontal cortex and influence thought processes.

Another example of a single-source divergent circuit involves the noradrenergic nucleus in the pons termed the **locus ceruleus** (Fig. 7-8B). Neurons originating in this nucleus widely innervate the cerebral cortex and cerebellum and maintain vigilance and responsiveness to unexpected stimuli. Thus, drugs such as **cocaine,** which inhibits the reuptake of catecholamines such as norepinephrine, can activate this system and cause hypervigilance (see Chapter 17).

TABLE 7-1	Single-Source Divergent Neuronal Systems	
ORIGIN	**NEUROTRANSMITTER**	**FUNCTIONS**
Substantia nigra (midbrain)	Dopamine	Enable intended movement; emotion, thought, memory storage
Locus ceruleus (pons)	Norepinephrine	Vigilance; responsiveness to unexpected stimuli
Raphé nuclei (medulla, pons, and midbrain)	Serotonin	Perception of pain; responsiveness of cortical neurons; mood (?)
Basal nucleus of Meynert	Acetylcholine	Alertness
Pedunculopontine nucleus	Acetylcholine	Sleep/wake cycles
Tuberomamillary nucleus (hypothalamus)	Histamine	Forebrain arousal

A Dopaminergic and cholinergic pathways

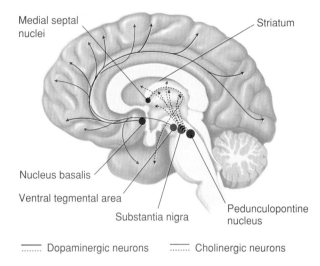

Dopaminergic neurons ······   Cholinergic neurons ······

B Noradrenergic and serotonergic pathways

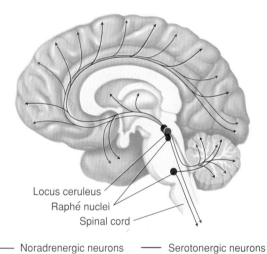

—— Noradrenergic neurons   —— Serotonergic neurons

Figure 7-8. Diffuse neuronal systems. A. Dopaminergic neurons (*black*) arise in the substantia nigra and the ventral tegmental area and project to the striatum and the cerebral cortex, respectively. These neurons are associated with the initiation of movement and the brain reward pathways. Cholinergic neurons (*blue*) arise in the nucleus basalis, pedunculopontine nucleus, and medial septal nuclei. These neurons, which project widely throughout the brain, are responsible for maintaining sleep-wake cycles and regulating sensory transmission. **B.** Noradrenergic neurons (*black*) arise in the locus ceruleus and innervate the entire brain. These neurons are responsible for maintaining alertness. Serotonergic neurons (*blue*) arise in the raphé nuclei and project to the diencephalon, to the basal ganglia, and, via the basal forebrain, to the cerebral hemispheres as well as the cerebellum and spinal cord. Serotonergic neurons are believed to have a role in modulating affect and pain.

Neurons that originate in the raphé nucleus in the caudal brainstem use the neurotransmitter **serotonin** and are responsible for modulating pain signals in the spinal cord and locus ceruleus (Fig. 7-8B). Other neurons originating in the raphé nucleus widely innervate the forebrain, modulating the responsiveness of neurons in the cortex. Serotonergic neurons regulate wakefulness and sleep, and dysfunction of the serotonergic system is hypothesized to be a cause of depression. Because antidepressants block the reuptake of serotonin, this class of drugs may activate the serotonergic raphé pathway (see Chapter 13, Pharmacology of Serotonergic and Central Adrenergic Neurotransmission).

Three other important nuclei that widely innervate the cortex are the **basal nucleus of Meynert,** the **pedunculopontine nucleus,** and the **tuberomamillary nucleus.** The basal nucleus and the pedunculopontine nucleus use **acetylcholine** as a neurotransmitter (Fig. 7-8A). The former nucleus projects to the cortex and regulates alertness, while the latter nucleus controls sleep-wake cycles and arousal. Cells in the basal forebrain that receive inputs from the pedunculopontine nucleus degenerate in several diseases, including Alzheimer's disease. The tuberomamillary nucleus uses the neurotransmitter **histamine** (see below) and may help maintain arousal through its actions on the forebrain. The somnolence induced by first-generation antihistamines—histamine H1 receptor antagonists used to treat allergies (see Chapter 42, Histamine Pharmacology)—may be caused by inhibition of transmission involving tuberomamillary nucleus neurons.

NEUROPHYSIOLOGY

NEUROTRANSMITTERS

The peripheral nervous system uses only two neurotransmitters, acetylcholine and norepinephrine (Fig. 7-9). In contrast, the CNS uses not only a wide variety of small molecule neurotransmitters, including acetylcholine and norepinephrine (Table 7-2), but also many **neuroactive peptides.** These peptides may be transmitted concurrently with the small molecule neurotransmitters, and they generally have a neuromodulatory role.

The small molecule neurotransmitters can be organized into several broad categories, based on both their structure and function (Fig. 7-10). The first category, the **amino acid** neurotransmitters, includes **glutamate, aspartate, GABA,** and **glycine.** The **biogenic amine** neurotransmitters, which are derived from decarboxylated amino acids, include **norepinephrine, dopamine, epinephrine, serotonin,** and **histamine. Acetylcholine,** which is neither an amino acid nor a biogenic amine, is used as a neurotransmitter in both the CNS and the peripheral nervous system. The purines **adenosine** and **adenosine triphosphate** (ATP) are also used in central neurotransmission, although their roles have not been studied in as much detail as those of other neurotransmitters. The lipid-soluble gas **nitric oxide** (NO), which has many effects in peripheral tissues, has recently been shown to act as a diffusible neurotransmitter in the CNS.

Amino Acid Neurotransmitters

The amino acid neurotransmitters are the primary excitatory and inhibitory neurotransmitters in the CNS. Two types of amino acid neurotransmitters are used: the acidic amino acids glutamate and aspartate, which are primarily excita-

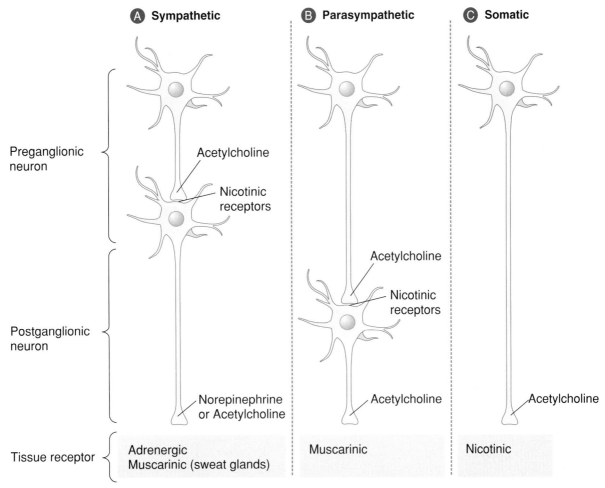

Figure 7-9. Neurotransmitters in the peripheral nervous system. Only two neurotransmitters are required to mediate neurotransmission in the peripheral nervous system. Acetylcholine is released by sympathetic and parasympathetic preganglionic neurons, parasympathetic postganglionic neurons, somatic motor neurons, and sympathetic postganglionic neurons that innervate sweat glands. All other sympathetic postganglionic neurons release norepinephrine. Acetylcholine stimulates nicotinic acetylcholine receptors on sympathetic and parasympathetic postganglionic neurons and at the neuromuscular junction. Acetylcholine stimulates muscarinic acetylcholine receptors on sweat glands and on tissues innervated by parasympathetic postganglionic neurons. Norepinephrine stimulates α- and β-adrenergic receptors on tissues (except for sweat glands) innervated by sympathetic postganglionic neurons.

tory, and the neutral amino acids GABA and glycine, which are primarily inhibitory. Glutamate, aspartate, and glycine are all alpha-amino acids that are also building blocks for protein synthesis. Glutamate is the primary excitatory neurotransmitter; it acts on both ionotropic (ligand-gated ion channels) and metabotropic (G protein-coupled) receptors (see Chapter 11). Excessive excitation of certain glutamate receptors is one of the mechanisms by which ischemic injury causes neuronal death. For this reason, glutamate receptors are a major target for pharmaceutical research. To date, however, there are few therapeutic agents in clinical use that bind selectively to glutamate receptors. GABA, which is also discussed in Chapter 11, is the primary inhibitory neurotransmitter in the CNS. Several classes of therapeutic agents, most notably the barbiturates and benzodiazepines, bind to GABA receptors and, by allosteric mechanisms, potentiate the effect of endogenous GABA.

Biogenic Amines

The biogenic amines (along with acetylcholine) are used by the diffuse neuronal systems to modulate complex central

nervous system functions such as alertness and consciousness. In the peripheral nervous system, norepinephrine is released by sympathetic postganglionic neurons to effect the sympathetic response. The adrenal medulla is a neuroendocrine tissue that releases the biogenic amine epinephrine into the circulation in response to stress.

The biogenic amines are all synthesized from amino acid precursors. Based on these precursors, the biogenic amines can be divided into three categories. The catecholamines (dopamine, norepinephrine, and epinephrine) are derivatives of tyrosine. The indoleamine serotonin is synthesized from tryptophan. **Histamine** is formed from histidine. These three categories are described briefly below.

The catecholamines are all derived from tyrosine in a series of biochemical reactions (Fig. 7-11). First, tyrosine is oxidized to **L-dihydroxyphenylalanine (L-DOPA)**. L-DOPA is then decarboxylated to dopamine. In the case of Ms. P, L-DOPA (levodopa) is one of the components of the medication used to compensate for the loss of dopaminergic neurons in the substantia nigra. (Dopamine is not an effective therapeutic for Parkinson's disease because it does not cross

TABLE 7-2	Small Molecule Neurotransmitters in the Central Nervous System		

NEUROTRANSMITTER	RECEPTOR SUBTYPE	RECEPTOR MOTIF	MECHANISM
GABA	$GABA_A$	Ionotropic	$\downarrow$ cAMP
	$GABA_B$	Metabotropic	$\uparrow$ Cl^- conductance
			$\uparrow$ K^+, Cl^- conductance
Glycine	α, β Subunits	Ionotropic	$\uparrow$ Cl^- conductance
Glutamate, Aspartate	AMPA	Ionotropic	$\uparrow$ Na^+, K^+ conductance
	Kainate	Ionotropic	$\uparrow$ Na^+, K^+ conductance
	NMDA	Ionotropic	$\uparrow$ Na^+, K^+, Ca^{2+} conductance
	mGlu (1–7)	Metabotropic	$\downarrow$ cAMP
			$\uparrow$ IP_3/DAG/Ca^{2+}
Dopamine	D1, D5	Metabotropic	$\uparrow$ cAMP
	D2, D3, D4	Metabotropic	$\downarrow$ cAMP; $\uparrow$ K^+, $\downarrow$ Ca^{2+} conductance
Norepinephrine	α_1	Metabotropic	$\uparrow$ IP_3/DAG/Ca^{2+}
	α_2	Metabotropic	$\downarrow$ cAMP; $\uparrow$ K^+, $\downarrow$ Ca^{2+} conductance
	β_1, β_2, β_3	Metabotropic	$\uparrow$ cAMP
Serotonin	$5-HT_1$	Metabotropic	$\downarrow$ cAMP; $\uparrow$ K^+ conductance
	$5-HT_2$	Metabotropic	$\uparrow$ IP_3/DAG/Ca^{2+}
	$5-HT_3$	Ionotropic	$\uparrow$ Na^+, K^+ conductance
	$5-HT_{4-7}$	Metabotropic	$\uparrow$ cAMP
Histamine	H_1	Metabotropic	$\uparrow$ IP_3/DAG/Ca^{2+}
	H_2	Metabotropic	$\uparrow$ cAMP
	H_3	Unknown	Unknown
Acetylcholine	Nicotinic	Ionotropic	$\uparrow$ Na^+, K^+, Ca^{2+} conductance
	Muscarinic	Metabotropic	$\uparrow$ IP_3/DAG/Ca^{2+}
			$\downarrow$ cAMP; $\uparrow$ K^+ conductance
Adenosine	P_1	Metabotropic	$\downarrow$ cAMP; $\downarrow$ Ca^{2+}, $\uparrow$ K^+ conductance
	P_{2X}	Ionotropic	$\uparrow$ Ca^{2+}, K^+, Na^+ conductance
	P_{2Y}	Metabotropic	$\uparrow$ IP_3/DAG/Ca^{2+}

Neurotransmitters can be organized into several categories, including the amino acids, biogenic amines, acetylcholine, adenosine, and nitric oxide. Each neurotransmitter can bind to one or more receptors. Except for the NO receptor, which is intracellular (not shown), the other small molecule receptors are all at the cell surface. These cell surface receptors may be ionotropic or metabotropic. The mechanism of action of each receptor is indicated. In addition to the small molecule neurotransmitters, more than 50 neuroactive peptides have been identified. AMPA, kainate, and NMDA receptors are named after agonists that selectively activate them. AMPA, α-amino-3-hydroxy-5-methylisoxazole-4-proprionic acid; NMDA, N-methyl-D-aspartate; cAMP, cyclic adenosine-3',5'-monophosphate; DAG, diacylglycerol; IP_3, inositol-1,4,5-trisphosphate.

the blood-brain barrier; see below.) Central dopaminergic receptors have been the target of a wide variety of therapeutics. For example, both dopamine precursors and direct dopamine receptor agonists are used in the treatment of Parkinson's disease, as discussed in Chapter 12. Dopamine receptor antagonists have been used with success in treating the psychotic symptoms of schizophrenia; this topic is also discussed in Chapter 12. Certain drugs of abuse, such as cocaine and the amphetamines, can activate brain reward pathways that depend on dopaminergic neurotransmission, as discussed in Chapter 17.

Dopamine is synthesized from tyrosine and L-DOPA in the cytoplasm, but is then transported into synaptic vesicles. In dopaminergic neurons, the dopamine contained in synaptic vesicles is released as the neurotransmitter. In adrenergic and noradrenergic neurons, the dopamine is converted to norepinephrine within the synaptic vesicles by the enzyme **dopamine-β-hydroxylase.** In a small number of neurons

and in the adrenal medulla, norepinephrine is then transported back into the cytoplasm, where it is methylated to form epinephrine. Chapter 9 discusses the pharmacology of drugs that target peripheral adrenergic receptors, including both agonists, such as bronchodilators and vasopressors, and antagonists, such as antihypertensives. Several classes of therapeutic agents act on central adrenergic receptors. **Clonidine** is a partial agonist that acts on presynaptic α_2-receptors.

Figure 7-10. Structures of the small molecule neurotransmitters. The principal small molecule neurotransmitters can be divided into two broad categories. Amino acids are the primary excitatory (glutamate and aspartate) and inhibitory (glycine and γ-aminobutyric acid) neurotransmitters in the CNS. Their amino and carboxylic acid groups are shown in blue. Biogenic amines are the primary modulatory neurotransmitters in the CNS. The amine moiety is shown in

Amino Acid Neurotransmitters

Aspartic acid

Glutamic acid

Glycine

γ-Aminobutyric acid (GABA)

Biogenic Amine Neurotransmitters

Dopamine

Epinephrine

Norepinephrine

Histamine

Serotonin

Other Neurotransmitters

Acetylcholine

Adenosine

NO
Nitric oxide

blue. Dopamine, norepinephrine, and epinephrine share a common catechol group; histamine has an imidazole group; and serotonin has an indole group. Acetylcholine (a neurotransmitter in diffuse modulatory systems in the CNS), adenosine, and nitric oxide (NO) do not fall into either structural category. The bond order is 2.5 for the nitrogen-oxygen bond in NO, intermediate in strength between a double bond and a triple bond.

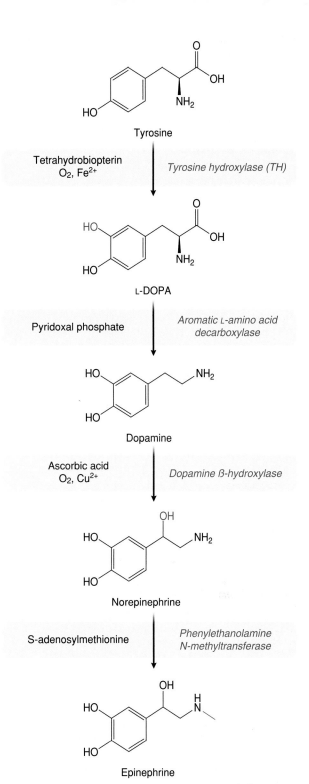

Tyrosine

Tetrahydrobiopterin
O_2, Fe^{2+}

Tyrosine hydroxylase (TH)

L-DOPA

Pyridoxal phosphate

Aromatic L-amino acid decarboxylase

Dopamine

Ascorbic acid
O_2, Cu^{2+}

Dopamine ß-hydroxylase

Norepinephrine

S-adenosylmethionine

Phenylethanolamine N-methyltransferase

Epinephrine

Figure 7-11. Synthesis of catecholamines. Catecholamines are all synthesized from tyrosine. Sequential enzymatic reactions result in hydroxylation of tyrosine to form L-DOPA, decarboxylation of L-DOPA to form dopamine, hydroxylation of dopamine to form norepinephrine, and methylation of norepinephrine to form epinephrine. Depending on the enzymes (*shown in blue lettering*) expressed in a particular type of presynaptic neuron, the reaction sequence may stop at any of the last three steps, so that dopamine, norepinephrine, or epinephrine can be the final product that is synthesized and used as a neurotransmitter.

Some **antidepressants** increase the synaptic concentration of norepinephrine by blocking its reuptake **(tricyclic antidepressants [TCAs])**, while others increase the intracellular pool of norepinephrine available for synaptic release by inhibiting its chemical degradation **(monoamine oxidase inhibitors [MAOIs])**.

5-Hydroxytryptamine (5-HT, also known as **serotonin**) is formed from the amino acid tryptophan by enzymatic oxidation at the 5 position followed by enzymatic decarboxylation. This sequence of reactions is similar to that used in the synthesis of dopamine, although the enzymes that carry out the reactions are different (Fig. 7-12). Several classes of drugs target serotonergic neurotransmission. Tricyclic antidepressants, which block norepinephrine reuptake, also block serotonin reuptake. **Selective serotonin reuptake inhibitors (SSRIs)**, which act more selectively on serotonin reuptake transporters, are also used to treat depression. The role of serotonergic neurons in depression, and the various therapies for depression that target serotonergic neurotransmission, are discussed in more detail in Chapter 13.

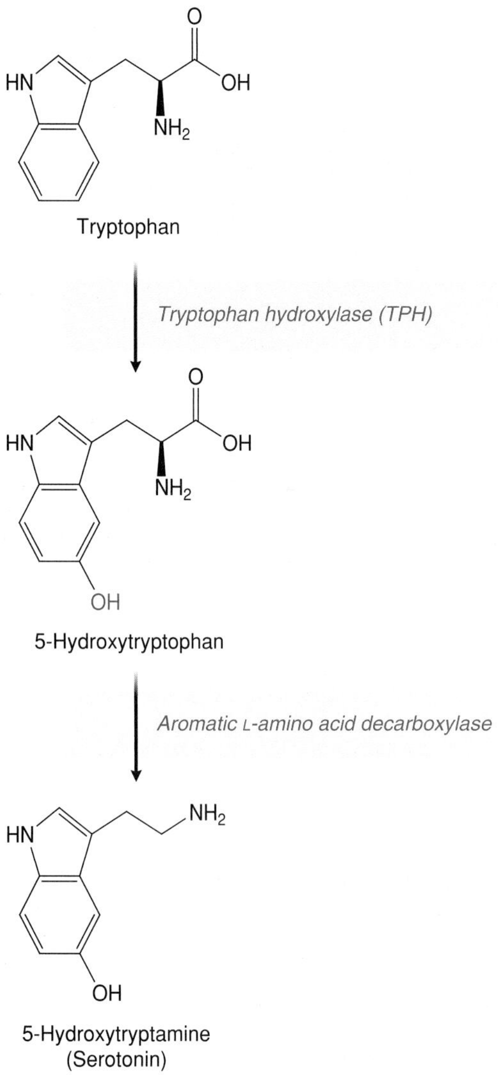

Histamine is formed by decarboxylation of the amino acid histidine. Histamine functions as a diffuse neurotransmitter in the CNS, although few therapeutics intentionally target central histaminergic neurotransmission. Many antihistamines are designed to act on peripheral histamine H1 receptors, at which histamine mediates the inflammatory response to allergic stimuli. Several therapeutics that target histamine H2 receptors are used in the treatment of peptic ulcer disease (see Chapters 42 and 45). As mentioned above, the action of histamine H1 receptor antagonists on central histamine receptors may produce the adverse effect of drowsiness.

Other Small Molecule Neurotransmitters

Acetylcholine plays a major role in peripheral neurotransmission. At the neuromuscular junction, this molecule is used by somatic motor neurons to depolarize striated muscle. In the autonomic nervous system, acetylcholine is the neurotransmitter used by all preganglionic neurons and by parasympathetic postganglionic neurons. The multiple functions of acetylcholine in the peripheral nervous system have spurred the development of a wide range of drugs that target peripheral cholinergic neurotransmission. These include muscle paralytics, which interfere with neurotransmission at the motor end plate, acetylcholinesterase inhibitors, which increase local acetylcholine concentration by interfering with the metabolic breakdown of the neurotransmitter, and receptor-specific agonists and antagonists.

In the CNS, acetylcholine acts as a diffuse system neurotransmitter. Like the biogenic amines, it is thought to regulate sleep and wakefulness. **Donepezil,** a reversible acetylcholinesterase inhibitor that acts at central cholinergic synapses, helps to ''brighten'' patients with dementia (see Chapter 8). Peripheral anticholinergic agents may cause central cholinergic blockade and thereby result in major adverse effects. For example, the antimuscarinic drug **scopolamine** can cause drowsiness, amnesia, fatigue, and dreamless sleep. In contrast, cholinergic agonists such as **pilocarpine** can induce adverse effects of cortical arousal and alertness.

The **purinergic** neurotransmitters adenosine and adenosine triphosphate have a role in central neurotransmission. This role is most evident in the effects of **caffeine,** which is a competitive antagonist at adenosine receptors and causes a mild stimulant effect. In this case, the adenosine receptors, which are located on *presynaptic* noradrenergic neurons, act to inhibit the release of norepinephrine. Antagonism of these adenosine receptors by caffeine causes the release of norepinephrine to be disinhibited, which causes the characteristic stimulatory effects of the drug.

Nitric oxide, which has generated significant interest as a peripheral vasodilator, acts in the brain as a neurotransmitter. Unlike the other small molecule neurotransmitters, NO diffuses through the neuronal membrane and binds to its receptors within the target cell. Receptors for NO are thought to reside in presynaptic neurons, allowing NO to act as a retrograde messenger. While many therapeutics target the

Figure 7-12. Synthesis of 5-hydroxytryptamine (serotonin). Tryptophan is first oxidized by tryptophan hydroxylase (TPH) and then decarboxylated by aromatic L-amino acid decarboxylase to yield serotonin.

peripheral vasodilatory effects of NO, none as of yet target its actions as a central neurotransmitter.

Neuropeptides

The neuroactive peptides are the last major class of neurotransmitters. Many neuropeptides also have endocrine, autocrine, and paracrine actions. Major examples of neuroactive peptide families are the **opioids, tachykinins, secretins, insulins,** and **gastrins.** Neuropeptides also include the pituitary hormone release and inhibiting factors, including **corticotropin-releasing hormone (CRH), gonadotropin-releasing hormone (GnRH), thyrotropin-releasing hormone (TRH), growth hormone-releasing hormone (GRH),** and **somatostatin.** The opioid peptide family includes the **enkephalins, dynorphins,** and **endorphins.** Opioid receptors, which are distributed widely in areas of the spinal cord and brain that are involved in pain sensation, are the principal pharmacologic targets of opioid analgesics such as morphine (see Chapter 16) and of some drugs of abuse such as heroin (see Chapter 17).

THE BLOOD-BRAIN BARRIER

In the case of Ms. P, L-DOPA, the immediate precursor of dopamine, is administered rather than the neurotransmitter itself. Unlike L-DOPA, which is able to cross from the blood to the brain tissue where it acts to treat Ms. P's Parkinson's disease, dopamine is unable to cross that boundary. The reason for this exclusion is the existence of a selective filter, termed the **blood-brain barrier,** which regulates the transport of many molecules from the blood into the brain (Fig. 7-13). The blood-brain barrier protects the brain tissue both from toxic substances that circulate in the blood and from neurotransmitters such as epinephrine, norepinephrine, glutamate, and dopamine that have systemic effects in body tissues but that would bind receptors in the CNS and cause undesirable effects if access were permitted.

The structural basis for the blood-brain barrier resides in the unique design of the cerebral microcirculation. In most tissues, there are small gaps, called **fenestrae,** between the endothelial cells that line the microvasculature. These gaps allow water and small molecules to diffuse across the lining without resistance but filter out large proteins and cells. In the CNS, the endothelial cells form tight junctions that prevent diffusion of small molecules across the vessel wall. Also, unlike peripheral endothelial cells, CNS endothelial cells do not generally have pinocytotic vesicles that transport fluid from the blood vessel lumen to the extracellular space. In addition, blood vessels in the CNS are covered by cellular processes derived from **astroglia.** These processes play an important role in selectively transporting certain nutrients from the blood to central neurons.

In the absence of a selective transport mechanism, the blood-brain barrier generally excludes water-soluble substances. In contrast, lipophilic substances, including important lipid-soluble gases such as oxygen and carbon dioxide, can usually diffuse across the endothelial membranes. The oil-water partition coefficient is a good indicator of the ease with which a small molecule can enter the CNS. Lipophilic

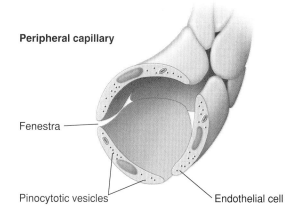

Peripheral capillary

Fenestra

Pinocytotic vesicles

Endothelial cell

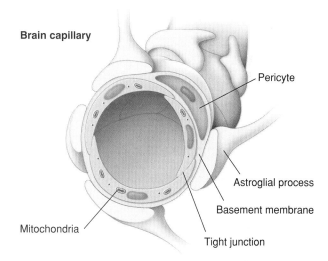

Brain capillary

Pericyte

Astroglial process

Basement membrane

Mitochondria

Tight junction

Figure 7-13. Features of capillaries in the central nervous system compared to the peripheral vasculature. In the periphery, capillary endothelial cells have gaps (termed *fenestrae*) between them and use intracellular pinocytic vesicles to facilitate the transcapillary transport of fluid and soluble molecules. In contrast, CNS vessels are sealed by tight junctions between the endothelial cells. The cells have fewer pinocytotic vesicles and are surrounded by pericytes and astroglial processes. In addition, capillary endothelial cells in the CNS have more mitochondria than those in systemic vessels; these mitochondria may reflect the energy requirements necessary for CNS endothelial cells to transport certain molecules into the CNS and transport other molecules out of the CNS.

substances with high oil-water partition coefficients can generally diffuse across the blood-brain barrier, whereas hydrophilic substances with low oil-water partition coefficients are typically excluded (Fig. 7-14).

Many important hydrophilic nutrients, such as glucose and a number of amino acids, would not be able to cross the blood-brain barrier without the existence of specific transporters. Glucose, for example, is transported across the barrier by a **hexose transporter** that allows this nutrient to move down its concentration gradient in a process called **facilitated diffusion.** Amino acids are transported by three

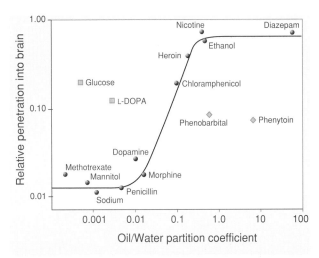

Figure 7-14.   Relative ability of compounds to enter the brain from the blood. In general, there is a correlation between the oil-water partition coefficient of a compound and its ability to enter the brain from the systemic circulation. Specific transporters facilitate the entry into the brain of certain compounds (*squares*), such as glucose (glucose transporter) and L-DOPA (large neutral L-amino acid transporter). Transporters also pump certain compounds out of the CNS (*diamonds*), such as phenobarbital and phenytoin. The metabolic blood-brain barrier, consisting of a number of drug-metabolizing enzymes, also limits the CNS concentration of certain drugs.

different transporters: one for large neutral amino acids such as valine and phenylalanine; one for smaller neutral amino acids and polar amino acids, such as glycine and glutamate, respectively; and one for alanine, serine, and cysteine. L-DOPA is transported by the large neutral amino acid transporter, but dopamine itself is excluded by the blood-brain barrier. For this reason, L-DOPA is administered in lieu of dopamine to patients with Parkinson's disease. After meals with a high protein content, however, the transporter can become overwhelmed, and its transport of L-DOPA can become ineffective. This explains Ms. P's complaint that her medication was less effective after she began a diet high in protein. The blood-brain barrier also contains a number of ion channels, which ensure that ion concentrations in the brain are maintained at homeostatic levels.

Just as certain vital hydrophilic nutrients are allowed access to the brain tissue via particular transporters, many potentially toxic lipophilic compounds can be excluded from the brain by a class of proteins known as **multiple drug resistance (MDR) transporters.** These transporters pump hydrophobic compounds out of the brain and back into the blood vessel lumen. (Note that MDR transporters are present in many cell types, playing an important role in processes such as the resistance of tumor cells to chemotherapeutic agents.) A **metabolic blood-brain barrier** adds a layer of protection against toxic compounds; this barrier is maintained by enzymes that metabolize compounds transported into CNS endothelial cells. One such enzyme, **aromatic L-amino acid decarboxylase** (sometimes called **DOPA decarboxylase**), metabolizes peripheral L-DOPA to dopamine, which is unable to cross the blood-brain barrier. For this reason, Ms. P's medication includes a second component, **carbidopa,** which is an inhibitor of

DOPA decarboxylase. Carbidopa ensures that L-DOPA is not metabolized to dopamine peripherally before crossing the blood-brain barrier. Importantly, carbidopa itself is unable to cross the blood-brain barrier and, therefore, does not interfere with the conversion of L-DOPA to dopamine in the CNS.

■ *Conclusion and Future Directions*

This chapter discusses the anatomical organization of the peripheral and central nervous systems, the transmission and processing of electric and chemical signals by neurons, the principal neurotransmitters used by CNS neurons, and the structure and function of the blood-brain barrier. Although this chapter introduces some specific drugs as examples, the focus is on the general principles of anatomy and neurotransmission that are important for understanding the action of all pharmacologic agents affecting the nervous system. The remaining chapters in this section discuss specific neurotransmitter systems and specific agents that act on the peripheral and central nervous systems. Thus, Chapters 8 and 9 describe peripheral cholinergic and adrenergic systems, and Chapter 10 discusses the production of local anesthesia by inhibition of electrical transmission through peripheral and spinal neurons. Chapter 11 describes central excitatory and inhibitory neurotransmission. Although few therapeutics currently take advantage of glutamatergic neurotransmission, two major classes of drugs, the benzodiazepines and the barbiturates, affect GABAergic neurotransmission by potentiating the effect of GABA at the GABA_A receptor. Chapter 12 discusses dopaminergic systems, describing in more detail the concept, introduced in the present chapter, that some of the symptoms of Parkinson's disease can be alleviated by drugs that increase dopaminergic transmission. Chapter 12 also explains how inhibiting dopaminergic transmission can alleviate some of the symptoms of schizophrenia, implying that dopamine may play a role in this disease. Chapter 13 discusses drugs that modify affect, the outward manifestations of mood. These agents include antidepressants, which block reuptake or inhibit metabolism of the biogenic amines norepinephrine and serotonin, as well as the "mood stabilizer" lithium, which is thought to affect a signal transduction pathway. Chapter 14 explores the pharmacology of abnormal electrical neurotransmission, including the action of channel blockers, such as **phenytoin,** which block the propagation of action potentials and thereby inhibit many types of seizures. Chapter 15 describes the pharmacology of general anesthetics, agents whose mechanism of action remains an area of active investigation. Chapter 16 discusses the pharmacology of analgesia, including opioid receptor agonists and nonopioid analgesics. To conclude, Chapter 17 focuses on mechanisms of drug dependence and addiction, major drugs of abuse, and treatments for addiction.

■ *Suggested Reading*

Kandel ER, Schwartz JH, Jessel TM, eds. *Principles of neural science.* 5th ed. New York: McGraw-Hill; 2006. *(Comprehensive textbook containing detailed information on human neuroanatomy and neurophysiology.)*

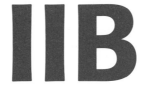

IIB

Principles of Autonomic and Peripheral Nervous System Pharmacology

8

Cholinergic Pharmacology

Alireza Atri, Michael S. Chang, and Gary R. Strichartz

INTRODUCTION

Cholinergic pharmacology is centered on the properties of the neurotransmitter **acetylcholine (ACh)**. The functions of cholinergic pathways are complex, but generally involve the neuromuscular junction (NMJ), the autonomic nervous system, and the central nervous system. Despite the many important physiologic actions of ACh, the current therapeutic uses for cholinergic and anticholinergic drugs are limited by the ubiquitous and complicated nature of cholinergic pathways, and thus, by the inherent difficulty in effecting a specific pharmacologic intervention without inducing adverse effects. Nonetheless, medications with somewhat targeted cholinomimetic and anticholinergic actions are in widespread clinical use for their effects on the brain (especially cognition and behavior), neuromuscular junction, heart, eyes, lungs, and genitourinary and gastrointestinal tracts.

Other relevant chapters discussing applications of cholinergic pharmacology are Chapter 16, Pharmacology of Analgesia; Chapter 45, Integrative Inflammation Pharmacology: Peptic Ulcer Disease; and Chapter 46, Integrative Inflammation Pharmacology: Asthma.

 Case

The year is 1744. Virginian settlers capture Chief Opechancanough, warrior chief of the Powhatans and uncle to Pocahontas. Opechancanough is considered a master tactician and has a reputation as a brutal warrior. One colonial correspondent portrays a different picture of the captured chief, however: "The excessive fatigues he encountered wrecked his constitution; his flesh became macerated; his sinews lost their tone and elasticity and his eyelids were so heavy that he could not see unless they were lifted up by his attendants ... he was unable to walk; but his spirit, rising above the ruins of his body, directed [his followers] from the litter on which he was carried by his Indians." While Opechancanough is confined to a prison in Jamestown, it is discovered that, after a period of inactivity, he is able to raise himself from the ground to a standing position.

It is thought that the story of Opechancanough provides the earliest recorded description of myasthenia gravis, a neuromuscular disease resulting from the autoimmune production of antibodies directed against cholinergic receptors at the neuromuscular junction. In 1934, almost 2 centuries later, the English physician Mary Broadfoot Walker encounters several patients with similar symptoms of muscle weakness, which remind her of the symptoms of patients with tubocurare poisoning. Given her findings, Dr. Walker administers an antidote, physostigmine, to her immobile patients. The results are startling — within minutes, her patients are able to rise and walk across the room. Dr. Walker has discovered the first truly effective medication for myasthenia gravis. Despite the significance of her accomplishment, it is largely ridiculed by the scientific community because the treatment improves the symptoms of myasthenia gravis too rapidly and effectively to be believable. It is not until many years later that the scientific community comes to accept her findings.

QUESTIONS

■ **1.** Why do tubocurare poisoning and myasthenia gravis produce similar symptoms?

■ **2.** What is the therapeutic use of tubocurare, if any?

■ **3.** How does physostigmine improve the symptoms of myasthenia gravis?

■ **4.** Why is it dangerous to administer physostigmine to every patient presenting with muscle weakness?

■ **5.** What are the other therapeutic uses of physostigmine?

BIOCHEMISTRY AND PHYSIOLOGY OF CHOLINERGIC NEUROTRANSMISSION

Acetylcholine synthesis, storage, and release follow a similar set of steps in all cholinergic neurons. The specific effects of ACh at a particular cholinergic synapse are largely determined by the ACh receptor type at that synapse. Cholinergic receptors are divided into two broad classes. **Muscarinic cholinergic receptors** (mAChR) are G protein-linked and expressed at the terminal synapses of all parasympathetic postganglionic fibers and a few sympathetic postganglionic fibers, at autonomic ganglia, and in the CNS. **Nicotinic cholinergic receptors** (nAChR) are ligand-gated ion channels that are concentrated postsynaptically at many excitatory synapses. **Acetylcholinesterase** (AChE), the enzyme responsible for acetylcholine degradation, is also an important pharmacologic target. In this section, a description of the biochemistry of each of these pharmacologic targets is followed by a discussion of the physiologic effects of acetylcholine at the neuromuscular junction, in the autonomic nervous system, and in the CNS.

SYNTHESIS OF ACETYLCHOLINE

Acetylcholine is synthesized in a single step from choline and acetyl coenzyme A (acetyl CoA) by the enzyme **choline acetyltransferase** (**ChAT**):

$$\text{Acetyl Coenzyme A} + \text{Choline} \xrightarrow{\text{ChAT}}$$
$$\text{Acetylcholine} + \text{Coenzyme A} + H_2O \qquad \text{Equation 8-1}$$

In the CNS, choline used for the synthesis of acetylcholine arises from one of three sources. Approximately 35% to 50% of the choline generated by acetylcholinesterase in the synaptic cleft (see below) is transported back into the axon terminal, where it comprises about half of the choline used in ACh synthesis. Plasma-based stores of choline may also be transported to the brain as the lipid phosphatidylcholine, which is then metabolized to free choline. (The incorporation of choline into phosphatidylcholine is essential, because choline itself cannot cross the blood–brain barrier.) Choline is also stored in phospholipids as phosphorylcholine, where it can be used when needed.

Acetyl CoA for the reaction is derived mainly from glycolysis and is ultimately produced by the enzyme pyruvate dehydrogenase. Although the synthesis of acetyl CoA occurs at the inner membrane of mitochondria, choline acetyltransferase is located in the cytoplasm. It is hypothesized that citrate serves as the carrier for acetyl CoA from the mitochondrion to the cytoplasm, where the citrate is freed by citrate lyase.

The rate-limiting step of ACh synthesis is mediated not by choline acetyltransferase, but rather by the uptake of choline into the neuron. There are two processes responsible for choline transport. The first is low-affinity ($K_m = 10\text{–}100$ μM) facilitated diffusion. This transport system is not saturable and is found in cells that synthesize choline-containing phospholipids, such as the corneal epithelium. Far more important is a sodium-dependent, high-affinity transport system ($K_m = 1\text{–}5$ μM) specific for cholinergic nerve terminals. Because the high-affinity transporter is easily saturated (at concentrations of choline >10 μM), it provides an upper limit on the supply of choline for ACh synthesis. As the rate-limiting component, this transporter is a target for several anticholinergic drugs (e.g., **hemicholinium-3,** see Fig. 8-1).

STORAGE AND RELEASE OF ACETYLCHOLINE

After its synthesis in the cytoplasm, ACh is transported into synaptic vesicles for storage. An ATPase that pumps protons into the vesicle provides the energy necessary for this process. Transport of protons out of the vesicle (i.e., down the H^+ concentration gradient) is coupled to uptake of ACh into the vesicle (i.e., against the ACh concentration gradient) via an ACh-H^+ antiport channel. This antiporter is a target for some anticholinergic drugs, such as **vesamicol,** and its inhibition results in a deficit of ACh storage and subsequent release (Fig. 8-1). Along with ACh, cholinergic vesicles contain ATP and heparan sulfate proteoglycans, both of which serve as counter-ions for ACh. By neutralizing the positive charge of ACh, these molecules disperse electrostatic forces that would otherwise prevent dense packing of ACh within the vesicle. (Released ATP also acts as a neurotransmitter, through purinergic receptors, to inhibit the release of ACh and norepinephrine from autonomic nerve endings.)

Release of ACh into the synaptic cleft occurs through fusion of the synaptic vesicle with the plasma membrane.

Figure 8-1. Acetylcholine synthesis, storage, release, and degradation pathways, and pharmacologic agents that act on these pathways. Choline is transported into the presynaptic cholinergic nerve terminal by a high-affinity Na^+-choline cotransporter. This transporter is inhibited by hemicholinium. The cytosolic enzyme choline acetyltransferase catalyzes the formation of acetylcholine (ACh) from acetyl coenzyme A (AcCoA) and choline. Newly synthesized ACh is packaged (together with ATP and proteoglycans) into vesicles for storage. Transport of ACh into the vesicle is mediated by a H^+-ACh antiporter, which is inhibited by vesamicol. The ACh-containing vesicles fuse with the plasma membrane when intracellular calcium levels rise in response to a presynaptic action potential, releasing the neurotransmitter into the synaptic cleft. Lambert–Eaton myasthenic syndrome (LEMS) results from an autoantibody that blocks the presynaptic Ca^{2+} channel. Botulinum toxin prevents the exocytosis of presynaptic vesicles, thereby blocking ACh release. Acetylcholine diffuses in the synaptic cleft and binds to postsynaptic and presynaptic receptors. Acetylcholine receptors are divided into nicotinic and muscarinic receptors. Nicotinic receptors are ligand-gated ion channels that are permeable to cations, while muscarinic receptors are G protein-coupled receptors that alter cell signaling pathways, including activation of phospholipase C (PLC) and opening of K^+ channels. Postsynaptic nicotinic receptors and M_1, M_3, and M_5 muscarinic receptors are excitatory; postsynaptic M_2 and M_4 muscarinic receptors are inhibitory. Presynaptic nicotinic receptors enhance Ca^{2+} entry into the presynaptic neuron, thereby increasing vesicle fusion and release of ACh; presynaptic M_2 and M_4 muscarinic receptors inhibit Ca^{2+} entry into the presynaptic neuron, thereby decreasing vesicle fusion and release of ACh. Acetylcholine in the synaptic cleft is degraded by membrane-bound acetylcholinesterase (AChE) into choline and acetate. Numerous inhibitors of AChE exist; most clinically relevant anticholinesterases are competitive inhibitors of the enzyme.

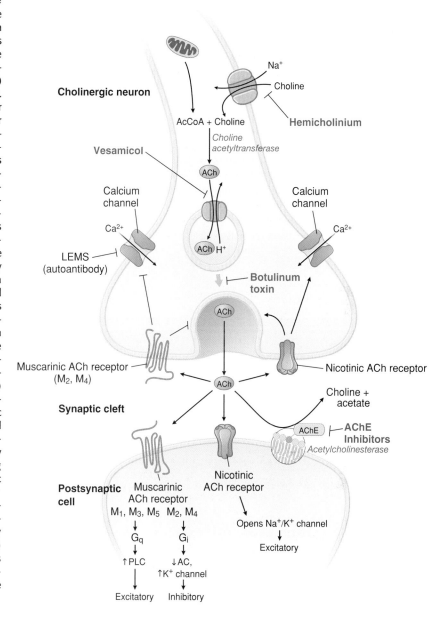

The process is dependent on axon terminal depolarization and the opening of voltage-dependent calcium channels. The increase in intracellular Ca^{2+} facilitates the binding of syntaxin and three SNARE (soluble N-ethylmaleimide-sensitive factor [NSF]-attachment protein receptor) proteins, which together mediate vesicle–membrane attachment and fusion. The result is that the contents of the vesicle are released into the synaptic cleft. (See Chapter 6, Principles of Cellular Excitability and Electrochemical Transmission, for additional details on electrochemical transmission.)

Two stores of ACh play distinct roles during the process of ACh release. One store, known as the "depot" pool, consists of vesicles positioned near the plasma membrane of the axon terminal. Axonal depolarization causes these vesicles to release ACh rapidly. The "reserve" pool serves to refill the depot pool as it is being used. An adequate rate of reserve pool mobilization is required to sustain ACh release for an extended period of time. Of the two stores, the depot pool is replenished first by vesicles loaded with newly synthesized ACh; this process displaces some of the older depot pool vesicles into the reserve pool.

CHOLINERGIC RECEPTORS

After ACh has been released into the synaptic cleft, it binds to one of two classes of receptors, usually on the membrane surface of the postsynaptic cell. **Muscarinic receptors (mAChR)** are seven transmembrane domain G protein-coupled receptors, and **nicotinic receptors (nAChR)** are ligand-gated ion channels. *Although muscarinic receptors are sensitive to the same neurotransmitter as nicotinic recep-*

tors, these two classes of cholinergic receptors share little structural similarity.

Muscarinic Receptors

Muscarinic cholinergic transmission occurs mainly at autonomic ganglia, at end organs innervated by the parasympathetic division of the autonomic nervous system, and in the CNS. Muscarinic receptors belong to the same family as a number of other cell surface receptors (such as the adrenergic receptors) that transduce signals across the cell membrane and interact with GTP-binding proteins. Because all the effects of muscarinic receptor activation occur through the actions of these G proteins, there is a latency of at least 100–250 ms associated with muscarinic responses. (In contrast, nicotinic channels have latencies on the order of 5 ms.)

G protein activation by agonist binding to muscarinic receptors has several effects on the cell. These include inhibition of adenylyl cyclase (via G_i) and stimulation of phospholipase C, both mediated by an α subunit of the G protein. (See Chapter 1, Drug–Receptor Interactions, for a discussion of these signaling mechanisms.) Muscarinic activation also influences ion channels via second messenger molecules. The predominant effect of mAChR stimulation is to increase the opening of specific potassium channels (G protein-modified inwardly rectifying K^+ channels, or GIRKs), thereby hyperpolarizing the cell. This effect is mediated through the $\beta\gamma$ subunit of a G protein (G_o), which binds to the channel and enhances its probability of being open.

Five distinct cDNAs for human muscarinic receptors, denoted M_1–M_5, have been isolated and detected in cells. These receptor types form two functionally distinct groups. M_1, M_3, and M_5 are coupled to G proteins responsible for the stimulation of phospholipase C. M_2 and M_4, on the other hand, are coupled to G proteins responsible for adenylyl cyclase inhibition and K^+ channel activation. The receptors of each functional group can be distinguished based on their

TABLE 8-1	**Characteristics of Cholinergic Receptor Subtypes**					
RECEPTOR	**TYPICAL LOCATIONS**	**RESPONSES**	**MECHANISM**	**PROTOTYPE AGONIST**	**PROTOTYPE ANTAGONIST**
Muscarinic M_1	Autonomic ganglia	Late excitatory postsynaptic potential (EPSP)	$G_{q/11} \rightarrow$ PLC $\rightarrow$ $\uparrow IP_3 + \uparrow$ DAG $\rightarrow$ $\uparrow Ca^{2+} + \uparrow$ PKC	Oxotremorine	Pirenzepine
	CNS	Complex: at least arousal, attention, analgesia			
Muscarinic M_2	Heart: SA node	Slowed spontaneous depolarization; hyperpolarization	$\beta\gamma$ of G-protein $\rightarrow$ inhibit AC and $\uparrow K^+$ channel opening		AF-DX 117
	Heart: AV node	$\downarrow$ conduction velocity			
	Heart: atrium	$\downarrow$ refractory period; $\downarrow$ contractile force			
	Heart: ventricle	Slight $\downarrow$ in contractility			
Muscarinic M_3	Smooth muscle	Contraction	As M_1		Hexahydro-siladifenidol
Muscarinic M_4	CNS		As M_2		Himbacine
Muscarinic M_5	CNS		As M_1		
Nicotinic N_M	Skeletal muscle at neuromuscular junction (NMJ)	End-plate depolarization; skeletal muscle contraction	Opening of Na^+/K^+ channels	Phenyltrimethyl-ammonium	Tubocurare
Nicotinic N_N	Autonomic ganglia	Depolarization and firing of postganglionic neuron	Opening of Na^+/K^+ channels	Dimethylphenyl-piperazinium	Trimethaphan
	Adrenal medulla	Secretion of catecholamines			
	CNS	Complex: at least arousal, attention, analgesia			

Cholinergic receptors are divided into nicotinic and muscarinic receptors. All nicotinic receptors are ligand-gated cation-selective channels, while muscarinic receptors are G protein-linked transmembrane receptors. Specific pharmacologic agonists and antagonists exist for most subclasses, although the majority of these agents are currently used only for experimental purposes.

responses to pharmacologic antagonists (Table 8-1). Generally, M_1 is expressed in cortical neurons and autonomic ganglia, M_2 in cardiac muscle, and M_3 in smooth muscle and glandular tissue. Because stimulation of M_1, M_3, and M_5 receptors facilitates excitation of the cell, while stimulation of M_2 and M_4 receptors suppresses cellular excitability, there is a predictable correlation between the receptor subtype and the effect of ACh on the cell. The various muscarinic receptor subtypes account for much of the diversity in cellular responses to mAChR agonists.

Nicotinic Receptors

Nicotinic cholinergic transmission results from the binding of ACh to the nAChR (Fig. 8-2). This phenomenon is known as *direct ligand-gated conductance*. The simultaneous binding of two ACh molecules to the nAChR elicits a conformational change in the receptor that, in turn, creates a monovalent cation-selective pore through the cell membrane.

Open channels of the activated nAChR are equally permeable to K^+ and Na^+ ions. Therefore, when open, these channels produce a net inward Na^+ current that depolarizes the cell. Stimulation of multiple nAChRs may result in the generation of action potentials and the opening of voltage-dependent calcium channels.

Because ACh dissociates rapidly from active-state receptor molecules and acetylcholinesterase rapidly degrades free (unbound) ACh in the synaptic cleft (see below), the depolarization mediated by nAChRs is brief (<10 ms). Although the simultaneous binding of two ACh molecules is required for channel opening, it is not necessary for both molecules to dissociate for the channel to open again; binding of a second ACh molecule to a receptor that still has one ACh bound may, once again, result in channel opening. The kinetics of nAChR binding and channel opening are detailed in Figure 8-3.

Structurally, the nicotinic acetylcholine receptor comprises five subunits, each of which has a mass of approximately 40 kilodaltons (Fig. 8-2A). Several types of subunits have been identified in the nAChR, designated α, β, γ, δ, and ϵ. All of these subunits share 35% to 50% homology with one another. Each receptor is composed of two α subunits, one β and one δ subunit, and either one γ or one ϵ subunit. (The $\alpha_2\beta\epsilon\delta$ form dominates at the neuromuscular junction in mature skeletal muscle, while the $\alpha_2\beta\gamma\delta$ form is expressed in embryonic muscle.) The α *subunits are responsible for binding ACh*—this is the structural basis for the binding of two ACh molecules to each receptor. The conformational change in the α subunits induced by the binding of ACh is responsible for permitting ion flow through the central pore of the receptor.

Beside simply opening and closing in response to ACh binding, nicotinic receptors also modulate their responses to various concentration profiles of ACh. The receptors react differently to discrete, brief pulses of ACh than to neurotransmitter that is present continuously. As noted above, under normal conditions a closed, resting-state channel responds to dual ACh binding by opening transiently, and the low affinity of the receptor for ACh causes rapid dissociation of ACh from the receptor and resumption of the receptor's resting state configuration. In comparison, continuous exposure of the receptor to ACh causes it to undergo a change to a "desensitized" conformation in which the channel is locked closed. The desensitized state is also characterized

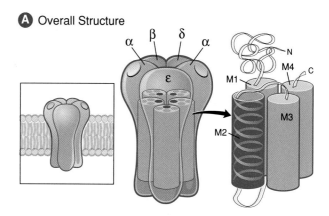

A Overall Structure

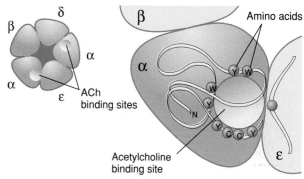

B Acetylcholine Binding Site

C Ion Channel

Figure 8-2. Structural biology of the nicotinic acetylcholine receptor. A. Overall structure of the nicotinic acetycholine receptor (N_M type) and its five subunits ($\alpha_2\beta\epsilon\delta$). Each subunit is composed of a transmembrane protein that has four membrane-spanning (hydrophobic) alpha-helical regions (M1, M2, M3, M4). The large hydrophilic N-terminal domains of the two α subunits contain the binding sites for acetylcholine. **B.** Acetylcholine binding site viewed from above (inset: lower magnification). The labeled amino acids of the α subunit hydrophilic domain are particularly important in binding acetylcholine. The conformational change that results from the binding of two acetylcholine molecules opens the channel. **C.** The M2 domains of the five subunits all face the interior of the protein, and together form the transmembrane channel (inset). Three negatively charged rings of five amino acids (one from each M2 subunit) draw positively charged ions through the channel. At the center, an uncharged leucine ring (gray) participates in closing the ion channel when the receptor becomes desensitized to acetylcholine.

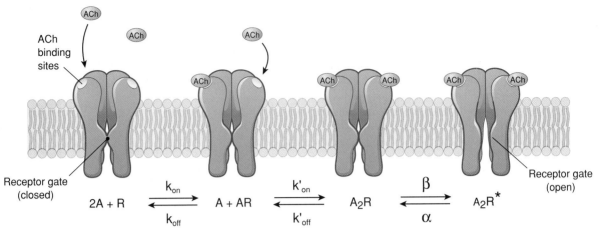

Figure 8-3. Kinetics of nicotinic acetylcholine receptor binding and channel Opening. Each transition between states of receptor binding and channel opening is completely reversible, and it is not necessary to go through all of the possible conformations before returning to a given state. For example, a receptor with two associated ligands may lose one and then gain another to return to its initial state, without the need for both ligands to dissociate. A = ligand (ACh), R = nicotinic ACh receptor (closed), R* = nicotinic ACh receptor (open), k_{on} = rate constant for association (binding) of the first ACh molecule to the receptor, k'_{on} = rate constant for association of the second ACh molecule to the receptor, k_{off} = rate constant for dissociation of the first ACh molecule from the receptor, k'_{off} = rate constant for dissociation of the second ACh molecule from the receptor, β = rate constant of channel opening after both ACh molecules have bound, α = rate constant of channel closure. Note that channel opening and closing are much slower events than binding of ACh to the receptor.

by a greatly increased affinity of the receptor for ACh, so that ACh remains bound to the receptor for a relatively long period of time. This prolonged binding of ACh to the desensitized conformation of the receptor delays the conversion of the receptor to its unstimulated, resting state.

Nicotinic cholinergic receptors at autonomic ganglia and in the central nervous system (termed N_2 or N_N) are similar to receptors at the neuromuscular junction (NMJ) (N_1 or N_M), with the exception that the subunits in N_N receptors are composed solely of α and β subunits. To complicate matters, however, seven different α subunit types (α_2–α_8) and three β subunit types (β_2–β_4) have been detected in neuronal tissues. (α_1 and β_1 refer to the distinct subunit types found at the NMJ.) This diversity of α and β subunit combinations is responsible for the variable responses of CNS and autonomic nAChRs to pharmacologic agents.

DEGRADATION OF ACETYLCHOLINE

In order for acetylcholine to be useful for rapid, repeated neurotransmission, there must exist a mechanism to limit the duration of action of the transmitter. Degradation of ACh is essential not only to prevent unwanted activation of neighboring neurons or muscle cells, but also to ensure proper timing of signaling at the postsynaptic cell. A single receptor molecule is typically capable of distinguishing between two sequential presynaptic release events because degradation of ACh in the synaptic cleft occurs faster than the time course of nAChR activation.

Enzymes collectively known as **cholinesterases** are responsible for degrading acetylcholine. The two types of cholinesterase, **AChE** and **butyrylcholinesterase (BuChE,** also known as pseudocholinesterase or nonspecific cholinesterase), are distributed widely throughout the body. AChE

is indispensable for the degradation of ACh and is capable of hydrolyzing about 4×10^5 molecules of ACh per enzyme molecule per minute; its turnover time of 150 μs makes it one of the most efficient hydrolytic enzymes known. BuChE plays a secondary role in ACh degradation. Recent evidence suggests that BuChE may play a minor role in early neural development as a co-regulator of ACh (it can hydrolyze ACh, but much less efficiently than AChE), and may be involved in the pathogenesis of Alzheimer's disease (AD). Because of its central importance to cholinergic transmission, an entire class of drugs known as acetylcholinesterase inhibitors has been designed to target AChE.

PHYSIOLOGIC EFFECTS OF CHOLINERGIC TRANSMISSION

Neuromuscular Junction

Acetylcholine is the principal neurotransmitter at the neuromuscular junction (Fig. 8-4). The binding of ACh released by α motor neurons to nicotinic receptors in the muscle cell membrane results in motor end-plate depolarization. The extent of depolarization depends on the quantity of ACh released into the synaptic cleft. Release of ACh is quantal in nature; that is, ACh is released in discrete quantities by the presynaptic motor neuron. Each quantum of ACh corresponds to the contents of a single synaptic vesicle and elicits a small depolarization in the motor end-plate termed a **miniature end-plate potential (MEPP).** Under resting conditions, sporadic MEPPs are detected at the motor end-plate, corresponding to a low baseline level of unstimulated ACh release that arises from spontaneous vesicle fusion with the motor axon's presynaptic membrane. In contrast, the arrival of an action potential at the motor axon terminal causes many more vesicles (up to thousands) to fuse with the neuronal membrane and release their ACh. At the motor end-plate, the result is a relatively large depolarization termed the **end-plate potential (EPP)** (Fig. 8-5). The magnitude of the EPP is more than sufficient to trigger a propagating action potential throughout the muscle fiber and, hence, to produce a single contraction or "twitch."

Acetylcholine not only triggers muscle contraction as its primary effect at the NMJ, but also modulates its own action at this site. Presynaptic cholinergic receptors, located on the axon terminal of the motor neuron, respond to ACh binding by *facilitating* the mobilization of synaptic vesicles from the reserve pool to the depot pool. This positive feedback loop, in which the release of ACh stimulates additional release, is necessary to ensure sufficient ACh release under high frequency stimulation of the nerve (approximately 100 Hz). Despite this mechanism, the ACh output per nerve impulse wanes rapidly during persistent high-frequency stimulation. Fortunately, because an excess of ACh is released, and an excess of ACh receptors is present, there is a large safety margin. Only when 50% or more of the postsynaptic receptors are desensitized is a decline in muscle tension observed during tetanic stimulation (a phenomenon known as **tetanic fade**). Importantly, selective blockade of the modulatory presynaptic cholinergic receptors by antagonists such as **hexamethonium** prevents facilitation and causes rapid tetanic fade to occur under otherwise normal conditions (Fig. 8-6).

Autonomic Effects

Neurotransmission through autonomic ganglia is complicated because several distinct receptor types mediate the complex changes in membrane potential observed in postganglionic neurons. The generalized postsynaptic response to presynaptic impulses can be separated into four distinct components (Fig. 8-7). *The primary event in the postsynaptic ganglionic response is a rapid depolarization mediated by nicotinic ACh receptors.* The mechanism is similar to that in the NMJ, in that an inward current elicits a near-immediate **excitatory postsynaptic potential (EPSP)** of 10–50 ms duration. Typically, the amplitude of such an EPSP is only a few millivolts, and many such events must sum for the postsynaptic cell membrane to reach the threshold for firing an action potential (Fig. 8-7A). The three remaining events of ganglionic transmission modulate this primary signal, and are known as the slow EPSP, the IPSP (inhibitory postsynaptic potential), and the late, slow EPSP. The **slow EPSP** occurs after a latency of 1 second and is mediated by M_1 muscarinic ACh receptors. The duration of this effect is 10–30 seconds (Fig. 8-7C). The **IPSP** is largely a product of catecholamine (i.e., dopamine and norepinephrine) stimulation of dopaminergic and α-adrenergic receptors (see Chapter 9, Adrenergic Pharmacology), although some IPSPs in a few ganglia are mediated by M_2 muscarinic receptors. The latency and duration of the IPSP generally vary between those of the fast and slow EPSPs. The **late, slow EPSP** is mediated by a decrease in potassium conductance induced by stimulation of receptors for peptide transmitters (i.e., angiotensin, substance P, and luteinizing hormone-releasing hormone). Lasting for several minutes, the late, slow EPSP is thought

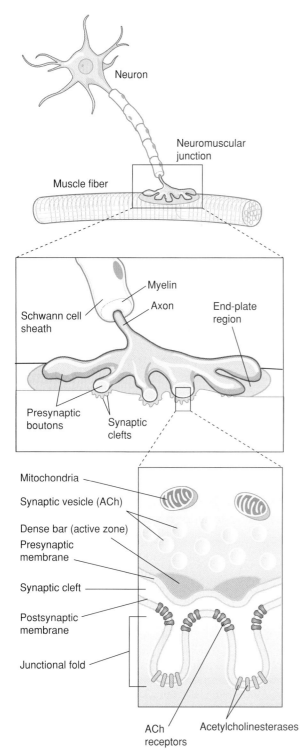

Figure 8-4. The neuromuscular junction (NMJ). At the neuromuscular junction, motor neurons innervate a group of muscle fibers. The area of muscle fibers innervated by an individual motor neuron is referred to as the **end-plate** region. Multiple presynaptic terminals extend from the axon of the motor neuron. When the motor neuron is depolarized, its synaptic vesicles fuse with the presynaptic membrane, releasing ACh into the synaptic cleft. ACh receptors of the neuromuscular junction are exclusively nicotinic, and stimulation of these receptors results in depolarization of the muscle cell membrane and generation of an end-plate potential.

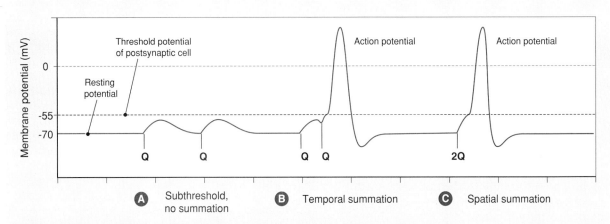

Figure 8-5. Quantal release of acetylcholine and muscle contraction. Muscle contraction relies on the accumulation of a sufficient concentration of acetylcholine at the motor end-plate to depolarize the muscle beyond the threshold potential (typically about −55 mV). After local depolarization occurs, a self-propagating action potential is generated that can spread along the muscle fiber and result in muscle contraction. **A.** As a single cholinergic vesicle releases its contents into the NMJ, a small depolarization (Q), otherwise known as a miniature end-plate potential (MEPP), occurs in the local region of the muscle. This MEPP is insufficient to generate an action potential. When a sufficient number of individual cholinergic vesicles empty their contents into the NMJ, either in quick succession **(B)** or simultaneously **(C),** sufficient depolarization occurs (termed the end-plate potential, or EPP) that the motor end-plate threshold for action potential generation is exceeded, and muscle contraction occurs. An isolated action potential produces a twitch, while a train of action potentials may produce sustained contraction of the muscle. Note that, although this example uses two MEPPs for simplicity, many more than two MEPPs are actually required to achieve threshold-level depolarization. In this figure, the x-axis is time.

to play a role in the long-term regulation of postsynaptic neuron sensitivity to repetitive depolarization.

One pharmacologic consequence of such a complex pattern of depolarization in autonomic ganglia is that drugs selective for the IPSP, slow EPSP, and late, slow EPSP are generally not capable of eliminating ganglionic transmission. Instead, such agents alter only the efficiency of transmission. For example, **methacholine,** a muscarinic receptor agonist, has modulatory effects on autonomic ganglia that resemble the stimulation of slow EPSPs (see below).

The overall effect of ganglionic blockade is complex, and depends on the relative predominance of sympathetic and parasympathetic tone at the various end-organs (Table 8-2). For example, the heart is influenced at rest primarily by the parasympathetic system. Thus, blockade of autonomic ganglia that innervate the heart by moderate to high doses of the antimuscarinic agent **atropine** results in blockade of vagal slowing of the sinoatrial node and hence in relative *tachycardia*. It should be noted that in low doses, the central parasympathetic stimulating effects of atropine predominate, initially resulting in *bradycardia* prior to its peripheral vagolytic action. Blood vessels, in contrast, are innervated only by the sympathetic system. Because the normal effect of sympathetic stimulation is to cause vasoconstriction, ganglionic blockade results in vasodilation. It is important to realize, however, that the responses described above ignore the presence of muscarinic ACh receptors at many of the end organs. When stimulated directly by cholinergic agents, such receptors often mediate a response that overrides the response produced by ganglionic blockade. In general, the expected net cardiovascular effects of muscarinic blockade produced by clinical doses of atropine in a healthy adult with a normal hemodynamic state are mild tachycardia, with or without flushing of the skin, and no profound effect on blood pressure.

The muscarinic receptor subtypes expressed in visceral smooth muscle, cardiac muscle, secretory glands, and endothelial cells mediate highly diverse responses to cholinergic stimulation. These effects are detailed in Table 8-3. In general, these end-organ effects tend to predominate over ganglionic influences. That is, for systemically administered cholinergic agents, the overall response is generally similar to that caused by direct stimulation of these postganglionic effector sites, and often different from that caused by ganglionic stimulation.

CNS Effects

CNS functions of ACh include modulation of sleep, wakefulness, learning, and memory; suppression of pain at the spinal cord level; and essential roles in neural plasticity, early neural development, immunosuppression, and epilepsy. While the past 2 decades have brought greater understanding of the diverse and complex roles of cholinergic neurotransmission, our knowledge remains far from complete, and this remains an active area of basic and translational research.

As part of the ascending **reticular activating system**, cholinergic neurons play an important role in arousal and attention (Fig. 7-8). Levels of ACh throughout the brain increase during wakefulness and REM sleep and decrease during inattentive states and non-REM/slow-wave sleep (SWS). During an awake or aroused state, cholinergic projections from the pedunculopontine nucleus, the lateral tegmental nucleus, and the nucleus basalis of Meynert (NBM) are all active. Because the NBM projects diffusely throughout the cortex and hippocampus (Fig. 7-8), activation of the NBM causes a global increase in ACh levels. Acetylcholine markedly potentiates the excitatory effects of other inputs to its cortical target cells, without affecting the baseline activity

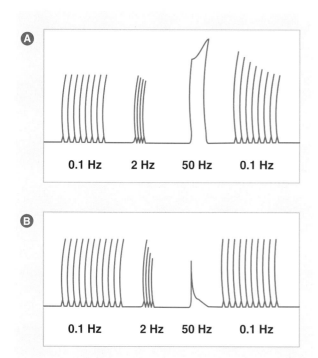

Figure 8-6. Tetanic fade and the effects of hexamethonium.
A. Control stimulation. Rapid stimulation of muscle contraction relies upon presynaptic acetylcholine autoreceptors that provide positive feedback and thereby increase the amount of acetylcholine released with each depolarization. The diagram shows control muscle responses to single shock stimulation (0.1 Hz), a train of four stimulations (2 Hz), or tetanic stimulation (50 Hz). Positive feedback increases the amount of ACh released with each depolarization during tetanic stimulation, providing enhanced muscle contraction that gradually fades back to baseline during subsequent single shock stimulation. **B.** Stimulation after the administration of hexamethonium. Note that, although the response to isolated (0.1 Hz) stimuli is unchanged in the presence of hexamethonium, the drug prevents the increased effect that normally occurs with higher-frequency (50 Hz) stimulation. This is a result of hexamethonium's antagonism of the acetylcholine autoreceptor on the presynaptic terminal that is normally responsible for positive feedback of ACh release.

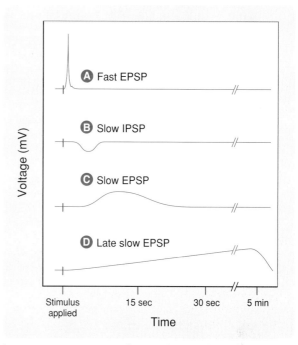

Figure 8-7. Four types of synaptic signals in an autonomic ganglion. The response of autonomic ganglia to neurotransmission is a complex event mediated by a number of different neurotransmitters and receptor types, and occurring on several distinct time scales. **A.** The primary mode of neurotransmission is the action potential, which is produced by a sufficiently strong (suprathreshold) excitatory postsynaptic potential (EPSP). The fast EPSP is mediated by acetylcholine acting on postsynaptic nicotinic ACh receptors. **B.** The slow inhibitory postsynaptic potential (IPSP) is a membrane hyperpolarization response. This response is thought to be mediated by several different postsynaptic receptor types, including modulatory dopamine receptors and α-adrenergic receptors as well as M_2 muscarinic ACh receptors. **C.** The slow EPSP is mediated by M_1 muscarinic receptors, has a latency of about 1 second after an initial depolarization, and lasts for 10–30 seconds. **D.** The late, slow EPSP occurs on the order of minutes after a depolarization event. This excitatory response may be mediated by peptides that are coreleased with acetylcholine.

of these neurons. This primed state is thought to improve the ability of such neurons to process incoming inputs. For the brain as a whole, the result is a heightened state of responsiveness.

The cholinergic link to memory processes is supported by evidence from diverse experimental models. Whereas elevated ACh levels during wakefulness appear to benefit memory encoding processes, consolidation of hippocampus-mediated, episodic, explicit memories benefit from SWS, when ACh levels are at their minimum. By artificially keeping ACh levels elevated during SWS (e.g., by administration of an AChE inhibitor), consolidation of newly acquired explicit learning and episodic memories can be disrupted. Current understanding of the interplay among ACh, sleep, and memory is as follows. During awake states, ACh prevents interference in the hippocampus during initial learning by suppressing retrieval of previously stored memories (to prevent them from interfering with new encoding), but release of this suppression is necessary to allow consolidation of new memories. During sleep (in particular, during SWS),

lower ACh levels are required for proper consolidation of newly acquired memories because stronger excitatory feedback transmission is needed to reactivate memories for consolidation within neocortical brain areas. Therefore, it may useful to remember to sleep, as sleep is needed to remember, or at least to remember better.

The clinical importance of ACh for cognitive function is illustrated by the pathophysiology and treatment of AD and other neurodegenerative dementias, including diffuse Lewy body (DLB) dementia and Parkinson's disease with dementia (PDD). Neurodegenerative dementias and brain injury produce central cholinergic dysfunction. Patients with these conditions manifest cognitive, functional, and behavioral deficits that are at least partially related to cholinergic deficits and amenable to symptomatic treatment with procholinergic medications. An example is the symptomatic treatment of AD with oral acetylcholinesterase inhibitors.

Acetylcholine also plays a role in pain modulation through inhibition of spinal nociceptive transmission. Cholinergic neurons located in the rostral ventromedial medulla extend processes to the superficial lamina of the dorsal horn

TABLE 8-2 **Effects of Autonomic Ganglionic Blockade on Tissues**

SITE	PREDOMINANT TONE	EFFECTS OF GANGLIONIC BLOCKADE
Arterioles	Sympathetic (adrenergic)	Vasodilation; ↑ peripheral blood flow; hypotension
Veins	Sympathetic (adrenergic)	Vasodilation; pooling of blood; ↓ venous return; ↓ cardiac output
Heart	Parasympathetic (cholinergic)	Tachycardia
Iris	Parasympathetic (cholinergic)	Mydriasis (pupil dilation)
Ciliary muscle	Parasympathetic (cholinergic)	Cycloplegia (focused to far vision)
Gastrointestinal tract	Parasympathetic (cholinergic)	↓ Tone and motility; constipation; ↓ secretions
Urinary bladder	Parasympathetic (cholinergic)	Urinary retention
Salivary glands	Parasympathetic (cholinergic)	Xerostomia (dry mouth)
Sweat glands	Sympathetic (cholinergic)	Anhidrosis (absence of sweating)

at all levels of the spinal cord, where secondary neurons in afferent sensory pathways are located. ACh released by the cholinergic neurons is believed to bind to muscarinic ACh receptors located on secondary sensory neurons specific for pain, resulting in suppression of action potential firing in these cells and consequently in analgesia (see Chapter 16). Clinically, the analgesic properties of ACh can be demonstrated by injecting AChE inhibitors into the spinal fluid.

Recent studies suggest that ACh may also have CNS effects unrelated to its role as a neurotransmitter. ACh has

TABLE 8-3 **Effects of Acetylcholine on Muscarinic Receptors in Peripheral Tissues**

TISSUE	EFFECTS OF ACETYLCHOLINE
Vasculature (endothelial cells)	Release of nitric oxide and vasodilation
Eye iris (pupillae sphincter muscle)	Contraction and miosis
Ciliary muscle	Contraction and accommodation of lens to near vision
Salivary and lacrimal glands	Thin and watery secretions
Bronchi	Constriction; ↑ secretions
Heart	Bradycardia, ↓ conduction velocity, AV block at high doses, slight ↓ in contractility
Gastrointestinal tract	↑ Tone, secretions; relaxation of sphincters
Urinary bladder	Contraction of detrusor muscle; relaxation of sphincter
Sweat glands	Diaphoresis
Reproductive tract, male	Erection
Uterus	Variable

been observed to inhibit neurite growth. During the early phases of neural development, when such growth is essential, AChE levels are increased. The presence of ACh in chick limb buds and myotomes suggests other, morphogenetic roles for this compound. Lesioning of rat cholinergic neurons during development results in cortical abnormalities, including aberrant growth and positioning of pyramidal cell dendrites, altered cortical connectivity, and gross cognitive defects. These abnormal findings are observed in the fetal alcohol syndrome and Rett syndrome, both of which demonstrate dramatically reduced numbers of cholinergic neurons in the brain. There is also some evidence for an immunomodulatory role for ACh, as many cells of the immune system both release ACh and possess ACh receptors. Finally, mutations in nicotinic ACh receptor genes responsible for autosomal dominant nocturnal frontal lobe epilepsy (ADNFLE) have been identified; this milestone in epilepsy research is the first demonstration that alterations in a ligand-gated ion channel can cause epilepsy.

PHARMACOLOGIC CLASSES AND AGENTS

Pharmacologic manipulation of ACh metabolism has met with only limited success because the complex actions of ACh make it difficult to obtain selective effects. For example, many cholinergic agents are capable of both stimulating and blocking cholinergic receptors through a process known as depolarizing blockade (see below). Therefore, only a relatively small fraction of the many cholinergic and anticholinergic agents discovered over the past century are used in clinical practice. These drugs are used primarily for (1) modulation of gastrointestinal motility, (2) xerostomia (dry mouth), (3) glaucoma, (4) motion sickness and anti-emesis,

(5) neuromuscular diseases such as myasthenia gravis and Eaton–Lambert syndrome, (6) acute neuromuscular blockade and reversal, (7) ganglionic blockade during aortic dissection, (8) dystonias (e.g., torticollis), headache, and pain syndromes, (9) reversal of vagal-mediated bradycardia, (10) mydriasis, (11) bronchodilators in chronic obstructive pulmonary disease, (12) bladder spasms and urinary incontinence, (13) cosmetic effects on skin lines and wrinkles, and (14) treatment of symptoms of Alzheimer's disease, cognitive dysfunction, and dementia.

Slight variations in the pharmacologic properties of individual cholinergic and anticholinergic agents are responsible for their large differences in therapeutic utility. The relative selectivity of action of the most useful agents depends on both pharmacodynamic and pharmacokinetic factors, including inherent differences in receptor binding affinity, bioavailability, tissue localization, and resistance to degradation. These variations, in turn, derive from the molecular structure and charge of the drug. The structure of **pirenzepine,** for example, allows the drug to bind M_1 muscarinic receptors (located in autonomic ganglia) with higher affinity than M_2 and M_3 receptors (located at parasympathetic end organs). As a result, the drug's predominant effect at clinically used doses is ganglionic blockade (see Table 8-1). Similarly, the addition of a methyl group to acetylcholine yields **methacholine,** which is more resistant to degradation by AChE and, hence, possesses a longer duration of action. Charged agents such as muscarine generally do not cross membrane barriers. The absorption of such drugs through both the gastrointestinal (GI) mucosa and the blood–brain barrier is significantly impaired, unless specific carriers are available to transport the drug; therefore, such drugs typically have little or no effect on the CNS. In contrast, lipophilic agents have excellent CNS penetration. As one example, the high CNS penetration of **physostigmine** makes this drug the agent of choice for treating the CNS effects of anticholinergic overdose.

The following discussion is ordered mechanistically. For each class of drugs, the selectivity of individual agents within the class is used as a basis to explain the therapeutic uses of each agent.

INHIBITORS OF ACETYLCHOLINE SYNTHESIS, STORAGE, AND RELEASE

Drugs that inhibit the synthesis, storage, or release of ACh have only recently begun to have clinical use (Fig. 8-1). **Hemicholinium-3** blocks the high-affinity transporter for choline, and thus prevents the uptake of choline required for ACh synthesis. **Vesamicol** blocks the ACh-H$^+$ antiporter that is used to transport ACh into vesicles, thereby preventing the storage of ACh. Both of these compounds are utilized only in research settings, however. **Botulinum toxin,** produced by *Clostridium botulinum,* degrades synaptobrevin and thus prevents synaptic vesicle fusion with the axon terminal (presynaptic) membrane. This paralysis-inducing property is currently used in the treatment of several diseases associated with increased muscle tone, such as torticollis, achalasia, strabismus, blepharospasm, and other focal dystonias. Botulinum toxin has also recently been approved for cosmetic treatment of facial lines or wrinkles, and is being

increasingly used to treat various headache and pain syndromes.

ACETYLCHOLINESTERASE INHIBITORS

Agents in this class bind to and inhibit AChE, thereby elevating the concentration of endogenously released ACh in the synaptic cleft. The accumulated ACh subsequently activates nearby cholinergic receptors. Agents in this class are also referred to as *indirectly acting* ACh receptor agonists because they generally do not activate receptors directly. It is important to note that a few AChE inhibitors have a direct action as well. For example, **neostigmine,** a quaternary carbamate, not only blocks AChE but also binds to and activates nAChRs at the neuromuscular junction.

Structural Classes

All indirectly acting cholinergic agonists interfere with the function of AChE by binding to the active site of the enzyme. There are three chemical classes of such agents, including (1) simple alcohols with a quaternary ammonium group, (2) carbamic acid esters of alcohols bearing either quaternary or tertiary ammonium groups, and (3) organic derivatives of phosphoric acid (Fig. 8-8). The most important functional difference among these classes is pharmacokinetic.

Edrophonium is a simple alcohol that inhibits AChE by reversibly associating with the active site of the enzyme. Because of the noncovalent nature of the interaction between the alcohol and AChE, the enzyme–inhibitor complex lasts for only 2–10 minutes, resulting in a relatively rapid but completely reversible block.

The carbamic acid esters **neostigmine** and **physostigmine** are hydrolyzed by AChE, so a labile covalent bond is formed between the drug and the enzyme. However, *the rate at which this reaction occurs is many orders of magnitude slower than for ACh.* The resulting enzyme–inhibitor complex has a half-life of approximately 15–30 minutes, corresponding to an effective inhibition lasting 3–8 hours.

Organophosphates such as **diisopropyl fluorophosphate** have a molecular structure that resembles the transition state formed in carboxyl ester hydrolysis. These compounds are hydrolyzed by AChE, but the resulting phosphorylated enzyme complex is extremely stable and dissociates with a half-life of hundreds of hours. Furthermore, the enzyme–organophosphate complex is subject to a process known as **aging,** in which oxygen–phosphorus bonds within the inhibitor are broken spontaneously in favor of stronger bonds between the enzyme and the inhibitor. Once aging occurs, the duration of AChE inhibition is increased even further. Thus, organophosphate inhibition is essentially irreversible, and the body must synthesize new AChE molecules to restore AChE activity. However, if strong nucleophiles (such as **pralidoxime**) are administered before aging has occurred, it is possible to recover enzymatic function from the inhibited AChE.

Clinical Applications

Acetylcholinesterase inhibitors have a number of clinical applications, including (1) increasing transmission at the

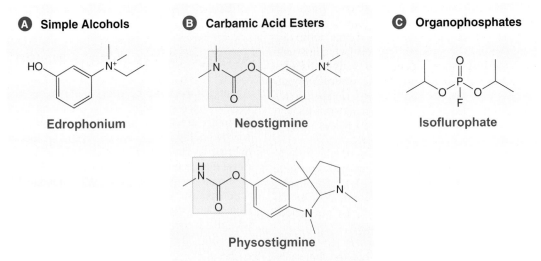

Figure 8-8.   Structural Classes of Acetylcholinesterase Inhibitors. Acetylcholinesterase (AChE) inhibitors are divided into three structural classes. **A.** Simple alcohols such as edrophonium have a short half-time of AChE inhibition. Edrophonium is used in the diagnosis of myasthenia gravis and other diseases of the neuromuscular junction. **B.** Carbamic acid esters are hydrolyzed by AChE. This results in the formation of a covalent bond between the carbamic acid ester (boxed) and AChE, and a consequently long half-time of AChE inhibition. Neostigmine is used to treat myasthenia gravis and, during or after surgery, to reverse paralysis induced by nicotinic acetylcholine receptor antagonists. Physostigmine, because it has good CNS penetration, is the agent of choice for treating anticholinergic poisoning. **C.** Organophosphates form an extremely stable phosphorus-carbon bond with AChE. This results in irreversible inactivation of AChE. As a result, many organophosphates are extremely toxic.

neuromuscular junction, (2) increasing parasympathetic tone, and (3) increasing central cholinergic activity (e.g., to treat symptoms of AD).

Because of their ability to increase the activity of endogenous ACh, AChEs are especially useful in diseases of the neuromuscular junction, where the primary defect is an insufficient quantity of either ACh or AChR. In myasthenia gravis, autoantibodies are generated against N_M receptors. These antibodies both induce N_M receptor internalization and block the ability of ACh to activate the receptors. As a result, patients with myasthenia gravis present with significant weakness (recall the description of Chief Opechancanough in the introductory case). Eaton–Lambert syndrome is also characterized by muscle weakness, but this disorder is caused by autoantibodies generated against Ca^{2+} channels; both presynaptic Ca^{2+} entry and the subsequent release of ACh in response to axon terminal depolarization are attenuated. Certain anticholinergic drugs (such as tubocurare) also cause weakness, or even paralysis, by acting as competitive antagonists at the nAChR. Acetylcholinesterase inhibitors (such as the physostigmine used in the introductory case) improve all three of these conditions by increasing the concentration of endogenously released ACh at the neuromuscular junction and thereby increasing ACh signaling.

Because the binding of ACh to N_M receptors results in muscle cell depolarization, *AChE inhibitors are ineffective at reversing the action of agents that cause paralysis by inducing sustained depolarization, such as succinylcholine* (see below). In fact, AChEs in sufficiently high doses can exacerbate existing weakness and paralysis because of depolarizing blockade. Thus, it is of fundamental importance that the cause of the muscle weakness should be determined before treatment is initiated. Short-acting AChEs such as edrophonium are ideal for such diagnostic purposes. **Edropho-**

nium will mitigate weakness if the blockade is attributable to competitive AChR antagonists or to diseases such as myasthenia gravis or Eaton–Lambert syndrome. In contrast, if muscle strength decreases further with edrophonium administration, then depolarizing blockade may be suspected. The short half-life of edrophonium ensures that exacerbation of the latter condition will last for a minimal amount of time. For chronic treatment of myasthenia gravis, longer-acting AChEs such as **pyridostigmine, neostigmine,** and **ambenonium** are the preferred agents.

AChE inhibitors mediate other therapeutic effects by potentiating parasympathetic actions in target tissues. Topical application of AChEs to the cornea of the eye decreases intraocular pressure by facilitating the outflow of aqueous humor. The main effect of AChE inhibitors on the GI system is an increase in smooth muscle motility because of enhancement of ganglionic transmission at Auerbach's plexus, although these agents also cause increased secretion of gastric acid and saliva. Neostigmine, the most popular drug for this application, is typically used for relief of abdominal distention. The use of anticholinesterases in reversing anticholinergic drug poisoning is also well established. The agent of choice for this indication is typically **physostigmine;** its tertiary amine structure allows it ready access to the brain and spinal cord, where it can counteract the CNS effects of anticholinergic toxicity.

Oral AChE inhibitors are also used to treat the symptoms of AD and other conditions that produce cognitive dysfunction and dementia. **Tacrine, donepezil, rivastigmine,** and **galantamine** are approved for the treatment of mild to moderate AD but have been shown to produce only modest symptomatic benefits in slowing the progression of cognitive, functional, and behavioral deficits. There are some mechanistic and pharmacokinetic differences among these

TABLE 8-4	Pharmacokinetic and Mechanistic Characteristics of Donepezil, Rivastigmine, and Galantamine					
DRUG	BIOAVAILABILITY (%)	t_{max} (h)	ELIMINATION HALF-LIFE (h)	HEPATIC METABOLISM	REVERSIBLE INHIBITION OF AChE	OTHER CHOLINOMIMETIC EFFECTS
Donepezil	100	3–5	60–90	Yes	Yes	
Rivastigmine	40	0.8–1.8	2	No	No*	BuChEI
Galantamine	85–100	0.5–1.5	5–8	Yes	Yes	nAChR agonist

t_{max} = time to maximum plasma concentration; * Rivastigmine is a "pseudo-irreversible" inhibitor of AChE and BuChE; AChE = acetylcholinesterase; BuChEI = butyrylcholinesterase inhibitor; nAChR agonist = non-potentiating ligand of the nicotinic receptor.

drugs (Table 8-4). For example, rivastigmine is a "pseudo-irreversible" cholinesterase inhibitor because it forms a temporary covalent bond with AChE, inactivating it until the covalent bond is broken. Rivastigmine affects both AChE and BuChE by forming a carbamoylate complex with the enzymes. Galantamine, in addition to being a reversible AChE inhibitor, also acts as a non-potentiating ligand of nicotinic receptors. All drugs exhibit linear kinetics and their t_{max} values and elimination half-lives are prolonged in elderly patients.

With slow and careful titration, these medications are generally tolerated well and have a favorable adverse effect profile (with the exception of tacrine, which is now rarely used due to reports of hepatotoxicity). While these medications are somewhat selective for CNS AChE, the most common adverse effects — including nausea, vomiting, anorexia, flatulence, loose stools, diarrhea, and abdominal cramping — are related to peripheral cholinomimetic effects on the GI tract. These adverse effects may occur in 5% to 20% of patients, are usually mild and transient, are related to the dose and rate of dose escalation, and can be minimized by administering the drug after a meal. Use of these agents is contraindicated in patients with unstable or severe cardiac disease, uncontrolled epilepsy, or active peptic ulcer disease.

RECEPTOR AGONISTS

All cholinergic receptor agonists bind to the ACh binding site of cholinergic receptors. Receptor agonists can be divided into muscarinic and nicotinic receptor-selective agents, although some cross-reactivity exists with virtually all of these agents. Muscarinic receptor agonists are used clinically in the diagnosis of asthma and as miotics (agents that cause pupil constriction). Nicotinic receptor agonists are used clinically for induction of muscle paralysis.

Muscarinic Receptor Agonists

Agents in this class are divided structurally into choline esters and alkaloids (Fig. 8-9). The choline esters are charged, highly hydrophilic molecules that are poorly absorbed by the oral route and inefficiently distributed to the CNS. Choline esters include acetylcholine, methacholine, carbachol, and bethanechol (Table 8-5). Acetylcholine is not administered in clinical settings because of its broad actions and its extremely rapid hydrolysis by AChE and pseudocholinesterase.

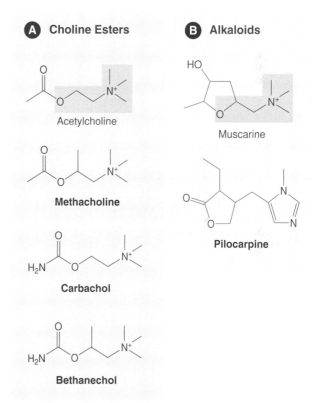

Figure 8-9. Structural Classes of Muscarinic Receptor Agonists. Muscarinic receptor agonists are divided into choline esters and alkaloids. **A.** Choline esters are all charged molecules and therefore have little CNS penetration. Methacholine is highly resistant to AChE and is used in the diagnosis of asthma. Carbachol has both nicotinic and muscarinic receptor activity; it is only used topically for treatment of glaucoma. Bethanechol is highly selective for muscarinic receptors; it is used to promote GI and bladder motility. Shown in blue are groups in the drug molecules that differ from acetylcholine. **B.** Alkaloids have highly variable structures; some have excellent CNS penetration. Muscarine, the prototypical muscarinic receptor agonist, is an alkaloid that is structurally similar to acetylcholine (boxed areas). Until recently, pilocarpine was the only alkaloid muscarinic receptor agonist used clinically. It is used to treat xerostomia (dry mouth) in patients with Sjogren's syndrome and post-radiation syndromes. Cevimeline, an M_1 and M_3 agonist, is also effective in xerostomia related to Sjogren's syndrome (not shown).

| TABLE 8-5 | Relative Pharmacologic Properties of Choline Esters |

ESTER	SUSCEPTIBILITY TO AChE	CARDIAC ACTIVITY	GI ACTIVITY	URINARY ACTIVITY	EYE ACTIVITY (TOPICAL)	ATROPINE ANTAGONISM	NICOTINIC ACTIVITY
Acetylcholine	+ + +	+ +	+ +	+ +	+	+ + +	+ +
Methacholine	+	+ + +	+ +	+ +	+	+ + +	+
Carbachol	−	+	+ + +	+ + +	+ +	+	+ + +
Bethanechol	−	±	+ + +	+ + +	+ +	+ + +	−

Note that all actions are mediated by muscarinic receptors, with the exception of nicotinic activity. " − ": negligible activity. " ± ": unpredictable.

Methacholine is at least three times more resistant to hydrolysis by AChE than is ACh. This agent is relatively selective for cardiovascular muscarinic cholinergic receptors, and it possesses relatively little affinity for nicotinic cholinergic receptors. Although methacholine can stimulate receptors expressed on cardiovascular tissue, the magnitude of its response is unpredictable. This fact has limited its use as a vasodilator or cardiac **vagomimetic** (i.e., a drug that mimics the cardiac response to vagus nerve [parasympathetic] stimulation, which typically involves bradycardia, decreased contractility, and compensatory sympathetic reflexes). Currently, methacholine is used only in the diagnosis of asthma; in this application, the bronchial hyperreactivity that is characteristic of asthma causes an exaggerated bronchoconstriction response to parasympathomimetics (see Chapter 46).

Both carbachol and bethanechol are resistant to cholinesterases because, in these drugs, a carbamoyl group is substituted for the acetyl group of ACh (Fig. 8-9). This resistance to AChE extends their duration of action and allows time for distribution to areas of lower blood flow. **Carbachol** has enhanced nicotinic action relative to other choline esters. This agent cannot be used systemically because its nicotinic action at autonomic ganglia leads to unpredictable responses. Instead, the agent is used principally as a topical miotic agent, typically in the treatment of glaucoma. Local application of the drug to the cornea of the eye results in both pupillary constriction (miosis) and decreased intraocular pressure.

Bethanechol is almost completely selective for muscarinic receptors. It is an agent of choice for promoting GI and urinary tract motility, particularly for post-operative, post-partum, and drug-related urinary retention and for hypotonic neurogenic bladder.

In contrast to the choline esters, the alkaloids vary greatly in structure. Some are amphipathic while others are highly charged. Most of these agents are tertiary amines, although a few are quaternary amines with protonated or permanently charged nitrogens substituting for the choline-centered N of ACh. The amphipathic nature of the tertiary amine alkaloids permits absorption through the GI mucosa and penetration into the CNS. **Muscarine** is an example of a quaternary amine alkaloid that has poorer bioavailability because of its permanently charged nature.

Most alkaloids are primarily of value in pharmacologic research. The most clinically used alkaloid is **pilocarpine,** a miotic agent and a sialagogue (saliva-inducing agent) used to treat xerostomia (dryness of the mouth secondary to reduced salivary secretion). **Cevimeline**, an M1 and M3 agonist, is used to treat xerostomia in Sjogren's syndrome.

Nicotinic Receptor Agonists

Succinylcholine is a choline ester that has a high affinity for nicotinic receptors and is resistant to AChE. It is used to induce paralysis during surgery by means of **depolarizing blockade.** This effect can be caused by any direct nAChR *agonist* because such drugs activate cholinergic channels and produce depolarization of the cell membrane. To produce depolarizing blockade, the agent must persist at the neuroeffector junction and activate the nicotinic receptor channels continuously. (Note that this effect is unlike the depolarization pattern seen in the generation of a standard action potential or end-plate potential, in which ACh is present at the neuroeffector junction for only a brief period of time.) The result is a brief period of excitation, manifested by widespread fasciculations in muscle cells, followed by flaccid paralysis. The paralysis occurs because the open cholinergic channels maintain the cell membrane in a depolarized condition, effecting inactivation of voltage-gated sodium channels so that they cannot open to support further action potentials. Because of this mechanism, *any nAChR agonist, including ACh, is capable of producing depolarizing blockade at sufficiently high concentrations.* Generally, depolarizing blockade with succinylcholine is used for only short durations because prolonged depolarization can lead to life-threatening electrolyte imbalances (caused by prolonged Na^+ influx and K^+ efflux). Table 8-6 compares the effects of depolarizing and nondepolarizing NMJ-blocking agents.

The concept of depolarizing blockade pertains to *all* cholinergic receptors, and is *not strictly limited to the NMJ.* For example, this mechanism accounts for the paradoxical suppression of parasympathomimetic activity at autonomic ganglia by high levels of agonists, such as nicotine, that are selective for nicotinic receptors. The potential for inducing depolarizing blockade is partially responsible for the unpredictable effects of nAChR agonists. Although muscarinic receptor agonists can also cause depolarizing blockade at autonomic ganglia, this effect is obscured by the overwhelmingly parasympathomimetic responses seen at other neuroeffector sites.

RECEPTOR ANTAGONISTS

Antagonists of AChRs act by binding directly to the agonist site and competitively blocking stimulation of the receptor by endogenous ACh or exogenously administered receptor agonists.

TABLE 8-6	Comparison of Nondepolarizing and Depolarizing NMJ-Blocking Agents	
EFFECT	NONDEPOLARIZING	DEPOLARIZING
Effect of previous administration of a competitive NMJ-blocking agent	Additive	Antagonistic effect
Effect of previous administration of a depolarizing NMJ-blocking agent	No effect or antagonistic	No effect or additive
Effect on motor end-plate	Elevated activation threshold to ACh; no depolarization	Partial; persisting depolarization
Initial excitatory effect on muscle	None	Transient fasciculations
Muscle response to tetanic stimulation during partial block	Poorly sustained contraction	Well-sustained contraction

Muscarinic Receptor Antagonists

Anticholinergic compounds that act on muscarinic receptors are used to produce a parasympatholytic effect in target organs. By blocking normal cholinergic tone, these compounds allow sympathetic responses to predominate (Table 8-2). The most commonly encountered anticholinergics are either naturally occurring alkaloids or synthetic quaternary ammonium compounds. The alkaloids are relatively selective for antagonist activity at muscarinic receptors, whereas the synthetic compounds also demonstrate significant antagonism at nicotinic receptors.

The prototypical muscarinic receptor antagonist is **atropine,** a naturally occurring alkaloid found in the plant *Atropa belladonna*, or deadly nightshade. Belladonna derived its name from Italian for ''beautiful woman''—during the Renaissance, women in Italy ingested or applied extracts and juices of berries from the plant to their eyes to cause dilation of the pupils, which was considered a mark of beauty. Atropine is used clinically to induce mydriasis (pupil dilation) for ophthalmologic examinations, to reverse symptomatic sinus bradycardia, to inhibit excessive salivation and mucus secretion during surgery, to prevent vagal reflexes induced by surgical trauma of visceral organs, and to counteract the effects of muscarine poisoning from certain mushrooms. Because of its marginal activity at nicotinic receptors, extremely high doses of atropine are required for any effects to be seen at the NMJ. Similarly, because nicotinic receptors are primarily responsible for excitatory transmission at autonomic ganglia, atropine produces partial block at these sites only at relatively high doses.

Scopolamine (hyoscine hydrobromide), a tertiary amine, differs from atropine by virtue of its significant CNS effects. Scopolamine is frequently used for the prevention and treatment of motion sickness. To effect slow absorption and long duration of the anti-motion sickness effect while avoiding a rapid rise in plasma levels and undesirable CNS side effects (e.g., anterograde disruption of novel learning and memory encoding, inattention, and slowing of psychomotor speed), a transdermal patch system has been developed. Scopolamine can also be used to ameliorate nausea, particularly that associated with chemotherapy, and can be given intravenously during procedures in which minimizing oral secretions is desirable.

Methscopolamine and **glycopyrrolate** are quaternary amine antimuscarinics with low CNS penetration that are used for their peripheral effects to decrease oral secretions, treat peptic ulcer disease, decrease GI spasms, and, in the case of glycopyrrolate, prevent bradycardia during surgical procedures. Both drugs have delayed but measurable CNS and cognitive anticholinergic effects. **Pirenzepine,** which is selective for M_1 and M_4 receptors, is an alternative to H_2-receptor antagonists in the treatment of peptic ulcers (see Chapter 45).

Ipratropium, a synthetic quaternary ammonium compound, is more effective than β-adrenergic agonists in the treatment of chronic obstructive pulmonary disease, but less effective in treating asthma (see Chapter 46). **Tiotropium** has recently been shown to have similar, and possibly superior, efficacy to ipratropium as a bronchodilator in the treatment of chronic obstructive pulmonary disease.

A number of antimuscarinic medications are used for the treatment of urinary incontinence and overactive bladder syndrome. Muscarinic stimulation promotes voiding by promoting (1) detrusor muscle contraction, and (2) bladder trigone and sphincter muscle relaxation. Antimuscarinics produce the opposite effects by promoting detrusor relaxation and tightening of the bladder sphincter, and thereby causing urinary retention. Currently approved antimuscarinics used in the treatment of overactive bladder include **oxybutynin, propantheline, terodiline, tolterodine, trospium, darifenacin,** and **solifenacin.** Among these agents, oxybutynin, propantheline, tolterodine, and trospium are nonspecific muscarinic receptor antagonists, whereas darifenacin and solifenacin are selective M_3 receptor antagonists. Each of these agents appears to have similar clinical efficacy. Clinical trials have suggested that tolterodine may cause less dry mouth than oxybutynin, and that the newer M_3-selective agents solifenacin and darifenacin may cause less dry mouth and constipation than the nonselective agents.

Antimuscarinic medications are contraindicated in patients with glaucoma, particularly in angle-closure glaucoma, which may be precipitated in patients with shallow

---

BOX 8-1.   Potential Adverse Effects of Drugs with Anticholinergic Properties in Geriatric and Cognitively Impaired Patients

Drug-related anticholinergic adverse effects are potentially hazardous to elderly patients, especially those with cognitive impairment, and cause significant morbidity in this population. Additive anticholinergic effects from medications can compromise the safety of geriatric patients because (1) many common drugs possess at least a small measure of anticholinergic activity; (2) the elderly, and especially the cognitively impaired elderly, are exquisitely sensitive to cholinergic blockade (due to central cholinergic hypofunction and dysfunction in aging and dementia, respectively); and (3) polypharmacy is a common practice in the geriatric population. Adverse effects from anticholinergic drugs in the elderly may include acute encephalopathy (delirium, confusional state), falls, urinary retention, constipation, and exacerbation and decompensation of underlying cognitive, functional, and behavioral deficits (particularly in patients with dementia), and may necessitate increased care and hospitalization. It should be noted that many over-the-counter medications have anticholinergic effects. For example, a common offender in causing confusion and cognitive dysfunction in the elderly and cognitively impaired individuals is **diphenhydramine**, a common antihistamine with anticholinergic properties, which is often also used as a hypnotic either alone or in combination with acetaminophen. Clinicians and pharmacists should be vigilant to minimize polypharmacy in the geriatric population and to monitor for and prevent medication-related anticholinergic adverse events.

---

anterior chambers. Antimuscarinics should also be used with caution in patients with prostatic hypertrophy and in the elderly (see Box 8-1). Depending on the dose, antimuscarinic agents such as atropine and scopolamine may cause bradycardia and sedation at low-to-medium levels of muscarinic blockade, and tachycardia and CNS hyperexcitation with delirium, hallucinations, and seizures at higher levels of blockade. Other adverse effects are predictable, and may include blurred vision (cycloplegia and mydriasis), dry mouth, ileus, urinary retention, flushing and fever, agitation, and tachycardia.

Nicotinic Receptor Antagonists

Selective nicotinic receptor antagonists are used primarily to produce **nondepolarizing (competitive) neuromuscular blockade** during surgical procedures. Non-depolarizing NMJ blocking agents act by antagonizing nicotinic ACh receptors directly, thus preventing endogenous ACh binding and subsequent muscle cell depolarization. This leads to a flaccid paralysis similar in presentation to that of myasthenia gravis. The primary consideration used in selecting a specific agent is its duration of action, from the very long-lasting agents (**d-tubocurarine, pancuronium**) to those in the intermediate range (**vecuronium, rocuronium**) to the rapidly degraded compounds (**mivacurium**). Because nicotinic receptors are expressed in autonomic ganglia as well as the NMJ, nondepolarizing blocking agents often have variable adverse effects associated with ganglionic blockade. These effects, as with the muscular paralysis, can be reversed by administration of AChE inhibitors.

Compounds with relatively selective antagonist activity at nAChRs are also used to induce autonomic blockade. The general effects of autonomic ganglionic blockade are discussed above and are listed in Table 8-2. Most commonly, **mecamylamine** and **trimethaphan** are administered when ganglionic blockade is desired. The only current use for these agents is in the treatment of hypertension in patients with acute aortic dissection, because the drugs lower blood pressure while simultaneously blunting the sympathetic reflexes that would normally cause a deleterious rise in pressure at the site of the tear.

Conclusion and Future Directions

There are two major classes of cholinergic receptors — nicotinic and muscarinic. Nicotinic receptors are ligand-gated channels that require the direct binding of two acetylcholine molecules to open. These receptors comprise all of the cholinergic receptors at the neuromuscular junction (N_M), and they predominate at the autonomic ganglia (N_N). Thus, the primary cholinergic functions mediated by the nAChR include skeletal muscle contraction and autonomic activity. The predominant applications of pharmacologic agents directed at nAChRs are (1) neuromuscular blockade through competitive antagonists and depolarizing blockers, and (2) ganglionic blockade resulting in effector organ responses that are opposite to those produced by normal autonomic tone.

Muscarinic receptors are G protein-coupled receptors that bind acetylcholine and initiate signaling through several intracellular pathways. These receptors are expressed in the autonomic ganglia and effector organs, where they mediate a parasympathetic response. The primary uses of muscarinic receptor agonists and antagonists are to modulate autonomic responses of effector organs. Both nicotinic and muscarinic receptors are ubiquitous in the CNS, where the effects of acetylcholine include analgesia, arousal, and attention. Because the relative roles of mAChRs and nAChRs in the brain and spinal cord are not fully understood, the most effective currently available CNS drugs increase endogenous cholinergic transmission by inhibiting the action of acetylcholinesterase, the enzyme that hydrolyzes ACh.

Although cholinergic pharmacology is a relatively mature field with a number of receptor-selective agents, the specificity of action of the various agents continues to be refined. The discovery of muscarinic receptor subtype diversity may lead to the development of agents specific for subtypes that are expressed in a tissue-specific pattern. Similarly, elucidation of the role of nicotinic receptor subunit diversity in the CNS may spur the development of more selective agents that modulate the activity of these receptor subtypes. Acetylcholinesterase inhibitors are now widely used in clinical practice and are standard of care in the treatment of AD and other dementias. While these medications provide modest symptomatic benefits, nicotinic and muscarinic agonists are in clinical development for the treatment of AD. Nicotinic receptors may also provide targets for future treatment approaches in epilepsy.

 ## *Suggested Reading*

Andersson KE. Antimuscarinics for treatment of overactive bladder. *Lancet Neurol* 2004;3:46–53. *(Review of overactive bladder pathophysiology and pharmacology.)*

Atri A, Sherman S, Norman KA, et al. Blockade of central cholinergic receptors impairs new learning and increases proactive interference in a word paired-associate memory task. *Behav Neurosci* 2004;118:223–236. *(Reviews the theoretic and experimental basis of cholinergic influences on learning and memory, and the effects of central blockade on cognitive processes.)*

Bartus RT. On neurodegenerative diseases, models, and treatment strategies: Lessons learned and lessons forgotten a generation following the cholinergic hypothesis. *Exp Neurol* 2000;163: 495–529. *(Reviews basis for the cholinergic hypothesis of cognitive aging and dementia.)*

Bertrand D, Elmslie F, Hughes E, et al. The CHRNB2 mutation I312M is associated with epilepsy and distinct memory deficits. *Neurobiol Dis* 2005;20:799–804. *(Reviews role of alterations in nicotinic ACh receptors in genetic epilepsy.)*

Darvesh S, Hopkins DA, Geula C. Neurobiology of butyrylcholinesterase. *Nat Rev Neurosci* 2003;4:131–138. *(Discusses characteristics and functions of butyrylcholinesterase in the nervous system.)*

Jann MW, Shirly KL, Small GW. Clinical pharmacokinetics and pharmacodynamics of cholinesterase inhibitors. *Clin Pharmacokinet* 2002;41:719–739. *(Review of clinical pharmacology of oral cholinesterase inhibitors.)*

Sabbagh MN, Farlow MR, Relkin N, et al. Do cholinergic therapies have disease-modifying effects in Alzheimer's disease? *Alzheimer's & Dementia* 2006;2:118–125. *(Review of clinical evidence for symptomatic and disease-modifying treatment effects of oral acetylcholinesterase inhibitors in Alzheimer's disease.)*

Drug Summary Table   Chapter 8 Cholinergic Pharmacology

INHIBITORS OF ACETYLCHOLINE SYNTHESIS, STORAGE, AND RELEASE
Mechanism—Inhibit the synthesis, storage, or release of acetylcholine

Drug	Clinical Applications	*Serious* and Common Adverse Effects	Contraindications	Therapeutic Considerations
Hemicholinium-3 Vesamicol	None (used experimentally only)	Not applicable		Hemicholinium-3 blocks the high-affinity transporter for choline and thereby prevents the uptake of choline required for ACh synthesis. Vesamicol blocks the ACh-H$^+$ antiporter that is used to transport ACh into vesicles. Both of these compounds are utilized only in research settings
Botulinum toxin	Focal dystonias Torticollis Achalasia Strabismus Blepharospasm Pain syndromes Wrinkles Hyperhidrosis	*Cardiac arrhythmia, syncope, hepatotoxicity, anaphylaxis* Injection-site pain, dyspepsia, dysphagia, muscle weakness, neck pain, eyelid ptosis, fever	Hypersensitivity to botulinum toxin Infection at the proposed injection site	Botulinum toxin, produced by *Clostridium botulinum*, degrades synaptobrevin and thus prevents synaptic vesicle fusion with the axon terminal (presynaptic) membrane

INHIBITORS OF ACETYLCHOLINE DEGRADATION
Mechanism—Inhibit acetylcholinesterase (AChE) by binding to the enzyme's active site

Drug	Clinical Applications	*Serious* and Common Adverse Effects	Contraindications	Therapeutic Considerations
Edrophonium Neostigmine Pyridostigmine Ambenonium Physostigmine	Diagnosis of myasthenia gravis, Eaton-Lambert syndrome, and disorders resulting in muscle weakness (edrophonium) Urinary or gastrointestinal motility agent, glaucoma, neuromuscular junction diseases such as myasthenia gravis (neostigmine, pyridostigmine, ambenonium) Reversal of anticholinergic toxicity or induced paralysis in surgery (physostigmine)	*Seizure, bronchospasm, cardiac arrhythmia, bradycardia, cardiac arrest* Hypotension or hypertension, salivation, lacrimation, diaphoresis, vomiting, diarrhea, miosis	Mechanical intestinal or urinary obstruction Concomitant choline ester or depolarizing neuromuscular blocker use Cardiovascular disease	Edrophonium is short-acting (2–10 minutes); rapid onset of action makes edrophonium useful for diagnosis of muscle weakness For chronic treatment of myasthenia gravis, longer-acting cholinesterase inhibitors such as pyridostigmine, neostigmine, and ambenonium are preferred Neostigmine also has direct cholinergic agonist effect at N$_M$ receptors Topical application of cholinesterase inhibitors to the cornea of the eye decreases intraocular pressure by facilitating the outflow of aqueous humor Non-polar structure makes physostigmine useful for combating CNS anticholinergic toxicity
Diisopropyl fluorophosphate	Not applicable (sometimes encountered as a toxin)	*Respiratory paralysis* Bradycardia, bronchospasm, fasciculations, muscle cramps, weakness, CNS depression, agitation, confusion, delirium, coma, bronchorrhea, salivation, lacrimation, diaphoresis, vomiting, diarrhea, miosis	Not applicable	An organophosphate compound used as an insecticide, as a substrate for the production of organophosphate chemical weapons (nerve gases), and formerly as a topical miotic medication in ophthalmology

Drug	Uses	Side Effects	Cautions / Contraindications	Notes
Tacrine **Donepezil** **Rivastigmine** **Galantamine**	Mild to moderate Alzheimer's disease Dementia	Diarrhea, nausea, vomiting, cramps, anorexia, vivid dreams	Treatment-associated liver function test abnormalities (contraindication for tacrine)	Tacrine, donepezil, rivastigmine, and galantamine produce modest symptomatic benefits in Alzheimer's disease Rivastigmine affects both acetylcholinesterase and butyrylcholinesterase by forming a carbamoylate complex with the enzymes Galantamine also acts as a non-potentiating ligand of nicotinic receptors

MUSCARINIC RECEPTOR AGONISTS
Mechanism—Stimulate muscarinic receptor activity

Drug	Uses	Side Effects	Cautions / Contraindications	Notes
Methacholine	Diagnosis of asthma	*Dyspnea* Lightheadedness, headache, pruritus, throat irritation	Recent heart attack or stroke Aortic aneurysm Uncontrolled hypertension	Methacholine is highly resistant to acetylcholinesterase; it is relatively selective for cardiovascular muscarinic cholinergic receptors
Carbachol **Bethanechol** **Cevimeline** **Pilocarpine**	Glaucoma (carbachol) Urinary tract motility agent (bethanechol) Xerostomia in Sjögren's syndrome (cevimeline and pilocarpine)	Sweating, shivering, nausea, dizziness, increased frequency of urination, rhinitis (oral formulations)	Acute iritis or glaucoma after cataract extraction Narrow-angle (angle-closure) glaucoma	Carbachol has enhanced nicotinic action relative to other choline esters; carbachol cannot be used systemically because of its unpredictable nicotinic action at autonomic ganglia; topical application of carbachol to the cornea of the eye results in both pupillary constriction (miosis) and decreased intraocular pressure Bethanechol is almost completely selective for muscarinic receptors Pilocarpine and cevimeline (an M1 and M3 agonist) are used to treat xerostomia in Sjögren's syndrome

NICOTINIC RECEPTOR AGONISTS
Mechanism—Stimulate opening of nicotinic ACh receptor channel and produce depolarization of the cell membrane; succinylcholine persists at the neuroeffector junction and activates the nicotinic receptor channels continuously, which results in inactivation of voltage-gated sodium channels so that they cannot open to support further action potentials (sometimes called ''depolarizing blockade'')

Drug	Uses	Side Effects	Cautions / Contraindications	Notes
Succinylcholine	Induction of neuromuscular blockade in surgery Intubation	*Bradyarrhythmia, cardiac arrest, cardiac arrhythmia, malignant hyperthermia, rhabdomyolysis, respiratory depression* Muscle rigidity, myalgia, raised intraocular pressure	Personal or family history of malignant hyperthermia Skeletal muscle myopathies Upper motor neuron injury Extensive denervation of skeletal muscle	Short duration of action makes succinylcholine drug of choice for paralysis during intubation. Causes transient fasciculations

MUSCARINIC RECEPTOR ANTAGONISTS
Mechanism—Selectively antagonize muscarinic receptors

Drug	Uses	Side Effects	Cautions / Contraindications	Notes
Atropine	Anticholinesterase overdose Acute, symptomatic bradycardia Premedication for anesthetic procedure Excessive salivation and mucus secretion during surgery Antidote to mushroom poisoning	*Cardiac arrhythmia, coma, respiratory depression, raised intraocular pressure* Tachycardia, constipation, xerostomia, blurred vision	Narrow-angle glaucoma	A naturally occurring alkaloid found in the plant *Atropa belladonna* Mainly muscarinic activity, marginal nicotinic effect More effective at reversal of exogenous rather than endogenous cholinergic activity

(Continued)

Drug Summary Table **Chapter 8 Cholinergic Pharmacology** (*Continued*)

Drug	Clinical Applications	Serious and Common Adverse Effects	Contraindications	Therapeutic Considerations
Scopolamine	Motion sickness Nausea and vomiting	*Alteration in heart rate, drug-induced psychosis* Somnolence, xerostomia, blurred vision	Narrow-angle glaucoma	Significant CNS effects Delivered via transdermal patch
Pirenzepine Methscopolamine Glycopyrrolate	Peptic ulcer disease Surgically-induced or vagally-induced bradycardia (glycopyrrolate)	*Cardiac arrhythmia, malignant hyperthermia, anaphylaxis; seizure* Constipation, xerostomia, urinary retention, decreased sweating	Gastrointestinal obstruction Narrow-angle glaucoma	Alternative or additive agents to standard peptic ulcer disease therapies Methscopolamine and glycopyrrolate have delayed but measurable CNS and cognitive anticholinergic effects
Ipratropium Tiotropium	Chronic obstructive pulmonary disease (COPD) Asthma	*Paralytic ileus, anaphylaxis, oropharyngeal edema* Abnormal taste in mouth, xerostomia (nasal spray)	Hypersensitivity to ipratropium or tiotropium	Ipratropium is more effective than β-adrenergic agonists in the treatment of COPD, but less effective in treating asthma Relative to ipratropium, tiotropium has been shown to have similar, and possibly superior, efficacy as a bronchodilator in the treatment of COPD
Oxybutynin Propantheline Terodiline Tolterodine Trospium Darifenacin Solifenacin	Hyperreflexic and overactive bladder Urge incontinence	Constipation, diarrhea, nausea, dry mouth, application-site erythema, pruritus	Narrow-angle glaucoma	Oxybutynin, propantheline, tolterodine, and trospium are nonspecific muscarinic receptor antagonists, whereas darifenacin and solifenacin are selective M3 receptor antagonists Tolterodine may cause less dry mouth than oxybutynin, and the newer M3-selective agents darifenacin and solifenacin may cause less dry mouth and constipation than nonselective agents

NICOTINIC RECEPTOR ANTAGONISTS
Mechanism—Selectively antagonize nicotinic receptors, thus preventing endogenous ACh binding and subsequent muscle cell depolarization (sometimes called "nondepolarizing blockade")

Drug	Clinical Applications	Serious and Common Adverse Effects	Contraindications	Therapeutic Considerations
Pancuronium Tubocurarine Vecuronium Rocuronium Mivacurium	Induction of neuromuscular blockade in surgery Intubation	*Hypertension, tachyarrhythmia, apnea, bronchospasm, respiratory failure* Salivation, flushing (mivacurium)	Hypersensitivity to pancuronium, tubocurarine, vecuronium, rocuronium, or mivacurium	Pancuronium and tubocurarine are long-acting agents; vecuronium and rocuronium are intermediate-acting agents; mivacurium is a short-acting agent. Nondepolarizing blocking agents have variable adverse effects associated with ganglionic blockade, which can be reversed by administration of AChE inhibitors
Trimethaphan Mecamylamine	Hypertension in patients with acute aortic dissection	*Paralytic ileus, urinary retention, respiratory arrest, syncope* Orthostatic hypotension, dyspepsia, diplopia, sedation	Contraindications for trimethaphan: asphyxia, uncorrected respiratory insufficiency, neonates at risk for paralytic or meconium ileus, shock Contraindications for mecamylamine: coronary insufficiency, glaucoma, recent myocardial infarction, pyloric stenosis, renal insufficiency, patients treated with sulfonamides	Mecamylamine and trimethaphan are administered when ganglionic blockade is desired; these drugs lower blood pressure while simultaneously blunting the sympathetic reflexes that would normally cause a deleterious rise in pressure at the site of the tear in cases of aortic dissection

9

Adrenergic Pharmacology

Freddie M. Williams and Timothy J. Turner

INTRODUCTION

Adrenergic pharmacology involves the study of agents that act on pathways mediated by the endogenous catecholamines norepinephrine, epinephrine, and dopamine. These neurotransmitters modulate many vital functions, including the rate and force of cardiac contraction, the resistance (constriction and dilation) of blood vessels and bronchioles, the release of insulin, and the breakdown of fat. Drugs that target the synthesis, storage, release, and reuptake of norepinephrine and epinephrine, and that target the postsynaptic receptors for these transmitters, are frequent therapies for hypertension, depression, shock, asthma, angina, and many other disorders. This chapter examines the biochemical and physiologic basis for adrenergic action and then discusses the action of the different classes of adrenergic drugs.

Case

The year is 1960. Ms. S has felt depressed for a number of years. She has tried several different medications to alleviate her feelings of hopelessness and lack of motivation, but nothing seems to help. Recently, however, her doctor has prescribed iproniazid, a new medication reported to be of benefit in many cases of depression. He tells her that researchers think the drug acts by inhibiting an enzyme in the brain called monoamine oxidase (MAO). MAO is one of the enzymes responsible for catecholamine degradation. Because it is a new drug, its potential adverse effects are not well defined, so her doctor advises Ms. S to report any unusual effects of the medication.

Hopeful, but not expecting significant changes, Ms. S begins taking the medication. Within a few weeks, she begins to feel motivated and energetic for the first time in 20 years. Exuberant at her newly found sense of energy, Ms.

S reclaims her past life as a debutante and socialite by hosting a gala wine and cheese reception. The best and brightest of the city are invited, and the party is looking to be a success. As she stands up to give thanks to her attendees, Ms. S celebrates with a large swig of her favorite 1954 Chianti. By the end of the party, Ms. S has a severe headache and nausea. Recalling her doctor's warning, Ms. S has a friend rush her to the nearest hospital. In the emergency department, the attending physician records a blood pressure of 230/160 mm Hg. Recognizing that Ms. S is experiencing a hypertensive emergency, the doctor quickly administers phentolamine (an α-adrenoceptor antagonist). Ms. S's blood pressure quickly normalizes, and the doctor's subsequent clinical investigation identifies a new, and now-famous, drug–food interaction involving MAO inhibitors.

QUESTIONS

■ **1.** What is the mechanistic explanation for the interaction of MAO inhibitors with red wine and aged cheese?

■ **2.** How does phentolamine act, and why was it useful in this clinical circumstance?

■ **3.** Why didn't her physician use a β-adrenoceptor antagonist to treat Ms. S' hypertension?

BIOCHEMISTRY AND PHYSIOLOGY OF ADRENERGIC FUNCTION

The autonomic nervous system maintains homeostasis through the concerted action of its sympathetic and parasympathetic branches. The sympathetic nervous system prevails under conditions of stress, producing a "fight-or-flight" response that aids the organism in surviving such challenges. The following discussion presents the biochemistry of catecholamine action, from synthesis to metabolism to receptor activation. Then the physiologic roles of the endogenous catecholamines epinephrine, norepinephrine, and dopamine are discussed, with emphasis on the specificity of receptor expression in different organ systems.

CATECHOLAMINE SYNTHESIS, STORAGE, AND RELEASE

Catecholamines are synthesized by oxidation of the amino acid tyrosine. This synthesis occurs primarily at sympathetic nerve endings, but also to some degree in neuronal cell bodies. Epinephrine synthesis predominates in adrenal medullary cells, while most adrenergic neurons produce norepinephrine (Fig. 9-1). Tyrosine, the precursor for catecholamine synthesis, is transported into neurons via an aromatic amino acid transporter that uses the Na$^+$ gradient across the neuronal membrane to concentrate tyrosine, phenylalanine, tryptophan, and histidine. The first step in catecholamine synthesis, the oxidation of tyrosine to **dihydroxy-**

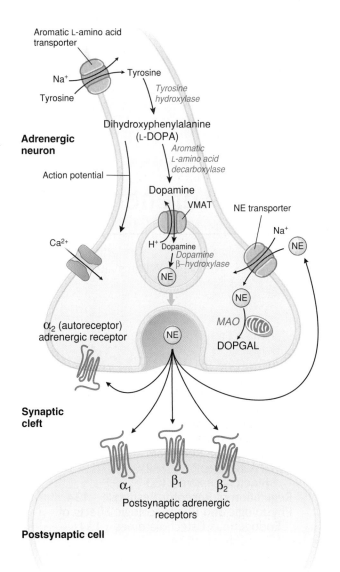

Figure 9-1. Catecholamine synthesis, storage, release, and reuptake pathways. The endogenous catecholamines dopamine, norepinephrine, and epinephrine are all synthesized from tyrosine. The rate-limiting step in catecholamine synthesis, the oxidation of cytoplasmic tyrosine to dihydroxyphenylalanine (L-DOPA), is catalyzed by the enzyme tyrosine hydroxylase. Aromatic L-amino acid decarboxylase then converts L-DOPA to dopamine. Vesicular monoamine transporter (VMAT) translocates dopamine (and other monoamines) into synaptic vesicles. In adrenergic neurons, intravesicular dopamine-β-hydroxylase converts dopamine to norepinephrine (NE). Norepinephrine is then stored in the vesicle until release. In adrenal medullary cells, norepinephrine returns to the cytosol, where phenylethanolamine N-methyltransferase (PNMT) converts norepinephrine to epinephrine. The epinephrine is then transported back into the vesicle for storage *(not shown)*. α-Methyltyrosine inhibits tyrosine hydroxylase, the rate-limiting enzyme in catecholamine synthesis *(not shown)*. Released norepinephrine can stimulate postsynaptic α$_1$-, β$_1$- or β$_2$- adrenergic receptors, or presynaptic α$_2$-adrenergic autoreceptors. Released norepinephrine can also be taken up into presynaptic terminals by the selective NE transporter. NE in the cytoplasm of the presynaptic neuron can be further taken up into synaptic vesicles by VMAT *(not shown)* or degraded to DOPGAL (see Fig. 9-3) by mitochondrion-associated monoamine oxidase (MAO).

phenylalanine (DOPA) by the enzyme **tyrosine hydroxylase** (TH), is the rate-limiting step. DOPA is converted to dopamine by a generic aromatic amino acid decarboxylase. Dopamine is then hydroxylated at the 9-position (or β-position) by **dopamine-β-hydroxylase** to yield norepinephrine. In tissues that produce epinephrine, norepinephrine is then methylated on its amino group by **phenylethanolamine-N-methyltransferase** (PNMT).

The subcellular localization of these various synthetic steps is tied to the eventual storage of neurotransmitter. The conversion of tyrosine to dopamine occurs within the cytoplasm of the neuron. Dopamine is then transported into synaptic vesicles by a 12-helix membrane-spanning proton antiporter called the **vesicular monoamine transporter (VMAT).** Dopamine inside the vesicle is converted to norepinephrine by dopamine-β-hydroxylase.

There are three distinct vesicular transporters that differ in substrate specificity and localization. VMAT1 and VMAT 2 (also known as Uptake 2 [Fig. 9-2]) both transport serotonin (5HT), histamine and all catecholamines, but they differ in that VMAT1 is expressed peripherally (adrenal, sympathetic ganglia) and VMAT2 is expressed primarily in the central nervous system (CNS). The vesicular acetylcholine transporter (VAChT) is expressed in cholinergic neurons, including motor nerves (see Chapter 8, Cholinergic Pharmacology). These antiporters use the proton gradient generated by a H^+-ATPase in the vesicular membrane to concentrate dopamine inside the vesicle. Norepinephrine concentrations within the vesicle can reach 100 mM. To stabilize the osmotic pressure resulting from the high concentration gradient for norepinephrine across the vesicle membrane, norepinephrine is thought to condense with ATP. Consequently, ATP and norepinephrine are coreleased upon vesicle exocytosis.

In adrenal medullary cells, norepinephrine is transported or diffuses from vesicles back into the cytoplasm, where PNMT converts it to epinephrine. Epinephrine is then transported back into vesicles for storage until its eventual release by exocytosis. The nonselective nature of VMAT1 and VMAT2 has important pharmacologic consequences, as discussed below.

Catecholamine release is initiated by signals originating in an array of processing areas in the CNS, especially the limbic system. These CNS neurons project axons that synapse on sympathetic preganglionic neurons in the intermediolateral columns of the spinal cord. The preganglionic axons project to the sympathetic ganglia, where they release acetylcholine. This neurotransmitter initiates excitatory postsynaptic potentials in postganglionic neurons by activating nicotinic acetylcholine (ACh) receptors (cation-selective channels that depolarize the neuronal membrane). Ganglionic blockers such as **hexamethonium** and **mecamylamine** block the ganglionic nicotinic ACh receptor, without significant effects on skeletal muscle ACh receptors (see Chapter 8). The sympathetic postganglionic axons form varicosities or *en passant* synapses in or on target organs. The arrival of an action potential at these endings opens voltage-gated Ca^{2+} channels, and the ensuing Ca^{2+} influx triggers exocytosis of the catecholamine-containing synaptic vesicles. Norepinephrine rapidly diffuses away from the presynaptic varicosity and locally regulates tissue responses (e.g., smooth muscle tone) by activating postsynaptic adrenergic

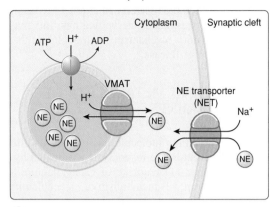

A Normal uptake of norepinephrine from synaptic cleft and concentration of NE in synaptic vesicle

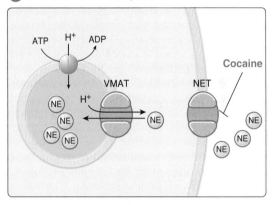

B Cocaine inhibits NE transporter

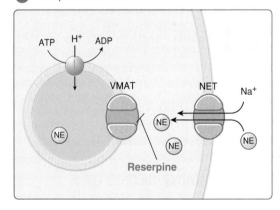

C Reserpine inhibits VMAT

Figure 9-2. Mechanisms of action of cocaine and reserpine. A. Norepinephrine (NE) that has been released into the synaptic cleft can be taken up into the cytoplasm of the presynaptic neuron by the selective NE transporter (NET), a Na^+-NE cotransporter. Cytoplasmic NE is concentrated in synaptic vesicles by the nonselective vesicular monoamine transporter (VMAT), an H^+-monoamine antiporter. An H^+-ATPase uses the energy of ATP hydrolysis to concentrate protons in synaptic vesicles, and thereby generates a transmembrane H^+ gradient. This H^+ gradient is used by VMAT to drive monoamine transport into the synaptic vesicle. **B.** Cocaine inhibits the NE transporter, allowing released NE to remain in the synaptic cleft for a longer period of time. By this mechanism, cocaine potentiates neurotransmission at adrenergic synapses. **C.** Reserpine inhibits the vesicular monoamine transporter, preventing the refilling of synaptic vesicles with NE and eventually depleting the adrenergic terminal of neurotransmitter. By this mechanism, reserpine inhibits neurotransmission at adrenergic synapses.

receptors (with the notable exception that ACh is the transmitter used at sympathetic nerve endings in sweat glands). It has recently been recognized that adrenergic receptors are also located on presynaptic nerve endings; this may serve as an autoregulatory mechanism for modulating the extent of neurotransmitter release.

REUPTAKE AND METABOLISM OF CATECHOLAMINES

Once a catecholamine molecule has exerted its effect at a postsynaptic receptor, the response is terminated by one of three mechanisms: (1) reuptake of catecholamine into the presynaptic neuron; (2) metabolism of catecholamine to an inactive metabolite; and (3) diffusion of the catecholamine away from the synaptic cleft. The first two of these mechanisms require specific transport proteins or enzymes and, therefore, are targets for pharmacologic intervention.

Reuptake of catecholamine into the neuronal cytoplasm is mediated by a selective catecholamine transporter (e.g., **norepinephrine transporter** or **NET**) that is also known as Uptake 1 (Fig. 9-2). This symporter uses the inward Na^+ gradient to concentrate catecholamines in the cytoplasm of sympathetic nerve endings, thus limiting the postsynaptic response and allowing neurons to recycle the transmitter for subsequent release. Inside the nerve terminal, catecholamines can be further concentrated in synaptic vesicles via VMAT, the same transporter used to transport dopamine into the vesicle for catecholamine synthesis. Thus, *the pool of catecholamines available for release comes from two sources: molecules that are synthesized de novo, and molecules that are recycled via neuronal reuptake.*

Catecholamine metabolism involves the two enzymes **MAO** and **catechol-O-methyltransferase (COMT)** (Fig. 9-3). MAO is a mitochondrial enzyme that is expressed in most neurons. It exists in two isoforms, MAO-A and MAO-B. The two isoforms have some degree of ligand specificity: MAO-A preferentially degrades serotonin, norepinephrine, and dopamine, while MAO-B degrades dopamine more rapidly than serotonin and norepinephrine. COMT is a cytosolic enzyme that is expressed primarily in the liver.

CATECHOLAMINE RECEPTORS

Adrenergic receptors (also called **adrenoceptors**) are selective for norepinephrine and epinephrine. Supraphysiologic concentrations of dopamine can also activate some adrenoceptors. These receptors are divided into two main classes, termed α and β. All of the catecholamine receptor classes and subclasses are members of the G protein-coupled receptor superfamily (see Chapter 1, Drug–Receptor Interactions).

Both α- and β-adrenoceptors are coupled to cytoplasmic scaffolding proteins that, in turn, couple to downstream signaling cascades. For example, $β_1$ receptors interact with an array of cytoskeletal elements called **PDZ proteins.** Members of the PDZ family mediate regulatory functions, including receptor internalization and coupling to adaptor proteins such as Grb2 or guanine-nucleotide exchange factors that regulate small monomeric G proteins. Second, a series of

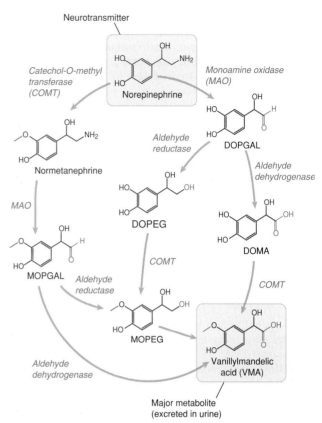

Figure 9-3. Norepinephrine metabolism. Norepinephrine is degraded to metabolites by two main enzymes. Catechol-O-methyl transferase (COMT) is a widely distributed cytosolic enzyme; COMT in the liver is particularly important in the metabolism of circulating catecholamines. Monoamine oxidase (MAO), which is localized to the outer surface of mitochondria, is found in many monoaminergic (including adrenergic) neurons. COMT, MAO, aldehyde reductase, and aldehyde dehydrogenase metabolize catecholamines to multiple intermediates that are eventually excreted. Vanillylmandelic acid (VMA) is the major metabolite excreted in urine.

biophysical, biochemical, and structural studies have revealed that many G protein-coupled receptors, including adrenoceptors, form functional dimers. For example, $β_1$ receptors can form homodimers as well as heterodimers with $β_2$ adrenoceptors, $α_2$ adrenoceptors, and δ-opiate receptors. The functional implications of these quaternary structures are unclear, but at a minimum the formation of heterodimers suggests a mechanism for heterologous receptor regulation.

α-Adrenoceptors

α-Adrenoceptors are divided into $α_1$ and $α_2$ subclasses (Table 9-1). The majority of $α_1$-receptors signal via G_q-mediated pathways that generate IP_3, which mobilizes intracellular Ca^{2+} stores, and DAG, which activates protein kinase C. α1-Receptors are expressed in vascular smooth muscle, genitourinary tract smooth muscle, intestinal smooth muscle, heart, and liver. In vascular smooth muscle cells, stimulation of $α_1$-receptors increases intracellular $[Ca^{2+}]$, activation of calmodulin, phosphorylation of myosin light chain, increased actin–myosin interaction, and muscle contraction (see Chapter 21, Pharmacology of Vascular Tone). The $α_1$-

TABLE 9-1	Adrenoceptor Actions		
RECEPTOR SUBTYPE	**SIGNALING MEDIATORS**	**TISSUE**	**EFFECTS**
α_1	$G_q/G_i/G_o$	Vascular smooth muscle	Contraction
		Genitourinary smooth muscle	Contraction
		Intestinal smooth muscle	Relaxation
		Heart	↑ Inotropy and excitability
		Liver	Glycogenolysis and gluconeogenesis
α_2	G_i/G_o	Pancreatic β-cells	↓ Insulin secretion
		Platelets	Aggregation
		Nerve	↓ Norepinephrine release
		Vascular smooth muscle	Contraction
β_1	G_s	Heart	↑ Chronotropy and inotropy
		Heart	↑ AV-node conduction velocity
		Renal juxtaglomerular cells	↑ Renin secretion
β_2	G_s	Smooth muscle	Relaxation
		Liver	Glycogenolysis and gluconeogenesis
		Skeletal muscle	Glycogenolysis and K^+ uptake
β_3	G_s	Adipose	Lipolysis

receptor subtype is, therefore, important for mediating increases in blood pressure, and α_1-receptor antagonists are logical therapies for hypertension. Because α_1-receptor activation also causes contraction of genitourinary smooth muscle, α_1-receptor antagonists are used clinically in the symptomatic treatment of prostatic hypertrophy (see below).

α2-Adrenoceptors activate G_i, an inhibitory G protein. G_i has multiple signaling actions, including inhibition of adenylyl cyclase (thus decreasing cAMP levels), activation of G protein-coupled inward rectifier K^+ channels (causing membrane hyperpolarization), and inhibition of neuronal Ca^{2+} channels. Each of these effects tends to decrease neurotransmitter release from the target neuron. α_2-Receptors are found on both presynaptic neurons and postsynaptic cells. *Presynaptic α_2-receptors function as autoreceptors to mediate feedback inhibition of sympathetic transmission.* α_2-Receptors are also expressed on pancreatic β-cells and platelets, where they mediate inhibition of insulin release and inhibition of platelet aggregation, respectively. The latter observation has led to the development of agents that are specific inhibitors of platelet α_2-receptors (see below). The main pharmacologic approach to α_2-receptors, however, has been in the treatment of hypertension. α_2-Receptor agonists act at CNS sites to decrease sympathetic outflow to the periphery, resulting in decreased norepinephrine release at sympathetic nerve terminals and, therefore, decreased vascular smooth muscle contraction.

β-Adrenoceptors

β-Adrenoceptors are divided into three subclasses, termed β_1, β_2, and β_3 (Table 9-1). All three subclasses activate a stimulatory G protein, G_s. G_s activates adenylyl cyclase, leading to an increase in the level of intracellular cAMP. Increased cAMP activates protein kinases (especially protein kinase A), which phosphorylate cellular proteins, including ion channels. The exact nature of the signaling differences among the β-adrenoceptor subtypes is unclear since they all

appear to couple efficiently to G_s. It has been suggested that specificity may be conferred by the exact G protein subunit composition found in the receptor complex. Thus, pharmacologic selectivity appears to reside in the tissue-specific distribution of each β-adrenoceptor subtype, and possibly in activation of tissue-specific downstream signaling pathways.

β_1-Adrenoceptors are localized primarily in the heart and kidney. In the kidney, they are present mainly on renal juxtaglomerular cells, where receptor activation causes renin release (see Chapter 20, Pharmacology of Volume Regulation). Stimulation of cardiac β_1-receptors causes an increase in both inotropy (force of contraction) and chronotropy (heart rate). The inotropic effect is mediated by increased phosphorylation of Ca^{2+} channels, including calcium channels in the sarcolemma and phospholamban in the sarcoplasmic reticulum (see Chapter 19, Pharmacology of Cardiac Contractility). The increased chronotropy results from a β_1-mediated increase in the rate of phase 4 depolarization of sinoatrial node pacemaker cells. Both effects contribute to increased cardiac output (recall that cardiac output = heart rate × stroke volume). Activation of β_1-receptors also increases conduction velocity in the atrioventricular (AV) node because the β_1-stimulated increase in Ca^{2+} entry increases the rate of depolarization of AV node cells.

The important effects of β_1-adrenoceptors on the force of contraction and heart rate make antagonists of this receptor subtype attractive agents in the treatment of hypertension and angina. β1-Adrenoceptor antagonists are also used to prevent a second myocardial infarction in patients who have already sustained one such event and in the treatment of mild-to-moderate heart failure. Because β_1-adrenoceptor antagonists slow AV-nodal conduction velocity, these agents are used to treat some forms of supraventricular tachycardia (see Chapter 18, Pharmacology of Cardiac Rhythm).

β2-Adrenoceptors are expressed in smooth muscle, liver, and skeletal muscle. In smooth muscle, receptor activation stimulates G_s, adenylyl cyclase, cAMP, and protein kinase

A. Protein kinase A phosphorylates several contractile proteins, especially myosin light chain kinase. Phosphorylation of myosin light chain kinase reduces its affinity for calcium-calmodulin, leading to relaxation of the contractile apparatus. Evidence also suggests that β_2-adrenoceptor activation may relax bronchial smooth muscle by G_s-independent activation of K^+ channels. Increased K^+ efflux leads to bronchial smooth muscle cell hyperpolarization and, therefore, opposes the depolarization necessary to elicit contraction. The powerful relaxation of bronchial smooth muscle mediated by β_2-receptors makes inhaled β_2-agonists especially useful agents in the treatment of asthma. In hepatocytes, activation of the G_s signaling cascade initiates a series of intracellular phosphorylation events that result in glycogen phosphorylase activation and glycogen catabolism. The outcome of β_2-adrenoceptor stimulation of hepatocytes is, therefore, an increase in plasma glucose. In skeletal muscle, activation of these same signaling pathways stimulates glycogenolysis and promotes K^+ uptake.

It has recently been discovered that β_3-adrenoceptors are expressed specifically in adipose tissue. Stimulation of β_3-receptors leads to an increase in lipolysis. This physiologic action has led to speculation that β_3-agonists may be useful in the treatment of obesity and noninsulin-dependent diabetes mellitus, but such selective pharmacologic agents remain to be developed for clinical use.

REGULATION OF RECEPTOR RESPONSE

The ability of receptor agonists to initiate downstream signaling is proportional to the number of receptors activated. Accordingly, changes in the density of receptors on the cell surface will alter the apparent efficacy of an agonist. Thus, both short-term (desensitization) and long-term (down-regulation) changes in the number of functional adrenoceptors are important in regulating tissue response.

When an agonist activates an adrenoceptor, the dissociation of heterotrimeric G proteins leads to downstream signaling as well as a negative feedback mechanism that limits tissue responses. The accumulation of the $\beta\gamma$ subunits in the membrane recruits a **G protein receptor kinase** (GRK), which phosphorylates the receptor at residues in the C-terminus that are important targets for inactivator proteins. Alternatively, protein kinase A and protein kinase C can phosphorylate G proteins. The phosphorylated state of a G protein can bind to another protein called **β-arrestin** that sterically inhibits the receptor-G protein interaction, effectively silencing receptor signaling. On a longer time scale, the receptor-β-arrestin complex is sequestered, in a clathrin-dependent manner, into an endocytic compartment for internalization, a process called **down-regulation.** Each of these processes is important in regulating tissue responsiveness on a short- or long-term basis.

PHYSIOLOGIC AND PHARMACOLOGIC EFFECTS OF ENDOGENOUS CATECHOLAMINES

The endogenous catecholamines epinephrine and norepinephrine act as agonists at both α- and β-adrenoceptors. At supraphysiologic concentrations, dopamine can also act as an agonist at α- and β-receptors. The overall effect of each catecholamine is complex and depends on the concentration of the agent and on tissue–specific receptor expression.

Epinephrine

Epinephrine is an agonist at both α- and β-adrenoceptors. *At low concentrations, epinephrine has predominantly β_1 and β_2 effects, while at high concentrations, its α_1 effects predominate.* Acting at β_1-receptors, epinephrine increases cardiac contractile force and cardiac output, with consequent increases in cardiac oxygen consumption and systolic blood pressure. Vasodilation mediated by β_2-receptors causes a decrease in peripheral resistance and a decrease in diastolic blood pressure. Stimulation of β_2-receptors also increases blood flow to skeletal muscle, relaxes bronchial smooth muscle, and increases the concentrations of glucose and free fatty acids in the blood. These β_1 and β_2 effects are all components of the ''fight-or-flight'' response. Epinephrine is used to treat an acute asthmatic attack and anaphylaxis; high doses of locally applied epinephrine cause vasoconstriction and prolong the action of local anesthetics. Epinephrine has a rapid onset and a brief duration of action, and is ineffective orally. The increased cardiac excitability induced by epinephrine can lead to cardiac arrhythmias, and the sharp rise in blood pressure can provoke cerebral hemorrhage.

Norepinephrine

Norepinephrine is an agonist at α_1- and β_1-receptors, but has relatively little effect at β_2-receptors. Because of the lack of action at β_2-receptors, systemic administration of norepinephrine increases not only systolic blood pressure (β_1 effect) but also diastolic blood pressure and total peripheral resistance. Norepinephrine also increases heart rate, but this effect is typically overcome by reflex vagal activity in response to increased blood pressure. Therefore, norepinephrine increases stroke volume, but cardiac output remains unchanged because heart rate is ultimately decreased. Norepinephrine is frequently used in the emergency treatment of distributive shock.

Dopamine

Although dopamine is a prominent CNS neurotransmitter, systemic administration has few CNS effects because it does not readily cross the blood–brain barrier. Dopamine activates one or more subtypes of catecholamine receptor in peripheral tissues, and the predominant effect is dependent on the local concentration of the compound. At low doses (< 2 μg/kg per min), a continuous intravenous infusion of dopamine acts predominately on D1 dopaminergic receptors in renal, mesenteric, and coronary vascular beds. D1 dopaminergic receptors activate adenylyl cyclase in vascular smooth muscle cells, leading to increased cAMP levels and vasodilation. At suprafisiologic rates of infusion (2–10 μg/kg per min), dopamine is a positive inotrope via its activation of β_1-adrenergic receptors. At still higher rates of infusion (>10 μg/kg per min), dopamine acts on vascular α_1-adrenergic receptors to cause vasoconstriction. Dopamine is used in the treatment of shock, particularly in states of shock caused by low cardiac output and accompanied by compromised renal function leading to oliguria.

PHARMACOLOGIC CLASSES AND AGENTS

Pharmacologic intervention is possible at each of the major steps in catecholamine synthesis, storage, reuptake, metabolism, and receptor activation. The following discussion presents the various classes of agents in the order of their action on adrenergic pathways, from neurotransmitter synthesis to receptor activation.

INHIBITORS OF CATECHOLAMINE SYNTHESIS

Inhibitors of catecholamine synthesis have limited clinical utility because such agents nonspecifically inhibit the formation of all catecholamines (see Fig. 9-1). α-**Methyltyrosine** is a structural analogue of tyrosine that is transported into nerve terminals, where it inhibits tyrosine hydroxylase, the first enzyme in the catecholamine biosynthesis pathway. This agent is used occasionally in the treatment of hypertension associated with pheochromocytoma (a tumor of the enterochromaffin cells of the adrenal medulla that produces norepinephrine and epinephrine).

INHIBITORS OF CATECHOLAMINE STORAGE

Catecholamines originate from two pools—de novo synthesis and recycled transmitter. An agent that inhibits catecholamine storage in vesicles can have two effects. In the short term, the agent can increase the net release of catecholamine from the synaptic terminal, and thus mimic sympathetic stimulation (''**sympathomimetic**''). Over a longer time period, however, the agent depletes the pool of available catecholamine and thus acts as a **sympatholytic** (inhibitor of sympathetic activity) (Fig. 9-4).

Reserpine binds tightly to the vesicular antiporter VMAT (see Figs. 9-1 and 9-2). The drug irreversibly damages VMAT, resulting in vesicles that lose their ability to concentrate and store norepinephrine and dopamine. At low doses, reserpine causes neurotransmitter leak into the cytoplasm, where the catecholamine is destroyed by MAO. At high doses, the rate of transmitter leak can be sufficiently high to overwhelm the MAO in the presynaptic neuron. Under these conditions, there is a high concentration of transmitter in the neuronal cytoplasm, and transmitter can exit from the cytoplasm to the synaptic space through NET acting in reverse. The efflux of catecholamine has a transient sympathomimetic effect. Because reserpine's inhibition of VMAT is irreversible, new storage vesicles must be synthesized and transported to the nerve terminal to restore proper vesicular function. The recovery phase may require days to weeks after an individual stops taking reserpine. Reserpine can also be used experimentally to assess whether drugs need to be

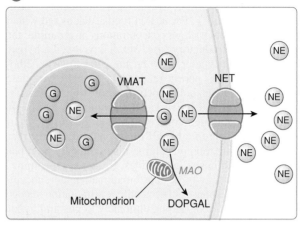

A Acute effect of indirect sympathomimetic

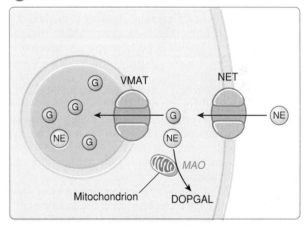

B Chronic effect of indirect sympathomimetic

Figure 9-4. Acute and chronic effects of indirect sympathomimetics. Indirect sympathomimetics have different effects on sympathetic outflow depending on whether they are administered acutely or chronically. **A.** Administered acutely, an indirect sympathomimetic such as guanethidine (G) displaces norepinephrine (NE) that is stored in the synaptic vesicles of adrenergic neurons. This results in a massive efflux of norepinephrine through the NE transporter acting in reverse; the resultant flooding of the synapse with norepinephrine causes marked sympathetic stimulation. **B.** Administered chronically, an indirect sympathomimetic such as guanethidine (G) is concentrated in synaptic vesicles and replaces norepinephrine. In addition, monoamine oxidase (MAO) degrades the small pool of norepinephrine that remains in the cytoplasm. Both of these effects contribute to decreased sympathetic stimulation.

concentrated in presynaptic terminals to exert their action. In the past, reserpine was used to treat hypertension. However, the irreversible nature of its action, and its association with psychotic depression, make it an unattractive agent now that safer, more efficacious drugs are available for the treatment of hypertension.

Tyramine is a dietary amine that is ordinarily metabolized in the gastrointestinal tract and liver by MAO. In patients taking MAO inhibitors (MAOIs, see below), tyramine is absorbed in the gut, transported through the blood, and taken up by sympathetic neurons, where it is transported into synaptic vesicles by VMAT. By this mechanism, an acute challenge with large amounts of tyramine can cause acute displacement of vesicular norepinephrine and massive nonvesicular release of norepinephrine from the nerve terminal via reversal of NET. Fermented foods such as red wine and aged cheese possess high concentrations of tyramine; this is why, in the introductory case, Ms. S developed a hypertensive crisis shortly after her wine and cheese party. Although tyramine itself is poorly retained in synaptic vesicles, its hydroxylated metabolite **octopamine** (the synthesis of which is catalyzed by vesicular dopamine β-hydroxylase) can be stored at high concentrations in the vesicles. Under conditions of chronic MAOI treatment and modest dietary tyramine intake, norepinephrine may gradually be replaced by octopamine in storage vesicles. Because octopamine has little agonist activity at most mammalian adrenoceptors, postsynaptic responses to sympathetic stimulation may gradually be diminished, leading ultimately to postural hypotension.

Guanethidine (like tyramine) is actively transported into neurons by NET, where it concentrates in transmitter vesicles and displaces norepinephrine, leading to gradual depletion of norepinephrine (Fig. 9-4). Guanethidine (like octopamine) is not an agonist at postsynaptic adrenoceptors, so its vesicular release upon sympathetic stimulation does not elicit a postsynaptic response. In the past, guanethidine was used to treat uncontrolled hypertension. Guanethidine inhibits cardiac sympathetic nerves, leading to reduced cardiac output, and it blocks sympathetically-mediated vasoconstriction, leading to reduced cardiac preload. Symptomatic hypotension following exercise or standing up (postural hypotension) may result from inhibition of these sympathetic responses by guanethidine.

Guanadrel also acts as a false neurotransmitter. As with guanethidine, this agent can be used in the treatment of hypertension, but it is no longer a first-line agent. The adverse effect profile of guanadrel is similar to that of guanethidine.

Amphetamine has several adrenergic actions: (1) it displaces endogenous catecholamines from storage vesicles (similar to tyramine); (2) it is a weak inhibitor of MAO; and (3) it blocks catecholamine reuptake mediated by NET and DAT. While amphetamine binds to postsynaptic adrenergic receptors, it has little agonist action at α- or β-adrenoceptors. Amphetamine has marked behavioral effects including increased alertness, decreased fatigue, depressed appetite, and insomnia. Thus, it has been used to treat depression and narcolepsy (recurrent attacks of drowsiness and sleep during the daytime) and to suppress appetite. Its adverse effects can be substantial, including fatigue and depression following the period of central stimulation.

Ephedrine, pseudoephedrine, and **phenylpropanolamine** are structurally related agents with actions less marked than those of amphetamine. While ephedrine and phenylpropanolamine are now restricted in the United States, pseudoephedrine is widely used as an over-the-counter decongestant and is found in some cold remedies and appetite suppressants.

Methylphenidate, a structural analogue of amphetamine, is widely used in psychiatry to treat attention-deficit hyperactivity disorder (ADHD) in children; its major effect is thought to be related to enhanced attention.

For all of the amphetamine-related agents, psychological and physiological dependence and tolerance can occur. These agents increase both systolic and diastolic blood pressure, and individuals taking these drugs may experience rest-lessness, dizziness, tremor, irritability, confusion, aggressiveness, erectile dysfunction, anxiety, paranoid hallucinations, panic, and suicidal or homicidal ideations. The severity of the adverse effect profile is related to the efficacy of the individual agent as a CNS stimulant. **Methamphetamine** ("crank" or "crystal meth") is a major drug of abuse.

INHIBITORS OF CATECHOLAMINE REUPTAKE

Inhibitors of catecholamine reuptake can exert an acute and powerful sympathomimetic effect by prolonging the time that released neurotransmitter remains in the synaptic cleft. **Cocaine** is a potent inhibitor of NET; unlike other uptake inhibitors (such as imipramine and fluoxetine), cocaine essentially eliminates catecholamine transport (see Fig. 9-2). Cocaine is a controlled substance with high abuse potential. It is used occasionally as a local anesthetic (see Chapter 10, Local Anesthetic Pharmacology), but its most important role is as an agent of abuse (see Chapter 17, Pharmacology of Drug Dependence and Addiction).

The **tricyclic antidepressants** (**TCAs**), such as **imipramine** and **amitriptyline,** inhibit NET-mediated reuptake of norepinephrine into presynaptic terminals, and thus allow accumulation of norepinephrine in the synaptic cleft. The TCAs are promiscuous, however, inhibiting serotonin as well as norepinephrine reuptake into presynaptic terminals and blocking serotonergic, α-adrenergic, histaminergic, and muscarinic receptors at therapeutic doses. Not surprisingly, therefore, the TCAs display a prominent adverse effect profile. One hallmark of TCA therapy for depression is that, although these drugs begin inhibiting norepinephrine and serotonin reuptake immediately, there is a latency period of several weeks before improvement in symptoms is seen. The molecular mechanism responsible for this delayed onset of benefit remains the subject of investigation. Paradoxically, the tricyclics may cause both postural hypotension (through α-adrenergic blockade) and sinus tachycardia (through potentiation of norepinephrine action on cardiac sympathetic nerves). At high doses or in overdose, TCAs can have a quinidine-like effect on cardiac ion channels and thereby induce arrhythmia (see Chapter 18). Because of their important role in the treatment of depression, TCAs and other inhibitors of reuptake, including **duloxetine**, a mixed serotonergic and norepinephrine reuptake inhibitor, are discussed in more detail in Chapter 13, Pharmacology of Serotonergic and Central Adrenergic Neurotransmission.

INHIBITORS OF CATECHOLAMINE METABOLISM

Monoamine oxidase inhibitors (MAOIs) prevent secondary deamination following reuptake of catecholamines into presynaptic terminals. Therefore, more catecholamine accumulates in presynaptic vesicles for release during each action potential. Most MAOIs are oxidized by MAO to reactive intermediates, which then act as irreversible inhibitors of MAO. Nonselective agents in this class (i.e., agents that inhibit both MAO-A and MAO-B) include **phenelzine, ipro-**

niazid (the drug used in the introductory case), and **tranyl-cypromine.** Selective inhibitors include **clorgyline,** which is selective for MAO-A and **selegiline,** which is selective for MAO-B. **Brofaromine, befloxatone,** and **moclobemide** are newer, reversible inhibitors of MAO-A.

As with the tricyclic antidepressants, MAOIs are used to treat depression. Selegiline is also approved for the treatment of Parkinson's disease; its mechanism of action may include both potentiation of dopamine in the remaining nigrostriatal neurons and decreased formation of neurotoxic intermediates. As noted above, patients taking MAOIs should avoid eating certain fermented foods containing large amounts of tyramine and other monoamines, because MAOIs block oxidative deamination of these monoamines in the gastrointestinal tract and liver, allowing them to enter the circulation and precipitate a hypertensive crisis. Concomitant use of MAOIs and selective serotonin reuptake inhibitors (SSRIs) is also contraindicated because it may precipitate the **serotonin syndrome,** characterized by restlessness, tremors, seizures, and possibly coma and death. The reversible inhibitors of MAO-A may be less prone to adverse effects and interactions. MAOIs and SSRIs are also discussed in Chapters 12 and 13.

RECEPTOR AGONISTS

Because of the important role that adrenoceptors play in mediating vascular tone, smooth muscle tone, and cardiac contractility, selective agonists and antagonists of these receptors are mainstays of therapy for hypertension, asthma, and myocardial infarction. In the following discussion, the agents are organized according to receptor subtype specificity (see Table 9-1 for an overview of the relevant receptor subtypes).

α-Adrenergic Agonists

The α_1-selective adrenergic agonists increase peripheral vascular resistance and thereby maintain or elevate blood pressure. These drugs may also cause sinus bradycardia through activation of reflex vagal responses. Systemically administered α_1-agonists, such as **methoxamine,** have limited clinical use, but are sometimes employed in the treatment of shock. A number of topically administered α_1-agonists, such as **phenylephrine, oxymetazoline,** and **tetrahydrazoline,** are used in the nonprescription remedies Afrin® and Visine® (and others) to constrict vascular smooth muscle in the symptomatic relief of nasal congestion and ophthalmic hyperemia. Unfortunately, rebound hypersensitivity and return of symptoms often accompany use of these remedies. Phenylephrine is also used intravenously in the treatment of shock.

Clonidine is the best characterized α_2-agonist. This drug is prescribed commonly for treatment of hypertension; it is also used as a sympatholytic to treat symptoms associated with drug withdrawal. Adverse effects include bradycardia caused by decreased sympathetic activity and increased vagal activity, as well as dry mouth and sedation. Other centrally acting α_2-agonists include the seldom-used agents **guanabenz** and **guanfacine.** These agents have adverse effect profiles similar to that of clonidine.

α-Methyldopa is a precursor (prodrug) to the α_2-agonist α-methylnorepinephrine. Endogenous enzymes catalyze the metabolism of methyldopa to methylnorepinephrine, and the α-methylnorepinephrine is then released by the adrenergic nerve terminal, where it can act presynaptically as an α_2-agonist. This action results in decreased sympathetic outflow from the CNS and consequent lowering of blood pressure in hypertensive patients. Because α-methyldopa use can be associated with rare hepatotoxicity and autoimmune hemolytic anemia, this drug is not a first-line agent in the treatment of hypertension. Because it has proved to be safer than other antihypertensive agents in pregnancy, however, it is often the drug of choice for the treatment of hypertension during pregnancy.

β-Adrenergic Agonists

Stimulation of β_1-adrenergic receptors causes an increase in heart rate and the force of contraction, resulting in increased cardiac output, while stimulation of β_2-adrenergic receptors causes relaxation of vascular, bronchial, and gastrointestinal smooth muscle. **Isoproterenol** is a nonselective β-agonist that can be used to relieve bronchoconstriction. This drug lowers peripheral vascular resistance and diastolic blood pressure (a β_2 effect), while systolic blood pressure remains unchanged or slightly increased (a β_1 effect). Because isoproterenol is a positive inotrope (increases cardiac contractility) and chronotrope (increases heart rate), cardiac output is increased. Isoproterenol causes less hyperglycemia than does epinephrine, because the former agent stimulates β-adrenergic activation of insulin secretion. Because isoproterenol is a nonselective activator of β_1- and β_2-adrenoceptors, and its use for relief of bronchoconstriction in asthma is often accompanied by unwanted cardiac side effects, use of this drug has been mostly supplanted by newer β_2-selective agonists (see below).

Dobutamine has classically been described as a β_1-selective agonist. It is now appreciated, however, that the overall effect of dobutamine depends on the differential effects of the two stereoisomers contained in the racemic mixture (see Chapter 1 for a discussion of stereoisomers). The $(-)$ isomer acts as both an α_1-agonist and a weak β_1-agonist, whereas the $(+)$ isomer acts as both an α_1-antagonist and a potent β_1-agonist. The α_1-agonist and antagonist properties effectively cancel each other out when the racemic mixture is administered, and the observed clinical result is that of a selective β_1-agonist. This agent has more prominent inotropic than chronotropic effects, resulting in increased contractility and cardiac output. Dobutamine is used clinically in the acute management of heart failure.

β_2-selective agonists are valuable in the treatment of asthma, because stimulation of β_1-adrenoceptors in the heart by nonselective β-agonists causes uncomfortable (and occasionally dangerous) cardiac side effects. Drug delivery devices have further facilitated selective stimulation of β_2-adrenoceptors in the target tissue of interest. For example, the use of aerosolizing inhalers allows dosing at the distal airways, where the drug is most needed. Pulmonary delivery also lowers the amount of drug that is delivered systemically, thus limiting the activation of cardiac β_1-receptors and skeletal muscle β_2-receptors. The most important effects of these agents are relaxation of bronchial smooth muscle and decrease in airway resistance. β_2-Selective agonists are not completely specific for β_2-receptors, however, and adverse effects can include skeletal muscle tremor (through β_2-stimulation) and tachycardia (through β_1-stimulation).

Metaproterenol is the prototype β_2-selective agonist. This drug is used to treat obstructive airway disease and acute bronchospasm. **Terbutaline** and **albuterol** are two other agents in this class that have similar efficacy and duration of action. **Salmeterol** is a long-acting β_2-agonist — its effects last for about 12 hours. The clinical utility of β_2-selective agonists is discussed more fully in Chapter 46, Integrative Inflammation Pharmacology: Asthma.

RECEPTOR ANTAGONISTS

Because of the wide spectrum of disease states that respond to modulation of adrenoceptor activity, antagonists at α- and β-adrenoceptors are among the most widely used medications in clinical practice.

α-Adrenergic Antagonists

α-Adrenergic antagonists block endogenous catecholamines from binding to α_1- and α_2-adrenoceptors. These agents cause vasodilation, decreased blood pressure, and decreased peripheral resistance. The baroreceptor reflex usually attempts to compensate for the fall in blood pressure, resulting in reflex increases in heart rate and cardiac output. **Phenoxybenzamine** blocks both α_1- and α_2-receptors irreversibly. A progressive decrease in peripheral resistance results from the block of α_1-receptors. This, in turn, leads to an increase in cardiac output through reflex sympathetic nerve stimulation. Blockade of α_2-autoreceptors allows more norepinephrine to be released by noradrenergic neurons, and tachycardia ensues from the resulting increase in β_1-receptor stimulation. In addition, phenoxybenzamine inhibits catecholamine uptake into both adrenergic nerve terminals and extraneuronal tissues. Because of its many direct and indirect effects on the sympathetic nervous system, phenoxybenzamine is generally employed only in the preoperative management of pheochromocytoma. **Phentolamine** is a reversible, nonselective α-adrenoceptor antagonist. This drug can also be used in the preoperative management of pheochromocytoma. Phentolamine was the ideal agent for use in introductory case, because it blocked the α-adrenergic–mediated vasoconstriction that caused Ms. S's hypertension.

Prazosin has a 1,000-fold greater affinity for α_1-receptors than for α_2-receptors. Its selective blockade of α_1-receptors in arterioles and veins results in decreased peripheral vascular resistance and dilation of the venous (capacitance) vessels. The latter effect decreases venous return to the heart; because of this reduction in cardiac preload, prazosin has little tendency to increase cardiac output and heart rate. Thus, reflex tachycardia does not typically occur. Prazosin is occasionally used as an antihypertensive. Because patients may experience marked postural hypotension and syncope with the first dose, this dose is generally prescribed in small quantities at bedtime (to ensure that the patient remains supine). Other agents in this class include **terazosin** and **doxazosin;** these agents have a longer half-life than prazosin, allowing less frequent dosing.

Because α_1-adrenoceptors mediate contraction of genitourinary as well as vascular smooth muscle, α_1-antagonists have found clinical application in the symptomatic treatment of benign prostatic hyperplasia (BPH). α1-Adrenoceptor antagonists may be more efficacious than finasteride (a 5α-reductase inhibitor; see Chapter 28, Pharmacology of Reproduction) in the medical treatment of BPH. It has recently been discovered that three subtypes of the α_1-receptor exist, termed α_{1A}, α_{1B}, and α_{1C}. Evidence points to preferential expression of the α_{1A}-receptor in genitourinary smooth muscle. **Tamsulosin** is a specific antagonist at α_{1A}-receptors; this agent has little effect at α_{1B}- or α_{1C}-subtypes. The increased specificity of tamsulosin for α_{1A}-receptors may decrease the incidence of orthostatic hypotension relative to that associated with prazosin and other nonsubtype selective α_1-adrenoceptor antagonists.

Selective blockade of α_2-autoreceptors by drugs such as **yohimbine** leads to increased release of norepinephrine, with subsequent stimulation of cardiac β_1-receptors and peripheral vasculature α_1-receptors. α_2-Selective antagonists also cause increased insulin release through blockade of α_2-receptors in the pancreatic islets, which suppress insulin secretion. Yohimbine was used in the past to treat erectile dysfunction, but the phosphodiesterase type 5 inhibitors have widely replaced its use.

β-Adrenergic Antagonists

β-Adrenergic antagonists block the positive chronotropic and inotropic actions of endogenous catecholamines at β_1-receptors, resulting in decreased heart rate and myocardial contractility. These drugs decrease blood pressure in hypertensive patients, but have no effect in normotensive individuals. Long-term use of β-adrenoceptor blockers causes a fall in peripheral vascular resistance, although the mechanism of this effect remains unclear. The decreases in peripheral vascular resistance and cardiac output both contribute to the antihypertensive effect of these drugs. Nonselective β-adrenoceptor antagonists also block β_2-receptors in bronchial smooth muscle, which can cause life-threatening bronchoconstriction in patients with asthma or chronic obstructive pulmonary disease. In addition, nonselective β-receptor blockade may mask symptoms of hypoglycemia in diabetic patients. For these reasons, selective inhibitors of β_1-adrenoceptors have been developed.

Pharmacologic antagonists at β-adrenergic receptors can be divided into nonselective β-antagonists, nonselective β- and α_1-antagonists, partial agonists, and β_1-selective antagonists (Table 9-2). Selective blockers of β_2-adrenergic receptors do not have clinical utility.

Propranolol, nadolol, and **timolol** interact with β_1- and β_2-receptors equally and do not block α-receptors. These agents are used in the treatment of hypertension and angina. Propranolol is extremely lipophilic; at therapeutic plasma levels, its CNS concentration is sufficiently high that sedation and decreased libido may result. An ocular formulation of timolol is used in the treatment of glaucoma.

Labetalol and **carvedilol** block α_1-, β_1-, and β_2-receptors (labetalol also acts as a weak partial agonist at β_2-receptors, but has a 5- to 10-fold greater effect as a β-blocker). The α_1-receptor blockade results in vasodilation, and the β_1-blockade prevents a reflex sympathetic increase in heart rate; both of these effects contribute to a decrease in blood pres-

TABLE 9-2	Selectivity of Beta-Adrenoceptor Antagonists
DRUG	**NOTES**
Nonselective β-Adrenergic Antagonists	
Propranolol	Short half-life
Nadolol	Long half-life
Timolol	Lipophilic, high CNS penetration
Nonselective β- and α_1-Antagonists	
Labetalol	Also partial agonist at β_2-receptors
Carvedilol	Intermediate half-life
β-Adrenergic Partial Agonists	
Pindolol	β-nonselective
Acebutolol	β_1-selective
β_1-Selective Adrenergic Antagonists	
Esmolol	Short half-life (4 minutes)
Metoprolol	Intermediate half-life
Atenolol	Intermediate half-life
Celiprolol	Also agonist at β_2-receptors

CNS, central nervous system.

sure. Because labetalol may cause liver damage, liver function tests should be performed regularly in patients receiving this drug. Both labetalol and carvedilol are used to treat hypertension; the long-term advantages and disadvantages of these drugs relative to those of other β-blockers have not yet been demonstrated.

Pindolol is a partial agonist at β_1- and β_2-receptors. The drug blocks the action of endogenous norepinephrine at β_1-receptors and is useful in treating hypertension. As a partial agonist, pindolol also causes partial stimulation of β_1-receptors, leading to overall smaller decreases in resting heart rate and blood pressure than those caused by pure β-antagonists. Therefore, the drug may be preferable in hypertensive patients who have bradycardia or decreased cardiac reserve. **Acebutolol** is a partial agonist at β_1-adrenoceptors but has no effect at β_2-receptors. This agent is also used to treat hypertension.

Esmolol, metoprolol, and **atenolol** are β_1-selective adrenergic antagonists. The elimination half-life is the main feature that distinguishes among these agents. Esmolol has

an extremely short half-life (3–4 min); metoprolol and atenolol have intermediate half-lives (4–9 hours). Because of its short half-life, esmolol is used for emergency β-blockade, as in thyroid storm (see Chapter 26, Pharmacology of the Thyroid Gland). Clinical trials have suggested that β-blockers, especially metoprolol, prolong life expectancy in patients with moderate to mild heart failure and in patients who have survived a first myocardial infarction (see Chapter 24, Integrative Cardiovascular Pharmacology: Hypertension, Ischemic Heart Disease, and Heart Failure). **Celiprolol** is a β_1-selective antagonist and β_2-selective agonist.

 Conclusion and Future Directions

Adrenergic pharmacology involves drugs that act at every step of adrenergic neurotransmission, from synthesis of catecholamines to stimulation of α- and β-receptors. The drugs discussed in this chapter are mainstays of therapy for psychiatric disorders, hypertension, angina, shock, asthma, pheochromocytoma, and other conditions. The beneficial pharmacologic actions of these drugs, as well as their important adverse effects, can be anticipated from knowledge of their molecular and cellular mechanisms of action and how these actions affect the processes of adrenergic neurotransmission. For example, gene cloning experiments have identified three subtypes of α_1-receptors and three subtypes of α_2-receptors. The clinical relevance of these subtypes has not yet been fully determined, but the development of more selective agonists and antagonists may lead to more effective (and less toxic) therapies for hypertension and prostatic hypertrophy. Although a wide variety of β-blockers currently exists for clinical use, the functional consequence of using a particular β-blocker in a particular clinical situation has often not been delineated. Future research will determine, for example, whether use of a partial agonist is more efficacious in certain patient populations, and the specific parameters for use of β-adrenoceptor antagonists in patients with heart failure.

Suggested Reading

Kirstein SL, Insel PA. Autonomic nervous system pharmacogenomics: a progress report. *Pharmacol Rev* 2004;56:31–52. (*Review of current concepts in pharmacogenomics as applied to adrenoceptor pharmacology.*)

Lefkowitz RJ, Shenoy SK. Transduction of receptor signals by beta-arrestins. *Science* 2005;308:512–517. (*Review of recent advances in adrenergic signaling.*)

Drug Summary Table	Chapter 9 Adrenergic Pharmacology

Drug	Clinical Applications	Serious and Common Adverse Effects	Contraindications	Therapeutic Considerations
INHIBITORS OF CATECHOLAMINE SYNTHESIS				
Mechanism—Inhibit tyrosine hydroxylase, the rate-limiting enzyme in the catecholamine biosynthesis pathway				
α-Methyltyrosine	Pheochromocytoma-associated hypertension	Orthostatic hypotension, sedation	Hypersensitivity to α-methyltyrosine	Used rarely
INHIBITORS OF CATECHOLAMINE STORAGE				
Mechanism—Inhibit catecholamine storage in vesicles, resulting in short-term increase in release of catecholamines from the synaptic terminal but long-term depletion of available pool of catecholamines				
Reserpine	Hypertension	*Cardiac arrhythmia, gastrointestinal hemorrhage, thrombocytopenia, dream anxiety disorder, impotence, psychotic depression* Dizziness, nasal congestion	Active gastrointestinal disease Depression, electroshock therapy Renal failure	Irreversibly damages VMAT, resulting in vesicles that lose the ability to concentrate and store norepinephrine and dopamine Used experimentally to assess whether effect of drug requires its concentration in presynaptic terminals Rarely used as a therapeutic agent due to its irreversible action and its association with psychotic depression
Guanethidine Guanadrel	Hypertension	*Kidney disease, apnea* Orthostatic hypotension, fluid retention, dizziness, blurred vision, impotence	MAOI therapy Heart failure Pheochromocytoma	Guanethidine concentrates in transmitter vesicles and displaces norepinephrine, leading to gradual depletion of norepinephrine; guanadrel has similar mechanism of action as guanethidine Inhibition of cardiac sympathetic nerves leads to reduced cardiac output; inhibition of sympathetic response leads to symptomatic hypotension following exercise
Amphetamine Methylphenidate	Attention deficit hyperactivity disorder (ADHD) Narcolepsy (amphetamine only)	*Hypertension, tachyarrhythmia, Gilles de la Tourette's syndrome, seizure, psychotic disorder with prolonged use* Restlessness, dysphoric mood, rebound fatigue, addiction potential, loss of appetite, irritability, erectile dysfunction	Advanced cardiovascular disease Glaucoma Hyperthyroidism MAOI therapy Severe hypertension	Amphetamine and methylphenidate displace endogenous catecholamines from storage vesicles, weakly inhibit MAO, and block catecholamine reuptake mediated by NET and DAT; dependence and tolerance can occur
Pseudoephedrine	Allergic rhinitis Nasal congestion	*Atrial fibrillation, ventricular premature beats, myocardial ischemia* Hypertension, tachyarrhythmia, rebound congestion, insomnia	Advanced cardiovascular disease MAOI therapy Severe hypertension	Used as an over-the-counter decongestant; often found in cold remedies and appetite suppressants Ephedrine and phenylpropanolamine have been restricted in the US
INHIBITORS OF CATECHOLAMINE REUPTAKE				
Mechanism—Inhibit norepinephrine transporter (NET)-mediated reuptake of catecholamines, potentiating catecholamine action				
Cocaine Imipramine Amitriptyline	See Drug Summary Table: Chapter 10 Local Anesthetic Pharmacology See Drug Summary Table: Chapter 13 Pharmacology of Serotonergic and Central Adrenergic Neurotransmission			

MONOAMINE OXIDASE (MAO) INHIBITORS

Mechanism—Inhibit MAO, increasing catecholamine levels by blocking catecholamine degradation

Drug	Serious and Common Adverse Effects	Clinical Applications
Phenelzine Iproniazid Tranylcypromine Clorgyline Brofaromine Befloxatone Moclobemide Selegiline		See Drug Summary Table: Chapter 13 Pharmacology of Serotonergic and Central Adrenergic Neurotransmission

α1-ADRENERGIC AGONISTS

Mechanism—Selectively activate α1-adrenergic receptors to increase peripheral vascular resistance

Drug	Serious and Common Adverse Effects	Contraindications	Clinical Applications
Methoxamine	*Bradycardia (vagal reflex), ventricular ectopic beat* Hypertension, vasoconstriction, nausea, headache, anxiety	Severe hypertension	Very limited clinical use in the treatment of shock
Phenylephrine Oxymetazoline Tetrahydrazoline	*Cardiac arrhythmia, hypertension* Headache, insomnia, nervousness, rebound nasal congestion	Narrow-angle glaucoma Severe hypertension or tachycardia (contraindication for IV form of phenylephrine)	Ophthalmic hyperemia Nasal congestion Hypotension (phenylephrine only) Used in the non-prescription remedies Afrin® and Visine® (and others) for relief of nasal congestion and ophthalmic hyperemia; rebound of symptoms often accompanies use of these drugs Phenylephrine is also used intravenously in the treatment of shock

α2-ADRENERGIC AGONISTS

Mechanism—Selectively activate central α2-adrenergic autoreceptors and thereby inhibit sympathetic outflow from CNS

Drug	Serious and Common Adverse Effects	Contraindications	Clinical Applications
Clonidine Guanabenz Guanfacine Methyldopa	*Bradycardia, heart failure, hepatotoxicity (methyldopa), autoimmune hemolytic anemia (methyldopa)* Hypotension, constipation, xerostomia, sedation, dizziness	MAO inhibitor therapy and active liver disease (contraindications for use of methyldopa)	Hypertension Opioid withdrawal (clonidine only) Cancer pain (clonidine only) Clonidine is used for treatment of hypertension and symptoms associated with opioid withdrawal Methyldopa is drug of choice for treatment of hypertension during pregnancy

β-ADRENERGIC AGONISTS

Mechanism—Activate β-adrenergic receptors

Drug	Clinical Applications
Isoproterenol Dobutamine	See Drug Summary Table: Chapter 19 Pharmacology of Cardiac Contractility
Metaproterenol Terbutaline Albuterol Salmeterol	See Drug Summary Table: Chapter 46 Integrative Inflammation Pharamacology: Asthma

(Continued)

Drug Summary Table | **Chapter 9 Adrenergic Pharmacology** *(Continued)*

α-ADRENERGIC ANTAGONISTS
Mechanism—Block endogenous catecholamines from binding to α1- and α2-adrenoceptors, causing vasodilation, decreased blood pressure, and decreased peripheral resistance

Drug	Clinical Applications	Serious and Common Adverse Effects	Contraindications	Therapeutic Considerations
Phenoxybenzamine Phentolamine	Pheochromocytoma-associated hypertension and sweating	*Seizure* Postural hypotension, tachycardia, palpitations, xerostomia, sedation, miosis, absence of ejaculation	Severe hypotension Coronary artery disease (phentolamine)	Phenoxybenzamine blocks both α1 and α2 receptors irreversibly Phentolamine is a reversible, non-selective α-adrenoceptor antagonist Used in preoperative management of pheochromocytoma
Prazosin Terazosin Doxazosin	Hypertension Benign prostatic hyperplasia	*Pancreatitis, hepatotoxicity, systemic lupus erythematosus* Marked first-dose postural hypotension, palpitations, dyspepsia, dizziness, sedation, increased urinary frequency, nasal congestion	Hypersensitivity to prazosin, terazosin, or doxazosin	Prazosin, terazosin, and doxazosin are nonsubtype selective antagonists of α1-receptors in arterioles and veins Reflex tachycardia does not usually occur Due to potential severe postural hypotension, first dose is generally prescribed in small quantities at bedtime (to ensure that the patient remains supine) Terazosin and doxazosin have a longer half-life than prazosin Tricylic antidepressants may increase the risk of postural hypotension
Tamsulosin	Benign prostatic hyperplasia	Same as prazosin, except less postural hypotension	Hypersensitivity to tamsulosin	Tamsulosin is a subtype-selective α1A-receptor antagonist that has more specificity toward smooth muscle in genitourinary tract; thus, tamsulosin has lower incidence of orthostatic hypotension
Yohimbine	Organic and psychogenic impotence	Bronchospasm, nervousness, tremor, anxiety, agitation, increased blood pressure, antidiuresis	Chronic inflammation of sexual organs or prostate gland Concurrent use with mood altering drugs Gastric and duodenal ulcers Pregnancy Psychiatric patients Renal and liver disease	Yohimbine is an α2-selective antagonist that leads to increased release of norepinephrine, which stimulates cardiac β1-receptors and peripheral vascular α1-receptors Also leads to increased insulin release due to blockade of α2-receptors in pancreatic islets

β-ADRENERGIC ANTAGONISTS

Mechanism—Block β-adrenergic receptors; this class of drugs can be divided into nonselective β antagonists, nonselective β and α1 antagonists, partial agonists, and β1-selective antagonists

Drugs	Clinical Applications	Adverse Effects	Contraindications	Therapeutic Considerations
Propranolol Nadolol Timolol	Hypertension Angina Heart failure Pheochromocytoma Glaucoma (timolol ocular formulation)	*Bronchospasm, atrioventricular block, bradyarrhythmia* Sedation, decreased libido, mask symptoms of hypoglycemia, depression, dyspnea, wheezing	Bronchial asthma or chronic obstructive pulmonary disease Cardiogenic shock Uncompensated cardiac failure Second- and third-degree AV block Severe sinus bradycardia	Propranolol, nadolol, and timolol block β1- and β2-receptors equally Propranolol is extremely lipophilic; its CNS concentration is sufficiently high that sedation and decreased libido may result An ocular formulation of timolol is used in the treatment of glaucoma
Labetalol Carvedilol	Hypertension Angina	Same as propranolol Additionally, labetalol can cause hepatotoxicity	Same as propranolol	Labetalol and carvedilol block α1-, β1-, and β2-receptors Labetalol may cause liver damage; liver function tests must be monitored
Pindolol Acebutolol	Hypertension Angina	Same as propranolol	Same as propranolol	Pindolol is a partial agonist at β1- and β2-receptors; it is preferred in hypertensive patients who have bradycardia or decreased cardiac reserve Acebutolol is a partial agonist at β1-adrenoceptors but has no effect at β2-receptors
Esmolol Metoprolol Atenolol Celiprolol	Hypertension Angina Heart failure Thyroid storm (esmolol)	Same as propranolol, except less bronchospasm	Same as propranolol	Esmolol, metoprolol, and atenolol are β1-selective adrenergic antagonists Esmolol has an extremely short half-life (3–4 min) and thus is used for emergency β blockade, as in thyroid storm; celiprolol is a β1-selective antagonist and β2-selective agonist

10

Local Anesthetic Pharmacology

Joshua M. Schulman and Gary R. Strichartz

INTRODUCTION

The word *"anesthesia"* comes directly from the Greek: "an" meaning without, and "aisthesis" meaning feeling or sensation. **Local anesthetics (LAs)** are a set of locally applied chemicals, with similar molecular structures, that can both inhibit the perception of sensations (importantly pain) and prevent movement. They are used in a variety of situations, ranging from topical application for burns and small cuts, to injections during dental care, to epidural and intrathecal ("spinal") blocks during obstetric procedures and major surgery.

Cocaine, the first local anesthetic, comes from the leaves of the coca shrub (*Erythroxylon coca*). It was first isolated in 1860 by Albert Niemann, who noted its numbing powers. In 1886, Carl Koller introduced cocaine into clinical practice as a topical ophthalmic anesthetic. However, its addictive properties and toxicity prompted the search for substitutes. **Procaine,** the first of these substitutes, was synthesized in 1905. Known as Novocain®, it is still used today, although less frequently than some more recently developed LAs.

Local anesthetics exert their effect by blocking voltage-gated sodium channels, thus inhibiting the propagation of action potentials along neurons (see Chapter 6, Principles of Cellular Excitability and Electrochemical Transmission). By inhibiting action potential propagation, LAs prevent transmission of information to and from the central nervous system (CNS). LAs are not selective for pain fibers; they can also block other sensory, motor, and autonomic fibers, as well as action potentials in skeletal and cardiac muscle. This nonselective blockade can serve other useful functions (see Chapter 18, Pharmacology of Cardiac Rhythm) or can be a source of toxicity.

 Case

EM is a 24-year-old graduate student in organic chemistry. While working in the lab one evening, he spills a beaker of hydrofluoric acid (HF) in the fume hood. Although he reflexively jerks his hand away, some of the liquid falls on the fingertips of his left hand. Some minutes later, EM feels a stinging pain, which increases in intensity and is followed by a burning, throbbing ache. Realizing the corrosiveness of the acid, EM begins rinsing his hand with water and a magnesium sulfate solution (the magnesium chelates the toxic fluoride ions). He also telephones 911 and is transported to the Emergency Department.

The resident notes that the acid has penetrated the nail beds of the affected fingers, and that EM is in severe pain. She commends him on his timely and appropriate actions, and decides on treatment with calcium gluconate (another fluoride chelator) to neutralize the remaining HF, in conjunction with a digital nerve block to reduce the pain. Lidocaine without epinephrine is injected into the fingers, followed by calcium gluconate. EM first notices a relief of the stinging, although the ache takes somewhat longer to fade. By the time his wounds are dressed, he cannot feel any sensation in his fingers. Over the next 2 weeks, EM's wounds heal spontaneously and the pain, now well controlled with ibuprofen, abates. He is able to plunge back into lab work, but his brush with serious injury affects him in an unforeseen way: he begins to contemplate applying to medical school.

QUESTIONS

■ **1.** What is lidocaine's mechanism of action? To which broader class of drugs does it belong?

■ **2.** Why did EM initially experience a stinging pain before the dull aching pain, and why did the stinging pain resolve more quickly than the dull pain after lidocaine administration?

■ **3.** Why is epinephrine sometimes administered with lidocaine, and why was it not co-administered in this case?

PHYSIOLOGY OF NOCICEPTION

Nociception is the activation of primary sensory nerve fibers (nociceptors) by noxious stimuli, that is, stimuli that are potentially tissue damaging. These include high temperatures, intense mechanical perturbations, and harsh chemicals. Nociceptors have free nerve endings located in the skin, deep soma, and viscera. Nociceptor cell bodies are located in the dorsal root ganglia close to the spinal cord or in the trigeminal ganglion for innervation of the face (Fig. 10-1). Nociceptors transmit impulses from the periphery to the dorsal horn of the spinal cord, where the information is subsequently processed through synaptic circuitry and transmitted to various parts of the brain. Thus, nociceptors are the first in a chain of neurons responsible for pain perception. Because nociceptors transmit information toward the brain, they are termed **afferent neurons.**

Tissue damage is the primary stimulus for nociceptor ac-

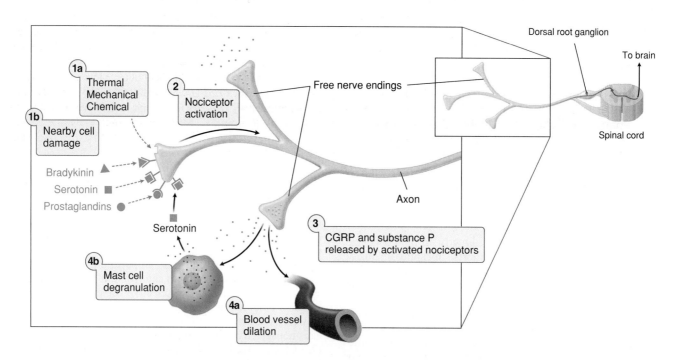

Figure 10-1. Nociceptor activation. Nociceptors transmit pain information using a variety of mechanisms. Some receptors transduce noxious stimuli (thermal, mechanical, or chemical) into electric potentials. Other receptors are stimulated by substances that are released when nearby cells are injured (bradykinin, serotonin, prostaglandins). The release of K$^+$ from nearby damaged cells directly depolarizes nociceptor membranes. All of these stimuli cause nociceptor "sensitization," which decreases the threshold for activation. **1a.** A noxious stimulus leads to nociceptor activation and action potential generation **(2). 1b.** Concurrent nearby cell damage causes nociceptor sensitization. **3.** Activated nociceptors release substances, including substance P and calcitonin gene related peptide (CGRP), that contribute to further sensitization and that initiate inflammatory responses to promote healing. For example: **4a.** Blood vessel dilation promotes white blood cell recruitment to the area; and **4b.** Mast cell degranulation releases histamine and serotonin, thus increasing sensitization.

tivation. Nociceptors do not transmit information about a breeze against one's skin or a firm touch, for example (the nerves that do this are termed **tactile** or **low-threshold mechanoreceptors**). Rather, nociceptors are activated when, for example, one touches a hot stove or slams a door on one's fingers (or spills acid on them). Nociceptors have receptors in their cell membranes for substances, such as **bradykinin,** that are released when nearby cells are injured. These transducing receptors convert noxious stimuli into "generator currents" that depolarize the neuron and can result in action potentials (Fig. 10-1).

For sensory stimuli whose intensity is above the nociceptor's threshold (e.g., above a certain temperature), the frequency of action potential generation increases as the stimulus intensity is elevated. If impulses in the nociceptive afferents are sufficiently frequent, they are perceived as "painful." In a local (or segmental) circuit response, nociceptive afferent axons also connect indirectly via interneurons to efferent (motor) neurons in the spinal cord, which then travel to the periphery and cause muscle movement. The motion of jerking one's hand away after touching a hot stove, which is a more complex response than the local circuit response described above, is nevertheless initiated in this manner by nociceptors and mediated by spinal circuits.

TRANSMISSION OF PAIN SENSATION

In their simplest form, neurons are composed of dendrites, a cell body, and an axon. Axons transmit information along the neuron from the cell body or from free nerve endings to dendrites, which synapse with other neurons. Depending on the diameter of the axons and their myelination status, axons are classified as **A-fibers, B-fibers,** or **C-fibers.** A-fibers and B-fibers are myelinated, while C-fibers are nonmyelinated (Table 10-1). Myelin is composed of the cell membranes of supportive cells in the nervous system, including Schwann cells in the peripheral nervous system and oligodendrocytes in the CNS. These supportive cell membranes wrap many times around neuronal axons to form an electrically insulating sheath that greatly increases the velocity of impulse transmission.

The most important fibers for pain perception are the axons of afferent nociceptors, including the anatomically classified **Aδ-fibers** and **C-fibers.** The afferent nociceptors comprise *thermal* nociceptors that are activated at temperatures above 45°C (C-fibers) or below 5°C (Aδ-fibers), *high-threshold mechanical* nociceptors that exclusively transmit information indicating injurious force on the skin (Aδ- and some Aβ-fibers), and *polymodal* nociceptors that are activated by thermal, chemical, and mechanical stimuli (C-fibers).

First Pain and Second Pain

The myelinated Aδ-fibers transmit impulses much faster than do the nonmyelinated C-fibers (Fig. 10-2). An Aδ-fiber transmits impulses along its axon at a rate of 5–25 meters per second (m/s), while C-fibers transmit impulses at roughly 1 m/s. Impulse transmission is slower in C-fibers primarily because these fibers are nonmyelinated.

The Aδ-fibers transmit what is called **first pain.** First pain is transmitted quickly, is sharp ("pinprick-like") in quality, and is highly localized on the body. The density of Aδ-fibers is high on the fingertips, face, and lips but relatively low on the back. Aδ-fibers require a weaker stimulus for excitation than do C-fibers.

C-fiber nociceptors are predominantly polymodal, which means that they can be activated by noxious thermal, chemical, and mechanical stimuli. Impulses in these C-fibers are responsible for what is called **second pain.** Second pain is slower to develop but longer lasting; it feels dull, throbbing or burning, is only diffusely localizable, and endures after the stimulus ends. In the case presented above, EM experienced an initial stinging first pain transmitted by myelinated Aδ-fibers, and a later burning and throbbing second pain transmitted by unmyelinated C-fibers.

TABLE 10-1	Types of Peripheral Nerve Fibers				
FIBER TYPE	**MYELINATED**	**DIAMETER (μm)**	**CONDUCTION VELOCITY (m/s)**	**FUNCTION**	**SENSITIVITY TO LIDOCAINE**
Aα, Aβ	Yes	6–22	10–85	Motor and proprioception (pressure, touch, position)	+, + +
Aγ	Yes	3–6	15–35	Muscle tone	+ +
Aδ	Yes	1–4	5–25	First pain and temperature	+ + +
B	Yes	<3	3–15	Vasomotor, visceromotor, sudomotor, pilomotor	+ + + +
C (sympathetic)	No	0.3–1.3	0.7–1.3	Vasomotor, visceromotor, sudomotor, pilomotor	+ + + +
C (dorsal root)	No	0.4–1.2	0.1–2.0	Second pain and temperature	+ + + +

Each peripheral nerve fiber type is responsible for transmitting one or more specific modalities. For example, the nociceptors (Aδ and C dorsal root fibers) are responsible for transmitting pain and temperature sensations. These fibers are not activated by pressure, light touch, or position changes. Myelin is an insulator that allows impulses to be conducted at faster speeds along axons. The nonmyelinated C-fibers have a slower conduction velocity than do the myelinated fibers. The different fiber types are affected by local anesthetics with different sensitivities.

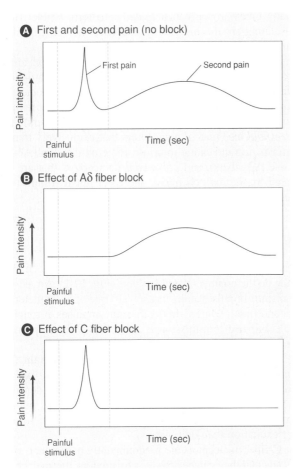

Figure 10-2.   First and second pain. First pain, which is transmitted by Aδ-fibers, is sharp and highly localizable. Second pain, which is transmitted by C-fibers, is slower in arriving, duller, and longer lasting **(A)**. First pain can be prevented by selective blockade of Aδ-fibers **(B)**, and second pain can be prevented by selective blockade of C-fibers **(C)**. Because Aδ-fibers are more susceptible than C-fibers to blockade by local anesthetics, first pain often disappears at concentrations of anesthetic lower than those required to eliminate second pain.

PAIN PERCEPTION

Impulses generated in the skin by nociceptor activation are carried by Aδ- and C-fibers to the dorsal horn of the spinal cord. In the dorsal horn, the nociceptors form synapses with interneurons and second-order neurons. The second-order neurons travel in the lateral areas of the spinal cord and project mainly to the thalamus, a gray-matter structure just superior to the brainstem. The thalamus has cells that project to the somatosensory cortex of the parietal lobe and to other areas of the cortex (Fig. 10-3). Pain perception is a complex process that normally results from the activation of non-nociceptive as well as nociceptive afferents, and can be altered depending on the situation, the person's state of mind, and other factors. The CNS uses efferent projections within the brain and spinal cord to modulate the incoming nociceptive signals, and thus to modify pain perception. For example, an athlete focused on an important game might not feel

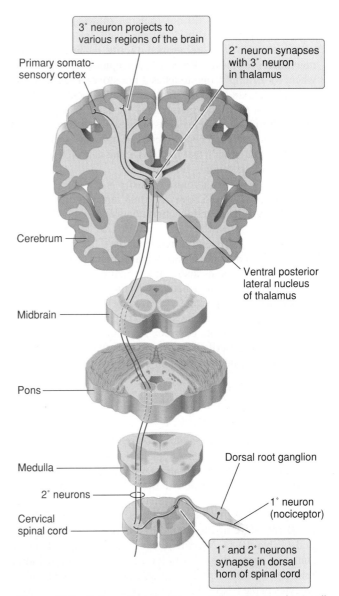

Figure 10-3.   Pain pathways. Primary (1°) nociceptors have cell bodies in the dorsal root ganglion, and synapse with secondary (2°) afferent neurons in the dorsal horn of the spinal cord. Primary afferents use the neurotransmitter glutamate. The 2° afferents travel in the lateral areas of the spinal cord and eventually reach the thalamus, where they synapse with tertiary (3°) afferent neurons. The processing of pain is complex, and 3° afferents have many destinations including the somatosensory cortex (localization of pain) and the limbic system (emotional aspects of pain).

the pain of an injury intensely until after the game is over. Her brain modulates the effect of the input so that the same stimulus is less painful at certain times than at others.

ANALGESIA AND ANESTHESIA

The terms "analgesic" and "anesthetic" are frequently confused. **Analgesics** are specific inhibitors of *pain* pathways, whereas **local anesthetics** are *nonspecific* inhibitors of peripheral sensory (including pain), motor, and autonomic pathways. Analgesics have actions at specific receptors on primary nociceptors and in the CNS (see Chapter 16, Pharmacology of Analgesia). For example, opioid analgesics activate opiate receptors, which signal cells to increase potassium conductance in postsynaptic neurons and to decrease calcium entry into presynaptic neurons. By these mechanisms, postsynaptic excitability and presynaptic transmitter release are reduced, and pain sensations are not transmitted as effectively to the brain (or within it). Importantly, the transmission of other sensations and motor information is not affected.

Local anesthetics act by a different mechanism. These agents inhibit conduction of action potentials in all afferent and efferent nerve fibers, usually in the peripheral nervous system. Thus, pain and other sensory modalities are not transmitted effectively to the brain, and motor impulses are not transmitted effectively to muscles in the periphery.

PHARMACOLOGIC CLASSES AND AGENTS

Local anesthetics can be classified as **ester-linked LAs** or **amide-linked LAs.** Because all LAs share similar properties, the next section highlights the general principles of LA pharmacology. Specific LA agents are discussed at the end of the chapter.

CHEMISTRY OF LOCAL ANESTHETICS

All local anesthetics have three structural domains: an aromatic group, an amine group, and an ester or amide linkage connecting these two groups (Fig. 10-4). As discussed below, the structure of the aromatic group influences the hydrophobicity of the drug, the nature of the amine group influences the rate of onset and potency of the drug, and the structure of the amide or ester group influences the duration of action and side effects of the drug.

Aromatic Group

All local anesthetics contain an aromatic group that gives the molecule much of its hydrophobic character. Adding substituents on the aromatic ring, or on the amino nitrogen, can alter the hydrophobicity of the drug.

Biological membranes have a hydrophobic interior because of their lipid bilayer structure. The hydrophobicity of a LA drug affects the ease with which the drug passes through nerve cell membranes to reach its target site, which is the cytoplasmic side of the voltage-gated sodium channel (Fig. 10-5). Molecules with low hydrophobicity partition very poorly into the membrane because their solubility in the lipid bilayer is so low; such molecules are largely restricted to the polar aqueous extracellular environment. As the hydrophobicity of a series of drugs increases, the permeability of those drugs through the cell membrane also increases. However, at a certain hydrophobicity this relationship reverses, and a further increase in hydrophobicity

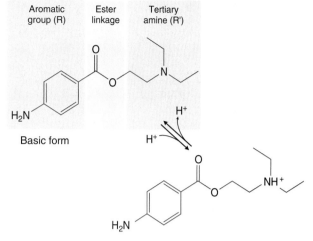

Ⓐ Ester-linked local anesthetic (procaine)

Basic form

Protonated (acidic) form

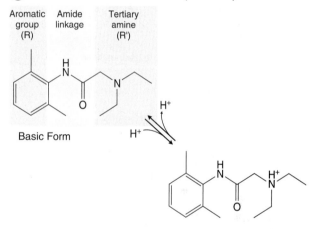

Ⓑ Amide-linked local anesthetic (lidocaine)

Basic Form

Protonated (acidic) form

Figure 10-4. Prototypical local anesthetics. Procaine **(A)** and lidocaine **(B)** are prototypical ester-linked and amide-linked local anesthetics, respectively. Local anesthetics have an aromatic group on one end and an amine on the other end of the molecule; these two groups are connected by an ester (-RCOOR′) or amide (-RHNCOR′) linkage. In solution at high pH, the equilibrium between the basic (neutral) and acidic (charged) forms of a local anesthetic favors the basic form. At low pH, the equilibrium favors the acidic form. At intermediate (physiological) pH, nearly equal concentrations of the basic and acidic forms are present. Generally, ester-linked local anesthetics are easily hydrolyzed to a carboxylic acid (RCOOH) and an alcohol (HOR′) in the presence of water and esterases. In comparison, amides are far more stable in solution. Consequently, amide-linked local anesthetics generally have a longer duration of action than do ester-linked anesthetics.

results in a decrease in permeability. This somewhat paradoxical behavior occurs because very hydrophobic molecules partition strongly into the cell membrane and remain there. Although such molecules are concentrated in the cell membrane, they dissociate from the membrane very slowly because of the hydrophobic interactions that stabilize them there. In other words, their free energy of partitioning into the membrane is so great that they are essentially trapped.

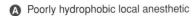

A Poorly hydrophobic local anesthetic

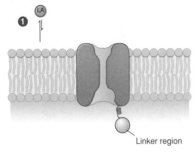

Linker region

B Moderately hydrophobic local anesthetic

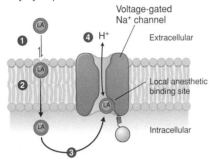

Voltage-gated
Na$^+$ channel

Extracellular

Local anesthetic
binding site

Intracellular

C Extremely hydrophobic local anesthetic

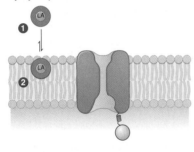

Figure 10-5. Local anesthetic hydrophobicity, diffusion, and binding. Local anesthetics act by binding to the cytoplasmic (intracellular) side of the voltage-gated Na$^+$ channel. The hydrophobicity of a local anesthetic determines how efficiently it diffuses across lipid membranes and how tightly it binds to the Na$^+$ channel, and therefore governs its potency. **A.** Poorly hydrophobic LAs are unable to cross the lipid bilayer efficiently: (1) Neutral LA cannot adsorb to or enter the neuronal cell membrane because the LA is very stable in the extracellular solution and has a very high activation energy for entering the hydrophobic membrane. **B.** Moderately hydrophobic local anesthetics (LAs) are the most effective agents: (1) Neutral LA adsorbs to the extracellular side of the neuronal cell membrane; (2) LA diffuses through the cell membrane to the cytoplasmic side; (3) LA diffuses and binds to its binding site on the voltage-gated sodium channel; (4) once bound, LA can switch between its neutral and protonated forms by binding and releasing protons. **C.** Extremely hydrophobic LAs become trapped in the lipid bilayer: (1) Neutral LA adsorbs to the neuronal cell membrane (2) where it is so stabilized that it cannot dissociate from or translocate across the membrane.

An effective local anesthetic must partition into, diffuse across, and finally dissociate from the membrane; the compounds most likely to do so have moderate hydrophobicity.

The LA binding site on the sodium channel also contains hydrophobic residues. Therefore, more hydrophobic drugs bind more tightly to the target site, increasing the potency of the drug. However, because of the practical need for the drug to diffuse across several membranes in order to reach the target site, LAs with moderate hydrophobicity are the clinically most effective forms. Excessively hydrophobic drugs have limited solubility in the aqueous environment around a nerve, and even the molecules that do dissolve remain in the first membrane that is encountered, never reaching the target site (despite their high affinity for that site).

Amine Group

The amine group of a local anesthetic molecule can exist in either the protonated (positively charged) form, also known as the *conjugate acid,* or the deprotonated (neutral) form, also known as the *conjugate base.*

The pKa is the pH at which the concentrations of a base and its conjugate acid are equal. LAs are weak bases; their pKa values range from about 8 to 10. Thus, at the physiologic pH of 7.4, both the protonated form and the neutral form exist in solution. As the pKa of a drug increases, a greater fraction of molecules exists in solution in the protonated form at physiologic pH (see Chapter 1, Drug–Receptor Interactions). Protonation and deprotonation reactions are very rapid in solution, but drugs in membranes are protonated and deprotonated more slowly.

The neutral forms of LAs cross membranes much more easily than do the positively charged forms. However, the positively charged forms bind with much higher affinity to the drugs' target binding site. This site is located in the pore of the voltage-gated sodium channel and is accessible from the intracellular entrance of the channel. This is why moderately hydrophobic weak bases are so effective as local anesthetics. At physiologic pH, a significant fraction of the weak base molecules are in the neutral form that, because of its moderate hydrophobicity, can cross membranes to enter nerve cells. Once the drug is inside the cell, it can then rapidly gain a proton, become positively charged, and bind with higher affinity to the sodium channel.

Surprisingly, the major path by which protons reach the drug molecules that bind to the Na$^+$ channel is through the channel's pore to the extracellular environment. As the extracellular pH becomes more acidic, there is a higher chance that the drug will become protonated at its binding site in the channel. Once protonated, the drug dissociates much more slowly from the channel. The pH inside the cell does not have an important effect on the protonation state of drug molecules that are already bound to the channel; this lack of effect is thought to be attributable to the orientation of the drug within the channel. Some nonionizable drugs, such as benzocaine, are permanently neutral but are still able to block sodium channels and action potentials. For these drugs, however, the block is weak and does not depend on extracellular pH.

MECHANISM OF ACTION OF LOCAL ANESTHETICS

Anatomic Considerations

The peripheral nerve is composed of a collection of different types of nerve fibers (A-, B-, and C-fibers) surrounded by three protective membranes, or "sheaths": the epineurium, perineurium, and endoneurium. Local anesthetic molecules

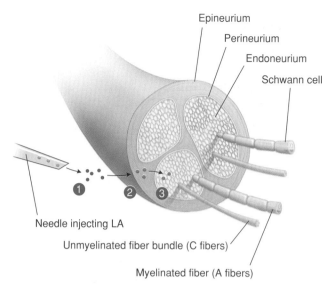

Figure 10-6. Peripheral nerve anatomy. 1. Local anesthetics (LAs) are injected or otherwise applied outside the peripheral nerve epineurium (the outermost sheath of connective tissue containing blood vessels, adipose tissue, fibroblasts, and mast cells). **2.** LA molecules must cross the epineurium to reach the perineurium, another epithelial membrane, which organizes nerve fibers into fascicles. The perineurium is the most difficult layer for local anesthetics to penetrate, because of the tight junctions between its cells. **3.** LAs then pass through the endoneurium, which envelops the myelinated and unmyelinated fibers, Schwann cells, and capillaries. Only LAs that have passed through these three sheaths can reach the neuronal membranes where the voltage-gated sodium channels reside. Clinically, a high concentration of local anesthetic must be applied because only a fraction of the molecules reach the target site.

must pass through these sheaths (presenting the same permeation-limiting barriers as the nerve cell membranes considered above) before they can reach the neuronal membranes (Fig. 10-6). The sheaths are made up of connective tissue and cellular membranes. LAs are injected outside the most external sheath, the epineurium, to avoid mechanical needle damage to the nerve, but the major barrier to LA penetration into the nerve is the perineurium, an epithelium-like tissue that bundles axons into separate fascicles. Recall that LAs affect not only nociceptors but also other afferent and efferent, somatic and autonomic nerve fibers. All of these fibers may be contained within a peripheral nerve, and conduction in all fibers can be blocked by local anesthetics. If the peripheral nerve is considered to represent a multilane road, then each fiber type can be considered a lane in this road. A blockade across the whole road (the blockade by a local anesthetic) will stop traffic in all lanes in both directions. This is why, in the introductory case, EM experienced not only loss of pain sensation, but also a more complete block of all sensation in his digits.

In general, more proximal regions of the body (shoulder, thigh) are innervated by axons traveling relatively superficially in a peripheral nerve, while more distal regions (hands, feet) are innervated by axons traveling closer to the core of the nerve. Because local anesthetics are applied to the outside of a peripheral nerve, external to the epineurium, the axons innervating more proximal areas are usually reached first by the local anesthetic diffusing into the nerve. Conse-

quently, *the anatomic progression of functional block shows that proximal areas are numbed before distal areas.* For example, if a nerve block is applied in the brachial plexus, the shoulder and upper arm are numbed before the forearm, hand, and fingers.

During the onset of local anesthesia, different fiber types within a peripheral nerve are also blocked at different times due to their intrinsic susceptibility to blockade and the LA's concentration gradient within the nerve. The general order in which functional deficits occur is as follows: first pain, second pain, temperature, touch, proprioception (pressure, position, or stretch), and finally skeletal muscle tone and voluntary tension. This phenomenon is referred to as **differential functional blockade.** In the introductory case, recall that EM's first pain was blocked before his second pain, and that block of both preceded the loss of his other sensory modalities. Clinically, if a patient is still able to feel the sharp pain of a pinprick, then the degree of anesthesia is unlikely to be sufficient to block the transmission of long-lasting second pain.

Because motor function is often the last ability to be lost, it is possible for some LAs to block nociception with relatively little effect on motor transmission. The concentration of local anesthetic required to block sensory impulses without inducing a large motor blockade varies for different agents. With lidocaine, for example, it is difficult to block Aδ-fibers without also blocking Aγ-motor fibers (Table 10-1); in contrast, epidural bupivacaine can achieve sensory block at low concentrations without significant motor block. For this reason, dilute epidural bupivacaine is frequently used during labor, as it relieves pain while still allowing the parturient woman to ambulate.

Voltage-Gated Sodium Channel

Local anesthetics prevent impulse transmission by blocking individual sodium channels in neuronal membranes. The sodium channel exists in three main conformational states: open, inactivated, and resting. In going from the resting to the open state, the channel also moves through several transient "closed" conformations. The resting neuronal membrane potential is −60 to −70 millivolts (mV). At this potential, the channels are in equilibrium between the resting state (majority) and the inactivated state (minority). During an action potential, the resting channels move through the closed conformations and finally open briefly to allow sodium ions to enter the cell. This sodium influx results in depolarization of the membrane. After a few milliseconds, the open channel spontaneously undergoes a conformational change to the inactivated state. This halts the influx of sodium, and the membrane repolarizes.

The inactivated state of the channel returns slowly to the resting state in the repolarized membrane. The time needed to make this transition largely determines the length of the refractory period. During the absolute refractory period, there are so few Na^+ channels in the resting state that, even if all of the resting-state channels were simultaneously activated to the open state, threshold would not be reached. Thus, no new action potentials can be generated during this period of time (Fig. 10-7A).

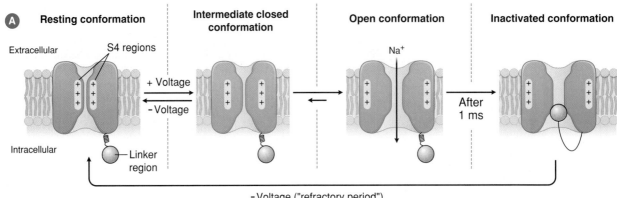

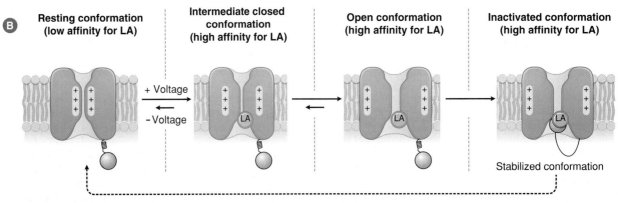

Figure 10-7.   Local anesthetic binding to different conformations (states) of the sodium channel. A. The sodium channel is composed of one polypeptide chain that has four repeating units. One region, known as the S4 region, has many positively charged amino acids (lysine and arginine). These residues give the channel its voltage dependence. At rest, the pore is closed. When the membrane is depolarized, the charged residues move in response to the change in the electric field. This results in several conformational changes (intermediate closed states) that culminate in channel opening. After about 1 ms (the channel open time), the 3–4 amino acid "linker region" plugs the open channel, yielding the inactivated conformation. The inactivated conformation returns to the resting state only when the membrane is repolarized; this conformational change involves the return of the S4 region to its original position and the expulsion of the linker region. The time required for the channel to return from the inactivated state to the resting state is known as the *refractory period;* during this period, the sodium channel is incapable of being activated. **B.** The binding of local anesthetic (LA) alters the properties of the intermediate forms assumed by the sodium channel. Sodium channels in any of the conformations (resting, closed, open, or inactivated) can bind local anesthetic molecules, although the resting state has a low affinity for LA, while the other three states have a high affinity for LA. LA can dissociate from the channel–LA complex in any conformational state, or the channel can undergo conformational changes while associated with the LA molecule. Ultimately, the channel–LA complex must dissociate, and the sodium channel must return to the resting state to become activated. LA binding extends the refractory period, including both the time required for dissociation of the LA molecule from the sodium channel and the time required for the channel to return to the resting state.

Modulated Receptor Hypothesis

The different conformational states of the sodium channel (resting, various closed, open, and inactivated) bind local anesthetics with different affinities. This concept is known as the **modulated receptor hypothesis** (Fig. 10-7B and Table 10-2).

Local anesthetics have a higher affinity for the closed, open, and inactivated states of the sodium channel than for the resting state. Although the LA binds at a site in the channel's pore, the molecular mechanism of channel inhibition involves not only the physical occlusion of the pore, but also the restriction of activation of the channel. The binding of drug to the closed states that occur during the sequential activation process seems to limit the conformational

changes of the sodium channel, so that a drug-bound channel cannot undergo the full range of conformational changes necessary to open the channel.

For a drug-bound channel to reopen, the LA must dissociate from the channel and, thus, allow the channel to return to its resting state. This dissociation of drug (the rate of which varies among the different LAs) is slower than the normal recovery from the inactivated to the resting channel conformation in the absence of LA. Thus, LAs extend the refractory period of the neuron by delaying the inactivated channel's return to the resting state by about 50-fold to 100-fold. At high concentrations, LAs bind to a sufficient number of low-affinity resting channels that impulse conduction is prevented altogether. In fact, this is almost certainly the situ-

TABLE 10-2	Modulated Receptor Hypothesis	
CHANNEL STATE	**AFFINITY FOR LA**	**RELATIVE EFFECT ON CHANNEL**
Resting	Low	Prevents channel opening (only at high LA concentrations)
Closed (several)	High	Prevents channel opening (major effect)
Open	High	Blocks channel pore (minor effect)
Inactive	High	Extends refractory period (major effect)

The voltage-gated sodium channel can assume several different conformations. Local anesthetics have different affinities for different conformations of the channel; this differential affinity alters the kinetics of sodium channel activation (see Fig. 10-7).

ation that occurs during a complete clinical block of peripheral nerve.

Tonic and Phasic Inhibition

The differential affinity of local anesthetics for different states of the voltage-gated sodium channel has an important pharmacologic consequence: the degree of inhibition of sodium current by the LA depends on the frequency of impulses in the nerve. When there is a long interval between action potentials, the level of inhibition of each impulse is the same, and the inhibition is said to be tonic. But when the interval between action potentials is short, the level of inhibition increases with each successive impulse, and the inhibition is said to be phasic, or use-dependent (Fig. 10-8).

Tonic inhibition occurs when the time between action potentials is long compared to the time for dissociation of the LA from the sodium channel. Assume, for example, that before an action potential arrives, an equilibrium has been established where 5% of the sodium channels are bound by local anesthetic molecules. When an action potential arrives, the other 95% of the channels are available to open and subsequently to inactivate. During the impulse, some of these channels become bound by local anesthetic molecules. However, there is sufficient time before the next impulse arrives at the LA-exposed region for many of the LA-sodium channel complexes to dissociate and for those channels to return to the resting state. Thus, before the next action potential arrives, the 5% binding equilibrium is re-established. The next action potential will, therefore, be blocked to the same extent as the previous one.

Phasic inhibition occurs when there is not enough time between action potentials for this equilibrium to be re-established. Rapidly arriving action potentials cause resting sodium channels to open and then inactivate, and some of these channels will be bound by LAs. However, because there is not enough time between impulses for all of the newly formed LA-sodium channel complexes to dissociate, only some of the channels are able to return to the resting state. With each arriving action potential, more and more channels are blocked until a new steady state of LA-sodium channel binding is reached. This is the phenomenon of phasic, or use-dependent, inhibition. As more of the channels are converted to LA-bound complexes, fewer and fewer channels are available to open when the next action potential arrives. Consequently, *action potential conduction is increasingly inhibited at higher frequencies of impulses.*

The clinical importance of this phenomenon is that tissue injury or trauma causes nociceptors in the area of injury to fire at high rates. Therefore, application of a local anesthetic will tend to block local nociceptors in a phasic manner, inhibiting pain transmission to a greater extent than other local sensory or motor impulses that are blocked only tonically.

Other Receptors for Local Anesthetics

In addition to blocking sodium channels, local anesthetics can have a wide range of other biochemical and physiologic effects. LAs can interact with potassium channels, calcium channels, ligand-gated channels (such as the nicotinic acetylcholine receptor), transient receptor potential (trp) channels, and several G protein-coupled receptors (including muscarinic cholinergic receptors, β-adrenergic receptors, and receptors for substance P). LAs can also uncouple some G proteins from their cell surface receptors, and thus inhibit signal transduction. In most cases, these effects are not significant because LAs have lower affinity for these other receptors than for the sodium channel. But for some types of local anesthetics in some clinical situations, these alternate targets may have important therapeutic and toxic consequences.

For example, in spinal anesthesia, a high concentration of local anesthetic is injected into the cerebrospinal fluid, from which the LA then diffuses into the spinal cord. Neuropeptides (such as **substance P**) and small organic neurotransmitters (such as glutamate) mediate the transmission of nociceptive impulses between the primary and secondary afferent neurons in the dorsal horn of the spinal cord (see above). Evidence from in vivo and in vitro studies indicates that receptors for substance P (NK-1) and bradykinin (B2), and the ligand-gated, ionotropic receptors for glutamate (AMPA and NMDA receptors; see Chapter 11, Pharmacology of GABAergic and Glutamatergic Neurotransmission), are all inhibited directly by local anesthetics. Combined with the analgesic action that results from the sodium channel-blocking effect of the LA, the overall result is a significantly increased pain threshold.

PHARMACOKINETICS OF LOCAL ANESTHETICS

Systemic Absorption

After administration by injection or topical application, local anesthetics diffuse to their sites of action. LA molecules are

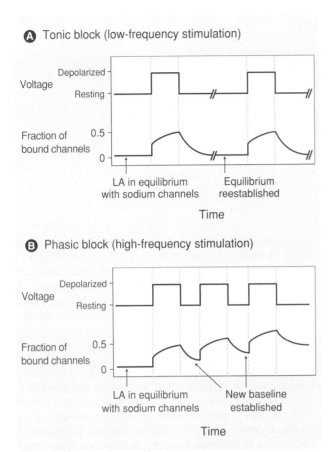

A Tonic block (low-frequency stimulation)

B Phasic block (high-frequency stimulation)

Figure 10-8. Tonic and phasic (use-dependent) inhibition. A. In tonic block, depolarizations occur with low frequency, and there is sufficient time between depolarizations for equilibrium binding of local anesthetic (LA) molecules to the various states of the sodium channel to be re-established. When a depolarization occurs, resting channels (which have low affinity for LA) are converted into open channels and inactivated channels (both of which have high affinity for LA). Thus, there is an increase in the number of LA-bound channels. Once the depolarization ends, there is enough time before the next depolarization for equilibrium between LA molecules and sodium channels to be re-established, and virtually all of the channels return to the resting and unbound state. **B.** In phasic block, depolarizations occur with high frequency, and there is not sufficient time between depolarizations for equilibrium to be re-established. After each depolarization, a new baseline is established that has more LA-bound channels than the previous baseline, leading eventually to conduction failure. Because high-frequency stimulation of nociceptors occurs in areas of tissue damage, phasic (use-dependent) block causes actively firing nociceptors to be inhibited more effectively than nerve fibers that are only occasionally firing. The frequency dependence of phasic block depends on the rate at which LA dissociates from its binding site on the channel.

also taken up by the local tissues and removed from the site of administration by the systemic circulation. The amount of local anesthetic that enters the systemic circulation and the potency of the LA together determine the systemic toxicity of the agent. Ideally, systemic absorption is minimized to avoid unnecessary toxicity. The vascularity of the injection site, the drug concentration, the addition of a vasoconstrictor, and properties of the injected solution (such as its viscosity) all influence the rate and extent of systemic absorption of local anesthetics. Absorption is greater from densely perfused tissues or following multiple administrations. For example, intratracheal administration of vaporized local anesthetic leads to rapid and nearly complete systemic absorption because of local anesthetic contact with the highly perfused lung parenchyma.

Vasoconstrictors (such as epinephrine) are often administered together with many short-acting or medium-acting local anesthetics. These adjunctive agents reduce blood flow to the area of injection by causing the smooth muscles of the vessels to contract, and thereby slow the rate of removal of the LA. In doing so, vasoconstrictors both increase the concentration of anesthetic around the nerve and decrease the maximal concentration that is reached in the systemic circulation. The former effect enhances the duration of action of the LA, and the latter effect decreases the LA's systemic toxicity. However, vasoconstriction can also lead to tissue hypoxia and damage if the oxygen supply to the area is reduced too severely. Thus, *vasoconstrictors are not used when LAs are administered in the extremities, because there is limited circulation to these areas.* In the introductory case, EM was given lidocaine without epinephrine to avoid tissue hypoxia in his digits.

Distribution

Local anesthetics diverted into the systemic circulation travel in the venous system to the capillary bed of the lung. As the first capillary bed reached by the drug, the lung "cushions" the impact of the drug on the brain and other organs. The lung also plays a role in metabolizing amide-linked LAs.

While traveling in the circulation, local anesthetics bind reversibly to two major plasma proteins: α-1 acid glycoprotein (an acute-phase protein) and albumin. LAs can also bind to erythrocytes. Binding to plasma proteins decreases as pH decreases, suggesting that the neutral form binds these proteins with higher affinity. Tissue binding occurs at the site of injection as well as other sites. The more hydrophobic the agent, the greater the tissue binding.

The volume of distribution (V_d) indicates the extent to which a drug distributes to the tissues from the systemic circulation. For the same amount of administered drug, a less hydrophobic LA (e.g., procaine) has a higher plasma concentration (i.e., less is stored in tissues) and therefore a smaller V_d. A more hydrophobic LA (e.g., bupivacaine) has a lower plasma concentration (i.e., more is stored in tissues) and therefore a larger V_d. Local anesthetics with a larger V_d are eliminated more slowly. (See Chapter 3, Pharmacokinetics, for a detailed discussion of the inverse relationship between V_d and the elimination half-life of a drug.)

Metabolism and Excretion

Ester-linked LAs are metabolized by tissue and plasma esterases (pseudocholinesterases). This process is fast (on the order of minutes), and the resulting products are excreted via the kidney.

Amide-linked LAs are primarily metabolized in the liver by P450 enzymes. The three major routes of hepatic metabolism are aromatic hydroxylation, N-dealkylation, and amide hydrolysis. Metabolites of amide-linked LAs are returned to the circulation and excreted by the kidney. Alterations in liver perfusion or in the maximum velocity of the liver enzymes can change the rate at which these agents are metabolized. Metabolism is slowed in patients with cirrhosis or other liver diseases, and a standard dose of an amide-linked LA can lead to toxicity in such a patient. Some metabolism of amide-linked LAs can also occur extrahepatically, for example, in the lung and kidney.

ADMINISTRATION OF LOCAL ANESTHETICS

The method of administration of local anesthetics can determine both the therapeutic effect and the extent of systemic toxicity. The following is an overview of the most common methods for administering local anesthetics.

Topical Anesthesia

Topical anesthetics provide short-term pain relief when applied to mucous membranes or skin. The drug must cross the epidermal barrier, with the stratum corneum (outermost layer of the epidermis) presenting the major obstacle, to reach the endings of Aδ-fibers and C-fibers in the dermis. Once across the epidermis, local anesthetics are absorbed rapidly into the circulation, increasing the risk of systemic toxicity. A mixture of tetracaine, adrenaline (epinephrine), and cocaine, known as **TAC,** is sometimes used before suturing small cuts. Because of concern about cocaine toxicity and/or addiction from this formulation, alternatives such as **EMLA** are now used (see below).

Infiltration Anesthesia

Infiltration anesthesia is used to numb an area of skin (or a mucosal surface) via an injection. The local anesthetic is injected intradermally or subcutaneously, often at several neighboring sites near the area to be anesthetized. This technique produces numbness much faster than does topical anesthesia, because the agent does not have to cross the epidermis. However, the injection can be painful because of the sting of the solution, which is usually kept at an acidic pH to maintain the drug in an ionized, soluble form. Neutralization of the solution by addition of sodium bicarbonate can reduce the injection pain. The local anesthetics most commonly used for infiltration anesthesia are lidocaine, procaine, and bupivacaine. Injection uses of local anesthetics for dental procedures are discussed in Box 10-1.

Peripheral Nerve Blockade

Peripheral nerve blockade can be subdivided into minor and major nerve blocks. For example, a minor nerve block for a distal extremity could involve the radial nerve, while a major nerve block for the entire arm would involve the brachial plexus. In both cases, local anesthetics are usually injected percutaneously. The amount injected is much more than would be necessary to block impulses in an unsheathed isolated nerve in vitro, because the anesthetic must cross several layers of membranes before it reaches the target site (as discussed above) and most of the drug is removed by the local circulation. Therefore, only a small fraction of the

---

> **BOX 10-1.** Local Anesthetics in Dentistry
>
> Modern dentistry is predicated on the action of local anesthetics: without adequate pain control, patients could not comfortably undergo the majority of dental procedures. Not surprisingly, then, local anesthetics are the most commonly used drugs in dentistry.
>
> Often, both an injected and a topical anesthetic agent are used in dental procedures; the injected agent blocks the sensation of pain during (and sometimes after) the procedure, while the topical agent allows for painless needle penetration when the injected agent is administered.
>
> Topical anesthetics are applied to mucus membranes and penetrate to a depth of 2 to 3 millimeters. Because topical anesthetics must diffuse across this distance, relatively high concentrations are used, and care must be taken to avoid local and systemic toxicity. Benzocaine and lidocaine—two commonly used topical anesthetics—are insoluble in water and poorly absorbed into the circulation, decreasing the likelihood of systemic toxicity.
>
> Injected anesthetics are administered either as local infiltrations or as field or nerve blocks. In a local infiltration, the anesthetic solution is deposited at the site where the dental procedure will be performed. The solution bathes free nerve endings at that site, blocking pain perception. In field and nerve blocks, the anesthetic solution is deposited more proximally along the nerve, away from the site of incision. These techniques are used when larger regions of the mouth must be anesthetized.
>
> Numerous injected anesthetics are used in dental practice, and the choice of which agent to use for a given procedure reflects factors such as the rate of onset, the duration of action, and the vasodilatory properties of the agent. Lidocaine is the most widely used injected anesthetic; it is notable for a rapid rate of onset, long duration of action, and extremely low incidence of allergic reaction. Mepivacaine is less vasodilating than most other local anesthetics, allowing it to be administered without a vasoconstrictor. This property makes mepivacaine ideally suited for pediatric dentistry, because it is "washed out" of the area of administration more rapidly than many agents given with vasoconstrictors. As a result, mepivacaine provides a relatively short period of soft-tissue anesthesia, minimizing the risk of inadvertent, self-inflicted trauma from biting or chewing on anesthetized tissue. Bupivacaine is a more potent and longer-acting anesthetic than lidocaine or mepivacaine. It is used for lengthy dental procedures and for the management of postoperative pain.

---

injected drug actually reaches the nerve membrane. The choice of anesthetic typically depends on the desired duration of action. Epinephrine helps extend the duration of action of peripheral nerve blocks (but can also cause tissue hypoxia, as described above).

Brachial plexus blocks are particularly useful in the upper extremity because the entire arm can be anesthetized. Other useful peripheral blocks include intercostal blocks for the anterior abdominal wall, cervical plexus blocks for neck surgery, and sciatic and femoral blocks for the distal lower limb. In the introductory case, EM was administered a digital nerve block, a type of peripheral block.

Central Nerve Blockade

This type of blockade, where drug is delivered near the spinal cord, includes both epidural anesthesia and intrathecal (spinal) anesthesia. The early effects of these procedures result primarily from impulse blockade in spinal roots, but in later phases, anesthetic drug penetrates and may act within the spinal cord. Bupivacaine is particularly useful as an epidural anesthetic during labor because, at low concentrations, it provides adequate pain relief without significant motor block. Reports of bupivacaine cardiotoxicity have led to decreased use of this agent in high concentrations (>0.5% weight/volume), although the dilute solutions used in obstetrics are rarely toxic. Newer, chemically similar drugs such as **ropivacaine** and **levobupivacaine** may be safer.

Intravenous Regional Anesthesia

This type of local anesthesia is also called Bier's block. Both a tourniquet and a distally located elastic band are applied to an elevated extremity, leading to partial exsanguination of the limb. The tourniquet is then inflated and the band removed. The LA is then injected into a vein in the extremity to provide local anesthesia, and the tourniquet prevents systemic toxicity by limiting blood flow to and from the extremity. Intravenous regional anesthesia is occasionally used for arm and hand surgery.

MAJOR TOXICITIES

Local anesthetics can have many potential toxicities, including effects on local tissues, peripheral vasculature, the heart, and the CNS. Hypersensitivity reactions are also possible. Administration of drug to a defined area usually limits the systemic side effects, but it is important to consider these potential toxicities whenever one is administering a local anesthetic.

Local anesthetics can cause local irritation. Skeletal muscle seems to be most sensitive to irritation from local anesthetic administration. Plasma levels of creatine kinase are elevated after intramuscular injection of LAs, indicating damage to muscle cells. This effect is usually reversible, and muscle regeneration is complete within a few weeks of the injection.

Local anesthetics have complex effects on the peripheral vasculature. Lidocaine, for example, initially causes vasoconstriction, but at later times it produces vasodilation. Such biphasic actions may be attributable to separate effects on the vascular smooth muscle and on sympathetic nerves that innervate resistance arterioles. Bronchial smooth muscle is also affected in a biphasic manner. Initially, local anesthetics cause bronchoconstriction, but at later times, bronchorelaxa-

tion. The early event may reflect LA-induced release of calcium ions into the cytoplasm from intracellular stores, while the later effect may be caused by LA inhibition of plasma membrane sodium and calcium channels (see below).

The cardiac effect of LAs is primarily to reduce the conduction velocity of the cardiac action potential. Local anesthetics can act as antiarrhythmic drugs because of their ability to prevent ventricular tachycardia and ventricular fibrillation (this is an example of use-dependent block; see above). Lidocaine, for example, acts as both a local anesthetic and a class I antiarrhythmic (see Chapter 18). Local anesthetics also cause a dose-dependent decrease in cardiac contractility (a negative inotropic effect). The mechanism of this effect is not entirely understood, but may be caused by LA-mediated slow release of calcium from the sarcoplasmic reticulum, with a consequent reduction in the stores of calcium available to drive subsequent contractions. LAs can also directly inhibit calcium channels in the plasma membrane. The combination of reduced intracellular calcium storage and decreased calcium entry leads to decreased myocardial contractility.

Local anesthetics can have serious effects on the CNS. LAs are small amphipathic molecules that can rapidly cross the blood–brain barrier. Initially, LAs produce signs of CNS excitement, including tremors, tinnitus (ringing in the ears), shivering, twitching, and sometimes generalized convulsions. CNS excitation is followed by depression. It is hypothesized that, initially, local anesthetics selectively block inhibitory pathways in the cerebral cortex, resulting in the excitatory phase of CNS toxicity. As the concentration of LA increases in the CNS, all neuronal pathways—excitatory as well as inhibitory—are blocked, leading to CNS depression. Death can ultimately result from respiratory failure.

Hypersensitivity to local anesthetics is rare. This adverse effect is usually manifested as allergic dermatitis or asthma. LA-induced hypersensitivity occurs almost exclusively with ester-linked LAs. For example, a metabolite of procaine, para-aminobenzoic acid (PABA), is a known allergen (as well as the active agent in many sunscreens).

INDIVIDUAL AGENTS

Having discussed the general properties of local anesthetics, this section briefly presents the individual anesthetics in current clinical use, with an emphasis on the agents' differences in potency and half-life.

Ester-Linked Local Anesthetics

Procaine

Procaine (Novocain®) is a short-acting, ester-linked LA. Its low hydrophobicity allows for rapid removal of drug from the site of administration via the circulation, and results in little sequestration of drug in the local tissue surrounding the nerve. In the bloodstream, procaine is degraded rapidly by plasma pseudocholinesterases, and the metabolites are subsequently excreted in the urine. Procaine's low hydrophobicity also causes it to dissociate rapidly from its binding site on the sodium channel, accounting for the low potency of this agent.

Procaine's primary use is in infiltration anesthesia and in dental procedures. Occasionally it is used in diagnostic nerve blocks. Procaine is rarely used for peripheral nerve block because of its low potency, slow onset, and short duration of action. However, the rapidly hydrolyzed, short-acting homolog of procaine, **2-chloroprocaine** (Nesacaine®), is popular as an obstetric anesthetic that is sometimes given epidurally just before delivery to control pain.

One of the metabolites of procaine is PABA, a compound required by some bacteria for purine and nucleic acid synthesis. The antibacterial sulfonamides are structural analogues of PABA that competitively inhibit the synthesis of an essential metabolite in folate biosynthesis (see Chapter 31, Principles of Antimicrobial and Antineoplastic Pharmacology). Excess PABA can reduce the effectiveness of sulfonamides and therefore exacerbate bacterial infections. As mentioned above, PABA is also an allergen.

Tetracaine

Tetracaine is a long-acting, highly potent, ester-linked LA. Its long duration of action is caused by its high hydrophobicity—it has a butyl group attached to its aromatic group—which allows tetracaine to remain in the tissue surrounding a nerve for an extended period of time. Tetracaine's hydrophobicity also promotes prolonged interaction with its binding site on the sodium channel, accounting for its greater potency than lidocaine and procaine. It is mainly used in spinal and topical anesthesia. Its effective metabolism is slow, despite the potential for rapid hydrolysis by esterases, because it is released only gradually from tissues into the bloodstream.

Cocaine

Cocaine, the prototypical and only naturally occurring LA, is ester-linked. It has a medium potency (one-half that of lidocaine) and a medium duration of action. Cocaine's structure is slightly unusual for local anesthetics. Its tertiary amine is part of a complex cyclic structure to which a secondary ester group is attached.

Cocaine's primary therapeutic uses are in ophthalmic anesthesia and as part of the topical anesthetic TAC (tetracaine, adrenaline, cocaine; see above). Like prilocaine (see below), cocaine has a marked vasoconstrictive action that results from its inhibition of catecholamine uptake in synaptic terminals of both the peripheral and central nervous systems (see Chapter 9, Adrenergic Pharmacology). Inhibition of this uptake system is also the mechanism for cocaine's profound cardiotoxic potential, and for the ''high'' associated with cocaine use. Cardiotoxicity and euphoria limit the value of cocaine as a local anesthetic.

Amide-Linked Local Anesthetics

Lidocaine and Prilocaine

Lidocaine, the most commonly used LA and the one used in EM's case, is an amide-linked drug of moderate hydrophobicity. It has a rapid onset of action and a medium duration of action (about 1–2 hours) and is moderately potent.

Lidocaine has two methyl groups on its aromatic ring, which enhance its hydrophobicity relative to procaine and slow its rate of hydrolysis.

Lidocaine has a relatively low pKa, and a large fraction of the drug is present in neutral form at physiologic pH. This results in rapid diffusion of the drug through membranes and a rapid block. Lidocaine's duration of action is based on two factors: its moderate hydrophobicity and its amide linkage. The amide linkage prevents degradation of the drug by esterases, and its hydrophobicity allows the drug to remain near the area of administration (i.e., in local tissue) for a long time. The hydrophobicity also allows lidocaine to bind more tightly than procaine to the LA binding site on the sodium channel, enhancing its potency. The vasoconstrictive effects of co-administered epinephrine can extend lidocaine's duration of action significantly.

Lidocaine is used in infiltration, peripheral nerve block, epidural, spinal, and topical anesthesia. It is also used as a Class I antiarrhythmic. The mechanism of antiarrhythmic action is its blocking of sodium channels in cardiac myocytes. Lidocaine's slow metabolism in the circulation makes it a useful antiarrhythmic (see Chapter 18). More potent amide-linked LAs, such as bupivacaine, bind too tightly to cardiac sodium channels to serve as useful antiarrhythmics; such drugs cause either conduction blocks or tachyarrhythmias (see below).

Lidocaine undergoes metabolism in the liver, where it is first N-dealkylated by P450 enzymes (see Chapter 4, Drug Metabolism). Subsequently, it undergoes hydrolysis and hydroxylation. Lidocaine's metabolites have only weak anesthetic activity.

The toxic effects of lidocaine are manifested mainly in the CNS and heart. Adverse effects can include drowsiness, tinnitus, twitching, and even seizures. CNS depression and cardiotoxicity occur at high plasma levels of the drug.

Prilocaine is similar to lidocaine, except that it has vasoconstrictive activity as well as local anesthetic activity. Because prilocaine does not require concurrent administration of epinephrine to prolong its duration of action, this drug is a good choice for patients in whom epinephrine is contraindicated.

Bupivacaine

Bupivacaine is an amide-linked LA with a long duration of action. It is highly hydrophobic (and, therefore, highly potent) as a result of a butyl group attached to the tertiary nitrogen. Dilute bupivacaine, applied epidurally, has more effect on nociception than on locomotor activity. This property, combined with the drug's long duration of action and high potency, has made bupivacaine useful in spinal, epidural, and peripheral nerve block, and in infiltration anesthesia. Bupivacaine is metabolized in the liver, where it undergoes N-dealkylation by P450 enzymes. It has been used widely in low concentrations for labor and post-operative anesthesia because it provides 2–3 hours of pain relief without immobilizing motor blockade. However, because of its cardiotoxicity at higher concentrations, bupivacaine is no longer used as commonly for these purposes. (The drug blocks cardiac myocyte sodium channels during systole, but is very slow to dissociate during diastole. Thus, it can trigger arrhythmias through the promotion of re-entry pathways.)

Because bupivacaine contains a chiral center, it exists as a racemic mixture of mirror-image R-enantiomers and S-enantiomers. The R-enantiomers and S-enantiomers have different affinities for the sodium channel and, therefore, different cardiovascular effects. The S-enantiomer has been separated and marketed as the safer and less cardiotoxic **levobupivacaine,** as has its structurally homologous relative **ropivacaine.**

Articaine

Articaine is an amide-linked LA that was approved for clinical use in the United States in 2000. Along with **prilocaine,** articaine is unique among local anesthetics because of its secondary amine group. (Virtually all other LAs have a tertiary amine group.) Articaine is also structurally unique because it contains an ester group bound to a thiophene ring; the presence of the ester group means that articaine can be partially metabolized in the plasma by cholinesterases, as well as in the liver. Its rapid metabolism in the plasma may minimize the potential toxicity of articaine. Articaine is currently used in dentistry, but it may find additional applications as more studies of its clinical properties are performed.

EMLA

EMLA (Eutectic Mixture of Local Anesthetic) is a combination of lidocaine and prilocaine that is delivered topically as a cream or patch. EMLA is useful clinically because it has a higher concentration of local anesthetic per drop contacting the skin than standard topical preparations. It is effective in a number of situations including venipuncture, arterial cannulation, lumbar puncture, and dental procedures, particularly in children who dread the pain of injections.

Conclusion and Future Directions

Local anesthetics are vital to the practice of medicine and surgery because they can block pain sensations regionally. Their clinical actions involve blocking pain neurons called nociceptors. Nociceptors are afferent neurons whose axons are classified as either Aδ- or C-fibers. Local anesthetics block all types of nerve fibers running in peripheral nerves, including those of nociceptors, by blocking voltage-gated sodium channels in neuronal membranes. LAs act on sodium channels from the cytoplasmic side of the membrane.

In general, local anesthetics have an aromatic group that is connected to an ionizable amine via an ester or amide linkage. This structure is common to almost all local anesthetics and contributes to their function. Both the hydrophobicity, attributable in large part to the aromatic ring and its substituents, and the ionizability (pKa) of the amine determine the potency of the LA and the kinetics of local anesthetic action. Molecules with pKa values of 8–10 (weak bases) are the most effective as local anesthetics. The neutral form can cross membranes to reach the LA binding site on the sodium channel, and the protonated form is available to bind with high affinity to the target site.

The sodium channel exists in three forms: open, inactivated, and resting. There are also several transient "closed" forms between the resting and open states. Local anesthetics bind strongly to the closed, open, and inactivated conformations of the sodium channel. This tight binding inhibits the return of the channel to the resting state, extends the refractory period, and inhibits the transmission of action potentials.

Local anesthetics seem to have effects beyond their inhibition of sodium channels in nerve fibers. Some of these ancillary effects show therapeutic promise and could potentially lead to other indications for LAs. For example, LAs have been reported to affect wound healing, thrombosis, hypoxia/ischemia-induced brain injury, and bronchial hyperactivity. LAs are also being investigated for use in chronic and neuropathic pain management, such as that seen in patients with diabetic neuropathy, post-herpetic neuralgia, burns, cancer, and strokes. The development of ultralong-acting LAs (whose effects could last for days) is continuing to be investigated; these studies involve altering LA structure at the molecular level, using a variety of drug delivery systems, and discovering different classes of neuronal impulse blockers.

One exciting area of research is the potential effect of LAs on the inflammatory response. LAs have been found to inhibit the recruitment and function of polymorphonuclear granulocytes (PMNs). Because PMNs do not express sodium channels, the mechanism of inhibition likely differs from the mechanism of LA-induced anesthesia. Preliminary studies have found that LAs affect several steps in inflammation, including cytokine release, PMN migration to the site of injury, PMN accumulation at the site, and free radical release at the site. Applications to diseases in which the inflammatory response is overactive—such as acute respiratory distress syndrome (ARDS), inflammatory bowel disease, and myocardial infarction and reperfusion injury—are being investigated.

Suggested Reading

Cousins MJ, Bridenbaugh PO. *Neural blockade.* 3rd ed. New York: Lippincott-Raven; 1998. (*A detailed but readable textbook. A good follow-up reference to concepts discussed in this chapter.*)

McLure HA, Rubin AP. Review of local anaesthetic agents. *Minerva Anestesiol* 2005;71:59–74. (*A clear discussion of both general concepts and individual agents.*)

Strichartz GR, Berde CB. Local anesthetics. In: Miller RD, et al, eds. *Miller's anesthesia.* Philadelphia: Elsevier Churchill Livingstone; 2005. (*A more complete mechanistic and, primarily, clinical summary.*)

Ulbricht W. Sodium channel inactivation: molecular determinants and modulation. *Physiol Rev* 2005;85:1271–1301. (*A thorough, highly technical review.*)

Yanagidate F, Strichartz G. Local anesthetics. In: Stein C, ed. *Analgesia: handbook of experimental pharmacology,* vol. 177. Berlin: Springer-Verlag; 2006. (*A detailed and complex review for those who want to delve deeper.*)

Drug Summary Table | **Chapter 10 Local Anesthetic Pharmacology**

ESTER-LINKED LOCAL ANESTHETICS
Mechanism—Inhibit voltage-gated sodium channels in excitable cell membranes

Drug	Clinical Applications	Serious and Common Adverse Effects	Contraindications	Therapeutic Considerations
Procaine 2-chloroprocaine	Infiltration anesthesia Obstetrical anesthesia, given epidurally before delivery (2-chloroprocaine)	*Cardiac arrest and hypotension from excessive systemic absorption, CNS depression or excitation, respiratory arrest* Contact dermatitis	Use epidural anesthesia with extreme caution in patients with neurological disease, spinal deformities, septicemia, or severe hypertension	Procaine's low hydrophobicity allows for rapid drug removal from administration site via circulation but also accounts for its low potency and short half-life Excess PABA (metabolite of procaine) can reduce the effectiveness of sulfonamides
Tetracaine	Topical anesthesia Spinal anesthesia	*Same as procaine* Additionally; drug-induced keratoconjunctivitis	Localized infection at proposed site of topical application	High hydrophobicity confers longer duration of action and higher potency; tetracaine is more potent than lidocaine and procaine Do not inject large doses in patients with heart block
Cocaine	Mucosal and ophthalmic local anesthetic Diagnosis of Horner's syndrome pupil	*Accelerates coronary atherosclerosis, tachycardia, seizure* CNS depression or excitation, anxiety	Hypersensitivity to cocaine-containing products	Medium potency (one-half that of lidocaine), medium duration of action, marked vasoconstrictive action, cardiotoxic Cardiotoxicity and euphoria limit the value of cocaine as a local anesthetic

AMIDE-LINKED LOCAL ANESTHETICS
Mechanism—Inhibit voltage-gated sodium channels in excitable cell membranes

Drug	Clinical Applications	Serious and Common Adverse Effects	Contraindications	Therapeutic Considerations
Lidocaine	Infiltration anesthesia Peripheral nerve block Epidural, spinal, and topical anesthesia Class I antiarrhythmic	*Cardiac and respiratory arrest, arrhythmias, decreased myocardial contractility, methemoglobinemia, seizure* Tinnitus, dizziness, paresthesia, tremor, somnolence, hypotension, skin irritation, constipation	Hypersensitivity to amide-linked local anesthetics Congenital or idiopathic methemoglobinemia	Lidocaine has a rapid onset of action, a medium duration of action (about 1–2 hours), and is moderately potent, due to its moderate hydrophobicity May require concurrent administration of epinephrine to prolong its duration of action
Prilocaine	Dental infiltration anesthesia and nerve block	*Same as lidocaine*	Same as lidocaine	Prilocaine does not require epinephrine to prolong its duration of action, which makes it a good choice for patients in whom epinephrine is contraindicated

(Continued)

Drug Summary Table | **Chapter 10 Local Anesthetic Pharmacology** *(Continued)*

Drug	Clinical Applications	*Serious and Common* Adverse Effects	Contraindications	Therapeutic Considerations
Bupivacaine	Infiltration, regional, epidural, and spinal anesthesia Sympathetic nerve block	*Same as lidocaine Additionally, cardiotoxicity at higher concentrations*	Local infection at the proposed site of spinal anesthesia Contraindicated for use in spinal anesthesia in the presence of septicemia, severe hemorrhage, shock, or arrhythmias such as complete heart block	Highly hydrophobic, high potency, long duration of action Cardiotoxicity at higher concentrations limits its use The R-enantiomer and S-enantiomer have different affinities for the sodium channel and, therefore, different cardiovascular effects; the S-enantiomer is levobupivacaine; its structural homologue is ropivacaine
Articaine	Dental anesthesia Epidural, spinal, and regional anesthesia	*Same as lidocaine*	Infection at site of injection (especially lumbar puncture sites) Shock	Articaine's current clinical application is largely in dentistry
EMLA (eutectic mixture of lidocaine and prilocaine)	Topical local anesthetic for normal intact skin, mucosal membranes, and dental procedures	*Same as lidocaine*	Hypersensitivity to amide-linked local anesthetics	Delivered topically as a cream, swab, or patch Useful clinically due to higher concentration of local anesthetic per drop contacting the tissue than standard topical preparations

IIC

Principles of Central Nervous System Pharmacology

11

Pharmacology of GABAergic and Glutamatergic Neurotransmission

Stuart A. Forman, Janet Chou, Gary R. Strichartz, and Eng H. Lo

INTRODUCTION

Inhibitory and excitatory neurotransmitters regulate a diverse array of behavioral processes including sleep, learning, memory, and pain sensation. Inhibitory and excitatory neurotransmitters are also implicated in pathologic processes such as epilepsy and neurotoxicity. The interactions among ion channels, the receptors that regulate these channels, and amino acid neurotransmitters in the central nervous system (CNS) constitute the molecular basis for these processes. This chapter discusses the physiology, pathophysiology, and pharmacology of the two most important amino acid neurotransmission systems in the CNS, those involving **γ-aminobutyric acid (GABA)** and **glutamate**.

Case

S.B., a 70-year-old man, is having trouble sleeping. He recalls that his sister has been prescribed phenobarbital, a barbiturate, to control her epileptic seizures, and that barbiturates are sometimes also prescribed as sleeping pills. He decides to take "just a few" with some alcohol to help him sleep. Shortly afterward, Mr. B is rushed to the emergency department after his sister finds him minimally responsive. On examination, he is difficult to arouse and dysarthric, with an unsteady gait and impaired attention and memory. His respiratory rate is approximately six shallow breaths per minute. The patient is subsequently intubated to protect him from aspirating gastric contents. Activated charcoal is administered through a nasogastric tube to limit further absorption of phenobarbital. He also receives intravenous sodium bicarbonate to alkalinize his urine to a pH of 7.5 to facilitate renal drug excretion. Three days later, he has recovered sufficiently to return home.

QUESTIONS

■ **1.** How do barbiturates act to control epileptic seizures and to induce sleep?

■ **2.** How does the patient's age affect the extent of CNS depression caused by barbiturates?

■ **3.** What is the interaction of barbiturates and ethanol that results in profound CNS and respiratory depression?

■ **4.** What are the signs of barbiturate poisoning, and how are these signs explained by the drugs' mechanism of action?

OVERVIEW OF GABAERGIC AND GLUTAMATERGIC NEUROTRANSMISSION

The CNS has high concentrations of certain amino acids that bind to postsynaptic receptors and thereby act as inhibitory or excitatory neurotransmitters. Of the two main classes of neuroactive amino acids, **γ-aminobutyric acid (GABA)** is the major inhibitory amino acid, and **glutamate** is the primary excitatory amino acid.

Amino acid neurotransmitters elicit inhibitory or excitatory responses by altering the conductance of one or more ion-selective channels. Inhibitory neurotransmitters trigger a selective outward current. For example, inhibitory neurotransmitters may open K^+ channels or Cl^- channels to induce K^+ efflux or Cl^- influx, respectively. Either type of ion movement—the loss of intracellular cations or the gain of intracellular anions—results in membrane hyperpolarization and decreased membrane resistance (Fig. 11-1).

In contrast, an excitatory neurotransmitter may open a cation-specific channel, such as a sodium channel, and thereby cause a net influx of sodium ions that depolarizes the membrane. Alternatively, an excitatory (depolarizing) response could result if a neurotransmitter closes potassium "leak channels" to reduce the outward flow of potassium ions (see Chapter 6, Principles of Cellular Excitability and Electrochemical Transmission). Notice that, in both of these examples, excitatory amino acid neurotransmitters cause a net inward current.

Pharmacologic agents that modulate GABAergic neurotransmission, including **benzodiazepines** and **barbiturates**, are drug classes of major clinical importance. In comparison, pharmacologic agents targeting glutamatergic neurotransmission remain largely experimental. The balance of the discussion is, therefore, addressed at GABAergic physiology and pharmacology; the pathophysiology and pharmacology of glutamatergic neurotransmission is discussed at the end of the chapter.

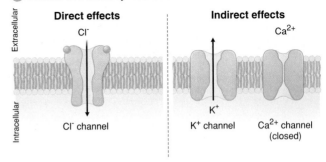

Ⓐ Effects of inhibitory neurotransmitters

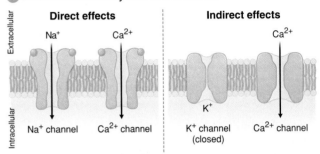

Ⓑ Effects of excitatory neurotransmitters

Figure 11-1. **Effects of inhibitory and excitatory neurotransmitters on ion conductances. A.** Inhibitory neurotransmitters hyperpolarize membranes by inducing a net outward current, by promoting either an influx of anions (for example, opening a Cl^- channel) or an efflux of cations (for example, opening a K^+ channel). Opening of chloride or potassium channels also decreases the membrane resistance and thereby lowers the ΔV_m response to excitatory currents. The decreased membrane resistance results in lower responsiveness (i.e., a smaller change in V_m per change in current) because $\Delta V_m = \Delta i_m \times r_m$, where V_m is the membrane potential, i_m is the excitatory current, and r_m is the membrane resistance. **B.** Excitatory neurotransmitters depolarize membranes by inducing a net inward current, either by enhancing inward current (for example, opening a Na^+ channel) or by reducing outward current (for example, closing a K^+ channel). Potassium channel closure also increases the resting membrane resistance and renders the cell more responsive to excitatory postsynaptic currents.

PHYSIOLOGY OF GABAERGIC NEUROTRANSMISSION

GABA functions as the primary inhibitory neurotransmitter in the mammalian CNS. The cell membranes of most vertebrate CNS neurons and astrocytes express GABA receptors, which decrease neuronal excitability through several types of mechanisms. Because of their widespread distribution, GABA receptors influence many neural circuits and functions. Drugs that modulate GABA receptors affect arousal and attention, memory formation, anxiety, sleep, and muscle tone. Modulation of GABA signaling is also an important mechanism for treatment of focal or widespread neuronal hyperactivity in epilepsy.

GABA METABOLISM

The synthesis of GABA is mediated by **glutamic acid decarboxylase (GAD)**, which catalyzes the decarboxylation of glutamate to GABA in GABAergic nerve terminals (Fig. 11-2A). Thus, the amount of GABA in brain tissue correlates with the amount of functional GAD. GAD requires pyridoxal phosphate (vitamin B_6) as a cofactor. GABA is packaged into pre-synaptic vesicles by a transporter (**VGAT**), which is the same transporter expressed in nerve terminals that release glycine, another inhibitory neurotransmitter. In response to an action potential, GABA is released into the synaptic cleft by fusion of GABA-containing vesicles with the pre-synaptic membrane.

Termination of GABA action at the synapse depends on the removal of GABA from the extracellular space. Neurons and glia take up GABA via specific **GABA transporters (GATs)**. Four GATs, GAT-1 through GAT-4, have been

identified, each with a characteristic distribution in the CNS. Within cells, the widely distributed mitochondrial enzyme **GABA-transaminase (GABA-T)** catalyzes the conversion of GABA to succinic semialdehyde (SSA), which is subsequently oxidized to succinic acid by SSA dehydrogenase and then enters the Krebs cycle to become α-ketoglutarate. GABA-T then regenerates glutamate from α-ketoglutarate (Fig. 11-2A).

GABA RECEPTORS

GABA mediates its neurophysiologic effects by binding to GABA receptors. There are two types of GABA receptors. **Ionotropic GABA receptors (GABA$_A$ and GABA$_C$)** are multi-subunit membrane proteins that bind GABA and open an intrinsic chloride ion channel. **Metabotropic GABA receptors (GABA$_B$)** are heterodimeric G protein-coupled re-

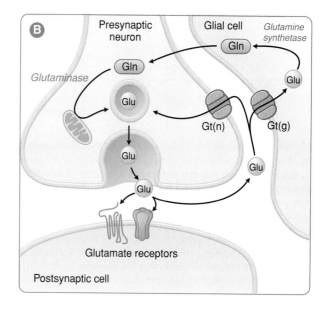

Figure 11-2. Glutamate and GABA synthesis and metabolism. A. Glutamate synthesis and metabolism are intertwined with GABA synthesis and metabolism. In one pathway for glutamate synthesis, α-ketoglutarate produced by the Krebs cycle serves as a substrate for the enzyme GABA transaminase (GABA-T), which reductively transaminates intraneuronal α-ketoglutarate to glutamate. The same enzyme also converts GABA to succinic semialdehyde. Alternatively, glutamate is converted to GABA by the enzyme glutamic acid decarboxylase (GAD), changing the major excitatory neurotransmitter to the major inhibitory transmitter. GABA-T is irreversibly inhibited by vigabatrin; by blocking the conversion of GABA to succinic semialdehyde, this drug increases the amount of GABA available for release at inhibitory synapses. *GABA-T:* GABA transaminase; *SSADH:* succinic semialdehyde dehydrogenase; *GAD:* glutamic acid decarboxylase. **B.** Glutamate transporters present in neurons [Gt(n)] and glial cells [Gt(g)] sequester glutamate (Glu) from the synaptic cleft into their respective cells. In the glial cell, the enzyme glutamine synthetase transforms glutamate into glutamine (Gln). Glutamine is then transferred to the neuron, which converts it back to glutamate via mitochondria-associated glutaminase.

ceptors that affect neuronal ion currents through second messengers.

Ionotropic GABA Receptors: GABA_A and GABA_C

The most abundant GABA receptors in the CNS are ionotropic **GABA_A** receptors, which are members of the superfamily of fast neurotransmitter-gated ion channels including peripheral and neuronal nicotinic acetylcholine receptors (nAChRs), serotonin type-3A/B ($5HT_{3A/B}$) receptors, and glycine receptors. Like other members of this superfamily, GABA_A receptors are pentameric transmembrane glycoproteins assembled to form a central ion pore surrounded by five subunits, each of which has four membrane-spanning domains (Fig. 11-3A). Sixteen different GABA_A receptor subunits, (α1-6, β1-3, γ1-3, δ, ϵ, π, θ) are currently known. The number of pentameric ion channels formed by potential combinations of 16 subunits is very large, but only about

20 different subunit combinations have been identified in native GABA_A receptors. Importantly, receptors containing different subunit combinations display distinct distributions at the cellular and tissue levels, and evidence is accumulating that different GABA_A receptor subtypes play distinct roles in specific neural circuits. Most synaptic GABA_A receptors consist of two α, two β, and one γ subunit. ''Extrasynaptic'' GABA_A receptors have also been identified on dendrites, axons, and neuronal cell bodies. These often contain δ or ϵ subunits instead of a γ subunit.

The five subunits of GABA_A receptors surround a central chloride-selective ion pore that opens in the presence of GABA. GABA and other agonists bind to two sites, which are located in extracellular portions of the receptor-channel complex at the interface between α and β subunits. GABA_A receptors also contain a number of modulatory sites where other endogenous ligands and/or drugs bind (Fig. 11-3B). In many cases, the presence of these sites and the impact of ligand binding depend on the receptor subunit composition.

GABA_A receptor channel-activation follows the binding of two molecules of GABA, one to each of the receptor's agonist sites (Fig. 11-3). Fast **inhibitory post-synaptic currents** (IPSCs) are responses activated by very brief (high-frequency) bursts of GABA release at synapses. Uptake by GAT removes GABA from the synapse in under 1 ms, while IPSCs deactivate over about 11–20 ms, a rate determined by both closure of the GABA_A receptor ion channel and dissociation of GABA from the receptor. Prolonged occupation of the agonist sites by GABA also leads to GABA_A receptor **desensitization**, a transition to an inactive agonist-bound state (Fig. 11-4). During burst (or ''phasic'') firing, the presynaptic nerve membrane releases ''quanta'' ($\sim$ 1 mM) of GABA by exocytosis of synaptic vesicles, resulting in large-amplitude **inhibitory post-synaptic potentials (IPSPs)**. Low levels of GABA can also cause a baseline inhibitory current in many neurons. Recent studies suggest that basal inhibitory currents are caused by extrasynaptic GABA_A receptors, which are activated by low micromolar concentrations of GABA that diffuse into cerebrospinal fluid and interstitial spaces.

Because the internal chloride concentration $[Cl^-]_i$ of mature neurons is lower than extracellular Cl^-, activation of chloride-selective channels (increasing conductance) shifts

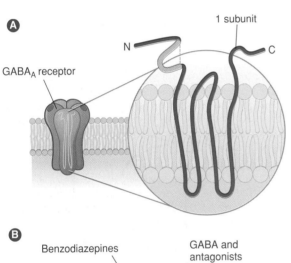

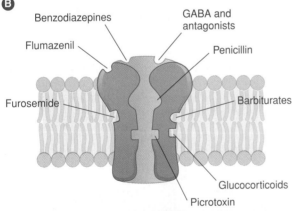

Figure 11-3. Schematic representation of the GABA_A receptor. A. The pentameric structure of the GABA_A receptor. Each receptor is made up of five subunits, and each subunit is of one of three predominant subtypes: α, β, or γ. Activation requires the binding of two GABA molecules to the receptor, one to each of the two α subunits. Each subunit of the GABA_A receptor has four membrane-spanning regions and a cysteine loop in the extracellular N-terminal domain *(depicted as a dashed line)*. **B.** Major binding sites on the GABA_A receptor. Although there is indirect evidence for the location of many of the drug binding sites that are schematically indicated in this diagram, the definitive localization of these sites remains to be determined.

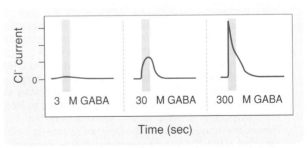

Figure 11-4. Effects of GABA on GABA_A-Mediated chloride conductance. Increasing concentrations of GABA induce both greater Cl^- currents and more rapid receptor desensitization. The latter phenomenon can be observed as the rapid decline from the peak current during continuous exposure to 300 μM GABA **(right panel)**. In each panel, the shaded bar indicates the time during which GABA was applied.

the neuronal transmembrane voltage towards the Cl^- equilibrium potential ($E_{Cl} \sim -70$ mV). This Cl^- flux *hyperpolarizes* or stabilizes the post-synaptic cell near its normal resting membrane potential ($V_m \sim -65$ mV), reducing the chance that excitatory stimuli will initiate action potentials. Open Cl^- channels attenuate the change in membrane potential caused by excitatory synaptic currents, an effect called **shunting.** This is the molecular explanation for the inhibitory effects of GABA signaling via GABA$_A$ receptors.

Certain endogenous molecules allosterically modulate GABA$_A$ receptor activity. Metabolism of these molecules in the brain produces **neurosteroids** such as pregnenolone, dehydroepiandrosterone (DHEA), 5α-dihydrodeoxycorticosterone (DHDOC), 5α-tetrahydrodeoxycorticosterone (THDOC), and allopregnanolone. Rather than acting through nuclear receptors as many steroid hormones do, these compounds alter GABA$_A$ receptor function by binding to allosteric sites on the receptor protein, causing increased GABA$_A$ receptor activation. DHDOC and THDOC are thought to modulate brain activity during stress. Menstrual variations in allopregnanolone, a metabolite of progesterone, contribute to perimenstrual (catamenial) epilepsy. Sulfation of pregnenolone and DHEA results in neurosteroids that inhibit GABA$_A$ receptors. Another endogenous substance that enhances GABA$_A$ receptor activity is **oleamide**, a fatty acid amide found in the cerebrospinal fluid of sleep-deprived animals. Injection of oleamide into normal animals induces sleep, in part through potentiation of GABA$_A$ receptors.

Another group of ionotropic GABA receptors, **GABA$_C$**, are formed by three subunits that are not found in GABA$_A$ receptors (ρ1-3). GABA$_C$ receptors are also pentameric ligand-gated chloride channels, but their distribution in the CNS is restricted. They are expressed primarily in the retina. GABA$_C$ receptors display distinct pharmacologic properties that differ from most GABA$_A$ receptors. There are no drugs currently in use that target GABA$_C$ receptors.

Metabotropic GABA Receptors: GABA$_B$

GABA$_B$ receptors are G protein-coupled receptors (Fig. 11-5). GABA$_B$ receptors are expressed at lower levels than GABA$_A$ receptors, principally in the spinal cord. GABA$_B$ receptors function as heterodimers of GABA$_{B1}$ and GABA$_{B2}$ subunits. The GABA$_B$ receptor interacts with heterotrimeric

G proteins containing $G_{\alpha i}$ and $G_{\alpha o}$, which inhibit adenylyl cyclase, activate K^+ ion channels, and inhibit voltage-gated Ca^{2+} channels. At GABAergic synapses, GABA$_B$ receptors are expressed both pre-synaptically and post-synaptically. Pre-synaptic "autoreceptors" modulate neurotransmitter release by reducing Ca^{2+} influx, while post-synaptic GABA$_B$ receptors produce slow IPSPs, through activation of G protein-activated K^+ channels (GIRKS). The slower rates of activation and deactivation for GABA$_B$ currents in comparison with GABA$_A$ currents appear to be due to the relatively slow second messenger signal transduction mechanism.

Activation of K^+ channels by $G_{\alpha i}$ and $G_{\alpha o}$ inhibits neuronal firing, because K^+ has an equilibrium potential near -70 mV. Thus, increased K^+ conductance, like increased Cl^- conductance, drives the neuronal transmembrane voltage toward "resting" potentials that reduce the frequency of action potential initiation, and also shunts excitatory currents.

PHARMACOLOGIC CLASSES AND AGENTS AFFECTING GABAERGIC NEUROTRANSMISSION

Pharmacologic agents acting on GABAergic neurotransmission affect GABA metabolism or receptor activity. The majority of pharmacologic agents affecting GABAergic neurotransmission act on the ionotropic GABA$_A$ receptor. GABA$_A$ receptors are regulated by several drug classes that interact with the GABA binding sites or with allosteric sites (Fig. 11-3). Therapeutic agents that activate GABA$_A$ receptors are used for sedation, anxiolysis, hypnosis, neuro-protection following stroke or head trauma, and control of epilepsy. A number of other agents are used for purely experimental purposes (Table 11-1).

INHIBITORS OF GABA METABOLISM

Tiagabine is a competitive inhibitor of the GABA transporters in neurons and glia, where it may act selectivity on GAT-1. The major clinical indication for tiagabine is in the treatment of epilepsy. By inhibiting GABA re-uptake, tiagabine

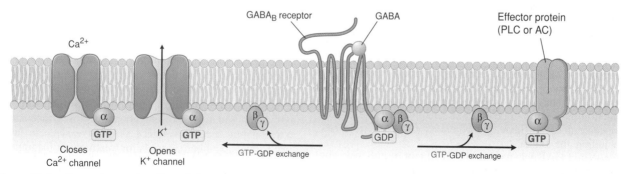

Figure 11-5. Downstream signaling of the GABA$_B$ receptor. GABA$_B$ receptors activate G proteins that are either coupled to K^+ or Ca^{2+} channels directly *(leftward arrow)* or linked to second messenger systems such as adenylyl cyclase (AC) or phospholipase C (PLC) *(rightward arrow)*. The increased K^+ efflux leads to slow, long-lasting inhibitory postsynaptic potentials. The reduced Ca^{2+} influx may enable GABA$_B$ autoreceptors to inhibit presynaptic neurotransmitter release.

DRUG CLASS	PRESUMED MECHANISM	EFFECTS
GABA Synthesis		
Allylglycine	Inhibits glutamic acid decarboxylase	Convulsant
Isoniazid	Inhibits pyridoxal kinase (antivitamin B_6 effect)	Convulsant at high doses
GABA Release		
Tetanus toxin	Inhibits GABA and glycine release	Convulsant
GABA Metabolism		
Tiagabine	Inhibits GAT-1	Anticonvulsant
Vigabatrin	Inhibits GABA transaminase	Anticonvulsant
GABA$_A$ Receptor Agonists		
Muscimol	GABA$_A$ receptor agonist	Mimics psychosis
Gaboxadol	GABA$_A$ receptor agonist	Anticonvulsant
GABA$_A$ Receptor Antagonists		
Bicuculline	Competitive antagonist	Convulsant
Gabazine		
Picrotoxin	Noncompetitive antagonist, pore blocker, occludes the chloride channel	Convulsant
GABA$_A$ Receptor Modulators		
Benzodiazepines	Potentiate GABA binding	Anticonvulsant, anxiolytic
Barbiturates	Increase GABA efficacy, weak agonist	Anticonvulsant, anesthetic
GABA$_B$ Receptor Agonists		
Baclofen	GABA$_B$ receptor agonist	Muscle relaxant

increases both synaptic and extrasynaptic GABA concentrations. The result is non-specific agonism of both ionotropic and metabotropic GABA receptors, with the major effects being at GABA$_A$ receptors.

Tiagabine is an oral medication that is rapidly absorbed with 90% bioavailability and is highly protein bound. Metabolism is hepatic, primarily by CYP3A4. Tiagabine does not induce cytochrome P450 enzymes, but its metabolism is influenced by concomitant use of either inducers or inhibitors of CYP3A4. Adverse effects of tiagabine are those of high GABA activity, including confusion, sedation, amnesia, and ataxia. Tiagabine potentiates the action of GABA$_A$ receptor modulators such as ethanol, benzodiazepines, and barbiturates.

γ-Vinyl GABA (**vigabatrin**) is a "suicide inhibitor" of GABA transaminase (GABA-T, see Fig. 11-2). Administration of this drug blocks the conversion of GABA to succinic semialdehyde, resulting in high intracellular GABA concentrations and increased synaptic GABA release. Like tiagabine, enhancement of GABA receptor function by γ-vinyl GABA is not selective because GABA concentrations are increased wherever GABA is released, including the retina.

γ-Vinyl GABA is used in the treatment of epilepsy, and it is being investigated for treatment of drug addiction, panic disorder, and obsessive-compulsive disorder. Adverse effects of γ-vinyl GABA include drowsiness, confusion, and headache. The drug has been reported to cause bilateral visual field defects associated with irreversible diffuse atrophy of the peripheral retinal nerve fiber layer. This appears to result from accumulation of the drug in retinal nerves.

GABA$_A$ RECEPTOR AGONISTS AND ANTAGONISTS

Agonists such as **muscimol** and **gaboxadol** activate the GABA$_A$ receptor by binding directly to the GABA binding site. Muscimol, first derived from hallucinogenic *Amanita muscaria* mushrooms, is a full agonist at many GABA$_A$ receptor subtypes and is used primarily as a research tool. Purified muscimol (as well as other GABA$_A$ receptor agonists) does not induce hallucinations, which are probably caused by other factors from *Amanita muscaria*. Gaboxadol at high concentrations is a partial agonist at synaptic GABA$_A$ receptors; at low concentrations, gaboxadol selectively activates extrasynaptic receptors containing α4, β3, and δ subunits. Gaboxadol was initially approved for treatment of epilepsy and anxiety, but therapeutic doses were associated with ataxia and sedation. Lower gaboxadol doses that activate extrasynaptic receptors induce slow-wave sleep in laboratory animals, and human trials for treatment of insomnia are in progress. Potential but unproven advantages with low-dose gaboxadol for treatment of insomnia include a lower potential for developing tolerance and few interactions with benzodiazepines and alcohol, which act at different GABA$_A$ receptor subtypes.

Bicuculline and **gabazine** are competitive antagonists that bind at the GABA sites on GABA$_A$ receptors. **Picrotoxin**, derived from a poisonous plant, is a non-competitive inhibitor of GABA$_A$ receptors. All of these GABA$_A$ antagonists produce epileptic convulsions and are used exclusively for research.

GABA$_A$ RECEPTOR MODULATORS

Benzodiazepines and barbiturates are modulators of GABA$_A$ receptors that act at allosteric binding sites to enhance GABAergic neurotransmission. **Benzodiazepines** have sedative, hypnotic, muscle relaxant, amnestic, and anxiolytic effects. At high doses, benzodiazepines can cause hypnosis and stupor. However, when used alone, these drugs rarely cause fatal CNS depression. **Barbiturates** constitute a large group of drugs that were first introduced in the mid-twentieth century and which continue to be used for control of epilepsy, as general anesthetic induction agents, and for control of intracranial hypertension.

Benzodiazepines

Benzodiazepines are high-affinity, highly selective drugs that bind at a single site on GABA$_A$ receptors containing α1, α2, α3, or α5 subunits and a γ subunit. Benzodiazepines act as positive allosteric modulators by enhancing channel gating in the presence of GABA (Fig. 11-6). Benzodiazepines do not activate native GABA$_A$ receptors directly in the absence of GABA, but they do activate certain mutant receptors, indicating that they are **weak allosteric agonists** (Fig. 11-7). This mechanism is consistent with the known location of the benzodiazepine-binding site at the interface between the external domains of α and γ subunits. This site is a structural homolog of the two GABA agonist sites at the interfaces between β and α subunits. Benzodiazepines increase the *frequency* of channel openings at low GABA concentrations. At GABA concentrations similar to those in synapses, receptor *deactivation is prolonged*, indicating either enhanced GABA binding and/or increased channel opening probability. The resulting increased Cl$^-$ influx causes membrane hyperpolarization and decreases neuronal excitability.

In GABA dose-response studies, benzodiazepines shift the response curve to the left, increasing the apparent potency of GABA up to three-fold (Fig. 11-6B). This is a smaller allosteric effect than that caused by other modulators, such as general anesthetics (see etomidate, below). The limited efficacy of benzodiazepines is therefore associated with a reduced potential for fatal overdose. However, the margin of safety decreases when benzodiazepines are administered together with other sedative/hypnotics.

Clinical Applications

Benzodiazepines are used as anxiolytics, sedatives, anti-epileptics, muscle relaxants, and for treatment of ethanol withdrawal symptoms (Table 11-2). Benzodiazepines achieve an anxiolytic effect by inhibiting synapses in the limbic system, a CNS region that controls emotional behavior and is characterized by a high density of GABA$_A$ receptors. Benzodiazepines such as **diazepam** and **alprazolam** are used to mitigate chronic, severe anxiety, and the anxiety associated with

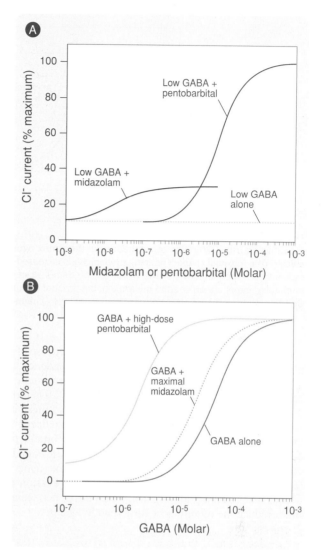

Figure 11-6. Effects of benzodiazepines and barbiturates on GABA$_A$ receptor activity. A. Both benzodiazepines and barbiturates enhance GABA$_A$ receptor activation (measured experimentally by Cl$^-$ current), but with different potencies and efficacies. Midazolam (a benzodiazepine) at 1 μM enhances by nearly three-fold the current evoked by 10 μM GABA. In contrast, the anesthetic barbiturate pentobarbital enhances the current evoked by 10 μM GABA to a much greater degree (near that of a maximal GABA response), but its maximal effect requires concentrations over 100 μM. Thus, benzodiazepines such as midazolam are high-potency, low-efficacy modulators of GABA$_A$ receptor activity, while barbiturates such as phenobarbital are low-potency, high-efficacy modulators. **B.** Another way to compare the efficacy of benzodiazepines and barbiturates is to measure the degree to which they enhance the sensitivity of GABA$_A$ receptors to GABA. Maximally effective concentrations of midazolam shift the GABA concentration–response curve modestly to the left, reducing the EC$_{50}$ of GABA by about two-fold. In contrast, high-dose pentobarbital causes a much greater shift to the left, reducing the EC$_{50}$ of GABA by approximately 20-fold. Pentobarbital at high concentrations also directly activates GABA$_A$ receptors, even in the absence of GABA (note the nonzero Cl$^-$ current at *); in contrast, the benzodiazepines do not show direct agonist activity.

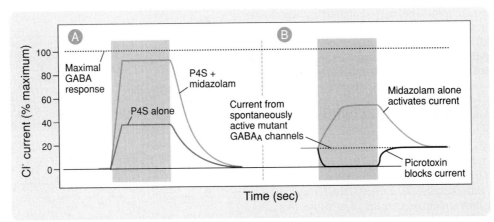

Figure 11-7. **Evidence that benzodiazepines enhance the GABA_A receptor channel opening probability.** **A.** When GABA_A receptors are activated using saturating concentrations of the partial agonist P4S, midazolam increases the peak current. This indicates that the P4S efficacy (the maximal channel opening probability) is increased by the addition of midazolam. **B.** GABA_A receptors containing a single point mutation are spontaneously active, which can be demonstrated by the addition of picrotoxin (a GABA_A receptor antagonist). When these mutant receptors are exposed to midazolam, the amount of current increases, indicating that midazolam directly influences the opening of GABA_A receptors. This effect is not observed in wild-type channels, which exhibit only rare spontaneous openings.

some forms of depression and schizophrenia. Because of the potential for the development of tolerance, dependence, and addiction, benzodiazepines use should be intermittent. In acute-care settings, such as in preparation for invasive procedures, **midazolam** is frequently used as a rapid-onset and short-acting anxiolytic/sedative/amnestic. Benzodiazepines are often adequate as sedatives for brief, uncomfortable procedures associated with minimal sharp pain, such as endoscopy. If combined with opioids, however, a synergistic potentiation of both sedation and respiratory depression can occur. When given prior to general anesthesia, benzodiazepines reduce the requirement for hypnotic agents.

Many benzodiazepines, including **estazolam, flurazepam, quazepam, temazepam, triazolam**, and **zolpidem,** are prescribed for treatment of insomnia. Benzodiazepines both facilitate sleep onset and increase the overall duration of sleep. They also alter the proportion of the various sleep stages: they increase the length of stage 2 non-REM sleep (the light sleep that normally comprises approximately half of sleeping time), and decrease the lengths of REM sleep (the period characterized by frequent dreams) and slow-wave sleep (the deepest level of sleep). After extended use these effects may diminish because of tolerance. In a healthy individual, hypnotic doses of benzodiazepines induce respi-

TABLE 11-2	Clinical Uses and Relative Duration of Action of Several Benzodiazepines	
BENZODIAZEPINE	**CLINICAL USES**	**DURATION OF ACTION**
Midazolam	Preanesthetic, IV general anesthetic	Short-acting (3–8 hours)
Clorazepate	Anxiety disorders, seizures	Short-acting (3–8 hours)
Alprazolam	Anxiety disorders, phobias	Intermediate-acting (11–20 hours)
Lorazepam	Anxiety disorders, status epilepticus, IV general anesthetic	Intermediate-acting (11–20 hours)
Chlordiazepoxide	Anxiety disorders, alcohol withdrawal	Long-acting (1–3 days)
Clonazepam	Seizures	Long-acting (1–3 days)
Diazepam	Anxiety disorders, status epilepticus, muscle relaxant, IV general anesthetic, alcohol withdrawal	Long-acting (1–3 days)
Triazolam	Insomnia	Short-acting (3–8 hours)
Estazolam	Insomnia	Intermediate-acting (11–20 hours)
Temazepam	Insomnia	Intermediate-acting (11–20 hours)
Flurazepam	Insomnia	Long-acting (1–3 days)
Quazepam	Insomnia	Long-acting (1–3 days)

ratory changes comparable to those present during natural sleep, and do not cause significant cardiovascular changes. Patients with either pulmonary or cardiovascular disease may experience significant respiratory or cardiovascular depression because of medullary depression from otherwise therapeutic doses of these drugs. Patients who have suffered brain damage from stroke or head trauma may also become profoundly sedated with these drugs.

The sedative benzodiazepines differ in their rates of onset, durations of effect, and tendencies to cause rebound insomnia when withdrawn. For example, **flurazepam** is a long-acting benzodiazepine that facilitates sleep onset and maintenance and increases sleep duration. Although it does not cause significant rebound insomnia, its long elimination half-life (about 74 hours) and the accumulation of active metabolites may cause daytime sedation. **Triazolam** is a fast-onset benzodiazepine that also decreases the time needed to fall asleep. Intermittent rather than chronic administration of this drug is recommended to lessen the rebound insomnia associated with its discontinuation. **Zolpidem** is unique among sedatives used for insomnia in selectively interacting with GABA$_A$ receptors containing α1 subunits. This selectivity is associated with reduced muscle relaxant and anxiolytic actions, but tolerance and amnesia remain as reported adverse effects.

Benzodiazepines also have antiepileptic effects. **Clonazepam** is frequently used for this indication, because the anticonvulsant effects of clonazepam are not accompanied by significant psychomotor impairment. Drugs used in the treatment of epilepsy are discussed further in Chapter 14, Pharmacology of Abnormal Electrical Neurotransmission in the Central Nervous System.

Benzodiazepines reduce skeletal muscle spasticity by enhancing the activity of inhibitory interneurons in the spinal cord. **Diazepam** is used to alleviate muscle spasms caused by physical trauma as well as the muscle spasticity associated with neuromuscular degenerative disorders such as multiple sclerosis. The high doses required for these effects also frequently cause sedation.

Pharmacokinetics and Metabolism

Benzodiazepines can be administered via oral, transmucosal, intravenous, and intramuscular routes. The lipophilic nature of benzodiazepines explains their rapid and complete absorption. Although these drugs and their active metabolites are bound to plasma proteins, they do not compete with other protein-bound drugs. Benzodiazepines are metabolized by hepatic microsomal cytochrome P450 enzymes, specifically CYP3A4, and subsequently excreted in the urine as glucuronides or oxidized metabolites. Prolonged benzodiazepine administration does not significantly induce hepatic drug-metabolizing enzyme activity. However, other drugs that inhibit CYP3A4 activity (e.g., ketoconazole and macrolide antibiotics) may enhance the effects of benzodiazepines, while drugs that induce CYP3A4 (e.g., rifampicin, omeprazole, nifedipine) may reduce their effectiveness. Patients with impaired hepatic function, including the elderly and the very young, may experience prolonged effects from benzodiazepine administration. Some benzodiazepine metabolites (e.g., **desmethyldiazepam**) remain pharmacologically active and are cleared more slowly than the original drug.

Adverse Effects

The relative safety of benzodiazepines derives from their limited efficacy in modulating GABA$_A$ receptors. High doses of benzodiazepines rarely cause death unless administered with other drugs, such as ethanol, CNS depressants, opioid analgesics, or tricyclic antidepressants. The enhanced CNS depression seen with concomitant ethanol and benzodiazepine use is due to both synergistic effects on GABA$_A$ receptors and ethanol-mediated inhibition of CYP3A4. This effect occurs when ethanol is consumed rapidly, decreasing benzodiazepine clearance.

Benzodiazepine overdose can be reversed by a benzodiazepine antagonist such as **flumazenil.** Although flumazenil has minimal clinical effects on its own, it antagonizes the effects of benzodiazepine agonists by competing for occupancy of high affinity benzodiazepine sites on GABA$_A$ receptors (Fig. 11-3B). In patients with benzodiazepine dependence, flumazenil can cause a severe withdrawal syndrome. This drug does not block the effects of barbiturates or ethanol.

Tolerance and Dependence

Chronic benzodiazepine use induces tolerance, which is manifested as a decrease in the efficacy of both benzodiazepines and barbiturates. Animal models suggest that tolerance to benzodiazepines results from decreased expression of benzodiazepine (GABA$_A$) receptors at synapses. Another proposed mechanism for tolerance involves uncoupling of the benzodiazepine-binding site from the GABA site. Sudden cessation after chronic benzodiazepine administration can result in a withdrawal syndrome characterized by confusion, anxiety, agitation, and insomnia.

Barbiturates

The CNS sites affected by **barbiturates** are widespread and include the spinal cord, the brainstem (cuneate nucleus, substantia nigra, reticular activating system), and the brain (cortex, thalamus, cerebellum). Barbiturates reduce neuronal excitability primarily by increasing GABA-mediated inhibition via GABA$_A$ receptors. Barbiturate-enhanced GABAergic transmission in the brainstem suppresses the reticular activating system (discussed in Chapter 7, Principles of Nervous System Physiology and Pharmacology), causing sedation, amnesia, and loss of consciousness. Heightened GABAergic transmission at motor neurons in the spinal cord relaxes muscles and suppresses reflexes. Selectivity for GABA$_A$ receptor subtypes containing specific subunit combinations has not been demonstrated for barbiturates. The number of barbiturate binding sites on GABA$_A$ receptors is uncertain.

The anesthetic barbiturates **thiopental, pentobarbital,** and **methohexital** act as agonists at GABA$_A$ receptors and also act to enhance receptor responses to GABA. Anticonvulsant barbiturates such as **phenobarbital** produce far less direct agonism on native GABA$_A$ receptors. The direct GABA$_A$ receptor activation is not mediated by GABA binding sites, but depends on specific sites in the β subunits.

At clinically relevant concentrations of barbiturates, the

degree of membrane hyperpolarization due to direct activation of GABA$_A$ receptors is far less than that from enhancement of GABA agonism. *The major action of the barbiturates is to enhance the efficacy of GABA by increasing the time that the Cl$^-$ channel stays open, permitting a much greater influx of Cl$^-$ ions for each activated channel* (Fig. 11-6). This leads to a greater degree of hyperpolarization and to decreased excitability of the target cell. The GABA-enhancing action of barbiturates is greater than that of the benzodiazepines. The direct-activating and GABA-enhancing actions of barbiturates may be associated with different types of binding sites, or as shown for etomidate (see below), may reflect actions at a single class of sites. As correlated with their relative efficacy for GABA potentiation, overdoses of the low-efficacy benzodiazepines are deeply sedating but rarely dangerous, whereas barbiturate overdose may produce profound hypnosis or coma, respiratory depression, and death if supportive therapy is not provided.

Barbiturates affect not only GABA$_A$ receptors, but also receptors involved in excitatory neurotransmission. Barbiturates decrease activation of the AMPA receptor by glutamate (see Fig. 11-8), thereby reducing both membrane depolarization and neuronal excitability. At anesthetic concentrations, pentobarbital also decreases the activity of voltage-dependent Na$^+$ channels, inhibiting high-frequency neuronal firing.

Clinical Applications

Before the discovery of benzodiazepines, the sedative/hypnotic effects of barbiturates were commonly used to treat insomnia or anxiety. Benzodiazepines have largely replaced barbiturates in most clinical applications, because benzodiazepines are safer, cause less tolerance, have fewer withdrawal symptoms, and induce less profound effects on drug-metabolizing enzymes. Barbiturates are still used for induction of general anesthesia, as antiepileptic agents, and for neuro-protection (Table 11-3).

The lipid-soluble barbiturates, such as **thiopental, pentobarbital** and **methohexital,** are used to induce general anes-thesia. These drugs enter the brain rapidly after intravenous administration and then redistribute to less highly perfused tissues. This redistribution produces a short duration of action after a single bolus administration. The anesthetic drugs are also discussed in Chapter 15, General Anesthetic Pharmacology.

Barbiturates such as **phenobarbital** serve as effective antiepileptics. As discussed in Chapter 14, seizures are characterized by rapidly depolarizing CNS neurons that repeatedly fire action potentials. Barbiturates reduce epileptic activity both by enhancing GABA-mediated synaptic inhibition and by inhibiting AMPA receptor-mediated excitatory transmission. Phenobarbital is used to treat partial and tonic–clonic seizures at concentrations that produce minimal sedation.

The profound suppression of neuronal activity by barbiturates can produce electroencephalographic silence, known as barbiturate coma. This state is associated with significantly reduced brain oxygen consumption and reduced cerebral blood flow. These effects can protect the brain from ischemic damage in pathologic conditions associated with reduced oxygen delivery (e.g., hypoxia, profound anemia, shock, brain edema) or increased oxygen demand (e.g., status epilepticus). To produce barbiturate coma, bolus administration is followed by infusion (or multiple additional boluses) to maintain the CNS concentration of drug at therapeutic levels.

Pharmacokinetics and Metabolism

Barbiturates, like benzodiazepines, can be administered orally or intravenously. Oral administration may be associated with significant first-pass metabolism and reduced bioavailability. **Methohexital** can also be absorbed transmucosally. The ability of a barbiturate to cross the blood–brain barrier and enter the CNS is largely determined by its lipid solubility. Consequently, termination of the drug's acute CNS effects depends primarily on its redistribution from the brain, first to such highly perfused areas as the splanchnic circulation, then to skeletal muscle, and, finally, to poorly perfused adipose tissue. As a result, bolus administration of a barbiturate that redistributes rapidly causes only a short-lived effect

TABLE 11-3	Clinical Uses and Relative Duration of Action of Several Barbiturates	
BARBITURATE	**CLINICAL USES**	**DURATION OF ACTION**
Thiopental	Anesthesia induction and short-term maintenance, emergency seizure treatment	Ultrashort-acting (5–15 minutes)
Methohexital	Anesthesia induction and short-term maintenance	
Pentobarbital	Insomnia, preoperative sedation, emergency seizure treatment	Short-acting (3–8 hours)
Secobarbital	Insomnia, preoperative sedation, emergency seizure treatment	
Amobarbital	Insomnia, preoperative sedation, emergency seizure treatment	
Phenobarbital	Treatment of seizures, status epilepticus	Long-acting (days)

A barbiturate's duration of action is determined by the rapidity with which it is redistributed from the brain to other, less vascular compartments, particularly to muscle and fat.

on the CNS. Chronic administration of the lipophilic barbiturates may have a prolonged effect because of the high capacity of adipose tissue, which leads to a high volume of distribution and to a long elimination half-life.

Barbiturates undergo extensive hepatic metabolism before renal excretion. The cytochrome P450 enzymes that metabolize barbiturates are CYP3A4, CYP3A5, and CYP3A7. Chronic barbiturate use up-regulates the expression of these enzymes, thereby accelerating the metabolism of barbiturates (contributing to tolerance) and other substrates for these enzymes. Barbiturates enhance the metabolism of other sedative/hypnotics, as well as benzodiazepines, phenytoin, digoxin, oral contraceptives, steroid hormones, bile salts, cholesterol, and vitamins D and K. Elderly patients (who often have impaired liver function) and patients with severe liver disease have reduced barbiturate clearance; even normal doses of sedative–hypnotics may have significantly greater CNS effects in these patients, as experienced by Mr. B. Because acidic compounds such as phenobarbital are excreted faster in alkaline urine, administration of intravenous sodium bicarbonate increases clearance.

Adverse Effects

The multiplicity of sites at which barbiturates act, coupled with their low selectivity and high efficacy for enhancing GABA$_A$ receptor activation, contributes to the relatively low therapeutic index of these drugs. Unlike benzodiazepines, high doses of barbiturates can cause fatal CNS depression. The anesthetic barbiturates such as pentobarbital are more likely to induce profound CNS depression than anticonvulsants such as phenobarbital (Table 11-4). In addition, as exemplified by the case of Mr. B, the concomitant administration of barbiturates and other CNS depressants, often ethanol, results in CNS depression more severe than that caused by barbiturates alone.

Tolerance and Dependence

Repeated and extended misuse of barbiturates induces tolerance and physiologic dependence. Prolonged barbiturate use increases the activity of the cytochrome P450 enzymes and accelerates barbiturate metabolism, thereby contributing to the development of tolerance to barbiturates and cross-tolerance to benzodiazepines, other sedative/hypnotics, and ethanol. Development of physiologic dependence results in a drug withdrawal syndrome characterized by tremors, anxiety, insomnia, and CNS excitability. If left untreated, these withdrawal signs may progress to seizures and cardiac arrest.

Etomidate, Propofol, and Alphaxalone

Etomidate, **propofol**, and **alphaxalone** are drugs used for induction of general anesthesia. Etomidate and propofol are also discussed in Chapter 15. Like barbiturates, these intravenous anesthetics act primarily on GABA$_A$ receptors. Etomidate is particularly useful during induction of anesthesia in hemodynamically unstable patients. Propofol is the most widely used anesthetic induction agent in the United States. It is used both for single-bolus induction of anesthesia and for maintenance via continuous intravenous infusion. Alphaxalone is a **neuro-active steroid** but is rarely used clinically.

Mechanisms of Action

Like barbiturates, etomidate, propofol, and alphaxalone enhance activation of GABA$_A$ receptors by GABA and, at high concentrations, can act as agonists. For etomidate, both of these actions display similar stereoselectivity. Quantitative analysis indicates that both actions are caused by etomidate binding at a single set of two identical allosteric sites per receptor. It is unknown whether a similar mechanism accounts for the actions of propofol and alphaxalone.

TABLE 11-4	Comparison of Pentobarbital and Phenobarbital	
	PENTOBARBITAL	**PHENOBARBITAL**
Routes of administration	Oral, IM, IV, rectal	Oral, IM, IV
Duration of action	Short-acting (1–4 hours)	Long-acting (days)
Suppression of spontaneous neuronal activity	Yes	Minimal
Activity at GABA$_A$ receptor	Major: Increases efficacy of GABA by increasing open time of Cl$^-$ channel. Minor: Direct GABA$_A$ receptor activation	Increases efficacy of GABA by increasing open time of Cl$^-$ channel
Activity at glutamate receptor	Noncompetitive antagonist at AMPA receptor (2–3 times more potent than phenobarbital)	Noncompetitive antagonist at AMPA receptor
Therapeutic uses	Preoperative sedation Emergency treatment for seizures	Anticonvulsant

Etomidate and propofol act selectively at GABA$_A$ receptors that contain β2 and β3 subunits. Based on knock-in animal experiments, where β3 subunits are expressed as transgenes, β3-containing receptors are the most important for the hypnosis and muscle relaxation associated with general anesthesia. Alphaxalone shows little selectivity among synaptic GABA$_A$ receptors, but is more potent at extrasynaptic receptors that contain δ subunits.

Pharmacokinetics and Metabolism

Etomidate and propofol both induce anesthesia rapidly following bolus intravenous injection. Like barbiturates, these hydrophobic drugs cross the blood-brain barrier rapidly. The CNS effect of a bolus dose lasts for only several minutes, because redistribution to muscle and other tissues rapidly reduces the CNS drug concentrations. Propofol has an extremely large volume of distribution, so that prolonged continuous infusions may be used without large increases in the apparent clearance time. Metabolism of etomidate and propofol is primarily hepatic.

Adverse Effects

Etomidate inhibits the synthesis of cortisol and aldosterone. Suppression of cortisol production is thought to contribute to mortality among critically ill patients who receive prolonged etomidate infusions, and administration of exogenous glucocorticoids is effective in preventing this complication. As a result, etomidate is only used for single-dose induction of anesthesia, and rarely at sub-hypnotic doses for treatment of metastatic cortisol-producing tumors.

The major toxicity of propofol as a general anesthetic is depression of cardiac output and vascular tone. Hypotension is observed in patients who are hypovolemic or, as with many elderly patients, dependent on vascular tone to maintain blood pressure. Propofol is formulated in a lipid emulsion and hyperlipidemia has been reported in patients receiving prolonged infusions for sedation.

GABA$_B$ RECEPTOR AGONISTS AND ANTAGONISTS

Baclofen is the only compound currently in clinical use that targets GABA$_B$ receptors. It was first synthesized as a GABA analogue and screened for anti-spastic action before GABA$_B$ receptors were discovered. Subsequently, it was found that baclofen is a selective GABA$_B$ receptor agonist. It is used primarily for treatment of spasticity associated with motor neuron diseases (e.g., multiple sclerosis) or spinal cord injury. Oral baclofen is effective for mild spasticity. Severe spasticity may be treated with intrathecal baclofen therapy using doses that are far lower than those required systemically. By activating metabotropic GABA receptors in the spinal cord, baclofen stimulates downstream second messengers to act on Ca^{2+} and K$^+$ channels. Although baclofen is prescribed primarily for treatment of spasticity, clinical observations suggest that it also modulates pain and cognition, and it is being investigated as a therapy for drug addiction.

Baclofen is absorbed slowly after oral administration with peak plasma concentrations after 90 minutes. It has a modest volume of distribution and does not readily cross the blood-brain barrier. Clearance from the circulation is primarily renal in an unmodified form and about 15% of the drug is metabolized by the liver before excretion in bile. The elimination half-time is about 5 hours in patients with normal renal function, and dosing is typically three times daily. Following intrathecal injection and infusion, spasmolytic effects are observed after one hour and peak at four hours.

Adverse effects of baclofen include sedation, somnolence, and ataxia. These are worsened when baclofen is taken with other sedative drugs. Reductions in renal function may precipitate toxicity as drug levels rise. Baclofen overdose can produce blurry vision, hypotension, cardiac and respiratory depression, and coma.

Tolerance apparently does not develop to oral baclofen. In contrast, dosing requirements after initiation of intrathecal baclofen often increase over the first one to two years. Withdrawal from baclofen therapy, especially intrathecal infusion, can precipitate acute hyperspasticity, rhabdomyolsis, pruritis, delirium, and fever. Withdrawal has also led to multi-organ failure, coagulation abnormalities, shock, and death. Symptoms may persist and effective treatments reportedly include administration of benzodiazepines, propofol, intrathecal opioids, and re-starting baclofen.

NONPRESCRIPTION USES OF DRUGS THAT ALTER GABA PHYSIOLOGY

Ethanol

Ethanol acts as an anxiolytic and sedative by causing CNS depression, but not without significant potential toxicity. Ethanol appears to exert its effects by acting on multiple targets, including GABA$_A$ and glutamate receptors. Ethanol increases GABA$_A$-mediated Cl$^-$ influx and inhibits the excitatory effects of glutamate at NMDA receptors. Ethanol interacts synergistically with other sedatives, hypnotics, antidepressants, anxiolytics, anticonvulsants, and opioids.

Ethanol tolerance and dependence are associated with changes in GABA$_A$ receptor function. In animal models, chronic ethanol administration blunts the ethanol-mediated potentiation of GABA-induced Cl$^-$ influx in the cerebral cortex and cerebellum. Acute tolerance to ethanol occurs without a change in the number of GABA$_A$ receptors, but chronic ethanol exposure alters GABA$_A$ receptor subunit expression in the cortex and cerebellum. Changes in the subunit composition of GABA$_A$ receptors may be responsible for the changes in receptor function associated with chronic ethanol use. Other mechanisms proposed for the development of tolerance to ethanol include post-translational modifications of GABA$_A$ receptors or changes in second messenger systems; for example, alterations in the expression patterns of different isoforms of protein kinase C (PKC). The upregulation of NMDA receptor expression that occurs with prolonged ethanol use may account for the hyperexcitability associated with ethanol withdrawal. Benzodiazepines, such as **diazepam** and **chlordiazepoxide,** reduce the tremors, agitation, and other effects of acute alcohol withdrawal. Use of these medications in a patient experiencing withdrawal from chronic alcohol abuse can also prevent the development of withdrawal seizures (delirium tremens).

Chloral Hydrate and Flunitrazepam

Chloral hydrate is an older sedative–hypnotic rarely used today to alleviate insomnia. It has occasionally been employed to incapacitate individuals against their will; for example, to facilitate the commission of a crime. **Flunitrazepam** (Rohypnol®) is a fast-acting benzodiazepine that can cause amnesia and thereby prevent an individual's recall of events that occurred under the drug's influence. This drug has been reported to facilitate "date rape."

PHYSIOLOGY OF GLUTAMATERGIC NEUROTRANSMISSION

Glutamatergic synapses exist throughout the CNS. The binding of glutamate to its receptors initiates molecular and cellular events associated with numerous physiologic and pathophysiologic pathways, including the development of elevated pain sensation (hyperalgesia), cerebral neurotoxicity, and synaptic changes involved in certain types of memory formation. Although the clinical applications of glutamate pharmacology are currently limited, it is anticipated that glutamate pharmacology will become an increasingly important area of neuropharmacology.

GLUTAMATE METABOLISM

Glutamate synthesis occurs via two distinct pathways. In one pathway, α-ketoglutarate formed in the Krebs cycle is transaminated to glutamate in CNS nerve terminals (Fig. 11-2A). Alternatively, glutamine produced and secreted by glial cells is transported into nerve terminals and converted to glutamate by **glutaminase** (Fig. 11-2B).

Glutamate is released via calcium-dependent exocytosis of transmitter-containing vesicles. Glutamate is removed from the synaptic cleft by glutamate reuptake transporters located on presynaptic nerve terminals and on the plasma membranes of glial cells. These transporters are Na^+ dependent and have a high affinity for glutamate. In glial cells, the enzyme **glutamine synthetase** converts glutamate to glutamine, which is recycled into adjacent nerve terminals for conversion back to glutamate. Glutamine generated in glial cells can also enter the Krebs cycle and undergo oxidation; the resulting α-ketoglutarate enters neurons to replenish the α-ketoglutarate consumed during glutamate synthesis (Fig. 11-2B).

GLUTAMATE RECEPTORS

As with GABA receptors, glutamate receptors are divided into **ionotropic** and **metabotropic** subgroups.

Ionotropic Glutamate Receptors

Ionotropic glutamate receptors mediate fast excitatory synaptic responses. These receptors are multi-subunit, cation-selective channels that, on activation, permit the flow of Na^+, K^+, and, in some instances, Ca^{2+} ions across plasma

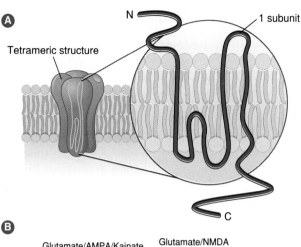

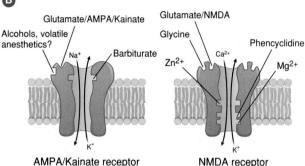

Figure 11-8. Schematic representation of the ionotropic glutamate receptors. A. All three ionotropic glutamate recaeptors are tetrameric complexes composed of the same (termed **homomeric**) or different (termed **heteromeric**) subunits. The structure on the right shows one ionotropic glutamate receptor subunit, which spans the membrane three times and has a hairpin turn that, when juxtaposed with homologous turns from the other three subunits, forms the lining of the ion channel's pore. **B.** Major binding sites on the AMPA/kainate and NMDA classes of ionotropic glutamate receptors are shown. Although there is indirect evidence for the location of many of the drug binding sites that are schematically indicated in this diagram, the definitive localization of these sites remains to be determined.

membranes. Ionotropic glutamate receptors are thought to be tetramers composed of different subunits, with each subunit containing helical domains that span the membrane three times, in addition to a short sequence that forms the channel's pore when the entire tetramer is assembled (Fig. 11-8A).

There are three main subtypes of glutamate-gated ion channels, classified according to their activation by the selective agonists **AMPA, kainate,** and **NMDA.** The diversity of ionotropic receptors arises from differences in amino acid sequence because of alternative mRNA splicing and post-transcriptional mRNA editing, and from the use of different combinations of subunits to form the receptors (Table 11-5).

AMPA (α-amino-3-hydroxy-5-methyl-4-isoxazole proprionic acid) **receptors** are located throughout the CNS, particularly in the hippocampus and cerebral cortex. Four AMPA receptor subunits (GluR1 $-$ GluR4) have been identified (Table 11-5). AMPA receptor activation results primarily in Na^+ influx (as well as some K^+ efflux), allowing these receptors to regulate fast, excitatory postsynaptic depo-

| TABLE 11-5 | Classification of Ionotropic Glutamate Receptor Subtypes |

IONOTROPIC GLUTAMATE RECEPTOR SUBTYPE	SUBUNITS	AGONISTS	ACTIONS
AMPA	GluR1 GluR2 GluR3 GluR4	Glutamate or AMPA	Increase Na^+ and Ca^{2+} influx, increase K^+ efflux (N.B. receptors with GluR2 have ion channels with decreased Ca^{2+} permeability)
Kainate	GluR5 GluR6 GluR7 KA1 KA2	Glutamate or kainate	Increase Na^+ influx, increase K^+ efflux
NMDA	NR1 NR2A NR2B NR2C NR2D	Glutamate or NMDA and glycine and membrane depolarization	Increase Ca^{2+} influx, increase K^+ efflux

larization at glutamatergic synapses (Fig. 11-8B). Although most AMPA receptors in the CNS have low Ca^{2+} permeability, the absence of certain subunits (such as GluR2) in the receptor complex increases the Ca^{2+} permeability of the channel. Calcium entry through AMPA receptors may play a role in neuronal damage.

Kainate receptors are expressed throughout the CNS, particularly in the hippocampus and cerebellum. Five kainate receptor subunits have been identified (Table 11-5). Like AMPA receptors, kainate receptors allow Na^+ influx and K^+ efflux through channels that possess rapid activation and deactivation kinetics. The combination of subunits in the kainate receptor complex determines whether the channel is also permeable to Ca^{2+}. Experiments using receptor-selective agents have allowed the assignment of specific functions to kainate receptors. For example, in the spinal cord, kainate receptors participate in pain transmission.

NMDA (N-methyl-D aspartate) **receptors** are expressed primarily in the hippocampus, cerebral cortex, and spinal cord. These receptors consist of multisubunit oligomeric transmembrane complexes. NMDA receptor activation, which requires simultaneous binding of glutamate and glycine, opens a channel that allows K^+ efflux as well as Na^+ and Ca^{2+} influx (Fig. 11-8B). In NMDA receptors that are occupied by glutamate and glycine, Mg^{2+} ions block the channel pore in the resting membrane (Figure 11-8B). Depolarization of the membrane concurrent with agonist binding is required to relieve this voltage-dependent Mg^{2+} block. Either trains of postsynaptic action potentials or activation of AMPA/kainate receptors in adjacent regions of the membrane can cause postsynaptic membrane depolarization that unblocks the Mg^{2+}-bound NMDA receptor. Therefore, NMDA receptors differ from the other ionotropic glutamate receptors in two important respects—they require the binding of multiple ligands for channel activation, and their gating depends on more intense pre-synaptic activity than that required to open AMPA or kainate receptors.

Metabotropic Glutamate Receptors

Metabotropic glutamate receptors (mGluR) consist of a seven transmembrane-spanning domain coupled via G proteins to various effector mechanisms (Fig. 11-9). At least eight subtypes of metabotropic glutamate receptors exist; each belongs to one of three groups (groups I, II, and III) according to its sequence homology, signal transduction mechanism, and pharmacology (Table 11-6).

Group I receptors cause neuronal excitation either through phospholipase C (PLC) activation and IP_3-mediated intracellular Ca^{2+} release, or through adenylyl cyclase activation and cAMP generation. Group II and III receptors inhibit adenylyl cyclase and decrease cAMP production (Table 11-6). These second messenger pathways regulate ion fluxes of other channels. For example, metabotropic glutamate receptor activation in the hippocampus, neocortex, and cerebellum increases neuronal firing rates by inhibiting a hyperpolarizing K^+ current. Presynaptic mGluRs, such as group II and III receptors in the hippocampus, can operate as inhibitory autoreceptors that inhibit presynaptic Ca^{2+} channels and thereby limit presynaptic release of glutamate.

PATHOPHYSIOLOGY AND PHARMACOLOGY OF GLUTAMATERGIC NEUROTRANSMISSION

Normally, termination of glutamate receptor activation occurs via transmitter reuptake by presynaptic and glial transporters, transmitter diffusion out of the synaptic cleft, or receptor desensitization. As described below, however, increased release or decreased reuptake of glutamate in pathologic states can lead to a positive feedback cycle involving increased intracellular Ca^{2+} levels, cellular damage, and fur-

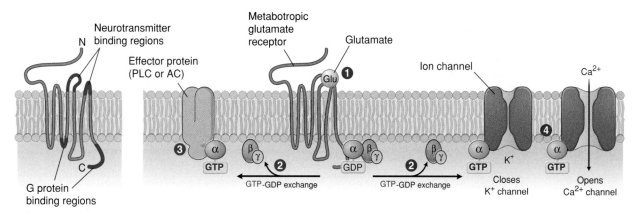

Figure 11-9. Schematic representation and downstream signaling of metabotropic glutamate receptors. Metabotropic glutamate receptors are seven transmembrane-spanning proteins with an extracellular ligand binding site and an intracellular G protein binding site **(left).** Ligand binding to the metabotropic glutamate receptor results in GTP association with the α-subunit of the G protein (*1;* **right**). The GTP-associated α subunit then dissociates from the βγ dimer *(2)*. G_{α} and $G_{\beta\gamma}$ can then activate effector proteins such as adenylyl cyclase *(AC)* and phospholipase C *(PLC; 3)*. G proteins can also open or close ion channels directly *(4)*.

ther glutamate release. Together, these processes can lead to **excitotoxicity**, defined as neuronal death caused by excessive cellular excitation.

Excitotoxicity has been implicated as a pathophysiologic mechanism in many diseases, including neurodegenerative syndromes, stroke and trauma, hyperalgesia, and epilepsy. Although the clinical applications of interrupting excitotoxicity remain limited, it is hoped that better understanding of glutamate-induced excitotoxicity will lead to the development of new approaches to treatment of these diseases.

TABLE 11-6	Metabotropic Glutamate Receptor (mGluR) Subtypes and Their Actions

GROUP	SUBTYPE	ACTIONS
I	mGluR1 mGluR5	Activates adenylyl cyclase → increases cAMP (mGluR1 only) Increases PLC activity → PIP_2 hydrolysis → increases IP_3 and DAG → increases Ca^{2+} levels, stimulates PKC Inhibits K^+ channels
II	mGluR2 mGluR3	Inhibits adenylyl cyclase → decreases cAMP Inhibits voltage-sensitive Ca^{2+} channels Activates K^+ channels
III	mGluR4 mGluR6 mGluR7 mGluR8	Inhibits adenylyl cyclase → decreases cAMP Inhibits voltage-sensitive Ca^{2+} channels

Group I mGluRs activate adenylyl cyclase and phospholipase C (PLC), while group II and group III mGluRs inhibit adenylyl cyclase. The downstream effects of mGluRs on ion channels are complex and varied. Some of the main actions on ion channels are listed. Note that the actions of group I receptors are generally excitatory, while those of groups II and III receptors are generally inhibitory.

NEURODEGENERATIVE DISEASES

Excessive glutamate receptor activation may contribute to the pathophysiology of certain neurodegenerative diseases, including amyotrophic lateral sclerosis (ALS), dementia, and Parkinson's disease.

In ALS, motor neurons degenerate in the ventral horn of the spinal cord, brainstem, and motor cortex, resulting in weakness and atrophy of skeletal muscles. The pathogenesis of this disease and the reasons for the selective pattern of neurodegeneration remain uncertain, but mechanisms currently proposed for cell death in ALS include excitotoxicity and oxidative stress. The CNS areas affected in ALS express diverse populations of AMPA and NMDA receptors as well as glutamate reuptake transporters. Patients with ALS have impaired glutamate transporters in the spinal cord and motor cortex. These abnormal glutamate transporters permit the accumulation of high glutamate concentrations in the synaptic cleft, possibly leading to motor neuron death via excitotoxicity.

Riluzole is a voltage-gated sodium channel blocker that prolongs survival and decreases disease progression in ALS. Although the exact mechanism of action is uncertain, it appears that riluzole acts in part by reducing Na^+ conductance and thereby decreasing glutamate release. It may also directly antagonize NMDA receptors.

Excitotoxicity from excessive glutamate release has also been implicated in progression of dementia in Alzheimer's disease. **Memantine** is a noncompetitive NMDA receptor antagonist used in the treatment of Alzheimer's disease. In clinical studies, memantine appears to slow the rate of clinical deterioration in patients with moderate to severe Alzheimer's disease.

In Parkinson's disease, reduced dopaminergic transmission to the striatum results in the overactivation of glutamatergic synapses in the CNS. Thus, glutamatergic neurotransmission contributes to the clinical signs of Parkinson's disease, as discussed in Chapter 12. The drug **amantadine** is a noncompetitive blocker of NMDA receptor channels, similar in action to memantine. Although amantadine is not an effective treatment as a single agent, the combination of amantadine and **levodopa** reduces the severity of dyskinesia in Parkinson's disease by 60%. It is not clear however, whether this effect derives solely from NMDA receptor blockade.

STROKE AND TRAUMA

In ischemic stroke, interruption of blood flow to the brain provides the initial insults in oxygen supply and glucose metabolism that trigger excitotoxicity (Fig. 11-10). In hemorrhagic strokes, high concentrations of glutamate are found in blood leaking into the brain. In traumatic brain injury the direct rupture of brain cells can release high intracellular stores of glutamate and of K^+ into the restricted extracellular space.

Once excitatory transmitters such as glutamate become unbalanced, widespread membrane depolarization and elevation of intracellular Na^+ and Ca^{2+} concentrations propagate, and more glutamate is released from adjacent neurons. Rising glutamate levels activate Ca^{2+}-permeable NMDA and AMPA receptor-coupled channels. Ultimately, the resultant accumulation of intracellular Ca^{2+} activates many Ca^{2+}-dependent degradation enzymes (e.g., DNAses, proteases, phosphatases, phospholipases) that lead to neuronal cell death.

Although the highly Ca^{2+}-permeable NMDA receptor was originally viewed as the major contributor to neuronal cell death caused by Ca^{2+} overload, AMPA receptors have also been implicated. Clinical trials of NMDA and AMPA receptor antagonists in patients with stroke have not, however, been successful, and in some cases led to schizophrenia-like effects, memory impairment, and neurotoxic reactions. Future pharmacologic research will be directed at the development of drugs with fewer adverse effects, such as the noncompetitive NMDA receptor antagonist **memantine**, or drugs targeted to specific subunits of the NMDA or AMPA receptor complex.

Glutamate released during ischemic or traumatic brain damage can also activate metabotropic receptors. In animal models of stroke, pharmacologic antagonism of the mGluR1 receptor subtype facilitates recovery and survival of hippocampal neurons and also prevents memory and motor loss caused by trauma. These findings suggest that the mGluR1 subunit may represent another target for future pharmacologic intervention (Figs. 11-10 and 11-11).

HYPERALGESIA

Hyperalgesia is the elevated perception of pain due to stimuli that, under normal conditions, cause little or no pain. It occurs in the presence of peripheral nerve injury, inflammation, surgery, and diseases such as diabetes. Although in most cases hyperalgesia is reversed when the underlying pathophysiology has resolved, it may persist even in the absence of an identified organic source, leading to chronic pain that is physically crippling and psychologically debilitating.

There is accumulating evidence that various forms of glutamatergic transmission contribute to the development and/

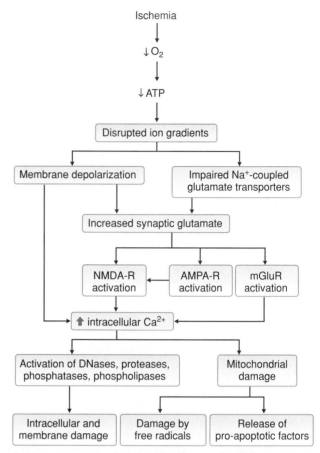

Figure 11-10. Role of glutamate receptors in excitotoxicity. Although a multiplicity of damaging cellular processes occur as a consequence of the decreased ATP levels that result from impaired oxidative metabolism, only glutamate-mediated processes are depicted here.

or the maintenance of hyperalgesia. NMDA receptors are known to enhance synaptic transmission between nociceptive afferent fibers and dorsal horn neurons. As discussed in Chapter 16, Pharmacology of Analgesia, experimental hyperalgesia often involves a phenomenon called **central sensitization**, in which repeated nociceptive stimuli in the periphery lead to progressively increasing excitatory postsynaptic responses in post-synaptic pain neurons in the superficial dorsal horn of the spinal cord. One mechanism by which this synaptic potentiation occurs involves postsynaptic NMDA receptors that, when stimulated chronically, appear to increase the strength of excitatory connections between pre- and post-synaptic neurons in spinal pain circuits. Experimental NMDA receptor antagonists can both prevent and reverse central sensitization in patients. Many of these antagonists, however, also inhibit a wide range of fast excitatory synaptic pathways in the CNS. For this reason, current NMDA receptor drug development focuses on intraspinal or extradural administration of NMDA receptor antagonists to limit the effects of the drug to the dorsal horn of the spinal cord. The high density of kainate receptors in sensory neurons may also modulate transmitter release, providing another future pharmacologic target for the relief of chronic pain.

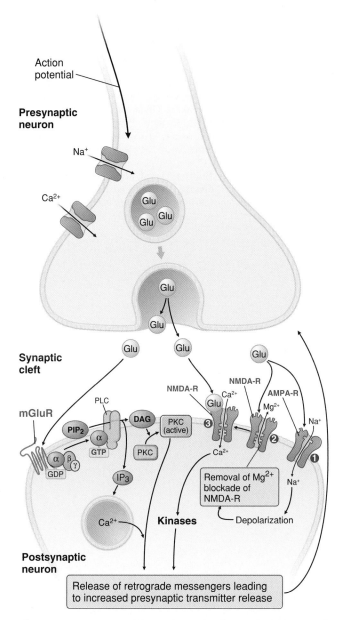

Figure 11-11. Interactions among metabotropic, AMPA, and NMDA classes of glutamate receptors. Action potentials depolarize the plasma membrane of presynaptic neurons, leading to opening of voltage-gated Ca^{2+} channels and ultimately to glutamate release into the synaptic cleft. Studies have proposed a "tonic" physiologic role for activation of the metabotropic glutamate receptor (mGluR) during low-frequency stimulation of postsynaptic neurons by glutamate. In contrast, high-frequency stimulation "phasically" activates AMPA receptors *(1)* and thereby induces the prolonged membrane depolarization required to relieve the Mg^{2+} blockade of NMDA receptors *(2)*. The activated NMDA receptor *(3)* is then able to activate downstream kinases independently of the mGluR. AMPA-R, AMPA receptor; DAG, diacylglycerol; IP_3, inositol-1,4,5-trisphosphate; mGluR, metabotropic glutamate receptor; NMDA-R, NMDA receptor; PIP_2, phosphatidylinositol-4,5-bisphosphate; PKC, protein kinase C; PLC, phospholipase C.

EPILEPSY

Seizures can result from overstimulation of glutamatergic pathways, beginning with overactivation of AMPA receptors and progressing to overactivation of NMDA receptors. In animal models, inhibition of AMPA receptor activation prevents seizure onset, whereas NMDA receptor antagonists decrease seizure intensity and duration. **Lamotrigine,** a drug used in the treatment of refractory complex partial seizures (see Chapter 14), stabilizes the inactivated state of the voltage-gated Na^+ channel, and thereby reduces membrane excitability, the number of action potentials in a burst, glutamate release, and glutamate receptor activation. **Felbamate** is another antiepileptic that has a variety of actions, including the inhibition of NMDA receptors. Because of associated aplastic anemia and hepatotoxicity, its use is restricted to patients with refractory seizures.

Conclusion and Future Directions

GABA and glutamate represent the major inhibitory and excitatory neurotransmitters in the CNS, respectively. Most drugs that act on GABAergic neurotransmission enhance GABAergic activity and thereby depress CNS functions. Modulation of GABAergic transmission can occur either pre-synaptically or post-synaptically. Drugs acting at pre-synaptic sites primarily target GABA synthesis, degradation, and reuptake. Drugs acting post-synaptically affect GABA receptors directly, either by occupying the GABA binding site or by an allosteric mechanism. Each of the three main GABA receptor types has a distinct pharmacology. The $GABA_A$ receptor is targeted by the largest number of drugs, including GABA binding site agonists, benzodiazepines, barbiturates, general anesthetics, and neuroactive steroids. $GABA_B$ receptors are currently targeted by only a few therapeutic agents, which are used to treat spasticity. Recently, $GABA_B$ receptors have been found to influence pain, cognition, and addictive behavior, so interest is growing in drugs that modulate these receptors. $GABA_C$ receptors have not yet been developed as a target of pharmacologic agents.

To improve safety and reduce adverse effects, including ataxia, tolerance, and physical dependence, development of new anxiolytics and sedatives has aimed for low-efficacy compounds (e.g., benzodiazepines) as well as compounds with selective activity at $GABA_A$ receptor subtypes. Animal models with selectively mutated $GABA_A$ receptor subunits have revealed that sedation/hypnosis is produced by enhancing the activity of receptors containing α1 subunits. In contrast, anxiolysis is produced by modulation of α2- or α3-containing receptors and amnesia is associated with α5-containing receptors. There is also evidence for distinct pharmacology and physiology of synaptic $GABA_A$ receptors containing different β subunits.

Because of the potential role of excitatory neurotransmission in a number of pathologic processes, such as neurodegenerative diseases, stroke, trauma, hyperalgesia, and epilepsy, glutamate receptors have become important targets for drug development. The diversity of glutamate receptors and receptor subunits constitutes a potential advantage for the development of glutamate receptor antagonists that are selective for a particular receptor subtype. In the future, highly specific antagonists for glutamate receptor subtypes could potentially protect the CNS in stroke, prevent hyperalgesia after tissue trauma, and treat epileptic seizures.

Suggested Reading

Bowery NG. GABA$_B$ receptor: a site of therapeutic benefit. *Curr Opin Pharmacol* 2006;6:37–43. (*Experimental approaches to targeting GABA$_B$ receptors.*)

Foster AC, Kemp JA. Glutamate- and GABA-based CNS therapeutics. *Curr Opin Pharmacol* 2006;6:7–17. (*General overview of pharmacologic strategies in GABAergic and glutamatergic neurotransmission.*)

Hardingham GE, Bading H. The yin and yang of NMDA receptor signaling. *Trends Neurosci* 2003;26:81–89. (*Physiology and pathophysiology of NMDA receptors.*)

Lo EH, Dalkara T, Moskowitz MA. Mechanisms, challenges and opportunities in stroke. *Nature Rev Neurosci* 2003;4:399–415. (*Advances in pathophysiology of excitotoxicity in stroke.*)

Mohler H, Fritschy JM, Rudolph U. A new benzodiazepine pharmacology. *J Pharmacol Exp Ther* 2002;300:2–8. (*Discusses pharmacologic agents targeting GABA receptor subtypes.*)

Ozawa S, Kamiya H, Tsuzuki K. Glutamate receptors in the mammalian central nervous system. *Prog Neurobiol* 1998;54:581–618. (*A thorough review of ionotropic and metabotropic glutamate receptor physiology, pathophysiology, and pharmacology.*)

Reisberg B, Doody R, Stöffler A, et al. Memantine in moderate-to-severe Alzheimer's disease. *N Engl J Med* 2003;348:1333–1341. (*Clinical trial demonstrating therapeutic benefit of memantine.*)

| Drug Summary Table | **Chapter 11 Pharmacology of GABAergic and Glutamatergic Neurotransmission** | | | |

Drug	Clinical Applications	*Serious* and Common Adverse Effects	Contraindications	Therapeutic Considerations
INHIBITORS OF GABA METABOLISM				
Mechanism—Inhibit GAT-1 (tiagabine) or GABA transaminase (vigabatrin)				
Tiagabine	Partial and tonic–clonic seizures (adjunct therapy)	*Unexplained sudden death* Confusion, sedation, dizziness, depression, psychosis, gastrointestinal irritation	Hypersensitivity to tiagabine	Enhances GABA activity by blocking GABA reuptake into presynaptic neurons Tiagabine potentiates the action of GABA-A receptor modulators such as ethanol, benzodiazepines, and barbiturates
Vigabatrin	Partial and tonic–clonic seizures (adjunct therapy)	*Retinal atrophy, angioedema* Fatigue, headache, ataxia, weight gain	Hypersensitivity to vigabatrin	Blocks conversion of GABA to succinic semialdehyde, resulting in high intracellular GABA concentrations and increased synaptic GABA release Transfer across the blood-brain barrier is slow, and the drug is cleared mainly by renal excretion with a half-life of 5–6 hours
GABA-A RECEPTOR AGONISTS AND ANTAGONISTS				
Mechanism—Directly activate GABA-A receptor (muscimol, gaboxadol), competitive antagonist of GABA-A receptor (bicuculline, gabazine), noncompetitive antagonist of GABA-A receptor (picrotoxin)				
Muscimol	None (used experimentally only)	Not applicable	Not applicable	Derived from hallucinogenic *Amanita muscaria* mushrooms
Gaboxadol	Investigational	Not applicable	Not applicable	Investigational agent for treatment of insomnia
Bicuculline Gabazine Picrotoxin	None (used experimentally only)	Not applicable	Not applicable	Produce epileptic convulsions
GABA-A RECEPTOR MODULATORS: BENZODIAZEPINES				
Mechanism—Weak allosteric agonists of the GABA-A receptor that act to increase the frequency of receptor opening and potentiate effects of GABA				
Short Acting: Midazolam Clorazepate Triazolam Zolpidem *Intermediate Acting:* Alprazolam Lorazepam Estazolam Temazepam *Long Acting:* Chlordiazepoxide Clonazepam Diazepam Flurazepam Quazepam	Partial and tonic–clonic seizures (diazepam, lorazepam, midazolam) Absence seizures (clonazepam) Status epilepticus (midazolam, lorazepam) Amnesia induction (midazolam, lorazepam, diazepam) Anxiety (clorazepate, alprazolam, lorazepam, chlordiazepoxide, clonazepam, diazepam) Alcohol withdrawal (clorazepate, chlordiazepoxide, diazepam) Insomnia (triazolam, zolpidem, lorazepam, estazolam, temazepam, flurazepam, quazepam)	*Respiratory depression, apnea, desaturation in pediatric patients, agitation* Excessive somnolence, headache, fatigue	Acute narrow-angle glaucoma Untreated open-angle glaucoma	Metabolized by P450 3A4 and excreted in the urine as glucuronides or oxidized metabolites Benzodiazepine levels are decreased by carbamazepine or phenobarbital Patients with impaired hepatic function, including the elderly and the very young, may experience prolonged effects from benzodiazepine administration Zolpidem is not technically a benzodiazepine, but binds to the same site on GABA-A receptors as benzodiazepines

(Continued)

Drug Summary Table   Chapter 11 Pharmacology of GABAergic and Glutamatergic Neurotransmission (Continued)

Drug	Clinical Applications	Serious and Common Adverse Effects	Contraindications	Therapeutic Considerations
Flumazenil	Reversal of benzodiazepine activity	*Seizures, cardiac arrhythmias* Dizziness, blurred vision, diaphoresis, agitation	Patient being given a benzodiazepine for intracranial hypertension or status epilepticus Patient with serious tricyclic antidepressant overdose	In patients with benzodiazepine dependence, flumazenil can induce a severe withdrawal syndrome

GABA-A RECEPTOR MODULATORS: BARBITURATES
Mechanism—Enhance GABA activity at GABA-A receptors. At high concentrations, act as direct agonists at GABA-A receptors. May also antagonize AMPA receptor.

Drug	Clinical Applications	Serious and Common Adverse Effects	Contraindications	Therapeutic Considerations
Methohexital Pentobarbital Thiopental Secobarbital Amobarbital	Induction and maintenance of anesthesia (methohexital, thiopental) Insomnia (pentobarbital, thiopental) Status epilepticus (pentobarbital, amobarbital) Raised intracranial pressure (thiopental) Insomnia (secobarbital, amobarbital)	*Stevens–Johnson syndrome, bone marrow suppression, hepatotoxicity, osteopenia* Sedation, ataxia, confusion, dizziness, decreased libido, depression	Porphyria Severe liver dysfunction Respiratory disease	Lipid-soluble barbiturates that enter the brain rapidly after intravenous administration and then redistribute to less highly perfused tissues Chronic use of P450 3A4 inducers such as phenytoin and rifampicin enhances barbiturate metabolism; conversely, P450 3A4 inhibitors such as ketoconazole, erythromycin, cimetidine, and certain SSRIs may reduce barbiturate metabolism, increasing sedative effects
Phenobarbital	Refractory epilepsy, especially partial and tonic–clonic seizures Insomnia	*Same as for other barbiturates*	Same as for other barbiturates	Phenobarbital is one of the few barbiturates that undergoes both renal and hepatic clearance Approximately 25% of a phenobarbital dose is cleared as the unchanged drug in the urine, while the liver metabolizes the remaining 75%

OTHER GABA-A RECEPTOR MODULATORS
Mechanism—Modulation of ligand-gated ion channels (most likely)

Drug	Clinical Applications	Serious and Common Adverse Effects	Contraindications	Therapeutic Considerations
Etomidate	Induction of anesthesia	*Cardiovascular and respiratory depression, injection-site reaction, myoclonus*	Hypersensitivity to etomidate	Causes minimal cardiopulmonary depression, possibly due to lack of effect on the sympathetic nervous system
Propofol	Induction and maintenance of anesthesia Sedation of mechanically ventilated patients	*Cardiovascular and respiratory depression* Injection-site reaction	Hypersensitivity to propofol	Useful especially in short day-surgery procedures because of its rapid elimination Tolerance to propofol has been reported in pediatric patients receiving frequent (daily) anesthetics for radiation therapy, possibly due to increased clearance rather than reduced sensitivity at the GABA-A receptor
Alphaxalone	None (used experimentally only)	*Not applicable*	Porphyria	Alphaxalone is a neuro-active steroid but is rarely used clinically

GABA-B RECEPTOR AGONIST
Mechanism—Activates metabotropic GABA-B receptor

Drug	Clinical Applications	Serious and Common Adverse Effects	Contraindications	Therapeutic Considerations
Baclofen	Spasticity	*Coma, seizure, death after abrupt withdrawal* Constipation, somnolence	Hypersensitivity to baclofen	Clearance is primarily renal in an unmodified form and about 15% of the drug is metabolized by the liver before excretion in bile Withdrawal from baclofen, especially intrathecal infusion, can precipitate acute hyperspasticity, rhabdomyolysis, pruritus, delirium, and fever

NMDA RECEPTOR ANTAGONISTS
Mechanism—Antagonize NMDA receptor

Drug	Clinical Applications	Serious and Common Adverse Effects	Contraindications	Therapeutic Considerations
Riluzole	Amyotrophic lateral sclerosis	*Neutropenia, cardiac arrest, hepatotoxicity, respiratory depression* Hypertension, tachycardia, arthralgias	Hypersensitivity to riluzole	Riluzole is thought to both block voltage-gated sodium channels (thereby reducing sodium conductance) and decrease glutamate release by directly antagonizing NMDA receptors Prolongs survival and decreases disease progression in ALS
Memantine	Alzheimer's disease	Hypertension, constipation, dizziness, headache	Hypersensitivity to memantine	Noncompetitive NMDA receptor antagonist Slows the rate of clinical progression of moderate to severe Alzheimer's disease
Amantadine	Parkinson's disease Influenza A prophylaxis and infection	*Neuroleptic malignant syndrome, suicidal ideation* Orthostatic hypotension, edema, insomnia, hallucinations	Hypersensitivity to amantadine	Noncompetitive NMDA receptor antagonist
Lamotrigine	Partial and tonic–clonic seizures Atypical absence seizures Bipolar I disorder	*Stevens-Johnson syndrome, toxic epidermal necrolysis, bone marrow suppression, hepatic necrosis, amnesia, angioedema* Rash, ataxia, somnolence, blurred vision	Hypersensitivity to lamotrigine	Lamotrigine is a useful alternative to phenytoin and carbamazepine as a treatment for partial and tonic–clonic seizures Lamotrigine is also effective in treating atypical absence seizures; it is the third drug of choice for treatment of absence seizures, after ethosuximide and valproic acid
Felbamate	Refractory epilepsy, especially partial and tonic–clonic seizures	*Aplastic anemia, bone marrow depression, hepatic failure, Stevens-Johnson syndrome* Photosensitivity, gastrointestinal irritation, abnormal gait, dizziness	Blood dyscrasia Liver disease	Felbamate lacks the behavioral effects observed with the other NMDA antagonists Felbamate is an extremely potent antiepileptic drug and has the additional benefit of lacking sedative effects It has been associated with a number of cases of fatal aplastic anemia and liver failure, and its use is restricted to patients with extremely refractory epilepsy

12

Pharmacology of Dopaminergic Neurotransmission

David G. Standaert and Joshua M. Galanter

INTRODUCTION

Dopamine (DA) is a catecholamine neurotransmitter that is the therapeutic target for a number of important central nervous system (CNS) disorders, including Parkinson's disease and schizophrenia. DA is also a precursor for the other catecholamine neurotransmitters norepinephrine and epinephrine. The machinery of catecholamine neurotransmission has a number of components that are shared among members of the class, including biosynthetic and metabolic enzymes. There are also components that are specialized for the individual members of the class, including reuptake pumps and presynaptic and postsynaptic receptors. This chapter presents the principles that underlie current therapies for diseases that directly or indirectly involve changes in dopaminergic neurotransmission. The chapter begins with a discussion of the biochemistry and cell biology of dopaminergic neurotransmission and the localization of the major DA systems in the brain. Following this background, the chapter explores the physiology, pathophysiology, and phar-

macology of **Parkinson's disease,** which results from the specific loss of neurons in one of these DA systems, and **schizophrenia,** which is currently treated, in part, with drugs that inhibit dopaminergic neurotransmission.

Case

Mark S is a 55-year-old man who goes to see his physician because he notices a tremor in his right hand that has developed gradually over a number of months. He finds he can keep the hand quiet if he concentrates on it, but the shaking quickly reappears if he is distracted. His handwriting has become small and difficult to read, and he has trouble using a computer mouse. His wife complains that he never smiles any more, and that his face is becoming expressionless. She also says that he walks more slowly and he has trouble keeping up with her. As Mr. S enters the examination room, his doctor notices that he is walking hunched over and has a short, shuffling gait. The doctor finds on physical examination that Mr. S has increased tone and cogwheel rigidity in his upper extremities, particularly on the right side, and that he is significantly slower than normal at performing rapid alternating movements. The physician determines that Mr. S's symptoms and signs most likely represent the early stages of Parkinson's disease, and she prescribes a trial of levodopa.

QUESTIONS

■ **1.** How does the selective loss of dopaminergic neurons result in symptoms such as those Mr. S is experiencing?

■ **2.** What will be the effect of levodopa on the course of Mr. S's disease?

■ **3.** How will Mr. S's response to levodopa change over time?

■ **4.** Is levodopa the best choice for Mr. S at this stage of his disease?

BIOCHEMISTRY AND CELL BIOLOGY OF DOPAMINERGIC NEUROTRANSMISSION

Dopamine belongs to the **catecholamine** family of neurotransmitters. In addition to dopamine, this family includes **norepinephrine** (NE) and **epinephrine** (EPI). As the name suggests, the basic structure of the catecholamines consists of a catechol (3,4-dihydroxybenzene) moiety connected to an amine group by an ethyl bridge (Fig. 12-1A). Recall from Chapter 7, Principles of Nervous System Physiology and Pharmacology, that catecholaminergic pathways in the brain have "single source-divergent" organization, in that they arise from small clusters of catecholamine neurons that give rise to widely divergent projections. CNS catecholamines modulate the function of point-to-point neurotransmission and affect complex processes such as mood, attentiveness, and emotion.

The neutral amino acid **tyrosine** is the precursor for all catecholamines (Fig. 12-1B). The majority of tyrosine is obtained from the diet; a small proportion may also be synthesized in the liver from **phenylalanine.** The first step in the synthesis of DA is the conversion of tyrosine to L-**DOPA** (L-3,4-dihydroxyphenylalanine, or levodopa) by oxidation of the 3 position on the benzene ring. This reaction is catalyzed by the enzyme **tyrosine hydroxylase** (TH), a ferro (iron containing)-enzyme that consists of four identical subunits of approximately 60 kDa each. In addition to Fe^{2+}, TH also requires the cofactor tetrahydrobiopterin, which is oxidized to dihydrobiopterin in the course of the reaction. Importantly, oxidation of tyrosine to L-DOPA is the rate-limiting step in the production not only of DA, but of all catecholamine neurotransmitters.

The next and final step in the synthesis of DA is the conversion of L-DOPA to DA by the enzyme **aromatic amino acid decarboxylase** (**AADC**). AADC cleaves the carboxyl group from the α-carbon of the ethylamine side chain, liberating carbon dioxide. AADC requires the cofactor pyridoxal phosphate. Although AADC is sometimes referred to as "DOPA decarboxylase," it is promiscuous in its ability to cleave carboxyl groups from the α-carbons of

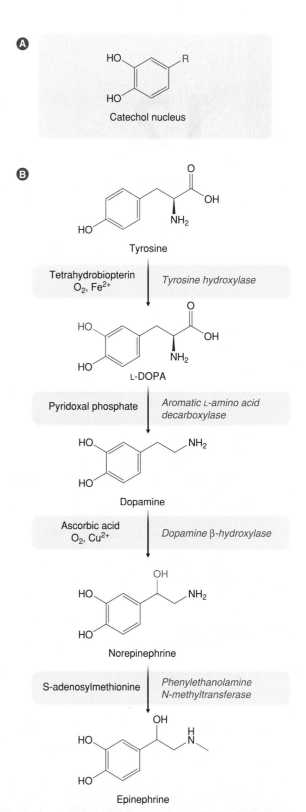

Figure 12-1. Catecholamine synthesis. A. Catecholamines consist of a catechol nucleus with an ethylamine side chain (R group). The R group is ethylamine in dopamine, hydroxyethylamine in norepinephrine, and N-methyl hydroxyethylamine in epinephrine. **B.** Dopamine is synthesized from the amino acid tyrosine in a series of stepwise reactions. In cells that contain dopamine β-hydroxylase, dopamine can be further converted to norepinephrine; in cells that also contain phenylethanolamine N-methyltransferase, norepinephrine can be converted to epinephrine.

all aromatic amino acids and is involved in the synthesis of non-catechol transmitters, such as serotonin. AADC is abundant in the brain. It is expressed by dopaminergic neurons, but it is also present in non-dopaminergic cells and glia. Furthermore, AADC is expressed throughout the body in almost all cell types.

In dopaminergic neurons the end product of the catecholamine synthetic pathway is dopamine. In cells that secrete the catecholamine NE, DA is converted to NE by the enzyme **dopamine β-hydroxylase.** In other cells, NE may subsequently be converted to epinephrine by **phenylethanolamine N-methyltransferase.** Dopaminergic neurons lack both of these enzymes, but it is important to keep in mind the entire pathway of catecholamine biosynthesis because pharmacologic manipulation of DA biosynthesis can also alter the production of NE and EPI. For a more complete discussion of the last two steps in NE and EPI synthesis, see Chapter 9, Adrenergic Pharmacology.

DOPAMINE STORAGE, RELEASE, REUPTAKE, AND INACTIVATION

DA is synthesized from tyrosine in the cytoplasm of the neuron, then transported into secretory vesicles for storage and release (Fig. 12-2). Two separate molecular pumps are required for the transport of DA into synaptic vesicles. A proton ATPase concentrates protons in the vesicle, creating an electrochemical gradient characterized by a low intravesicular pH (i.e., a high proton concentration) and an electropositive vesicle interior. This gradient is exploited by a proton antiporter, the **vesicular monoamine transporter (VMAT),** which allows protons to move down the gradient (out of the vesicle) while simultaneously transporting DA into the vesicle against its concentration gradient. Upon nerve cell stimulation, the DA storage vesicles fuse with the plasma membrane in a Ca^{2+}-dependent manner, releasing DA into the synaptic cleft. In the cleft, DA can bind to both postsynaptic DA receptors and presynaptic DA autoreceptors (see below).

Several mechanisms exist to remove synaptic DA and terminate the signaling produced by the neurotransmitter. Most of the DA released into the synaptic cleft is transported back into the presynaptic cell by an 11-transmembrane domain protein, the **dopamine transporter (DAT).** DAT belongs to the family of catecholamine reuptake pumps. DA reuptake involves transport of the neurotransmitter against its concentration gradient, and therefore requires an energy source. For this reason, the DAT couples dopamine reuptake to the cotransport of Na^+ down its concentration gradient into the cell. In fact, both Na^+ and Cl^- are cotransported with DA into the cell. Because the Na^+ gradient is maintained by the Na^+/K^+-ATPase pump, DA reuptake depends indirectly on the presence of a functioning Na^+/K^+ pump. DA taken up into the presynaptic cell can either be recycled into vesicles for further use in neurotransmission (by VMAT) or degraded by the action of the enzymes **monoamine oxidase (MAO)** or **catechol-O-methyl transferase (COMT)** (Fig. 12-3).

MAO is a key enzyme that functions to terminate the action of catecholamines in both the brain and the periphery. MAOs exist in two isoforms: MAO-A, which is expressed

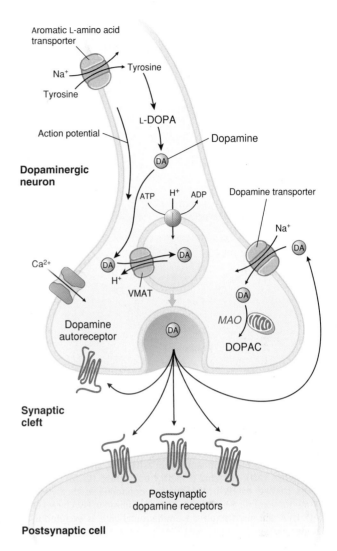

Figure 12-2. Dopaminergic neurotransmission. Dopamine (DA) is synthesized in the cytoplasm and transported into secretory vesicles by the action of a nonselective monoamine-proton antiporter (VMAT) that is powered by the electrochemical gradient created by a proton ATPase. Upon nerve cell stimulation, DA is released into the synaptic cleft, where the neurotransmitter can stimulate postsynaptic dopamine receptors and presynaptic dopamine autoreceptors. DA is transported out of the synaptic cleft by the selective, Na^+-coupled dopamine transporter (DAT). Cytoplasmic DA is re-transported into secretory vesicles by VMAT or degraded by the enzyme monoamine oxidase (MAO).

in the brain as well as the periphery, and MAO-B, which is concentrated in the CNS. Both isoforms of MAO can degrade dopamine as well as a wide range of monoamine compounds. Under normal conditions, MAO-B is responsible for catabolizing most CNS dopamine. The different roles played by the isoforms of MAO are therapeutically important. Selective inhibition of MAO-B is used to augment the function of CNS dopamine, and generally is well tolerated. Inhibition of MAO-A, on the other hand, retards the break-

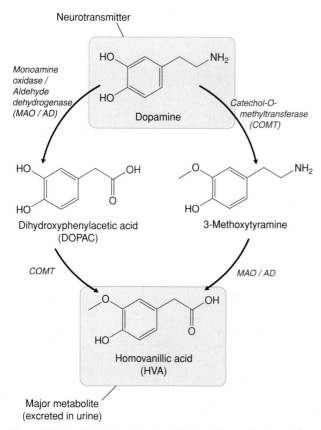

Figure 12-3.   Catecholamine metabolism. Dopamine is metabolized to homovanillic acid (HVA) in a series of reactions. Dopamine is oxidized to dihydroxyphenylacetic acid (DOPAC) by sequential action of the enzymes monoamine oxidase (MAO) and aldehyde dehydrogenase (AD). Catechol-O-methyl transferase (COMT) then oxidizes DOPAC to HVA. Alternatively, dopamine is methylated to 3-methoxytyramine by COMT, and then oxidized to HVA by MAO and AD. HVA, the most stable dopamine metabolite, is excreted in the urine.

down of all central and peripheral catecholamines; as noted in Chapter 9, MAO-A inhibition may lead to life-threatening toxicity when combined with catecholamine releasers such as the indirect-acting sympathomimetic **tyramine** found in certain wines and cheeses.

Synaptic DA that is not taken up into the presynaptic cell can either diffuse out of the synaptic cleft or be degraded by the action of COMT. COMT is expressed in the brain, liver, kidney, and heart; it inactivates catecholamines by adding a methyl group to the hydroxyl group at the 3 position of the benzene ring. In the CNS, COMT is expressed primarily by neurons. The sequential action of COMT and MAO degrades DA to the stable metabolite **homovanillic acid (HVA),** which is excreted in the urine (Fig. 12-3).

DOPAMINE RECEPTORS

Dopamine receptors are members of the G protein-coupled family of receptor proteins. The properties of dopamine receptors were originally classified by their effect on the formation of cyclic AMP (cAMP): activation of D1 class recep-

tors leads to increased cAMP, while activation of D2 class receptors inhibits cAMP generation (Fig. 12-4). Subsequent studies led to cloning of the receptor proteins, revealing five distinct receptors, each encoded by a separate gene. All known DA receptors have the typical structure of G protein-coupled receptors, with seven transmembrane domains. The **D1** class contains two dopamine receptors (D1 and D5) while the **D2** class contains three receptors (D2, D3, and D4). There are two alternative forms of the D2 protein, $D2_S$ (i.e., short) and $D2_L$ (i.e., long), which represent alternate splice variants of the same gene; their difference lies in the third cytoplasmic loop, which affects G protein interaction but not dopamine binding.

The five different dopamine receptor proteins have distinct distributions in the brain (Fig. 12-5). Both D1 and D2 receptors are expressed at high levels in the **striatum** (caudate and putamen), where they play a role in motor control by the **basal ganglia,** as well as in the **nucleus accumbens** (see Chapter 17, Pharmacology of Drug Dependence and Addiction) and **olfactory tubercle.** D2 receptors are also expressed at high levels on anterior pituitary gland **lactotrophs,** where they regulate prolactin secretion (see Chapter 25, Pharmacology of the Hypothalamus and Pituitary Gland). D2 receptors are thought to play a role in **schizophrenia** because many antipsychotic medications have high affinity for these receptors (see below), although the localization of the D2 receptors involved remains to be elucidated. D3 and D4 receptors are structurally and functionally related to D2 receptors, and may also be involved in the pathogenesis of schizophrenia. High levels of D3 receptors are expressed in the **limbic system,** including the nucleus accumbens and olfactory tubercle, while D4 receptors have been localized to the **frontal cortex, diencephalon,** and brainstem. D5 receptors are distributed sparsely and expressed at low levels, mainly in the **hippocampus, olfactory tubercle,** and **hypothalamus.**

Regulation of cAMP formation is the defining characteristic of the dopamine receptor classes, but dopamine receptors can also affect other aspects of cellular function depending on their localization and linkage to second messenger systems. Most dopamine receptors are expressed on the surface of postsynaptic neurons at dopaminergic synapses. The density of these receptors is tightly controlled through regulated insertion and removal of dopamine receptor proteins from the postsynaptic membrane. DA receptors are also expressed presynaptically on the terminals of dopaminergic neurons. Presynaptic dopamine receptors, most of which are of the D2 class, serve as **autoreceptors.** These autoreceptors sense dopamine overflow from the synapse and reduce dopaminergic tone, both by decreasing DA synthesis in the presynaptic neuron and by reducing the rate of neuronal firing and dopamine release. Inhibition of DA synthesis occurs through cAMP-dependent down-regulation of TH activity, while the inhibitory effect on DA release and neuronal firing is due, in part, to a separate mechanism involving the modulation of K^+ and Ca^{2+} channels. Increased K^+ channel opening results in a larger current that hyperpolarizes the neuron, so that a larger depolarization is needed to reach the firing threshold. Decreased Ca^{2+} channel opening results in decreased levels of intracellular Ca^{2+}. Because Ca^{2+} is required for synaptic vesicle trafficking to and fusion with the presynaptic membrane, decreases in intracellular Ca^{2+} levels result in decreased dopamine release.

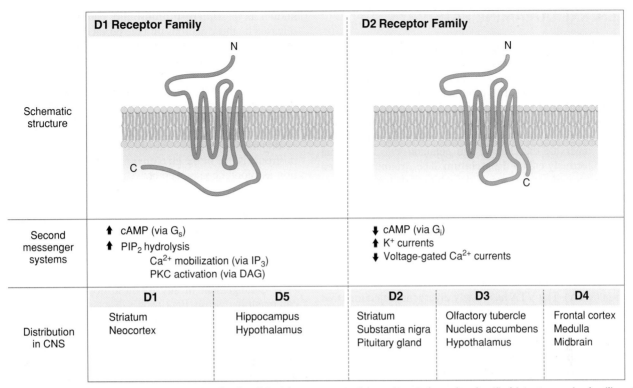

	D1 Receptor Family		D2 Receptor Family		
Schematic structure					
Second messenger systems	↑ cAMP (via G_s) ↑ PIP$_2$ hydrolysis Ca^{2+} mobilization (via IP$_3$) PKC activation (via DAG)		↓ cAMP (via G_i) ↑ K$^+$ currents ↓ Voltage-gated Ca^{2+} currents		
Distribution in CNS	**D1** Striatum Neocortex	**D5** Hippocampus Hypothalamus	**D2** Striatum Substantia nigra Pituitary gland	**D3** Olfactory tubercle Nucleus accumbens Hypothalamus	**D4** Frontal cortex Medulla Midbrain

Figure 12-4. Dopamine receptor families. The five dopamine receptor subtypes (D1–D5) can be classified into two major families of receptors. The D1 receptor family has a long C-terminal tail and a short cytoplasmic loop between transmembrane helices 5 and 6, whereas the D2 receptor family has a short C-terminal tail and a long cytoplasmic loop between helices 5 and 6. Stimulation of the D1 family is excitatory, increasing cAMP and intracellular Ca^{2+} levels and activating protein kinase C (PKC). Stimulation of the D2 family is inhibitory, decreasing cAMP and intracellular Ca^{2+} levels and hyperpolarizing the cell. The five receptor subtypes exhibit distinctive patterns of distribution in the central nervous system. Within the D2 receptor subtype, there are D2$_S$ and D2$_L$ isoforms *(not shown)*. IP$_3$, inositol trisphosphate; DAG, diacylglycerol.

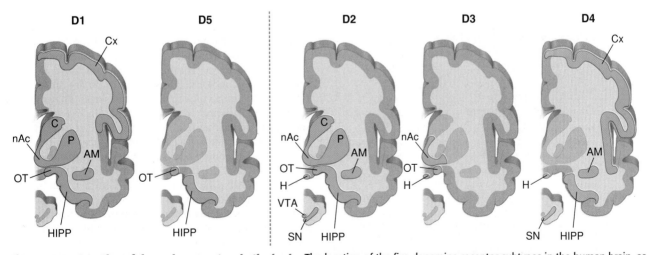

Figure 12-5. Location of dopamine receptors in the brain. The location of the five dopamine receptor subtypes in the human brain, as determined by localization of receptor mRNAs in corresponding regions of the rat brain, is shown in *blue* in coronal section. Both D1 and D2 receptors are localized in the caudate and putamen (the striatum), nucleus accumbens, amygdala, olfactory tubercle, and hippocampus. In addition, D1 receptors are present in the cerebral cortex, whereas D2 receptors are present in the substantia nigra, ventral tegmental area, and hypothalamus. Abbreviations: AM = amygdala, C = caudate, Cx = cerebral cortex, H = hypothalamus, HIPP = hippocampus, nAc = nucleus accumbens, OT = olfactory tubercle, P = putamen, SN = substantia nigra, VTA = ventral tegmental area.

CENTRAL DOPAMINE PATHWAYS

Most central dopaminergic neurons originate in discrete areas of the brain, as shown in Figure 12-6 (see also Fig. 7-8), and have divergent projections. Three major pathways can be distinguished. The largest DA tract in the brain is the **nigrostriatal** system, which contains about 80% of the brain's DA. This tract projects rostrally from cell bodies in the **pars compacta** of the **substantia nigra** to terminals that richly innervate the caudate and putamen, two nuclei that are collectively called the **striatum**. The striatum is named for the striped appearance of the white fiber tracts that run through it; the substantia nigra is named for the dark pigmentation that results from the decomposition of DA to melanin. Dopaminergic neurons of the nigrostriatal system are involved in the stimulation of purposeful movement. Their degeneration results in Parkinson's disease.

Medial to the substantia nigra is an area of dopaminergic cell bodies in the midbrain called the **ventral tegmental area (VTA)**. The VTA has widely divergent projections that innervate many forebrain areas, most notably the cerebral cortex, the nucleus accumbens, and other limbic structures. These systems play an important and complex (as yet poorly understood) role in motivation, goal-directed thinking, regulation of affect, and positive reinforcement (reward). Derangement of these pathways may be involved in the development of **schizophrenia**; as discussed below, the blocking of dopaminergic neurotransmission can lead to a remission in psychotic symptoms. (See Chapter 17 for a more complete discussion of the reward pathway.)

DA-containing cell bodies in the **arcuate** and **periventricular nuclei** of the hypothalamus project axons to the median eminence of the hypothalamus. This system is known as the **tubero-infundibular** pathway. Dopamine is released by these neurons into the portal circulation connecting the median eminence with the anterior pituitary gland, and tonically inhibits the release of prolactin by pituitary lactotrophs.

A fourth anatomic structure, the **area postrema** located in the floor of the fourth ventricle, is also a target of dopaminergic therapies. The area postrema contains only a modest number of intrinsic dopamine neurons, but a high density of dopamine receptors (mostly of the D2 class). The area postrema is one of the **circumventricular organs** that function as blood chemoreceptors. Unlike the rest of the brain, the blood vessels in the circumventricular organs are fenestrated, allowing communication between the blood and CNS (that is, the circumventricular organs are "outside" the blood–brain barrier (BBB)). Stimulation of DA receptors in the area postrema activates the vomiting centers of the brain and is one of the causes of **emesis.** Drugs that block dopamine D2 receptors are used to treat nausea and vomiting.

A derangement in any of these dopaminergic systems can result in disease. Parkinson's disease, which arises from dysregulated dopamine neurotransmission, and schizophrenia, which may also result from abnormal dopamine neurotransmission, are two such examples. These two diseases, and the pharmacologic interventions used to treat them, are highlighted below. Because the pharmacologic manipulation of dopaminergic systems is not always specific to one system, many of the adverse effects of drugs that act on these systems can be predicted based on their effects on the other dopaminergic systems.

DOPAMINE AND CONTROL OF MOVEMENT: PARKINSON'S DISEASE

PHYSIOLOGY OF NIGROSTRIATAL PATHWAYS

The basal ganglia have a crucial role in the regulation of purposeful movement and are the site of the pathology in Parkinson's disease. The basal ganglia do not connect directly to spinal motor neurons, and thus do not directly control the individual movements of muscles. They function instead by assisting in learning coordinated patterns of movement and by facilitating the execution of learned motor patterns. Dopamine has a central role in the operation of this system by signaling when desired movements are executed successfully and driving the learning process.

Anatomically, the basal ganglia form a re-entrant loop by receiving input from the cerebral cortex, processing this information in the context of dopaminergic input from the substantia nigra, and sending information back to the cortex by way of the thalamus. The internal circuitry of the basal ganglia consists of several components. The striatum (caudate and putamen) is the primary input nucleus of the system, while the globus pallidus pars interna and substantia nigra pars reticulata are the output nuclei. These are interconnected through two internuclei, the subthalamic nucleus and the globus pallidus pars externa.

Much of the information processing performed by the basal ganglia occurs in the striatum. The cortical inputs to

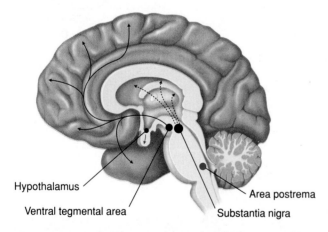

Hypothalamus

Ventral tegmental area

Area postrema

Substantia nigra

Figure 12-6. Central dopamine pathways. Dopaminergic neurons originate in a number of specific nuclei in the brain. Neurons that originate in the hypothalamus and project to the pituitary gland (*blue arrow*) are tonically active and inhibit prolactin secretion. Neurons that project from the substantia nigra to the striatum (*dashed arrows*) regulate movement. Dopaminergic neurons that project from the ventral tegmental area to the limbic system and prefrontal cortex (*solid black arrows*) are thought to have roles in the regulation of mood and behavior. The area postrema contains a high density of dopamine receptors, and stimulation of these receptors activates the vomiting centers of the brain.

this structure are excitatory and use glutamate as a transmitter. The striatum is also the target of the dopaminergic nigrostriatal pathway. The neurons in the striatum are of several types. The majority of neurons are "medium spiny" neurons. These cells are studded with spines that receive input from corticostriatal axons. These medium spiny neurons release the inhibitory transmitter GABA and send their projections to two downstream targets, forming the **direct pathway** and the **indirect pathways** (Fig. 12-7). The striatum also contains several small but important populations of interneurons, including neurons that release acetylcholine. These interneurons participate in the intercommunication between the direct and indirect pathways.

The balance of activity between the direct and indirect pathways regulates movement. The direct pathway, formed by striatal neurons expressing primarily dopamine D1 receptors, projects directly to the output of the basal ganglia, the internal segment of the **globus pallidus.** The latter neurons tonically inhibit the thalamus, which in turn, sends excitatory projections to the cortex that initiate movement. In this manner, activation of the direct pathway disinhibits the thalamus; that is, *the direct pathway stimulates movement.* The indirect pathway, formed by striatal neurons expressing predominantly D2 receptors, projects to the external segment of the globus pallidus, which in turn, inhibits neurons in the **subthalamic nucleus.** The neurons in the subthalamic nucleus are excitatory glutamatergic neurons that project to the internal segment of the globus pallidus. As a result of this multi-

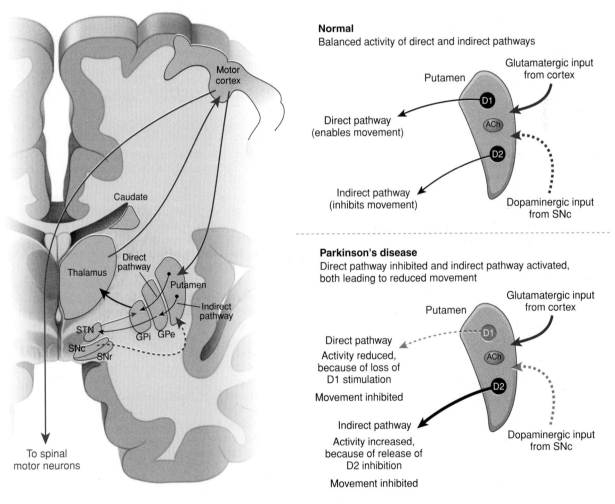

Figure 12-7. Effect of Parkinson's disease on dopaminergic pathways that regulate movement. Two principal pathways in the basal ganglia regulate movement: the indirect pathway, which inhibits movement, and the direct pathway, which enables movement. Dopamine inhibits the indirect pathway and stimulates the direct pathway, yielding a net bias that allows purposeful movement. Excitatory pathways are shown in *blue,* and inhibitory pathways are shown in *black.* The direct pathway signals from putamen to GPi to thalamus to cortex, while the indirect pathway signals from putamen to GPe to STN to GPi to thalamus to cortex. GPi, internal segment of the globus pallidus; GPe, external segment of the globus pallidus. SNc, substantia nigra pars compacta. SNr, substantia nigra pars reticulata. STN, subthalamic nucleus. **Inset:** Both direct and indirect pathway neurons in the putamen receive inputs from the nigrostriatal dopaminergic system *(dotted blue arrow)* and from cortical glutamatergic systems *(solid blue arrow),* process these inputs in the context of local cholinergic influences *(ACh),* and transmit a GABAergic output *(not shown).* Degeneration of dopaminergic neurons in the substantia nigra results in understimulation of the direct (movement-enabling) pathway and underinhibition of the indirect (movement-inhibiting) pathway. The net result is a paucity of movement. *Dotted gray arrow* indicates decreased activity caused by understimulation, and *thick black arrow* indicates increased activity caused by underinhibition.

step pathway, activation of the indirect pathway disinhibits neurons of the subthalamic nucleus, which in turn, stimulate neurons in the internal segment of the globus pallidus to inhibit the thalamus; that is, *the indirect pathway inhibits movement.*

The differential expression of D1 and D2 receptors within the two pathways leads to differing effects of dopaminergic stimulation. Increased levels of dopamine in the striatum tend to activate the D1-expressing neurons of the direct pathway while inhibiting the D2-expressing neurons of the indirect pathway. Notice that both of these effects promote movement. The opposite effect occurs in Parkinson's disease, a state of dopamine deficiency: the direct pathway shows reduced activity while the indirect pathway is overactive, leading to reduced movement.

This model of basal ganglia function is greatly simplified, of course, but it has been useful in developing a deeper understanding of how the basal ganglia work. An important prediction of the model is that, in Parkinson's disease, the indirect pathway (and, in particular, the subthalamic nucleus) should be overactive. This prediction has been proven directly by electrical recordings in living patients with Parkinson's disease. Furthermore, surgical therapies that target the subthalamic nucleus, such as deep brain stimulation in this location, are now often used to treat Parkinson's disease when pharmacologic treatments are inadequate.

PATHOPHYSIOLOGY

In Parkinson's disease, there is a selective loss of dopaminergic neurons in the **substantia nigra pars compacta** (Fig. 12-7).The extent of loss is profound, with at least 70% of the neurons destroyed at the time symptoms first appear; often, 95% of the neurons are missing at autopsy. The destruction of these neurons results in the core features of the disease: bradykinesia, or slowness of movement; rigidity, a resistance to passive movement of the limbs; impaired postural balance, which predisposes to falling; and a characteristic tremor when the limbs are at rest.

The mechanisms underlying the destruction of DA neurons in the substantia nigra in Parkinson's disease are not fully understood. Both environmental factors and genetic influences have been implicated. In 1983, the unexpected development of Parkinson's disease in abusers of the synthetic opioid meperidine (see Chapter 16, Pharmacology of Analgesia) yielded the first agent known to produce Parkinson's disease directly and the strongest evidence that environmental factors can cause Parkinson's disease. These individuals, who tended to be young and otherwise healthy, suddenly developed severe, levodopa-responsive parkinsonian symptoms. The cases were all linked to a single contaminated batch of meperidine that had been synthesized in a makeshift lab. The contaminant was found to be **1-methyl-4-phenyl-1,2,3,6-tetrahydropyridine (MPTP),** which forms as an impurity in the synthesis of meperidine when its manufacture is carried out for too long and at too high a temperature. Studies in nonhuman primates have shown that MPTP is oxidized in the brain to MPP^+ (1-methyl-4-phenyl-pyridinium), which is selectively toxic to neurons in the substantia nigra. Despite extensive searches, it does not appear that there is any significant amount of MPTP present in the everyday environment, and MPTP itself is not the cause of most cases of Parkinson's disease. There may, however, be other environmental factors that have a more subtle effect on development of the disease, such as exposure to certain pesticides.

Recent research has established that genetic factors may cause Parkinson's disease. The best studied examples are families with mutations in the protein α-synuclein, which lead to an autosomal dominant form of Parkinson's disease. While the function of this protein is not clear, it appears to be involved in the formation of neurotransmitter vesicles and the release of dopamine in the brain. At least four other genes have been identified as causing Parkinson's disease in one or more families. These genetic discoveries have provided important clues into the biology of Parkinson's disease and have allowed the development of transgenic mouse and fruit fly models that serve as a platform for developing new treatments. Although these genetic discoveries have provided insight into the biology of Parkinson's disease, it is important to note that all of the different genetic causes identified so far account for less than 5% of cases, and most cases are still of unknown cause. The etiology of Parkinson's disease in most patients is likely multifactorial, with contributions from both genetic and environmental factors.

PHARMACOLOGIC CLASSES AND AGENTS

Parkinson's disease is a progressive disorder. Loss of dopaminergic neurons begins a decade or more before the symptoms become apparent, and this loss continues relentlessly. All of the currently available treatments are *symptomatic,* meaning that they treat the symptoms but do not alter the underlying degenerative process. These symptomatic treatments are very useful, and can restore function and quality of life for many years, but ultimately the progress of the disease leads to increasing difficulty in managing the symptoms. In addition, some features of Parkinson's disease do not respond well to current medications, particularly the cognitive impairment and dementia that characterize the late stages of the disease and that result from an extension of the disease process from the dopaminergic system to other areas of the brain. The goal of much current research is the development of **neuroprotective** and **neurorestorative** therapies, which might delay or eliminate the need for symptomatic treatment and avoid the late complications of the disorder.

Most of the pharmacologic interventions currently used in Parkinson's disease are aimed at restoring DA levels in the brain. In general, medications used in the management of Parkinson's disease can be divided into DA precursors, DA receptor agonists, and inhibitors of DA degradation. There is a smaller but still useful role for the existing nondopaminergic therapies, such as anticholinergic agents that modify the function of striatal interneurons.

Dopamine Precursors

Levodopa was first used to treat Parkinson's disease over 30 years ago, and is still the most effective treatment for the disease. DA itself is not suitable because it cannot cross the BBB. However, DA's immediate precursor, L-DOPA (levodopa), is readily transported across the BBB by the neutral amino acid transporter (see Chapter 7); once in the CNS, L-DOPA is converted to dopamine by the enzyme AADC. Thus, L-DOPA must compete with other neutral amino acids for transport across the BBB, and its availability in the CNS may be compromised by recent protein meals (see the introductory case in Chapter 7).

Orally administered levodopa is readily converted into dopamine by AADC in the gastrointestinal tract. This metabolic process both diminishes the amount of levodopa that can reach the blood–brain barrier for transport into the CNS, and increases the peripheral adverse effects that result from the generation of dopamine in the peripheral circulation (predominantly nausea, due to binding of this dopamine to dopamine receptors in the area postrema). When levodopa is administered alone, only 1% to 3% of the administered dose reaches the CNS unchanged. In order to boost the levels of levodopa available to the brain and reduce the adverse effects of peripheral levodopa metabolism, levodopa is almost always administered in combination with **carbidopa,** an inhibitor of AADC (Fig. 12-8). *Carbidopa effectively prevents the conversion of levodopa to DA in the periphery.* Importantly, because carbidopa is not able to cross the BBB, it does not interfere with the conversion of levodopa to DA in the CNS. Carbidopa increases the fraction of orally administered levodopa available in the CNS from 1%–3% (without carbidopa) to 10% (with carbidopa), allowing a significant reduction in the dose of levodopa and reducing the incidence of peripheral adverse effects.

Many patients with Parkinson's disease show remarkable symptomatic improvement when prescribed the combination of levodopa and carbidopa, especially during the early phase of the disease. In fact, an improvement in symptoms following the initiation of levodopa therapy is considered diagnostic of Parkinson's disease. Over time, however, the effectiveness of levodopa declines. Continued use results in both tolerance and sensitization to the medication, manifested as

a drastic narrowing of the therapeutic window. As patients continue on levodopa therapy, they require more drug to produce a clinically significant improvement in symptoms. They develop fluctuations in motor function that include periods of freezing and increased rigidity, known as ''off'' periods, alternating with periods of normal or even dyskinetic movement, known as ''on'' periods. These ''on'' periods generally occur shortly after the administration of levodopa/carbidopa, when a large bolus of dopamine is delivered to the striatum. ''On'' periods can be overcome initially by taking smaller doses of medication, although this increases the likelihood of ''off'' periods. ''Off'' periods tend to occur as plasma levels of levodopa decline, and can be compensated for by increasing either the dose of levodopa or the frequency of dosing of the medication. As the disease progresses, these symptoms become increasingly difficult to manage.

The most profound adverse effect of levodopa is its propensity to cause **dyskinesias,** or uncontrollable rhythmic movements of the head and trunk. These appear in at least half of all patients within 5 years of starting the drug, and they generally worsen as the disease progresses. Similar to the ''on/off'' phenomenon, dyskinesias are usually linked to levodopa dosing, occurring at times of maximal levodopa plasma concentrations. Accordingly, dyskinesias can also be managed initially by using smaller doses of levodopa more frequently. Unfortunately, as the disease progresses, continued therapy leads to worsening of both the dyskinesias and the ''on/off'' phenomenon, to the point where one or the other is almost always present.

Although levodopa-induced dyskinesias and fluctuations in motor function are complex and poorly understood, at

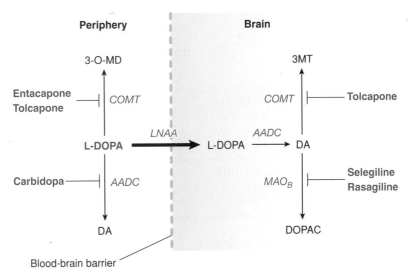

Figure 12-8. Effects of carbidopa, COMT inhibitors, and MAO_B inhibitors on the peripheral and central metabolism of levodopa. Orally administered levodopa (L-DOPA) is metabolized in the peripheral tissues and in the gastrointestinal (GI) tract by aromatic L-amino acid decarboxylase (AADC), catechol-O-methyltransferase (COMT), and monoamine oxidase A (MAO_A; *not shown*). This metabolism substantially reduces the effective dose of levodopa available to the brain and substantially increases the adverse peripheral effects of the drug. Carbidopa is an AADC inhibitor that cannot cross the blood–brain barrier. When levodopa is administered in combination with carbidopa, a greater fraction of the levodopa is available to the brain. Therefore, a smaller dose of levodopa is required for clinical efficacy, and the drug has less severe adverse effects in the periphery. By inhibiting COMT in the periphery, entacapone and tolcapone similarly increase the fraction of peripheral levodopa available to the brain. L-DOPA is transported across the blood–brain barrier by the L-neutral amino acid transporter (LNAA) and metabolized to dopamine (DA) by AADC. Within the brain, DA is metabolized by COMT and MAO_B. Tolcapone (COMT inhibitor) and selegiline and rasagiline (selective MAO_B inhibitors) augment the effectiveness of levodopa therapy by inhibiting the metabolism of DA in the brain. 3-O-MD, 3-O-methylDOPA. DOPAC, dihydroxyphenylacetic acid. 3MT, 3-methoxytyramine.

least two factors are thought to contribute to these adverse effects. First, the continued destruction of dopaminergic neurons as Parkinson's disease progresses results in the striatum's increasing inability to store dopamine effectively, and reduces the ability of dopamine terminals to buffer the synaptic concentrations of dopamine. Second, chronic therapy with levodopa appears to cause adaptations in postsynaptic neurons in the striatum. Dopamine concentrations in striatal synapses are normally tightly regulated. The large fluctuations in dopamine concentration produced by intermittent oral levodopa administration induce changes in the cell surface expression of dopamine receptors and in post-receptor signaling events. These postsynaptic adaptations alter the cell's sensitivity to synaptic dopamine levels, further accentuating responses associated with high ("on" period, dyskinesia) and low ("off" period, akinesia) transmitter concentrations.

The predictable decline in efficacy and increase in adverse effects that result from prolonged levodopa therapy have led to discussions about the appropriate time to begin treatment of Parkinson's disease with levodopa and the relative merits of delaying the use of this drug in the early stages of the disease. Recent studies have suggested that there may be advantages to initial treatment with therapies other than levodopa, particularly the dopamine receptor agonists (see below), but these alternatives may lead to more severe adverse effects than levodopa, at least in some patients. In addition, most patients who are initially treated with other therapies generally require levodopa treatment at some point. Levodopa remains the most effective therapy for Parkinson's disease, and should be initiated as soon as other therapies are unable to control parkinsonian symptoms effectively. Further delays in levodopa therapy are associated with reduced rates of symptom control and increased mortality.

Dopamine Receptor Agonists

Another strategy for enhancing dopaminergic neurotransmission is to target the postsynaptic DA receptor directly through the use of DA receptor agonists. Ergot derivatives, such as **bromocriptine** (D2 agonist) and **pergolide** (D1 and D2), and nonergot agonists, such as **pramipexole** (D3>D2) and **ropinirole** (D3>D2), have all been used successfully as adjuvants to treatment with levodopa. As a class, DA receptor agonists have several advantages. Because they are nonpeptide molecules, they do not compete with levodopa or other neutral amino acids for transport across the BBB. Furthermore, because they do not require enzymatic conversion by AADC, they remain effective late in the course of Parkinson's disease. All of the dopamine receptor agonists in current use have half-lives longer than that of levodopa, which allows for less frequent dosing and a more uniform response to the medications.

The major limitation on the use of the dopamine receptor agonists is their tendency to induce unwanted adverse effects. This is particularly true of the older ergot derivatives bromocriptine and pergolide. Both of these drugs can cause significant nausea, peripheral edema, and hypotension. The newer nonergot dopamine agonists pramipexole and ropinirole are less likely to produce these adverse effects; as a result, these drugs are much more commonly used than the ergot derivatives. All of the dopamine agonists may also produce a variety of cognitive side effects, including excessive sedation, vivid dreams, and hallucinations.

Recent studies have examined the use of pramipexole and ropinirole as initial monotherapy for Parkinson's disease. It was thought that, because the dopamine agonists have longer half-lives than levodopa, they might be less likely to induce "off" periods. These studies show that use of the dopamine receptor agonists as initial treatment for Parkinson's disease does delay the onset of "off" periods and dyskinesias, but there is also an increased rate of adverse effects compared to initial treatment with levodopa. At present, many practitioners use dopamine agonists as the initial treatment for Parkinson's disease, especially in younger individuals.

Inhibitors of Dopamine Metabolism

A third strategy that has been employed to treat Parkinson's disease involves the inhibition of DA breakdown. Inhibitors of both MAO-B (the isoform of MAO that predominates in the striatum) and COMT have been used as adjuvants to levodopa in clinical practice (Fig. 12-8). **Selegiline** is a MAO inhibitor that, in low doses, is selective for MAO-B. It does not interfere with the peripheral metabolism of monoamines by MAO-A, and it avoids the toxic effects of dietary tyramine and other sympathomimetic amines that are associated with nonselective MAO blockade (see Chapter 13, Pharmacology of Serotonergic and Central Adrenergic Neurotransmission). A drawback of selegiline is that this drug forms a potentially toxic metabolite, amphetamine, which can cause sleeplessness and confusion, especially in the elderly. **Rasagiline**, a newer MAO-B inhibitor that does not form toxic metabolites, has recently been approved in the US. Both rasagiline and selegiline improve motor function in Parkinson's disease when used alone, and both can augment the effectiveness of levodopa therapy.

Tolcapone and **entacapone** inhibit COMT, and thereby inhibit the degradation of DA. Tolcapone is a highly lipid-soluble agent that can cross the BBB, while entacapone distributes only to the periphery. Both drugs decrease the peripheral metabolism of levodopa and thereby make more levodopa available to the CNS. Because their mechanism of action is different from that of carbidopa (which blocks AADC), the COMT inhibitors can be used in combination with carbidopa to further extend the half-life of levodopa and facilitate entry of the drug into the brain. In clinical trials, these COMT inhibitors have been shown to reduce the "off" periods that are associated with decreasing plasma levodopa levels. Although tolcapone has a theoretical advantage over entacapone in that it can act both in the brain and periphery (Fig. 12-8), there have been several reports of fatal hepatic toxicity associated with tolcapone. In practice, therefore, entacapone is the more widely used COMT inhibitor.

Nondopaminergic Pharmacology in Parkinson's Disease

Amantadine, trihexyphenidyl, and benztropine are all drugs that do not affect dopaminergic pathways directly but are nonetheless effective in the treatment of Parkinson's disease. **Amantadine** was developed and is marketed primarily as an antiviral that reduces the length and severity of influenza A infections (see Chapter 36, Pharmacology of Viral Infections). In patients with Parkinson's disease, however, amantadine is used to treat levodopa-induced dyskinesias that develop late in the course of the disease. The mechanism by which amantadine reduces dyskinesia is thought to involve blockade of excitatory NMDA receptors. **Trihexyphenidyl** and **benztropine** are muscarinic receptor antagonists that reduce cholinergic tone in the CNS. They reduce tremor more than bradykinesia, and are therefore more effective in treating patients for whom tremor is the major clinical manifestation of Parkinson's disease. These anticholinergic drugs are thought to act by modifying the actions of striatal cholinergic interneurons, which regulate the interactions of direct and indirect pathway neurons.

DOPAMINE AND DISORDERS OF THOUGHT: SCHIZOPHRENIA

PATHOPHYSIOLOGY

Schizophrenia is a thought disorder characterized by one or more episodes of psychosis (impairment in reality testing).

Patients may manifest disorders of perception, thinking, speech, emotion, and/or physical activity. Schizophrenic symptoms are divided into two broad categories. **Positive symptoms** involve the development of abnormal functions; these symptoms include **delusions** (distorted or false beliefs and misinterpretation of perceptions), **hallucinations** (abnormal perceptions, especially auditory), **disorganized speech,** and **catatonic behavior. Negative symptoms** involve the reduction or loss of normal functions; these symptoms include **affective flattening** (decrease in the range or intensity of emotional expression), **alogia** (decrease in the fluency of speech), and **avolition** (decrease in the initiation of goal-directed behavior). The American Psychiatric Association criteria for schizophrenia are listed in Box 12-1.

Schizophrenia typically affects individuals in their late teens and early 20s. The disorder affects males and females equally. Approximately 4.75 million individuals suffer from schizophrenia in the United States, and 100,000 to 150,000 new cases are diagnosed annually. A genetic component of the disease has been demonstrated, but concordance among identical twins is only 50%. Schizophrenia, therefore, ap-

---

BOX 12-1. **Criteria for Schizophrenia, from the Diagnostic and Statistical Manual of Mental Disorders, Fourth Edition Text Revision**

A. Characteristic symptoms: Two (or more) of the following, each present for a significant portion of time during a 1-month period (or less if successfully treated):
   1. Delusions
   2. Hallucinations
   3. Disorganized speech (e.g., frequent derailment or incoherence)
   4. Grossly disorganized or catatonic behavior
   5. Negative symptoms (i.e., affective flattening, alogia, or avolition)
   Note: Only one Criterion A symptom is required if delusions are bizarre or hallucinations consist of a voice keeping up a running commentary on the person's behavior or thoughts, or two or more voices conversing with each other.
B. Social/occupational dysfunction: For a significant portion of the time since the onset of the disturbance, one or more major areas of functioning, such as work, interpersonal relations, or self-care, are markedly below the level achieved before the onset (or when the onset is in childhood or adolescence, failure to achieve expected level of interpersonal, academic, or occupational achievement).
C. Duration: Continuous signs of the disturbance persist for at least 6 months. This 6-month period must include at least 1 month of symptoms (or less if successfully treated) that meet Criterion A (i.e., active-phase symptoms) and may include periods of prodromal or residual symptoms. During these prodromal or residual periods, the signs of the disturbance may be manifested by only negative symptoms or two or more symptoms listed in Criterion A present in an attenuated form (e.g., odd beliefs, unusual perceptual experiences).

D. Schizoaffective and mood disorder exclusion: Schizoaffective disorder and mood disorder with psychotic features have been ruled out because either (1) no major depressive, manic, or mixed episodes have occurred concurrently with the active-phase symptoms, or (2) if mood episodes have occurred during active-phase symptoms, their total duration has been brief relative to the duration of the active and residual periods.
E. Substance/general medical condition exclusion: The disturbance is not attributable to the direct physiologic effects of a substance (e.g., a drug of abuse, a medication) or a general medical condition.
F. Relationship to a pervasive developmental disorder: If there is a history of autistic disorder or another pervasive developmental disorder, the additional diagnosis of schizophrenia is made only if prominent delusions or hallucinations are also present for at least 1 month (or less if successfully treated).

Classification of longitudinal course (can be applied only after at least 1 year has elapsed since the initial onset of active-phase symptoms):

Episodic with interepisode residual symptoms (episodes are defined by the re-emergence of prominent psychotic symptoms); also, specify if with prominent negative symptoms
Episodic with no interepisode residual symptoms
Continuous (prominent psychotic symptoms are present throughout the period of observation); also, specify if with prominent negative symptoms
Single episode in partial remission; also, specify if with prominent negative symptoms
Single episode in full remission

pears to have a multifactorial etiology, with both genetic and environmental components.

The model that is most commonly cited to explain the pathogenesis of schizophrenia is the **dopamine hypothesis,** which states that the illness is caused by increased and dysregulated levels of DA neurotransmission in the brain. This hypothesis arises from the empiric observation that treatment with DA receptor antagonists, specifically D2 antagonists, relieves a number of the symptoms of schizophrenia in many, but not all, patients with the disease. The DA hypothesis is supported by several additional clinical observations. First, some patients taking drugs that increase DA levels or that activate dopamine receptors in the CNS, including **amphetamines, cocaine,** and **apomorphine,** develop a schizophrenia-like state that subsides when the dose of the drug is lowered. Second, hallucinations are a known adverse effect of levodopa therapy for Parkinson's disease. Finally, because treatment with DA receptor-blocking antipsychotics changes the levels of the DA metabolite HVA in the plasma, urine, and CSF, researchers have been able to correlate decreased DA metabolite levels, and by extension decreased DA levels, with clinical improvement in schizophrenic symptoms.

The dysregulation of dopaminergic neurotransmission in schizophrenia is thought to occur at specific anatomic locations in the brain. The **mesolimbic system** is a dopaminergic tract that originates in the ventral tegmental area and projects to the nucleus accumbens, ventral striatum, parts of the amygdala and hippocampus, and other components of the limbic system. This system is involved in the development of emotions and memory, and some hypothesize that mesolimbic hyperactivity is responsible for the positive symptoms of schizophrenia. This hypothesis is supported by positron emission tomography (PET) scans of the brains of patients displaying the earliest signs of schizophrenia; these PET images show changes in blood flow to the mesolimbic system that represent changes in the level of functioning of this system. Dopaminergic neurons of the **mesocortical system** originate in the ventral tegmental area and project to regions of the cerebral cortex, particularly the prefrontal cortex. Because the prefrontal cortex is responsible for attention, planning, and motivated behavior, the hypothesis has been advanced that the mesocortical system plays a role in the negative symptoms of schizophrenia.

All of the evidence implicating DA in the pathogenesis of schizophrenia is circumstantial, however, and much of it is conflicting. Changes in DA levels, particularly in the mesolimbic and mesocortical systems, could simply reflect downstream consequences of a pathologic process in a heretofore undiscovered pathway. One hypothesis involving such an upstream process suggests that an imbalance in glutamatergic neurotransmission plays an important role in schizophrenia. This model is supported by the observation that phencyclidine (PCP) (see Chapter 17, Pharmacology of Drug Dependence and Addiction), an antagonist at NMDA receptors, causes symptoms similar to those of schizophrenia. In fact, the syndrome seen in patients taking PCP chronically—consisting of psychotic symptoms, visual and auditory hallucinations, disorganized thought, blunted affect, withdrawal, psychomotor retardation, and an amotivational state—has components of both the positive and negative symptoms of schizophrenia. Dopaminergic neurons and excitatory glutamatergic neurons often form reciprocal synaptic connections, which could account for the efficacy of DA receptor antagonists in schizophrenia. Even if this hypothesis is correct, at present there are no useful therapies for schizophrenia that act at glutamate receptors. Glutamate is the primary excitatory transmitter in the brain, and further research will be required to identify drugs that are selective enough for use in schizophrenia and that have an acceptable adverse effect profile.

PHARMACOLOGIC CLASSES AND AGENTS

Although the biological basis of schizophrenia remains controversial, a number of drugs are effective in treating the illness. When successful, these medications can lead to a remission of psychosis and allow the patient to integrate into society. Patients only rarely return completely to their premorbid state, however. Drugs used in the management of psychosis are often called **neuroleptics** or **antipsychotics.** Although these terms are frequently used interchangeably, they have slight yet important differences in connotation. The term *"neuroleptic"* emphasizes the drugs' neurological actions that are commonly manifested as adverse effects of treatment. These adverse effects, often called **extrapyramidal effects,** result from DA receptor blockade in the basal ganglia and include the parkinsonian symptoms of slowness, stiffness, and tremor. The term *"antipsychotic"* denotes the ability of these drugs to abrogate psychosis and alleviate disordered thinking in schizophrenic patients. The antipsychotics may be further divided into **typical antipsychotics**, older drugs with prominent actions at the D2 receptor, and **atypical antipsychotics**, a newer generation of drugs with less prominent D2 antagonism and consequently fewer extrapyramidal effects.

Typical Antipsychotic Agents

The history of the typical antipsychotic drugs dates back to the approval of **chlorpromazine** in 1954, based on observations of effectiveness in schizophrenia but little understanding of the mechanism of action. In the 1960s, as the role of DA in the brain became better understood, the ability of these drugs to block dopaminergic neurotransmission in the CNS was first elucidated. Affinity binding studies performed in the 1980s demonstrated that both therapeutic efficacy and extrapyramidal adverse effects of the typical antipsychotics correlate directly with the affinity of these drugs for D2 receptors. As shown in Figure 12-9, drugs with higher affinity for D2 receptors, as represented by lower dissociation constants, tend to require smaller doses to control psychotic symptoms and alleviate schizophrenia.

Mechanism of Action

Although the typical antipsychotics block D2 receptors in all of the CNS dopaminergic pathways, their mechanism of action as antipsychotics appears to involve antagonism of mesolimbic, and possibly mesocortical, D2 receptors. As described above, one hypothesis holds that the positive symptoms of schizophrenia correlate with hyperactivity of the mesolimbic system, and antagonism of mesolimbic dopamine receptors could alleviate these symptoms. The typical

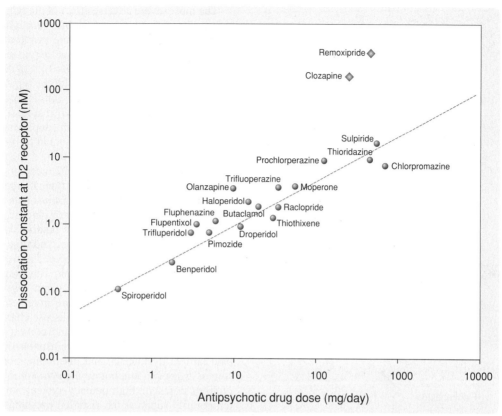

Figure 12-9. Antipsychotic potency of dopamine receptor antagonists. Over at least three orders of magnitude, the clinically effective dose of the typical antipsychotics is proportional to the dissociation constant of the drugs at D2 receptors. (Note that a higher dissociation constant represents a lower binding affinity.) Atypical antipsychotics such as clozapine and remoxipride *(blue diamonds)* are exceptions to this rule; these agents have clinical effects at a dose lower than that predicted by their dissociation constants. Data points represent the mean dissociation constant (averaged over multiple studies) at the most common clinically effective dose. The *dotted line* represents the best fit to the data for all of the typical antipsychotics *(blue circles)*.

antipsychotics are relatively less effective at controlling the negative symptoms of schizophrenia. This relative lack of efficacy at treating the negative symptoms could relate to the hypothesis that the negative symptoms correlate with hypoactivity of mesocortical neurons, because the antagonist action of the antipsychotics would not be expected to correct dopaminergic hypoactivity. Many of the adverse effects of the typical antipsychotics are likely mediated by binding of these drugs to D2 receptors in the basal ganglia (nigrostriatal pathway) and pituitary gland.

The typical antipsychotics fall into several structural classes, of which the most prominent are the **phenothiazines** and the **butyrophenones** (Fig. 12-10). **Chlorpromazine** is the prototypical phenothiazine, and **haloperidol** is the most widely used butyrophenone. Despite differences in structure and D2 receptor affinity, all typical antipsychotics have similar clinical efficacy at their standard doses. In general, aliphatic phenothiazines (such as chlorpromazine) are less potent antagonists at D2 receptors than are butyrophenones, **thioxanthenes** (phenothiazines in which a nitrogen in the phenothiazine nucleus is substituted by a carbon), or phenothiazines functionalized with a piperazine derivative (such as **fluphenazine**). For all of these drugs, the clinical dose can be adjusted to account for the in vitro D2 receptor binding affinity, so that effectiveness is unaffected by potency at clinically useful doses. However, the potency of the typical

antipsychotics is critical in determining the drugs' adverse effects profile.

Adverse Effects

The adverse effects of typical antipsychotic drugs can be divided into two broad categories: those caused by antagonist action at dopamine D2 receptors outside the mesolimbic and mesocortical systems (on-target effects) and those caused by nonspecific antagonist action at other receptor types (off-target effects). Given the broad distribution of dopamine receptors, it is not surprising that dopamine receptor antagonists have a wide range of on-target adverse effects. As noted above, the most prominent of these effects are often referred to as **extrapyramidal effects**. Because endogenous stimulation of dopamine D2 receptors inhibits the indirect pathway within the basal ganglia, antagonism of D2 receptors by typical antipsychotic drugs can disinhibit the indirect pathway and thereby induce parkinsonian symptoms. Such symptoms can sometimes be treated with the non-dopaminergic therapies for Parkinson's disease, such as amantadine and anticholinergic drugs. Dopaminergic drugs are often ineffective because of the high affinity of the antagonists for the D2 receptor and because, when used in this setting, dopaminergic drugs could cause a relapse of schizophrenia symptoms.

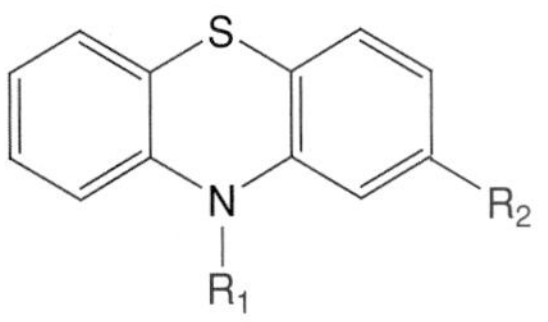

Phenothiazine skeleton

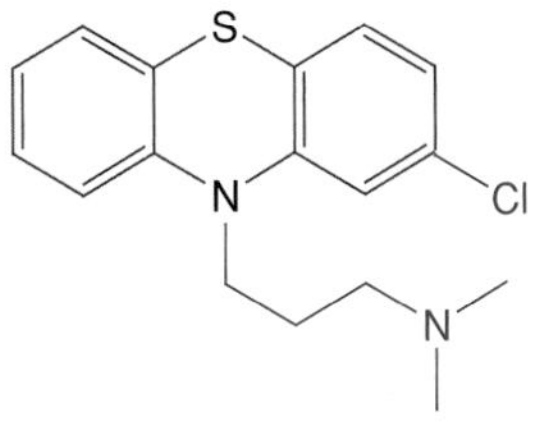

Chlorpromazine

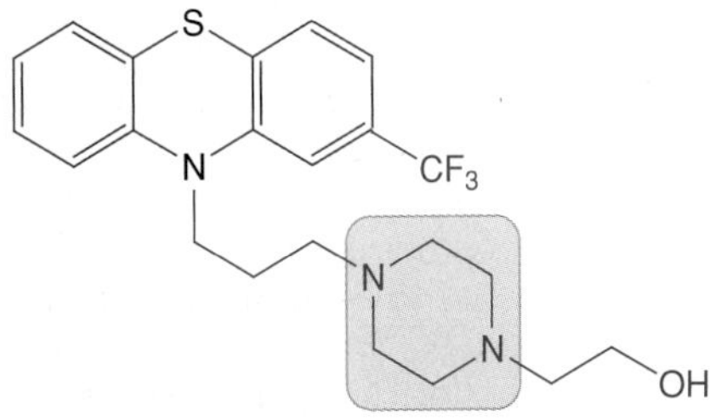

Fluphenazine

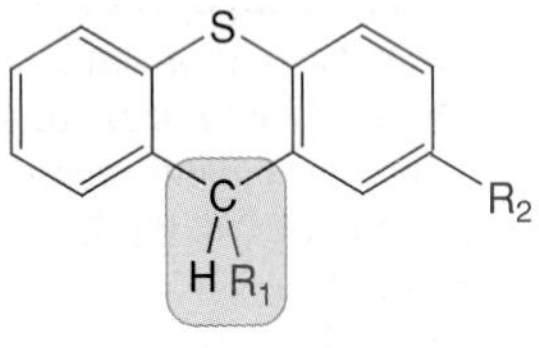

Thioxanthene skeleton

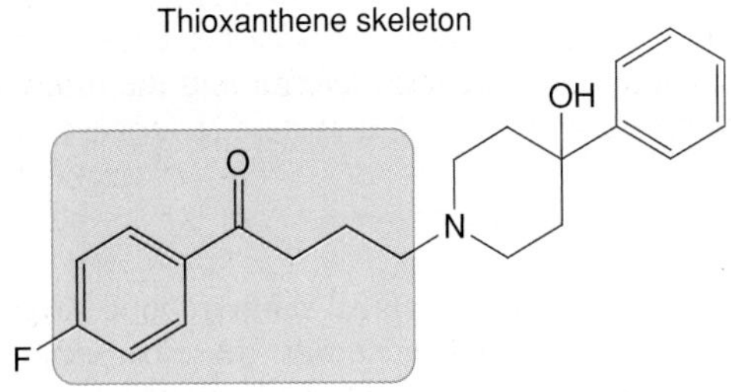

Haloperidol (a butyrophenone)

Figure 12-10. Chemical structures of the typical antipsychotics. The structure of the phenothiazines is based on a common skeleton, with two variable functional groups. Chlorpromazine, the first approved antipsychotic, has substituted aminopropyl (R_1) and chloride (R_2) side groups. Piperazine *(in blue box)*-substituted phenothiazines, such as fluphenazine, are significantly more potent than aliphatic-substituted phenothiazines, such as chlorpromazine. The fourth structure represents the skeleton of a thioxanthene, which substitutes a carbon *(in blue box)* for the phenothiazine nitrogen. As illustrated by the structure of haloperidol, butyrophenones *(in blue box)* are structurally distinct from phenothiazines and thioxanthenes.

The most severe adverse effect of the typical antipsychotics is the so-called **neuroleptic malignant syndrome (NMS),** a rare but life-threatening syndrome characterized by catatonia, stupor, fever, and autonomic instability; myoglobinemia and death occur in about 10% of these cases. NMS is most commonly associated with the typical antipsychotic drugs that have a high affinity for D2 receptors, such as haloperidol. NMS is thought to arise at least in part from the actions of the antipsychotics on the dopaminergic systems in the hypothalamus, which are essential for the body's ability to control temperature.

After some time, as striatal D2 receptors become supersensitized, most patients taking typical antipsychotic drugs experience an amelioration of parkinsonian adverse effects. However, after months to years of chronic typical antipsychotic use, a condition known as **tardive dyskinesia** develops in about 20% of patients. The syndrome is characterized by repetitive, involuntary, stereotyped movements of the facial musculature, arms, and trunk. The exact mechanism is unknown, but it is believed that adaptations resulting in excessive dopaminergic activity are involved. The condition mimics Huntington's chorea, a disease characterized by destruction of the basal ganglia and consequent involuntary choreiform movements. Antiparkinsonian drugs can exacerbate tardive dyskinesia, and discontinuation of antiparkinsonian drugs can ameliorate the symptoms. Administration of high doses of high-potency typical antipsychotics can temporarily suppress the disorder, presumably by overcoming the adaptive response in the striatal neurons, but may in the long run lead to worsening of symptoms. In many cases, cessation of all typical antipsychotic medications will lead to slow reversal of the adaptive hypersensitivity of D2 receptors in the striatum, with eventual improvement in the symptoms of tardive dyskinesia.

Some adverse effects of typical antipsychotics are thought to be caused by antagonist action at dopamine receptors in the pituitary gland, where dopamine tonically inhibits **prolactin** secretion. Antagonism of D2 receptors increases prolactin secretion, leading to amenorrhea, galactorrhea, and false-positive pregnancy tests in women, and to gynecomastia and decreased libido in men.

Other adverse effects of the typical antipsychotics result from nonspecific antagonism of muscarinic and α-adrenergic receptors. Antagonism of peripheral muscarinic pathways causes anticholinergic effects, including dry mouth, constipation, difficulty urinating, and loss of accommodation (see Chapter 8, Cholinergic Pharmacology). α-Adrenergic antagonism can cause orthostatic hypotension and, in men, failure to ejaculate. Sedation can also occur because of inhibition of central α-adrenergic pathways in the reticular activating system. When sedation interferes with normal functioning during chronic antipsychotic use, it is considered an adverse effect. In the acutely psychotic patient, however, sedation may be part of the drug's intended spectrum of action.

The adverse effect profiles of the typical antipsychotics depend on their potency. High-potency drugs (whose clinical doses are only a few milligrams) tend to have fewer sedative adverse effects and cause less postural hypotension than drugs with lower potency (i.e., drugs that require high doses to achieve a therapeutic effect). On the other hand, lower-potency typical antipsychotics tend to cause fewer extrapyramidal adverse effects. These observations can be rationalized by the fact that high-potency drugs have high affinity for D2 receptors and are therefore more selective in their action. Thus, these drugs are more likely to cause adverse effects mediated by dopamine D2 receptors (i.e., extrapyramidal effects), and fewer adverse effects mediated by muscarinic and α-adrenergic receptors (i.e., anticholinergic effects, sedation, and postural hypotension). Conversely, low-potency typical antipsychotics do not bind D2 receptors as tightly and cause fewer extrapyramidal effects, while their lower selectivity results in more prominent anticholinergic and antiadrenergic effects.

Pharmacokinetics, Metabolism, and Drug Interactions

As with many drugs active in the CNS, the typical antipsychotics are highly lipophilic. In part because of this lipophilicity, typical antipsychotics tend to be metabolized in the liver and to exhibit both high binding to plasma proteins and high first-pass metabolism. The drugs are generally formulated as oral or intramuscular dosage forms. The latter are useful in treating acutely psychotic patients who may be a danger to themselves or others, while the oral formulations are generally used for chronic therapy. Elimination half-lives of the typical antipsychotics are erratic because their kinetics of elimination typically follow a multiphasic pattern and are not strictly first-order. In general, however, the half-lives of most typical antipsychotics are on the order of one day, and it is common practice to follow a once-daily dosing regimen.

Two drugs, **haloperidol** and **fluphenazine,** are available as the decanoate esters. These highly lipophilic drugs are injected intramuscularly, where they are slowly hydrolyzed and released. The decanoate ester dosage forms provide a long-acting formulation that can be administered every 3 to 4 weeks. These formulations are particularly useful for treating poorly compliant patients.

Because typical antipsychotics are antagonists at dopamine receptors, it is logical that these drugs should interact prominently with antiparkinsonian drugs that act by increasing synaptic dopamine concentrations (levodopa) or by stimulating dopamine receptors directly (bromocriptine). Specifically, antipsychotics inhibit the action of both of the latter drug classes, and administration of typical antipsychotics to patients with Parkinson's disease often leads to a marked worsening of parkinsonian symptoms. In addition, typical antipsychotics potentiate the sedative effects of benzodiazepines and centrally active antihistamines. Because the latter are pharmacodynamic effects that result from the nonspecific binding of typical antipsychotics to cholinergic and adrenergic receptors, the low-potency typical antipsychotics tend to manifest more pronounced sedative effects than their high-potency counterparts.

Atypical Antipsychotic Agents

The so-called atypical antipsychotics have efficacy and adverse effect profiles that differ from those of the typical antipsychotics. The five principal atypical antipsychotics are **clozapine, olanzapine, quetapine, ziprasidone,** and **risperidone.** All of these drugs are more effective than typical antipsychotics at treating the ''negative'' symptoms of schizophrenia. In addition, direct comparisons of risperidone and haloperidol have shown that risperidone is more effective at combating the positive symptoms of schizophrenia and preventing a relapse of the active phase of the disease. Atypical antipsychotics cause significantly milder extrapyramidal symptoms than typical antipsychotics; this adverse effect generally appears only when the drugs are administered in high doses.

The atypical antipsychotics have a relatively low affinity for D2 receptors; unlike the typical antipsychotics, their affinity for D2 receptors does not correlate with their clinically effective dose (Fig. 12-9). Three main hypotheses have emerged to explain this discrepancy. The 5-HT$_2$ hypothesis states that antagonist action at the serotonin 5-HT$_2$ receptor (see Chapter 13), or antagonist action at both 5-HT$_2$ and D2 receptors, is critical for the antipsychotic effect of the atypical antipsychotics. This hypothesis is based on the finding that the FDA-approved atypical antipsychotics are all high-affinity 5-HT$_2$ receptor antagonists. It is not clear, however, how 5-HT$_2$ antagonism contributes to the antipsychotic effect. Moreover, **amisulpride,** an atypical antipsychotic not currently approved for use in the United States, is not a 5-HT$_2$ receptor antagonist. In addition, although some typical antipsychotics also act as antagonists at 5-HT$_2$ receptors, it appears that their clinical effectiveness can be explained based on their affinity for D2 receptors.

The second model, the D4 hypothesis, is based on the finding that many of the atypical antipsychotics are also dopamine D4 receptor antagonists. This model suggests that selective D4 antagonism, or a combination of D2 and D4 antagonism, is critical to the mechanism of action of the atypical antipsychotics. D4 receptors are localized to the frontal cortex, medulla, and midbrain (Figs. 12-4 and 12-5), and appear not to be involved in the regulation of movement. This observation is consistent with the clinical experience that atypical antipsychotics exhibit relatively few extrapyramidal adverse effects. Quetapine does not act as a D4 receptor antagonist, however, so the D4 hypothesis cannot account for the mechanism of action of all atypical antipsychotics.

The final hypothesis states that the atypical antipsychotics exhibit a milder adverse effect profile because of their relatively fast dissociation from the D2 receptor. As described in Chapter 2, Pharmacodynamics, the binding affinity (K_d) of a drug is equal to the ratio of its rate of dissociation from the receptor (k_{off}) to its rate of association to the receptor (k_{on}):

$$D + R \xrightarrow{k_{on}} DR \xrightarrow{k_{off}} D + R$$

$$K_d = \frac{k_{off}}{k_{on}} \qquad \text{Equation 12-1}$$

Because of their rapid off-rates, the atypical antipsychotics bind dopamine D2 receptors more transiently than do typical antipsychotics. This could allow the atypical antipsychotics to inhibit the low-level, tonic dopamine release that may occur in the mesolimbic system. However, the drugs would be displaced by a surge of dopamine, as would occur in the striatum during the initiation of movement. Thus, extrapyramidal adverse effects would be minimized. Because of their relatively high off-rates, the drugs tend to have a higher

K_d and a lower potency. As with the low-potency typical antipsychotics, this should result in relatively low selectivity. According to this **fast dissociation** hypothesis of atypical antipsychotic action, the 5-HT$_2$ and D4 antagonism exhibited by these drugs is an incidental observation related to the lower potency of the atypical antipsychotics, and has no bearing on their mechanism of antipsychotic action. Although this model is attractive in some respects, it fails to explain the atypical antipsychotics' relatively low incidence of prolactin-mediated adverse effects. Recall that prolactin is tonically inhibited by dopamine release in the pituitary gland. One might expect that, because prolactin inhibition is tonic, the atypical antipsychotics would interfere with this process and cause symptoms such as gynecomastia and galactorrhea.

The atypical antipsychotics comprise a structurally diverse set of drugs. Their receptor-binding profiles also differ, as summarized in the Drug Summary Table. As noted above, these agents all show combined antagonist properties at dopamine D2 and serotonin 5-HT$_2$ receptors, and most of the drugs are also dopamine D4 receptor antagonists.

Risperidone has combined antagonist properties at D2 and 5-HT$_2$ receptors, although it is a stronger serotonergic antagonist. The drug also antagonizes α_1-adrenergic, α_2-adrenergic, and histamine H$_1$ receptors with relatively high affinity. Its adverse effect profile is predictable from its broad pharmacologic profile.

Clozapine binds D1–D5 receptors as well as 5-HT$_2$ receptors; in addition, it blocks α_1-adrenergic, H$_1$, and muscarinic receptors. Clozapine has been used therapeutically in patients who have failed other antipsychotic drugs, whether for lack of efficacy or intolerable adverse effects. Clozapine has not been used as a first-line agent because of a small but significant risk of agranulocytosis (approximately 0.8% per year). Thus, the administration of clozapine requires frequent monitoring of white blood cell counts.

Olanzapine, ziprasidone, and quetapine are also combined D2 and 5-HT$_2$ receptor antagonists, and each binds a number of other receptors. Their pharmacologic profiles are summarized in the Drug Summary Table.

Conclusion and Future Directions

Treatments for both Parkinson's disease and schizophrenia modulate dopaminergic neurotransmission in the CNS. Parkinson's disease, which results from the degeneration of dopaminergic neurons that project to the striatum, causes resting tremor and bradykinesia. In this disease, the direct pathway—which enables movement—is understimulated, whereas the indirect pathway—which inhibits movement—is disinhibited. Pharmacologic treatment of Parkinson's disease depends on agents that increase dopamine release or activate dopamine receptors in the caudate and putamen, and thereby help restore the balance between the direct and indirect pathways.

Schizophrenia is treated by inhibiting dopamine receptors at various sites in the limbic system. The pathophysiology of schizophrenia is not fully understood, and this lack of knowledge about etiology limits rational drug development. The clinical effectiveness of the various antipsychotic agents has provided useful clues, however. In particular, the pharmacology of the typical antipsychotic agents has formed the basis of the dopamine model of schizophrenia, which argues that dysregulated levels of dopamine in the brain play a role in the pathophysiology of the disease. The effectiveness of the atypical antipsychotic agents, which affect the function of several different receptor types, has highlighted the fact that the dopamine hypothesis is a simplification. The atypical agents represent an attractive new modality for treating schizophrenia because they have fewer extrapyramidal effects and are more effective than the typical antipsychotics.

Future developments in the treatment of Parkinson's disease and schizophrenia are focused on creating more selective agents within the current drug classes and on better elucidating the underlying pathophysiology of the disorders. New dopamine receptor agonists with higher selectivity, particularly those that bind D1 receptors, may one day provide more effective treatment for Parkinson's disease with less severe adverse effects. The development of newer antipsychotics with increased receptor selectivity may similarly expand the therapeutic options for treating schizophrenia. Because Parkinson's disease results from the death of dopaminergic neurons, much effort is currently directed at neuroprotective drugs that may slow the progression of the disease. One such effort is focused on the use of trophic factors such as glial-cell–derived neurotrophic factor (GDNF), which has been shown to increase the survival of dopaminergic neurons in vitro and to improve parkinsonian symptoms in monkeys. Further research into a potential role for a glutamate deficit in the pathophysiology of schizophrenia may yield new therapeutics for this disorder. For example, the development of selective glutamate receptor agonists may one day complement or even replace the use of dopamine receptor antagonists. Another important advance in the treatment of schizophrenia will likely result from the elucidation of models for the mechanism of the atypical antipsychotics, which will allow rational development of more effective drugs.

Suggested Reading

Albin RL, Young AB, Penney JB. The functional anatomy of basal ganglia disorders. *Trends Neurosci* 1989;12:366–375. (*A classic article that describes the concept of "direct" and "indirect" pathways.*)

Farrer MJ. Genetics of Parkinson disease: paradigm shifts and future prospects. *Nat Rev Genet* 2006;7:306–318. (*A review of the rapidly evolving genetics of Parkinson's disease.*)

Freedman R. Drug therapy: schizophrenia. *N Engl J Med* 2003; 349:1738–1749. (*Discusses the clinical use of many of the drugs used to treat schizophrenia, including the atypical agents.*)

Kellendonk C, Simpson EH, Polan HJ, et al. Transient and selective overexpression of dopamine D2 receptors in the striatum causes persistent abnormalities in prefrontal cortex functioning. *Neuron* 2006;49:603–615. (*A new mouse model for schizophrenia suggesting a role for D2 receptors in cognitive impairment.*)

Langston JW. The Parkinson's complex: parkinsonism is just the tip of the iceberg. *Ann Neurol* 2006;59:591–596. (*A review that emphasizes the many aspects of Parkinson's disease beyond the motor abnormalities.*)

Mueser KT, McGurk SR. Schizophrenia. *Lancet* 2004;363: 2063–2072. (*General overview of schizophrenia pathophysiology and treatment.*)

Perlmutter JS, Mink JW. Deep brain stimulation. *Annu Rev Neurosci* 2006;29:229–257. (*A comprehensive review of deep brain stimulation, a non-pharmacologic alternative for treatment of Parkinson's disease.*)

Spooren W, Riemer C, Meltzer H. NK3 receptor antagonists: the next generation of antipsychotics? *Nat Rev Drug Discov* 2005; 4:967–975. (*Discusses pathophysiologic basis of potential antipsychotic agents.*)

Suchowersky O, Reich S, Perlmutter J, et al. Practice parameter: diagnosis and prognosis of new onset Parkinson disease (an evidence-based review). Report of the Quality Standards Subcommittee of the American Academy of Neurology. *Neurology* 2006;66:968–975. (*This "parameter," as well as several others published in the same issue, represents the product of a careful review of the evidence for the effectiveness of various treatments for Parkinson's disease.*)

Drug Summary Table Chapter 12 Pharmacology of Dopaminergic Neurotransmission

Drug	Clinical Applications	Serious and Common Adverse Effects	Contraindications	Therapeutic Considerations
DOPAMINE PRECURSORS				
Mechanism—Provide substrate for increased dopamine synthesis; levodopa is transported across the blood-brain barrier by the neutral amino acid transporter and then decarboxylated to dopamine by the enzyme aromatic L-amino acid decarboxylase (AADC).				
Levodopa	Parkinson's disease	Dyskinesia, heart disease, orthostatic hypotension, psychotic disorder Loss of appetite, nausea, vomiting	History of melanoma Narrow-angle glaucoma Concomitant use of MAO inhibitor	Levodopa, when administered alone, has low availability in CNS due to peripheral metabolism to dopamine; therefore, it is almost always administered in combination with carbidopa, an inhibitor of DOPA decarboxylase Continued use results in both tolerance and sensitization; patients develop periods of increased rigidity alternating with periods of normal or dyskinetic movement Dyskinesias are nearly ubiquitous in patients within 5 years of starting levodopa; as the disease progresses, continued levodopa therapy leads to worsening of both the dyskinesias and the "on/off" phenomenon
DOPAMINE RECEPTOR AGONISTS				
Mechanism—Ergot derivatives, such as bromocriptine (D2 agonist) and pergolide (D1 and D2), and nonergot agonists, such as pramipexole (D3 >D2) and ropinirole (D3 >D2), bind to and activate postsynaptic dopamine receptors directly				
Bromocriptine Pergolide	See Drug Summary Table: Chapter 25 Pharmacology of the Hypothalamus and Pituitary Gland			
Pramipexole Ropinirole	Parkinson's disease Restless leg syndrome (ropinirole)	Dyskinesia, orthostatic hypotension Extrapyramidal movements, somnolence, dizziness, hallucinations, dream disorder, asthenia, amnesia	Concomitant use of other sedating medications	Dopamine agonists have half-lives longer than that of levodopa, which allows for less frequent dosing The non-ergot dopamine agonists pramipexole and ropinirole produce fewer adverse effects than the ergot derivatives bromocriptine and pergolide Cognitive effects can include excessive sedation, vivid dreams, and hallucinations Some studies suggest that use of dopamine agonists rather than levodopa as initial treatment for Parkinson's disease delays the onset of "off" periods and dyskinesias, especially in younger individuals

INHIBITORS OF LEVODOPA OR DOPAMINE METABOLISM

Mechanism—Inhibit breakdown of dopamine in the CNS by inhibiting MAO-B (rasagiline and selegiline) or COMT (tolcapone); inhibit breakdown of levodopa by COMT in the periphery (entacapone and tolcapone)

Drug	Clinical Applications	Serious and Common Adverse Effects	Contraindications	Therapeutic Considerations
Rasagiline Selegiline	Parkinson's disease	*Bundle branch block, gastrointestinal hemorrhage* Orthostatic hypotension, dyskinesia, rash, dyspepsia, arthralgia, headache, weight loss, insomnia (selegiline), confusion (selegiline)	Concomitant use of cyclobenzaprine, mirtazapine, St. John's wort Concomitant use of dextromethorphan due to risk of psychosis Concomitant use of meperidine, methadone, propoxyphene, tramadol due to risk of severe hypertension or hypotension, malignant hyperpyrexia, or coma Concomitant use of other monoamine oxidase inhibitors (MAOI) or sympathomimetic amines due to risk of severe hypertensive reactions Concomitant use of cocaine or local anesthesia containing sympathomimetic vasoconstrictors Elective surgery requiring general anesthesia Pheochromocytoma	Selegiline in low doses is selective for MAO-B, which predominates in the striatum; higher doses inhibit MAO-A as well as MAO-B, with associated risks of toxicity Selegiline forms the potentially toxic metabolite amphetamine, which may lead to insomnia and confusion (especially in the elderly) Rasagiline does not form toxic metabolites Both rasagiline and selegiline improve motor function when used alone and can augment the effectiveness of levodopa
Tolcapone Entacapone	Parkinson's disease	*Dyskinesia, dystonia, hallucinations, orthostatic hypotension (tolcapone), hyperpyrexia (tolcapone), fulminant hepatic failure (tolcapone), rhabdomyolysis (tolcapone)* Dyspepsia, dream disorder, sleep disorder	History of rhabdomyolysis or hyperpyrexia related to tolcapone Liver disease (contraindication for tolcapone)	Tolcapone is a highly lipid-soluble agent that can cross the blood-brain barrier, while entacapone distributes only to the periphery COMT inhibitors can be used in combination with carbidopa to further enhance the plasma half-life of levodopa; COMT inhibitors have been shown in some trials to reduce the "off" periods that are associated with decreasing plasma levodopa levels Rare but fatal hepatic toxicity has been reported with tolcapone use Entacapone is the more widely used COMT inhibitor

MISCELLANEOUS ANTIPARKINSONIAN MEDICATIONS

Mechanism—Amantadine's therapeutic mechanism in the treatment of Parkinson's disease is thought to be related to antagonism of excitatory NMDA receptors; trihexyphenidyl and benztropine are muscarinic receptor antagonists that reduce cholinergic tone in the CNS by modifying the actions of striatal cholinergic interneurons

Drug	Clinical Applications	Serious and Common Adverse Effects	Contraindications	Therapeutic Considerations
Amantadine	Parkinson's disease Influenza A	*Neuroleptic malignant syndrome, exacerbation of mental disorder* Insomnia, dizziness, hallucinations, agitation, orthostatic hypotension, peripheral edema, dyspepsia, livedo reticularis	Hypersensitivity to amantadine	Amantadine was developed as an antiviral that reduces the length and severity of influenza A infections; in patients with Parkinson's disease, amantadine is used to treat levodopa-induced dyskinesias that develop late in the course of the disease May exacerbate mental illness in patients with psychiatric illness or substance abuse problems

(Continued)

| Drug Summary Table | **Chapter 12 Pharmacology of Dopaminergic Neurotransmission** (*Continued*) |

Drug	Clinical Applications	Serious and Common Adverse Effects	Contraindications	Therapeutic Considerations
Trihexyphenidyl Benztropine	Parkinson's disease	*Angle-closure glaucoma, increased intraocular pressure, psychosis, hyperpyrexia (benztropine), paralytic ileus (benztropine)* Dizziness, blurred vision, nervousness, nausea, xerostomia, urinary retention	Narrow-angle glaucoma Younger than 3 years Tardive dyskinesias (contraindication for trihexyphenidyl)	Trihexyphenidyl and benztropine reduce tremor more than bradykinesia and are therefore more effective in treating patients for whom tremor is the major clinical manifestation of Parkinson's disease May worsen dementia and cognitive impairment in the elderly

ANTIPSYCHOTIC AGENTS

Mechanism—Antagonize mesolimbic, and possibly mesocortical, D2 receptors; adverse effects are likely mediated by binding to D2 receptors in basal ganglia (nigrostriatal pathway) and pituitary gland

Drug	Clinical Applications	Serious and Common Adverse Effects	Contraindications	Therapeutic Considerations
Phenothiazines and derivatives: Chlorpromazine Thioridazine Mesoridazine Perphenazine Fluphenazine Thiothixene Trifluoperazine Chlorprothixene	Psychotic disorder Nausea and vomiting (chlorpromazine, perphenazine)	*Parkinsonian symptoms, neuroleptic malignant syndrome (characterized by catatonia, stupor, fever, and autonomic instability; also myoglobinemia and, potentially, death), tardive dyskinesia (characterized by repetitive, involuntary, stereotyped movements of the facial musculature, arms, and trunk)* Anticholinergic symptoms (dry mouth, constipation, urinary retention), orthostatic hypotension, failure to ejaculate, sedation	Myelosuppression Severe toxic central nervous system depression or comatose states Concomitant administration of drugs that prolong QT interval or patients with prolonged QT interval (contraindication for thioridazine and mesoridazine) Parkinson's disease	In general, aliphatic phenothiazines are less potent antagonists at D2 receptors than butyrophenones, thioxanthenes, or phenothiazines functionalized with a piperazine derivative The potency of the typical antipsychotics is critical in determining the drugs' adverse effect profile; high-potency drugs tend to have fewer sedative effects and cause less postural hypotension than drugs with lower potency; on the other hand, lower-potency typical antipsychotics tend to cause fewer extrapyramidal effects Fluphenazine is available as decanoate ester, delivered intramuscularly every 3 to 4 weeks Administration of typical antipsychotics to patients with Parkinson's disease often leads to marked worsening of parkinsonian symptoms Typical antipsychotics potentiate the sedative effects of benzodiazepines and centrally active antihistamines
Butyrophenones: Haloperidol Droperidol	Psychoses (haloperidol) Tourette's syndrome (haloperidol) Nausea and vomiting; anesthesia adjunct (droperidol)	*Same as phenothiazines*	Parkinson's disease Severe toxic central nervous system depression or comatose states	Haloperidol is the most widely used butyrophenone. Haloperidol is available as decanoate ester, delivered intramuscularly every 3 to 4 weeks; this formulation is useful for treating poorly compliant patients
Other typical antipsychotics: Loxapine Molindone Pimozide	Psychotic disorders Tourette's syndrome (pimozide)	*Parkinsonian symptoms, neuroleptic malignant syndrome, tardive dyskinesia, prolonged QT interval (pimozide)* Anticholinergic symptoms, sedation	Comatose or severe drug-induced depressed states Parkinson's disease *Contraindications unique to pimozide:* Concomitant pemoline, methylphenidate, or amphetamines that may cause motor and phonic tics Concomitant dofetilide, sotalol, quinidine, other Class Ia and III anti-arrhythmics, mesoridazine, thioridazine, chlorpromazine, or droperidol	Molindone exerts its antipsychotic effects on the ascending reticular activating system in the absence of muscle relaxation and incoordination effects Pimozide has more specific dopamine receptor antagonism and less alpha-adrenergic receptor blocking activity than other neuroleptic agents, which results in less potential for inducing sedation and hypotension

ATYPICAL ANTIPSYCHOTIC AGENTS

Mechanism—Combined antagonist properties at dopamine D2 and serotonin 5-HT2 receptors; clozapine and olanzapine are also dopamine D4 receptor antagonists

Drug	Clinical Applications	Serious and Common Toxicities	Contraindications	Hypersensitivity	Notes / Receptor Binding
Risperidone	Psychotic disorders Bipolar disorder	*Mild extrapyramidal symptoms, QT prolongation* Anticholinergic symptoms (dry mouth, constipation, urinary retention), sedation, weight gain	Concomitant sparfloxacin, gatifloxacin, moxifloxacin, halofantrine, mefloquine, pentamidine, arsenic trioxide, levomethadyl acetate, dolasetron mesylate, probucol, tacrolimus, ziprasidone, sertraline, or macrolide antibiotics Concurrent administration with drugs that have demonstrated QT prolongation and inhibitors of P450 3A4 (zileuton, fluvoxamine) History of cardiac arrhythmias	Hypersensitivity to risperidone	Atypical antipsychotics are more effective than typical antipsychotics at treating the "negative" symptoms of schizophrenia Atypical antipsychotics cause significantly milder extrapyramidal symptoms than typical antipsychotics Risperidone binds to D2, 5-HT2, α1, α2, H1 receptors
Clozapine	Schizophrenia refractory to other antipsychotics	*Mild extrapyramidal symptoms, agranulocytosis* Anticholinergic symptoms, sedation, weight gain	History of clozapine-induced agranulocytosis or severe granulocytopenia Myeloproliferative disorders		Clozapine has not been used as a first-line agent because of a small but significant risk of agranulocytosis Clozapine binds to D1–D5, 5-HT2, α1, H1, muscarinic receptors
Olanzapine	Psychotic disorders Bipolar disorder	*Mild extrapyramidal symptoms* Anticholinergic symptoms, sedation, weight gain		Hypersensitivity to olanzapine	Olanzapine binds to D1–D4, 5-HT2, α1, H1, M1–M5 receptors
Quetiapine	Psychotic disorders Bipolar disorder	Same as olanzapine		Hypersensitivity to quetiapine	Quetiapine binds to D1, D2, 5-HT1, 5-HT2, α1, α2, H1 receptors
Ziprasidone	Psychotic disorders Bipolar disorder	*Mild extrapyramidal symptoms, QT prolongation* Anticholinergic symptoms, sedation, weight gain	Concomitant arsenic trioxide, chlorpromazine, class Ia and III anti-arrhythmics, or other drugs that cause QT prolongation Concomitant mesoridazine, moxifloxacin, pentamidine, pimozide, probucol, sotalol, sparfloxacin, tacrolimus, or thioridazine QT prolongation history including congenital long-QT syndrome Cardiac arrhythmias Recent acute myocardial infarction Uncompensated heart failure	Hypersensitivity to ziprasidone	Ziprasidone binds to D2, 5-HT1, 5-HT2, α1, H1 receptors
Aripiprazole	Psychotic disorders Bipolar disorder	Same as risperidone		Hypersensitivity to aripiprazole	Aripiprazole is a D2 and 5-HT1A partial agonist and a 5-HT2A antagonist

13

Pharmacology of Serotonergic and Central Adrenergic Neurotransmission

Mireya Nadal-Vicens, Jay H. Chyung, and Timothy J. Turner

INTRODUCTION

This chapter introduces the neurotransmitter **serotonin** (5-hydroxytryptamine or 5-HT), which is the target for many of the drugs used to treat depression. Many of these antidepressant medications also affect **norepinephrine (NE)** neurotransmission; both neurotransmitter pathways are believed to be central to the modulation of mood. The different mechanisms by which medications can alter serotonin and norepinephrine signaling are discussed. Though many of the drugs presented function as antidepressants and hypnotics, other medications in this pharmacologic group are effective treatments for migraine headaches and irritable bowel syndrome. **Lithium** and other drugs used to treat bipolar affective disorder are also discussed briefly.

The major mood disorders are defined by the presence of depressive and/or manic episodes. Patients who have experienced at least one manic episode, with or without an additional history of depressive episodes, are said to have bipolar affective disorder (BPAD); patients with recurrent depressive episodes and no history of mania are said to have major depressive disorder (MDD). The lifetime prevalence

of MDD is approximately 17%, whereas that of BPAD is 1% to 2%. There is a particularly strong heritable risk in BPAD, even though environmental factors are often triggers for the manic or depressive episodes. Although mania is characteristic of BPAD, bipolar patients spend significant periods of their lives depressed, and the mortality of the disorder derives primarily from suicidal impulses. MDD can occur as an isolated illness or can be precipitated by other diseases such as stroke, dementia, diabetes, cancer, and coronary artery disease. Though there is some genetic predisposition for MDD, it is believed that stressful environments or disease may elicit MDD in the absence of genetic vulnerability. Aging and cerebral microvascular atherosclerosis are also associated with a late onset depression in the elderly. In addition to genetic and environmental triggers, many classes of drugs can exacerbate depression.

Both MDD and BPAD are major causes of morbidity worldwide, resulting in lost productivity and substantial use of medical resources. Affective illness is associated with an increased risk of suicide; rates of completed suicide are estimated to be as high as 15% among untreated patients. In the majority of suicides, a physician (not necessarily a psychiatrist) will have seen the patient less than 1 month before the suicide.

207

Case

Mary R. is a 27-year-old office worker who presents to her primary care physician, Dr. Lee, with an 18-lb. weight loss over the previous 2 months. Ms. R tearfully explains that she is plagued by near-constant feelings of sadness and by a sense of helplessness and inadequacy at work. She feels so terrible that she has not had a good night of sleep in more than a month. She no longer enjoys living and has recently become scared when new thoughts of suicide enter her mind. Ms. R tells Dr. Lee that she had felt like this once before, but that it had passed. Dr. Lee asks her about her sleep patterns, appetite levels, ability to concentrate, energy level, mood, interest level, and feelings of guilt. He asks her specific questions about thoughts of suicide, particularly whether she has formed a specific plan and whether she has ever attempted suicide. Dr. Lee explains to Ms. R that she has major depressive disorder, likely caused by a chemical imbalance in her brain, and he prescribes the antidepressant fluoxetine.

Two weeks later, Ms. R calls to indicate that the medicine is not working. Dr. Lee encourages her to continue taking the medicine, and after 2 more weeks, Ms. R begins to feel better. She no longer feels sad and demoralized; the feelings of helplessness and inadequacy that previously plagued her have diminished. In fact, when she returns to see Dr. Lee 6 weeks later, she reports feeling much better. She no longer needs much sleep, and is always full of energy. She is now convinced that she is the most intelligent person in her company. She proudly tells Dr. Lee that she has recently purchased a new sports car and gone on a large shopping spree. Dr. Lee tells Ms. R that she may be having a manic episode and, in consultation with a psychiatrist, prescribes lithium and tapers the fluoxetine. Ms. R is hesitant to take the new medication, arguing that she feels fine and that she is concerned about the adverse effects of lithium.

QUESTIONS

■ **1.** How is a depressive episode different from occasionally "feeling blue"?
■ **2.** How does fluoxetine work?
■ **3.** Why is there a delay in the onset of fluoxetine's therapeutic effect?
■ **4.** What caused Ms. R's hypomania? Why is it necessary to treat bipolar affective disorder if the patient "feels good"?
■ **5.** What specific concerns might Ms. R have about the adverse effects of lithium?

BIOCHEMISTRY AND PHYSIOLOGY OF SEROTONERGIC AND CENTRAL ADRENERGIC NEUROTRANSMISSION

Serotonin (5-hydroxytryptamine or 5HT) and norepinephrine (NE) play critical roles in modulating mood, the sleep–wake cycle, motivation, pain perception, and neuroen-docrine function. Serotonergic projections to the spinal cord are involved in pain perception, visceral regulation, and motor control, while projections to the forebrain are important for modulating mood, cognition, and neuroendocrine function. The noradrenergic system modulates vigilance, stress responses, neuroendocrine function, pain control, and sympathetic nervous system activity.

The primary mode of 5HT and NE release is from varicosities. Unlike synapses, which form tight contacts with specific target neurons, varicosities release large amounts of neurotransmitter from vesicles into the extracellular space, establishing concentration gradients of neurotransmitter in the projection areas of the varicosities. 5HT-containing cells within the **raphe nuclei** and NE-containing cells within the **locus ceruleus** project broadly throughout the cerebral cortex, while dopamine has a more focused pattern of projections. Each of these systems has prominent presynaptic autoreceptors that control local transmitter concentrations. This autoregulation results in coordinated firing, which causes spontaneous and synchronous waves of activity that can be measured as firing frequencies; for example, the cells within the raphe nuclei usually fire at rates between 0.3 and 7 spikes per second. Because the frequency of firing does not change rapidly and the quanta of neurotransmitter released with each discharge are fairly well conserved, the neurotransmitter concentration in the vicinity of the varicosities is maintained within a narrow range.

The mean concentration establishes the baseline **tone** of activity in the target neurons that receive 5HT and NE projections. In addition, specific stimuli can elicit rapid bursts of firing, superimposed on the baseline tonic activity, which provide additional information content. Diffusely projecting systems can thus provide two types of information: a rapid and discrete neuronal firing akin to more traditional neurotransmission, and a slower tonic firing frequency that presumably allows for integration of information over a longer period of time.

SEROTONIN SYNTHESIS AND REGULATION

Serotonin is synthesized from the amino acid tryptophan by the enzyme **tryptophan hydroxylase (TPH),** which converts tryptophan to **5-hydroxytryptophan. Aromatic L-amino acid decarboxylase** then converts 5-hydroxytryptophan to serotonin (Fig. 13-1A). These enzymes are present throughout the cytoplasm of serotonergic neurons, both in the cell body and in cell processes. Serotonin is concentrated and stored within vesicles located in axons, cell bodies, and dendrites.

The serotonin metabolic cycle (Fig. 13-2) involves synthesis, uptake into synaptic vesicles, exocytosis, reuptake into the cytoplasm, and then either uptake into vesicles or degradation. Importantly, regulation of the levels of 5HT and NE neurotransmission can occur at any of these steps.

The biochemistry of norepinephrine synthesis and regulation is discussed in Chapter 9, Adrenergic Pharmacology. For review, the synthesis of norepinephrine is summarized in Fig. 13-1B, and the metabolic cycle of norepinephrine is summarized in Figure 13-3.

For all monoamines, the first synthetic step is rate-limiting. Thus, DA and NE synthesis is rate-limited by **tyrosine hydroxylase** (TH), and 5HT synthesis by **tryptophan hydroxylase** (TPH). Both enzymes are tightly regulated by

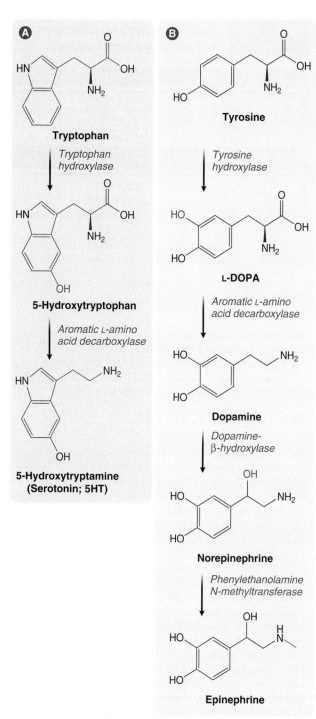

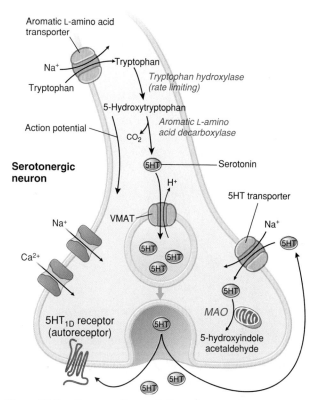

Figure 13-2. Presynaptic regulation of serotonin neurotransmission. Serotonin (5HT) is synthesized from tryptophan in a two-reaction pathway: the rate-limiting enzyme is tryptophan hydroxylase. Both newly synthesized and recycled 5HT are transported from the cytoplasm into synaptic vesicles by the vesicular monoamine transporter (VMAT). Neurotransmission is initiated by an action potential in the presynaptic neuron, which eventually causes synaptic vesicles to fuse with the plasma membrane in a Ca^{2+}-dependent manner. 5HT is removed from the synaptic cleft by a selective 5HT transporter as well as by nonselective reuptake transporters (not shown). 5HT can stimulate $5HT_{1D}$ autoreceptors to provide feedback inhibition. Cytoplasmic 5HT is either sequestered in synaptic vesicles by VMAT or degraded by mitochondrial MAO.

Figure 13-1. Synthesis of serotonin and norepinephrine. A. 5-Hydroxytryptamine (serotonin) is synthesized from the amino acid tryptophan in two steps: the hydroxylation of tryptophan to form 5-hydroxytryptophan, and the subsequent decarboxylation of this intermediate to produce 5-hydroxytryptamine (5HT). Tryptophan hydroxylase is the rate-limiting enzyme in this pathway. **B.** Norepinephrine is synthesized from the amino acid tyrosine in a three-step process similar to the synthetic pathway for serotonin. Tyrosine is first oxidized to L-DOPA by the enzyme tyrosine hydroxylase and then decarboxylated to dopamine. After dopamine is transported into the synaptic vesicle, it is hydroxylated by the enzyme dopamine β-hydroxylase to form norepinephrine. The same enzyme decarboxylates 5-hydroxytryptophan and L-DOPA; it is known generically as aromatic L-amino acid decarboxylase. Tyrosine hydroxylase is the rate-limiting enzyme in this pathway.

inhibitory feedback via autoreceptors. 5HT presynaptic autoreceptors respond to locally increased 5HT concentrations by G protein signaling, which leads to a decrease in the level of cAMP, resulting in decreased activity of protein kinase A and calcium-CaM kinase II. Because phosphorylation of TPH increases its activity, the decrease in kinase activity results in decreased 5HT synthesis. This autoregulatory loop may be an explanation for the observed time course of action of antidepressants clinically, as will be discussed in the section on the monoamine theory of depression.

5HT is transported into vesicles using the vesicular monoamine transporter (VMAT). The transporter is a nonspecific monoamine transporter that is important for the vesicular packaging of dopamine (DA) and epinephrine (EPI) as well as 5HT. **Reserpine** binds irreversibly to VMAT and thereby inhibits the packaging of DA, NE, EPI, and 5HT in vesicles.

Selective serotonin reuptake transporters recycle 5HT from the synaptic cleft back into the presynaptic neuron. Selective monoamine reuptake transporters are twelve-transmembrane–spanning proteins that couple neurotransmitter transport to the transmembrane sodium gradient. Unlike

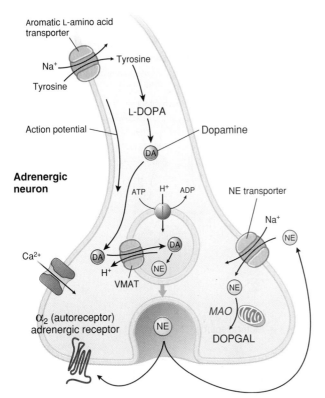

Figure 13-3. Presynaptic regulation of norepinephrine neurotransmission. Norepinephrine in the synaptic vesicle is derived from two sources. First, dopamine synthesized from tyrosine is transported into the vesicle by the vesicular monoamine transporter (VMAT). Inside the vesicle, dopamine is converted to norepinephrine by dopamine-β-hydroxylase. Second, recycled NE is transported from the cytoplasm into the vesicle, also by VMAT. Neurotransmission is initiated by an action potential in the presynaptic neuron, which eventually causes synaptic vesicles to fuse with the plasma membrane in a Ca^{2+}-dependent manner. NE is removed from the synaptic cleft by a selective norepinephrine transporter (NET) as well as by nonselective reuptake transporters *(not shown)*. NE can stimulate α_2-adrenergic autoreceptors to provide feedback inhibition. Cytoplasmic NE that is not sequestered in synaptic vesicles by VMAT is instead degraded by monoamine oxidase (MAO) on the outer mitochondrial membrane to 3,4-dihydroxyphenylglycoaldehyde (DOPGAL).

VMAT, which is a nonspecific monoamine transporter, the individual monoamine reuptake transporters show selectivity, high affinity, and low capacity for each specific monoamine. The selective monoamine transporters, which include the **serotonin transporter** (SERT), **norepinephrine transporter** (NET), and **dopamine transporter** (DAT), are also capable of transporting the other monoamines, although less efficiently.

Once 5HT is returned to the neuronal cytoplasm, the neurotransmitter is transported into vesicles via VMAT or degraded by the **monoamine oxidase** (MAO) system. MAOs are mitochondrial enzymes that regulate the levels of monoamines in neural tissues and inactivate circulating and dietary monoamines (such as tyramine) in the liver and gut. The two isoforms, MAO-A and MAO-B, differ according to substrate specificity such that MAO-A oxidizes 5HT, NE and DA, and MAO-B preferentially oxidizes DA. Monoamine oxidases inactivate monoamines by oxidative

TABLE 13-1 **Signaling Mechanisms of Norepinephrine and Serotonin Receptor Subtypes**

NE RECEPTOR SUBTYPE	SIGNALING MECHANISMS
α_1	$\uparrow$ IP$_3$, DAG
α_2*	$\downarrow$ cAMP
$\beta_{1,2}$	$\uparrow$ cAMP
5HT RECEPTOR SUBTYPE	
5HT$_{1A,B,D}$*$_{,E,F}$	$\downarrow$ cAMP
5HT$_{2A,B,C}$	$\uparrow$ IP$_3$, DAG
5HT$_3$	Ligand-gated ion channel
5HT$_{4,6,7}$	$\uparrow$ cAMP

Abbreviations: cAMP = cyclic AMP; IP$_3$ = inositol 1,4,5-trisphosphate; DAG = diacylglycerol
*α_2 adrenergic and 5HT$_{1D}$ are presynaptic autoreceptors important for feedback inhibition.

deamination, using a functional flavin moiety as an electron acceptor. **Catechol-O-methyltransferase** (COMT) in the extracellular space is another important degradation enzyme for monoamines, although COMT plays a less significant role in the CNS than it does peripherally.

SEROTONIN RECEPTORS

Multiple subtypes of 5HT receptors have been characterized and all but one are G protein-coupled (Table 13-1). In general, the 5HT$_1$ class of receptors inhibits adenylyl cyclase, the 5HT$_2$ class increases phosphotidylinositol turnover, and the 5HT$_4$, 5HT$_6$, and 5HT$_7$ classes stimulate adenylyl cyclase. The only known ligand-gated ion channel is the 5HT$_3$ receptor, although several 5HT receptor subtypes have yet to be fully characterized. 5HT$_{1A}$ is expressed both on serotonergic cell bodies in the raphe nuclei and on postsynaptic neurons in the hippocampus, and its activation results in decreased cAMP levels. Presynaptic 5HT$_{1D}$ mediates the autoinhibitory mechanisms of 5HT neurotransmission at axon terminals. 5HT$_{2A}$ and 5HT$_{2C}$ signaling is excitatory and lowers the threshold for neuronal firing. The various receptor subtypes are expressed differentially throughout the brain. For example, a subset of 5HT projections to the cortex stimulates postsynaptic 5HT$_2$ receptors, while other projections to the limbic system stimulate postsynaptic 5HT$_{1A}$ receptors. There is considerable overlap of receptor subtype expression, however, and the physiologic significance of this overlap is not well understood.

The signaling mechanisms of norepinephrine (adrenergic) receptor subtypes are discussed in Chapter 9 and reviewed in Table 13-1.

PATHOPHYSIOLOGY OF AFFECTIVE DISORDERS

Major depressive disorder (MDD) and bipolar affective disorder (BPAD) are characterized by mood dysregulation.

Major depressive disorder is typified by recurrent depressive episodes, whereas bipolar disorder is defined by the presence of mania or hypomania (although periods of depression are more common than periods of elevated mood in BPAD). In addition, a number of other disorders, such as dysthymia and cyclothymia, involve combinations or less extreme manifestations of depression and mania. Current molecular theories for the etiology of depression center on the **monoamine hypothesis**, and theories for the etiology of mania arise mainly from the inferred actions of lithium, a first-line agent used to treat mania. However, because the underlying etiologies of these disorders are still not well understood at a molecular level, the criteria for diagnosis rely primarily on clinical evaluation. The American Psychiatric Association diagnostic criteria for major depressive disorder and bipolar disorder are summarized in Boxes 13-1 and 13-2.

BOX 13-1. Diagnostic and Statistical Manual of Mental Disorders, Text Revision Criteria for Major Depressive Disorder (MDD)

A. At least one of the following three abnormal moods, which significantly interfered with the person's life:
   1. Abnormal depressed mood most of the day, nearly every day, for at least 2 weeks
   2. Abnormal loss of all interest and pleasure most of the day, nearly every day, for at least 2 weeks
   3. If 18 or younger, abnormal irritable mood most of the day, nearly every day, for at least 2 weeks
B. At least five of the following symptoms have been present during the same 2-week depressed period:
   1. Abnormal depressed mood (or irritable mood if a child or adolescent)
   2. Abnormal loss of all interest and pleasure
   3. Appetite or weight disturbance, either:
      • abnormal weight loss (when not dieting) or decrease in appetite, or
      • abnormal weight gain or increase in appetite
   4. Sleep disturbance, either abnormal insomnia or abnormal hypersomnia
   5. Activity disturbance, either abnormal agitation or abnormal slowing (observable by others)
   6. Abnormal fatigue or loss of energy
   7. Abnormal self-reproach or inappropriate guilt
   8. Abnormal poor concentration or indecisiveness
   9. Abnormal morbid thoughts of death (not just fear of dying) or suicide
C. The symptoms are not attributable to a mood-incongruent psychosis
D. There has never been a manic episode, a mixed episode, or a hypomanic episode
E. The symptoms are not attributable to physical illness, alcohol, medication, or street drugs
F. The symptoms are not attributable to normal bereavement

BOX 13-2. Diagnostic and Statistical Manual of Mental Disorders, Text Revision Criteria for Bipolar Disorder (abbreviated)

BIPOLAR I DISORDER
Single manic episode:
A. Presence of only one manic episode and no past major depressive episodes (Note: Recurrence is defined as either a change in polarity from depression or an interval of at least 2 months without manic symptoms)
B. The manic episode is not better accounted for by schizoaffective disorder and is not superimposed on schizophrenia, schizophreniform disorder, delusional disorder, or psychotic disorder not otherwise specified
In cases where a patient has had multiple mood episodes, bipolar I subtypes are defined by the most recent mood episode:
   • Most recent episode hypomanic
   • Most recent episode manic
   • Most recent episode mixed
   • Most recent episode depressed
   • Most recent episode unspecified

BIPOLAR II DISORDER
A. Presence (or history) of one or more major depressive episodes
B. Presence (or history) of at least one hypomanic episode
C. There has never been a manic episode or a mixed episode
D. The mood episodes in criteria A and B are not better accounted for by schizoaffective disorder and are not superimposed on schizophrenia, schizophreniform disorder, delusional disorder, or psychotic disorder not otherwise specified
E. The symptoms cause clinically significant distress or impairment in social, occupational, or other important areas of functioning

---

CLINICAL CHARACTERISTICS OF AFFECTIVE DISORDERS

Major depressive disorder is characterized by recurrent episodes of depressed mood together with increased social isolation (decreased interest or sense of pleasure, feelings of worthlessness) and characteristic somatic symptoms (decreased energy, changes in appetite and sleep, muscle pain and slowing of movement with speech latency). MDD may be precipitated by significant social stressors or may occur spontaneously due to biological predisposition. A single depressive episode must last 2 weeks or longer and must interfere significantly with the patient's daily functions, such as work and personal relationships. An episode is not considered to be MDD if it is due to bereavement (i.e., depressive symptoms within the first 2 months of the loss of a loved one is considered normal grief) or to a general medical condition such as hypothyroidism or the administration of high doses of β-adrenergic receptor blockers.

There are three clinical subtypes of MDD: typical depression, atypical depression (which is actually more common than typical depression) and melancholic depression. In all depressed patients, it is crucial to determine whether there is any suicidality and whether there is evidence of psychosis. Although psychosis is more typical of bipolar disorder, severely depressed patients may become psychotic, and either suicidality or psychosis are indications for prompt referral to a psychiatrist or psychiatric hospitalization.

Typical depression is characterized by early morning awakening (e.g., waking up spontaneously at 5AM with inability to return to sleep), decreased appetite with weight loss, and marked feelings of social disengagement. In the introductory case, Dr. Lee makes a clinical diagnosis of major depressive episode based on Ms. R having had essentially all these symptoms for more than a month. Typical depression generally responds well to selective serotonin reuptake inhibitors (**SSRIs**). Given that significant improvement may not be seen for 2 to 3 weeks, the short-term administration of a somnorific such as a benzodiazepine may be indicated to produce initial relief of symptoms.

Atypical depression is characterized by neurovegetative signs that are the reverse of those seen in typical depression. Patients have increased appetite, particularly for high fat/high carbohydrate "comfort" foods, and hypersomnia. They are also particularly sensitive to criticism (they view even innocent comments by others as intensely critical of their actions) but unlike typically depressed patients, they are capable of feeling brief periods of pleasure and indulge in pleasure-seeking behavior. Clinically, patients with atypical depression may not respond as well to SSRIs as patients with typical depression. Monoamine oxidase inhibitors (MAOIs) have been shown to be particularly effective for this group, but given the significant adverse effects of this class of medication, MAOIs are considered second- or third-line agents. However, the effectiveness of MAOIs, together with the pleasure-seeking behavior seen in this type of depressive (over-eating, indulgence in shopping), suggests that atypical depression results from a relative decrease in both serotonin and dopamine pathways. The most effective medications for this class of depression typically target the monoamines generally; such medications include **bupropion, venlafaxine**, and stimulants such as **methylphenidate**.

Melancholic depression is the least common subtype of depression and is often the most severe and disabling. Patients lose all interest in their surroundings and are often completely indifferent to criticism or concern. They are incapable of feeling pleasure even briefly. SSRIs or **mirtazapine** are considered first-line agents for this subtype of depression, but patients may require tricyclic antidepressants (**TCAs**) or even a trial of electroconvulsant therapy if the symptoms are refractory to first-line agents. Psychiatric hospitalization is often warranted even in the absence of a suicidal plan, because these patients are often so disabled they cannot formulate a plan despite intense feelings of emptiness.

A **manic episode** is the clinical inverse of a depressed episode. Though patients may feel irritable, there is usually a sense of elevated mood and an inflated sense of self-worth (termed **grandiosity**). Rather than speech latency and soft speech seen in depression, there is increased, rapid and

loud speech that is often difficult to interrupt. Rather than the sense of fatigue and need for sleep seen in depression, there is a decreased need for sleep. Patients may not need any sleep for days at a time, and rather than feeling tired, they feel energized. Usually there is some form of purposeful activity at nighttime when they should be asleep, for example, driving, cleaning, or working. Manic episodes are characterized by disorganized, racing thoughts, often to the point where patients cannot stay on topic for more than a few seconds, and may be associated with psychosis and auditory hallucinations. Mania usually results in some adverse outcome (traffic accidents, arrests, or psychiatric hospitalization) within a few days.

If a patient has manic symptoms for more than 4 days without such an adverse outcome, it is then by definition a **hypomanic episode** (literally, a "little mania"). In the introductory case, Ms. R had a hypomanic episode. If Dr. Lee had not intervened, her symptoms could have progressed to frank mania. When symptoms of a manic episode and a depressive episode are present simultaneously, it is referred to as a **mixed** episode, and these patients are at the highest risk for committing suicide (depressed patients often lack the energy needed to carry out a suicidal plan).

Though bipolar disorder is characterized by manic symptoms (either mania or hypomania), the disorder usually is dominated by periods of significant, debilitating depression. The depressive episodes often occur before any mania is experienced, and these patients are often mistakenly diagnosed with MDD. Patients with bipolar disorder often experience rapid and potentially life-threatening switches into mania when taking antidepressants (as in the case of Ms. R). However, if manic symptoms are experienced only when taking antidepressants or on stimulants, these symptoms do not technically meet criteria for bipolar disorder. The pharmacologic classes used to treat bipolar disorder are discussed at the end of the pharmacology section and are referred to as **mood stabilizers**. Often patients continue to suffer from depression when taking mood stabilizers, and adjunct treatment with antidepressants may be necessary (the risk of inducing mania is significantly reduced in the presence of a mood stabilizer).

THE MONOAMINE THEORY OF DEPRESSION

The biological basis for depression began to be understood in the 1940's and 1950's, when keen observers noticed that imipramine, iproniazid, and reserpine had unexpected effects on mood.

In the late 1940's the tricyclic drug **imipramine** was developed for use in the treatment of psychotic patients, but it was subsequently noted to have strong antidepressant effects. Imipramine preferentially blocks 5HT transporters, and its active metabolite desipramine preferentially blocks NE transporters. Thus, neurotransmitters persist in the synapse at higher concentrations and for longer durations, yielding greater activation of postsynaptic 5HT and NE receptors.

In 1951, the antituberculosis drug **iproniazid** was shown to have antidepressant effects. Iproniazid inhibits monoamine oxidase and thereby prevents the degradation of

5HT, NE, and DA. The resulting increase in cytosolic neurotransmitter leads to increased neurotransmitter uptake into vesicles and, consequently, to greater release of neurotransmitter after exocytosis.

In the 1950's, the antihypertensive agent **reserpine** was noted to induce depression in 10–15% of patients. Researchers then found that reserpine could induce depression in animal models as well as in humans. Reserpine depletes 5HT, NE, and DA in presynaptic neurons by inhibiting the transport of these neurotransmitters into synaptic vesicles. The drug binds irreversibly to VMAT and ultimately destroys the vesicles. The 5HT, NE, and DA that accumulate in the cytoplasm are degraded by mitochondrial MAO. The resulting decrease in monoamine neurotransmission is thought to be responsible for inducing a depressed mood.

The findings described above strongly suggested that the central monoaminergic serotonin and norepinephrine systems are intimately involved in the pathogenesis of depression. The **monoamine theory of depression** holds that depression results from pathologically decreased serotonin and/or norepinephrine neurotransmission. Based on this hypothesis, it follows that increasing serotonin and/or norepinephrine neurotransmission could ameliorate or reverse depression. As a biological disease related to long-term pathologic alterations in monoamine activity, MDD should thus be treatable by medications.

Limitations of the Monoamine Theory

Although nearly all the classes of antidepressants are pharmacologically active at their molecular and cellular sites of action almost immediately, their clinical antidepressant effects are generally not seen until 3 or more weeks of continuous treatment. Similarly, although reserpine rapidly depletes neurotransmitter in monoaminergic systems, it takes several weeks of continued treatment with reserpine to induce depression. The unexplained delay in the onset of action of these drugs remains a central conundrum in understanding the pathophysiology of depression.

In some patients, drugs that selectively increase 5HT neurotransmission eliminate depression, while drugs that selectively increase NE neurotransmission have little or no effect. In other patients, drugs affecting the NE system are more beneficial than those affecting the 5HT system. Overall, each individual drug is effective in about 70% of patients suffering from depression, and drugs that have markedly different efficacies in blocking the reuptake of NE and/or 5HT may have similar clinical effectiveness when tested in large clinical populations. These clinical observations are not easily explained by the monoamine theory.

The time lag in the clinical effectiveness of antidepressants may be explained by the autoregulatory mechanisms affecting presynaptic monoaminergic neurons. Somewhat paradoxically, treatment with a classical antidepressant drug produces an immediate decrease in the frequency of neuronal firing in the locus ceruleus and/or the raphe nucleus (depending on the drug), with a concomitant decrease in the synthesis and release of 5HT and NE. This observation suggests that the antidepressant-induced increase in synaptic cleft neurotransmitter concentration results in acute feedback inhibition of neuronal firing via $5HT_{1D}$ and α_2 autoreceptors for 5HT and NE, respectively. In response to the elevated levels of

neurotransmitter, inhibitory autoreceptor stimulation acutely down-regulates the activity of the rate-limiting enzymes TPH and TH, and acutely reduces the rate of neuronal firing. The net effect is that initial exposure to antidepressant drugs may not significantly increase postsynaptic signaling.

In contrast, chronic use of antidepressants causes the inhibitory autoreceptors themselves to be down-regulated, leading to enhancement of neurotransmission. (Note that postsynaptic 5HT and NE receptors are also down-regulated by changes in neurotransmitter release and reuptake, but to a lesser degree.) Chronic, but not acute, treatment increases the levels of cAMP in target neurons, indicating that the net effect of chronic treatment with antidepressants is to increase second messenger signaling through the 5HT and/or NE pathways. The change in autoreceptor sensitivity takes several weeks to occur, consistent with the time-course of the therapeutic response in patients. Therefore, the delay in onset of the therapeutic response could be caused by physiologic inhibitory feedback mechanisms; only after chronic drug therapy does gradual desensitization of autoreceptors allow increased neurotransmission (Fig. 13-4). Although speculative, this hypothesis regarding changes in monoamine receptor sensitivity offers an explanation for the delay in onset of the therapeutic action of fluoxetine experienced by Ms. R. It may also explain why some patients have an acute worsening of depression or suicidality in the first days of antidepressant treatment, and underscores the need for following patients closely during the initial weeks of treatment.

PHARMACOLOGIC CLASSES AND AGENTS

Serotonergic transmission is modulated by a broad range of agents that target neurotransmitter storage, degradation, uptake, and neurotransmitter receptors. Because serotonin is involved in a number of physiologic processes, both centrally and peripherally, agents that alter serotonergic tone have diverse actions on the brain (mood, sleep, migraines), on the gastrointestinal (GI) system, and on core temperature and hemodynamics (serotonin syndrome). Many of these biological effects are discussed as the pharmacologic agents are introduced, though the emphasis is on agents that regulate mood.

INHIBITORS OF SEROTONIN STORAGE

Amphetamine and related drugs interfere with the ability of synaptic vesicles to store monoamines such as serotonin. Thus, amphetamine, methamphetamine, and methylphenidate displace 5HT, DA, and NE from their storage vesicles. For atypical depression and for depression in the elderly, stimulants such as **amphetamine**, **methylphenidate** and **modafinil** have proved to be useful as second-line agents, in part because of their combined effects on serotonin, norepinephrine and dopamine. These agents can, however, induce psychosis in susceptible patients, thus caution should be used in bipolar disorder. In addition, **fenfluramine** and **dexfenfluramine** are halogenated amphetamine derivatives that are

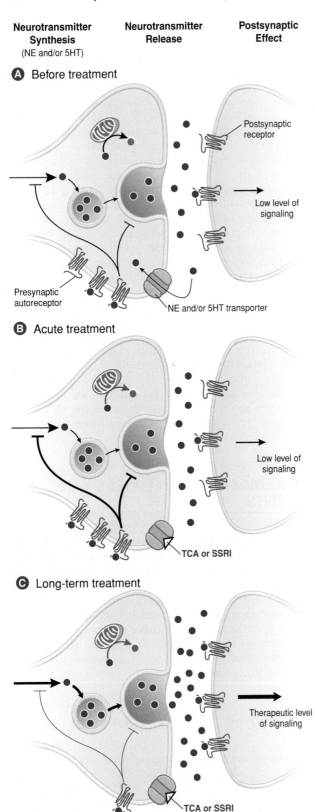

Neurotransmitter Synthesis (NE and/or 5HT) Neurotransmitter Release Postsynaptic Effect

A Before treatment

Postsynaptic receptor

Low level of signaling

Presynaptic autoreceptor

NE and/or 5HT transporter

B Acute treatment

Low level of signaling

TCA or SSRI

C Long-term treatment

Therapeutic level of signaling

TCA or SSRI

Figure 13-4. Postulated mechanism of the delay in onset of the therapeutic effect of antidepressant medications. A. Before treatment, neurotransmitters are released at pathologically low levels and exert steady-state levels of autoinhibitory feedback. The net effect is an abnormally low baseline level of postsynaptic receptor activity *(signaling).* **B.** Short-term use of antidepressant medication results in increased release of neurotransmitter and/or increased duration of neurotransmitter action in the synaptic cleft. Both effects

modestly selective for 5HT. This combination was used briefly in the U.S. for weight loss, but severe cardiac toxicity led to its withdrawal. Another amphetamine derivative, **methylenedioxymethamphetamine (MDMA),** is both a selective serotonin storage inhibitor as well as a 5HT receptor ligand. It is not approved for use in medical practice but is a significant clinical issue due to its illicit use (as "ecstasy").

INHIBITORS OF SEROTONIN DEGRADATION

The major pathway for serotonin degradation is mediated by MAO, and accordingly MAOIs have significant effects on serotonergic neurotransmission. The MAOIs are classified according to their specificity for the MAO-A and MAO-B isoenzymes and according to the reversibility or irreversibility of their binding. The older MAOIs are nonselective, and most older MAOIs, such as **iproniazid, phenelzine,** and **isocarboxazid,** are irreversible inhibitors. Newer MAOIs, such as **moclobemide, befloxatone,** and **brofaromine,** are selective for MAO-A and bind reversibly, and are thus called **reversible inhibitors of monoamine oxidase A** (RIMAs). **Selegiline,** a MAO-B inhibitor (see Chapter 12, Pharmacology of Dopaminergic Neurotransmission), also inhibits MAO-A at higher doses.

MAOIs block the deamination of monoamines by binding to and inhibiting the functional flavin moiety of MAO (Fig. 13-5). By inhibiting the degradation of monoamines, MAOIs increase the 5HT and NE available in the cytoplasm of presynaptic neurons. The increase in cytoplasmic levels of these monoamines leads not only to increased uptake and storage of 5HT and NE in synaptic vesicles, but also to some constitutive leakage of the monoamines into the synaptic cleft.

As noted in Chapter 9, the most toxic adverse effect of MAOI use is systemic **tyramine toxicity.** Because GI and hepatic MAO metabolizes tyramine, consumption of foods that contain tyramine, such as processed meats, aged cheese and red wine, can lead to excess levels of circulating tyramine. Tyramine is an indirect sympathomimetic that can stimulate the release of large amounts of stored catecholamines by reversing the reuptake transporters. This uncontrolled catecholamine release can induce a *hypertensive crisis* characterized by headache, tachycardia, nausea, cardiac arrhythmia, and stroke. The older MAOIs are no longer considered first-line therapy for depression because of the potential for systemic tyramine toxicity; they can be prescribed

cause increased stimulation of inhibitory autoreceptors, with increased inhibition of neurotransmitter synthesis and increased inhibition of exocytosis. The net effect is to dampen the initial effect of the medication, and postsynaptic receptor activity remains at pretreatment levels. **C.** Chronic use of antidepressant medication results in desensitization of the presynaptic autoreceptors. Thus, the inhibition of neurotransmitter synthesis and exocytosis is reduced. The net effect is enhanced postsynaptic receptor activity, leading to a therapeutic response. NE, norepinephrine. 5HT, serotonin. TCA, tricyclic antidepressant. SSRI, selective serotonin reuptake inhibitor.

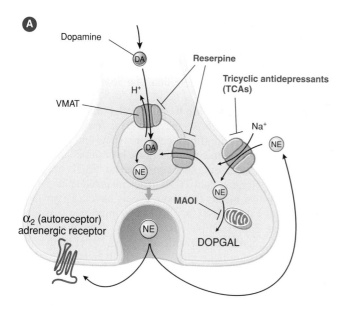

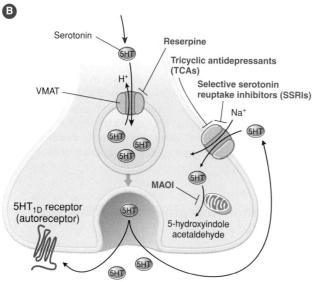

Figure 13-5.   Sites and mechanisms of action of antidepressant drugs. The sites of action of antidepressant drugs and of reserpine (which can induce depression) are indicated in noradrenergic neurons **(A)** and serotonergic neurons **(B)**. Monoamine oxidase inhibitors (MAOIs) inhibit the mitochondrial enzyme monoamine oxidase (MAO); the resulting increase in cytosolic monoamines leads to increased vesicular uptake of neurotransmitter and to increased release of neurotransmitter during exocytosis. Tricyclic antidepressants (TCAs) and heterocyclic antidepressants inhibit both the norepinephrine transporter (NET) and the serotonin transporter (SERT), causing increased levels of both NE and 5HT in the synaptic cleft. Selective serotonin reuptake inhibitors (SSRIs) specifically inhibit the SERT-mediated reuptake of 5HT. TCAs, heterocyclics, and SSRIs increase the duration of neurotransmitter action in the synaptic cleft, leading to increased downstream signaling. Reserpine, which can induce depression in humans and in animal models, blocks the VMAT-mediated uptake of monoamines into synaptic vesicles, which ultimately destroys the vesicles.

only to patients able to commit to a tyramine-free diet. The newer MAOIs (i.e., the RIMAs, which bind reversibly to MAO), are displaced by high concentrations of tyramine, resulting in significantly more tyramine metabolism and hence less tyramine toxicity. Selegiline (considered an MAO-B inhibitor but also capable of inhibiting brain MAO-A) has been recently approved as a transdermal patch, thus bypassing the GI system. Transdermal selegiline can maximally inhibit brain MAO-A at doses that reduce gastrointestinal MAO-A by only 30% to 40%, thus reducing the risk of a tyramine-induced hypertensive crisis and allowing patients greater freedom with their diet. MAOIs, as other antidepressants, can precipitate manic or hypomanic episodes in some bipolar patients.

All antidepressant drugs, including MAOIs, are hydrophobic and cross the blood–brain barrier. They are well absorbed orally and are metabolized to active metabolites by the liver. These metabolites are subsequently inactivated by acetylation, also in the liver. Excretion is primarily via renal clearance. The older, irreversibly binding MAOIs are cleared from the circulation as complexes with MAO, and are effectively inactivated only when a new enzyme is synthesized. Because of the extensive effects of MAOIs on cytochrome P450 enzymes in the liver, they can cause numerous drug-drug interactions. All members of a patient's medical team must prescribe other drugs with caution when a patient is taking a MAOI.

REUPTAKE INHIBITORS

Serotonergic tone is maintained at steady-state by the balance between transmitter release and reuptake. Thus, inhibitors of the serotonin reuptake transporter (SERT) typically increase the amount of 5HT in the extracellular space. These drugs alleviate the symptoms of a variety of common psychiatric conditions, including depression, anxiety, and obsessive-compulsive disorder. Three classes of reuptake inhibitors are in use; the non-selective **tricyclic antidepressants** (TCAs), **selective serotonin reuptake inhibitors** (SSRIs), and the newer **serotonin-norepinephrine reuptake inhibitors** (SNRIs). Each class is discussed below, followed by a discussion of atypical antidepressants that do not fall clearly into one of these three categories.

Tricyclic Antidepressants (TCAs)

The TCAs derive their name from their common chemical backbone, consisting of three rings that include two aromatic rings attached to a cycloheptane ring. The prototype TCA is **imipramine**, and other members of this class include **amitriptyline**, **desipramine**, **nortriptyline** and **clomipramine** (which is a first-line agent for obsessive-compulsive disorder). TCAs with secondary amines preferentially affect the NE system, whereas those with tertiary amines primarily affect the 5HT system. Tetracyclic antidepressants, which include **maprotiline**, have also been developed, but they are not widely used.

TCAs inhibit the reuptake of 5HT and NE from the synaptic cleft by blocking 5HT and NE reuptake transporters, respectively. These agents do not affect DA reuptake (Fig. 13-5). The molecular mechanism of transporter inhibition remains to be elucidated. Because the increased time spent by neurotransmitter in the synaptic cleft leads to increased receptor activation, the reuptake inhibitors cause enhancement of postsynaptic responses. Despite widely varying affinities for 5HT and NE reuptake transporters, the TCAs are markedly similar in their clinical efficacy. The TCAs are also useful for treating pain syndromes, and are often used for this indication at lower doses than those needed to produce antidepressant effects. They are particularly useful in the treatment of migraine headaches, other somatic pain disorders, and chronic fatigue syndrome.

The adverse effect profile of TCAs results from their ability to bind a number of channels and receptors in addition to their therapeutic targets. The most dangerous adverse effects of TCAs involve the cardiovascular system. TCAs appear to affect sodium channels in a quinidine-like manner. *The quinidine-like side effects of TCAs include potentially lethal conduction delays, such as first-degree atrioventricular and bundle branch blocks.* TCAs should thus always be prescribed with caution in patients at risk of attempting suicide, and an ECG should be done to rule out conduction system disease prior to starting TCAs.

TCAs can also act as antagonists at muscarinic (cholinergic), histamine, adrenergic, and dopamine receptors. The *anticholinergic effects* are most prominent and include symptoms typical of muscarinic acetylcholine receptor blockade: nausea, vomiting, anorexia, dry mouth, blurred vision, confusion, constipation, tachycardia, and urinary retention. The *antihistaminergic effects* include sedation, weight gain, and confusion (in the elderly). The *antiadrenergic effects* include orthostatic hypotension, reflex tachycardia, drowsiness, and dizziness. Orthostatic hypotension is an especially significant risk for elderly patients, and TCA use must be monitored carefully in such patients. Finally, TCAs may also precipitate mania in patients with bipolar affective disorder.

Selective Serotonin Reuptake Inhibitors (SSRIs)

In 1987, the treatment of depression was revolutionized with the introduction of **selective serotonin reuptake inhibitors** (SSRIs). The first SSRI to be introduced was **fluoxetine**; this drug is still one of the most widely prescribed SSRIs. Other SSRIs include **citalopram, fluvoxamine, paroxetine, sertraline,** and **escitalopram.** Although the effectiveness of the SSRIs is similar to that of the TCAs for the treatment of depression, their higher selectivity and reduced adverse effect profile has made them first-line agents for the treatment of depression, as well as for anxiety and obsessive-compulsive disorder. SSRIs are also used in the treatment of panic syndromes, obsessive-compulsive disorder, and posttraumatic stress disorder.

The SSRIs are similar to the TCAs in their mechanism of action, except that the SSRIs are significantly more selective for 5HT transporters (Fig. 13-5B). Inhibition of serotonin reuptake increases synaptic serotonin levels, causing increased 5HT receptor activation and enhanced postsynaptic responses. At low doses, SSRIs are believed to bind primarily to 5HT transporters, whereas at higher doses, they lose selectivity and also bind NE transporters. Despite widely varying chemical structures, the SSRIs have clinical effica-

cies similar to the TCAs and to one another. Thus, the choice of drug often depends on issues such as cost and tolerability of adverse effects. In addition, because of the variability of individual patient responses to individual antidepressants, a patient may need to try more than one SSRI to find the most effective drug.

Because the SSRIs are more selective than the TCAs at clinically effective doses, they have far fewer adverse effects. SSRIs lack significant cardiotoxicity, and do not bind as avidly to muscarinic (cholinergic), histamine, adrenergic, or dopamine receptors. As a consequence, SSRIs are generally better tolerated than TCAs. The enhanced selectivity of the SSRIs also means that these agents have a larger therapeutic index than the TCAs. This is an important consideration in the depressed patient, who may attempt to commit suicide by intentionally overdosing on his or her medication.

The SSRIs are not entirely without adverse effects, however. All SSRIs can cause some degree of sexual dysfunction. Another common adverse effect is GI distress; sertraline is more often associated with diarrhea, while paroxetine is associated with constipation. A more serious adverse effect of the SSRIs is **serotonin syndrome,** a rare but dangerous elevation of 5HT that can occur when both an SSRI and a monoamine oxidase inhibitor (MAOI; see below) are administered simultaneously. *The clinical manifestations of serotonin syndrome include hyperthermia, muscle rigidity, myoclonus, and rapid fluctuations in mental status and vital signs.* SSRIs can also cause vasospasm in a small percentage of patients. Finally, as with TCAs and MAOIs, SSRIs can cause a ''switch'' from depression to mania or hypomania in patients with bipolar disorder. The fluoxetine that Ms. R was prescribed for MDD was likely responsible for her subsequent manic episode. The mechanism of the SSRI-induced switch from depression to mania or hypomania is unknown.

Serotonin-Norepinephrine Reuptake Inhibitors (SNRIs)

Though SSRIs are useful first-line agents for the treatment of depression, there is a significant patient population that responds only partially to SSRIs, particularly when there are comorbid medical or psychiatric disorders. It is appreciated that TCAs are particularly useful in cases in which somatic pain is a significant concern, although the broad receptor profile of TCAs make them particularly difficult to prescribe in medically complicated or fragile patients. A newer class of drugs is proving to be particularly useful, the serotonin-norepinephrine reuptake inhibitors, which presently consist of **venlafaxine** and **duloxetine.** Venlafaxine blocks the 5HT reuptake transporter and the NE reuptake transporter in a concentration-dependent manner; at low concentrations, it behaves as an SSRI, but at high concentrations it also increases NE levels. Duloxetine also inhibits NE and 5HT reuptake specifically and has been approved for the treatment of neuropathic pain and other pain syndromes in addition to treating depression.

ATYPICAL ANTIDEPRESSANTS

Other drugs that interact with multiple targets are sometimes referred to as ''atypical antidepressants,'' and include bupropion, mirtazapine, nefazodone, and trazodone. They are categorized together here only because they do not fit conveniently into other categories. These agents are newer than TCAs and act by several different mechanisms, although some have unknown or incompletely characterized mechanisms of action.

Bupropion appears to act mechanistically like the amphetamines and is particularly useful for treatment of atypical depression because it increases both serotonin and dopamine levels in the brain. Bupropion is the antidepressant with the fewest sexual adverse effects. It is also believed to induce less switching into mania than the other antidepressants. The principal contraindication to the use of bupropion is a concurrent seizure disorder, since it lowers the seizure threshold.

Mirtazapine blocks $5HT_{2A}$, $5HT_{2C}$, and the α_2-adrenergic autoreceptor, and presumably decreases neurotransmission at $5HT_2$ synapses while increasing NE neurotransmission. Mirtazapine is a potent somnorific as well as an appetite stimulant, making it a particularly useful antidepressant for the elderly population (who often present with insomnia and weight loss).

Nefazodone and **trazodone** also block postsynaptic $5HT_2$ receptors and are discussed below.

Overall, the atypical antidepressants have relatively few adverse effects and demonstrate similar clinical efficacies despite their widely heterogeneous mechanisms of action and molecular targets.

SEROTONIN RECEPTOR AGONISTS

Ergots are naturally occurring serotonin receptor (5HTR) agonists. Several dozen structurally similar ergots are elaborated by the rye rust fungus *Claviceps purpurea*. Many naturally occurring ergot alkaloids produce intense vasoconstriction by acting as agonists of 5HTRs in vascular smooth muscle. This action was responsible for ergotism—described during the Middle Ages as "St. Anthony's Fire"—in which consumers of fungus-infected grains experienced severe peripheral vasoconstriction leading to necrosis and gangrene. In more modern times, a number of ergot alkaloids have been employed clinically. The semi-synthetic ergot lysergic acid diethylamide (LSD) has been of interest to psychiatrists (and others) due to the hallucinations and sensory dysfunction it produces at doses as small as 50 µg in humans.

5HTR subtype-selective agonists have become a therapeutic target of increasing interest in the past decade. These agents are used primarily to treat anxiety and migraine headaches. **Buspirone** is a non-benzodiazepine anxiolytic that does not bind to GABA receptors, but rather acts as a $5HT_{1A}$R-selective agonist. It is non-sedating with moderate anxiolytic properties. Although it is often not as effective clinically as a benzodiazepine, it is attractive given that it is non-addictive and does not have abuse potential.

Migraine headaches are believed to be precipitated by cerebral vasodilation with subsequent activation of small pain fibers. A class of selective serotonin agonists ($5HT_1$ agonists) have been found to be particularly effective in the treatment of migraine headaches, presumably because of their potent vasoconstrictive effects. **Sumatriptan** is the prototype $5HT_{1D}$R agonist of this group, known collectively as

the **triptans**, which also includes **rizatriptan**, **almotriptan**, **frovatriptan**, **eletriptan** and **zolmitriptan**. The triptans, as well as the less selective ergot alkaloid **ergotamine**, act on $5HT_1$R in the vasculature to alter intracranial blood flow. These agents are most useful for acute migraine attacks when taken at the onset of an episode rather than as prophylaxis. They must be taken early in a migraine (ideally at the time of the aura) to effectively block the activation of pain receptors. The triptans are thought to activate both $5HT_{1D}$R and $5HT_{1B}$R. In the CNS, both receptor subtypes are present on presynaptic endings of a variety of neurons in the vasculature.

There are relatively few $5HT_2$R agonists used clinically. **Trazodone** is a prodrug that is converted into meta-chlorophenylpiperazine (mCPP), a selective $5HT_{2A/2C}$R agonist used in the treatment of depression and insomnia. Trazadone is used principally as a somnorific because the higher doses required for antidepressant effects are usually over-sedating. The ergot derivative methysergide is a partial agonist of $5HT_2$R, but also has adrenergic and muscarinic effects and is no longer available in the U.S.

Serotonin and serotonin receptors are abundant in the GI tract. Serotonin is a critical mediator of GI motility, mediated in large part by $5HT_4$R. **Cisapride**, a $5HT_4$R agonist that also enhances acetylcholine release from the myenteric plexus, induces gastric motility. However, cisapride has been withdrawn in the U.S. due to safety concerns related to QT prolongation and cardiac arrhythmias.

SEROTONIN RECEPTOR ANTAGONISTS

Serotonin receptor antagonists are increasingly important therapeutics. Like many receptor ligands, these drugs show varying degrees of receptor subtype selectivity and often cross-react with adrenergic, histamine, and muscarinic receptors. This property is advantageous in some cases (e.g., the atypical antipsychotics), but can also limit their clinical utility because of intolerable adverse effects.

Ketanserin is a $5HT_{2A/2C}$R antagonist with substantial α-adrenergic activity. It reduces blood pressure to a similar degree as β-blockers, and has been used topically to reduce intraocular pressure in glaucoma.

Ondansetron is a $5HT_3$R antagonist. This drug is of interest because, of all the currently identified monoamine receptors, only $5HT_3$R is an ionotropic receptor belonging to the nicotinic acetylcholine superfamily of pentameric receptors. $5HT_3$Rs are expressed in the enteric nervous system, the nerve endings of the vagus, and in the CNS, particularly in the chemo-trigger zone. Ondansetron is a potent antiemetic, and is specifically used as an adjunct to cancer chemotherapy or in cases of refractory nausea. Due to its mechanism of action, it has little effect on nausea caused by vertigo.

Irritable bowel syndrome (IBS) is believed to be primarily a disorder of GI motility, particularly in the colon. Patients can suffer from episodes of diarrhea, constipation, or both, with significant GI cramping. The $5HT_4$R antagonists **tegaserod** and **prucalopride** enhance GI motility and are effective in treating the constipation associated with IBS. **Alosetron** is a $5HT_3$R antagonist that decreases serotonergic tone in intestinal cells, thus reducing motility. It is particularly useful for diarrhea associated with IBS.

MOOD STABILIZERS

In 1949, an Australian researcher noted that lithium had a calming effect on animals and hypothesized that lithium would have a similar effect on manic patients. Subsequent studies substantiated this hypothesis. This discovery sparked intense research on the biochemical effects of lithium and the mechanisms by which this drug exerts its antimanic effects. Although research on lithium has provided some insights, the mechanisms responsible for its psychiatric effects remain poorly understood. At about the same time, it was noted that antidepressant medications can precipitate manic episodes in some patients with MDD. The mechanism by which antidepressant drugs cause the switch from MDD to bipolar disorder is also poorly understood.

In the 1970's, some researchers considered the possibility that mania could be related to epilepsy, because both disorders exhibit episodic patterns involving brain overactivity. Subsequent research did not bear out this relationship, but anticonvulsants such as **carbamazepine** and **valproic acid** were found to have some efficacy in the treatment of BPAD. Carbamazepine, valproic acid, and **lamotrigine** (see Chapter 14, Pharmacology of Abnormal Electrical Neurotransmission in the Central Nervous System) are used to treat mania and bipolar depression and to prevent future episodes of mood disorder. Traditionally, the term **mood stabilizer** has been used to refer to both lithium and valproic acid. Lithium and lamotrigine are most useful for bipolar depression. Valproic acid is considered most useful for irritability and impulsivity.

Given the similarity in the psychotic symptoms experienced during mania and those seen in schizophrenia (auditory hallucinations, commands hallucinations, persecution paranoia, and hyperreligiosity) antipsychotics have also been used successfully to treat mania. Olanzapine, risperidone, and aripiprazole (discussed in Chapter 12) have specific indications for bipolar affective disorder, although they are not generally referred to as mood stabilizers.

Lithium

Lithium, commonly administered as lithium carbonate, is a small monovalent cation that is similar in electrochemical properties to sodium and potassium. At therapeutic concentrations, lithium enters cells via Na^+ channels. Because lithium can mimic other small monovalent cations, it has the potential to disrupt any number of proteins and transporters that require specific cation cofactors.

Lithium exerts numerous effects at the intracellular level. Its effect on the regeneration of inositol for second messenger signaling is particularly well studied, although this effect is not necessarily central to its therapeutic actions. In the inositol lipid pathway, G protein-coupled receptors (such as $5HT_2$ receptors) activate phospholipase C (PLC), which cleaves phosphatidylinositol 4,5-bisphosphate (PIP_2) to the signaling molecules diacylglycerol (DAG) and inositol 1,4,5-trisphosphate (IP_3). IP_3 signaling is terminated by conversion to inositol 4,5-bisphosphate (IP_2), either directly or via an IP_4 intermediate. Lithium inhibits both the inositol phosphatase that dephosphorylates IP_2 to inositol phosphate (IP_1), and the inositol phophatase that dephosphorylates IP_1 to free inositol. Because free inositol is essential for the regeneration of PIP_2, lithium effectively blocks the phosphatidylinositol signaling cascade in the brain. Though inositol circulates freely in blood, it cannot cross the blood–brain barrier. The two mechanisms of inositol synthesis in CNS neurons—regeneration from IP_3 and de novo synthesis from glucose-6-phosphate—are both inhibited by lithium. By blocking the regeneration of PIP_2, lithium inhibits central adrenergic, muscarinic, and serotonergic neurotransmission.

Disruption of the phosphatidylinositol signaling cascade was previously thought to be the primary mechanism of lithium's mood-stabilizing action. However, recent studies suggest that other actions of lithium may also be relevant. These actions include: increasing 5HT neurotransmission by increasing neurotransmitter synthesis and release; decreasing NE and DA neurotransmission by inhibiting neurotransmitter synthesis, storage, release, and reuptake; inhibiting adenylyl cyclase by decoupling G proteins from neurotransmitter receptors; and altering electrochemical gradients across cell membranes by substituting for Na^+ and/or blocking K^+ channels. Possible neurotrophic effects of lithium are also under investigation.

Lithium has a narrow therapeutic window and a wide range of adverse effects, leading patients such as Ms. R to be concerned about its potential adverse actions. **Acute lithium intoxication,** a clinical syndrome characterized by nausea, vomiting, diarrhea, renal failure, neuromuscular dysfunction, ataxia, tremor, confusion, delirium, and seizures, is a medical emergency and may require dialysis for treatment. Hyponatremia or the administration of non-steroidal anti-inflammatory drugs (NSAIDs) can lead to increased lithium reabsorption in the proximal tubule and elevation of plasma lithium concentration to toxic levels.

Lithium's inhibition of K^+ entry into myocytes leads to abnormalities in repolarization, resulting in abnormal T waves seen by ECG. In addition, the transmembrane electrical potential is shifted because inhibition of K^+ entry into cells leads to extracellular hyperkalemia and intracellular hypokalemia. This shift in transmembrane electrical potential exposes patients to a greater risk of sudden cardiac arrest from small changes in potassium balance.

Antidiuretic hormone and thyroid-stimulating hormone both activate adenylyl cyclase, which is inhibited by lithium. By this mechanism, lithium treatment can also lead to **nephrogenic diabetes insipidus** and to hypothyroidism and/or goiter.

Given the wide range of adverse effects that may accompany lithium treatment and the euphoria that may be associated with manic or hypomanic episodes, many patients are hesitant to begin treatment. However, lithium and a limited number of other mood-stabilizing drugs (see Drug Summary Table) help to prevent depressive episodes as well as mania. In addition, lithium is the only medication shown in clinical trials to reduce the risk of suicide in patients with bipolar disorder.

■ *Conclusion and Future Directions*

This chapter discusses central monoamine neurotransmission, primarily serotonin pathways, but also norepinephrine and, to a lesser extent, dopamine pathways. Serotonin is a critical mediator of mood and anxiety, and is also involved in the pathophysiology of migraine headaches and IBS. The focus of the chapter has been on the antidepressant class of medications. The monoamine theory of depression forms a framework for considering the pathophysiology and treatment of MDD, although this theory has inconsistencies that require further study. Therapy with drugs that increase synaptic concentrations of 5HT and NE is effective in many cases of MDD and forms the basis of treatment for this disorder. The delay between initiation of treatment and onset of clinical improvement may occur because of slow changes in presynaptic autoreceptor sensitivities.

TCAs, SSRIs, MAOIs, and other antidepressants have similar clinical efficacies when tested on groups of patients, although individual patients may respond to one drug and not to another. TCAs nonselectively inhibit 5HT and NE reuptake transporters (in addition to other receptors); SSRIs selectively block 5HT transporters; SNRIs selectively block 5HT and NE reuptake transporters; and MAOIs inhibit the degradation of both 5HT and NE. The choice of antidepressant medication for an individual patient depends on the two goals of finding an effective agent for that patient and minimizing adverse effects. The type of depressive symptoms may suggest one treatment modality over another. Given the favorable therapeutic index of SSRIs, they have become the most commonly prescribed antidepressants and are the first line choice for MDD, anxiety, obsessive-compulsive disorder, and post-traumatic stress disorder.

BPAD is less well understood than MDD in terms of both its pathophysiology and the mechanisms underlying effective therapies. Agents used to treat BPAD include lithium, anticonvulsants, and antipsychotics. Lithium and valproic acid are referred to as mood stabilizers because they limit the extremes of both mania and depression; however, their mechanisms of action are not well understood.

Recent advances in drug development for the treatment of MDD have focused on a deeper understanding of the mechanism of action of current drugs and the physiology of their molecular targets. Currently approved antidepressants are administered as racemic mixtures, and the isolation of active stereoisomers, such as S-citalopram, may yield drugs that are better tolerated. Pharmacogenomic approaches have uncovered polymorphisms in the 5HT reuptake transporter that could affect the likelihood of an individual's response to SSRI treatment. Thus, pharmacogenomics may lead to better matching of drugs to patients by identifying patients who are particularly likely or particularly unlikely to respond to or tolerate a specific drug. Other drug targets beyond the monoamine systems are also promising, including neuropeptide antagonists of substance P and corticotropin-releasing hormone.

Suggested Reading

Arane GW, Hyman SE, Rosenbaum JF. Handbook of Psychiatric Drug Therapy. 4th Ed. Philadelphia:Lippincott Williams & Wilkins, 2000. (*Psychiatric handbook that emphasizes the molecular understanding of psychiatric diseases, including MDD and bipolar disorder, and of the drugs used to treat those diseases.*)

Price LH, Heninger GR. Lithium in the treatment of mood disorders. *N Engl J Med* 1994;331:591–594. (*Review of lithium and its possible mechanisms of action in bipolar disorder.*)

Richelson E. Pharmacology of antidepressants. *Mayo Clin Proc* 2001;76:511–527. (*Broad and thorough overview of the molecular mechanisms and cellular targets of antidepressant medications.*)

Santarelli L, Saxe M, Gross C, et al. Requirement of hippocampal neurogenesis for the behavioral effects of antidepressants. *Science* 2003;301:805–809. (*Research article on MDD.*)

Tkachev D, Mimmack ML, Ryan MM, et al. Oligodendrocyte dysfunction in schizophrenia and bipolar disorder. *Lancet* 2003;362: 798–805. (*Research article on BPAD.*)

| Drug Summary Table | **Chapter 13 Pharmacology of Serotonergic and Central Adrenergic Neurotransmission** | | |

Drug	Clinical Applications	Serious and Common Adverse Effects	Contraindications	Therapeutic Considerations
INHIBITORS OF SEROTONIN STORAGE				
Mechanism—Interfere with the ability of synaptic vesicles to store monoamines; displace 5HT, DA, and NE from their storage vesicles in presynaptic nerve terminals				
Amphetamine Methylphenidate	See Drug Summary Table: Chapter 9 Adrenergic Pharmacology			
Modafinil	Atypical depression Narcolepsy Obstructive sleep apnea	Cardiac arrhythmia, hypertension Dizziness, insomnia, agitation, rhinitis	Hypersensitivity to modafinil	Useful as second-line agent for atypical depression and for depression in the elderly Can induce psychosis in susceptible patients, especially those with bipolar disorder
INHIBITORS OF SEROTONIN DEGRADATION				
Mechanism—Block deamination of monoamines by inhibiting the functional flavin moiety of MAO; increases the 5HT and NE available in the cytoplasm of presynaptic neurons, which leads to increased uptake and storage of 5HT and NE in synaptic vesicles and to some constitutive leakage of monoamines into the synaptic cleft				
Iproniazid Phenelzine Isocarboxazid	Depression	*Systemic tyramine toxicity from consumption of foods that contain tyramine (uncontrolled catecholamine release can induce a hypertensive crisis characterized by headache, tachycardia, nausea, cardiac arrhythmia, and stroke), fever associated with increased muscle tone, leukopenia, hepatic failure, drug-induced lupus, worsening depression* Dizziness, somnolence, orthostatic hypotension, weight gain, increased liver aminotransferase level, orgasm disorder	Concomitant use of sympathomimetic drugs Concomitant bupropion, buspirone, guanethidine, other MAOIs, serotonergic drugs Concomitant methyldopa, L-dopa, L-tryptophan, L-tyrosine, phenylalanine Concomitant CNS depressants, narcotics, dextromethorphan Concomitant, excessive coffee or chocolate intake Concomitant foods with high tyramine content (cheese, beer, wine, pickled herring, yogurt, liver, yeast extract) Liver disease Pheochromocytoma Heart failure General anesthesia, local anesthesia with vasoconstrictors	Due to the extensive effects of MAOIs on P450 enzymes, MAOIs can cause extensive drug-drug interactions; extreme caution must be used when prescribing medications to patients concurrently taking a MAOI Iproniazid, phenelzine, and isocarboxazid are irreversible, nonselective MAOIs The most toxic effect of MAOI use is systemic tyramine toxicity; the older, nonselective MAOIs are no longer considered first-line therapy for depression because of their significant potential for systemic tyramine toxicity MAOIs can precipitate manic or hypomanic episodes in some bipolar patients
Moclobemide Befloxatone Brofaromine	Depression	*Same as iproniazid, except less tyramine toxicity*	Same as iproniazid	Moclobemide, befloxatone, and brofaromine are reversible inhibitors of monoamine oxidase A (RIMAs) These RIMAs are displaced by high concentrations of tyramine, resulting in significantly more tyramine metabolism and thus less tyramine toxicity
Selegiline	Depression	*Same as iproniazid, except less tyramine toxicity*	Same as iproniazid except patients have greater freedom with their diet	Selegiline is a MAO-B inhibitor that also inhibits MAO-A at higher doses Transdermal selegiline reduces the risk of a tyramine-induced hypertensive crisis, allowing patients greater freedom with their diet

TRICYCLIC ANTIDEPRESSANTS (TCAs)

Mechanism—Inhibit reuptake of 5HT and NE from the synaptic cleft by respectively blocking 5HT and NE reuptake transporters, and thereby cause enhancement of postsynaptic responses

| Amitriptyline
Clomipramine
Desipramine
Doxepine
Imipramine
Nortriptyline
Protriptyline
Trimipramine | Depression
Pain syndromes such as migraine headaches, chronic fatigue syndrome, and other somatic pain disorders
Nocturnal enuresis (imipramine)
Obsessive-compulsive disorder (clomipramine) | Heart block, cardiac arrhythmia, orthostatic hypotension, myocardial infarction, agranulocytosis, jaundice, seizure, worsening depression with suicidal thoughts
Bloating, constipation, xerostomia, dizziness, somnolence, blurred vision, urinary retention | Concomitant use of monoamine oxidase inhibitors
Cardiac conduction system defects
Use in patients during acute recovery after a myocardial infarction | TCAs appear to affect cardiac sodium channels in a quinidine-like manner, leading to potentially lethal conduction delays; an ECG should be done to rule out conduction system disease prior to starting TCAs
Concurrent use of other agents that affect the cardiac conduction system requires careful monitoring
In patients taking TCAs, pressor response to IV epinephrine may be markedly enhanced
Orthostatic hypotension is a significant adverse effect for elderly patients
TCAs can precipitate mania in patients with bipolar disorder |

SELECTIVE SEROTONIN REUPTAKE INHIBITORS (SSRIs)

Mechanism—Selectively inhibit reuptake of serotonin and thereby increase synaptic serotonin levels; also cause increased 5HT receptor activation and enhanced postsynaptic responses. At high doses, also bind NE transporter.

| Citalopram
Fluoxetine
Fluvoxamine
Paroxetine
Sertraline | Depression
Anxiety
Obsessive compulsive disorder
Post-traumatic stress disorder
Pain syndromes | Serotonin syndrome from concomitant administration of MAOI (characterized by hyperthermia, muscle rigidity, myoclonus, and rapid fluctuations in mental status and vital signs); may precipitate mania in a bipolar patient
Sexual dysfunction, gastrointestinal distress (sertraline is more often associated with diarrhea, and paroxetine is associated with constipation), vasospasm, sweating, somnolence, anxiety | Concomitant use of monoamine oxidase inhibitors (MAOIs), pimozide, or thioridazine | First-line agents for the treatment of depression, anxiety, and obsessive-compulsive disorder
SSRIs are significantly more selective for 5HT transporters than TCAs, and therefore SSRIs have fewer adverse effects
SSRIs have a larger therapeutic index than the TCAs |

SEROTONIN–NOREPINEPHRINE REUPTAKE INHIBITORS (SNRIs)

Mechanism—Block 5HT reuptake transporter and NE reuptake transporter in a concentration-dependent manner

| Venlafaxine
Duloxetine | Depression
Anxiety
Panic disorder with or without agoraphobia
Pain syndromes (duloxetine) | Neuroleptic malignant syndrome, hepatitis, may exacerbate mania or depression in susceptible patients
Hypertension, sweating, weight loss, gastrointestinal distress, blurred vision, nervousness, sexual dysfunction | Concomitant use of monoamine oxidase inhibitors (MAOIs) | Venlafaxine at low concentrations acts as an SSRI by increasing serotonin levels, but at high concentrations it also increases NE levels
Duloxetine inhibits NE and 5HT reuptake and has been approved for treatment of neuropathic pain and other pain syndromes in addition to treatment of depression |

(Continued)

Drug Summary Table　**Chapter 13 Pharmacology of Serotonergic and Central Adrenergic Neurotransmission** (*Continued*)

Drug	Clinical Applications	Serious and Common Adverse Effects	Contraindications	Therapeutic Considerations
OTHER ATYPICAL ANTIDEPRESSANTS				
Mechanism—Bupropion is an aminoketone antidepressant that weakly inhibits neuronal uptake of 5HT, dopamine, and NE. Mirtazapine blocks 5HT2A, 5HT2C, and the α2-adrenergic autoreceptor, and presumably decreases neurotransmission at 5HT2 synapses while increasing NE neurotransmission. Nefazodone and trazodone block postsynaptic 5HT2 receptors.				
Bupropion	Depression Smoking cessation	*Tachyarrhythmia, hypertension especially when combined with nicotine patch, seizure, may exacerbate mania in susceptible patients (effect less than other antidepressants)* Pruritus, sweating, rash, dyspepsia, constipation, dizziness, tremor, blurred vision, agitation	Seizure Bulimia or anorexia Concomitant MAO inhibitor Concomitant use of other bupropion products Patients undergoing abrupt discontinuation of alcohol or sedatives (including benzodiazepines)	Has the fewest sexual effects among antidepressant agents Induces less mania than the other antidepressants
Mirtazapine	Depression	*Agranulocytosis, seizure, may exacerbate depression or mania in suspectible patients* Somnolence, increased appetite, hyperlipidemia, constipation, dizziness	Concomitant MAO inhibitor	Because mirtazapine is a potent somnorific as well as an appetite stimulant, it is useful in the elderly population in whom insomnia and weight loss are frequent presentations
Nefazodone Trazodone	Depression Insomnia (trazodone)	*Priapism (trazodone), orthostatic hypotension (nefazodone), liver failure (nefazodone), seizure, may worsen depression or mania* Sweating, weight change, dyspepsia, dizziness, somnolence, blurred vision	Coadministration of MAOI, pimozide, triazolam, or carbamazepine (contraindication for nefazodone) Hypersensitivity to nefazodone or trazodone	Trazodone is a prodrug that is converted into meta-chlorophenylpiperazine (mCPP), a selective 5HT2A/2CR agonist used in the treatment of depression and insomnia Trazodone is used principally as a somnorific because the higher doses required for antidepressant effects are usually oversedating
SEROTONIN RECEPTOR AGONISTS				
Mechanism—Buspirone is a 5HT1AR selective agonist and does not bind to GABA receptors; the vasoconstrictive therapeutic effect of triptans is mediated by the 5HT1Rs (both 5HT1DR and 5HT1BR) expressed in the cerebral vasculature				
Buspirone	Anxiety	*Myocardial ischemia or infarction, cerebrovascular accident* Dizziness, confusion, headache, excitement, blurred vision, hostile feeling and behavior, nervousness	Hypersensitivity to buspirone	Buspirone is non-sedating with moderate anxiolytic properties; although not as effective as benzodiazepines, it is attractive because of its non-addictive properties
Sumatriptan Rizatriptan Almotriptan Frovatriptan Eletriptan Zolmitriptan	Migraine headaches	*Coronary artery spasm, hypertensive crisis, myocardial ischemia or infarction, cerebrovascular accident, seizure* Chest pain, flushing, nausea, dizziness	Ergot agent or serotonin 5HT1 agonist within 24 hours Concomitant MAOI therapy Ischemic cardiac, cerebrovascular, or peripheral vascular syndromes Uncontrolled hypertension	Triptans are most useful for acute migraine attacks when taken at the onset of an episode rather than as prophylaxis

SEROTONIN RECEPTOR ANTAGONISTS

Mechanism—Serotonin receptor antagonists show varying degrees of receptor subtype selectivity and often cross-react with adrenergic, histamine, and muscarinic receptors

Drug	Clinical Applications	Adverse Effects	Contraindications	Therapeutic Considerations
Ketanserin	Glaucoma Hypertension	*Orthostatic hypotension, ventricular tachycardia* Flushing, rash, fluid retention, dyspepsia, dizziness, sedation	Hypersensitivity to ketanserin	5HT2A/2CR antagonist Primarily used topically to reduce intraocular pressure in glaucoma
Ondansetron	Nausea	*Cardia arrhythmia, bronchospasm* Increased liver enzymes, constipation, diarrhea, fatigue, headache	Hypersensitivity to ondansetron	5HT3R antagonist A potent anti-emetic that is frequently used as an adjunct to cancer chemotherapy or in cases of refractory nausea
Tegaserod Prucalopride	Irritable bowel syndrome with constipation predominance	*Hypotension, syncope* Diarrhea, dizziness, headache	History of bowel obstruction, abdominal adhesions or symptomatic gallbladder disease Moderate to severe hepatic impairment Severe renal impairment Suspected sphincter of Oddi dysfunction	5HT4R antagonists Enhance GI motility to treat constipation associated with IBS
Alosetron	Irritable bowel syndrome with diarrhea predominance	*Severe constipation, acute ischemic colitis* Abdominal pain, nausea, headache	Pre-existing constipation Concurrent use of fluvoxamine Crohn's disease, ulcerative colitis, diverticulitis Severe hepatic impairment History of hypercoagulable state History of impaired intestinal circulation, intestinal stricture, ischemic colitis, toxic megacolon	5HT3R antagonist Decreases serotonergic tone in intestinal cells, thus reducing intestinal motility Useful for diarrhea associated with IBS

MOOD STABILIZERS

Carbamazepine Valproic acid Lamotrigine	See Drug Summary Table: Chapter 14 Pharmacology of Abnormal Electrical Neurotransmission in the Central Nervous System

LITHIUM

Mechanism—Lithium can mimic other small monovalent cations and disrupt proteins and transporters that require cation cofactors. Lithium enters cells via Na$^+$ channels. Lithium inhibits both the inositol phosphatase that dephosphorylates IP2 to inositol phosphate (IP1), and the inositol phophatase that dephosphorylates IP1 to free inositol, thereby blocking the phosphatidylinositol signaling cascade in the brain. By blocking the regeneration of PIP2, lithium inhibits central adrenergic, muscarinic, and serotonergic neurotransmission. Other mechanisms of action include increasing 5HT neurotransmission, decreasing NE and DA neurotransmission, inhibiting adenylyl cyclase by decoupling G proteins from neurotransmitter receptors, and altering electrochemical gradients across cell membranes by substituting for Na$^+$ and/or blocking K$^+$ channels.

Drug	Clinical Applications	Adverse Effects	Contraindications	Therapeutic Considerations
Lithium	Bipolar affective disorder	*Acute lithium intoxication (characterized by nausea, vomiting, diarrhea, renal failure, neuromuscular dysfunction, ataxia, tremor, confusion, delirium, and seizures), severe bradyarrhythmia, hypotension, sinus node dysfunction, hyperkalemia, pseudotumor cerebri, increased intracranial pressure and papilledema, seizure, polyuria* Nephrogenic diabetes insipidus, hypothyroidism, goiter, ECG and EEG abnormalities, diarrhea, nausea, muscle weakness, transient visual field scotoma, renal impairment, acne	Severe debilitation, dehydration, or sodium depletion Significant cardiovascular disease Significant renal impairment Lactation	Lithium has a narrow therapeutic window and a wide range of adverse effects Acute lithium intoxication is a medical emergency and may require dialysis for treatment Non-steroidal anti-inflammatory drugs (NSAIDs) or hyponatremia can lead to increased lithium reabsorption in the proximal tubules and elevation of plasma lithium concentrations Lithium's inhibition of potassium entry into myocytes leads to abnormalities in myocyte repolarization, extracellular hyperkalemia, and intracellular hypokalemia Lithium has been shown to reduce the risk of suicide in patients with bipolar disorder

14

Pharmacology of Abnormal Electrical Neurotransmission in the Central Nervous System

Edmund A. Griffin, Jr., and Daniel H. Lowenstein

INTRODUCTION

With over 10 billion neurons and an estimated 10^{14} synaptic connections, the human brain boasts unparalleled electrical complexity. Unlike myocardial tissue, where electrical signals spread synchronously through a syncytium of cells, proper functioning of the brain requires distinct isolation of electrical signals, and thus demands a far higher level of regulation. Control of this complex function begins at the level of the ion channel and is further maintained through the effects of these ion channels on the activity of highly organized neuronal networks. Abnormal function of ion channels and neural networks can result in rapid, synchronous, and uncontrolled spread of electrical activity, which is the basis of a **seizure**.

The seizure disorders belong to a heterogeneous group comprising a variety of clinical presentations and many different causes. They represent clinical manifestations of abnormal electrical activity in the brain and should be distinguished from **epilepsy,** which refers to the condition where an individual has a tendency toward recurrent seizures (i.e., a patient who has had a single seizure does not necessarily have

epilepsy). Depending on the location of seizure activity in the central nervous system (CNS), a patient may experience a variety of symptoms. These symptoms include the relatively common, prominent motor symptoms and loss of consciousness seen in tonic–clonic seizures, as well as paroxysmal changes observed in a variety of nonmotor functions—such as sensation, olfaction, vision—and higher-order functions—such as emotion, memory, language, and insight.

This chapter explores the molecular mechanisms by which the brain maintains precise control over the spread of electrical activity and how various abnormalities can undermine these physiologic mechanisms and lead to seizures. The various classes of antiepileptic drugs are then discussed, with an emphasis on molecular mechanisms for restoring inhibitory function in the brain and suppressing seizure activity.

 Case

Jon arrives in the emergency department with his brother Rob at 9:12 PM. Because his brother is still too lethargic to speak, Jon relays most of the story to the attending physician. The two had been watching television when Jon noticed that his 40-year-old brother seemed to be daydreaming. Never missing an opportunity to tease, Jon began chiding his brother for "spacing out." But instead of the boisterous laugh that he was so used to, Jon observed only a confused, almost fearful stare.

Jon recalls that his brother's right hand suddenly began to bend into an awkward position and then to shake. The shaking grew worse, progressing gradually from the hand to the arm and then to the entire right side of the body. Jon then noticed that Rob's body stiffened, almost as if he were attempting to contract every muscle in his body. This sustained contraction lasted for about 15 seconds, and was followed by shaking movements of all four limbs that lasted another 30 seconds or so. The frequency of the shaking slowed after several minutes, and Rob then became limp, began breathing very heavily, and remained unresponsive. Rob regained consciousness on the way to the emergency department.

At the hospital, a magnetic resonance imaging (MRI) scan shows a small neoplasm in Rob's left temporal lobe. Because the neoplasm appears to be benign, Rob, following the advice of his physician, decides not to undergo surgery. The potential benefits and risks of various anticonvulsant drugs are discussed, including phenytoin, carbamazepine, valproic acid, and lamotrigine, and it is decided to start Rob on a regimen of carbamazepine to prevent further seizures.

QUESTIONS

■ **1.** What is the significance of the order of spread of the seizure from the hands to the arm and then to the leg?

■ **2.** The generalized seizure that followed the right-sided shaking included a tonic phase (stiffening) followed by a clonic phase (shaking). What occurs at the molecular level to cause these symptoms?

■ **3.** By what mechanisms can a focal neoplasm result in a seizure?

■ **4.** Is there any clinical significance to the fearful, blank stare?

■ **5.** How do drugs such as phenytoin, carbamazepine, valproic acid, and lamotrigine prevent seizures? Why was carbamazepine chosen for Rob?

PHYSIOLOGY

The normal human brain, in the absence of any lesions or genetic abnormalities, is capable of undergoing a seizure. Acute changes in the availability of excitatory neurotransmitters (e.g., caused by ingestion of the toxin **domoate,** which is a structural analogue of glutamate) or changes in the effect of inhibitory neurotransmitters (e.g., caused by injection of **penicillin,** a $GABA_A$ antagonist) can result in massive seizure activity in the otherwise healthy human brain. These examples demonstrate that the complex circuits within the brain exist in a balance between excitatory and

inhibitory factors, and that changes in either of these control mechanisms can lead to major dysfunction.

In the CNS, two important elements normally involved in the fine-tuning of neuronal signaling also function to prevent the repetitive and synchronous firing characteristic of a seizure. At the cellular level, a ''refractory period'' induced by Na^+ channel inactivation and K^+ channel-mediated hyperpolarization prevents abnormal repetitive firing in neuronal cells. As discussed in Chapter 6, Principles of Cellular Excitability and Electrochemical Transmission, action potentials are propagated by voltage-sensitive ion channels. After initiation in the axon hillock, the action potential is propagated by alternating currents of depolarizing Na^+ influx and hyperpolarizing K^+ efflux. Throughout the course of an action potential (Fig. 14-1), the Na^+ channels exist in three distinct states: (1) a **closed state** before activation, (2) an **open state** during depolarization, and (3) an **inactivated state** shortly after the peak of depolarization. Because Na^+ channels adopt the inactivated state in response to depolarization, action potentials are intrinsically self-limiting—Na^+ channels will not recover from the inactivated state until the membrane is sufficiently repolarized. K^+ channel opening repolarizes the cell, but the high K^+ efflux transiently hyperpolarizes the membrane beyond its resting potential, further

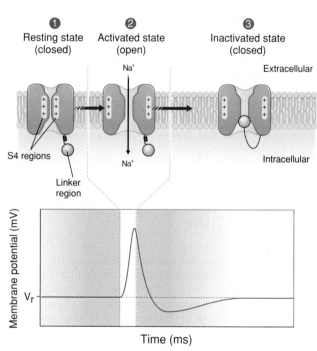

Figure 14-1. Duration and frequency of the action potential is limited by properties intrinsic to the sodium channel. The voltage-sensitive Na^+ channel exists in three different conformations during the course of an action potential. After opening transiently in response to membrane depolarization *(2)*, the Na^+ channel spontaneously inactivates *(3)*. This closure of the channel decreases the strength of the Na^+-mediated depolarization. Na^+ channels recover from inactivation only when the membrane potential is restored to its resting level (V_r). Membrane depolarization also has the effect of opening voltage-sensitive K^+ channels, which hyperpolarize the cell. Under hyperpolarizing conditions, the Na^+ channel adopts its resting (closed) conformation *(1)*. During these refractory periods of Na^+ channel inactivation and membrane hyperpolarization, the neuron is essentially insensitive to depolarizing signals (see also Fig. 10-7).

increasing the time before a new action potential can be generated. Thus, *the biochemical properties of Na^+ and K^+ channels, under physiologic conditions, impose a limit on the frequency of firing, helping prevent the repetitive firing characteristic of many seizure types.*

Beyond the single-cell level, **neural networks** ensure the specificity of neuronal signaling by restricting the effects of a given action potential to a defined area. Even a strong train of action potentials, if contained within about 1,000 neurons, will not generate seizure activity. This is quite a remarkable feat, given the close proximity of neurons in the CNS and the fact that a single neuron in the neocortex may have more than 1,000 postsynaptic connections. As seen in the simplified neural network in Figure 14-2, the firing neuron activates immediately neighboring neurons in addition to interneurons that transmit inhibitory **(GABA)** signals to surrounding neurons. This contrast of local amplification and surrounding cell inhibition results in what is referred to as **surround inhibition.** Surround inhibition is essential to the normal function of the nervous system, because this phenomenon not only amplifies local signals but also provides insulation and protection against synchronicity in surrounding areas. Many seizure disorders appear to result from disruption of this intricate balance.

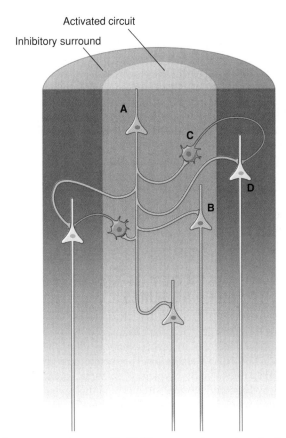

Figure 14-2. Surround inhibition prevents synchronization of adjacent neurons. In this simplified neuronal circuit, neuron *A* sends excitatory projections *(blue)* to proximal neurons such as *B.* In addition to activating nearby neurons, cell *A* also activates GABAergic interneurons *(C)* that send inhibitory projections *(gray)* to surrounding neurons *(D).* This type of circuit creates an "inhibitory surround" *(dark gray),* so that action potentials generated by neuron *A,* even if rapid and robust, are unable to activate surrounding circuits.

PATHOPHYSIOLOGY

Because the pathophysiologic mechanisms underlying seizure disorders are only beginning to be determined, seizures are still classified according to their clinical manifestations rather than their biologic underpinnings. Seizures that begin focally **(partial seizures)** are clinically distinct from seizures that begin generally and involve both hemispheres **(generalized seizures)** (Table 14-1). All seizures, however, share the common characteristic of abnormal synchronous discharge. For this to occur, protective mechanisms must be compromised at the cellular and network levels. The direct causes of these changes can be primary (e.g., genetic abnormalities such as channel defects), secondary (e.g., changes in the neuronal environment induced by toxins or acquired lesions such as strokes or neoplasms), or a combination of the two (e.g., febrile seizures in children). The following examples illustrate the mechanistic links between these initiating factors and subsequent seizure activity.

PATHOPHYSIOLOGY OF PARTIAL SEIZURES

The partial seizure (Fig. 14-3A) occurs in three specific steps: (1) initiation at the cellular level by an increase in electrical activity, (2) synchronization of surrounding neurons, and (3) spread to adjacent regions of the brain. Seizures are initiated by a sudden depolarization within a group of neurons. This sudden change, called a **paroxysmal depolarizing shift (PDS),** lasts up to 200 ms and results in the generation of an abnormally rapid train of action potentials. Changes in the extracellular milieu, attributable, for instance, to a space-occupying lesion (such as in the introductory case), can have major effects on neuronal burst activity. For example, an increase in extracellular K^+ would blunt the effects of K^+-mediated after-hyperpolarization by decreasing the magnitude of the K^+ gradient between the outside and inside of the cell. Similarly, an increase in excitatory neurotransmitters or modulation of excitatory receptors by other exogenous molecules could increase burst activity. Increased burst activity could also result from properties intrinsic to the cell, such as abnormal channel conductance or altered membrane characteristics.

Because of surround inhibition, local discharges are often contained within a so-called **focus,** and do not induce symptomatic pathology. These local discharges can be seen on an **electroencephalogram (EEG)** as sharp **interictal** spikes. Identification of these spikes can be useful in locating the seizure focus in a patient who is not actively undergoing a seizure. There are several pathways, however, whereby the seizure focus can override surround inhibition. Repetitive firing of neurons increases extracellular K^+. As described above, this weakens K^+-mediated hyperpolarization, allowing the seizure activity to spread. Rapidly firing neurons also open depolarization-sensitive NMDA channels (see Chapter 11, Pharmacology of GABAergic and Glutamatergic Neurotransmission) and accumulate Ca^{2+} in their synaptic terminals, both of which increase the likelihood of signal propagation and local synchronization. In many cases, however, it

| TABLE 14-1 | Classification of Epileptic Seizures |

TYPE OF SEIZURE	SYMPTOMS/KEY FEATURES
Partial Seizures	
Simple partial seizure	Symptoms vary depending on location of abnormal activity in the brain: involuntary, repetitive movement (motor cortex), paresthesias (sensory cortex), flashing lights (visual cortex), etc.
	Consciousness is preserved
	Spread to ipsilateral regions within cortex (e.g., ''Jacksonian march'')
Complex partial seizure (also known as *temporal lobe epilepsy*)	Symptoms typically result from abnormal activity in the temporal lobe (amygdala, hippocampus) or frontal lobe
	Altered consciousness (cessation of activity, loss of contact with reality)
	Often associated with involuntary ''automatisms'' ranging from simple repetitive movements (lip smacking, hand wringing) to highly skilled activity (driving, playing musical instrument)
	Impaired memory of ictal phase
	Classically preceded by an aura
Partial seizure with secondary generalization	Initially manifests with symptoms of simple or complex partial seizure
	Evolves into a tonic–clonic seizure with sustained contraction (tonic) followed by rhythmic movements (clonic) of all limbs
	Loss of consciousness
	Preceded by aura
Primary Generalized Seizures	
Absence seizure (petit mal)	Sudden, brief interruption of consciousness
	Blank stare
	Occasional motor symptoms such as lip smacking, rapid blinking
	Not preceded by an aura
Myoclonic seizure	Brief (1 second or less) muscle contraction; symptoms may occur in individual muscle or generalize to all muscle groups of the body (the latter can result in falling)
	Associated with systemic disease states such as uremia, hepatic failure, hereditary degenerative conditions, Creutzfeldt–Jakob disease
Tonic–clonic (grand mal) seizure	Symptoms as described above, but onset is abrupt and not preceded by symptoms of partial or complex seizure

appears that the most important compromise of surround inhibition occurs at the level of GABAergic transmission. *Decreases in GABA-mediated inhibition—because of exogenous factors, degeneration of GABAergic neurons, or changes at the receptor level—are major factors that aid in the synchronization of a seizure focus.*

If the synchronizing focus is sufficiently strong, the abnormal, synchronized firing from a small neural network will begin to spread to neighboring regions of the cortex. During this spread to neighboring areas, the patient may experience an **aura**, a conscious ''warning'' of the spread of the seizure. In the introductory case, Rob's aura manifested as a blank, fearful stare. Although the aura is usually stereotypical for a given patient, a wide variety of auras exist. These include a sense of fear and confusion, disturbances of memory (e.g., déjà vu) or language, altered sensations, or an olfactory hallucination. As the seizure continues to spread, it can lead to additional clinical manifestations; the specific manifestation depends on the brain regions that become involved. In the introductory case, the clinical symptoms initially started with shaking of the hands and progressed to the arm and then to the leg. This is a **Jacksonian march** (named after the English neurologist Hughlings Jackson,

who first described the symptoms), where the clinical symptoms result from spread of synchronous activity across the motor homunculus.

PATHOPHYSIOLOGY OF SECONDARY GENERALIZED SEIZURES

Partial seizures may become generalized by spreading along diffuse connections to involve both cerebral hemispheres. This is known as a **secondary (or secondarily) generalized seizure** (Fig. 14-3B). Typically, seizures spread to distant sites by following normal circuits, and this spread can occur through several pathways. **U fibers** connect various regions of the cortex; the **corpus callosum** allows for spread between hemispheres; and **thalamocortical projections** provide a pathway for diffuse synchronized spread throughout the brain. Once seizure activity spreads to involve both hemispheres, a patient usually loses consciousness.

Among the secondarily generalized seizures, the **tonic–clonic** subtype is the most common. In the introductory clinical case, Rob underwent a period where he appeared to be contracting every muscle in his body, followed

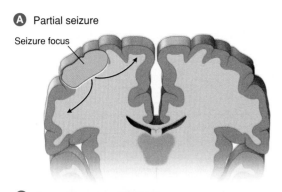

A Partial seizure

Seizure focus

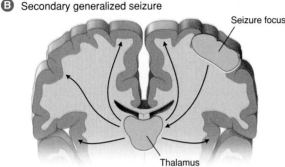

B Secondary generalized seizure

Seizure focus

Thalamus

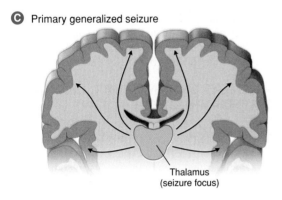

C Primary generalized seizure

Thalamus
(seizure focus)

Figure 14-3. Pathways of seizure propagation. A. In a partial seizure, paroxysmal activity begins in a seizure focus *(blue)* and spreads to adjacent areas via diffuse neuronal connections. When activity is confined to one region of the cortex that serves a basic function, such as motor movement or sensation, and there is no change in the patient's mental status, the seizure is referred to as a *simple partial seizure.* Seizures that involve brain regions serving more complex functions such as language, memory, and emotions are referred to as *complex partial seizures.* **B.** In a secondary generalized seizure, paroxysmal activity begins in a focus but then spreads to subcortical areas. Diffuse connections from the thalamus then synchronize the spread of activity to both hemispheres. **C.** Primary generalized seizures, such as the absence seizure, result from abnormal synchronization between thalamic and cortical cells (see Fig. 14-5B).

by an episode of uncontrolled shaking of all four limbs. These clinical symptoms can be understood at the level of abnormal channel activity (Fig. 14-4). The initial phase of the tonic–clonic seizure is associated with a sudden loss of GABA input, which leads to a long train of firing lasting for several seconds. This sustained, rapid firing manifests clinically as contraction of both agonist and antagonist muscles, and is referred to as the **tonic** phase. Eventually, as

GABA-mediated inhibition begins to be restored, AMPA-mediated and NMDA-mediated excitation starts to oscillate with the inhibitory component. This oscillatory pattern (when involving the motor cortex) results in **clonic** or shaking movements of the body. With time, the GABA-mediated inhibition prevails, and the patient becomes flaccid and remains unconscious during the **postictal** period until normal brain function returns.

PATHOPHYSIOLOGY OF PRIMARY GENERALIZED SEIZURES

Primary generalized seizures differ from partial seizures in both pathophysiology and etiology (Fig. 14-3C). In contrast to the partial seizure, where synchronicity begins with sudden trains of action potentials within an aggregate of neurons and subsequently spreads to adjacent regions, the primary generalized seizure emanates from central brain regions and then spreads rapidly to both hemispheres. These seizures do not necessarily begin with an aura (which is an important method of clinically distinguishing primary generalized seizures from partial seizures that secondarily generalize).

Currently, the best understood of the primary generalized seizures is the **absence seizure** (also known as the **petit mal seizure**). Absence seizures are characterized by sudden interruptions in consciousness that are often accompanied by a blank stare and occasional motor symptoms, such as rapid blinking and lip smacking. Absence seizures are thought to result from abnormal synchronization of thalamo-cortical and cortical cells. The underlying pathophysiology of absence seizures is based on the observation that patients experiencing absence seizures have EEG readings somewhat similar to the patterns generated during **slow-wave (stage 3) sleep.**

Relay neurons connecting the thalamus to the cortex exist in two different states depending on the level of wakefulness (Fig. 14-5A). During the awake state, these neurons function in **transmission mode,** whereby incoming sensory signals are faithfully transmitted to the cortex. During sleep, however, the transient, bursting activity of a unique, dendritic **T-type calcium channel** alters incoming signals so that output signals to the cortex have an oscillatory firing rate, which, on an EEG, has a characteristic ''spike and wave'' readout. In this slow-wave sleep state, sensory information is not transmitted to the cortex.

For reasons not yet understood, absence seizures are associated with activation of the T-type calcium channel during the awake state (Fig. 14-5B). Because this channel is active only when the cell is hyperpolarized, several factors can activate the channel during the awake state. These factors include an increase in intracellular K^+, an increase in GABAergic input from the reticular nucleus, or a loss of excitatory input. A variety of studies have shown that the activity of the T-type calcium channel in the relay neurons is essential to the 3-per-second spike-and-wave activity observed in absence seizures. Because of its important pathophysiologic role, the T-type calcium channel is a primary target in the pharmacologic treatment of absence seizures.

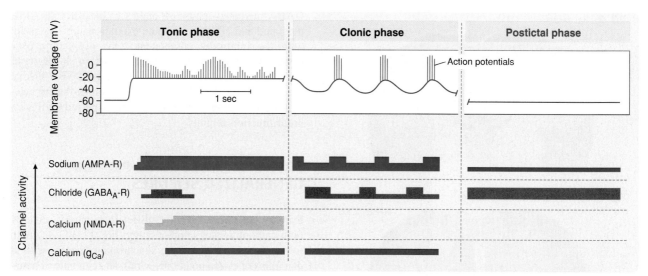

Figure 14-4. Abnormal channel activity in the tonic–clonic seizure. The tonic phase of the tonic–clonic seizure is initiated by a sudden loss of GABA-mediated surround inhibition. Loss of inhibition results in a rapid train of action potentials, which manifests clinically as tonic contraction of the muscles. As GABAergic innervation is restored, it begins to oscillate rhythmically with the excitatory component. The oscillation of excitatory and inhibitory components manifests clinically as clonic movements. The postictal phase is characterized by enhanced GABA-mediated inhibition.

PHARMACOLOGIC CLASSES AND AGENTS

The current approach to treating a patient with epilepsy depends in part on the type of seizure(s) experienced by the patient. Patients with partial seizures, with or without secondary generalization, are typically treated pharmacologically with antiepileptic drugs. In such patients, there is also an attempt to determine whether the seizures are caused by an identifiable focal lesion that can be removed surgically or ablated by other means. Antiepileptic drugs (AEDs) remain the mainstay of treatment for patients with generalized seizures as well.

Mechanistically, the efficacy of AEDs centers on manipulation of ion channel activity. As discussed above, physiologic protection against repetitive firing occurs via inhibition at two levels: the cellular level (e.g., Na$^+$ channel inactivation), and the network level (e.g., GABA-mediated inhibition). Accordingly, currently available AEDs fall into four main categories: (1) drugs that enhance Na$^+$ channel-mediated inhibition, (2) drugs that inhibit calcium channels, (3) drugs that enhance GABA-mediated inhibition, and (4) drugs that inhibit glutamate receptors.

Although AEDs fall into several different mechanistic classes, it is important to keep in mind that *the therapeutic efficacy of many of the AEDs is only partially explained by the known mechanisms described below, primarily because the AEDs act pleiotropically.* Valproic acid, for example, stabilizes Na$^+$ channels, but the drug also has an effect on T-type calcium channels and may have effects on GABA metabolism as well. Thus, although in vitro studies may suggest that a drug is best suited for the treatment of one particular type of seizure, other seizure types may also respond to the drug. (One benefit of this pleiotropy is that many of the drugs are interchangeable to the extent that minimization of adverse effects is often the main clinical criterion underlying

the choice of AED.) The classification below is shown only for simplicity and is based on the primary target of the drug. A list of the main drugs discussed here and their multiple mechanisms of action is provided in Table 14-2.

DRUGS THAT ENHANCE NA$^+$ CHANNEL-MEDIATED INHIBITION

Each neuron in the brain is equipped with the machinery to prevent rapid, repetitive firing. As discussed above, depolarization of the neuronal membrane results in sodium channel inactivation. This inactivation of the Na$^+$ channel provides a key checkpoint in the prevention of repetitive firing within a potential seizure focus. Although changes in the extracellular milieu, such as altered ion concentration, can override this checkpoint, the AEDs **phenytoin, carbamazepine, lamotrigine,** and **valproic acid** enhance inhibition at the single-cell level by acting directly on the Na$^+$ channel (Fig. 14-6A).

In general, *antiepileptic drugs that act on Na$^+$ channels show strong specificity for the treatment of partial and secondary generalized seizures.* This is consistent with their molecular profile. The Na$^+$ channel blockers act in a use-dependent manner, much like the action of lidocaine on peripheral nerves (see Chapter 10, Local Anesthetic Pharmacology). Thus, neurons that fire rapidly are particularly susceptible to inhibition by this class of drug. Conversely, many Na$^+$ channel blockers (particularly those that act only at the Na$^+$ channel, such as phenytoin) have little effect on absence seizures. Presumably, the rate of cyclical Na$^+$ channel opening and closing within the thalamocortical cells that are activated during absence seizures is too slow to be amenable to inhibition through use-dependent Na$^+$ channel inactivation.

Phenytoin

Phenytoin acts directly on the Na$^+$ channel to slow the rate of channel recovery from the inactivated state to the closed

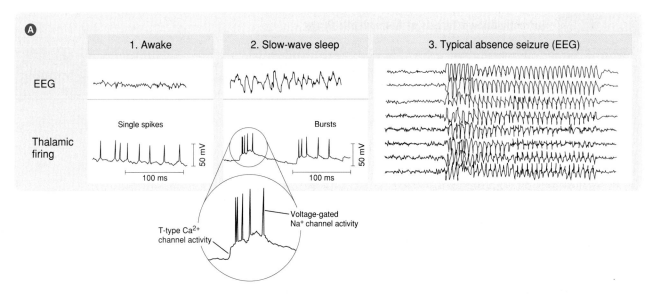

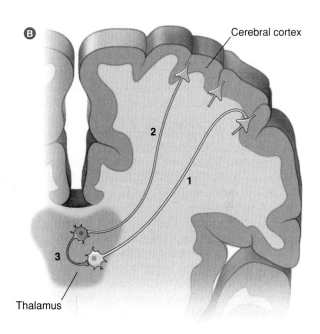

Figure 14-5. Mechanism of absence seizure. A. EEG recordings of patients experiencing absence seizures are similar to "sleep spindle" patterns generated during slow-wave sleep. The 3-per-second oscillatory pattern is generated by the burst activity of a dendritic T-type calcium channel in the thalamus. **1.** During the awake state, relay neurons of the thalamus are in "transmission mode," in which incoming signals are faithfully transmitted to the cortex as single spikes. These signals to the cortex register on the EEG as small, desynchronized, low voltage waves. **2.** During slow-wave sleep, signals relayed through the thalamus are altered because of the bursting activity of a dendritic T-type calcium channel (see below). During this stage, called "burst mode," sensory information is not transmitted to the cortex. **3.** Absence seizures result from abnormal activation of the T-type calcium channel during the awake state, resulting in a similar spike-and-wave EEG pattern. **B.** The absence seizure is generated by a self-sustaining cycle of activity between the thalamus and the cortex. Synchronicity is initiated by hyperpolarization of the thalamic relay neurons *(light gray)*. This occurs normally during slow-wave sleep and is caused by GABAergic input from the reticular thalamic nucleus *(dark gray)*. The factors that cause hyperpolarization in relay neurons during an absence seizure are poorly understood. **1.** Hyperpolarization of relay neurons induces burst activity of the T-type calcium channel, resulting in synchronous depolarization in the cortex via excitatory connections. This large depolarization in the cortex registers as a spike-and-wave pattern on the EEG. **2.** Excitatory input from the cortex activates the reticular thalamic neurons. **3.** The activated GABAergic reticular neurons hyperpolarize the thalamic relay neurons and reinitiate the cycle.

state. As described above, the Na$^+$ channel exists in three conformations—closed, open, and inactivated—and the probability of a channel existing in each state depends on the membrane potential (Fig. 14-1; see also Fig. 10-7). By slowing the rate of recovery from the inactivated state to the closed state, phenytoin increases the threshold for action potentials and prevents repetitive firing. This has the effect of stabilizing the seizure focus by preventing the paroxysmal depolarizing shift (PDS) that initiates the partial seizure. In addition, phenytoin prevents the rapid spread of seizure activity to other neurons, accounting for its efficacy in secondarily generalized seizures.

Importantly, phenytoin targets Na$^+$ channels in a use-dependent manner (see Fig. 10-8). Thus, only channels that are opened and closed at high frequency (i.e., those involved in the PDS) are likely to be inhibited. This use-dependency

lessens the effects of phenytoin on spontaneous neuronal activity and avoids many of the adverse effects observed with GABA$_A$ potentiators (which are not use-dependent).

Because of its use-dependent blockade, as well as its ability to prevent sudden rapid firing, phenytoin is a major drug of choice for partial seizures and tonic–clonic seizures. It is not used in absence seizures. The pharmacokinetics and drug interactions of phenytoin are complex and play a decisive role in the choice between phenytoin and similarly acting drugs such as carbamazepine.

Phenytoin is more than 95% bound to plasma albumin. Phenytoin is inactivated by metabolism in the liver and, at typical doses, has a plasma half-life of about 24 hours. Phenytoin metabolism shows properties of saturation kinetics, whereby small increases in dose can cause large and often unpredictable increases in plasma drug concentration (see

TABLE 14-2   Currently Known Targets of Antiepileptic Drugs

DRUG	SODIUM CHANNELS	T-TYPE CALCIUM CHANNELS	HIGH-VOLTAGE-ACTIVATED CALCIUM CHANNELS	GABA SYSTEM	GLUTAMATE RECEPTORS
Main effects on ion channels					
Phenytoin	✓				
Carbamazepine	✓				
Lamotrigine	✓		✓		
Zonisamide	✓	✓			
Ethosuximide		✓			
Main effects on GABA mechanisms					
Benzodiazepines				✓	
Tiagabine				✓	
Mixed actions					
Valproic acid	✓	✓		✓	
Gabapentin			✓	✓	
Levetiracetam			✓	✓	
Topiramate	✓		✓	✓	✓
Felbamate	✓		✓	✓	✓
Phenobarbital			✓	✓	✓

Chapter 3, Pharmacokinetics). These increases in plasma phenytoin concentration increase the risk of adverse effects, including ataxia, nystagmus, incoordination, confusion, gingival hyperplasia, megaloblastic anemia, hirsutism, facial coarsening, and a systemic skin rash.

Phenytoin inactivation by the hepatic microsomal P450 enzyme system is susceptible to alteration by several drugs. Drugs that inhibit the P450 system, such as chloramphenicol, cimetidine, disulfiram, and isoniazid, increase phenytoin plasma concentration. Carbamazepine, an antiepileptic drug (see below) that induces the liver P450 system, increases the metabolism of phenytoin, thereby lowering phenytoin plasma concentrations when these drugs are used concurrently. Similarly, phenytoin, because of its ability to induce the hepatic P450 system, increases the metabolism of drugs that are inactivated by this system. Some of these drugs include oral contraceptives, quinidine, doxycycline, cyclosporine, methadone, and levodopa.

Carbamazepine

Although structurally unrelated to phenytoin, carbamazepine appears to exert its antiseizure activity in a manner similar to phenytoin. That is, carbamazepine is a Na^+ channel blocker that slows the rate of recovery of Na^+ channels from the inactivated state to the closed state. This has the effect of suppressing a seizure focus (by preventing the PDS) as well as preventing rapid spread of activity from the seizure focus. A metabolite of carbamazepine, 10,11-epoxycarbamazepine, also acts to slow Na^+ channel recovery, and may be responsible for some of the therapeutic effects of the drug.

Carbamazepine is often the drug of choice for partial seizures (simple and complex) because of its dual action in the suppression of seizure foci and the prevention of spread of activity. The half-life of carbamazepine is initially between 10 and 20 hours and is further reduced with chronic treatment (because of P450 induction), requiring patients to take several doses daily. Metabolism of carbamazepine is linear (i.e., it exhibits first-order kinetics); this property makes carbamazepine a more attractive choice than phenytoin for patients with potential drug interactions.

Lamotrigine

As with phenytoin and carbamazepine, lamotrigine stabilizes the neuronal membrane by slowing Na^+ channel recovery from the inactivated state. Lamotrigine may also have other, undetermined, mechanisms of action; this hypothesis is based on the clinical observation that lamotrigine has wider clinical applications than the other Na^+ channel blockers.

Lamotrigine is a useful alternative to phenytoin and carbamazepine as a treatment for partial and tonic–clonic seizures. Surprisingly, and for reasons not correlated with its defined mechanism, lamotrigine has been shown to be effective in the treatment of atypical absence seizures. It is the third drug of choice for treatment of absence seizures, after ethosuximide and valproic acid (see below).

DRUGS THAT INHIBIT CALCIUM CHANNELS

Drugs used to treat epilepsy through inhibition of calcium channels fall into two main classes: those that inhibit the T-type calcium channel and those that inhibit the high-voltage-activated (HVA) calcium channel.

The T-type calcium channel is depolarized and inactive during the awake state (Fig. 14-5B). In absence (petit mal) seizures, paroxysmal hyperpolarization is thought to activate the channel during the awake state, initiating the spike and

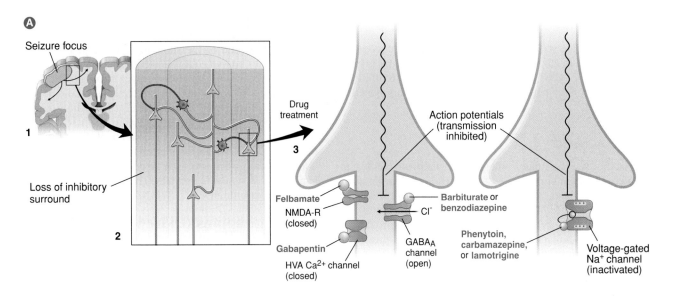

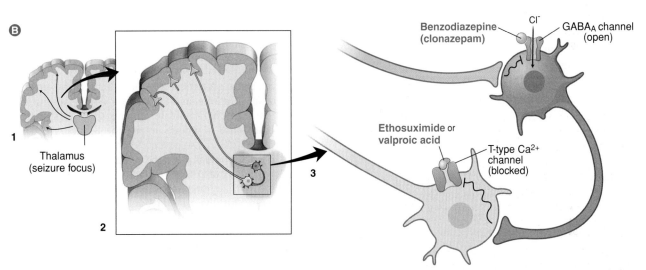

Figure 14-6. Mechanisms of pharmacotherapy for seizures. A. The partial seizure *(1)* results from rapid, uncontrolled neuronal firing and a loss of surround inhibition *(2)*. Antiepileptic drugs act at four molecular targets to enhance inhibition and prevent spread of synchronous activity *(3)*. Barbiturates and benzodiazepines prevent seizure spread by acting on the GABA$_A$ receptor to potentiate GABA-mediated inhibition. Na$^+$ channel inhibitors such as phenytoin, carbamazepine, and lamotrigine prevent rapid neuronal firing by selectively prolonging Na$^+$ channel inactivation in rapidly firing neurons (see Figs. 10-7, 10-8). Felbamate suppresses seizure activity by inhibiting the NMDA receptor and thereby decreasing glutamate-mediated excitation. Gabapentin decreases release of excitatory neurotransmitter by inhibiting the high-voltage-activated (HVA) calcium channel. **B.** The absence seizure *(1)* is caused by a self-sustaining cycle of activity generated between thalamic and cortical cells *(2)*. Antiepileptic drugs prevent this synchronous thalamocortical cycle *(3)* by acting at two molecular targets. Clonazepam, a benzodiazepine, potentiates GABA$_A$ channels in the reticular thalamic nucleus, thus decreasing the activation of the inhibitory reticular neurons and decreasing the hyperpolarization of the thalamic relay neurons. T-type calcium channel inhibitors such as ethosuximide and valproic acid prevent the burst activity of thalamic relay neurons that is required for synchronous activation of cortical cells.

wave discharges characteristic of this seizure type. Thus, *drugs inhibiting the T-type calcium channel are specifically used to treat absence seizures.*

HVA calcium channels play an important role in controlling the entry of calcium into the presynaptic terminal and therefore help to regulate neurotransmitter release. The HVA calcium channel is formed by an α1 protein that assembles into the channel pore, and it has several auxiliary subunits. Drugs that inhibit HVA calcium channels tend to have pleiotropic effects; although they are used primarily for partial seizures with or without secondary generalization, they can

also be used for generalized seizures other than absence seizures.

Ethosuximide

In vitro, **ethosuximide** has a highly specific molecular profile. In experiments on thalamocortical preparations from rats and hamsters, ethosuximide has been shown to reduce low-threshold T-type currents in a voltage-dependent manner. This inhibition occurs without altering the voltage dependence or recovery kinetics of the Na$^+$ channel. Ethosuximide does not have any effect on GABA-mediated inhibition.

Ethosuximide is often the first line therapy for uncomplicated absence seizures. Consistent with its molecular profile as a specific T-type Ca^{2+} channel blocker, ethosuximide is not effective in the treatment of partial or secondary generalized seizures.

Valproic Acid

As is the case for many other AEDs, **valproic acid** acts pleiotropically in vitro. Similar to phenytoin and carbamazepine, valproic acid slows the rate of Na^+ channel recovery from the inactivated state. At slightly higher concentrations than those necessary to limit repetitive firing, valproic acid has also been shown to limit the activity of the low-threshold T-type calcium channel.

Another proposed mechanism of valproic acid action occurs at the level of GABA metabolism. In vitro, valproic acid increases the activity of glutamic acid decarboxylase, the enzyme responsible for GABA synthesis, while it inhibits the activity of enzymes that degrade GABA. Taken together, these effects are thought to increase the availability of GABA in the synapse and thereby to increase GABA-mediated inhibition.

Perhaps because of its many potential sites of action, valproic acid is one of the most effective antiepileptic drugs for the treatment of patients with generalized epilepsy syndromes having mixed seizure types. Valproic acid is also the drug of choice for patients with idiopathic generalized seizures and is used for the treatment of absence seizures that do not respond to ethosuximide. Valproic acid is also commonly used as an alternative to phenytoin and carbamazepine for the treatment of partial seizures.

Gabapentin

Gabapentin was one of the first AEDs developed using the concept of "rational drug design." That is, with the recognition that GABA receptors play an important role in the control of seizure spread, gabapentin was synthesized as a structural analogue of GABA and was predicted to enhance GABA-mediated inhibition. Consistent with this hypothesis, gabapentin has been shown to increase the content of GABA in neurons and in glial cells in vitro. However, the main anti-seizure effect of gabapentin appears to be through its inhibition of HVA calcium channels, which results in decreased neurotransmitter release. A main advantage of gabapentin is that, because its structure is similar to that of endogenous amino acids, it has few interactions with other drugs. On the other hand, gabapentin does not appear to be a particularly effective antiepileptic drug for most patients.

DRUGS THAT ENHANCE GABA-MEDIATED INHIBITION

In contrast to Na^+ channel blockers and calcium channel inhibitors, whose mechanistic properties correlate well with their clinical activity, the enhancers of GABA-mediated inhibition have more varied effects and tend not to be as interchangeable. This is largely because of the diversity of GABA$_A$ receptors in the brain. The GABA$_A$ receptor channel has five subunits, with at least two alternative splice variants of several of the subunits (see Chapter 11). There are at least 10 known subtypes of the GABA$_A$ receptor, with varying distributions of these subtypes throughout the brain. Although barbiturates and benzodiazepines both increase Cl^- influx through GABA$_A$ channels, benzodiazepines act on a specific subset of GABA$_A$ channels whereas barbiturates appear to act on all GABA$_A$ channels. This difference in specificity results in distinct clinical profiles. Drugs that nonspecifically increase GABA content (e.g., through enhancement of synthetic pathways) tend to have a profile similar to the barbiturates.

Benzodiazepines (Diazepam, Lorazepam, Midazolam, Clonazepam)

Benzodiazepines increase the affinity of GABA for the GABA$_A$ receptor and enhance GABA$_A$ channel gating in the presence of GABA, and thereby increase Cl^- influx through the channel (see Chapter 11). This action has the dual effect of suppressing the seizure focus (by raising the threshold of the action potential) and strengthening surround inhibition. Thus, benzodiazepines such as **diazepam**, **lorazepam**, and **midazolam** are particularly well suited for the treatment of partial and tonic–clonic seizures. The benzodiazepines cause prominent adverse effects, however, including dizziness, ataxia, and drowsiness. Thus, these drugs are typically used only to ablate seizures acutely.

Clonazepam is unique among the benzodiazepines because it can inhibit T-type Ca^{2+} channel currents in in vitro preparations of thalamocortical circuits. In vivo, clonazepam acts specifically at GABA$_A$ receptors in the reticular nucleus (Fig. 14-5B), augmenting inhibition in these neurons and essentially "turning off" the nucleus. By this action, clonazepam prevents GABA-mediated hyperpolarization of the thalamus and thereby indirectly inactivates the T-type Ca^{2+} channel, which is the channel thought to be responsible for generating absence seizures (see above). However, as with diazepam, clonazepam use is limited because of its extensive side effects. Clonazepam is the fourth drug of choice in the treatment of absence seizures, after lamotrigine.

Barbiturates (Phenobarbital)

Phenobarbital binds to an allosteric site on the GABA$_A$ receptor and thereby potentiates the action of endogenous GABA by greatly increasing the duration of Cl^- channel opening. In the presence of phenobarbital, there is a much greater influx of Cl^- ions for each activation of the channel (see Chapter 11). Barbiturates also display weak agonist activity at the GABA$_A$ channel, perhaps furthering the ability of this drug to increase Cl^- influx. This enhancement of GABA-mediated inhibition, similar to that of the benzodiazepines, may explain the effectiveness of phenobarbital in the treatment of partial seizures and tonic–clonic seizures.

In contrast to the benzodiazepines, which are sometimes useful in treating the spike-wave discharges of the absence seizure, the barbiturates may actually exacerbate this type of seizure. This exacerbation may be caused by two important factors. First, barbiturates act at all GABA$_A$ receptors. Although benzodiazepines selectively augment GABA inhibition in the reticular nucleus, barbiturates potentiate GABA$_A$

receptors in both the reticular nucleus and the thalamic relay cells. Importantly, the latter effect enhances the T-type calcium currents that are responsible for the absence seizure (Fig. 14-5B). Second, unlike benzodiazepines, which are purely allosteric enhancers of endogenous GABA activity, barbiturates can also act on the GABA$_A$ channel in the absence of the native ligand. The latter property may function to increase nonspecific activity of the barbiturates.

Phenobarbital is used primarily as an alternative drug in the treatment of partial seizures and tonic–clonic seizures. Because of the pronounced sedative effects of this drug, however, its clinical use has been decreasing as more effective antiepileptic medications have become available.

DRUGS THAT INHIBIT GLUTAMATE RECEPTORS

The ionotropic glutamate receptors mediate the effects of glutamate, the principal excitatory neurotransmitter of the CNS (see Chapter 11). Not surprisingly, excessive activation of excitatory synapses is a key component of most forms of seizure activity. Numerous studies using animal models have shown that inhibition of the NMDA and AMPA subtypes of glutamate receptors can inhibit the generation of seizure activity and protect neurons from seizure-induced injury. However, none of the specific and potent glutamate receptor antagonists have been routinely used clinically for the treatment of seizures because of unacceptable behavioral adverse effects.

Felbamate

Felbamate has a variety of actions, including the inhibition of NMDA receptors. It appears to have some selectivity for NMDA receptors that include the NR2B subunit. Because this particular receptor subunit is not expressed ubiquitously throughout the brain, NMDA receptor antagonism by felbamate is not as widespread as that seen with other NMDA antagonists. This relative selectivity may explain why felbamate lacks the behavioral adverse effects observed with the other agents. Felbamate is an extremely potent antiepileptic drug, and has the additional benefit that it lacks the sedative effects common to many other drugs used for the treatment of epilepsy. However, shortly after it was made available for general use, felbamate was found to be associated with a number of cases of fatal aplastic anemia and liver failure, and its use is now restricted primarily to patients with extremely refractory epilepsy.

◗ Conclusion and Future Directions

In recent years, improved understanding of the physiology and pathophysiology of neuronal signaling in the CNS has led to a more thorough understanding of the current antiepileptic drugs (AEDs), as well as the design and discovery of novel agents. Under physiologic conditions, Na$^+$ channel inactivation and GABA-mediated surround inhibition prevent uncontrolled, rapid spread of electrical activity. There are, however, numerous potential alterations in the brain that can weaken these inhibitory forces, such as damage and degeneration of GABAergic neurons, abnormal ion gradients induced by space-occupying lesions, and gene mutations that alter channel function.

The AEDs described in this chapter restore the inherent inhibitory capacity of the brain. These include drugs such as phenytoin, which increases Na$^+$ channel inactivation, as well as drugs such as clonazepam, which enhances GABA-mediated inhibition. Newer classes of AEDs that have recently reached clinical application extend this repertoire by acting not only to decrease Na$^+$-dependent burst firing and GABA-mediated inhibition, but also through modulation of the Ca^{2+} channel required for neurotransmitter release and modulation of excitatory receptors such as the NMDA receptor.

Despite increased understanding of the mechanisms of certain seizure types, the efficacy of many of the anticonvulsants is only partially explained by their known molecular profile. Hence, current decisions about therapy are often driven more by empirical example than by known molecular mechanisms. As knowledge of the mechanisms of various seizure types and antiseizure drugs increases, the application of a more rational, mechanism-based pharmacology will become increasingly possible.

◗ Suggested Reading

Lowenstein DH. Seizures and epilepsy. In: *Harrison's principles of internal medicine.* 16th ed. New York: McGraw Hill; 2004. *(Discussion of seizure pathophysiology. Extensive discussion of clinical use of antiepileptic drugs.)*

Rogawski MA, Loscher W. The neurobiology of antiepileptic drugs. *Nat Rev Neurosci* 2004;5:553–564. *(Cellular biology of antiepileptic drugs and their targets.)*

Westbrook GL. Seizures and epilepsy. In: Kandel ER, Schwartz JH, Jessell TM, eds. *Principles of neural science.* 4th ed. New York: McGraw-Hill; 2000. *(Detailed description of normal electric signaling and seizure pathophysiology.)*

| Drug Summary Table | **Chapter 14** Pharmacology of Abnormal Electrical Neurotransmission in the Central Nervous System |

Drug	Clinical Applications	Serious and Common Adverse Effects	Contraindications	Therapeutic Considerations
SODIUM CHANNEL INHIBITORS				
Mechanism—Inhibit electrical neurotransmission by use-dependent block of neuronal voltage-gated sodium channel				
Phenytoin	Partial and secondary generalized (tonic–clonic) seizures, status epilepticus, non-epileptic seizures Seizures related to eclampsia Neuralgia Ventricular arrhythmias unresponsive to lidocaine or procainamide Arrhythmias induced by cardiac glycosides	_Agranulocytosis, leukopenia, pancytopenia, thrombocytopenia, megaloblastic anemia, hepatitis, Stevens-Johnson syndrome, toxic epidermal necrolysis_ Ataxia, nystagmus, incoordination, confusion, gingival hyperplasia, hirsutism, facial coarsening	Hydantoin hypersensitivity Sinus bradycardia, SA node block, second- or third-degree AV block Stokes-Adams syndrome	Phenytoin interacts with numerous drugs due to its hepatic metabolism. Phenytoin is metabolized by P450 2C9/10 and P450 2C19. Other drugs that are metabolized by these enzymes can increase or decrease plasma concentration of phenytoin. Phenytoin can also induce various P450s, such as P450 3A4, which can lead to increased metabolism of other drugs. Examples of these interactions include: phenytoin levels are increased by chloramphenicol, cimetidine, disulfiram, felbamate, and isoniazid; phenytoin levels are decreased by carbamazepine and phenobarbital. Phenytoin increases the metabolism of carbamazepine, cyclosporine, doxycyline, lamotrigine, levodopa, methadone, oral contraceptives, quinidine, warfarin At low doses, half-life is 24 h; at higher doses, phenytoin saturates the P450 system, such that small changes in dose can result in large changes in plasma concentration, thereby increasing the risk of adverse effects
Carbamazepine	Partial and tonic–clonic seizures Bipolar I disorder (see Box 13-2) Trigeminal neuralgia	_Aplastic anemia, agranulocytosis, thrombocytopenia, leukopenia, atrioventricular block, arrhythmia, Stevens-Johnson syndrome, toxic epidermal necrolysis, hyponatremia, hypocalcemia, SIADH, porphyria, hepatitis, nephrotoxicity_ Blood pressure lability, rash, confusion, nystagmus, blurred vision	Concomitant use of monoamine oxidase inhibitors History of bone marrow depression	A metabolite of carbamazepine, 10,11–epoxycarbamazepine, also acts to slow sodium channel recovery Drug of choice for partial seizures (simple and complex) The half-life of carbamazepine is reduced with chronic treatment, requiring patients to take several doses daily Linear metabolism of carbamazepine makes carbamazepine a more attractive choice than phenytoin for patients with potential drug interactions
Lamotrigine	Partial and tonic–clonic seizures Atypical absence seizures Bipolar I disorder (see Box 13-2)	_Stevens-Johnson syndrome, toxic epidermal necrolysis, bone marrow suppression, hepatic necrosis, amnesia, angioedema_ Rash, ataxia, somnolence, blurred vision	Hypersensitivity to lamotrigine	Lamotrigine is a useful alternative to phenytoin and carbamazepine as a treatment for partial and tonic–clonic seizures Lamotrigine is also effective in treating atypical absence seizures; it is third drug of choice for treatment of absence seizures, after ethosuximide and valproic acid

CALCIUM CHANNEL INHIBITORS
Mechanism—Ethosuximide and valproic acid inhibit the low-threshold T-type calcium channel; gabapentin inhibits the high-voltage-activated (HVA) calcium channel

Drug	Clinical uses	Side effects	Contraindications	Notes
Ethosuximide	Absence seizures	*Stevens-Johnson syndrome, bone marrow suppression, systemic lupus erythematosus, seizures* Gastrointestinal irritation, ataxia, somnolence	Hypersensitivity to ethosuximide	Ethosuximide reduces low-threshold T-type currents in a voltage-dependent manner without altering the voltage dependence or recovery kinetics of the sodium channel First-line therapy for uncomplicated absence seizures
Valproic acid	Tonic–clonic seizures, absence seizures, atypical absence seizures, partial seizures	*Hepatotoxicity, pancreatitis, thrombocytopenia, hyperammonemia* Gastrointestinal irritation, weight gain, ataxia, sedation, tremor	Liver disease Urea cycle disorders	Valproic acid acts pleiotropically in vitro: inhibits low-threshold T-type calcium channel, shows use-dependent block of voltage-gated sodium channel, increases activity of glutamic acid decarboxylase (enzyme responsible for GABA synthesis), inhibits activity of enzymes that degrade GABA Most effective for treatment of generalized epilepsy syndromes having mixed seizure types Also drug of choice for patients with idiopathic generalized seizures Used for treatment of absence seizures that do not respond to ethosuximide and as alternative to phenytoin and carbamazepine for treatment of partial seizures
Gabapentin	Partial seizures Diabetic peripheral neuropathy Prophylaxis of migraine	*Stevens-Johnson syndrome* Sedation, dizziness, ataxia, fatigue, gastrointestinal irritation	Hypersensitivity to gabapentin	Although gabapentin increases GABA content in neurons and glial cells in vitro, its main anti-seizure effect appears to be through its inhibition of HVA calcium channels Gabapentin has few interactions with other drugs Gabapentin does not appear to be a particularly effective antiepileptic drug for most patients

GABA CHANNEL POTENTIATORS
Mechanism—Potentiate GABA-mediated inhibition to increase chloride current through the channel

Drug	Clinical uses	Side effects	Contraindications	Notes
Benzodiazepines: **Diazepam** **Lorazepam** **Midazolam** **Clonazepam**	Partial and tonic–clonic seizures (diazepam, lorazepam, midazolam) Absence seizures (clonazepam) Status epilepticus Anxiety Alcohol withdrawal	Ataxia, dizziness, somnolence, fatigue	Acute narrow-angle glaucoma Untreated open-angle glaucoma	Benzodiazepines increase the affinity of the GABA receptor for GABA and thereby increase chloride current through the channel, resulting in suppression of the seizure focus and strengthening surround inhibition Benzodiazepines are typically used only to ablate seizures acutely Clonazepam acts specifically at GABA receptors in the reticular nucleus to "turn off" transmission in the nucleus, thereby inhibiting GABA-mediated hyperpolarization of the thalamus and indirectly inactivating the T-type calcium channel Clonazepam is the fourth drug of choice in treatment of absence seizures, after lamotrigine Benzodiazepine levels are decreased by carbamazepine or phenobarbital

(Continued)

Drug Summary Table   **Chapter 14 Pharmacology of Abnormal Electrical Neurotransmission in the Central Nervous System** (*Continued*)

Drug	Clinical Applications	Serious and Common Adverse Effects	Contraindications	Therapeutic Considerations
Barbiturates: Phenobarbital	Partial and tonic–clonic seizures Insomnia Preoperative sedation	*Stevens-Johnson syndrome, bone marrow suppression, hepatotoxicity, osteopenia* Sedation, ataxia, confusion, dizziness, decreased libido, depression	Porphyria Severe liver dysfunction Respiratory disease	Phenobarbital binds to an allosteric site on the GABA receptor and potentiates the action of endogenous GABA by greatly increasing the duration of chloride influx Barbiturates may exacerbate absence seizure Phenobarbital is used primarily as an alternative drug in the treatment of partial seizures and tonic–clonic seizures Phenobarbital levels can be increased by valproic acid or phenytoin

GLUTAMATE RECEPTOR INHIBITORS

Mechanism—Felbamate inhibits glycine binding site of NMDA receptor-ionophore complex, resulting in suppression of seizure activity

Drug	Clinical Applications	Serious and Common Adverse Effects	Contraindications	Therapeutic Considerations
Felbamate	Refractory epilepsy, especially partial and tonic–clonic seizures	*Aplastic anemia, bone marrow depression, hepatic failure, Stevens-Johnson syndrome* Photosensitivity, gastrointestinal irritation, abnormal gait, dizziness	Blood dyscrasia Liver disease	Felbamate lacks the behavioral adverse effects observed with the other NMDA antagonists Felbamate is an extremely potent antiepileptic drug and has the additional benefit of lacking sedative effects However, it has been associated with a number of cases of fatal aplastic anemia and liver failure, and its use is restricted to patients with refractory epilepsy

OTHER ANTIEPILEPTIC DRUGS

Mechanisms under investigation

Drug	Clinical Applications	Serious and Common Adverse Effects	Contraindications	Therapeutic Considerations
Tiagabine	Partial and tonic–clonic seizures (adjunct therapy)	*Unexplained sudden death* Confusion, sedation, dizziness, depression, psychosis, gastrointestinal irritation	Hypersensitivity to tiagabine	May enhance GABA activity by blocking GABA reuptake into presynaptic neurons Tiagabine levels are decreased by phenytoin, carbamazepine, or phenobarbital. Non-enzyme-inducing antiepileptic drugs (e.g., gabapentin) may require lower doses or slower titration of tiagabine for clinical response
Topiramate	Partial and tonic–clonic seizures (adjunct therapy)	Sedation, psychomotor slowing, fatigue, speech or language problems, renal stones	Hypersensitivity to topiramate	May inhibit sodium channel. May potentiate GABA activation of GABA-A channel. May antagonize AMPA receptor
Levetiracetam	Partial seizures (adjunct therapy)	*Anemia, leukopenia* Sedation, fatigue, incoordination, psychosis	Hypersensitivity to levetiracetam	Inhibits burst firing without affecting normal neuronal excitability
Zonisamide	Partial and tonic–clonic seizures (adjunct therapy)	Sedation, dizziness, confusion, headache, anorexia, renal stones	Hypersensitivity to zonisamide	May inhibit sodium channel Zonisamide levels are decreased by carbamazepine, phenytoin, or phenobarbital

15

General Anesthetic Pharmacology

Jacob Wouden and Keith W. Miller

INTRODUCTION

Before the discovery of **general anesthetics,** pain and shock severely limited the possibilities for surgical intervention. Postoperative mortality dropped dramatically following the first public demonstration of **diethyl ether** at Massachusetts General Hospital in 1846. Since then, the administration of agents for the induction and maintenance of anesthesia has become a separate medical specialty. The modern anesthesiologist is responsible for all aspects of patient health during surgery. As part of this process, the anesthesiologist controls the depth of anesthesia and maintains homeostatic equilibrium with an arsenal of inhaled and intravenous anesthetics as well as many adjuvant drugs.

General anesthetics induce a generalized, reversible depression of the central nervous system (CNS). Under gen-

eral anesthesia, there is a lack of perception of all sensations. The anesthetic state includes loss of consciousness, amnesia, and immobility (a lack of response to noxious stimuli), but not necessarily complete analgesia. Other desirable effects provided by anesthetics or adjuvants during surgery may include muscle relaxation, loss of autonomic reflexes, analgesia, and anxiolysis. All of these effects facilitate safe and painless completion of the procedure; some effects are more important in certain types of surgery than others. For example, abdominal surgery necessitates near complete relaxation of the abdominal muscles, whereas neurosurgery often requires light anesthesia that may be lifted rapidly when the neurosurgeon needs to judge the patient's ability to respond to commands.

This chapter provides a framework for understanding the pharmacodynamics and pharmacokinetics of general anesthetics in the context of physiologic and pathophysiologic variables. After discussing the pharmacology of specific agents and how a balanced anesthetic approach is achieved, the chapter considers what is currently known about the mechanism of action of general anesthetics.

■ Case

Matthew is a 7-year-old, 20-kg boy who has been undergoing multidrug chemotherapy for aggressive osteosarcoma of his right femur. The time has now come for a surgical resection.

- 8:00 PM (night before the operation): Dr. Snow, the anesthesiologist, provides reassurance and revisits the importance of fasting after midnight to prevent aspiration of gastric contents while under general anesthesia.
- 6:30 AM: Matthew clings to his mother and appears anxious, cachectic, and in some pain. His vital signs are stable with an elevated pulse of 120 and a blood pressure of 110/75. An oral dose of midazolam (a benzodiazepine; see Chapter 11, Pharmacology of GABAergic and Glutamatergic Neurotransmission) is given to relieve anxiety and to allow Matthew to separate from his parents.
- 7:00 AM: Dr. Snow injects a small amount of lidocaine subcutaneously (a local anesthetic; see Chapter 10, Local Anesthetic Pharmacology) before inserting an intravenous catheter (which he carefully conceals from Matthew until the last possible moment). Through the catheter, Dr. Snow delivers an infusion of morphine sulfate (an opioid; see Chapter 16, Pharmacology of Analgesia) for analgesia.
- 7:30 AM: Dr. Snow rapidly induces anesthesia with an intravenous bolus of 60 mg (3 mg/kg) of thiopental (a barbiturate; see Chapter 11). Within 45 seconds, Matthew is in a deep anesthetic state. The doctor adds a dose of intravenous succinylcholine (a depolarizing muscle relaxant; see Chapter 8, Cholinergic Pharmacology) to facilitate endotracheal intubation, and Matthew is placed on artificial respiration.
- 7:32 AM: A mixture of inhaled general anesthetics consisting of 2% isoflurane, 50% nitrous oxide, and 48% oxygen is provided through the ventilator to maintain the anesthetic state.
- 7:50 AM: Matthew shows no response, either through movement or increased sympathetic tone (e.g., increased heart rate, increased blood pressure), to the first surgical incision.
- 8:20 AM: Dr. Snow notices with a start that Matthew's pulse has fallen to 55 and his blood pressure to 85/45. Berating himself for forgetting to turn down the inspired partial pressure of the anesthetic as its mixed venous partial pressure increased, Dr. Snow reduces the inspired isoflurane level to 0.8% while keeping the nitrous oxide level at 50%. Within 15 minutes, Matthew's pulse and blood pressure rebound.
- 12:35 PM: After a long surgery, Dr. Snow stops the isoflurane and nitrous oxide and turns on pure oxygen for a few minutes.
- 12:45 PM: In less than 10 minutes, Matthew is breathing spontaneously and is able to respond to questions, although he is still somewhat groggy. Matthew's parents are relieved to find him awake and alert after more than 5 hours of anesthesia.

QUESTIONS

- **1.** What determines the rate of induction and recovery from anesthesia, and how does this differ for children as compared to adults?
- **2.** Why is it necessary to reduce the inspired partial pressure of isoflurane some minutes into the procedure (as Dr. Snow initially neglected to do)?
- **3.** What are the advantages of using a mixture of two anesthetics (in this example, nitrous oxide and isoflurane) instead of just one or the other?
- **4.** Why did Dr. Snow give pure oxygen for a few minutes following the cessation of anesthetic administration?

PHARMACODYNAMICS OF INHALED ANESTHETICS

General anesthetics distribute well to all parts of the body, becoming most concentrated in the fatty tissues. The CNS is the primary site of action of anesthetics. Most likely, loss of consciousness and amnesia ensue from supraspinal action (i.e., action in the brainstem, midbrain and cerebral cortex), while immobility in response to noxious stimuli is caused by depression of both supraspinal and spinal sensory and motor pathways. Different sites in the CNS are differentially affected by general anesthetics, giving rise to the classical stages observed with increasing anesthetic depth (Fig. 15-1).

THE MINIMUM ALVEOLAR CONCENTRATION (MAC)

To control the depth of anesthesia, the anesthesiologist must control rather precisely the level of anesthetic in the CNS. This level is denoted by the partial pressure of anesthetic in the CNS, also called the **CNS partial pressure,** P_{CNS}. (See Box 15-1 for a discussion of partial pressures versus concentrations and Appendix A for a glossary of abbreviations and symbols.) The anesthesiologist maintains P_{CNS} within the desired range by varying the **inspired partial pressure,** P_I. Because the value of P_{CNS} cannot be monitored directly, it is commonly inferred from the **alveolar partial pressure,** P_{alv}. The alveolar partial pressure is a useful substitute for P_{CNS}, because P_{CNS} tracks P_{alv} with only a small time lag (see below). P_{alv} may be measured directly as the partial pressure of anesthetic in the end-tidal exhaled gas, when the dead space no longer contributes to the exhaled gas.

The alveolar partial pressure that results in the lightest possible anesthesia is termed the **minimum alveolar concentration** (MAC). Specifically, MAC is the alveolar partial

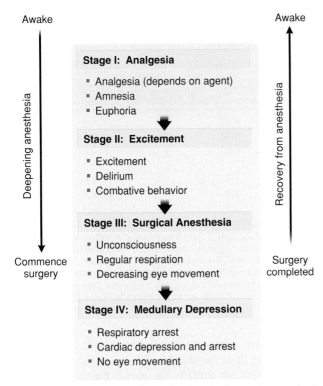

Figure 15-1. The stages of anesthesia. The deepening anesthetic state can be divided into four stages, based on observations with diethyl ether. The analgesia of stage I is variable and depends on the particular anesthetic agent. With fast induction, the patient passes rapidly through the undesirable "excitement" phase (stage II). Surgery is generally undertaken in stage III. The anesthesiologist must take care to avoid stage IV, which begins with respiratory arrest. Cardiac arrest occurs later in stage IV. During recovery from anesthesia, the patient progresses through the stages in reverse.

BOX 15-1. Partial Pressure Versus Concentration

The **partial pressure** of gas A in a mixture of gases is the portion of the total pressure that is supplied by gas A. For ideal gases, the partial pressure of gas A is obtained by multiplying the total pressure by the mole fraction of A in the mixture (i.e., the fraction of molecules in the mixture represented by gas A). The concentration of gas A in the mixture ($[A]_{\text{mixture}}$) is the number of moles of gas A (n_A) divided by the volume (V); $[A]_{\text{mixture}}$ can also be obtained from the ideal gas equation by dividing the partial pressure of gas A (P_A) by the temperature (T) and the universal gas constant (R).

$$[A]_{\text{mixture}} = n_A / V = P_A / RT$$

Inhaled anesthetics dissolve in the tissues of the body, such as the blood and the brain. The partial pressure of a gas dissolved in a liquid is equal to the partial pressure of free gas in equilibrium with that liquid. For gases, partial pressures are convenient because the partial pressures in all compartments are equal at equilibrium. This is true, independent of whether the compartments contain gas that is in the gaseous (alveoli) or the dissolved (tissues) form. In contrast, the concentrations within different compartments will not be equal at equilibrium. To convert the partial pressure of a dissolved gas to its concentration within the solvent, the partial pressure is multiplied by a measure of solubility known as the **solvent/gas partition coefficient.**

---

pressure that abolishes a movement response to a surgical incision in 50% of patients. The potency of an anesthetic is related inversely to its MAC. If the MAC is small, then the potency is high, and a relatively low partial pressure will be sufficient to cause anesthesia. For example, **isoflurane**—which has a MAC of 0.0114 atm—is much more potent than **nitrous oxide**—which has a MAC of 1.01 atm (Table 15-1).

THERAPEUTIC AND ANALGESIC INDICES

Loss of response to extremely noxious stimuli, such as endotracheal intubation, requires a higher partial pressure of anesthetic than is required for loss of response to a surgical incision (Fig. 15-2). Still higher partial pressures of anesthetic cause medullary depression. In general, however, anesthetics have steep **dose–response curves** and low therapeutic indices, defined as the ratio of **LD$_{50}$** (the partial pressure that is lethal in 50% of subjects) to MAC (which is analogous to ED$_{50}$; see Chapter 2, Pharmacodynamics). Furthermore, the variability among patients in their response to a given dose of anesthetic is small. Therefore, for all patients, the levels of anesthetic that cause respiratory and cardiac arrest are not much higher than the levels that cause general anes-

thesia. It should also be noted that no pharmacologic antagonists of general anesthetics exist to counteract inadvertently high levels of anesthetic. Although these disadvantages are partially offset by the ability to control P_{CNS} through control of P_I, the combination of low therapeutic index and lack of antagonist means that anesthetics are dangerous drugs that demand specialty training for their proper and safe administration.

Pain relief (analgesia) may or may not occur at a partial pressure lower than that required for surgical anesthesia. The partial pressure at which 50% of persons lose nociception is the AP$_{50}$ (partial pressure that results in analgesia in 50% of patients), and the **analgesic index** is the ratio of MAC to AP$_{50}$. A high analgesic index implies that analgesia is induced at a partial pressure of anesthetic significantly lower than that required for surgical anesthesia. For example, nitrous oxide has a high analgesic index and is a good analgesic, whereas **halothane** has a low analgesic index and is a poor analgesic.

THE MEYER–OVERTON RULE

The potency of an anesthetic can be predicted from its physicochemical characteristics. The most reliable predictor has been the anesthetic's solubility in olive oil (or in another lipophilic solvent, such as octanol), as denoted by the **oil/gas partition coefficient, λ(oil/gas)** (Box 15-2). Specifi-

TABLE 15-1   Properties of Inhaled Anesthetics

| ANESTHETIC | MAC (atm) | SOLVENT/GAS PARTITION COEFFICIENTS | | CONCENTRATION IN OIL AT 1 MAC |
		λ(oil/gas) ($L_{gas} L_{tissue}^{-1} atm^{-1}$)	λ(blood/gas) ($L_{gas} L_{tissue}^{-1} atm^{-1}$)	λ(oil/gas) $\times$ MAC ($L_{gas} L_{tissue}^{-1}$)
Nitrous oxide	1.01	1.4	0.47	1.4
Desflurane	0.06	19	0.45	1.1
Sevoflurane	0.02	51	0.65	1.0
Diethyl ether	0.019	65	12	1.2
Enflurane	0.0168	98	1.8	1.6
Isoflurane	0.0114	98	1.4	1.1
Halothane	0.0077	224	2.3	1.7

The commonly used inhaled anesthetics are listed in order of increasing potency (or decreasing MAC). Also listed are the important solvent/gas partition coefficients λ(oil/gas) and λ(blood/gas). λ(oil/gas) defines the potency of the anesthetic (larger is more potent), while λ(blood/gas) defines the rate of induction and recovery of anesthesia (smaller is faster). The product of λ(oil/gas) and MAC for these anesthetics has a rather constant value of 1.3 $L_{gas} L_{tissue}^{-1}$ (with a standard deviation of 0.27). This is an illustration of the Meyer–Overton Rule; another illustration of the rule is shown in Figure 15-3. Also note the general trend that anesthetics with larger λ(oil/gas) tend to have larger λ(blood/gas); this means that there is frequently a trade-off between potency and speed of induction among the inhaled anesthetics. The structures of these agents are shown in Figure 15-14.

cally, *the potency of an anesthetic increases as its solubility in oil increases.* That is, *as λ(oil/gas) increases, MAC decreases.*

The relationship between MAC and λ(oil/gas) is such that MAC multiplied by λ(oil/gas) is nearly constant, independent of the identity of the anesthetic. Because multiplication of the partition coefficient by the partial pressure yields the concentration of anesthetic (Box 15-2), this is equivalent to saying that, at 1 MAC, the concentration of anesthetic in a

lipophilic solvent (such as olive oil) is nearly constant for all anesthetics. Thus, the MAC, which varies with the identity of the anesthetic, is actually the partial pressure required to generate a particular concentration of anesthetic in a lipophilic medium, such as the lipid bilayers in the CNS. This correlation, known as the **Meyer–Overton Rule,** holds over at least five orders of magnitude of anesthetic potency (Fig. 15-3). The constant that represents the concentration of anesthetic at 1 MAC is 1.3 liters of gas per liter of oil (L_{gas} /

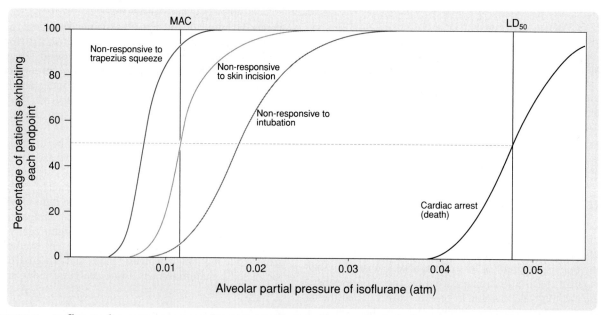

Figure 15-2.   Isoflurane dose-response curves for various endpoints. These curves depict the percentage of patients exhibiting endpoints of nonresponsiveness to a set of stimuli and of cardiac arrest as the alveolar partial pressure of isoflurane is increased. Note that the dose-response curves are quite steep, especially for mild stimuli, and that higher partial pressures are required to achieve lack of response to stronger stimuli. In the example shown, lack of response to intubation in 50% of patients requires nearly 0.02 atm isoflurane, while lack of response to a squeeze of the trapezius muscle requires only 0.008 atm. The MAC is defined as the alveolar partial pressure at which 50% of patients do not respond to a skin incision. The therapeutic index is defined as the LD_{50} divided by the MAC. The theoretical curve for cardiac arrest is derived from a known therapeutic index of about 4 for isoflurane. Accordingly, the anesthesiologist must carefully monitor each individual patient to achieve the desired effect while avoiding cardiac depression.

BOX 15-2. Partition Coefficients

The **solvent/gas partition coefficient, λ(solvent/gas),** defines the solubility of a gas in a solvent or, in other words, how the gas "partitions" between its gaseous state and the solution. More specifically, λ(solvent/gas) is the ratio of the amount of gas dissolved in a given volume of solvent to the amount of free gas that would occupy the same volume of space, all at standard temperature (25°C) and pressure (1.0 atm) (STP). The solvent could be olive oil, blood, or brain tissue, for example.

Dissolved amounts of gas are typically given not in terms of moles but in terms of the volume that the gas would occupy at STP in a gaseous state. Recall that, to convert from moles to liters at STP, one multiplies by the volume of one mole of gas at 25°C and 1.0 atm (i.e., by 24.5 L/mol). Thus, λ(solvent/gas) is the number of liters of gas that will dissolve in one liter of solvent per atmosphere of partial pressure. (Note that the units of λ(solvent/gas) are $L_{gas} L_{solvent}^{-1} atm^{-1}$, or simply atm^{-1}.)

For a particular solvent, a gas with a larger λ(solvent/gas) is more soluble in that solvent. For example, diethyl ether has a λ(blood/gas) of about 12 $L_{diethyl\ ether} L_{blood}^{-1} atm^{-1}$, so diethyl ether is relatively soluble in blood. In contrast, nitrous oxide has a λ(blood/gas) of about 0.47 $L_{nitrous\ oxide} L_{blood}^{-1} atm^{-1}$, so nitrous oxide is relatively insoluble in blood (see Table 15-1 and Fig. 15-8, for examples).

Likewise, a gas may have different solubilities in different solvents. Solvents or tissues in which a gas has a large partition coefficient (high solubility) will dissolve large amounts of the gas at a given partial pressure, resulting in a high concentration of the gas in that solvent or tissue. Thus, large amounts of gas must be transferred to change the partial pressure by an appreciable amount.

In contrast, solvents or tissues in which a gas has a small partition coefficient (low solubility) will dissolve only small amounts of the gas at a given partial pressure. In this case, transferring a small amount of the gas will significantly change the partial pressure (Fig. 15-8).

For any given partial pressure, Henry's law for dilute solutions allows the concentration of gas A in a solvent ($[A]_{solution}$) to be calculated from λ(solvent/gas). The partial pressure is multiplied by the partition coefficient to calculate the concentration in terms of L_{gas} per $L_{solvent}$. The result is divided by the volume of one mole of gas at 25°C at 1.0 atm (24.5 L/mol) to get the molar concentration.

$$[A]_{solution} = P_{solvent} \times \lambda(solvent/gas) \text{ \{in terms of } L_{gas}/L_{solvent}\}$$
$$= P_{solvent} \times \lambda(solvent/gas)/(24.5\ L/mol) \text{ \{in terms of } mol_{gas}/L_{solvent}\}$$

For example, because the λ(blood/gas) of nitrous oxide is 0.47 $L_{nitrous\ oxide} L_{blood}^{-1} atm^{-1}$, if the partial pressure of nitrous oxide in the blood is 0.50 atm, then the concentration is 0.50 atm $\times$ 0.47 $L_{nitrous\ oxide} L_{blood}^{-1} atm^{-1} = 0.24$ $L_{nitrous\ oxide} L_{blood}^{-1}$ or 9.6 mM (after dividing by 24.5 L/mol). Also note that doubling the partial pressure will double the concentration.

A partition coefficient can also be defined for the partitioning of a gas between two solvents. For example, the tissue/blood partition coefficient, λ(tissue/blood), is the ratio of the molar concentration of gas in the tissue ($[A]_{tissue}$) to the molar concentration of gas in the blood ($[A]_{blood}$) at equilibrium (note that this coefficient is unitless). From the previous equation defining concentration and, the fact that partial pressures are equal at equilibrium, it follows that

$$\lambda(tissue/blood) = [A]_{tissue}/[A]_{blood}$$
$$= \lambda(tissue/gas)/\lambda(blood/gas)$$

L_{oil}), or 0.05 M after dividing by the volume of one mole (see Box 15-2). Thus, if one knows the oil/gas partition coefficient of an anesthetic, one can estimate its MAC from the following equation (see also Table 15-1):

$$MAC \approx 1.3/\lambda(oil/gas) \qquad \text{Equation 15-1}$$

PHARMACOKINETICS OF INHALED ANESTHETICS

A cardiopulmonary model of the **uptake** of anesthetic from the alveoli into the circulation and the **distribution** of anesthetic from the circulation to the tissues allows determination of the rate at which the partial pressure of anesthetic rises within the CNS. The anesthesiologist must navigate the small space between allowing a patient to awaken and causing medullary depression by predicting the effects of various

physiologic responses and disease states on the depth of anesthesia. For example, an understanding of the distribution characteristics of anesthetics enabled Dr. Snow to respond appropriately to Matthew's hypotension by lowering the P_I of isoflurane without overcorrecting and causing him to awaken.

The anesthesiologist must also be aware of how anesthetics differ in their pharmacokinetics. The pharmacokinetic characteristics of an ideal general anesthetic would be such that the anesthetic provides a rapid and pleasant induction of surgical anesthesia, followed by a smooth and rapid recovery to a fully functional and conscious state. The pharmacokinetics of individual agents are discussed below; this section deals with general principles of the **uptake model,** which uses basic respiratory and cardiovascular physiology to predict the pharmacokinetics of the inhaled anesthetics. As discussed below, the uptake model depends on calculations of the time required for the equilibration of anesthetic partial pressures in the tissues with the inspired anesthetic partial pressure.

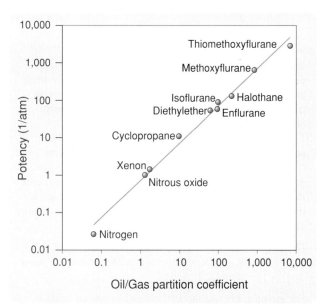

Figure 15-3. The Meyer-Overton rule. Molecules with a larger oil/gas partition coefficient (λ(oil/gas)) are more potent general anesthetics. This log–log plot shows the very tight correlation between lipid solubility (λ(oil/gas)) and anesthetic potency over five orders of magnitude. Note that even such gases as xenon and nitrogen can act as general anesthetics when breathed at high enough partial pressures. The equation describing the line is: Potency = λ(oil/gas) / 1.3. Recall that Potency = 1/MAC.

CONCEPTS FROM RESPIRATORY PHYSIOLOGY

Local Equilibration

During general anesthesia, the patient breathes, either spontaneously or via a ventilator, an anesthetic or mixture of anesthetics together with oxygen and/or normal air. Once the anesthetic gas reaches the alveoli, it must diffuse across the respiratory epithelium into the alveolar capillary bed. According to Fick's law, the rate of diffusion of gas through a sheet of tissue down its partial pressure gradient is proportional to the tissue area and the partial pressure difference between the two sides, and is inversely proportional to the thickness of the sheet:

$$\text{Diffusion rate} = D \times (A/l) \times \Delta P \qquad \text{Equation 15-2}$$

where D = diffusion constant; A = surface area; l = thickness; and ΔP = partial pressure difference.

One principle evident from Fick's Law is that the equalization of the partial pressure of the gas, not its concentration, defines the approach to equilibrium across a boundary sheet. Thus, at equilibrium (i.e., when the net diffusion rate is zero), the partial pressure in the two compartments is the same, even though the concentration in the two compartments may be different.

With its enormous alveolar surface area (~75 m², or nearly half a tennis court) and thin epithelium (~0.3 μm, which is less than 1/20th the diameter of a red blood cell), the lung optimizes the rate of gas diffusion. Accordingly, the alveolar partial pressure P_{alv} and the systemic arterial partial pressure P_{art} are nearly the same at all times. (In

normal individuals, small amounts of physiologic shunting keep P_{art} slightly lower than P_{alv}). By using the lungs as an uptake system for inhaled anesthetics, anesthesiologists take advantage of the body's system for absorbing oxygen.

Similarly, the capillary beds in tissues have evolved to deliver oxygen rapidly to all cells in the body. The distances between arterioles are small, and diffusion pathways are on the order of one cell diameter. Consequently, the arterial partial pressure of a general anesthetic can equilibrate completely with tissues in the time required for blood to traverse the capillary bed. Likewise, the partial pressure in the post-capillary venules P_{venule} equals the partial pressure in the tissue P_{tissue}.

Another way of stating the above conclusion is that *the transfer of anesthetic in both the lungs and the tissues is limited by perfusion rather than diffusion*. Because perfusion is rate-limiting, increasing the rate of diffusion (e.g., by using a lower molecular weight anesthetic) will not, by itself, increase the rate of induction of anesthesia.

Global Equilibration

If an anesthetic is inspired for a long enough period of time, all compartments in the body will equilibrate to the same partial pressure (equal to P_I). This global equilibration may be divided into a series of partial pressure equilibrations between each successive compartment and its incoming flow of anesthetic. In the case of the tissues, the incoming flow is the arterial blood flow, with partial pressure approximately equal to P_{alv}. In the case of the alveoli, the incoming flow is the alveolar ventilation with partial pressure P_I.

The **time constant** τ describes the rate of approach of a compartment's partial pressure to that of its incoming flow. Specifically, τ is the time required for equilibration to be 63% complete. This time constant is convenient because it can be calculated by dividing the compartment's **volume capacity** (relative to the delivering medium; see below) by the **flow rate.** In other words, once a volume of flow equal to the capacity of a compartment has gone through that compartment, the partial pressure of anesthetic in the compartment (i.e., in the tissues or alveoli) will be 63% of the partial pressure in the incoming flow (i.e., in the arterial blood flow or alveolar ventilation, respectively). Equilibration is 95% complete after three time constants.

$$\tau = \text{Volume Capacity / Flow Rate} \qquad \text{Equation 15-3}$$

$$P_{compartment} = P_{flow}[1 - e^{-(t/\tau)}] \qquad \text{Equation 15-4}$$

where t = elapsed time.

These equations describe what should make intuitive sense: equilibration of the partial pressure of the compartment with the incoming flow takes place more quickly (i.e., the time constant is smaller) when the inflow is larger or the compartment capacity is smaller.

THE UPTAKE MODEL

For simplicity, the model of anesthetic uptake and distribution organizes the tissues of the body into groups based on

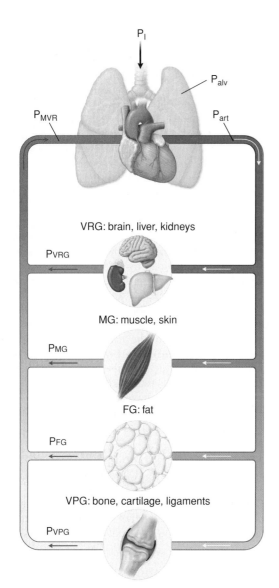

Tissue group	% Cardiac output	% Body weight	Vol. cap. for N$_2$O at P$_{alv}$ = 0.8atm	Vol. cap. for halo. at P$_{alv}$ = 0.8atm
VRG	75%	9%	2.6 L	0.30 L
MG	18%	50%	16 L	3.0 L
FG	5.5%	19%	12 L	17 L
VPG	1.5%	22%	7.0 L	1.3 L

Figure 15-4. Distribution of cardiac output and volume capacity for general anesthetics among the major tissue compartments. The tissues of the body can be divided into four groups based on their level of perfusion and their capacity to take up anesthetic. These include the Vessel-Rich Group (VRG), Muscle Group (MG), Fat Group (FG), and Vessel-Poor Group (VPG). (The contribution of the VPG is generally ignored in most pharmacokinetic models of anesthesia.) The VRG, which contains the internal organs including the brain, constitutes a small percentage of the total body weight (9%), has the lowest capacity for anesthetic, and receives most of the cardiac output (75%). The high perfusion and low capacity allow P_{VRG} to equilibrate rapidly with P_{art}. Also, the VRG makes the largest contribution to the mixed venous return partial pressure P_{MVR}, which is equal to (0.75 P_{VRG} + 0.18 P_{MG} + 0.055 P_{FG} + 0.015 P_{VPG}).

similar characteristics. Each group can be modeled as a container with a particular capacity for anesthetic and a particular level of blood flow delivering anesthetic. An adequate approximation groups the tissues into three main compartments that are perfused in parallel (Fig. 15-4). The **vessel-rich group (VRG)**, which consists of the CNS and visceral organs, has a low capacity and high flow. The **muscle group (MG)**, which consists of muscle and skin, has a high capacity and moderate flow. The **fat group (FG)** has a very high capacity and low flow. (A fourth group, the **vessel-poor group [VPG]**, which consists of bone, cartilage, and ligaments, has a negligible flow and capacity, and its omission does not significantly affect the model.)

The rate of increase of the partial pressure in the VRG (P_{VRG}) is of the greatest interest because the VRG includes the CNS. The overall equilibration of P_{VRG} with the inspired partial pressure occurs in two steps, either of which may be rate limiting. First, the alveolar and inspired partial pressures equilibrate (P_{alv} approaches P_I, or $P_{alv} \rightarrow P_I$). Second, P_{VRG} (and specifically P_{CNS}) equilibrates with the arterial partial pressure (which is essentially equal to the alveolar partial pressure) ($P_{VRG} \rightarrow P_{art}$). The discussion will now consider the time constant for each of these two steps, and define conditions under which one or the other is rate-limiting.

Equilibration of Alveolar with Inspired Partial Pressure

The equilibration of P_{alv} with P_I is conceptually the first step of the equilibration of P_{VRG} with P_I. During induction of anesthesia, P_{VRG} can never be higher than P_{alv}; if P_{alv} rises slowly, then P_{VRG} must also rise slowly.

To calculate the time constant for the approach of P_{alv} to P_I, $\tau\{P_{alv} \to P_I\}$, the flow rate and volume capacity must be defined. The delivering medium is free gas arriving through the airways, and the compartment is the lung and alveoli. The volume capacity is simply the volume of gas that remains in the lungs after normal exhalation, or the **functional residual capacity** (FRC, typically ~3 L for an average adult). Assume initially that the only component of the flow rate is the rate of **alveolar ventilation,** which delivers the anesthetic ($V_{alv} = \{$Tidal Volume $-$ Dead Space$\} \times$ Respiratory Rate; for an average adult, $V_{alv} = \{0.5\ L - 0.125\ L\} \times 16\ min^{-1} \approx 6$ L/min). Then, because

$$\tau\{P_{alv} \to P_I\} = FRC/V_{alv} \qquad \text{Equation 15-5}$$

a typical value for $\tau\{P_{alv} \to P_I\}$ is 3 L / 6 L/min, or 0.5 min—independent of the particular gas being inhaled. In children, the increased alveolar ventilation rate and decreased FRC (smaller lungs) both tend to shorten the time constant and to accelerate equilibration between the alveolar and inspired partial pressures.

The assumption to this point has been that no uptake of anesthetic into the bloodstream occurs, as would be the case if the solubility of the anesthetic in blood were zero. In practice, at the same time that alveolar ventilation is delivering anesthetic to the alveoli, anesthetic is also being removed from the alveoli by diffusion into the bloodstream. The balance between delivery and removal is analogous to adding water into a leaky bucket (Fig. 15-5). The level of water in

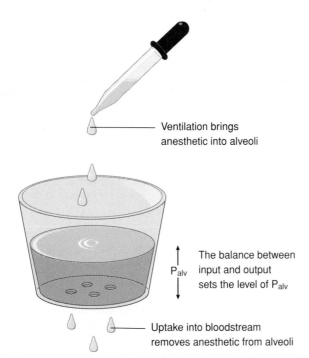

Ventilation brings anesthetic into alveoli

P_{alv} The balance between input and output sets the level of P_{alv}

Uptake into bloodstream removes anesthetic from alveoli

Figure 15-5. Determinants of the alveolar partial pressure of an inhaled anesthetic. The alveolar partial pressure, represented by the depth of fluid in the bucket, results from the balance between delivery by ventilation and removal by uptake into the bloodstream. Increased delivery of anesthetic, resulting from either increased ventilation or an increased inspired partial pressure of anesthetic, raises P_{alv}. In contrast, increased uptake into the bloodstream, caused by a large λ(blood/gas) or increased cardiac output, lowers P_{alv}.

the bucket (which represents the alveolar partial pressure) is determined both by the rate at which the water is added (the minute ventilation) and the size of the leak (the rate of anesthetic uptake from the alveoli into the bloodstream). Increasing anesthetic delivery (for example, by using a higher ventilation rate or a higher inspired partial pressure) will increase the alveolar partial pressure of the gas, just as adding water faster will increase the level of water in the bucket. Conversely, increasing anesthetic removal (for example, by increasing the perfusion rate or using a more blood-soluble anesthetic) will decrease the alveolar partial pressure of the gas; this is analogous to increasing the leakiness of the bucket. Thus, uptake of anesthetic from the alveoli into the bloodstream constitutes a negative component to the flow (i.e., a flow out of the lungs), which makes the time constant longer than the theoretical case where $\tau\{P_{alv} \to P_I\}$ equals FRC divided by V_{alv}.

The magnitude of the increase in the time constant compared to the limiting case depends on the rate of uptake of anesthetic by the blood, with longer $\tau\{P_{alv} \to P_I\}$ resulting from greater uptake. If one knows the cardiac output (i.e., the volume of blood pumped by the heart in 1 minute) and the value of the instantaneous difference between the pulmonary arterial partial pressure (which equals the systemic partial pressure of the mixed venous return, P_{MVR}) and the pulmonary venous partial pressure (which equals the systemic arterial partial pressure, P_{art}), then one can calculate the rate of uptake of a gas from the alveoli:

Rate of uptake $\{$in $L_{gas}/min\}$

$$= \lambda(\text{blood/gas}) \times (P_{art} - P_{MVR}) \times CO \qquad \text{Equation 15-6}$$

where CO = cardiac output in liters of blood per minute. Equation 15-7 follows from Equation 15-6 because the anesthetic concentration $[A]_{blood}$ is equal to λ(blood/gas) $\times P_{blood}$ (see Box 15-2):

$$\text{Rate of uptake} = ([A]_{art} - [A]_{MVR}) \times CO \qquad \text{Equation 15-7}$$

If any of the components of these equations approaches zero, the rate of uptake becomes small, and the delivery of anesthetic by ventilation drives the alveolar partial pressure toward the inspired partial pressure. In other words, equilibration of alveolar with inspired partial pressure is faster (i.e., $\tau\{P_{alv} \to P_I\}$ is smaller) with lower blood solubility of the anesthetic [smaller λ(blood/gas)], lower cardiac output, or smaller arterial ($\sim$alveolar) to venous partial pressure difference.

Equilibration of Tissue with Alveolar Partial Pressure

In addition to the equilibration between P_{alv} and P_I, equilibration between P_{tissue} and P_{art} (which is nearly equal to P_{alv}) must occur for P_{tissue} to equilibrate with P_I. Changes in P_{alv} are transmitted rapidly to systemic arterioles, because equilibration across the pulmonary epithelium is fast and the circulation time from pulmonary veins to tissue capillaries is generally less than 10 seconds. Thus, the time constant for equilibration between P_{tissue} and P_{alv} can be approximated as the time constant for equilibration between P_{tissue} and P_{art}. To calculate the time constant $\tau\{P_{tissue} \to P_{art}\}$, one must define the capacity of the compartment and the flow rate of the delivering medium. The flow rate is simply the rate at which blood perfuses the tissue. Recall that capacity is a volume capacity relative to the delivering medium. Specifically, *the capacity is the volume that the tissue would need to contain all of its gas if the solubility of the gas in the tissue were the same as that in the blood.* (This definition is similar to that of the volume of distribution of a drug; see Chapter 3, Pharmacokinetics):

Relative Volume Capacity of Tissue

$$= ([A]_{\text{tissue}} \times \text{Vol}_{\text{tissue}})/[A]_{\text{blood}} \qquad \text{Equation 15-8}$$

where $\text{Vol}_{\text{tissue}}$ is the volume of tissue. Equation 15-9 follows from Equation 15-8 because $[A]_{\text{tissue}} / [A]_{\text{blood}}$ at equilibrium is equal to $\lambda(\text{tissue/blood})$ (see Box 15-2):

Relative Volume Capacity of Tissue

$$= \lambda(\text{tissue/blood}) \times \text{Vol}_{\text{tissue}} \qquad \text{Equation 15-9}$$

Then, using Equation 15-3, we can write

$$\tau\{P_{\text{tissue}} \rightarrow P_{\text{art}}\} \approx \tau\{P_{\text{tissue}} \rightarrow P_{\text{alv}}\}$$
$$= \text{Relative Vol. Cap. of Tissue} /Q_{\text{tissue}} \qquad \text{Equation 15-10}$$

$$\tau\{P_{\text{tissue}} \rightarrow P_{\text{art}}\}$$
$$= \lambda(\text{tissue/blood}) \times \text{Vol}_{\text{tissue}}/Q_{\text{tissue}} \qquad \text{Equation 15-11}$$

where Q_{tissue} is tissue perfusion in L/min.

The tissue groups differ greatly in their capacities for anesthetic and in the time constants for their equilibration with arterial (and thus alveolar) partial pressure. With a small $\lambda(\text{tissue/blood})$ (Table 15-2) and a small volume ($\sim$6 L), the VRG has a low capacity for anesthetic. The combination of low capacity and high blood flow (75% of cardiac output) results in a very short equilibration time constant ($\tau\{P_{\text{VRG}} \rightarrow P_{\text{alv}}\}$) for the VRG. With a slightly higher $\lambda(\text{tissue/blood})$, a much larger volume ($\sim$33 L), and only moderate blood flow, the MG has a longer equilibration time constant ($\tau\{P_{\text{MG}} \rightarrow P_{\text{art}}\}$). Finally, with an extremely high $\lambda(\text{tissue/blood})$, a large volume, and low blood flow, the FG has an extremely long equilibration time constant ($\tau\{P_{\text{FG}} \rightarrow P_{\text{art}}\}$) (Table 15-3 and Fig. 15-6).

Because the anesthesiologist seeks to control P_{CNS}, the time constant for equilibration of the brain partial pressure P_{brain} with the arterial partial pressure P_{art} (which is nearly equal to P_{alv}) is of particular interest. The volume of the brain is approximately 1.4 L, the blood flow to the brain is about 0.9 L/min, and an average $\lambda(\text{brain/blood})$ for most anesthetics is about 1.6. Then, because

Relative Volume Capacity of Brain

$$= \lambda(\text{brain/blood}) \times \text{Vol}_{\text{brain}} \qquad \text{Equation 15-12}$$

$$\tau\{P_{\text{brain}} \rightarrow P_{\text{art}}\} = \lambda(\text{brain/blood}) \times \text{Vol}_{\text{brain}}/Q_{\text{brain}}$$

$$\tau\{P_{\text{brain}} \rightarrow P_{\text{art}}\} = (1.6 \times 1.4 \text{ L})/(0.9 \text{ L/min})$$
$$= 2.5 \text{ min} \qquad \text{Equation 15-13}$$

where $\text{Vol}_{\text{brain}}$ is the volume of the brain and Q_{brain} is the blood flow to the brain.

Variations in $\lambda(\text{brain/blood})$ among the different anesthetic agents cause $\tau\{P_{\text{brain}} \rightarrow P_{\text{art}}\}$ to range from 1.5 min for nitrous oxide [$\lambda(\text{brain/blood}) = 1.1$] to 2.7 min for diethyl ether [$\lambda(\text{brain/blood}) = 2.0$] (Table 15-3). Of course, variability in blood flow to the brain also affects $\tau\{P_{\text{brain}} \rightarrow P_{\text{art}}\}$. In summary, *the time constant for equilibration of the CNS with the alveolar partial pressure is short, and relatively independent of the particular anesthetic being used.*

The Rate-Limiting Step

As described above, the equilibration of the CNS with the inspired partial pressure occurs in two steps. Unlike $\tau\{P_{\text{brain}} \rightarrow P_{\text{art}}\}$, which is relatively independent of the particular anesthetic being used, $\tau\{P_{\text{alv}} \rightarrow P_{\text{I}}\}$ varies greatly among different anesthetics. On this basis, inhaled anesthetics can be divided into two broad categories:

- Ventilation-limited anesthetics, such as **diethyl ether, enflurane, isoflurane,** and **halothane;** and

TABLE 15-2 **Tissue/Blood Partition Coefficients**

	TISSUE/BLOOD PARTITION COEFFICIENTS		
ANESTHETIC	λ(brain/blood) (unitless)	λ(muscle/blood) (unitless)	λ(fat/blood) (unitless)
Nitrous oxide	1.1	1.2	2.3
Diethyl ether	2.0	1.3	5
Desflurane	1.3	2.0	27
Enflurane	1.4	1.7	36
Isoflurane	1.6	2.9	45
Sevoflurane	1.7	3.1	48
Halothane	1.9	3.4	51

The tissue/blood partition coefficient describes the comparative solubility of an anesthetic in a tissue compared to blood. λ(tissue/blood) is obtained from the ratio of the concentration of anesthetic in the tissue to the concentration in the blood at equilibrium (i.e., when the partial pressure is the same in both tissues). Alternatively, one may calculate λ(tissue/blood) from the equation λ(tissue/blood) = λ(tissue/gas)/λ(blood/gas) (see Box 15-2). With very few minor exceptions, the general trend is λ(fat/blood) $>>$ λ(muscle/blood) $>$ λ(brain/blood). High values of λ(fat/blood) give the FG a very high capacity for the inhaled anesthetics.

TABLE 15-3	Time Constants for Equilibration of Tissue with Arterial Partial Pressure		
ANESTHETIC	TIME CONSTANT FOR EQUILIBRATION OF TISSUE WITH ARTERIAL PARTIAL PRESSURE, $\tau\{P_{tissue} \rightarrow P_{art}\}$		
	VRG (min)	MG (min)	FG (min)
Nitrous oxide	1.5	36	104
Diethyl ether	2.7	39	227
Desflurane	1.7	61	1223
Enflurane	1.9	51	1631
Isoflurane	2.1	88	2039
Sevoflurane	2.3	94	2175
Halothane	2.5	103	2311

The time constants $\tau\{P_{tissue} \rightarrow P_{art}\}$ describe the time for 63% equilibration of the tissue with arterial (and therefore alveolar) partial pressure. Notice the very small time constants for equilibration of the VRG, in contrast to the large time constants for MG equilibration and very large time constants for FG equilibration. For all anesthetics except nitrous oxide, the partial pressure of the FG remains far below that of the alveolus for even the longest surgical procedures. Conversely, the VRG partial pressure is nearly in equilibrium with the alveolus from almost the start of anesthetic administration. The values in this table were calculated from the equation $\tau\{P_{tissue} \rightarrow P_{art}\} = \lambda(tissue/blood) \times$ Volume of tissue / Blood flow to tissue.

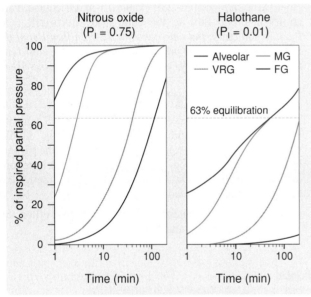

Figure 15-6. Equilibration of the tissue groups with the inspired partial pressure. These curves show, as a function of time, the approach of the partial pressures in the alveoli and in the three major tissue groups toward the inspired partial pressure. The partial pressure in the VRG equilibrates rapidly with the alveolar partial pressure, while the MG equilibrates more slowly, and the FG much more slowly. For a perfusion-limited anesthetic such as nitrous oxide, the alveolar partial pressure rises so quickly that the rate of rise of the VRG partial pressure is as much limited by its rise toward the alveolar partial pressure as by the rise of P_{alv} toward P_I. For a ventilation-limited anesthetic such as halothane, the rate at which the partial pressure in the VRG rises is limited not by its approach to the alveolar partial pressure, but rather by the rise of the alveolar toward the inspired partial pressure. In other words, the rate-limiting step is the equilibration of the alveolar partial pressure with the inspired partial pressure. The *dashed line* shows the point at which the partial pressure is 63% of P_I; the time constant for equilibration of each tissue group with P_I is approximated by the time at which each curve crosses this line.

• Perfusion-limited anesthetics, such as **nitrous oxide, desflurane,** and **sevoflurane.**

Ventilation-limited anesthetics have a long, rate-limiting $\tau\{P_{alv} \rightarrow P_I\}$ because of their high $\lambda(blood/gas)$: the high rate of uptake of anesthetic into the bloodstream prevents P_{alv} from rising rapidly. Thus, the slow and rate-limiting equilibration of alveolar with inspired partial pressure results in slow induction of anesthesia and slow recovery from anesthesia. Accordingly, for these anesthetics, physiologic or pathologic changes that act to increase the rate of rise of the alveolar partial pressure will speed induction. Conversely, because equilibration of the tissue with the arterial partial pressure is not rate limiting, physiologic or pathologic changes that shorten $\tau\{P_{VRG} \rightarrow P_{art}\}$ will have little effect on induction time (see below).

Perfusion-limited anesthetics have a $\tau\{P_{alv} \rightarrow P_I\}$ that is similar in magnitude to $\tau\{P_{VRG} \rightarrow P_{art}\}$ because their $\lambda(blood/gas)$ is small. Induction and recovery occur quickly, and neither $\tau\{P_{alv} \rightarrow P_I\}$ nor $\tau\{P_{VRG} \rightarrow P_{art}\}$ may be clearly rate-limiting. Accordingly, induction time may be affected by changes in either the rate of rise of alveolar partial pressure or the rate at which P_{CNS} approaches P_{art} (e.g., see the discussion of hyperventilation below). Physiologic changes may alter the balance between $\tau\{P_{alv} \rightarrow P_I\}$ and $\tau\{P_{VRG} \rightarrow P_{art}\}$. See Figure 15-6 for a graphic comparison of the kinetics of ventilation-limited and perfusion-limited anesthetics.

The characteristic that distinguishes perfusion-limited from ventilation-limited anesthetics is the blood/gas partition coefficient, $\lambda(blood/gas)$. With the smaller $\lambda(blood/gas)$ of perfusion-limited anesthetics, the bloodstream removes less anesthetic from the alveoli; thus, the alveolar partial pressure rises more quickly and induction is faster (Fig. 15-7). This is the key point, although the correlation may seem paradoxical at first: *agents that are less soluble in the blood induce anesthesia faster.*

To clarify, consider two hypothetical anesthetics that differ solely in $\lambda(blood/gas)$: Anesthetic A has a small $\lambda(blood/gas)$; while Anesthetic B has a large $\lambda(blood/gas)$. Because Anesthetics A and B are identical in $\lambda(oil/gas)$, they have the

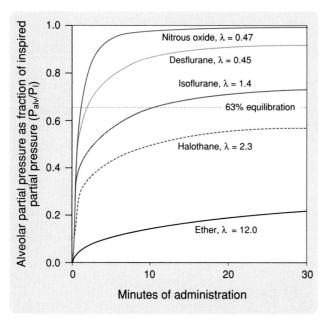

Figure 15-7. Rate of approach of the alveolar toward the inspired partial pressure. For agents with smaller λ(blood/gas) such as nitrous oxide, the alveolar partial pressure approaches the inspired partial pressure quickly, while for agents with larger λ(blood/gas) such as ether, the alveolar partial pressure approaches the inspired partial pressure much more slowly. The *dashed line* shows the point at which $P_{alv}/P_I = 0.63$; the time constant $\tau\{P_{alv}{\rightarrow}P_I\}$ is approximated by the time at which each curve crosses this line. λ = λ(blood/gas).

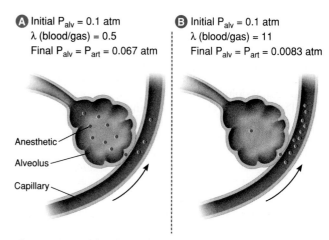

Figure 15-8. Why do anesthetics with smaller λ(blood/gas) have shorter induction times? Consider two equally potent anesthetics inspired at the same partial pressure, P_I. Before any anesthetic molecules have been taken up from the alveolus into the blood, the alveolar partial pressure, P_{alv}, of each anesthetic is 0.1 atm. This partial pressure would be represented in the diagram by 12 anesthetic "spheres" in each alveolus. For each anesthetic, equilibration of the partial pressures in the alveolus and the capillary then takes place. For a relatively blood-insoluble agent with λ(blood/gas) = 0.5 (**Anesthetic A,** which closely resembles nitrous oxide, desflurane, sevoflurane, and cyclopropane), the transfer of a small amount of anesthetic from the alveolus significantly raises the partial pressure in the capillary. To illustrate, consider a time, t_v, when the volume of blood that has flowed past the alveolar wall is equal to the volume of the alveolus. At that time, the concentration in the alveolus will be twice that in the capillary (because λ (blood/gas) = 0.5; see Box 15-2) when four of the "spheres" have been transferred from the alveolus to the capillary and eight "spheres" remain in the alveolus. The partial pressure in the alveolus will now have dropped to (8/12) × 0.1 = 0.067 atm. This is also the partial pressure in the capillary. In contrast, for a very blood-soluble agent with λ(blood/gas) = 11 (**Anesthetic B,** which closely resembles diethyl ether), much larger amounts of anesthetic must dissolve in the blood to raise the partial pressure in the capillary. Using the same illustration as above, at t_v, 11 of the 12 "spheres" will have been transferred from the alveolus to the capillary, and the remaining P_{alv} will be given by (1/12) × 0.1 = 0.0083 atm. Thus, although the inspired partial pressure of the two anesthetics is the same, at time t_v, the P_{alv} and P_{art} of Anesthetic A will be eight times higher than that of Anesthetic B. Within approximately 1 minute, P_{brain} will also reach these values. Thus, the brain partial pressure rises toward the inspired partial pressure much more rapidly for Anesthetic A than for Anesthetic B (i.e., the induction time for Anesthetic A is much shorter than that for Anesthetic B). If the reader is confused by the fact that more molecules of Anesthetic B are being carried to the brain, recall that λ(brain/blood) is ~1 for all of the commonly used anesthetics (that is, for each agent, λ(blood/gas) is approximately equal to λ(brain/gas); see Table 15-2). Thus, proportionally many more molecules of Anesthetic B than Anesthetic A must be delivered to the brain in order to raise the partial pressure of each anesthetic by an equivalent amount. See Boxes 15-1 and 15-2 and the Appendix for definitions.

same MAC. They also have identical λ(brain/blood), so their $\tau\{P_{brain}{\rightarrow}P_{alv}\}$ is the same (see Equations 15-12 and 15-13). To cause anesthesia, both must achieve the same partial pressure in the CNS. At any particular partial pressure, however, the blood and CNS contain more moles of Anesthetic B than Anesthetic A because Anesthetic B is more soluble than Anesthetic A in the blood and CNS. The transfer of a larger number of moles of Anesthetic B out of the lungs slows the rate of rise of P_{alv}, so a longer period is necessary for Anesthetic B than for Anesthetic A to achieve the anesthetic partial pressure in the CNS (Fig. 15-8).[a]

---

[a]In this hypothetical model, one may correctly note that the *concentration* of Anesthetic B in the CNS *as a whole* will be higher than that of Anesthetic A at any particular time point. One may, therefore, wonder how Anesthetic B can have a slower induction, if anesthesia results when a particular concentration (0.05 M) is reached at the site of action (see Pharmacodynamics, above). At this point, one must recognize that the brain is primarily aqueous, but that anesthetics are likely to have a *hydrophobic* site of action, and that both Anesthetic A and Anesthetic B must have the same concentration (0.05 M) in the key hydrophobic portions of the brain at their anesthetic partial pressures. However, Anesthetic B, with its larger aqueous solubility (λ(blood/gas)), will partition relatively more than Anesthetic A into the aqueous portions of the brain. To provide the higher aqueous concentrations, many more moles of Anesthetic B than Anesthetic A must be transferred from the lungs.

The overall conclusion still holds if λ(oil/gas) and thus MAC differ for the two hypothetical anesthetics. P_{alv} for a less blood-soluble agent will rise proportionally faster toward its P_I than a more blood-soluble agent, independent of what that P_I is (note that P_I will be larger for the less oil-soluble anesthetic). A larger λ(oil/gas) allows the anesthetic to cause anesthesia at a lower partial pressure, but does not affect the proportional rate at which the partial pressure rises.

APPLICATIONS OF THE UPTAKE MODEL

Throughout the following discussion, it is critical to remember that the primary responsibility of the anesthesiologist is to keep the patient well oxygenated and the vital signs stable while manipulating the inspired partial pressure of anesthetic to maintain the desired depth of anesthesia.

Armed with the uptake model, the anesthesiologist can predict the effects of cardiopulmonary changes and pathologic states on the depth of anesthesia. Changes in ventilation and cardiac output may be caused by the general anesthetic itself, by the trauma of surgery, or by some other physiologic or pathophysiologic process.

The effects of changes in both ventilation and cardiac output on P_{CNS} are greatest when the difference between P_I and P_{alv} is greatest; that is, early in the course of anesthesia (Fig. 15-6). To understand this, consider the partial pressure in the mixed venous return (MVR), P_{MVR}, which is a weighted average of the partial pressures in each of the tissue groups, with P_{VRG} making the largest contribution because the VRG receives the majority of the cardiac output (Fig. 15-4). When P_{alv} (and thus P_{VRG}) is much less than P_I, P_{MVR} is low, and the bloodstream is capable of carrying large amounts of anesthetic away from the alveoli to the tissues. Under these conditions, the rate of uptake of anesthetic from the alveoli into the bloodstream can be greatly modified by cardiopulmonary changes, and P_{CNS} can be greatly affected by changes in ventilation and cardiac output. As each successive tissue group approaches saturation with anesthetic, P_{MVR} approaches P_I. When P_{MVR} is nearly equal to P_I, the bloodstream cannot remove much anesthetic from the lungs under any circumstances, and changes in ventilation or cardiac output have little effect on P_{CNS}.

Upon commencement of anesthetic administration, the length of time during which there is a significant difference between P_I and P_{alv} increases with λ(blood/gas). With ventilation-limited anesthetics, such as diethyl ether and halothane, the prolonged time during which P_{alv} lags behind P_I allows cardiopulmonary changes to modulate P_{alv} significantly, potentially leading to unexpected CNS partial pressures. With perfusion-limited anesthetics, such as nitrous oxide, however, the alveolar partial pressure rises so rapidly that P_{alv} is significantly less than P_I for only a short time, minimizing the time during which cardiopulmonary changes could have a significant effect on P_{CNS} (Fig. 15-6).

Effects of Changes in Ventilation

Hypoventilation decreases the delivery of anesthetic to the alveoli. Meanwhile, removal of anesthetic from the alveoli continues provided that cardiac output is maintained. Consequently, the alveolar partial pressure rises more slowly, and $\tau\{P_{alv}{\rightarrow}P_I\}$ is prolonged. In other words, *hypoventilation slows induction*. This effect is greater with ventilation-limited than with perfusion-limited anesthetics (Fig. 15-9A).

General anesthetics themselves can cause hypoventilation by depressing the medullary respiratory center. In this manner, anesthetic-induced hypoventilation sets up a beneficial negative feedback loop on the depth of anesthesia. Increasing anesthetic depth leads to medullary depression, which, in turn, depresses respiration. The beneficial effect of this physiologic response is that the depressed ventilation slows the rate of rise of the alveolar partial pressure, while perfusion continues to remove anesthetic from the lung at the same rate (Fig. 15-5). Thus, P_{alv} falls, and shortly thereafter, the partial pressure of anesthetic in the medulla falls as well. This decrease in P_{CNS} relieves the respiratory depression. In the extreme example of a full respiratory arrest, there is no ventilation to deliver anesthetic to the alveoli, but cardiac output continues to distribute anesthetic from the alveoli and

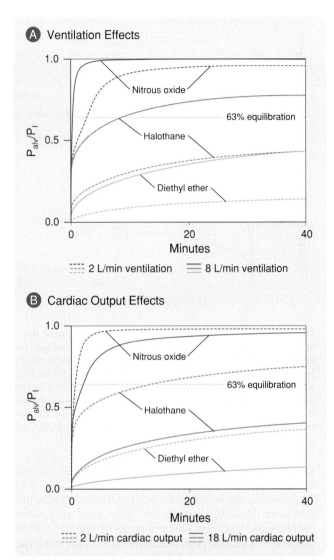

Figure 15-9. Effects of changes in ventilation and cardiac output on the rate at which alveolar partial pressure rises toward inspired partial pressure. The rate of equilibration of the alveolar partial pressure with the inspired partial pressure can be affected by changes in ventilation **(A)** and cardiac output **(B)**. Increasing ventilation from 2 L/min *(dashed lines)* to 8 L/min *(solid lines)* accelerates equilibration. On the other hand, increasing cardiac output from 2 L/min *(dashed lines)* to 18 L/min *(solid lines)* slows equilibration. Both effects are much larger for more blood-soluble gases, such as halothane and diethyl ether, which have rather slow induction times. For nitrous oxide, the rate of equilibration is so fast that any changes caused by hyperventilation or decreased cardiac output are small. The *dashed horizontal line* represents 63% equilibration of P_{alv} with P_I; the time required for each curve to cross this line represents $\tau\{P_{alv}{\rightarrow}P_I\}$.

VRG to the MG and FG. In the case of diethyl ether, the decrease in P_{CNS} can be of a sufficient magnitude that spontaneous ventilation resumes.

Hyperventilation delivers anesthetic more quickly to the alveoli. This decreases the time constant for equilibration of the alveolar with the inspired partial pressure (recall that $\tau\{P_{alv}{\rightarrow}P_I\}$ = FRC / V_{alv}, in the limiting case). The hyperventilation-induced hypocapnia may concomitantly decrease cerebral blood flow, however, increasing $\tau\{P_{CNS}{\rightarrow}P_{art}\}$.

Thus, while the partial pressure in the alveoli rises faster, the rate of equilibration between the CNS and the alveoli could be slower. The net effect depends on which of these two steps is rate-limiting. For perfusion-limited anesthetics such as nitrous oxide, the decrease in cerebral blood flow results in a slower induction. For the most soluble ventilation-limited anesthetics such as diethyl ether, the faster delivery of anesthetic to the alveoli hastens induction. For less soluble ventilation-limited anesthetics such as isoflurane, the effects roughly balance and induction is not significantly affected.

Effects of Changes in Cardiac Output

At anesthetic partial pressures higher than those required to depress the respiratory center, cardiac output falls. When cardiac output falls, the bloodstream removes anesthetic from the alveoli at a slower rate. Consequently, the alveolar partial pressure rises faster (Fig. 15-9B). Because the alveolar partial pressure equilibrates relatively quickly with the VRG (even at the lower cardiac output), the partial pressure in the CNS also rises more rapidly. In other words, *decreased cardiac output speeds induction*. This effect is more marked with ventilation-limited than with perfusion-limited anesthetics.

Moreover, cardiac depression by anesthetics sets up a harmful positive feedback loop on the depth of anesthesia. Increasing P_{CNS} depresses cardiac function, which further increases P_{alv}, which further increases P_{CNS}, which further depresses cardiac function. If cardiac arrest occurs, then positive measures must be taken to restore the circulation (e.g., CPR) while reducing the alveolar partial pressure through controlled breathing with oxygen.

Increased cardiac output increases perfusion to the lungs and accelerates equilibration between the alveoli and the tissues. However, because the increased blood flow to the lungs removes anesthetic from the alveoli at a faster rate, the rate of rise of the alveolar partial pressure is slowed. Thus, *increased cardiac output slows induction*. This effect is greater with ventilation-limited than with perfusion-limited agents.

Effects of Age

Relative to their body weight, young children such as Matthew have higher ventilation than do adults. This effect tends to speed induction. However, young children also have relatively higher cardiac output than do adults; this effect tends to slow induction. Although one might expect that these effects would cancel out, there are two additional factors to consider. First, the partial pressure of anesthetic in the mixed venous return rises more rapidly in children. This is because, relative to adults, a greater proportion of the blood flow serves the VRG in children, resulting in a higher partial pressure of anesthetic in the mixed venous return early in the course of anesthesia. Second, the increased cardiac output and the lower capacity of the tissues for anesthetic in children relative to adults both accelerate the rate at which the tissues become saturated with anesthetic. Both effects lead to a decreased alveolar-to-venous partial pressure difference, blunting the removal of anesthetic by the pulmonary circulation and moderating the extent to which cardiac output slows the rise in alveolar partial pressure.

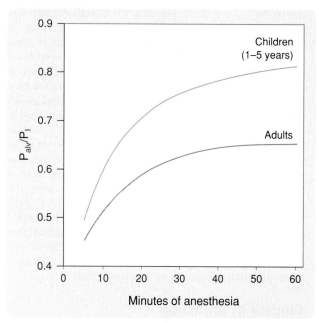

Figure 15-10. Anesthesia induction in children. Using halothane as an example, the alveolar partial pressure of anesthetic rises more quickly in children than in adults. The faster induction time in children results from a balance between children's increased respiration (favoring faster induction) and increased cardiac output (favoring slower induction); the time-dependent increase in the mixed venous partial pressure of anesthetic limits anesthetic uptake from the lungs, dampening the effect of increased cardiac output on induction time.

Thus, proportional increases in ventilation and cardiac output result in an accelerated rise of alveolar partial pressure and faster induction in children than in adults (Fig. 15-10). Ventilation-limited anesthetics, which are most affected by cardiopulmonary changes, have a markedly faster induction in children. Therefore, care must be taken to guard against the attainment of unexpectedly high (toxic) levels of anesthetic during anesthesia induction in children.

Effects of Abnormal States

In hemorrhagic shock, perfusion to the CNS may be maintained in the face of decreased cardiac output and hyperventilation. The decreased cardiac output and hyperventilation both accelerate the rise in alveolar partial pressure of anesthetic. P_{MVR} also rises faster because of the relatively greater perfusion to the VRG, lowering the ability of the pulmonary circulation to remove anesthetic from the alveoli and further accelerating the rise in the alveolar partial pressure. In patients with hemorrhagic shock, the additive combination of these effects can speed induction to a significant degree. In such cases, perfusion-limited anesthetics, whose kinetics are not greatly affected by cardiopulmonary changes, are preferred over ventilation-limited agents (Fig. 15-9).

In ventilation/perfusion (V/Q) mismatch (e.g., in chronic obstructive pulmonary disease [COPD]), some alveoli are underventilated and overperfused, while others may be adequately ventilated but underperfused. Because the alveolar partial pressure of anesthetic rises more slowly in the underventilated alveoli, the anesthetic partial pressure in the arterial blood leaving these alveoli is lower than normal. Conversely, the partial pressure of anesthetic leaving the adequately ventilated but underperfused alveoli is higher than normal. Because the former (overperfused) alveoli contribute a larger percentage to the overall perfusion, the weighted average partial pressure of anesthetic in the blood leaving the lung is decreased. Thus, P_{CNS} equilibrates with a lower than normal arterial partial pressure and may not achieve the level required to induce anesthesia. Therefore, higher inspired partial pressures are necessary to compensate for the effects of V/Q mismatch. This effect is mitigated somewhat with ventilation-limited anesthetics because the partial pressure in the underperfused but overventilated alveoli rises much faster than normal. For this reason, perfusion-limited anesthetics are most affected by V/Q mismatch.

Based on the principles and examples discussed above and summarized in Table 15-4, it should be possible to make reasonable predictions about the effect of other changes in cardiopulmonary function on anesthesia induction.

Control of Induction

An anesthesiologist can decrease induction time by setting the initial P_I higher than the final desired P_{CNS}. (This concept is similar to that of a loading dose, which is discussed in Chapter 3.) Because the time constant for equilibration of P_{CNS} with P_I does not depend on the absolute level of P_I, administration of anesthetic for a given amount of time always results in the same proportional equilibration of P_{CNS} with P_I. Consequently, a given absolute P_{CNS} is reached faster when P_I is higher because that P_{CNS} is a smaller fraction of the higher P_I. Dr. Snow took advantage of this concept by starting isoflurane at a P_I of 0.02 atm, even though the MAC of isoflurane is only 0.0114 atm. However, the anesthesiologist must remember to reduce P_I as P_{alv} approaches the target value, or, as demonstrated by Dr. Snow, P_{CNS} will equilibrate with this higher P_I and cause cardiopulmonary depression (Fig. 15-11).

RECOVERY

It is desirable that recovery from general anesthesia proceed quickly, so that patients can maintain their own airways as soon as possible following surgery. In general, the stages of recovery from anesthesia occur in the opposite sequence from those of anesthesia induction, including the unpleasant excitement stage (Fig. 15-1). During recovery, the partial pressure of anesthetic in the mixed venous return (P_{MVR}) is the weighted average of the partial pressures in the VRG, MG, and FG, with the VRG making the largest contribution (see Fig. 15-4). Ventilation removes anesthetic from the bloodstream into the exhaled air, and therefore, increased ventilation always accelerates recovery. As is the case with induction, recovery from anesthesia with perfusion-limited agents is rapid, whereas recovery from ventilation-limited agents is more prolonged.

Recovery differs from induction in several important ways, however. First, the anesthesiologist can increase the inspired partial pressure of anesthetic to speed the process of induction, whereas during recovery, the inspired partial pressure cannot be decreased below zero. Second, during induction, all of the tissue compartments start out at the same partial pressure (zero). In contrast, at the start of recovery, the compartments may have very different partial pressures depending on the duration of anesthesia and the characteristics of the anesthetic. The VRG quickly equilibrates with the alveolar partial pressure during most surgical procedures, but the MG may or may not equilibrate, and the FG equilibrates so slowly that, in all but the longest procedures, P_{FG} is far from equilibrium. Consequently, during recovery, perfusion **redistributes** anesthetic down its partial pressure gradient from the VRG to the MG and FG as well as to the lung. Because of this redistribution, the initial decrease in alveolar partial pressure during recovery is more rapid than the corresponding increase during induction. This initial decrease in alveolar partial pressure is dominated by the decrease in the VRG partial pressure. When the alveolar pressure falls to the level of the MG, then the decrease in the partial pressure of the MG becomes rate-limiting, and likewise subsequently for the FG. If the MG or both the MG and FG are heavily saturated following prolonged administration of anesthetic, then recovery will also be prolonged (Fig. 15-12).

Third, although anesthetic is delivered by one route, ventilation, it can be eliminated by both ventilation and metabo-

TABLE 15-4	Summary of the Effects of Physiologic, Pathophysiologic, and Clinical Variables on Rate of Induction of Anesthesia
CAUSE FASTER THAN USUAL INDUCTION	**CAUSE SLOWER THAN USUAL INDUCTION**
Hyperventilation (ventilation-limited anesthetics)	Hyperventilation (perfusion-limited anesthetics)
Decreased cardiac output	Hypoventilation
Young age (i.e., children)	Increased cardiac output
Shock	Chronic obstructive pulmonary disease
Thyrotoxicosis	Right-to-left shunt
Initial P_I higher than final desired P_{CNS}	

Based on the uptake model for inhaled anesthetics, the effect of changes in physiologic variables on the rate of induction can be predicted. Entities in the column on the *left* speed induction, while entities on the *right* slow induction, as discussed in the text. Note that the effect of hyperventilation depends on whether a ventilation-limited or perfusion-limited anesthetic is being administered (see text).

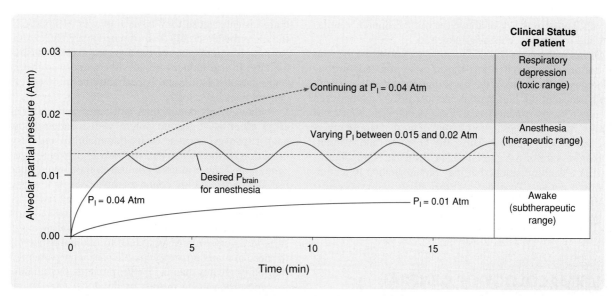

Figure 15-11. Applying overpressure to speed induction. Using halothane as an example, the anesthesiologist can use an initial P_I greater than the final desired P_{brain} to speed induction. If the desired partial pressure of anesthetic in the brain is about 0.01 atm, then the anesthesiologist could initially administer the inspired anesthetic at a higher partial pressure, for example, 0.04 atm. This method is effective because the time constant for $P_{alv} \rightarrow P_I$ is independent of the absolute value of P_I. In other words, if P_I is increased, then the ratio P_{alv}/P_I will increase proportionally at the same rate, resulting in a greater absolute rise in P_{alv} in a given amount of time. The anesthesiologist must be sure to decrease the inspired partial pressure in a timely manner, however, or the desired P_{brain} for anesthesia can be overshot and, instead, partial pressures capable of causing respiratory depression can be reached. On the other hand, if the inspired partial pressure is reduced too rapidly, the patient may awaken as P_{alv} is decreased because of uptake of anesthetic from the alveoli into the bloodstream *(not shown)*.

lism. In most cases, metabolism is not a significant route of anesthetic elimination. Halothane is an exception because metabolism may account for 20% of its elimination.

Finally, the outflow of high partial pressures of nitrous oxide into the lungs can cause an effect called **diffusion hypoxia.** To understand this, it is helpful first to understand

an effect on anesthetic induction called the **concentration effect.** When high partial pressures of nitrous oxide are administered, the rate of anesthetic uptake by the blood may be quite large, on the order of 1 L/min for a 75% nitrous oxide mixture. The absorbed gas is rapidly replaced by inspired gas flowing into the lung, effectively increasing alveo-

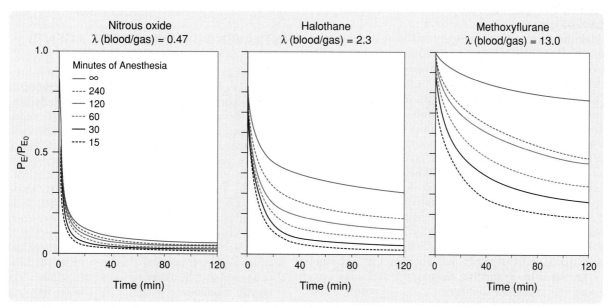

Figure 15-12. Recovery from inhaled anesthetics. These curves show, as a function of time, the exhaled partial pressure of anesthetic (P_E) as a fraction of the exhaled partial pressure at the moment administration of the anesthetic is stopped (P_{E0}). The rate of recovery is inversely proportional to the λ(blood/gas) of the anesthetic, because anesthetics with smaller λ(blood/gas) values equilibrate faster between alveolar and inspired partial pressures (the latter being zero after anesthetic administration is stopped). The rate of recovery is also proportional to the duration of anesthesia because the partial pressures of anesthetic in the muscle group and fat group increase with duration. During recovery, anesthetic redistributes from these slowly equilibrating, high-capacity tissues to the vessel-rich group, thus slowing the rate of fall of P_{brain}.

lar ventilation by 1 L/min above the normal minute ventilation and thereby accelerating induction.

Diffusion hypoxia is conceptually the opposite of the concentration effect. When anesthesia is terminated, nitrous oxide gas diffuses out of the blood into the alveoli at a high rate because of the high partial pressure difference between these two compartments (recall Fick's law). This volume of nitrous oxide displaces up to 1 L/min of air that would otherwise have been inhaled. Thus, the alveolar (and arterial) partial pressure of oxygen falls. The decrease is not significant for a healthy patient, but may be threatening to a compromised patient. To counteract this effect, pure oxygen is routinely administered for a few minutes following anesthesia with nitrous oxide, as Dr. Snow did for Matthew.

PHARMACOLOGY OF GENERAL ANESTHETICS AND ADJUVANTS

INHALED ANESTHETIC AGENTS

From the preceding analysis, we can distill two physicochemical properties of inhaled anesthetics that predict their behavior. First, the oil/gas partition coefficient predicts potency; *an anesthetic with a larger λ(oil/gas) is more potent and causes anesthesia at lower partial pressures.* Second, the blood/gas partition coefficient predicts the rate of induction; *an anesthetic with a smaller λ(blood/gas) has a shorter induction time.* Typically, there is a trade-off between fast induction and high potency. An anesthetic that has a rapid induction, as denoted by a small λ(blood/gas), typically has a low potency, represented by a small λ(oil/gas). Conversely, a very potent anesthetic with a large λ(oil/gas) typically has a large λ(blood/gas) and, thus, a long induction time (see Table 15-1).

Halothane has a high λ(oil/gas), providing high potency and, thus, low MAC; however, halothane also has a high λ(blood/gas), causing slow induction and recovery. The nonirritating smell of halothane makes it useful in pediatric anesthesia, but **sevoflurane** is increasingly replacing halothane for use in pediatric anesthesia (see below). One disadvantage of halothane is that toxic metabolites can result in fatal hepatotoxicity. The incidence of this serious adverse effect is approximately 1 in 35,000 in adult populations but much lower in pediatric populations; this is another reason for its continuing role in pediatric anesthesia. Another rare but potentially lethal adverse effect, seen most often with halothane but occasionally with the other halogenated anesthetics, is **malignant hyperthermia.** The susceptibility for this adverse reaction is inherited, typically as an autosomal dominant mutation in the sarcoplasmic reticulum Ca^{2+} channel (also known as the **ryanodine receptor**). In individuals expressing this mutation, halothane causes uncontrolled calcium efflux from the sarcoplasmic reticulum, with subsequent tetany and heat production. Malignant hyperthermia is treated with **dantrolene,** an agent that blocks calcium release from the sarcoplasmic reticulum.

Isoflurane and **enflurane** are somewhat less potent than halothane (they have a smaller λ(oil/gas)), but they equili-

brate faster because they have a smaller λ(blood/gas). Enflurane is metabolically defluorinated to a greater extent than isoflurane, and may thus have a greater risk of causing renal toxicity. It also induces seizure-like activity in the EEG of some patients. Isoflurane is probably the most widely used general anesthetic today.

Although less potent than isoflurane and enflurane, **diethyl ether** is still quite potent with a rather high λ(oil/gas). However, because of its flammability and very slow induction attributable to its extremely high λ(blood/gas), this agent is no longer in common use in the United States and Europe. In developing countries, however, its low price and simplicity of application favor its continued use.

Nitrous oxide has a very low λ(blood/gas) and thus equilibrates extremely rapidly. However, its low λ(oil/gas) results in a very high MAC, close to one atmosphere. Thus, the need to maintain an acceptable partial pressure of oxygen (normally greater than 0.21 atm) prevents the attainment of full anesthesia using nitrous oxide alone, and this agent is commonly employed in combination with other agents (see Balanced Anesthesia below).

Desflurane and **sevoflurane** are newer anesthetics that, by design, have low λ(blood/gas); times of equilibration between their alveolar and inspired partial pressures are nearly as short as that of nitrous oxide. Furthermore, they are much more potent than nitrous oxide because their oil/gas partition coefficients are higher. Thus, these agents offer great improvements over earlier agents. However, desflurane is a poor induction agent because its pungency irritates the airway, potentially causing cough or laryngospasm. Sevoflurane is sweet-tasting, but can be chemically unstable when exposed to some carbon dioxide adsorbents in anesthetic machinery, degrading to an olefinic compound that is potentially nephrotoxic. These disadvantages are being overcome with improved machinery, and sevoflurane is gaining in popularity.

INTRAVENOUS ANESTHETIC AGENTS

Intravenous anesthetics, such as **barbiturates** (see also Chapter 11), allow for rapid induction. Ultrashort-acting barbiturates, such as **thiopental,** are capable of inducing surgical anesthesia within seconds. As nonvolatile compounds, intravenous agents differ from inhaled anesthetics in that they cannot be removed from the body by ventilation. Accordingly, one must take great care during their administration to avoid severe medullary depression that is not easily reversible. The primary method of removal of these agents from the CNS is by redistribution from the VRG to the MG and finally to the FG. Metabolism and/or excretion then slowly decrease the overall body levels of drug (Fig. 15-13).

Propofol is an important intravenous anesthetic prepared in an intralipid formulation. This agent produces anesthesia at a rate similar to the ultrashort-acting barbiturates. Propofol is rapidly metabolized, resulting in a faster recovery than for barbiturates. Propofol is used both for induction and for maintenance, especially in short day-surgery procedures where its fast elimination favors prompt recovery and early discharge. The intralipid preparation of propofol can rarely be a source of infection, and the lipid preparation provides a large caloric source; these considerations can be important

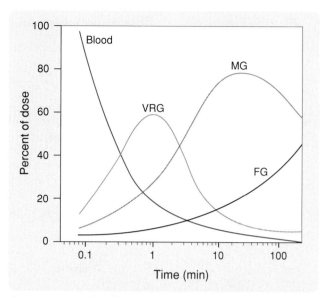

Figure 15-13. Distribution of a bolus of intravenous anesthetic. When a bolus of intravenous anesthetic is administered, it is initially transported through the vascular system to the heart and then distributed to the tissues. The vessel rich group (VRG) receives the highest percentage of the cardiac output; its anesthetic concentration rises rapidly, reaching a peak within 1 minute. Redistribution of anesthetic to the muscle group (MG) then quickly decreases the anesthetic level in the VRG. Because of very low fat group (FG) perfusion, redistribution from the MG to the FG does not occur until much later. Note that rapid redistribution from the VRG to the MG does not occur if the MG has previously approached saturation through prolonged administration of anesthetic *(not shown);* this can lead to significant toxicity if intravenous barbiturates are administered continuously for long periods of time. Newer agents, such as propofol, are designed to be eliminated by rapid metabolism and, therefore, can be used safely for longer periods of time.

in critically ill patients who may receive prolonged propofol infusions.

Etomidate is an imidazole that is used for induction of anesthesia because its kinetics are similar to those of propofol. This agent causes minimal cardiopulmonary depression, perhaps because of its unique lack of effect on the sympathetic nervous system.

Unlike the above agents, **ketamine** produces dissociative anesthesia, in which the patient seems to be awake but is actually in an analgesic and amnesic state. Ketamine has the unusual property that it increases cardiac output by increasing sympathetic outflow; for this reason, it is occasionally useful in emergency trauma situations. However, it can also produce unpleasant hallucinations. This agent is rarely used today.

ADJUVANT DRUGS

Adjuvant drugs provide additional effects that are desirable during surgery but are not necessarily provided by the general anesthetics. Benzodiazepines (see Chapter 11), such as **diazepam, lorazepam,** and **midazolam,** are often given for their anxiolytic and anterograde amnesic properties. These agents are administered 15 to 60 minutes before the induction of anesthesia to calm the patient and obliterate memory

of the induction, although they may also be used for intraoperative sedation. If necessary, benzodiazepine effects can be reversed with the antagonist **flumazenil.**

Opioids (see Chapter 16) such as **morphine** and **fentanyl** are used for their ability to produce analgesia. Their action can be reversed by an antagonist such as **naltrexone.** Opioids are poor amnesics, however, and are typically used in combination with a general anesthetic.

The combination of fentanyl and **droperidol** produces both analgesia and amnesia. This combination together with nitrous oxide is called neuroleptanesthesia (the prefix ''neurolept'' is added because droperidol is a butyrophenone antipsychotic related to haloperidol; see Chapter 12).

Nicotinic acetylcholine receptor blockers, such as the competitive inhibitors **tubocurarine** and **pancuronium** or the depolarizing inhibitor **succinylcholine,** are commonly used to achieve muscle relaxation (see Chapter 8). The effects of the competitive inhibitors can be reversed by an acetylcholinesterase inhibitor such as **neostigmine.**

BALANCED ANESTHESIA

No single drug achieves all of the desired goals of anesthesia. Accordingly, in a method termed **balanced anesthesia,** several inhaled and/or intravenous drugs are used in combination to produce the anesthetic state. The effects of simultaneously administered general anesthetics are additive. That is, 0.5 MAC of one inhaled anesthetic in combination with 0.5 MAC of another is equivalent in terms of potency to 1 MAC of either anesthetic as a single agent.

Using a mixture of inhaled anesthetics allows the two goals of potency and rapid recovery to be achieved. For example, although using nitrous oxide alone is generally impractical because the MAC of this gas is higher than atmospheric pressure, nitrous oxide is desirable for its fast induction and recovery characteristics and its high analgesic index. If nitrous oxide is part of the anesthetic mixture, then the nitrous oxide component of the anesthesia can be rapidly removed by ventilation during recovery or in an emergency situation. Matthew was able to awaken quickly from anesthesia because nitrous oxide was responsible for about half of his anesthetic state. He remained groggy because of the lingering isoflurane. The advantages of using isoflurane in combination with nitrous oxide include isoflurane's low cost and relatively low incidence of adverse effects (especially hepatic and renal toxicity) as compared to other anesthetics.

Dr. Snow's use of the intravenous agent thiopental in combination with inhaled anesthetic agents has a similar rationale. Short-acting intravenous agents can be used to induce stage III surgical anesthesia quickly, allowing the patient to pass through the undesirable excitement of stage II rapidly. Subsequently, the anesthetic depth can be maintained with inhaled anesthetics that could be removed by ventilation if necessary. Because intravenous agents act additively with inhaled anesthetics, less than 1 MAC of inhaled anesthetic will be required for as long as the intravenous agent is acting. As another example, the use of high concentrations of opioids in cardiac surgery allows the partial pressure of the inhaled anesthetic to be lowered significantly, reducing the risk of cardiovascular and respiratory depression.

Finally, balanced anesthesia is clinically useful because the anesthesiologist has more control if a separate drug is used to mediate each desired effect. For example, if the surgeon requires more muscle relaxation, the anesthesiologist can administer more of a neuromuscular blocking agent without having to increase the depth of anesthesia and potentially cause cardiopulmonary depression. Similarly, a bolus of a short-acting opioid can be administered immediately before a particularly painful surgical maneuver.

MECHANISM OF ACTION OF GENERAL ANESTHETICS

Despite intensive research, the exact mechanism of anesthetic action remains elusive. The **unitary hypothesis** states that a common mechanism accounts for the action of all anesthetics. Alternatively, each anesthetic, or each class of anesthetic, could have its own mechanism of action. The unitary hypothesis has been traditionally assumed, but recent research has shown that the situation is more complex.

A related question asks whether anesthetics have specific binding sites or act nonspecifically. Traditionally, several clues have suggested the absence of a specific site of action. First, molecules of disparate sizes and structures are capable of causing anesthesia (Fig. 15-14). Assuming the unitary hypothesis, it is difficult to imagine a specific binding site or receptor molecule capable of accommodating such an array of compounds. Second, stereoisomers of volatile anesthetics have generally been found to have equal potency. One criteria for specific binding is that stereoisomers should have different binding constants and, thus, different potencies. Finally, no pharmacologic antagonists of general anesthetics have been discovered to date, suggesting the lack of a specific site at which an antagonist could compete with a general anesthetic.

THE MEYER–OVERTON RULE AND THE LIPID SOLUBILITY HYPOTHESIS

Any proposed mechanism of anesthetic action should be consistent with the Meyer–Overton Rule, which suggests a hydrophobic site of action. The **lipid solubility hypothesis,** which postulates that this hydrophobic site of action is the lipid bilayer of a cell membrane, could account for both the Meyer–Overton Rule and the apparent nonspecificity of anesthetic action. According to this hypothesis, general anesthesia results when a sufficient amount of the anesthetic dissolves in the lipid bilayer and a fixed (''anesthetic'') concentration is reached. Most lipid theories postulate that the dissolved anesthetic perturbs the physical properties of the lipid bilayer, which in turn modifies the function of an excitable membrane protein.

Hyperbaric pressure, applied using a nonanesthetic gas (e.g., helium), can reverse anesthesia. This observation supports the lipid perturbation hypotheses, because anesthetics that dissolve in a membrane increase the membrane's volume (by approximately 0.5%) and fluidity. If this volume expansion is the mechanism of general anesthesia, perhaps

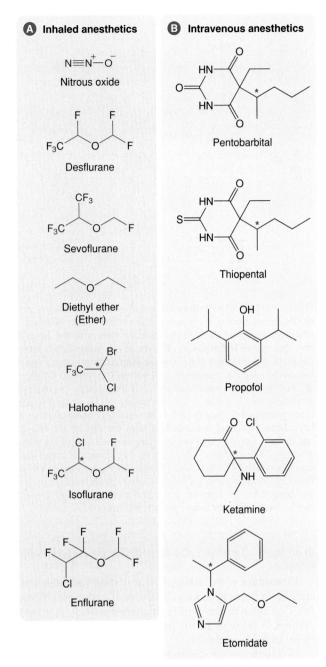

Figure 15-14. Structures of general anesthetics. A. Structures of some inhaled anesthetics. **B.** Structures of some intravenous anesthetics. The extreme variability in the structures of these molecules, all of which are capable of causing general anesthesia, suggests that not all general anesthetics interact with a single receptor site. * Indicates carbons where asymmetry results in enantiomeric structures.

by affecting excitable transmembrane proteins, then reversal of the volume and fluidity changes with pressure could reverse the anesthesia (this is called the critical volume hypothesis).

The main weakness in the lipid perturbation hypotheses is that no mechanism has been discovered that explains how the small magnitude of the predicted volume or fluidity change would alter the excitability of the cell membrane. The hypothesis has several more specific weaknesses. First, recent studies have shown that several potent intravenous anesthetics (such as barbiturates, etomidate, and anesthetic steroids) do exhibit significant stereoselectivity. That is, one enantiomer is more potent than the other. Second, many so-called **non-anesthetics** or **nonimmobilizers** are chemically similar to known anesthetics but do not cause anesthesia. For example, straight-chain alcohols with more than 12 carbons lack anesthetic activity, even though their λ(oil/gas) is larger than the shorter alcohols. Other compounds, called **transitional anesthetics,** have a much higher MAC than that predicted by the Meyer–Overton Rule.

Recently, refinements to the Meyer–Overton Rule have been proposed to account for some of the weaknesses listed above. If interfacial solubilities (i.e., the solubility of a compound at an aqueous–lipid interface) are considered instead of simple lipid solubilities, the Meyer–Overton Rule is much more successful at explaining the activity of transitional and nonanesthetic compounds. This finding is likely to mean that anesthetics act at a hydrophobic–hydrophilic interface. Examples of such an interface could include a water–membrane interface, a protein–membrane interface, or an interface between a hydrophobic protein pocket and the hydrophilic lumen of an ion-conducting pore.

EFFECTS ON ION CHANNELS

Current research has focused on proteins that may alter neuronal excitability when acted on by anesthetics, either directly or indirectly. Anesthetics affect both axonal conduction and synaptic transmission, but modulation of synaptic transmission occurs at lower anesthetic concentrations and is, therefore, likely to be the pharmacologically relevant action. Accordingly, anesthetics are thought to act on ligand-gated ion channels at lower concentrations than on voltage-gated ion channels. Both presynaptic and postsynaptic modulation occur, although the postsynaptic actions seem to dominate.

A superfamily of genetically and structurally related ligand-gated channels is sensitive to modulation by anesthetics at clinically relevant concentrations. Members of this superfamily have five homologous subunits, each with four transmembrane regions. The sensitivity of these ligand-gated ion channels to anesthetics can vary with their subunit composition. The superfamily includes the excitatory nicotinic acetylcholine and 5-HT$_3$ receptors, as well as the inhibitory GABA$_A$ and glycine receptors (see Fig. 8-2 and Fig. 11-8). Although receptors for glutamate, the major excitatory neurotransmitter in the brain, do not belong to this superfamily, NMDA glutamate receptors are also modulated by some anesthetics (e.g., ketamine and nitrous oxide).

Excitatory receptors (nicotinic acetylcholine, 5-HT$_3$, and NMDA) are inhibited by anesthetics. The binding of anesthetic to these receptors lowers their maximum activation, without changing the concentration of agonist required to achieve a half-maximal effect (EC$_{50}$) (Fig. 15-15). This action is consistent with noncompetitive inhibition and an allosteric site of action (see also Chapter 2).

In contrast, inhibitory receptors (GABA$_A$ and glycine) are potentiated by anesthetics. The binding of anesthetic to these receptors decreases the concentration of agonist required to achieve a maximum response, and thereby prolongs

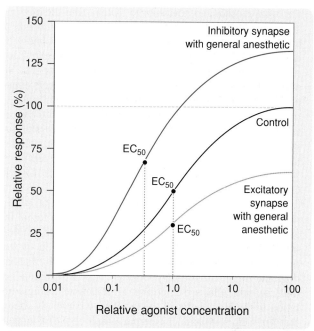

Figure 15-15. Actions of anesthetics on ligand-gated ion channels. Anesthetics potentiate the action of endogenous agonists at inhibitory receptors, such as GABA$_A$ and glycine receptors, and inhibit the action of endogenous agonists at excitatory receptors, such as nicotinic acetylcholine, 5-HT$_3$, and NMDA glutamate receptors. At GABA$_A$ receptors, anesthetics both decrease the EC$_{50}$ of GABA (i.e., GABA becomes more potent) and increase the maximum response (i.e., GABA becomes more efficacious). The latter effect is thought to be due to the ability of anesthetics to stabilize the open state of the receptor channel. At excitatory receptors, anesthetics decrease the maximum response while leaving the EC$_{50}$ unchanged; these are the pharmacologic hallmarks of noncompetitive inhibition.

the synaptic current. The activation curves for these receptors are shifted to the left (lower EC$_{50}$), and the maximal response often increases as well because the anesthetics stabilize the open state of the receptor (Fig. 15-15).

Until recently, GABA$_A$ receptors seemed to be the most relevant receptors for general anesthetic action, based on the sensitivity of GABA$_A$ receptors to clinical concentrations of anesthetics and the wide range of agents that act on these receptors. However, it now seems that glycine receptors and some neuronal acetylcholine receptors are equally sensitive to many anesthetics, and that nonpolar anesthetics such as xenon and cyclopropane (both of which have been used in clinical practice) as well as nitrous oxide and ketamine act by inhibiting nicotinic acetylcholine and NMDA glutamate receptors. Thus, it currently appears that an agent must cause either sufficient enhancement of inhibition (e.g., etomidate) or inhibition of excitation (e.g., ketamine), or a mixture of the two (e.g., volatile anesthetics), to cause anesthesia. This hypothesis also suggests that surgical anesthesia may not represent only one neurological state.

Direct anesthetic–protein interactions are probably responsible for the effects of anesthetics on ligand-gated ion channels. If anesthetics bind in the pore of excitatory channels, they could directly plug the channel. Alternatively, anesthetics could bind elsewhere on the protein and affect the channel's conformation (and, thereby, its equilibrium among the open, closed, and desensitized states). Site-directed mutagenesis, photolabeling, and kinetic studies suggest that inhibition of excitatory acetylcholine receptors probably occurs at a site in the ion channel that is on the central axis of symmetry and in contact with all five subunits. The site of anesthetic binding to inhibitory $GABA_A$ receptors cannot be in the ion pore because potentiation, not inhibition, is observed at clinical concentrations. Indeed, $GABA_A$ receptors lack a stretch of hydrophobic amino acids that is present in the pore of excitatory receptors. Instead, site-directed mutagenesis suggests an anesthetic binding site located on the "outside" of one of several alpha helices that line the $GABA_A$ ion channel.

Although the emphasis of current research is on protein sites of anesthetic action, no single site has been found that accounts for the Meyer–Overton Rule or the pharmacology of all general anesthetics. Consequently, adoption of such protein site theories may have to be accompanied by an abandonment of the unitary hypothesis. However, some new unifying principles are emerging. For example, a single mutation in the alpha helix of the $GABA_A$ receptor β_2 subunit that lines the ion channel (see paragraph above) attenuates the action of etomidate on this receptor. This mutation has no effect on the potency of volatile anesthetics. In contrast, the equivalent mutation in the α subunit attenuates the channel's response to volatile anesthetics but not to etomidate. Thus, although different classes of anesthetics act on different $GABA_A$ receptor subunits, it is possible that each class acts in a similar manner on the subunit to which it binds, and that selectivity is a function of the detailed architecture of each subunit at that site.

Conclusion and Future Directions

Inhaled and intravenous anesthetics provide the components of general anesthesia, including unconsciousness, immobility, and amnesia. The pharmacodynamics of general anesthetics are unique. Anesthetics have steep dose-response curves and small therapeutic indices, and they lack a pharmacologic antagonist. According to the Meyer–Overton Rule, the potency of a general anesthetic can be predicted simply from its oil/gas partition coefficient.

The pharmacokinetics of inhaled anesthetics can be modeled assuming three principal tissue compartments that are perfused in parallel. Equilibration of the partial pressure of anesthetic in the CNS with the inspired partial pressure proceeds in two steps: (1) equilibration between the alveolar partial pressure and the inspired partial pressure; and (2) equilibration between the CNS partial pressure and the alve-

olar partial pressure. With ventilation-limited anesthetics, which have a large blood/gas partition coefficient, the first of these steps is slow and rate-limiting. With perfusion-limited anesthetics, which have a small blood/gas partition coefficient, both steps are rapid and neither is clearly rate-limiting; changes in either can affect induction time. Recovery occurs roughly as the opposite of induction, except that redistribution of anesthetic from the vessel-rich group to the muscle group and fat group can also occur.

The "ideal" inhaled anesthetic has not yet been found. Future researchers may attempt to identify a nonflammable anesthetic with high λ(oil/gas), low λ(blood/gas), high therapeutic index, good vapor pressure, and few or no significant side effects. Currently, the combined use of adjuvants and balanced anesthesia with multiple inhaled and/or intravenous anesthetics achieves all of the goals of general anesthesia, including fast induction and a state of analgesia, amnesia, and muscle relaxation.

The exact mechanism of action of general anesthetics remains a mystery. Although the site of action was formerly thought to reside in lipid bilayers, direct interactions with several ligand-gated ion channels—members of the four-transmembrane–helices, Cys-loop superfamily and the glutamate receptor family—now seem to be more likely. More research is required to elucidate the mechanisms of action of general anesthetics. Once discovered, however, these mechanisms could shed light on such far-reaching issues as the generation of consciousness itself.

Suggested Reading

Campagna JA, Miller KW, Forman SA. The mechanisms of volatile anesthetic actions. *N Engl J Med* 2003;348:2110–2124. (*Article reviews how general anesthetics act.*)

Eger EI. Uptake and distribution. In: Miller RD, ed. *Anesthesia.* Philadelphia: Churchill Livingstone; 2000:74–95. (*Chapter covers the pharmacokinetics and uptake of inhaled anesthetics.*)

Rudolph U, Antkowiak B. Molecular and neuronal substrates for general anesthetics. *Nat Rev Neurosci* 2004;5:709–720. (*A short review with good diagrams.*)

Various authors. Molecular and basic mechanisms of anaesthesia. In: Hopkins PM, Lambert DG, Urban BW, eds. *Brit J Anesth* 2002;89:1–183. (*Postgraduate Educational Issue is a compilation of detailed reviews relating to all major current theories on the mechanism of action of general anesthetics.*)

Wiklund RA, Rosenbaum SH. Anesthesiology. *N Engl J Med* 1997; 337:1132–1151, 1215–1219. (*Two-part review covers many aspects of the modern practice of anesthesiology.*)

Winter PM, Miller JN. Anesthesiology. *Sci Am* 1985;252:124–131. (*Article is a good account of the clinical approach of the anesthesiologist.*)

APPENDIX A
Abbreviations and Symbols

P_I = inspired partial pressure

P_E = exhaled partial pressure

P_{alv} = alveolar partial pressure

P_{art} = arterial partial pressure

P_{tissue} = partial pressure in a tissue

P_{venule} = partial pressure in a venule

P_{MVR} = mixed venous partial pressure

$P_{solvent}$ = partial pressure in a solvent

P_{CNS} = partial pressure in the central nervous system

P_{VRG} = partial pressure in the vessel-rich group

λ(oil/gas) = partition coefficient defining solubility of a gas in a lipophilic solvent such as oil

λ(blood/gas) = partition coefficient defining solubility of a gas in blood

λ(tissue/gas) = partition coefficient defining solubility of a gas in a tissue

λ(tissue/blood) = partition coefficient describing ratio of solubility in tissue to solubility in blood

= λ(tissue/gas) / λ(blood/gas)

τ = time constant for 63% equilibration

$\tau\{P_{alv} \rightarrow P_I\}$ = time constant for 63% equilibration of P_{alv} with P_I

$\tau\{P_{tissue} \rightarrow P_{alv}\}$ = time constant for 63% equilibration of P_{tissue} with P_{alv}

[A] = concentration of gas A, in terms of either $L_{gas}/L_{solvent}$ or $mol/L_{solvent}$

CNS = central nervous system

VRG = vessel-rich group (includes CNS, liver, kidney)

MG = muscle group (includes muscle, skin)

FG = fat group (includes adipose tissue)

VPG = vessel-poor group (includes bone, cartilage, ligaments, tendons)

FRC = functional residual capacity of lung

V_{alv} = alveolar ventilation

CO = cardiac output

Q = perfusion rate

Vol_{tissue} = volume of tissue

MAC = minimum (or median) alveolar concentration

P_{50} = alveolar partial pressure sufficient for immobility in 50% of patients $\equiv$ MAC

AP_{50} = alveolar partial pressure sufficient to cause analgesia in 50% of patients

LP_{50} = alveolar partial pressure sufficient to cause death in 50% of subjects

EC_{50} = concentration of agonist required to activate 50% of channels

APPENDIX B
Equations

Gas Concentrations

In an ideal gas mixture: $[A]_{\text{mixture}} = n_A / V = P_A / RT$ {in terms of mol/L}

In solution (Henry's Law):

$[A]_{\text{solution}} = P_{\text{solvent}} \times \lambda(\text{solvent/gas})$ {in terms of $L_{\text{gas}}/L_{\text{solvent}}$}

$= P_{\text{solvent}} \times \lambda(\text{solvent/gas}) / 24.5$ {in terms of mol/L_{solvent}}

{where n_A = moles of gas A, V = total volume, P_A = partial pressure of A, R = universal gas constant, T = temperature in degrees Kelvin}

Meyer–Overton Rule

$MAC \approx 1.3 / \lambda(\text{oil/gas})$

Fick's Law for Diffusion Across a Boundary

Rate of diffusion = $D \times (A / l) \times \Delta P$

{where D = Diffusion constant; A = Surface area; l = Thickness; ΔP = Partial pressure difference}

Alveolar Capillary Rate of Uptake

Rate of uptake = $([A]_{\text{art}} - [A]_{\text{MVR}}) \times CO$ {in L_{gas}/min}

Rate of uptake = $\lambda(\text{blood/gas}) \times (P_{\text{art}} - P_{\text{MVR}}) \times CO$

{where CO = cardiac output}

Equilibration Time Constants (for 63% equilibration)

τ = Volume Capacity / Flow Rate

$\tau\{P_{\text{tissue}} \rightarrow P_{\text{alv}}\} \approx \tau\{P_{\text{tissue}} \rightarrow P_{\text{art}}\}$

= Volume Capacity of Tissue / Tissue Blood Flow

= $\lambda(\text{tissue/blood}) \times$ Volume of Tissue / Tissue Blood Flow

$\tau\{P_{\text{brain}} \rightarrow P_{\text{art}}\} = \lambda(\text{brain/blood}) \times$ Volume of brain / Blood flow to brain

$P_{\text{container}} = P_{\text{flow}} [1 - e^{-(t/\tau)}]$

Volume Capacity

Volume Capacity = $([A]_{\text{compartment}} \times$ Volume of compartment) / $[A]_{\text{medium}}$ {at equilibrium}

= $\lambda(\text{compartment/medium}) \times$ Volume of Compartment

Mixed Venous Partial Pressure

$P_{\text{Venous}} = 0.75 \, P_{\text{VRG}} + 0.18 \, P_{\text{MG}} + 0.055 \, P_{\text{FG}} + 0.015 \, P_{\text{VPG}}$

Drug Summary Table Chapter 15 General Anesthetic Pharmacology

INHALED GENERAL ANESTHETICS
Mechanism—Modulation of ligand-gated ion channels (most likely)

Drug	Clinical Applications	Serious and Common Adverse Effects	Contraindications	Therapeutic Considerations
Isoflurane Enflurane	General anesthesia Supplement to other anesthetic agents during obstetrical anesthesia	*Cardiovascular and respiratory depression, arrhythmias* Malignant hyperthermia Seizure (with enflurane)	Susceptibility to malignant hyperthermia Seizure (contraindication of enflurane only)	Less potent than halothane, but faster induction Pungency irritates respiratory tract Malignant hyperthermia is treated with dantrolene Enflurane has greater risk of causing renal toxicity than isoflurane
Halothane	General anesthesia	*Same as isoflurane. Additionally, can cause hepatitis and fatal hepatic necrosis*	Obstetrical anesthesia Susceptibility to malignant hyperthermia History of hepatic damage from previous halothane exposure	Less pungent than isoflurane; useful in pediatric anesthesia due to its non-irritating smell Toxic metabolites can result in fatal hepatotoxicity in adults High potency but slow induction and recovery
Diethyl ether	General anesthesia	*Same as isoflurane*	Susceptibility to malignant hyperthermia	Relatively high potency but very slow induction Pungency irritates respiratory tract Flammable; not in common use in the U.S.
Nitrous oxide	General anesthesia (usually used in combination with other agents)	*Can cause expansion of air collections such as pneumothorax, obstructed middle ear, obstructed loop of bowel, and intracranial air*	Should not be administered without oxygen Should not be administered continuously for more than 24 hours Pre-existing air collection	Rapid induction and recovery, but low potency Analgesia in subhypnotic concentrations The need to maintain an acceptable partial pressure of oxygen prevents the attainment of full anesthesia using nitrous oxide alone
Desflurane Sevoflurane	General anesthesia	*Same as isoflurane. Additionally, desflurane can cause laryngeal spasm*	Susceptibility to malignant hyperthermia	Newer anesthetic agents with relatively high potency as well as rapid induction and recovery Desflurane irritates the airway. Sevoflurane can be chemically unstable when exposed to carbon dioxide adsorbents in some anesthetic machinery

INTRAVENOUS GENERAL ANESTHETICS
Mechanism—Modulation of ligand-gated ion channels (most likely)

Drug	Clinical Applications	Serious and Common Adverse Effects	Contraindications	Therapeutic Considerations
Propofol	Induction and maintenance of anesthesia Sedation of mechanically ventilated patients	*Cardiovascular and respiratory depression* Injection-site reaction	Hypersensitivity to propofol	Induces anesthesia at a rate similar to the ultra-short-acting barbiturates and has a faster recovery than barbiturates; useful especially in short day-surgery procedures because of its rapid elimination
Thiopental	Induction of anesthesia Narcoanalysis Elevated intracranial pressure Seizure	*Same as propofol. Additionally, can cause laryngeal spasm, hemolytic anemia, and radial neuropathy* No injection-site reaction	Acute intermittent porphyria or variegate porphyria	Ultrashort-acting barbiturate capable of inducing surgical anesthesia within seconds
Etomidate	Induction of anesthesia	*Same as propofol. Additionally, can cause myoclonus*	Hypersensitivity to etomidate	Causes minimal cardiopulmonary depression, possibly due to lack of effect on the sympathetic nervous system

(Continued)

Drug Summary Table	**Chapter 15 General Anesthetic Pharmacology** (*Continued*)			
Drug	**Clinical Applications**	***Serious* and Common Adverse Effects**	**Contraindications**	**Therapeutic Considerations**
Ketamine	Dissociative anesthesia/ analgesia Sole anesthetic agent for procedures that do not require skeletal muscle relaxation	*Hypertension, tachyarrhythmia, myoclonus, respiratory depression, increased intracranial pressure* Hallucinations, vivid dreams, psychiatric symptoms	Hypersensitivity to ketamine Severe hypertension	Antagonizes NMDA receptor Increases cardiac output by increasing sympathetic outflow

BENZODIAZEPINES
Mechanism—Potentiation of GABA_A receptors

Diazepam Lorazepam Midazolam	See Drug Summary Table: Chapter 11 Pharmacology of GABAergic and Glutamatergic Neurotransmission			

OPIOIDS
Mechanism—Opioid receptor agonists

Morphine Meperidine Fentanyl Remifentanil	See Drug Summary Table: Chapter 16 Pharmacology of Analgesia			

NEUROMUSCULAR BLOCKERS
Mechanism—Depolarizing or non-depolarizing inhibition of nicotinic acetylcholine receptors

Tubocurarine Pancuronium Vecuronium Cisatracurium Mivacurium Succinylcholine	See Drug Summary Table: Chapter 8 Cholinergic Pharmacology			

16

Pharmacology of Analgesia

Robert S. Griffin and Clifford J. Woolf

INTRODUCTION

Everyone has experienced pain in response to an intense or noxious stimulus. This physiologic ''ouch'' pain helps us to avoid potential damage by acting as an early warning or protective signal. Pain can, however, also be incapacitating, as after trauma, during recovery from surgery, or in association with medical conditions that are characterized by inflammation, such as rheumatoid arthritis. Under circumstances where tissue injury and inflammation are present, noxious stimuli elicit more severe pain than normal because of increases in the excitability of the somatosensory system, and stimuli that would not normally cause pain become painful. In addition, nerve injury produced by disease or trauma, as in amputation, HIV infection, varicella zoster (VZV) infection, cytotoxic treatment, and diabetes mellitus, produces

pain that persists long after the initiating cause has disappeared. In these conditions, pathologic and sometimes irreversible alterations in the structure and function of the nervous system lead to severe and intractable pain. For such patients, the pain is the pathology rather than a physiologic defense mechanism. Finally, there are patients with no noxious stimuli and no inflammation or lesions to the nervous system, but who experience considerable pain. This dysfunctional pain, as in tension-type headache, fibromyalgia, or irritable bowel syndrome, results from an abnormal function of the nervous system.

These categories of pain—physiologic, inflammatory, neuropathic, and dysfunctional —are produced by a number of different mechanisms. Ideally, treatment should be targeted at specific mechanisms rather than at suppressing the symptom of pain. A number of pharmacologic agents are currently available to relieve pain. These drugs have mechanisms of action that interfere with the response of primary sensory neurons to somatic or visceral sensory stimuli, with the relaying of information to the brain, and with the perceptual response to a painful stimulus. The following discussion of pain and analgesic pharmacology begins by describing the mechanisms by which noxious stimuli lead to the perception of pain. The chapter continues by considering the processes responsible for the heightened pain sensitivity that occurs in response to inflammation and lesions of the nervous system. The chapter concludes by describing the mechanisms of action of the major drug classes used for clinical pain relief.

■ Case

JD, a 15-year-old boy, receives severe burns while escaping from a building fire. The extensive burns include first and second degree burns covering much of his body and a local, full-thickness burn on his right forearm. He reaches the emergency department in severe pain, and is treated with intravenous morphine in increasing quantities until he reports that the pain has subsided. This dose of morphine is then maintained. The next day, he receives a skin graft covering the region of his full-thickness burn. During the operation, an anesthesiologist provides a continuous intravenous infusion of remifentanil, with a bolus dose of morphine added 15 minutes before the end of the operation. At the end of the operation, and for 4 days thereafter, JD receives intravenous morphine through a patient-controlled analgesia device. As the burns heal, the morphine dose is tapered and eventually replaced with an oral codeine/acetaminophen combination tablet. Three months later, JD reports severe loss of sensation to touch in the area of the skin graft. He also describes a persistent tingling sensation in this area, with occasional bursts of sharp, knife-like pain. After referral to a pain clinic, JD is prescribed oral gabapentin, which partially reduces his symptoms. However, he reports to the pain clinic again 2 months later, still in severe pain. At this time, amitriptyline is added to the gabapentin, and the pain is further relieved. Three years later, JD's lingering pain has resolved and he no longer requires medication, but the lack of forearm sensation persists.

QUESTIONS

■ **1.** What mechanisms produced and sustained the pain that lasted from JD's exposure to the fire until his initial treatment?

■ **2.** What was the rationale for the sequence of medications used during the skin graft operation?

■ **3.** Why was morphine tapered gradually and replaced with a combination codeine/acetaminophen tablet?

■ **4.** Explain the mechanisms that could produce spontaneous pain in the region of the full-thickness burn months to years after healing of the skin graft, and the rationale for using gabapentin to treat JD's chronic pain.

PHYSIOLOGY

Pain is the end perceptual consequence of the neural processing of particular sensory information. The initial stimulus usually arises in the periphery and is transferred under multiple controls through sensory relays in the central nervous system (CNS) to the cortex. This system can be usefully analyzed in terms of the sites of action at which drugs intervene to produce analgesia. First, transduction of intense external, noxious stimuli depolarizes the peripheral terminals of "high-threshold" primary sensory neurons. The primary sensory neurons, called **nociceptors** because they respond to noxious stimuli, are high-threshold because they require a strong, potentially tissue-damaging stimulus to depolarize their terminals. The resulting action potentials are conducted to the CNS by the axons of the primary afferent sensory neurons, running first in peripheral nerves and then in dorsal roots, which then synapse on neurons in the dorsal horn of the spinal cord. The secondary projection neurons transmit information to the brainstem and thalamus, which then relay signals to the cortex, hypothalamus, and limbic system. Transmission is modulated at all levels of the nervous system by remote and local-circuit inhibitory and excitatory interneurons (Fig. 16-1).

SENSORY TRANSDUCTION: EXCITATION OF PRIMARY AFFERENT NEURONS

The peripheral terminals of primary afferent somatic and visceral sensory nociceptor fibers respond to thermal, mechanical, and chemical stimuli (Fig. 16-2). Highly specialized ion channels/receptors undergo conformational changes in response to one or more of these stimuli, and thereby mediate the depolarization (generator potential) necessary to initiate an action potential. The frequency and duration of the action potentials in the activated fiber then transfer to the CNS information about the onset, intensity, and duration of the stimulus.

Thermal pain sensitivity depends on distinct populations of primary sensory neurons: some become active at cold temperatures ($<16°C$), whereas others respond to heat. Heat pain-sensing neurons produce action potentials at temperatures above $42°C$. Responses to noxious heat involve thermosensitive non-selective cation channels, particularly **TRPV1**, which is a member of the transient receptor potential (TRP) family of ion channels. This channel becomes active in response to low extracellular pH, vanilloid chemical ligands such as capsaicin (the pungent ingredient in chili peppers), or heat in excess of $42°C$. In addition to TRPV1, a second vanilloid receptor, **TRPV2**, is activated only above $50°C$. Warm stimuli are transduced by TRPV3 and TRPV4 channels. TRPV heat-sensitive ion channels represent targets for the development of new drugs to interfere with peripheral heat sensation. In JD's case, the initial experience of pain was mediated by heat-activation of thermosensitive high-threshold peripheral neurons expressing TRPV1 or TRPV2. Cold is detected by two other TRP channels, TRPM8 for cool and TRPA1 for intense cold stimuli. TRPM8 is also

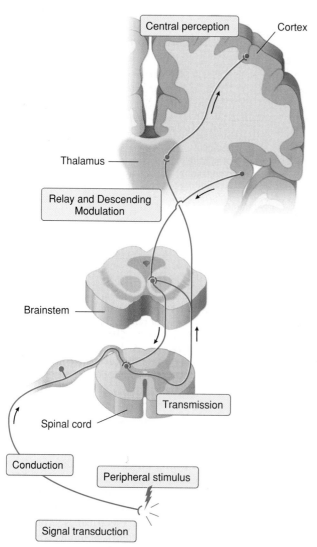

Figure 16-1. Overview of the nociceptive circuit. Activation of the peripheral terminal by a noxious stimulus leads to the generation of action potentials, which are conducted to the dorsal horn of the spinal cord. Neurotransmission in the dorsal horn relays the signal to CNS neurons, which send the signal to the brain. This circuit is also subject to descending modulatory control.

activated by menthol and TRPA1 by mustard oil, the pungent ingredient in mustard and wasabi.

Similarly, a specific subpopulation of primary afferent terminals (the high-threshold mechanonociceptors) is excited by relatively intense mechanical stimuli, such as a pinch or a pin-prick. This excitation is likely to be mediated both by TRPA1 and a family of cation channels, the degenerin epithelial sodium channels (ENaC).

The peripheral terminals of **nociceptor neurons** respond not only to thermal and mechanical stimuli, but also to multiple chemical signals. Some chemical agents directly excite peripheral terminals (**chemical activators**), whereas others increase the sensitivity of the peripheral terminals (**sensitizing agents**). Most known chemical ligands that evoke a somatosensory response are associated with cell injury or inflammation. These chemical ligands include protons, potassium ions, ATP, amines, cytokines, nerve growth factor

and bradykinin. For example, cardiac angina is a nociceptive event that involves activation of visceral chemotransducers in nociceptor neurons innervating the heart. These chemotransducers are activated by protons that are released by inadequately perfused myocardial tissue.

Several different types of chemical stimuli can excite nociceptor neurons (Table 16-1). First, low extracellular pH, which occurs in ischemia and inflammation, produces depolarizing cation influx through both TRPV1 and **acid sensitive ion channels (ASICs).** The acid-sensing sodium ion channels belong to a single superfamily, **degenerin/ENaC.** Second, elevated extracellular ATP concentration also signals cell injury, because cell rupture releases millimolar concentrations of ATP into the extracellular space (where the ATP concentration is normally very low). There are two major classes of ATP receptor, the **P2X** ligand-gated channels and the **P2Y** G protein-coupled ATP receptors.

Kinins are a third set of chemical stimuli that excite the peripheral terminals of sensory neurons. Kinin peptides are produced from kininogens by serine protease kallikreins; this process usually occurs in the setting of inflammation and tissue damage. Kinins act by stimulating **bradykinin B1** and **B2** receptors. The B2 receptor is constitutively expressed throughout the nervous system, while expression of the B1 receptor is induced in response to bacterial lipopolysaccharide and to the inflammatory cytokines IL-1β, TNF-α, IL-2, and IL-9. Both kinin receptors are G protein-coupled and increase intracellular calcium by production of inositol 1,4,5-trisphosphate. Activation of the B2 receptor also leads to the formation of prostaglandins E_2 and I_2. In the introductory case, as the heat sensation was followed by burn injury, these chemical mediators further contributed to JD's pain.

Each of these chemosensitive receptors represents a potential target for future drug development. Antagonists of the ASICs or P2X/P2Y channels and antagonists of the B1 or B2 receptors could be useful for reducing acute pain caused by tissue damage and inflammation. In addition, such antagonists could have a role in preventing peripheral sensitization during inflammatory pain (see below).

CONDUCTION FROM THE PERIPHERY TO THE SPINAL CORD

The axons of primary afferent neurons conduct information from the peripheral terminal to the CNS. These neurons can be classified into three major groups according to their conduction velocity and caliber; these groups also have distinct stimulus sensitivities and distinct central termination patterns. The first group (**Aβ**) consists of rapidly conducting fibers that respond with a low stimulus threshold to mechanical stimuli and are activated by light touch, vibration, or movement of hairs. Aβ fibers synapse on CNS neurons located in the dorsal horn of the spinal cord and in dorsal column nuclei of the brainstem. The second population (**Aδ**) includes fibers that conduct with intermediate velocity and respond to cold, heat, and high-intensity mechanical stimuli. The third group (**C fibers**) conduct slowly, synapse in the spinal cord, and typically respond multimodally; they are capable of producing action potentials in response to heat, warmth, intense mechanical stimuli, or chemical irritants (polymodal nociceptors). Some C-fiber afferents (referred

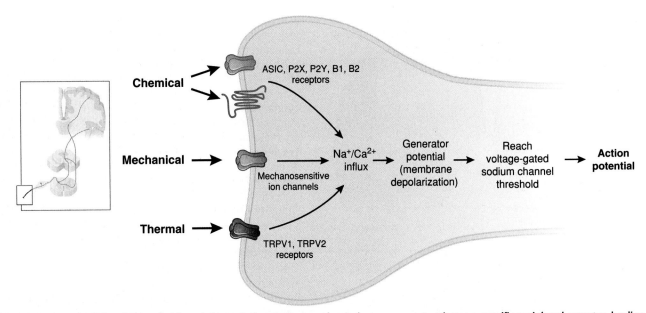

Figure 16-2. Peripheral transduction. A thermal, chemical, or mechanical sensory event activates a specific peripheral receptor, leading to ion influx and depolarization of the peripheral terminal. Thermal stimuli activate the transient receptor potential (TRP) vanilloid receptor 1 (TRPV1), or the TRP vanilloid-receptor like protein 1 (TRPV2), both of which are heat-sensitive cation channels. Chemical stimuli can activate acid sensitive ion channels (ASIC), ATP-sensitive P2X or P2Y channels, or kinin-sensitive B1 or B2 receptors. Mechanical stimuli can also lead to ion influx and depolarization, but the molecular identity of the relevant channels is not certain. In each case, the generator potential induced by the nociceptive signal leads to action potential production if the threshold for activation of the voltage-sensitive sodium channel is reached.

to as *silent,* or *sleeping* fibers) cannot be activated normally, but only become responsive during inflammation. Aδ and C fibers terminate in the most superficial laminae of the dorsal horn (lamina I and II).

For conduction to occur, voltage-gated sodium ion channels must convert depolarization of the peripheral terminal into an action potential. Six types of voltage-gated sodium channels are expressed in primary afferent neurons, of which four, $Na_v1.7$, $Na_v1.8$, $Na_v1.9$, and Na_x, are expressed uniquely in primary afferents. A gain of function mutation in $Na_v1.7$ contributes to erythromelalgia, an inherited condition associated with severe burning pain in response to mild thermal stimuli, by producing hyperexcitability of nociceptors. $Na_v1.8$ and $Na_v1.9$ are selectively expressed in small caliber neurons, most of which respond only to high-threshold peripheral stimuli (nociceptors). These two channel types also have higher activation thresholds and inactivate more slowly than other neuronal voltage-gated sodium channels. Because of their specific expression pattern in pain fibers, $Na_v1.8$ and $Na_v1.9$ represent pharmacologic targets of particular interest.

Selective blockade of these sensory neuron-specific sodium channels may inhibit pain induced in the periphery without blocking tactile sensibility or somatic or autonomic motor function and without acting on CNS or cardiovascular sodium channels. Currently, the use of sodium channel blocking drugs, such as local anesthetics (see Chapter 10, Local Anesthetic Pharmacology) and anticonvulsants (see Chapter 14, Pharmacology of Abnormal Electrical Neurotransmission in the Central Nervous System), is limited by the adverse effects associated with nonselective blockade of voltage-gated sodium channels.

TRANSMISSION IN THE DORSAL HORN OF THE SPINAL CORD

Action potentials generated in primary afferents induce neurotransmitter release upon reaching their central axon terminals in the dorsal horn of the spinal cord. **N-type voltage-gated calcium channels** have a substantial role in control-

TABLE 16-1	Chemosensitive Transduction Receptors Expressed by Nociceptor Neurons	
NOCICEPTIVE STIMULUS	**RECEPTORS**	**TYPE OF RECEPTOR**
Low pH (H^+)	ASIC	pH-gated ion channel
ATP	P2X	Ligand-gated ion channel
	P2Y	G protein-coupled receptor
Kinin peptides	B1	G_q protein-coupled receptor
	B2	G_q protein-coupled receptor

ling this neurotransmitter release from synaptic vesicles. A naturally occurring snail poison, omega-conotoxin, acts as a selective N-type calcium channel blocker; a synthetic mimic of this peptide **ziconitide** is currently used to treat severe pain conditions. However, such calcium channel blockers also alter the function of sympathetic neurons (producing hypotension) and many central neurons (affecting cognitive function). Thus, the use of these agents is limited to intrathecal administration, in an effort to localize their effects to the spinal cord. Use-dependent N-type calcium channel blockers may have a greater therapeutic index with less severe adverse effects. Drugs that bind to the $\alpha_2\delta$ subunit of calcium channels, such as gabapentin and pregabalin, may also produce their analgesic action by reducing transmitter release.

Synaptic transmission in the dorsal horn, between C-fiber primary afferents and secondary projection neurons, has fast and slow components (Fig. 16-3). Glutamate mediates fast excitatory transmission between primary and secondary sensory neurons. **Neuropeptides,** such as the tachykinins **substance P** and **calcitonin gene-related peptide (CGRP),** as well as other **synaptic neuromodulators,** including the neurotrophin **brain-derived neurotrophic factor (BDNF),** are co-released with glutamate and produce slower synaptic effects by acting on metabotropic G protein-coupled receptors and receptor tyrosine kinases. The presence of these co-released peptides allows considerable use-dependent functional plasticity of pain transmission. The physiologic function of the neuropeptides in synaptic transmission involves signaling responses to stimuli of particularly high intensity, because release of neuropeptide-containing synaptic vesicles requires higher-frequency and longer-lasting action potential trains than release of glutamate-containing vesicles.

DESCENDING AND LOCAL INHIBITORY REGULATION IN THE SPINAL CORD

Synaptic transmission in the spinal cord is regulated by the actions of both local inhibitory interneurons and projections that descend from the brainstem to the dorsal horn. Because these systems can limit transfer of incoming sensory information to the brain, they represent an important site for pharmacologic intervention. The major inhibitory neurotransmitters in the dorsal horn of the spinal cord are **opioid** peptides, **norepinephrine, serotonin (5-HT), glycine,** and **GABA** (Fig. 16-4). The physiology of GABA receptors is discussed in Chapter 11, Pharmacology of GABAergic and Glutamatergic Neurotransmission.

The opioid peptides inhibit synaptic transmission, and are released at several CNS sites in response to noxious stimuli. All endogenous opioid peptides, which include **β-endorphin,** the **enkephalins,** and the **dynorphins,** share the N-terminal sequence Tyr-Gly-Gly-Phe-Met/Leu. The opioids are proteolytically released from the larger precursor proteins pro-opiomelanocortin, proenkephalin, and prodynorphin. Opioid receptors fall into three classes, designated **μ, δ,** and **κ,** all of which are seven transmembrane G protein-coupled receptors. The μ-opioid receptors mediate morphine-induced analgesia. This conclusion is based on the observation that the μ-opioid receptor knockout mouse exhibits neither analgesia nor side effects in response to **mor-**

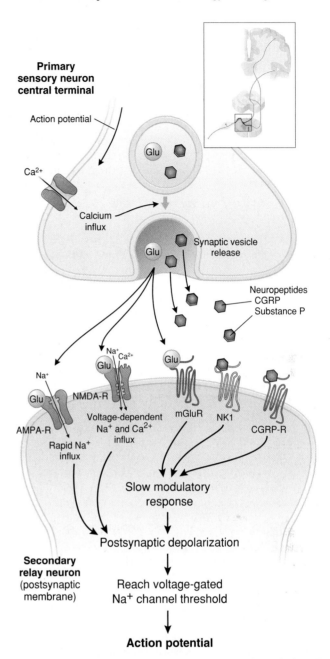

Figure 16-3. Neurotransmission in the spinal cord dorsal horn. An incoming action potential from the periphery activates presynaptic voltage-sensitive calcium channels, leading to calcium influx and subsequent synaptic vesicle release. The released neurotransmitters (i.e., glutamate and neuropeptides, such as calcitonin gene-related peptide [CGRP] and substance P) then act on postsynaptic receptors. Stimulation of ionotropic glutamate receptors leads to fast postsynaptic depolarization, while activation of other modulatory receptors mediates slower depolarization. Postsynaptic depolarization, if sufficient, leads to action potential production (signal generation) in the secondary relay neuron.

phine administration. The endogenous opioid peptides are receptor-selective; the dynorphins act primarily on κ receptors, while both enkephalins and β-endorphin act on μ and δ receptors. The effects of opioid receptor signaling include reduced presynaptic calcium conductance, enhanced postsynaptic potassium conductance, and reduced adenylyl cyclase

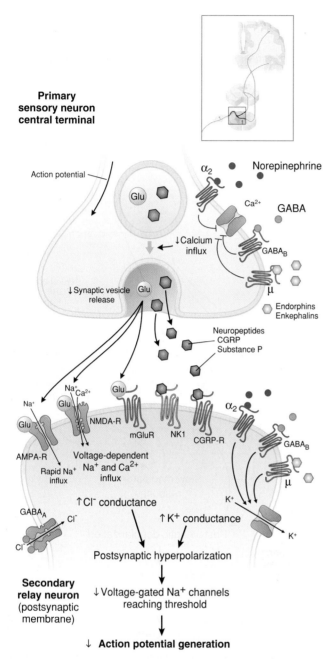

Figure 16-4. Inhibitory regulation of neurotransmission. Norepinephrine, GABA, and opioids, released by descending and/or local-circuit inhibitory neurons, act both presynaptically and postsynaptically to inhibit neurotransmission. Presynaptic inhibition is mediated through reduced activity of voltage-sensitive calcium channels, whereas postsynaptic inhibition is mediated primarily by enhanced chloride influx and potassium efflux.

activity. The first function impedes presynaptic neurotransmitter release; the second reduces postsynaptic neuronal responses to excitatory neurotransmitters; the physiologic role of the last remains unknown.

Opioids produce analgesia because of their action in the brain, brainstem, spinal cord, and peripheral terminals of primary afferent neurons. In the brain, opioids alter mood, produce sedation, and reduce the emotional reaction to pain. In the brainstem, opioids increase the activity of cells that

provide descending inhibitory innervation to the spinal cord; here, opioids also produce nausea and respiratory depression. Spinal opioids inhibit synaptic vesicle release from primary afferents and hyperpolarize postsynaptic neurons. There is also evidence that peripheral opioid receptor stimulation reduces the activation of primary afferents. Action of opioids at these serially located sites is thought to have a synergistic effect to inhibit information flow from the periphery to the brain.

Norepinephrine is released by projections that descend from the brainstem to the spinal cord. The α_2-adrenergic receptor, a seven transmembrane G protein-coupled receptor (see Chapter 9, Adrenergic Pharmacology), is the primary receptor for norepinephrine in the spinal cord. As with opioid receptor activation, α_2-adrenergic receptor activation opens postsynaptic potassium channels, inhibits presynaptic voltage-gated calcium channels, and inhibits adenylyl cyclase. Because α_2-adrenergic receptors are expressed both presynaptically and postsynaptically, spinal norepinephrine release can both reduce presynaptic vesicle release and decrease postsynaptic excitation. The α_2-adrenergic receptor agonist **clonidine** is sometimes used to treat pain, although this application is limited by adverse effects that include sedation and postural hypotension. Serotonin is also released in the spinal cord by projections that descend from the brainstem. This neurotransmitter acts on several receptor subtypes that mediate both excitatory and inhibitory effects on nociception. The 5-HT3 ligand-gated channel may be responsible for the excitatory actions of serotonin in the spinal cord; several of the 5-HT G protein-coupled receptors may mediate the inhibitory actions of 5-HT. Given this complexity, the mechanism of the analgesic effect is not fully understood. Selective serotonin reuptake inhibitors have been tested in the treatment of pain but generally have had little beneficial effect. Selective norepinephrine (NE) reuptake inhibitors do have an analgesic action, as do dual NE/5-HT reuptake inhibitors such as **duloxetine**. **Tramadol**, a weak centrally acting opioid, also has monoaminergic actions and is widely used to treat mild pain. Its relatively weak efficacy as a single agent is increased when combined with acetaminophen, and its lack of abuse potential makes the drug attractive to prescribers.

Other compounds also have regulatory roles in the spinal cord. The **cannabinoid receptors** and the endogenous cannabinoids have recently become a focus for research on pain regulation. There are two cannabinoid receptors, both of which are G protein-coupled: CB1, expressed in the brain, spinal cord, and sensory neurons; and CB2, expressed in non-neural tissues, largely in immune cells including microglia. Several endogenous cannabinoids, including members of the **anandamide** and **2-arachidonylglycerol** (2AG) families, have been identified. Anandamide and 2-AG are synthesized via separate pathways for immediate use without storage. Anandamide has relatively low efficacy at CB1 and CB2, whereas 2-AG has high efficacy at both receptors. Clearance of anandamide is mediated by fatty acid amino hydrolase (FAAH); 2-AG is cleared via monacylglycerol lipase. Anecdotal evidence suggests that marijuana has an analgesic effect in patients with AIDS neuropathy or multiple sclerosis. Selective cannabinoid receptor agonists and FAAH inhibitors under development may prove useful for pain management. Preclinical data have specifically implicated the CB1 receptor as a mediator of analgesia following a stressor, whereas CB2 receptors are up-regulated in spinal cord microglia after peripheral nerve injury.

Endogenous cannabinoids could modulate pain via cannabinoid receptors that are located peripherally or in the spinal cord and that affect nociceptive transmission, or via receptors in the periaqueductal gray that affect descending inhibitory projections. Centrally acting CB1 agonists could have psychotropic effects and may have abuse potential. CB receptor antagonists may be useful in the management of opioid-seeking behavior, and the CB1 receptor antagonist **rimonabant** has been shown safe and effective for the treatment of obesity in phase III clinical trials. Theoretically, CB receptor antagonists could have a pain-enhancing action by removing endocannabinoid tone.

PATHOPHYSIOLOGY

The pain processing circuit described above is responsible for producing acute **nociceptive pain,** a physiologic, adaptive sensation elicited only by noxious stimuli that acts as a warning or protective signal. There are some clinical situations, such as in acute trauma, labor, or surgery, in which it is necessary to control nociceptive pain. In these cases, the pain pathway can be interrupted either by blocking transmission with local anesthetics (see Chapter 10) or by administering high-dose opioids. The opioids may be rapidly acting, such as **remifentanil** for intraoperative use, or more slowly acting, such as **morphine**; administered perioperatively, morphine retains activity for postoperative pain control.

Both peripheral inflammation and nervous system damage produce pain that is characterized by **hypersensitivity** to noxious and innocuous stimuli and by **spontaneous pain** that arises in the absence of any obvious stimulus. Understanding the mechanisms responsible for these types of clinical pain will facilitate both the appropriate use of currently available drugs and the development of novel therapeutic agents.

CLINICAL PAIN

The ideal treatment of pain would be based on identifying and targeting the precise pain mechanisms operative in a particular patient. Clinical pain syndromes may involve a combination of mechanisms, however, and there are few diagnostic tools to identify which particular mechanisms are responsible. Chronic pain conditions can be complicated to treat, and effective treatment usually demands multiple drugs (polypharmacy) to obtain the optimal therapeutic effect while reducing adverse effects. Chronic inflammatory pain conditions require the use of drugs that reduce the inflammatory response; such drugs may both correct the underlying inflammatory condition (disease-modifying therapy) and reduce the pain. For example, the **non-steroidal anti-inflammatory drugs (NSAIDs)** (see Chapter 41, Pharmacology of Eicosanoids) are the first line of treatment for rheumatoid arthritis. By reducing inflammation, this intervention can decrease the release of chemical ligands that sensitize pe-

ripheral nerve terminals and thereby prevent peripheral sensitization (see below). Other disease-modifying anti-inflammatory treatments that may also reduce pain include cytokine inhibitors or sequestering agents such as TNF-α inhibitors, and immunosuppressants.

The major agents used to treat most noninflammatory neuropathic or dysfunctional pain conditions are generally not disease-modifying because the underlying disease processes are either not known (e.g., fibromyalgia) or refractory to currently available treatments (e.g., neuropathic pain). Neuropathic pain associated with peripheral nervous tissue damage, spinal cord injury, or stroke commonly requires the use of several agents to alleviate pain symptoms. Generally, in nonmalignant pain, opioids have been used as a matter of last resort because of their adverse effects and the potential for the development of tolerance and physical dependence (see Chapter 17, Pharmacology of Drug Dependence and Addiction). However, in recent years, opioids have increasingly been used for the management of chronic noncancer pain, albeit with the risks of producing drug-seeking behavior in a sizable proportion of patients as well as creating opportunity for diversion of the drugs for illicit use.

Severe acute pain due to injury or inflammation is usually treated with opioids, tramadol and fast-acting NSAIDs. For example, the pain of setting a fracture can be ameliorated effectively by the opioid remifentanil, which acts rapidly and is cleared rapidly. A more serious operative procedure, involving tissue damage that takes time to heal, may call for longer-acting agents to control postoperative pain. Acute inflammatory pain conditions, such as pancreatitis, are often treated with morphine. Gout, a second example of an acute inflammatory condition producing severe pain, is usually treated with indomethacin (an NSAID) to reduce the pain rapidly, whereas more specific disease-modifying agents are used to correct the underlying disorder over the longer term (see Chapter 47, Integrative Inflammation Pharmacology: Gout).

PERIPHERAL SENSITIZATION

Several peripheral stimuli can induce primary afferent neurons to lower their activation thresholds and increase their responsiveness (Fig. 16-5). These alterations, which constitute **peripheral sensitization,** can result in **allodynia,** in which normally innocuous stimuli are perceived as painful, and **hyperalgesia,** in which high-intensity stimuli are perceived as more painful than usual at the site of injury (zone of primary hyperalgesia). The mechanisms responsible for primary hyperalgesia involve both direct changes in transduction and indirect changes induced by the release of effector molecules. An example of altered transduction is the repeated heat activation of the TRPV1 receptor, which reduces its activation threshold so that it can be activated by warm stimuli (38–40°C) that are normally not painful. The major known effectors that produce peripheral sensitization are the inflammatory mediators bradykinin, protons, histamine, prostaglandin E_2, and nerve growth factor (NGF). Prostaglandin E_2 acts on EP receptors, of which there are four types, while NGF acts on TrkA receptors. The actions of histamine are more prominent on sensory neurons that contribute to itch.

Sensitizing chemical mediators act on G protein-coupled

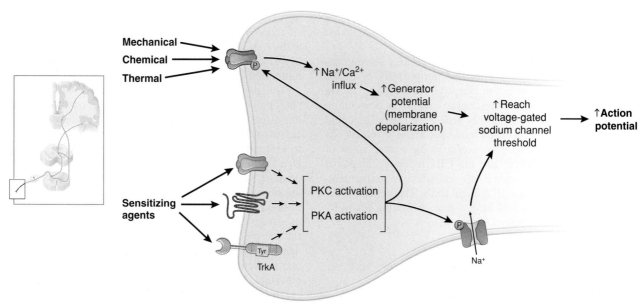

Figure 16-5. Peripheral sensitization. Peripherally released sensitizing agents activate signal transduction that can increase sensitivity of the peripheral nerve terminal. Mechanisms mediating increased sensitivity include: (1) enhancement of ion influx in response to a noxious stimulus, and (2) reduction of the activation threshold of the voltage-sensitive sodium channels responsible for initiating and propagating action potentials. In the example shown, a sensitizing agent activates its G protein-coupled receptor. This receptor initiates two parallel signaling cascades. One branch activates the phospholipase C (PLC) pathway, which results in increased release of calcium from intracellular stores and in activation of protein kinase C (PKC). Both of these effects increase the ion influx in response to a nociceptive stimulus. The second branch of the signaling cascade activates adenylyl cyclase (AC), leading to increased formation of cAMP, activation of protein kinase A (PKA), and ion channel phosphorylation. Both signaling cascades serve to increase the likelihood of action potential initiation and propagation.

receptors or receptor tyrosine kinases expressed on the peripheral terminals of nociceptor neurons. Activation of phospholipase C, phospholipase A_2, and adenylyl cyclase occurs in response to the activation of G protein-coupled receptors, such as those for bradykinin, prostaglandin E2, and adenosine. In turn, these signaling enzymes generate mediators that activate protein kinase A (PKA) or protein kinase C (PKC). Protein kinase A phosphorylates the voltage-gated sodium channel $Na_v1.8$, resulting in both a decrease in its activation threshold and an increase in the current passed when the channel opens. Protein kinase C phosphorylates TRPV1, thus reducing its threshold and thereby increasing the response of peripheral terminals to heat stimuli.

In addition to the enhancement of peripheral response caused by an outside event that produces inflammation, the peripheral terminals themselves can contribute to inflammation (the neurogenic component of inflammation). Depolarization and chemical stimuli induce the release of neuropeptides, such as substance P and CGRP, from the peripheral terminals of primary afferents. This peripheral neuropeptide release produces vasodilation and increases capillary permeability, contributing to the wheal and flare response to tissue injury. In addition, neuropeptides induce the release of histamine and TNF-α from inflammatory cells. The recruitment and activation of granulocytes, as well as the increase in local capillary diameter and permeability to plasma, results in a local inflammatory response at the site of the excited peripheral terminal.

Peripheral sensitization is an important target for clinical pain pharmacology. The NSAIDs are the most widely used pain treatment. By inhibiting the activity of cyclooxygenase enzymes, NSAIDs reduce prostaglandin production and,

hence, the local inflammatory response and peripheral sensitization. There are two isoforms of cyclooxygenase, COX-1 and COX-2 (see Chapter 41). The former is constitutively active and is important in a variety of physiologic functions, such as maintenance of gastric mucosal integrity and normal platelet function. COX-2 is selectively up-regulated at the site of inflammation in response to local secretion of cytokines, particularly IL-1β and TNF-α acting via the transcription factor NF-κB. Selective inhibitors of COX-2, such as **celecoxib, rofecoxib** and **valdecoxib,** were developed in an attempt to control inflammatory pain while decreasing some of the dangerous adverse effects of the nonselective NSAIDs, such as gastrointestinal bleeding. However, large post-marketing trials have revealed an increased incidence of serious cardiovascular effects, including an increased risk of myocardial infarction, associated with COX-2 inhibitor therapy. This has led to the withdrawal of several COX-2 selective inhibitors. It is not clear whether the cardiovascular effects are a class effect for all NSAIDs or all COX-2 inhibitors, or specific to some compounds within the class. In addition to the cyclooxygenases, the transduction molecules, signaling intermediates, and sodium channels expressed at peripheral terminals may all represent targets for the development of new analgesic drugs that reduce peripheral pain hypersensitivity.

In the case of JD, peripheral sensitization was induced at the burn site. The high-intensity stimulus led to neurogenic inflammation. The associated tissue damage further potentiated inflammatory mediator release, leading to the activation of second messenger cascades that heightened peripheral terminal excitability over time.

CENTRAL SENSITIZATION

Frequently, hyperalgesia and allodynia extend beyond the primary area of inflammation and tissue damage. Pain hypersensitivity in this region, described as the area of secondary hyperalgesia and/or allodynia, depends on alterations in sensory processing in the dorsal horn of the spinal cord. These alterations, which are a form of neuronal plasticity termed **central sensitization,** occur when repetitive, usually high-intensity, synaptic transmission activates intracellular signal transduction cascades in dorsal horn neurons that enhance the response to subsequent stimuli.

Several of the postsynaptic receptors expressed by dorsal horn neurons are involved in the induction of central sensitization (Fig. 16-6). These receptors include AMPA, NMDA, and metabotropic glutamate receptors, as well the substance P (neurokinin) receptor NK1 and the BDNF (neurotrophin) receptor TrkB. Upon activation of metabotropic receptors or calcium influx through NMDA channels, intracellular protein kinases, such as calcium/calmodulin kinase, PKC, and extracellular signal-related protein kinase (ERK), are activated. In turn, these effectors can alter the function of existing membrane proteins by post-translational processing, usually by phosphorylation. For example, after NMDA receptors are phosphorylated, they open more rapidly and for longer periods in response to glutamate. Phosphorylation of AMPA receptors results in their translocation from cytosolic stores to the membrane, thus increasing synaptic efficacy. Activation of ERKs leads to a reduction in potassium channel activity in dorsal horn neurons; the decreased potassium current increases neuronal excitability. Most often, central sensitization slowly subsides after the inducing stimulus ceases. However, chronic injury or inflammation can produce a state of central sensitization that persists over time.

NMDA receptor blockade can prevent both the induction and maintenance of central sensitization. For example, NMDA receptor blockade instituted preoperatively has been shown to reduce pain experienced postoperatively. A component of postoperative pain is likely attributable to NMDA receptor-dependent central sensitization associated with the intense peripheral stimulation that occurs during surgery. The NMDA receptor blocker **ketamine** can be used in burn patients to oppose activation of sensitized NMDA receptors. NMDA receptors are widely expressed, however, and NMDA blockers such as ketamine and **dextromethorphan** produce significant psychotropic effects, including amnesia and hallucinations. Protein kinase C or ERK are alternative targets. Although many of the signaling proteins involved in dorsal horn sensitization are expressed in all cells, it may be possible to target treatment to the spinal cord by intrathecal or epidural injection.

The intense peripheral activation produced by JD's burn injury also led to the development of central sensitization. This effect further enhanced the lingering pain he felt at the burn site and also produced pain surrounding the burn site, outside the primary area of tissue damage and inflammation.

NEUROPATHIC PAIN

The mechanisms responsible for the persistent pain that can occur following nerve injury involve both functional and

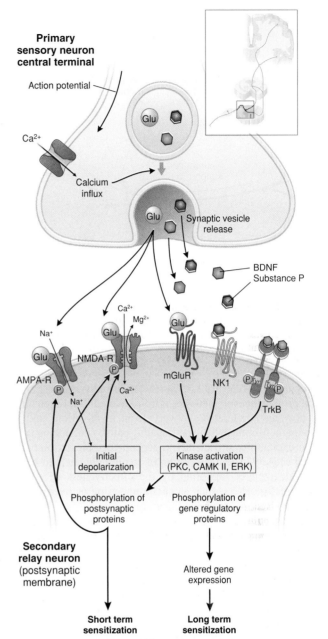

Figure 16-6. Central sensitization. Sustained or intense activation of central transmission can lead to postsynaptic calcium influx, primarily through NMDA receptors. Together with a variety of neuromodulatory signals, calcium influx activates signal transduction cascades that can enhance both short-term and long-term excitability of the synapse.

structural alterations in the nervous system, and occur in both primary afferent neurons and the CNS (Fig. 16-7). In the periphery, changes in the physiology and transcriptional profile of primary afferent sensory neurons occur after nerve damage, contributing to neuropathic pain. These alterations are induced by combinations of positive signals, such as inflammatory cytokine release by macrophages and Schwann cells, and negative signals, such as the loss of peripheral support from neurotrophic factors. In addition, the expression pattern of sodium channels changes in injured primary sensory neurons: $Na_v1.8$ and $Na_v1.9$ are down-

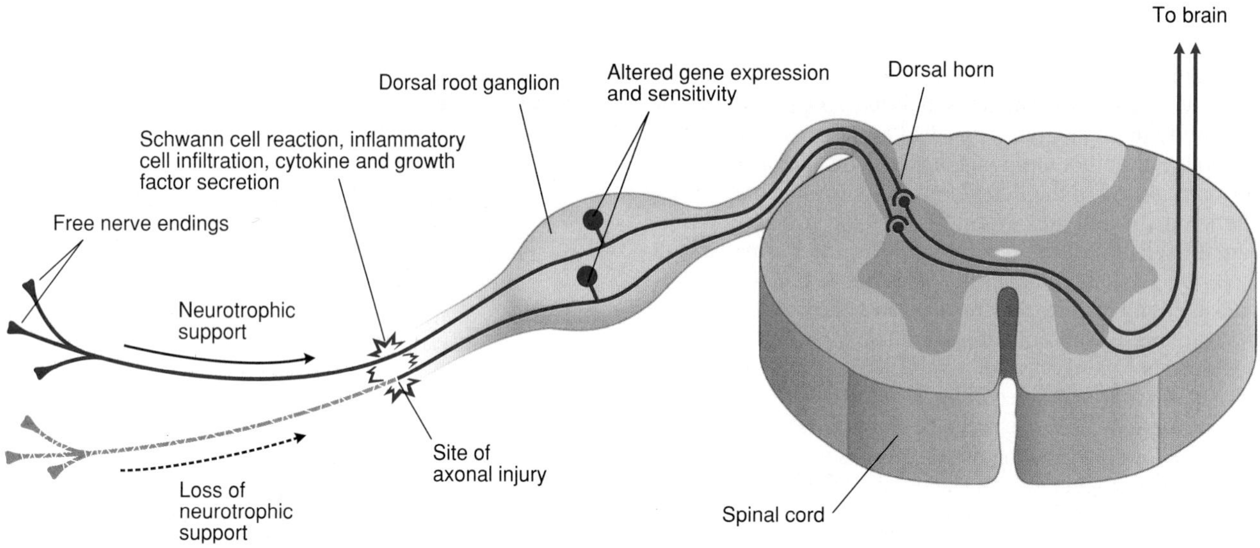

Figure 16-7. Schematization of neuropathic pain. Nerve injury results in a combination of negative signals and positive signals that alter the physiology of the nociceptive system. The loss of neurotrophic support alters gene expression in the injured nerve fiber, whereas the release of inflammatory cytokines alters gene expression in both the injured and adjacent uninjured nerve fibers. These changes in gene expression can lead to altered sensitivity and activity of nociceptive fibers, and, thus, to the continued perception of injury that is characteristic of neuropathic pain.

regulated, while $Na_v1.3$, which is normally not detectable in primary sensory neurons, is up-regulated. $Na_v1.3$ channels show an accelerated recovery from inactivation, and are thought to contribute to neuropathic pain by enhancing cellular excitability sufficiently to generate ectopic action potential activity. The contribution of sodium channels to neuropathic pain is supported by the effectiveness of sodium channel blockers, such as **carbamazepine** or **oxcarbazepine,** in treating trigeminal neuralgia.

Nerve damage also promotes reorganization of synaptic connection patterns within the dorsal horn of the spinal cord. Peripheral nerve injury leads to a regenerative response. Because primarily C fibers are lost upon the withdrawal of peripheral trophic support, regenerating central terminals of Aβ fibers are free to invade the area normally occupied by the central terminals of C fibers. Another structural change is an excitotoxic loss of inhibitory neurons in the dorsal horn after peripheral nerve injury. The loss of inhibition (disinhibition) contributes to the heightened pain sensitivity. Neuroprotective treatment designed to prevent transynaptic neurodegeneration might represent an opportunity for a disease-modifying approach to neuropathic pain, particularly when the time of nerve damage can be identified (e.g., after surgery). It may be possible to treat both the transcriptional changes and some of the structural alterations in circuitry with neurotrophic factors. A combination of these mechanisms would have been involved in maintaining JD's pain over the years following his operation.

MIGRAINE

Migraine headaches, a highly prevalent spontaneous pain condition, involve certain unique pathophysiologic mechanisms that are not completely understood. The leading theory for the pathophysiology of these headaches involves four events. First, before the headache occurs, a region of neural activation followed by inactivation travels across the cortex. This phenomenon is termed **cortical spreading depression** and is correlated with the sensory disturbances of the migraine aura such as scotoma (visual field disturbances). Second, neuropeptide (particularly CGRP) release, possibly evoked by the cortical excitation, occurs in the dural vasculature. Third, trigeminal afferents from the dural vasculature are activated and sensitized by the local release of neuropeptides and inflammatory mediators. Fourth, the high degree of activity in trigeminal afferent high-threshold fibers produces central sensitization, leading to secondary hyperalgesia and tactile allodynia. Thus, a migraine attack can be considered the acute manifestation of abnormal intermittent peripheral and central excitability.

PHARMACOLOGIC CLASSES AND AGENTS

Several drug classes are widely used for pain relief. These include **opioid receptor agonists, NSAIDs** (see Chapter 41), **tricyclic antidepressants** (see Chapter 13, Pharmacology of Serotonergic and Central Adrenergic Neurotransmission), **anticonvulsants** (sodium channel blockers) (see Chapter 14, Pharmacology of Abnormal Electrical Neurotransmission in the Central Nervous System), **NMDA receptor antagonists** (see Chapter 11, Pharmacology of GABAergic and Glutamatergic Neurotransmission), and **adrenergic agonists.** In addition, **$5HT_1$ receptor agonists** have specific applications in the acute treatment of migraine.

OPIOID RECEPTOR AGONISTS

Opioid receptor agonists are the primary drug class used in the acute management of moderate to severe pain. The naturally occurring opioid receptor agonist **morphine** has the greatest historical importance and remains in wide use, but synthetic and semisynthetic opioids add pharmacokinetic versatility. Historically, opioids have been most widely used to treat acute and cancer-related pain, but in recent years they have become one component of the management of chronic noncancer pain as well.

Mechanism of Action and Major Adverse Effects

Opioid receptor agonists produce both analgesia and other effects by acting on μ-opioid receptors (Fig. 16-8). Sites of analgesic action include the brain, brainstem, spinal cord, and primary afferent peripheral terminals, as described previously. Through receptors in the medullary respiratory control center, the medullary chemoreceptor zone, and the gastrointestinal tract, opioids also produce respiratory depression, nausea and vomiting, and constipation, respectively. In addition, opioids can cause sedation, confusion, dizziness, and euphoria.

Opioid use is often associated with the development of **tolerance,** in which repeated use of a constant dose of a drug results in a decreased therapeutic effect (see Chapter 17, Pharmacology of Drug Dependence and Addiction). The molecular mechanisms responsible for tolerance remain a matter of debate, and may involve a combination of gene regulation and post-translational modification of opioid receptor activity. The development of tolerance requires either a change of analgesic drug or an increase in the dose or frequency of administration to maintain analgesia. **Physical dependence** can also occur, such that abrupt cessation of treatment results in a characteristic withdrawal syndrome. **Addiction,** in which physical dependence is accompanied by substance abuse or drug-seeking behavior, is a potential adverse effect of opioid administration. The incidence and prevalence of opioid addiction in patients receiving opioids for therapeutic reasons remain unknown, but is not negligible. Balancing the risk of opioid addiction against the undertreatment of pain is a complex issue in pain management and a topic of considerable debate. In JD's case, intravenous morphine was tapered and replaced with a combined oral analgesic to prevent the onset of opioid withdrawal symptoms.

Morphine, Codeine, and Derivatives

Morphine, **codeine (methylmorphine),** and their semisynthetic derivatives are the most widely used opioids for pain control. Morphine is typically considered the reference opioid against which others are compared. It is metabolized in the liver, and its first-pass metabolism reduces its oral availability. In the liver, morphine undergoes glucuronidation at either the 3 position (M3G) or the 6 position (M6G). While M3G is inactive, M6G has analgesic activity. M6G is excreted by the kidney, and its accumulation in patients with chronic kidney disease may contribute to opioid toxicity.

To meet the needs of its diverse indications, several different routes are available for administering morphine. Controlled-release oral preparations are marketed to reduce the number of daily doses required for analgesia. These formulations contain a high dose of opioid designed for release over

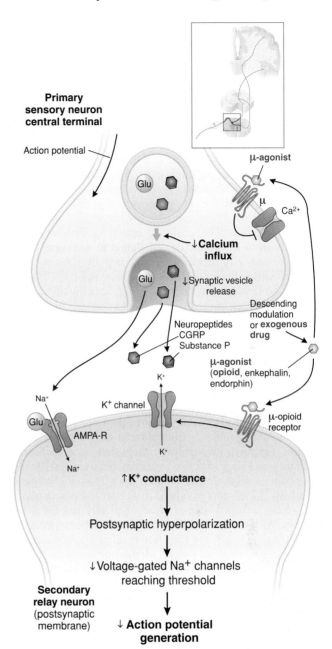

Figure 16-8. Mechanism of action of μ-opioid receptor agonists in the spinal cord. Activation of both presynaptic and postsynaptic μ-opioid receptors by descending and local-circuit inhibitory neurons inhibits central relaying of nociceptive stimuli. In the presynaptic terminal, μ-opioid receptor activation decreases Ca^{2+} influx in response to an incoming action potential. Post-synaptic μ-opioid receptor activation increases K^+ conductance and thereby decreases the postsynaptic response to excitatory neurotransmission.

the course of 12–24 hours. Unfortunately, because they contain high doses and are in widespread use, sustained release formulations have been associated with a high abuse potential, especially when they are illegally reformulated to deliver the entire dose at once rather than over the course of hours. Abusers of these formulations seek a ''high'' from a rapid increase in plasma levels. Intravenous or subcutaneous morphine is commonly administered in patient-controlled analgesia devices, which are used in treating cancer pain and the severe acute pains of trauma, burn, surgical operation, and vaso-occlusive crisis in sickle cell disease. Epidural or intrathecal morphine can produce highly effective analgesia by achieving locally high concentrations in the dorsal horn of the spinal cord. Epidural administration of the drug results in a much longer duration of action than does parenteral administration, because of the time required for morphine, a relatively hydrophilic compound, to diffuse out of the CNS into the systemic circulation.

Codeine, like morphine, is a naturally occurring opioid receptor agonist. Although much less effective than morphine for the treatment of pain, codeine is commonly used for its antitussive (i.e., cough-suppressing) and antidiarrheal effects because it has considerably higher oral availability than morphine. The analgesic action of codeine results largely from its hepatic demethylation to morphine, which has substantially greater μ-agonist activity. Genetic polymorphisms in the cytochrome P450 enzymes P450 2D6 and P450 3A4, which are responsible for demethylation of codeine, may determine the individual variations in response to codeine treatment. The semisynthetic compounds **oxycodone** and **hydrocodone** are more effective analogues of codeine that are also orally available and are widely used, often in combination with acetaminophen

Synthetic Agonists

The two major classes of synthetic μ-receptor agonists are the phenylheptylamines (**methadone**) and the phenylpiperidines (**fentanyl, meperidine**). Methadone is most familiar for its use in drug addiction treatment, but it can also be used for pain management. Methadone has a 24-hour elimination half-life, which may be related to its interaction with plasma proteins, and its analgesic effects typically last for 4 to 8 hours. As a result of its long duration of action, methadone is often used to achieve long-lasting relief of chronic pain in patients with terminal cancer. Methadone has some NMDA receptor antagonist activity as well, but this mechanism is unlikely to be relevant clinically.

Fentanyl, an example of a short-acting synthetic opioid agonist with an elimination half-life comparable to that of morphine, is 75 to 100 times more potent than morphine. Because of its high lipophilicity, fentanyl is bioavailable through several unique routes. For example, fentanyl has been formulated as a lozenge for buccal transmucosal administration, which is particularly valuable for avoiding parenteral treatment in pediatric patients. Fentanyl can also be administered transdermally in the form of a patch that releases the drug slowly over time to provide long-acting systemic analgesia. **Alfentanil,** which is even more potent than fentanyl, and **sufentanil,** which is less potent, are structurally related to fentanyl.

Remifentanil, the most recently developed phenylpiperidine, exhibits distinct pharmacokinetic behavior. Remifentanil contains a methyl ester moiety that is essential for activity, but that is also the substrate for the action of numerous nonspecific tissue esterases. Thus, it has unusually rapid metabolism and elimination. When administered as a continuous infusion during anesthesia, remifentanil permits precise matching of the drug dose to the clinical response (see Chapter 15, General Anesthetic Pharmacology). However, the rapid offset of action demands that the use of remifentanil

during anesthesia be coupled with the administration of a longer-acting drug to maintain analgesia postoperatively. In the introductory case, remifentanil was used for intraoperative analgesia during the skin graft procedure to ensure that JD did not experience pain during surgery. Morphine was added before the end of the operation to provide postoperative pain coverage. Because of remifentanil's short half-life, pain associated with surgical tissue damage would have returned immediately after surgery if morphine had not been added.

Another phenylpiperidine is **meperidine**, which is a μ-agonist with analgesic efficacy similar to morphine; 75–100 mg of meperidine is equivalent to 10 mg of morphine. Its analgesic activity is reduced by half when taken orally, and it often produces dysphoria. The toxic meperidine metabolite normeperidine can cause increased CNS excitability and seizures. Normeperidine is excreted by the kidney and its elimination half-life is longer than that of meperidine; therefore, meperidine toxicity is a particular problem with repeated dosing of the drug or in patients with chronic kidney disease. Unlike other opioids, meperidine causes mydriasis rather than miosis.

Partial and Mixed Agonists

Although opioid receptor agonists are predominantly μ agonists, a number of drugs have also been developed as partial and mixed μ or κ agonists. These include the partial μ agonists **butorphanol** and **buprenorphine,** as well as nalbuphine, a κ agonist with μ antagonist activity. Butorphanol and buprenorphine produce morphine-like analgesia, but with milder euphoric symptoms. Nalbuphine and similar compounds are effective analgesics because of their action at κ receptors, but are also associated with undesirable psychological dysphoria. The reduced tendency of these agents to produce euphoria may diminish the likelihood of substance abuse behavior in susceptible individuals.

Opioid Receptor Antagonists

μ-Opioid receptor antagonists are used to reverse life-threatening side effects of opioid administration, specifically respiratory depression. **Naloxone,** one such antagonist, is a synthetic derivative of oxymorphone that is administered parenterally. Because the half-life of naloxone is shorter than that of morphine, it is not safe to leave the patient unattended immediately after successful treatment of an episode of respiratory depression with naloxone; monitoring can be relaxed only when it is certain that morphine no longer remains in the system. The orally administered antagonist **naltrexone** is primarily used in outpatient settings, typically for detoxification of individuals addicted to opioids (see Chapter 17). Combinations of opioid agonists and antagonists are being developed to reduce illicit drug use. Antagonists restricted to the periphery, such as **alvimopan,** have been developed to reduce post-operative ileus and to ameliorate the gastrointestinal effects of chronic opioid use.

NONSTEROIDAL ANTI-INFLAMMATORY DRUGS AND NONOPIOID ANALGESICS

General Features

Nonsteroidal anti-inflammatory agents inhibit the activity of **cyclooxygenase** enzymes (**COX-1** and **COX-2**) that are necessary for the production of prostaglandins (see Chapter 41). NSAIDs affect pain pathways in at least three different ways. First, prostaglandins reduce the activation threshold at the peripheral terminals of primary afferent nociceptor neurons (Fig. 16-9). By reducing prostaglandin synthesis, NSAIDs decrease inflammatory hyperalgesia and allodynia. Second, NSAIDs decrease the recruitment of leukocytes and, thereby, the production of leukocyte-derived inflammatory mediators. Third, NSAIDs that cross the blood-brain barrier prevent the generation of prostaglandins that act as pain-producing neuromodulators in the spinal cord dorsal horn. Because **acetaminophen** and NSAIDs act through mechanisms different from the opioids, NSAID–opioid or acetaminophen–opioid combinations can act synergistically to reduce pain. NSAIDs and COX-2 inhibitors act both peripherally and centrally, whereas acetaminophen acts only centrally. Preclinical data suggest that, while the acute action of NSAIDs is peripheral, much of their analgesic effect derives from their central action to prevent a PGE2-induced reduction in glycinergic inhibition. Like the opioids, nonselective COX-inhibiting NSAIDs have some deleterious side effects, particularly injury to the gastric mucosa and the kidneys. In some settings, these side effects can be minimized by co-treatment with other drugs such as **misoprostol**; this agent helps to replace the prostaglandin activity essential for the normal function of the gastric mucosa, although it carries its own set of adverse effects (diarrhea, uterine contraction). It had been thought that the anti-inflammatory and analgesic effects of the NSAIDs are primarily attributable to inhibition of COX-2, an inducible enzyme active in inflammatory states, whereas the adverse effects are primarily attributable to inhibition of COX-1, a constitutive enzyme responsible for the production of prostanoids involved in physiologic tissue maintenance and vascular regulation. However, this view may be an oversimplification because COX-2 may be induced to support COX-1 activity in the setting of gastric mucosal injury, and COX-1 may produce prostaglandins in tandem with COX-2 in inflammatory states. There is also concern that COX-2 inhibition may promote thrombosis and reduce or delay wound healing (see below).

Specific Agents

There are several major classes of NSAIDs, including the salicylates (**aspirin** or **acetylsalicylate),** indole acetic acid derivatives (**indomethacin**), pyrrole acetic acid derivatives (**diclofenac**), propionic acid derivatives (**ibuprofen),** and benzothiazines (**piroxicam**). The para-aminophenols (**acetaminophen**) are a related class of compounds with analgesic and antipyretic activity, but not anti-inflammatory activity. The COX-2 selective inhibitors **celecoxib, rofecoxib,** and **valdecoxib** were designed to produce analgesia equivalent to that of the NSAIDs while decreasing the adverse effects associated with chronic NSAID use. This has turned out to be a disappointment, and both rofecoxib and valdecoxib have been withdrawn from the market because of an increased risk of cardiovascular effects and skin reactions. Representative agents are discussed here; further information on their anti-inflammatory uses and side effects is discussed in Chapter 41.

- **Acetylsalicylic acid (aspirin)** acts by covalently acetylating the cyclooxygenase active site in both COX-1 and COX-2. Aspirin is rapidly absorbed and distributed throughout the body. Chronic aspirin use can produce gastric irritation and erosion, hemorrhage, vomiting, and renal tubular necrosis. Aspirin is of great value in the treatment of mild or moderate pain.
- The coxibs are COX-2 selective enzyme inhibitors. Currently, only **celecoxib** remains in clinical use in the U.S. This class of drugs was originally reserved for patients who required NSAIDs but were at high risk for developing gastrointestinal, renal, or hematologic side effects.
- The widely used compound **ibuprofen** is a derivative of propionic acid. Used primarily for analgesia and anti-inflammatory action, it also is an antipyretic, and it has a lower incidence of adverse effects than aspirin. Another common propionic acid derivative is **naproxen.** Compared to ibuprofen, naproxen is more potent and has a longer half-life; therefore, it can be administered less frequently with equivalent analgesic efficacy. Its adverse effect profile is similar to ibuprofen and it is generally well tolerated. As with all NSAIDs, ibuprofen and naproxen can cause GI complications ranging from dyspepsia to gastric bleeding.
- The pyrrole acetic acid derivatives **diclofenac** and **ketorolac** are used to treat moderate to severe pain. Ketorolac can be administered orally or parenterally, while diclofenac is

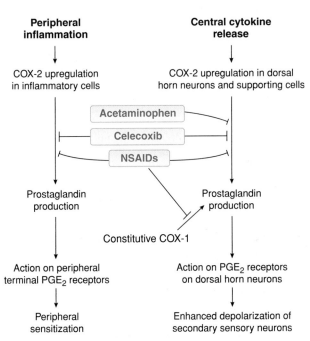

Figure 16-9. Mechanism of analgesic action of cyclo-oxygenase inhibitors. Inflammatory states are often associated with the production of prostaglandins, which are important mediators of both peripheral **(left)** and central **(right)** pain sensitization. In the periphery, prostaglandins produced by inflammatory cells sensitize peripheral nerve terminal prostaglandin *(EP)* receptors, making them more responsive to a painful stimulus. In central pain pathways, cytokines released in response to inflammation induce prostaglandin production in the dorsal horn of the spinal cord. These prostaglandins sensitize secondary nociceptive neurons and thereby increase the perception of pain. Nonsteroidal anti-inflammatory drugs (NSAIDs) block peripheral and central sensitization mediated by prostanoids that are released in inflammation; NSAIDs also reduce the extent of inflammation.

available in oral formulations. Both agents carry a risk of severe adverse effects, including anaphylaxis, acute renal failure, Stevens–Johnson syndrome (a diffuse life-threatening rash involving the skin and mucous membranes), and gastrointestinal bleeding.

- **Acetaminophen** (paracetamol) preferentially reduces central prostaglandin synthesis by an uncertain mechanism; as a result, the drug produces analgesia and antipyresis but has little anti-inflammatory efficacy. Acetaminophen is frequently combined with weak opioids for the treatment of moderate pain, and preparations featuring acetaminophen combined with codeine, hydrocodone, oxycodone, pentazocine, or propoxyphene are available. Following deacetylation to its primary amine, acetaminophen is conjugated to arachidonic acid by fatty acid amide hydrolase in the brain and spinal cord; the product of this reaction, N-arachidonoylphenolamine, may inhibit COX-1 and COX-2 in the CNS. N-arachidonoylphenolamine is an endogenous cannabinoid and an agonist at TRPV1 receptors, suggesting that direct or indirect activation of TRPV1 and/or cannabinoid CB1 receptors could also be involved in the mechanism of acetaminophen action.

Tramadol is a centrally acting analgesic. Analgesia apparently results from a monoaminergic effect within the CNS, as well as an opioid effect mediated by a metabolite that is formed by O-demethylation of the parent drug by P450 2D6. Tramadol has minimal abuse liability but it does cause nausea, dizziness and constipation. Administration of the drug in combination with acetaminophen improves its analgesic efficacy.

ANTIDEPRESSANTS

Drugs originally developed for treating depression are widely used as adjuvant therapy in pain management, particularly for treatment of chronic pain conditions. It is thought that tricyclic antidepressants produce analgesia both by blocking sodium channels and by increasing the activity of anti-nociceptive noradrenergic and serotonergic projections descending from the brain to the spinal cord. In general, the least selective agents (i.e., those with the broadest neurochemical effects), such as the tricyclics **amitriptyline, nortriptyline,** and **imipramine,** have been more effective than the selective norepinephrine reuptake blockers **desipramine** and **maprotiline,** while serotonin-selective reuptake inhibitors (SSRIs) such as **paroxetine, fluoxetine,** and **citalopram** are the least effective. The use of these drugs in mood disorders is discussed in Chapter 13.

Venlafaxine and **duloxetine** are dual norepinephrine/serotonin reuptake inhibitors with actions as both antidepressants and analgesics. These agents are used in the treatment of neuropathic pain and fibromyalgia. Duloxetine has a balanced action on NE and 5-HT reuptake and a weak action on dopamine reuptake as well. Although SSRIs have minimal analgesic action by themselves, inhibition of the serotonin reuptake transporter appears to produce some analgesic effect when NE reuptake is also blocked.

While patients with chronic pain are commonly depressed, and reducing depression may improve quality of life, antidepressants have an analgesic action distinct from their antidepressant effect. Based on results from animal models, the analgesic action appears to be mediated mainly

in the spinal cord and to involve the reduction of central sensitization.

ANTICONVULSANTS AND ANTIARRHYTHMICS

A number of pharmacologic agents used to control the excessive cellular excitability that leads to seizures (see Chapter 14) or cardiac arrhythmias (see Chapter 18) can also be used to manage the symptoms of some chronic pain conditions. In the search for drugs that produce analgesia, a number of these agents have been tested on the basis of their ability to reduce neuronal excitability. Of these, the most clinically valuable are the anticonvulsants **gabapentin, pregabalin, lamotrigine,** and **carbamazepine.**

Gabapentin has become widely used for the management of chronic pain. It was originally developed as a structural analogue of GABA, but it does not bind to the GABA receptor and does not affect the metabolism or reuptake of GABA. Gabapentin binds to the $\alpha 2\delta$ subunit of voltage-dependent calcium channels, but it remains to be determined exactly how binding to this site reduces neuronal activity and pain in patients. Randomized clinical trials in diabetic neuropathy and trigeminal neuralgia show that gabapentin is superior to placebo in reducing subjectively reported pain. Gabapentin also has some efficacy in reducing postoperative pain. Gabapentin is associated with several adverse effects, particularly dizziness, somnolence, confusion, and ataxia. It is widely thought that gabapentin's adverse effects are milder than those of amitriptyline, but this has not yet been proven in a clinical trial. In the introductory case, gabapentin reduced JD's spontaneous paroxysmal pain, probably by reducing aberrant neuronal excitability. However, the exact molecular mechanism of gabapentin's action remains in question.

One problem with gabapentin is that its oral bioavailability is not predictable or linear. Some patients require 10 times as much drug as others to achieve a similar effect. A newer antiepileptic drug with a similar structure is **pregabalin**; this substituted GABA analogue is more potent and it has a faster onset of action and more predictable bioavailability than gabapentin. Pregabalin produces an analgesic effect similar to that of gabapentin in patients with neuropathic pain and fibromyalgia, and the two drugs have similar CNS side effects. Pregabalin also produces a mild euphoric effect in some patients. Because of its increased potency, it is claimed that dose-related adverse effects may be lower with pregabalin than gabapentin.

Carbamazepine acts to block sodium channels; the drug is used primarily to treat trigeminal neuralgia but it has a relatively high adverse effect profile. **Oxcarbazepine** is a close structural derivative of carbamazepine with an additional oxygen atom decorating the benzylcarboxamide group. This difference alters metabolism of the drug in the liver. More importantly, it reduces the risk of aplastic anemia, which is a serious side effect occasionally associated with carbamazepine. **Lamotrigine**, an antiepileptic drug that is also a sodium channel blocker, reduces the painful sensory symptoms that can occur in neuropathy, stroke, multiple sclerosis, and phantom limb; however, it has a high incidence of skin reactions. The use of **mexiletine**, an antiarrhythmic, is limited by gastrointestinal effects caused by paralysis of the gastrointestinal tract. **Lidocaine**, a use-dependent sodium channel blocker, is typically used as a local anesthetic for regional anesthesia (see Chapter 10); this drug is also used topically in patches for patients with cutaneous pain, as in patients with post-herpetic neuralgia. Lidocaine can also be used for regional pain management when administered intravenously.

NMDA RECEPTOR ANTAGONISTS

Because of the critical role of NMDA receptors in the induction and maintenance of central sensitization, NMDA receptor antagonists are currently under investigation for use in pain treatment. Two currently available drugs act as antagonists at the NMDA receptor, and both of these drugs, the anesthetic **ketamine** and the antitussive **dextromethorphan,** effectively reduce chronic pain symptoms and postoperative pain. Ketamine use is severely limited by its psychomimetic effects. Dextromethorphan, when used at the relatively high doses required for analgesia, also produces dizziness, fatigue, confusion, and psychomimetic effects. Ketamine has particular utility for acute severe pain, such as battlefield injury, because there is minimal risk of respiratory depression. NMDA receptor subtype selective antagonists may have a greater therapeutic index.

ADRENERGIC AGONISTS

Stimulation of α_2-adrenergic receptors in the dorsal horn of the spinal cord produces an anti-nociceptive state. Therefore, α_2-adrenergic agonists may have therapeutic utility as analgesics. The α_2-agonist **clonidine** has been used systemically, epidurally, intrathecally, and topically, and appears to produce analgesia in both acute and chronic pain states. Clonidine does, however, cause postural hypotension; this effect limits its usefulness in pain control.

MIGRAINE THERAPY

The treatment of pain associated with migraine has features distinct from the treatment of other pain conditions. In many but not all patients, an effective treatment for migraine is the **triptan** class of serotonin receptor agonists; the most well-studied example is **sumatriptan.** The triptans are selective for the $5-HT_{1B}$ and $5-HT_{1D}$ receptor subtypes. These drugs reduce both sensory activation in the periphery and nociceptive transmission in the brainstem trigeminal nucleus, where they diminish central sensitization. The triptans also cause vasoconstriction, opposing the vasodilation thought to be involved in the pathophysiology of migraine attacks. It remains unclear whether the vasoconstriction is helpful in producing the antimigraine actions of these drugs, however. Furthermore, as a result of this vasoconstrictive effect, the triptans can be dangerous in patients with coronary heart disease. The triptans can reduce the pain and other symptoms associated with acute migraine attack, and have replaced the vasoconstrictive agent **ergotamine tartrate** in the treatment of migraine. Sumatriptan can be administered subcutaneously, orally, or by nasal inhalation. Several other orally administered agents in the triptan class are also available, including **zolmitriptan, naratriptan,** and **rizatriptan** (see Drug Summary Table). NSAIDs and opioids also have

activity and some utility for treatment of acute migraine headaches. During an attack, migraine patients often experience gastric stasis that can reduce the bioavailability of oral medications. CGRP receptor antagonists are promising candidates for migraine therapy.

Although the triptans are relatively effective in ameliorating the acute symptoms of migraine, other classes of drugs are used to reduce the frequency of attacks. Numerous drugs are used for migraine prophylaxis, including β-adrenergic blockers, valproic acid, serotonin antagonists, and calcium channel blockers. These agents are generally chosen based on the severity and frequency of the migraine attacks, the cost of the drug, and the adverse effects of the drug in the context of the individual patient. None has been shown to have a high level of efficacy, and new drugs need to be developed for more effective migraine prophylaxis.

Conclusion and Future Directions

Because of the limited efficacy of any single drug, it is common in clinical practice to use a polypharmacy approach to manage pain. In combination, several drugs that are only moderately effective as single agents can have additive or supra-additive effects. This is largely a consequence of the multiple processing events and mechanisms responsible for producing pain: intervention at several steps may be required to achieve adequate analgesia (Fig. 16-10). Because many drugs used to treat pain are also active systemically and/or in parts of the nervous system that are not related to somatic sensation, analgesics can produce deleterious adverse effects. One approach to limiting toxicity is to use localized (nonsystemic) forms of drug delivery. In particular, epidural and topical delivery limit the drug to a local site of action. Many of the opioids are short-acting and must be administered frequently to patients in severe pain. Modes of drug delivery have also been developed to optimize the pharmacokinetics of the short-acting opioids; these methods include transdermal and buccal dosage forms, patient-controlled analgesia devices, and controlled-release oral preparations. Patient-controlled devices ensure that patients do not suffer pain because of waning drug effects, and instrumental controls can effectively prevent overdose. At the present time, however, patient-controlled technologies are suitable only for inpatient treatment.

Most of the currently available analgesics have been identified by empirical observation (opioids, NSAIDs, and local anesthetics) or serendipity (anticonvulsants). Now that the mechanisms responsible for pain are being explored at a molecular level, many new targets are being revealed that are likely to lead to new and different classes of analgesics. It is hoped that drugs active at these targets will achieve greater efficacy and have fewer adverse effects than current therapies. Effective pain management approaches must rely not only on pharmacologic intervention; physical therapy and rehabilitation, and, in some very limited situations, surgical approaches may also have a role. The placebo reaction produces analgesia and may explain the limited success produced by treatments such as acupuncture and homeopathy. These effects are usually unpredictable, modest, and of short duration. The growing complexity of pain management has spawned specialized pain services for inpatient pain control,

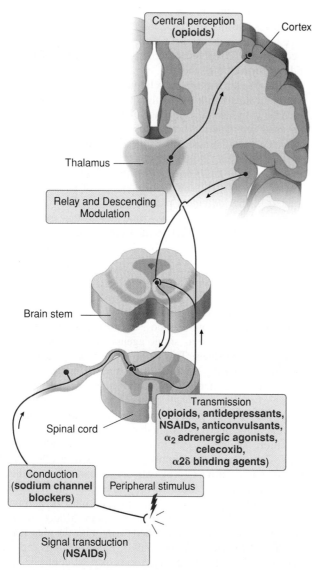

Figure 16-10. Summary of the sites of action of the major drug classes used for pain management. Analgesics target various steps in pain perception, from the initiation of a pain stimulus to the central perception of that pain. NSAIDs modulate the initial membrane depolarization (signal transduction) in response to a peripheral stimulus. Sodium channel blockers decrease action potential conduction in nociceptive fibers. Opioids, antidepressants, NSAIDs, anticonvulsants, and α_2-adrenergic agonists all modulate transmission of pain sensation in the spinal cord by decreasing the signal relayed from peripheral to central pain pathways. Opioids also modulate the central perception of painful stimuli. The multiple sites of action of analgesics allow a combination drug approach to be used in pain management. For example, moderate pain is often treated with combinations of opioids and NSAIDs. Because these drugs have different mechanisms and sites of action, the combination of the drugs is more effective than one drug alone.

as well as pain clinics and centers for the outpatient management of chronic pain.

Acknowledgments

The authors thank Salahadin Abdi, MD, Rami Burstein, PhD, Carl Rosow, MD, PhD, and Joachim Scholz, MD, for their valuable comments.

Suggested Reading

Bertolini A, Ferrari A, Ottani A, et al. Paracetamol: new vistas of an old drug. *CNS Drug Rev* 2006;12:250–275. (*Discusses new concepts in acetaminophen pharmacology.*)

Eisenberg E, McNicol ED, Carr DB. Efficacy and safety of opioid agonists in the treatment of neuropathic pain of nonmalignant origin. *JAMA* 2005;293:3043–3052. (*A systematic review of published randomized controlled trials using opioids for nonmalignant neuropathic pain.*)

Finnerup NB, Otto M, McQuay HJ, et al. Algorithm for neuropathic pain treatment: an evidence-based proposal. *Pain* 2005;118: 289–305. (*Clinical approach to management of neuropathic pain.*)

Julius D, Basbaum AI. Molecular mechanisms of nociception. *Nature* 2001;413:203–210. (*Discussion of pain mechanisms, focusing on the peripheral terminal.*)

Mackie K. Cannabinoid receptors as therapeutic targets. *Ann Rev Pharmacol Toxicol* 2006;46:101–122. (*Review of cannabinoid pharmacology.*)

Mendell JR, Sahenk Z. Painful sensory neuropathy. *N Engl J Med* 2003;348:1243–1255. (*Clinically oriented discussion of the diagnosis, pathophysiology, and treatment of painful sensory neuropathy.*)

Scholz J, Woolf CJ. Can we conquer pain? *Nature Neurosci* 2002; 5 Suppl:1062–1067.

Waxman SG. Transcriptional channelopathies: an emerging class of disorders. *Nature Rev Neurosci* 2001;2:652–659. (*Reviews pathologic states associated with transcriptional changes in ion channel gene expression; pain is included as an example.*)

Woolf CJ. Pain: moving from symptom control toward mechanism-specific pharmacologic management. *Ann Intern Med* 2004;140: 441–451. (*Advances in molecular understanding of pain pathways.*)

Woolf CJ, Salter MW. Neuronal plasticity: increasing the gain in pain. *Science* 2000;288:1765–1769. (*Discusses regulated sensitivity of the nociceptive system.*)

Yaksh TL. Central pharmacology of nociceptive transmission. In: McMahon SB, Koltzenburg M, eds. *Wall and Melzack's textbook of pain.* 5th ed. New York: Churchill Livingstone; 2006. (*Contains a discussion of dorsal horn neurotransmission as it relates to pain.*)

Drug Summary Table | **Chapter 16 Pharmacology of Analgesia**

Drug	Clinical Applications	Serious and Common Adverse Effects	Contraindications	Therapeutic Considerations
μ-OPIOID RECEPTOR AGONISTS				
Morphine, Codeine, and Semisynthetic Derivatives				
Mechanism—Natural or semisynthetic agonists of the μ-opioid receptor that result in inhibition of neurotransmission				
Morphine	Pain (moderate to severe) Analgesia for a mechanically ventilated patient	*Respiratory depression, hypotension, confusion, and abuse potential* Constipation, nausea, vomiting, dizziness, headache, sedation, urinary retention, and pruritus	Severe asthma Paralytic ileus Respiratory depression/hypoventilation Upper airway obstruction	Morphine is metabolized in the liver, and its active metabolite M6G is excreted in kidney; dose adjustment may be required in patients with renal disease Controlled-release oral preparations reduce the number of daily doses, but these formulations are associated with abuse potential Intravenous or subcutaneous morphine is commonly used in patient-controlled analgesia devices Epidural or intrathecal morphine can produce highly effective analgesia by achieving locally high concentrations in the dorsal horn of the spinal cord
Codeine	Pain (mild to moderate)	*Same as morphine. Additionally, seizure with excessive dose*	During delivery of a premature infant Premature infants	Much less effective than morphine in pain treatment Used for its antitussive and antidiarrheal effects Quinidine reduces analgesic effects of codeine by inhibiting bioactivation of codeine to morphine
Oxycodone Hydrocodone	Pain (moderate to severe)	*Same as morphine*	Same as morphine	More effective analogues of codeine in the treatment of pain
Synthetic Agonists				
Mechanism—Synthetic agonists of the μ-opioid receptor that result in inhibition of neurotransmission				
Methadone	Detoxification of patients with opioid addiction Severe pain	*Same as morphine*	Hypersensitivity to methadone	Due to its long duration of action, methadone is used to achieve long-lasting pain relief in cancer patients
Fentanyl Alfentanil Sufentanil	Pain (moderate to severe)	*Same as morphine*	Same as morphine	Fentanyl is more potent than morphine and is bioavailable through several routes. Transmucosal administration (as lozenge) is useful in pediatric patients. A transdermal (patch) formulation releases the drug slowly over time Alfentanil and sufentanil are structurally related to fentanyl; alfentanil is more potent than fentanyl, whereas sufentanil is less potent than fentanyl

(Continued)

Drug Summary Table | **Chapter 16 Pharmacology of Analgesia** (*Continued*)

Drug	Clinical Applications	Serious and Common Adverse Effects	Contraindications	Therapeutic Considerations
Remifentanil	Pain (moderate to severe) Adjunct to general anesthesia	*Same as morphine. Additionally, muscle rigidity is observed*	Do not use for epidural or intrathecal administration because the glycine in the formulation may cause neurotoxicity	Remifentanil has unusually rapid metabolism and elimination. Remifentanil permits precise matching of the drug dose to the clinical response. However, remifentanil's rapid offset of action during anesthesia requires co-administration of a longer-acting drug to maintain analgesia postoperatively
Meperidine	Pain (moderate to severe)	*Same as morphine. Additionally, euphoria and mydriasis are observed*	Recent or concomitant MAOI	The toxic metabolite normeperidine can cause increased CNS excitability and seizures. Renal excretion of normeperidine makes toxicity a problem in either repeated dosing or in patients with kidney disease. Unlike other opioids, meperidine causes mydriasis rather than miosis Recent or concomitant MAOI is an absolute contraindication due to the risk of life-threatening serotonin syndrome Coadministration with selegiline or sibutramine is usually avoided due to the theoretical risk of serotonin syndrome
Levorphanol	Pain (moderate to severe)	*Same as morphine*	Hypersensitivity to levorphanol	Like other opioids, exerts analgesic effects through receptors in periventricular and periaqueductal gray matter in brain and spinal cord, thereby altering pain perception and transmission Available in IV and oral forms
Propoxyphene	Pain (mild to moderate)	*Same as morphine*	Hypersensitivity to propoxyphene	Structurally related to methadone. Mild centrally-acting analgesia Propoxyphene markedly increases serum level of carbamazepine

Partial and Mixed Agonists
Mechanism—Partial μ-receptor agonists (butorphanol and buprenorphine) and a κ-agonist with partial μ-antagonist activity (nalbuphine)

Drug	Clinical Applications	Serious and Common Adverse Effects	Contraindications	Therapeutic Considerations
Butorphanol Buprenorphine	Pain (moderate to severe) Adjunct to balanced anesthesia	Hypotension, palpitations, tinnitus, respiratory depression, upper respiratory infection Dizziness, sedation, insomnia and nasal congestion with long-term intranasal administration	Hypersensitivity to either medication	Produce morphine-like analgesia, but with milder euphoric symptoms Available in intranasal spray and IV formulations
Nalbuphine	Pain (moderate to severe) Adjunct to balanced anesthesia	Respiratory depression, hypersensitivity (frequent) Sweating, nausea, vomiting, dizziness, sedation	Hypersensitivity to nalbuphine	Its μ-antagonist activity may precipitate withdrawal in patients who have received opioids chronically

OPIOID RECEPTOR ANTAGONISTS

Mechanism—Antagonists of μ-opioid receptor, thereby blocking endogenous or exogenous opioid effects

Drug	Clinical Applications	Serious and Common Adverse Effects	Contraindications	Therapeutic Considerations
Naloxone Naltrexone	Acute opioid toxicity (Naloxone) Opioid, alcohol addiction (Naltrexone)	*Cardiac arrhythmia, hypertension, hypotension, hepatotoxicity, pulmonary edema, opioid withdrawal* Deep vein thrombosis and pulmonary embolism (naltrexone)	Acute hepatitis or liver failure (naltrexone)	Combination of yohimbine and naloxone results in greater anxiety, tremors, palpitations, hot and cold flashes, as well as elevated plasma cortisol levels
Alvimopan	Post-operative ileus and opioid-mediated bowel dysfunction	Diarrhea, flatulence, abdominal pain, nervousness, polyuria, elevated LFTs	Hypersensitivity to alvimopan	Alvimopan is a potent antagonist of *peripheral* μ-opioid receptors Limited human studies show that alvimopan prevents morphine-induced constipation, but has no effect on morphine analgesia

NON-STEROIDAL ANALGESICS

Mechanism—Affect prostaglandin synthetic pathway

Drug				
Acetaminophen Aspirin Naproxen Ibuprofen Indomethacin Diclofenac Piroxicam Celecoxib	See Drug Summary Table: Chapter 41 Pharmacology of Eicosanoids			

TRICYCLIC ANTIDEPRESSANTS

Mechanism—Promote serotonergic and noradrenergic neurotransmission by inhibiting neurotransmitter reuptake

Drug				
Amitriptyline Nortriptyline Imipramine Desipramine Duloxetine Venlafaxine	See Drug Summary Table: Chapter 13 Pharmacology of Serotonergic and Central Adrenergic Neurotransmission			

ANTICONVULSANTS AND ANTIARRHYTHMICS

Mechanism—Inhibit action potential initiation or conduction

Drug				
Carbamazepine Oxcarbazepine Gabapentin Pregabalin Lamotrigine	See Drug Summary Table: Chapter 14 Pharmacology of Abnormal Electrical Neurotransmission in the Central Nervous System			
Mexiletine	See Drug Summary Table: Chapter 18 Pharmacology of Cardiac Rhythm			

(Continued)

| Drug Summary Table | Chapter 16 Pharmacology of Analgesia (Continued) |

Drug	Clinical Applications	Serious and Common Adverse Effects	Contraindications	Therapeutic Considerations
NMDA RECEPTOR ANTAGONISTS *Mechanism—Block NMDA receptor-dependent post-synaptic depolarization*				
Ketamine	Analgesia Dissociative anesthesia Sole anesthetic agent for procedures that do not require skeletal muscle relaxation	*Hypertension, tachyarrhythmia, myoclonus, respiratory depression, increased intracranial pressure* Hallucinations, vivid dreams, psychiatric symptoms	Hypersensitivity to ketamine Severe hypertension	Useful in acute severe pain, such as battlefield injury, due to minimal risk of respiratory depression. Wider application of ketamine is limited by its psychomimetic effects Increases cardiac output by increasing sympathetic outflow
Dextromethorphan	Cough Neuropathic pain	Dizziness, somnolence, fatigue	Coadministration of MAOI	Dextromethorphan, when used at the relatively high doses required for analgesia, also produces dizziness, fatigue, confusion, and psychomimetic effects Coadministration of MAOI is absolutely contraindicated due to the risk of serotonin syndrome Coadministration with selegiline or sibutramine is usually avoided
5-HT₁D SEROTONIN RECEPTOR AGONISTS *Mechanism—Induce cerebrovascular vasoconstriction, reduce nociceptive transmission*				
Sumatriptan Rizatriptan Naratriptan Zolmitriptan Almotriptan Electriptan	See Drug Summary Table: Chapter 13 Pharmacology of Serotonergic and Central Adrenergic Neurotransmission			

17

Pharmacology of Drug Dependence and Addiction

Robert M. Swift and David C. Lewis

INTRODUCTION

This chapter considers pharmacologic agents implicated in drug misuse, abuse, and dependence. While understanding the neuropharmacology of these agents is important to understanding their effects on behavior and the risks of addiction, their pharmacology is by no means the only determinant of the drug experience or behavior. Personality characteristics, such as risk-taking behavior, may contribute to the risk of developing drug abuse. Age of first use, prior drug experience, the anticipated effects of the drug experience, nutritional status, and social factors may also influence risk of abuse and dependence.

There is also some overlap between alcohol and drug problems and psychiatric disease. Alcohol is widely used as a self-medication for anxiety (i.e., as an anxiolytic), and amphetamines may be used to self-medicate for attention deficit hyperactivity disorder. However, it is often difficult to determine whether such illnesses are the cause of drug abuse or its effect, because the actions of the drugs themselves, as well as drug withdrawal and dependence, can unmask psychiatric illness in a previously compensated individual.

Environmental variables have a strong influence on the development of addiction. For example, societal attitudes toward drug-taking behavior often influence the likelihood that a drug will be taken in the first place. The availability and cost of the drug may also be affected by its legal and tax status. The availability of other, nondrug alternatives may be a key factor in determining the likelihood of drug use and addiction.

Although this chapter does not describe exhaustively the mechanisms of action of all drugs of abuse, selected representative drugs are considered mechanistically, and the mechanisms of the important remaining drugs are summarized in Table 17-1. Finally, the therapeutic strategies—both pharmacologic and psychosocial—used to treat drug dependence are discussed.

| TABLE 17-1 | Major Drugs of Abuse |

DRUG CLASS	EXAMPLES	RECEPTOR (ACTION)	CLINICAL SIGNS	NOTES
Opioids	Morphine Heroin Codeine Oxycodone	μ-Opioid (agonist)	Euphoria, followed by sedation, respiratory depression	Used therapeutically as analgesics (except for heroin)
Benzodiazepines	Triazolam Lorazapam Diazepam	$GABA_A$ (modulator)	Sedation, respiratory depression	Used therapeutically as anxiolytics, sedatives
Barbiturates	Phenobarbital Pentobarbital	$GABA_A$ (modulator)	Sedation, respiratory depression	Used therapeutically as anxiolytics and sedatives; greater danger of overdose than benzodiazepines
Alcohol	Ethanol	$GABA_A$ (modulator), NMDA antagonist	Intoxication, sedation, memory loss	Legal in many countries
Nicotine	Tobacco	Nicotinic ACh (agonist)	Alertness, muscle relaxation	Legal in many countries
Psychostimulants	Cocaine Amphetamine	Dopamine, adrenergic, serotonin (reuptake inhibitor)	Euphoria, alertness, hypertension, paranoia	Amphetamines also reverse the reuptake transporter and release neurotransmitter from synaptic vesicles into the cytosol
Caffeine	Coffee	Adenosine (antagonist)	Alertness, tremulousness	Generally legal, addiction rare
Cannabinoids	Cannabis	CB1, CB2 (agonist)	Changes in mood, hunger, giddiness	
Phencyclidine (PCP)	N/A	NMDA (antagonist)	Hallucinations, hostile behavior	
Phenylethylamines	MDMA (Ecstasy), MDA	Serotonin, dopamine, adrenergic (reuptake inhibitors, multiple actions)	Euphoria, alertness, hypertension, hallucinations	Structurally related to amphetamines, effects similar to psychedelic agents
Psychedelic agents	LSD DMT Psilocybin	$5-HT_2$ (partial agonist)	Hallucinations	
Inhalants	Toluene Amyl nitrate Nitrous oxide	Unknown	Dizziness, intoxication	

MDMA, methylenedioxymethamphetamine; MDA, methylenedioxyamphetamine; LSD, lysergic acid diethylamide; DMT, dimethyltryptamine; NMDA, N-methyl-D-aspartate.

■ Case

J.B., a 25-year-old man with a history of heavy heroin use, is brought to the emergency department of a suburban Phoenix hospital with an 8-hour history of increasing nausea, vomiting, diarrhea, muscle aches, and anxiety. Mr. B explains that he is trying to "kick the habit" and that his last "hit" was approximately 24 hours ago. He expresses an intense craving for heroin and is extremely fidgety and uncomfortable. On physical examination, he has a temperature of 103°F, enlarged pupils, a blood pressure of 170/95 mm Hg, and a heart rate of 108 beats/min. He is irritable and exquisitely sensitive to touch, and his responses

to painful stimuli, such as a pinprick, are out of proportion to the intensity of the stimulus. Mr. B is given 20 mg of methadone, a long-acting opioid. He becomes slightly more comfortable and is given a second dose of 20 mg, after which he is noticeably more comfortable and the worst of his symptoms abate. Mr. B is then admitted to an inpatient detoxification center to complete a 28-day treatment program. Over the course of the next week, his methadone dose is decreased by approximately 20% each day. Mr. B is enrolled in a Narcotics Anonymous (NA) program, where he tells the tale of his addiction. It had started out slowly, with only a few hits of heroin each month, "on special occasions," as he puts it. Over time, however, he had found that the high he got from the drug wasn't as intense as it had been when he first started, and he had found himself shooting (injecting intravenously) both larger amounts and more frequently. Eventually, he was shooting twice a day and felt as if he were "trapped" by the drug.

Although Mr. B finds the sessions at NA useful, his attendance is sporadic. Over the next few weeks he experiences cyclical changes in weight, alternating periods of insomnia and anxiety, and craving for heroin despite opioid-free urine tests. Two months later he relapses, and is again shooting heroin.

QUESTIONS

■ **1.** What caused Mr. B's physical symptoms and signs (i.e., nausea, vomiting, fever, enlarged pupils, and hypertension) on his initial visit to the emergency department?

■ **2.** Why was Mr. B treated for heroin withdrawal with another opioid (methadone)?

■ **3.** Why did Mr. B find that, over time, the effect of heroin was less intense than when he first started using it?

■ **4.** Why did Mr. B experience intense cravings for heroin after his physiologic symptoms abated?

■ **5.** How can programs such as Narcotics Anonymous help treat addiction, and why are such programs incompletely successful?

DEFINITIONS

Before describing the various drugs of abuse and the possible mechanisms of action, it is important to define terms. Many medical journals use the empirically-based nomenclature developed by the American Psychiatric Association (APA) in a volume entitled DSM-IV (Box 17-1). Therein, **substance dependence (addiction)** is defined as "a maladaptive pattern of substance use, leading to clinically significant impairment or distress, as manifested by three (or more)" characteristics including tolerance, withdrawal, and giving up or reducing "important social, occupational, or recreational activities . . . because of substance abuse," over a 12-month period. The term **"abuse"** applies specifically to *nonprescribed* substances. Thus, ethanol and cocaine, which are not commonly prescribed, are considered drugs of abuse.

Drug misuse commonly refers to the improper use of *prescribed* compounds, or the use of such compounds for nontherapeutic purposes. The use of prescribed morphine or a benzodiazepine for purposes other than its therapeutic indication, or at a higher or more frequent dose than indicated, constitutes a misuse of that drug.

The line between abuse and misuse is sometimes indistinct. For example, marijuana, long considered a drug of abuse, is now finding legitimate therapeutic use as an antiemetic for patients undergoing cancer chemotherapy; several states permit health care professionals to prescribe marijuana for that purpose. Moreover, nicotine (technically a drug of abuse)—in the form of a patch or a gum—can combat the effects of nicotine withdrawal in tobacco users attempting to overcome their addiction. Even the distinction between a "therapeutic" and a "nontherapeutic" use of a drug may

> **BOX 17-1. Diagnostic and Statistical Manual of Mental Disorders (DSM-IV) Criteria for Substance Dependence (Addiction)**
>
> A maladaptive pattern of substance use, leading to clinically significant impairment or distress, as manifested by three (or more) of the following, occurring at any time in the same 12-month period:
>
> 1. Tolerance, as defined by either of the following:
>   a. A need for markedly increased amounts of the substance to achieve intoxication or the desired effect.
>   b. Markedly diminished effect with continued use of the same amount of substance.
> 2. Withdrawal, as manifested by either of the following:
>   a. The characteristic withdrawal syndrome for the substance (as defined by the APA criteria for withdrawal for a specific substance).
>   b. The same (or closely related) substance is taken to relieve or avoid withdrawal symptoms.
> 3. The substance is often taken in larger amounts or over a longer period than was intended.
> 4. A persistent desire or unsuccessful efforts to cut down or control substance use.
> 5. A great deal of time is spent in activities necessary to obtain the substance (e.g., visiting multiple doctors or driving long distances), to use the substance (e.g., chain-smoking), or to recover from its effects.
> 6. Important social, occupational, or recreational activities are given up or reduced because of substance use.
>
> The substance use is continued despite knowledge of having a persistent or recurrent physical or psychological problem that is likely to have been caused or exacerbated by the substance (e.g., current cocaine use despite recognition of cocaine-induced depression, or continued drinking despite recognition that an ulcer was made worse by alcohol consumption).

be imprecise, since much drug abuse is rooted in attempts to self-medicate. Thus, ethanol may be self-administered as an anxiolytic, even though such use is not monitored or endorsed by a physician, whereas caffeine, perhaps the most widely used substance that is active in the central nervous system (CNS), is self-administered as a stimulant to combat drowsiness.

The terms *tolerance, dependence,* and *withdrawal* may be defined based on their physiologic actions. These terms apply equally to physician-prescribed and nonprescribed drugs. **Tolerance** refers to the decreased effect of a drug that develops with continued use. The first administration of a drug produces a characteristic dose–response curve; after repeated administration of the same drug, however, the dose–response curve shifts to the right as *larger doses are needed to produce the same response* (Fig. 17-1), as happened in the case of Mr. B. The drug toxicity profile and the drug lethality profile do not always shift in the same way or to the same degree as the "therapeutic" profile, so that

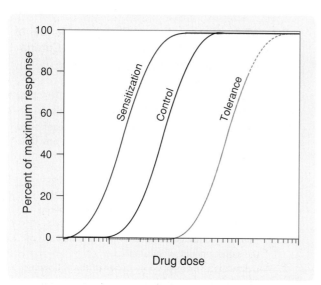

Figure 17-1. Effects of tolerance and sensitization on the dose-response curve. The first administration of a drug produces a certain dose–response curve *(black)*. Repeated administrations of the drug can lead to the development of tolerance, in which the dose–response curve shifts to the right *(light blue)*. A higher dose is required to produce the same effect, and it is not always possible to achieve the same maximal effect *(dashed portion of curve)*. Sensitization to the effects of a drug means that the dose–response curve shifts to the left *(dark blue)*, and a lower dose is needed to elicit the same response. In addition to the illustrated changes in the apparent potency of the drug, tolerance and sensitization can also be associated with changes in the maximal response produced by the drug.

repeated administrations may decrease the therapeutic index of the drug. Thus, it is likely that Mr. B developed less tolerance to the side effects of constipation and pupillary constriction than he did to the heroin "high." For the same reason, he was at greater risk of a lethal overdose as his heroin requirement increased. The opposite effect, termed **sensitization** (also called **inverse tolerance**), refers to a shift of the dose-response curve to the left, so that repeated administrations of a drug result in a greater effect of a given dose or require a lower dose to achieve the same effect. Interestingly, tolerance and sensitization to a drug may occur concurrently. The mechanisms that underlie tolerance and sensitization have been the subject of significant research, as described below.

Physical dependence (or **physiologic dependence**) refers to the adverse physical symptoms and signs that result from the **withdrawal** of a drug. In Mr. B's case, his initial symptoms in the emergency room were caused by heroin withdrawal, and his need to continue taking heroin to prevent those symptoms indicated a physical dependence. Physical dependence results from many of the same mechanisms that produce tolerance. As with tolerance, homeostatic set-points are altered to compensate for the presence of the drug. If the drug is withdrawn, the altered set-points produce effects opposite to those manifested in the presence of the drug. For example, abrupt withdrawal from an opioid analgesic produces hypersensitivity to painful stimuli (as well as other symptoms), whereas abrupt withdrawal from a barbiturate sedative/hypnotic produces insomnia, anxiety, and agitation (among other symptoms).

Psychological dependence is a more complex phenomenon that can occur even with drugs that do not produce tolerance and physical dependence. Psychological dependence occurs when a drug affects the **reward system** of the brain. The resulting pleasurable sensations cause the user to want to continue taking the drug. When the drug is withheld, adaptations in the brain reward system manifest as dysphoria and drug craving, as Mr. B experienced. Thus, both physical and psychological dependence result from alterations in homeostatic processes, but these processes occur in different regions of the brain.

This chapter will use the term **addiction** interchangeably with dependence. As noted in the DSM criteria (Box 17-1), addiction often involves *compulsive drug-using (and drug-seeking) behavior that interferes with normal functioning and causes the addict to continue using the drug despite increasingly damaging consequences.* Because Mr. B felt that he was "trapped" by the drug and was compelled to continue using it, it is likely that he was addicted to heroin.

Addiction may coexist with tolerance and dependence, but the presence of the latter does not necessarily imply addiction. For example, a patient given an opioid for chronic pain will likely develop tolerance to the drug and require larger doses over time. The patient has not necessarily become addicted to the opioid, however, and it will likely be possible to taper and eventually eliminate the analgesic once the pain abates. In this case, the patient is considered to be tolerant and dependent to the opioid, but not addicted. Tolerance and dependence are normal physiologic adaptations to the continued use of a drug, whereas addiction represents a maladaptive state. A more detailed examination of the mechanisms and factors that affect the likelihood of addiction is presented below.

MECHANISMS OF TOLERANCE, DEPENDENCE, AND ADDICTION

MECHANISMS OF TOLERANCE

Tolerance results when repeated administration of a drug results in a shift of the drug's dose–response curve to the right, so that a larger dose (concentration) of the drug is required to produce the same effect. There are multiple mechanisms by which a drug can cause tolerance. **Innate tolerance** refers to interindividual variations in sensitivity to the drug that are present before its first administration. These variations in sensitivity can arise from polymorphisms in the genes for the drug's receptor or the genes that affect the drug's absorption, metabolism, or excretion. As with any multifactorial trait, genetic variability is likely modified by the environment. An example of innate tolerance is observed with alcohol. Individuals vary in their sensitivity to the behavioral effects of alcohol; people with high sensitivity experience pleasurable effects and or sedation after one or two drinks, while others with low sensitivity require several drinks to feel an effect of alcohol. Those with low sensitivity as young adults are at higher risk for becoming alcoholics later in life.

Tolerance that develops over time is termed **acquired tolerance.** Three classes of mechanism govern the development of acquired tolerance: pharmacokinetic, pharmacodynamic, and learned. **Pharmacokinetic tolerance** develops when the ability to metabolize or excrete the drug increases over time. Increased metabolism is most commonly attributable to the induced synthesis of metabolic enzymes such as the cytochrome P450s (see Chapter 4, Drug Metabolism). In such cases, pharmacokinetic tolerance results in a lower plasma drug concentration for any given dose of drug (Fig. 17-2).

Pharmacodynamic tolerance, the most important mechanism of tolerance, results from changes in the drug–receptor interaction. These changes may involve a decrease in the number of receptors or a change in the signal transduction pathway (Fig. 17-3). In the short term, changes in receptor number or binding affinity can be caused by inactivation of receptors (e.g., through phosphorylation), internalization, and degradation of cell surface receptors, or other mechanisms. For example, a kinase present in the cytoplasm may phosphorylate (and, thereby, inactivate) only the agonist-bound form of a membrane receptor. For some metabotropic G protein-coupled receptors, short-term adaptations can include mechanisms that interfere with the coupling between G protein and receptor, for example, by phosphorylation of the receptor or the G protein subunits. Alteration in the conductance of an ion channel by receptor-mediated phosphorylation provides yet another mechanism of tolerance.

In the long term, changes in the number of receptors or other signaling molecules are typically caused by regulation of the genes encoding these proteins. For example, the cellular effects of opioids are mediated through a G protein-coupled metabotropic receptor. Among other effects, opioid binding to the receptor inhibits the activity of adenylyl cyclase (see Chapter 16, Pharmacology of Analgesia). Short-term administration of an opioid such as morphine, therefore, causes a decrease in cellular cyclic adenosine monophosphate (cAMP). With continued administration of the drug, however, downstream activation of a transcription factor(s) increases the transcription of the adenylyl cyclase gene and, thereby, reduces the cellular response to a given dose of morphine (Fig. 17-4). Even longer-lasting effects are postulated to result from certain mechanisms that underlie long-term memory. For example, long-term changes in the pattern of gene expression can alter the expression of AMPA glutamate receptors (see Chapter 11, Pharmacology of GABAergic and Glutamatergic Neurotransmission). In addition, long-lasting cellular adaptations caused by the release of neurotrophic factors may produce persistent adaptations to drug use by modifying existing synapses and creating new synapses, thus effectively ''rewiring'' the brain. Such long-lasting molecular and cellular adaptations are likely to explain the cravings and relapses that can occur long after drug use has been discontinued, as in the case of Mr. B.

Another form of tolerance is termed **learned tolerance.** In learned tolerance, a drug produces compensatory changes that are unrelated to its action. The most common mechanism of learned tolerance is behavioral tolerance, in which a person learns to alter his or her behavior to hide the effects of the drug. For example, someone who has been repeatedly intoxicated with alcohol can learn to hide the symptoms of intoxication, such as slurred speech and lack of coordination, and, thus, appear less intoxicated. **Conditioned tolerance** (a type of learned tolerance) occurs when environmental cues associated with exposure to a drug induce pre-emptive compensatory changes, called a **conditioned opponent response.** This mechanism of conditioning is an unconscious phenomenon. For example, seeing paraphernalia associated with use of a drug such as cocaine (which produces tachycardia) may elicit a preemptive bradycardia.

MECHANISMS OF PHYSICAL DEPENDENCE

Physical dependence is a phenomenon that is usually associated with tolerance and that typically results from mechanisms similar to those that produce pharmacodynamic tolerance. Physical dependence is the need for the drug to be present to maintain ''normal'' functioning. If the drug is not present, the adaptations that produced the tolerance are unmasked. *The hallmark of physical dependence is the manifestation of withdrawal symptoms in the absence of the drug.*

As with tolerance, dependence can result from changes in cellular signaling pathways. For example, a drug that produces pharmacodynamic tolerance by up-regulating the cAMP pathway also produces dependence because the abrupt withdrawal of the drug allows the up-regulated adenylyl cyclase to affect a ''supranormal'' response. Conversely, a drug that decreases receptor number or decreases receptor sensitivity produces dependence because withdrawal of the drug leaves the down-regulated receptors understimulated. These effects are often visible because the receptor has an endogenous agonist, such that receptor activation is a part of normal physiologic processes. When a second messenger system is up-regulated or a cell surface receptor is down-regulated, a ''normal'' amount of endogenous agonist can effect a supranormal or a subnormal response, respectively. For exam-

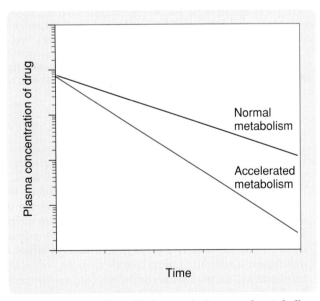

Figure 17-2. Induction of tolerance by increased metabolism of drug. Upon initial administration, a drug that is metabolized by hepatic microsomal enzymes exhibits first-order elimination kinetics *(black curve)*. Upon repeated administrations of the drug, induction of these enzymes causes accelerated metabolism of the drug and a decreased plasma half-life *(blue curve)*. Because the drug is eliminated more rapidly, a higher dose of drug is required to elicit the same response.

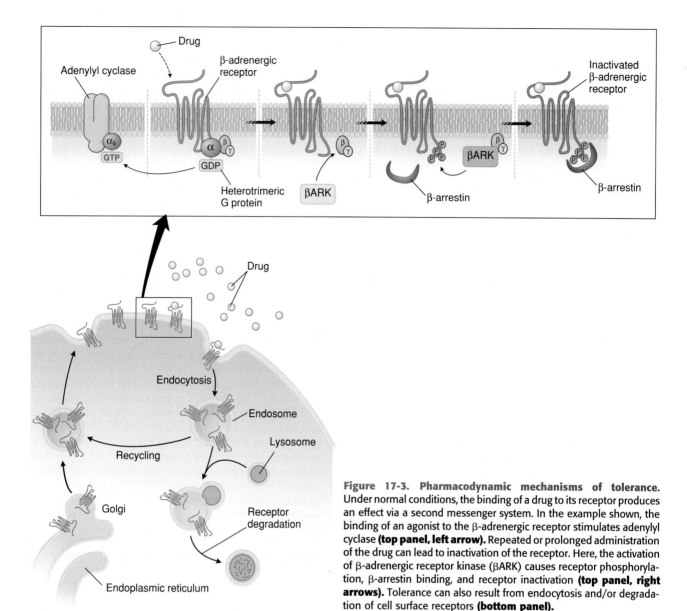

Figure 17-3. Pharmacodynamic mechanisms of tolerance. Under normal conditions, the binding of a drug to its receptor produces an effect via a second messenger system. In the example shown, the binding of an agonist to the β-adrenergic receptor stimulates adenylyl cyclase **(top panel, left arrow)**. Repeated or prolonged administration of the drug can lead to inactivation of the receptor. Here, the activation of β-adrenergic receptor kinase (βARK) causes receptor phosphorylation, β-arrestin binding, and receptor inactivation **(top panel, right arrows)**. Tolerance can also result from endocytosis and/or degradation of cell surface receptors **(bottom panel)**.

ple, acute alcohol intake facilitates the inhibitory activity of GABA at its receptors causing sedation. Over time, the GABA receptors become down-regulated, decreasing the level of inhibition to counter the sedative effects of alcohol. If the alcohol is abruptly removed, the decreased GABAergic inhibition results in a state of central nervous system hyperactivity, which characterizes alcohol withdrawal. Thus, tolerance and physical dependence arise from similar mechanisms, although because it is possible to have dependence without tolerance and vice versa, it is clear that our understanding of these phenomena is incomplete.

MECHANISMS OF PSYCHOLOGICAL DEPENDENCE

Although the mechanisms of physical dependence are relatively well characterized, the causes of psychological dependence are still controversial, despite much work in this area.

In the 1950's, Olds and Milner implanted electrodes in various regions of the rat brain to determine which neuroanatomic areas mediate rewarded behavior. The rats learned to perform an act (such as pressing a lever) that resulted in a short pulse of nondestructive stimulation in the brain at the site of the electrode. The **medial forebrain bundles** and the **ventral tegmental area** (VTA) in the midbrain were found to be particularly effective brain reward sites. A subset of dopaminergic neurons projects directly from the ventral tegmental area to the **nucleus accumbens** (NAc) via the medial forebrain bundle. It is believed that these neurons are crucial for the brain reward pathway, because severing this pathway, or blocking dopamine receptors in the nucleus accumbens with a dopamine receptor antagonist (such as haloperidol; see Chapter 12, Pharmacology of Dopaminergic Neurotransmission), decreases the rewarding effects of stimulating the ventral tegmental area. Moreover, release of dopamine in the nucleus accumbens can be detected using the technique

A Acute administration of morphine decreases cellular activity

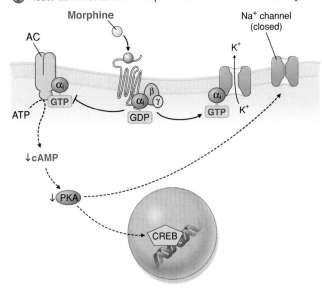

B Chronic administration of morphine induces tolerance

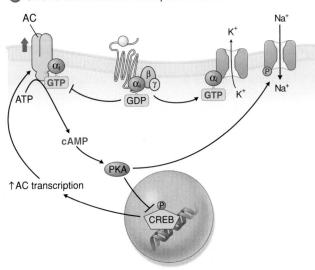

Figure 17-4. Induction of tolerance to morphine. A. The μ-opioid receptor is coupled to a G protein that activates potassium channels and inhibits adenylyl cyclase (AC), resulting in membrane hyperpolarization and in decreased production of cAMP. Because cAMP activates protein kinase A (PKA), which in turn regulates the threshold of the voltage-gated sodium channel, the decreased cAMP levels indirectly decrease sodium channel conductance. Decreased cAMP also decreases activation of the transcription factor cAMP response element-binding protein (CREB), which regulates the level of AC expression. **B.** Chronic administration of morphine up-regulates CREB, which stimulates the transcription of adenylyl cyclase, which, in turn, restores cAMP production toward normal levels. The increased cAMP stimulates PKA, which phosphorylates (and thereby activates) both CREB and the voltage-gated sodium channel. Therefore, up-regulation of the cAMP pathway counteracts the acute effects of the drug, resulting in tolerance.

of microdialysis. These measurements show that dopaminergic synapses of the nucleus accumbens are active during stimulation of the brain reward pathway and that dopamine in the nucleus accumbens is necessary for reward. Drugs capable of causing psychological dependence induce the greatest dependence when administered directly to the ventral tegmental area, the nucleus accumbens, or the cortical or subcortical areas that innervate these two areas.

Although the dopaminergic pathway is associated with reward, dopamine may also increase the salience of stimuli and alert the animal or person to its importance. As discussed above, the dopamine pathway is activated during drug use. It is known that dopamine is released in the nucleus accumbens of rats while the animals are eating after a fast or eating particularly palatable food. (Thus, the assertion that chocolate is "addictive" has a mechanistic rationale, even though most "chocoholics" would not meet the DSM-IV criteria in Box 17-1.) The reward pathway is also activated in rats during mating behaviors and certain social interactions. With repeated experiences, however, this dopamine pathway is also activated during anticipation of the reward. The nucleus accumbens receives inputs from a number of brain regions in addition to the dopaminergic ventral tegmental area. Pathways have been found from several areas of the cortex, hippocampus, thalamus, and amygdala, and from serotonergic nuclei; these pathways may mediate reward-associated learning and association.

Although the discovery that drugs of abuse activate the brain reward pathway offers an easy explanation for psychological dependence (i.e., that administration of a drug is associated with reward), recent literature has suggested that psychological dependence is more complicated. It is likely that many of the molecular mechanisms that mediate physical dependence, such as the up-regulation of second messenger signaling pathways and alterations in receptor sensitivity, are also important in psychological dependence. In this formulation, the distinction between physical and psychological dependence arises not because different molecular mechanisms are operative, but because drug-induced changes affect neurons having different functions. For example, a drug could be acutely euphorigenic because it activates the dopaminergic brain reward pathway, but the euphoria could be followed by a period of dysphoria. If the brain reward pathway undergoes adaptations after repeated administration of the drug, then these adaptations would be unmasked during withdrawal from the drug, resulting in a state of psychological dependence.

MECHANISMS OF ADDICTION

Addiction was originally thought to depend primarily on the physical or psychological effects of withdrawal. Because withdrawal is an aversive event, the need to maintain blood levels of the drug was thought to be a compelling reason for continued use of the drug. Although this mechanism may be operative in the short run, it does not explain the observation that the effects of addiction are felt long after the physical symptoms of withdrawal have abated. Years after an addict has discontinued use of a substance, the addict can experience intense **cravings** for the drug (i.e., an intense preoccupation with obtaining the drug), suggesting that a form of psychological dependence may be long-lasting. Thus, addicts are prone to **relapse,** even after years of sobriety. The likelihood of relapse is especially strong in situations in which individuals simultaneously encounter both stress and the context in which the drug was previously used. In part, this increased likelihood of relapse may result from an interplay between reward circuitry and memory circuitry in the brain that, under normal circumstances, assigns emotional value to certain memories.

Physical dependence is unlikely to be the primary mechanism of addiction for drugs such as cocaine and amphetamines, which cause few symptoms of physical dependence but are nonetheless highly addictive. Most interviews with addicts in recovery suggest that they used to arrange their priorities to obtain more drug, not for fear of the physical symptoms associated with withdrawal, but because they are constantly striving to feel more normal. These observations suggest that chronic drug use causes a long-lasting change in the underlying brain reward system and/or in memory systems related to the reward system.

The concept of **allostasis** has provided a useful explanation for the persistence of addiction. Allostasis is a long-lasting brain adaptation to the chronic presence of a drug, which establishes an altered homeostasis that depends on continued presence of the drug. When the addict is abstinent and the drug is removed, the addict doesn't feel ''normal'' and will seek and reuse the drug to re-establish the drug-dependent homeostasis. Human and animal studies have found evidence for these long-term neuroadaptations in altered neurotransmitter levels (e.g., dopamine depletion after chronic alcohol or stimulant use), increased stress reactivity, altered signal transduction mechanisms, changes in gene expression, and altered synaptic configurations and function. Clinically, abstinent patients report dysphoria, sleep disturbances, and heightened stress responses that can last for weeks to months after detoxification.

Current thinking about addiction recognizes the heterogeneity of the addictive process. For some individuals, reward factors may predominate, and getting high or feeling euphoric motivates drug use. For others, relief factors predominate, such as drinking to reduce stress, to reduce the dysphoria of protracted withdrawal and feel normal, or to treat withdrawal. Still others may self-medicate to the reduce psychiatric symptoms of a co-occurring disorder.

Variables Affecting the Development of Addiction

The development of addiction is dependent on a number of variables, including the nature of the drug, genetic and other traits of the drug user, and environmental factors.

As noted above, the ability of a drug to produce psychological dependence is strongly correlated with its ability to cause addiction. Pharmacokinetic properties of the drug also affect its propensity to cause addiction. In general, short-acting drugs are more addictive than long-acting drugs because the clearance of a long-acting drug results in a slow decrease in drug concentration over time, preventing acute withdrawal. In addition, the more rapid the rise in drug concentration at the target neurons, the greater the potential for addiction. Direct injection or rapid absorption of drug through a large surface area (e.g., the lungs via smoking) is more highly addictive than slower absorption through the intestinal or nasal mucosa. The importance of this effect is demonstrated by the potential for abuse of various forms of cocaine (Fig. 17-5). The use of coca leaves as a chew or in teas is widely practiced among people living in the Andean mountains: this has a relatively low potential for addiction, because of the slow rate of rise and low peak concentration of drug attained by absorption through the buccal or intestinal mucosa. The rapid absorption of extracted cocaine hydrochloride through the nasal mucosa is significantly more addictive. The most addictive forms of cocaine are intravenous injections and inhalation of smoked freebase (crack cocaine), both of which result in a very rapid rise in plasma concentration and a high peak concentration of drug.

Different people react differently to drugs. Some individuals use a drug once and never use it again; others use a drug repeatedly in moderate amounts without developing an addiction; in others, the first use of a drug produces such an intense euphoric feeling that the likelihood of addiction is high. The factors discussed above (i.e., the chemistry of the molecule and its site of action; the peak and rate of rise of drug concentration; the context in which the drug is used; previous experiences; and the ease with which the experience can be repeated) all interact with the genetics, personality, and environment of the individual to affect the probability of drug addiction.

Genetic influences have been best studied in individuals with alcohol abuse. Alcohol abuse and dependence are complex phenotypes determined by multiple genes, environmental exposures throughout the lifespan, gene-environment interactions, gene-behavior interactions, and gene-gene interactions. Heritability estimates suggest that genetic factors account for 50% to 60% of the variance associated with alcohol abuse.

The best known examples of candidate genes that alter risk for alcohol dependence are the alcohol metabolism genes, including those encoding the alcohol dehydrogenases ADH1B*2, ADH2 and ADH3 that metabolize alcohol more rapidly, and those encoding certain aldehyde dehydrogenases (particularly ALDH2*2). Polymorphisms in these genes alter enzymatic activity and result in increases in the levels of acetaldehyde, which causes aversive symptoms that act as a deterrent to drinking alcohol and development of alcohol dependence.

Sensitivity to alcohol is also a physiologically-based trait influenced by genetic inheritance. Low sensitivity to alcohol (high innate tolerance) is associated with an increased risk for developing alcoholism. Schuckit and colleagues found evidence for genetic linkage of the ''low level of response'' phenotype with the same region on chromosome 1 that was linked with the ''alcohol dependence'' phenotype. However, subjective response to alcohol is a complex trait affected by several neurotransmitters. For example, individuals with the alcohol dependence-associated GABRA2 allele have a blunted subjective response to alcohol, and individuals carrying the ASP40 variant of the μ-opioid receptor or those with a certain single nucleotide polymorphism of the cannabinoid receptor appear to have an enhanced euphoric response to alcohol.

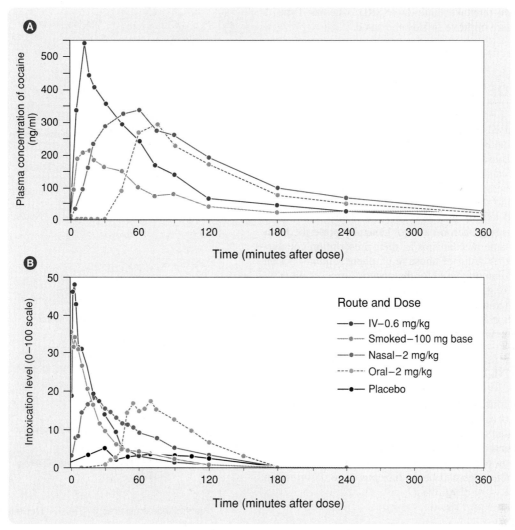

Figure 17-5. Plasma cocaine concentrations and levels of intoxication as a function of route of administration of the drug. The pharmacokinetics **(A)** and pharmacodynamics **(B)** of cocaine are highly dependent on the route of administration of the drug. Intravenous (IV) cocaine and smoked free-base cocaine are associated with very rapid attainment of peak plasma drug concentrations **(A)** and high levels of intoxication **(B)**. In contrast, the nasal and oral routes of administration are associated with a slower rise in plasma drug concentrations **(A)** and lower levels of intoxication **(B)**. Because of the very rapid rise in plasma drug concentration and very high intoxication levels, smoked and intravenous cocaine carry a higher risk of addiction than cocaine taken nasally or orally.

Alcohol and Drug User Subtypes

Alcoholics differ with regard to patterns of drinking and drinking outcomes. The first classification of alcoholic subtypes related to genetic and neurobiological differences was the distinction between Type 1 and Type 2 alcoholism. Type 1 is characterized by ''late'' onset of alcohol-related problems after 25 years of age, less antisocial behavior, infrequent spontaneous alcohol seeking and loss of control, and guilt and fear about alcohol. Type 1 alcoholics are low in novelty seeking and high in harm avoidance and reward dependence. In contrast, Type 2 is characterized by early onset of alcohol problems (before age 25), antisocial behavior when drinking, frequent spontaneous alcohol seeking and loss of control, and infrequent guilt and fear about drinking.

The Lesch Typology, used in Europe, envisions four alco-

holism subtypes: Type 1 exhibits early withdrawal and frequent alcohol-related psychoses and convulsions; Type 2 exhibits pre-morbid conflicts and anxiety; Type 3 emerges from a permissive alcoholic milieu and shows mood changes; Type 4 has pre-morbid cerebral injuries and social problems.

A third classification system consists of Type A and Type B alcoholics. Type A is characterized by later onset, fewer childhood risk factors such as attention deficit hyperactivity disorder (ADHD) or conduct disorder, less severe dependence, fewer alcohol problems, less alcoholism treatment, and less psychopathology. Type B is characterized by early onset, childhood conduct disorder, more severe dependence, more treatment, and more psychopathology. Recently, alcohol subtype has been shown to be a predictor of treatment response to serotonergic medications. For example, Type B alcoholics may worsen their drinking in response to a selective serotonin reuptake inhibitor (SSRI), whereas Type A alcoholics may improve or stay the same.

DRUGS OF ABUSE

Having focused on the mechanisms by which drugs cause dependence and addiction, the discussion now turns to some commonly abused classes of drugs. Several drugs with the potential to cause dependence and addiction are commonly prescribed therapeutics (e.g., opioids, barbiturates, benzodiazepines), and their mechanisms of action have been discussed in detail in previous chapters. Other commonly abused drugs (e.g., heroin) are not generally prescribed, but act via the same mechanisms as their prescription counterparts. Yet other drugs of abuse (e.g., phencyclidine) act on targets not commonly used for therapeutic purposes. Finally, some drugs (e.g., cannabis) affect receptors that are not yet targets for therapeutic intervention. Nonetheless, the mechanisms of action of these drugs have many parallels to receptors and systems that have been described in earlier chapters.

COMMONLY PRESCRIBED THERAPEUTICS

Many commonly prescribed therapeutics can cause dependence and, occasionally, addiction. This category includes three important classes of drugs: **opioids, benzodiazepines,** and **barbiturates.** The mechanisms of action and general pharmacology of opioids are described in Chapter 16, and those of barbiturates and benzodiazepines are described in Chapter 11.

Opioids

As the case of Mr. B illustrates, chronic opioid use can lead to a significant probability of relapse that persists long after the physical symptoms of dependence have abated. There appear to be two pathways by which opioids interact with the brain reward system. One site of action lies in the ventral tegmental area, where GABAergic interneurons tonically inhibit the dopaminergic neurons responsible for activating the brain reward pathway in the nucleus accumbens. These GABAergic interneurons can be inhibited by endogenous enkephalins, which bind to μ-opioid receptors on the GABAergic terminals. Because exogenous opioids, such as morphine, also bind to and activate μ-opioid receptors (see Chapter 16), it follows that an exogenously administered opioid could activate the brain reward pathway by disinhibiting dopaminergic neurons in the ventral tegmental area (Fig. 17-6). The second pathway, which has not been as well studied, is localized in the nucleus accumbens. Opioids acting in this region may inhibit GABAergic neurons that project back to the ventral tegmental area, perhaps as part of an inhibitory feedback loop. The relative importance of these two pathways is still being debated.

Although all opioids have the potential to cause tolerance and physical dependence, certain opioids are more likely than others to cause addiction. Opioids associated with the fastest rise in brain concentration of drug, including those

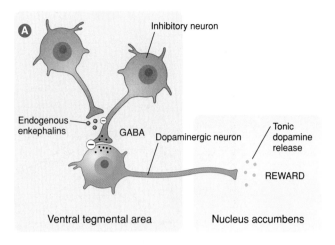

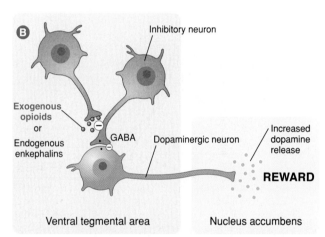

Figure 17-6.   Role of opioids in the brain reward pathway. A. GABAergic neurons tonically inhibit the dopaminergic neurons that arise in the ventral tegmental area and are responsible for reward. These GABAergic neurons can be inhibited by endogenous enkephalins, which locally modulate the release of neurotransmitter at the GABAergic nerve terminal. **B.** Administration of exogenous opioids results in decreased GABA release and disinhibition of the dopaminergic reward neurons. The increased release of dopamine in the nucleus accumbens signals a strong reward.

injected intravenously, have the highest likelihood for abuse. Likewise, abuse of the drug oxycodone (sold as a slow release OxyContin®), which is commonly prescribed for moderate or severe pain, has received much recent publicity because of misuse and cases of addiction. One reason for the highly addictive nature of oxycodone is that the oral tablets can be broken up, dissolved, and injected. This form of administration results in a much more rapid rise in plasma (and hence brain) concentrations of drug, a more intense feeling of euphoria, and a greater addiction potential as compared to the normally prescribed, slow-release oral form of the drug.

Benzodiazepines and Barbiturates

Benzodiazepines and barbiturates can cause both physical dependence and addiction, although addiction is rare. Because benzodiazepines and barbiturates increase the efficiency of GABAergic pathways, chronic use of these drugs can induce down-regulation of these pathways by a compensatory mechanism. One possible mechanism of down-regulation is the uncoupling of the benzodiazepine site from the GABA site on GABA$_A$ receptors (see Chapter 11). Thus, the binding of benzodiazepines to GABA$_A$ would remain unchanged, but the drug would have little or no potentiating effect on the binding of GABA to the receptor. Down-regulation of inhibitory GABAergic pathways would be expected to leave the brain "underinhibited," increasing the possibility of seizures (see Chapter 14), delirium, and occasionally death upon abrupt withdrawal of the benzodiazepine or barbiturate. Underinhibition of pathways involving central sympathetic activity can lead to physical symptoms such as anxiety, sleep disturbance, and dizziness. Similarly, underinhibition of pathways governing anxiety, fear, confusion, and panic can cause psychological dependence and lead to addiction. Clearly, the potential consequences of benzodiazepine and barbiturate withdrawal should not be ignored.

It is important to note that most prescribed therapeutics cause addiction only rarely, and that the potential for addiction should not deter physicians or other health professionals from prescribing a drug for legitimate medical purposes. Unfortunately, opioids are often underprescribed for the treatment of pain because tolerance (manifested as a request for higher and higher doses of drug) is mistaken for addiction. This condition is often referred to as **pseudoaddiction.** Because tolerance is an expected effect of the drug, physicians should be prepared to increase the dose, if necessary, to control the patient's pain. Because of the high potential for withdrawal symptoms upon discontinuation of therapy, physicians should also be careful to taper the dose of such a medication that has been prescribed for an extended period and to explain to the patient the rationale for the taper.

This is not to say that opioids, benzodiazepines, and barbiturates cannot be misused. For example, a patient in possession of medication left over from a previous prescription may use it inappropriately for another indication. Similarly, a patient may "share" medication with someone else outside a physician's supervision. For a variety of reasons, especially an inability to obtain more of the drug, this type of drug misuse rarely leads to addiction. In contrast, some patients may exhibit drug-seeking behavior and resort to forging prescriptions or obtaining prescriptions from multiple physicians, especially after suboptimal management of the underlying condition (e.g., failing to taper slowly a drug that has resulted in dependence). In some cases, a "black market" for the drug may develop (note the example of oxycodone cited above). It bears repeating, however, that, although cases of addiction receive much publicity, undermedication of pain is far more common than addiction to pain medication.

Another serious concern is the misuse of prescription opioids (or, less commonly, benzodiazepines or barbiturates) by health professionals. For at least two reasons, health professionals who misuse prescription medications are at greater risk for developing addiction. First, they have more ready access to prescription medication. Second, they may mistakenly believe that, because they understand a drug's effects, they will be able to control its use more easily.

DRUGS RELATED TO THERAPEUTICS

The second category of commonly abused drugs consists of agents that bind to the same receptors as commonly prescribed therapeutics, but that are not themselves used as therapeutic agents. For example, **heroin** binds to the same receptor as **morphine. Alcohol,** which binds to the GABA$_A$ receptor, and **nicotine,** which binds to the nicotinic acetylcholine receptor, mimic other GABAergic and cholinergic agonists, respectively. **Cocaine** and **amphetamine** have actions similar to those of other drugs that inhibit monoamine reuptake transporters. For these drugs, it is possible to understand their effects by understanding the effects of their prescribed counterparts.

Heroin

As with morphine, heroin exerts its effects by binding to the μ-opioid receptor. The difference in the action of the two drugs is due primarily to differences in their pharmacokinetics. The two drugs are close structural analogues (heroin is deacetylated to 6-monoacetylmorphine, and morphine is acetylated to the same compound), but heroin is more hydrophobic than morphine. Because of this property, heroin crosses the blood–brain barrier more rapidly. The more rapid increase in brain concentrations of heroin produces a sharper "high," which explains why heroin is typically preferred over morphine as a drug of abuse. The mechanism by which heroin produces dependence and addiction is identical to that of morphine and the other opioids.

Alcohol

Alcohol (specifically, ethanol) affects a number of different receptors, including GABA$_A$ receptors, NMDA glutamate receptors, and cannabinoid receptors. Although the specific sites of action are unknown, GABA$_A$ channels are believed to mediate the anxiolytic and sedative effects of alcohol, as well as the effects of alcohol on motor coordination, tolerance, dependence, and self-administration. Alcohol increases GABA-mediated chloride conductance and enhances hyperpolarization of the neuron. Its mechanisms of dependence and addiction are likely to be similar to those of other drugs affecting the GABA neurotransmission system.

Evidence also points to a role for NMDA receptors in the development of tolerance and dependence to alcohol, and NMDA receptors may have a role in the alcohol withdrawal syndrome. Specifically, alcohol inhibits subtypes of NMDA receptors that seem to be capable of long-term potentiation. Thus, although GABA receptors play a vital role in mediating the effects of alcohol, the ability of alcohol to interact with a number of different receptor types suggests that our understanding of its mechanisms of action remains incomplete.

Nicotine

Nicotine directly activates nicotinic acetylcholine receptors that are located centrally, peripherally, and at the neuromuscular junction. Centrally, nicotine produces a strong depen-

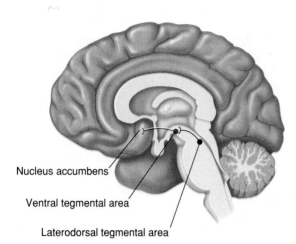

Figure 17-7. Role of cholinergic neurotransmission in the brain reward pathway. Nicotinic neurons *(black)* arising in the laterodorsal tegmental area (DTA) activate dopaminergic neurons *(blue)* in the ventral tegmental area (VTA). These neurons, which make up the brain reward pathway, release dopamine in the nucleus accumbens (NAc).

dence, and the craving for cigarettes is directly tied to decreases in the plasma levels of nicotine. Cholinergic neurons arising from the **laterodorsal tegmental area** (near the border of the midbrain and pons) activate nicotinic and muscarinic acetylcholine receptors on dopaminergic neurons in the ventral tegmental area; stimulation of these nicotinic receptors by nicotine activates the dopaminergic brain reward pathway (Fig. 17-7). This strong and direct effect on the reward pathway explains the high addiction potential of nicotine, and hence of cigarettes and other forms of tobacco.

Cocaine and Amphetamine

By blocking or reversing the direction of the neurotransmitter transporters that mediate reuptake of the monoamines dopamine, norepinephrine, and serotonin into presynaptic terminals, **cocaine** and **amphetamine** potentiate dopaminergic, adrenergic, and serotonergic neurotransmission. Cocaine is most potent at blocking the dopamine transporter (DAT), although higher concentrations block the serotonin and norepinephrine transporters (5HTT and NET, respectively). Recall that the tricyclic antidepressants (TCAs) and selective serotonin reuptake inhibitors (SSRIs) function in a similar manner, blocking reuptake of norepinephrine and serotonin (TCAs) or serotonin alone (SSRIs) into presynaptic neurons. Amphetamine reverses the direction of all three monoamine transporters, although this drug is more effective at the norepinephrine transporter. Amphetamine also releases vesicular transmitter stores into the cytoplasm; these combined actions cause the catecholamine neurotransmitter to be transported into, rather than out of, the synaptic cleft. By these actions, cocaine and amphetamine increase the concentration of monoamine neurotransmitters in the synaptic cleft, potentiating neurotransmission (Fig. 17-8).

Although cocaine and amphetamine act on monoamine neurons throughout the body, it is the action of these drugs

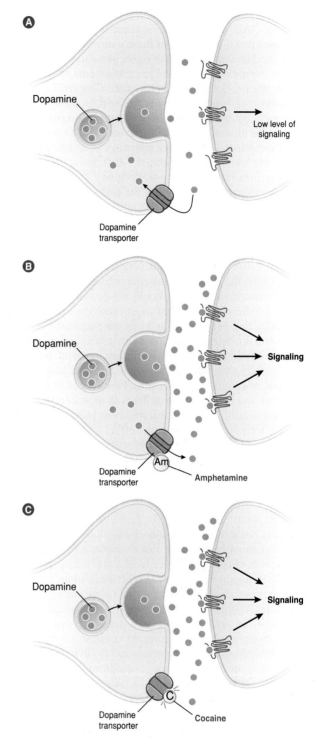

Figure 17-8. Mechanism of action of amphetamine and cocaine. A. In normal dopaminergic neurotransmission, dopamine released from synaptic vesicles is cleared from the synapse by dopamine reuptake transporters in the presynaptic membrane. **B.** Amphetamine *(Am)* releases dopamine from synaptic vesicles into the cytosol *(not shown)* and reverses the direction of dopamine transport through the dopamine transporter. Together, these actions increase the concentration of dopamine in the synaptic cleft, and thereby potentiate neurotransmission. **C.** Cocaine *(C)* potentiates dopaminergic neurotransmission by blocking the dopamine reuptake transporter and thereby increasing synaptic dopamine concentration. Amphetamine and cocaine have similar effects at noradrenergic and serotonergic nerve terminals.

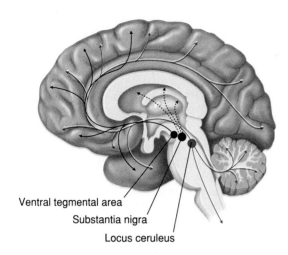

Ventral tegmental area
Substantia nigra
Locus ceruleus

——— Noradrenergic neurons ······· Dopaminergic neurons

Figure 17-9. Locus of action of amphetamine and cocaine. Amphetamine and cocaine act on noradrenergic neurons originating in the locus ceruleus and projecting throughout the cerebral cortex, hypothalamus, cerebellum and spinal cord (blue). Noradrenergic neurons that terminate in the cerebral cortex maintain alertness. Amphetamine and cocaine also act on dopaminergic neurons originating in the ventral tegmental area and projecting to the cerebral cortex, hypothalamus, and nucleus accumbens (black solid lines). Dopaminergic neurons that terminate in the nucleus accumbens are an important component of the brain reward pathway (see Figs. 17-6, 17-7). Other dopaminergic neurons originating in the substantia nigra and projecting to the striatum (black dashed lines) help initiate intended movement.

on neurons in two major centers in the brain that likely governs their potential for abuse (Fig. 17-9). The first set of neurons, in the **locus ceruleus** in the pons, sends ascending adrenergic projections throughout the hypothalamus, thalamus, cerebral cortex and cerebellum, and descending projections to the medulla and spinal cord. These projections maintain alertness and responsiveness to unexpected stimuli (see Chapter 9, Adrenergic Pharmacology). Thus, drugs such as cocaine and amphetamine, which potentiate the actions of norepinephrine by inhibiting neurotransmitter reuptake, produce enhanced arousal and vigilance. For this reason, cocaine and amphetamine are considered psychostimulants.

The second major site at which cocaine and amphetamine act is on midbrain dopaminergic neurons, the axons of which terminate in the nucleus accumbens, striatum, and cortex. These dopaminergic terminals in the nucleus accumbens are a critical component of the brain's reward pathway.

Given the widespread distribution of monoamine neurons in the CNS, it is not surprising that cocaine and amphetamine have a number of effects in addition to psychostimulation. These drugs can cause paranoia and delusions, effects that may be related to potentiation of neurotransmission in the dopaminergic projections to the cortex, thalamus, and amygdala that may be involved in schizophrenia. Cocaine and amphetamine can also cause involuntary movements through their action on the basal ganglia, in much the same way that the anti-Parkinsonian dopaminergic drugs can cause dyskinesias associated with ''on periods.''

Because there is an extensive distribution of adrenergic

neurons in the peripheral nervous system, cocaine and amphetamine have widespread actions in peripheral tissues. These potentiators of norepinephrine neurotransmission increase heart rate and blood pressure through the increased action of norepinephrine on adrenergic receptors. Cocaine, in particular, can cause vasospasm leading to stroke, myocardial infarction, or aortic dissection.

It was long believed that the psychostimulants do not cause physical dependence. However, cocaine use can be associated with withdrawal symptoms such as bradycardia, sleepiness, and fatigue. Withdrawal from cocaine or amphetamine also causes psychological symptoms, such as dysphoria and anhedonia (an inability to experience pleasure), that are opposite to the euphoria experienced immediately following administration of the drug. Many of these symptoms are not strictly attributable to withdrawal because they cannot be alleviated by the administration of more cocaine or amphetamine. In fact, symptoms of withdrawal can appear even when psychostimulant levels in the plasma are still high. This is because the drugs cause **tachyphylaxis**, an acute process in which the target tissue becomes less and less responsive to constant concentrations of a drug. In the case of cocaine and amphetamine, tachyphylaxis may be caused by depletion of the neurotransmitter. Because the drugs block presynaptic neurotransmitter reuptake, over time the transmitter diffuses away from the synaptic cleft and neurotransmitter stores in the presynaptic terminal are depleted. This may explain why administering a dopamine receptor agonist such as **bromocriptine** (a semi-synthetic ergot alkaloid) can alleviate the symptoms of withdrawal.

DRUGS OF ABUSE AFFECTING NON-THERAPEUTIC RECEPTORS

A number of commonly abused drugs bind to receptors that have yet to be exploited therapeutically. One such drug, **phencyclidine** (PCP), blocks NMDA-type glutamate receptors. NMDA receptors mediate excitatory synaptic transmission and are involved in synaptic plasticity and memory. PCP interferes with these processes, producing complex effects such as anesthesia, delirium, hallucinations, and amnesia.

The drug **methylenedioxymethamphetamine** (MDMA), known colloquially as ecstasy, has received recent attention because of its increased use and the unfortunate perception that it is a ''safe'' drug. Although it is chemically related to methamphetamine and has similar dopaminergic effects, the primary effect of MDMA is on serotonergic neurotransmission. MDMA causes serotonin release into the synaptic cleft, inhibition of serotonin synthesis, and block of serotonin reuptake. Together, these complex actions of MDMA increase serotonin in the synaptic cleft while depleting presynaptic stores of the neurotransmitter. The drug causes a central stimulant effect like cocaine and amphetamine but, unlike those drugs, it also has hallucinogenic properties. Like cocaine and amphetamine, MDMA affects the brain reward pathway through dopaminergic stimulation. Finally, MDMA may be neurotoxic to a subpopulation of serotonergic neurons when the drug is administered repeatedly or in large amounts.

Cannabinoids are compounds found in cannabis (marijuana). These natural products bind to cannabinoid receptors, which are G protein-coupled receptors whose endogenous ligand is the arachidonic acid derivative **anandamide.** The two known cannabinoid receptors, CB1 and CB2, are widely distributed in the basal ganglia (including the substantia nigra pars reticulata and globus pallidus), the hippocampus, and the brainstem, and the effects of cannabis are correspondingly diffuse. Endogenous cannabinoids appear to be involved in the mediation of a variety of appetitive (reinforcing and consumptive) behaviors including eating, smoking and alcohol drinking. Cannabinoid use causes a prompt and generalized ''high'' characterized by euphoria, laughter, giddiness, and depersonalization. After 1–2 hours, cognitive functions such as memory, reaction time, coordination, and alertness are compromised, and the user has difficulty concentrating. This effect corresponds to a ''mellowing'' phase, which results in relaxation and even sleep. In rats, the administration of natural and synthetic cannabinoids causes dopamine release in the nucleus accumbens of the brain reward pathway, although the specific pathway involved is not yet known.

Cannabis use induces tolerance; the mechanism of this effect remains to be elucidated. Discontinuation of cannabis is followed by a withdrawal syndrome that includes restlessness, irritability, agitation, insomnia, and nausea. There is evidence that enkephalins are involved in this withdrawal syndrome.

Caffeine and the related methylxanthines theophylline and theobromine are ubiquitous drugs occurring in coffee, tea, cola, and other carbonated drinks, chocolate, and in many prescribed and over-the-counter medications. Methylxanthines act by blocking adenosine receptors that are expressed presynaptically on many neurons, including adrenergic neurons. Because activation of adenosine receptors inhibits norepinephrine release, competitive antagonism of the receptors by caffeine disinhibits norepinephrine release and, thus, acts as a stimulant. Caffeine may also block adenosine receptors on cortical neurons, and thereby disinhibit these neurons. Additionally, CNS adenosine is a natural promoter of sleep and drowsiness; by blocking adenosine receptors, caffeine has alerting effects and produces insomnia. Caffeine can cause withdrawal effects such as lethargy, irritability, and a characteristic headache, but addiction, though documented, is rare. Clinically significant caffeine withdrawal symptoms are commonly observed in even low to moderate users of caffeine.

Inhalants are volatile organic compounds that are inhaled (sometimes called *huffing*) for their psychotropic effects. The typical user of inhalants is a male teenager. Inhalants include organic solvents, such as gasoline, toluene, ethyl ether, fluorocarbons, and volatile nitrates, including nitrous oxide and butyl nitrate. Inhalants are readily available in many households and workplaces. At low doses, inhalants produce mood changes and ataxia; at high doses, they may produce dissociative states and hallucinosis. Dangers of organic solvent use include suffocation and organ damage, especially hepatotoxicity and neurotoxicity in the central and peripheral nervous systems. Cardiac arrhythmias and sudden death may occur. Inhaled nitrates may produce hypotension and methemoglobinemia. Hydrocarbon inhalants do not appear to act at a specific receptor, but rather disrupt cell functions by binding non-specifically to hydrophobic sites on receptors, signal transduction proteins, and other macromolecules. Nitrates, however, act at receptors for nitric oxide, a small molecule neuromodulator (see Chapter 21, Pharmacology of Vascular Tone).

MEDICAL COMPLICATIONS OF DRUG ABUSE AND DEPENDENCE

Given the multiplicity of drugs, the means by which they are obtained, and the variety of routes of administration, complications may be secondary to tissue toxicity, induced metabolic changes, adulterants mixed with the drugs, or infection from needle administration.

Many patients who abuse drugs use more than one substance. Little is known regarding the complex pharmacodynamic and pharmacokinetic effects of polysubstance abuse. For example, research has revealed a potentially dangerous interaction between cocaine and alcohol. When taken together, the two drugs are converted to **cocaethylene.** Cocaethylene has a longer duration of action in the brain and is more toxic than either drug alone. It is noteworthy that the mixture of cocaine and alcohol is the most common two-drug combination that results in drug-related death.

Other drugs may cause significant organ dysfunction. With repeated high doses of ethanol (alcohol) as seen in alcoholism, decreased left ventricular function with cardiomegaly can be life-threatening. Here, ethanol is directly toxic to heart muscle cells, affecting contractility of the myocytes and inhibiting the repair of injury to these cells. There is some suggestion that the mechanism of myocyte damage may be the overproduction of oxygen-containing molecules secondary to alcohol metabolism, with damage to the plasma membrane of the myocyte.

With moderate drinking, there is typically an increase in systolic blood pressure. Alcohol withdrawal also plays a role in hypertension because sympathetic activity is increased during withdrawal. Stress appears to cause a greater rise in blood pressure in drinkers than non-drinkers.

There appears to be a protective effect of drinking on coronary artery disease, at least in older individuals and those otherwise at risk for coronary disease. The so-called J-shaped mortality curve shows that these populations have decreased mortality with low to moderate drinking (generally 0.5 to 2 drinks/day) and increased mortality with heavy drinking. The mechanism of this protection involves beneficial effects of ethanol on lipoprotein metabolism and thrombosis: ethanol increases high-density lipoprotein (HDL) levels in a dose-dependent manner, and ethanol inhibits platelet aggregation and lowers plasma fibrinogen levels.

TREATMENTS FOR ADDICTION

In spite of the high prevalence of alcohol and drug problems in medical practice (10% to 15% in ambulatory care; 30% to 50% in emergency departments, and 30% to 60% in general hospital settings), the diagnosis is often overlooked. As is the case with other stigmatized diseases, specialized services are often inaccessible. A recent report of the Institute of Medicine points the way toward a renewed medical response to these health problems.

Treatments for addiction can be divided into two broad approaches, pharmacologic and psychosocial. Traditionally, pharmacologic treatments for addiction have focused on acute detoxification to relieve the withdrawal symptoms that accompany the cessation of drug use. It has been increasingly recognized, however, that detoxification does not affect the long-term course of addiction. Based on this understanding, new pharmacologic agents are being developed not just for detoxification but also to treat the chronic condition of addiction. These agents are summarized in the Drug Summary Table at the end of this chapter.

Pharmacologic agents for addiction assist in reducing harmful alcohol and drug use. These agents help the patient achieve prolonged abstinence. Thus, drug addiction is considered a chronic medical problem, and therapy must include long-term as well as short-term management. Psychosocial treatment approaches—for example, counseling techniques such as cognitive-behavioral therapy—have been effective when used alone or in combination with pharmacologic treatment. Often, the use of both approaches increases the positive outcomes of treatment. In addition, 12-step participation often improves outcomes, either utilized alone or when 12-step messages are incorporated into treatment programs (see below).

Although counseling typically focuses on an individual patient's psychological needs, effective treatment must also address the underlying factors that impede long-term recovery, such as unemployment, family disruption, and lack of access to health care.

Treatment outcomes in drug dependence and addiction are comparable to those in other chronic diseases, such as diabetes, hypertension, and asthma. Although some treatments are more effective in some patients than in others, the best predictor of positive outcomes is participation in treatment.

DETOXIFICATION

The first step in the treatment of dependence is **detoxification.** The goals of detoxification are to allow blood levels of the drug to fall to near zero and to allow the body to adapt to the absence of drug. Although detoxification may be achieved technically within a few days, for most drug dependence, withdrawal symptoms such as anxiety and insomnia may persist, requiring prolonged medication assistance. Psychosocial counseling should begin at the outset of the detoxification program and proceed with more intensity following detoxification. For example, Mr. B completed a 28-day inpatient rehabilitation protocol after acute detoxification.

The manifestations of drug withdrawal depend on the type of drug abused and can range from mild dysphoria to life-threatening seizures. The most commonly employed strategies for alleviating withdrawal are to taper the dose of the drug slowly and/or to use a long-acting drug in the same class. For example, a common treatment for nicotine withdrawal is the administration of nicotine via a sustained re-

lease transdermal patch or via a chewing gum. The dose is tapered slowly to allow the patient to avoid many of the unpleasant effects of nicotine withdrawal. Another example is the use of **methadone** for the treatment of addiction to an opioid, such as heroin. Methadone is a long-acting opioid that is administered as an oral tablet and hence has a much slower uptake than heroin. The combination of the slow onset and long plasma half-life cause the plasma levels of methadone to remain fairly constant, and the drug can be tapered slowly while avoiding the acute effects of opioid withdrawal (Fig. 17-10). Withdrawal symptoms from alcohol and benzodiazepines can be severe, in some cases even life-threatening. In these cases, administration of a long-acting benzodiazepine (such as **diazepam**) is indicated to prevent withdrawal seizures. Antiepileptic medications also suppress CNS hyperactivity due to sedative withdrawal and are efficacious as a primary treatment in alcohol and benzodiazepine withdrawal.

Another method of detoxification is to utilize medications from a different class to block the signs and symptoms of withdrawal. For example, α_2-adrenergic agonists such as **clonidine** and **lofexidine** can block the sympathetic hyperactivity and, to some extent, the gastrointestinal hyperactivity in opioid withdrawal. α_2-Receptors inhibit the stimulation of noradrenergic neurons in the brain and cholinergic neurons in the gut associated with opioid withdrawal, and α_2-agonists partially block opioid withdrawal symptoms.

A somewhat radical variant of the symptom-blockade technique uses general anesthesia to suppress opioid withdrawal. This technique has been adapted into a **rapid-detox** protocol for the treatment of opioid addiction. This protocol involves placing the patient under general anesthesia for up to 24 hours, during which an opioid antagonist such as **naltrexone** is administered. The antagonist effectively displaces the bound opioid from its receptor, hastening the elimination of opioid from the body. Massive withdrawal would normally be induced by such treatment, but these symptoms are suppressed by the anesthesia. This approach is not widely used and has not been endorsed by professional addiction societies. It does not assure long term recovery, and the risks of general anesthesia in this population are significant.

TWELVE-STEP SELF- AND MUTUAL-HELP APPROACHES

As the case of Mr. B illustrates, detoxifying a patient is not sufficient to ensure long-term abstinence. The risk of relapse is high, and long-term management of addiction is needed to achieve continued sobriety. While not acceptable or helpful to all patients, 12-step programs have played a prominent role in successful recovery for millions of individuals. These approaches are modeled after **Alcoholics Anonymous** (AA), which emphasizes 12 specific positive steps that foster continued sobriety (Box 17-2). Foremost among these steps is the admission by the patient that the problem is drinking, and that the only way to prevent a relapse is to maintain abstinence. AA and related programs such as Narcotics Anonymous (NA) and Cocaine Anonymous (CA) provide community support groups and mentoring. The presence of such help mitigates the sense of alienation and loneliness often felt by abusers of drugs and alcohol. Participation is

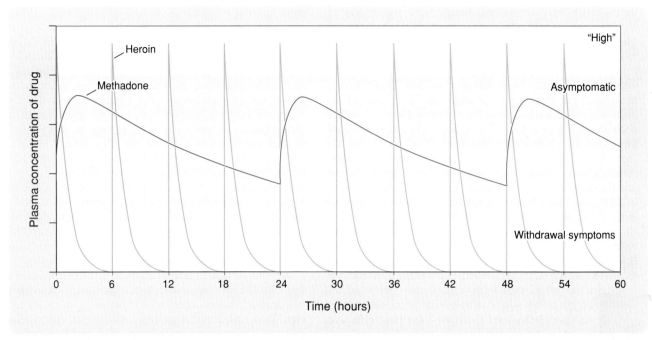

Figure 17-10.   Pharmacokinetics and pharmacodynamics of a fast-acting opioid (heroin) compared to a slow-acting opioid (methadone). The plasma concentration of a fast-acting opioid such as heroin rises rapidly after intravenous administration, generating a "high," but also falls quickly, producing withdrawal symptoms. On the other hand, the plasma concentration of a slow-acting, long half-life drug such as methadone remains in the asymptomatic range for a period of over 24 hours, so that the patient does not experience either the "high" or the withdrawal symptoms. Moreover, because of its long plasma half-life, methadone needs to be administered only once daily.

free and readily available. Related mutual support groups such as Al-Anon for spouses and Al-teen for teenage family members provide important support for recovery. All health professional students are encouraged and are welcome to attend an open AA meeting in their community.

Another therapeutic stance toward alcohol abuse, much less frequently utilized than AA, emphasizes moderation rather than abstinence. **Moderation management** focuses on establishing boundaries to drinking and on taking steps to ensure that the patient stays within those boundaries. This is accomplished by helping the patient understand the context under which alcohol is being used and avoid situations, such as drinking under excessive stress, that lead to problem drinking. Although there is much controversy over the effectiveness of moderation management in individuals who are clearly dependent on alcohol, this strategy has proved to be an effective way of managing alcohol use for some "problem drinkers"—patients who often overindulge but are not yet dependent.

PHARMACOLOGIC TREATMENT OF DEPENDENCE

The recognition that addiction is caused by fundamental changes in brain reward pathways indicates that pharmacotherapy could have an important role in the management of addiction. To date, several pharmacologic strategies have been employed.

The first of these strategies is the chronic administration of an agent that causes unpleasant adverse effects when the drug of abuse is used. For example, **disulfiram** inhibits alde-

hyde dehydrogenase, a critical enzyme in the alcohol metabolism pathway. In an individual who ingests ethanol while taking disulfiram, alcohol dehydrogenase oxidizes the ethanol to acetaldehyde, but disulfiram prevents aldehyde dehydrogenase from metabolizing the acetaldehyde. Therefore, this toxic metabolite accumulates in the blood. Acetaldehyde causes a number of unpleasant symptoms, including facial flushing, headache, nausea, vomiting, weakness, orthostatic hypotension, and respiratory difficulty. These symptoms can last from 30 minutes to several hours and are followed by exhaustion and fatigue. The unpleasant effects of alcohol consumption in the presence of disulfiram are intended as a deterrent to further drinking. Unfortunately, the effectiveness of disulfiram is limited by failures in compliance.

A second strategy used to treat addiction is to block the effects of the drug of abuse. **Naltrexone** is an opioid antagonist that competitively blocks the binding of opioids to the opioid receptor. Thus, a patient who injects an opioid, such as heroin, while taking naltrexone will not experience the "high" that normally accompanies drug use. Studies have shown that naltrexone also acts as an opioid inhibitor in the brain reward pathway. Thus, the effects of a drug such as ethanol, which releases endogenous opioids resulting in a disinhibition (or stimulation) of mesolimbic dopamine, share a final common reward pathway involving the opioid receptor and dopamine and are therefore also inhibited by naltrexone. For this reason, naltrexone has been used to treat alcohol addiction. Although not all randomized, placebo-controlled clinical trials have shown efficacy of naltrexone compared to placebo, meta-analyses of several studies do show an overall positive effect, particularly in reducing relapse to heavy

The 12-Step Program

The relative success of the Alcoholics Anonymous (AA) program seems to be attributable to the fact that an alcoholic in recovery (i.e., one who no longer drinks) has an exceptional faculty for "reaching out" and helping an uncontrolled drinker.

In its simplest form, the AA program operates when a recovered alcoholic passes along the story of his or her own problem drinking, describes the sobriety he or she has found in AA, and invites the newcomer to join the informal fellowship.

The heart of the suggested program of personal recovery is contained in twelve steps describing the experience of the earliest members of the society.

1. We admitted we were powerless over alcohol—that our lives had become unmanageable.
2. Came to believe that a power greater than ourselves could restore us to sanity.
3. Made a decision to turn our will and our lives over to the care of God *as we understood Him.*
4. Made a searching and fearless moral inventory of ourselves.
5. Admitted to God, to ourselves, and to another human being the exact nature of our wrongs.
6. Were entirely ready to have God remove all these defects of character.
7. Humbly asked Him to remove our shortcomings.
8. Made a list of all persons we had harmed and became willing to make amends to them all.
9. Made direct amends to such people wherever possible, except when to do so would injure them or others.
10. Continued to take personal inventory and when we were wrong promptly admitted it.
11. Sought through prayer and meditation to improve our conscious contact with God *as we understood Him,* praying only for knowledge of His will for us and the power to carry that out.
12. Having had a spiritual awakening as the result of these steps, we tried to carry this message to alcoholics and to practice these principles in all our affairs.

Newcomers are not asked to accept or follow these twelve steps in their entirety if they feel unwilling or unable to do so. Instead, they are asked to keep an open mind, to attend meetings where recovered alcoholics describe their personal experiences in achieving sobriety, and to read AA literature describing and interpreting the AA program.

AA members usually emphasize to newcomers that only problem drinkers themselves, individually, can determine whether or not they are, in fact, alcoholics.

At the same time, all available medical testimony indicating that alcoholism is a progressive illness is pointed out, that it cannot be cured in the ordinary sense of the term, but that it can be arrested through total abstinence from alcohol in any form. (Adapted from "The Twelve Steps of Alcoholics Anonymous.")

drinking. Naltrexone is not generally administered when there are traces of exogenous opioids in the system, because antagonism of remaining drug by naltrexone can lead to the development or exacerbation of withdrawal symptoms. Although naltrexone can effectively prevent the "high" associated with opioid abuse, it does not alleviate cravings or withdrawal effects, and there is a relatively high likelihood of non-compliance. Therefore, naltrexone has been effective only in individuals addicted to opioids or alcohol who have a high motivation to stay drug-free. An injectable long-acting naltrexone preparation has been approved by the U.S. Food and Drug Administration (FDA) for the treatment of alcohol dependence. This sustained-release naltrexone is injected intramuscularly once a month and has been demonstrated to reduce heavy alcohol consumption and increase alcohol abstinence.

The blockade approach may be efficacious for the treatment of other drug addictions as well. The CB1 cannabinoid receptor antagonist **rimonabant** has been developed to block the effects of exogenous cannabinoids and prevent cannabis users from becoming intoxicated. Because endogenous cannabinoids appear to be involved in nicotine dependence and alcohol dependence, rimonabant is also being studied as a potential treatment of these addictions.

A third pharmacologic approach has been the use of a slow-acting agonist for medication maintenance. **Methadone,** as discussed above, is a slow-acting opioid agonist. Because it is taken orally, it does not produce the sharp increases in plasma levels required to elicit a "high" such as that accompanying the injection of heroin or other opioids. Methadone also has a long half-life compared to heroin or morphine. Thus, once-daily administration of methadone produces plasma opioid levels that remain relatively constant over time and, therefore, mitigate cravings and prevent the emergence of withdrawal signs and symptoms (Fig.17-10). Moreover, methadone produces cross-tolerance to other opioids, so that a patient who injects heroin or another opioid while taking methadone experiences a reduced effect of the injected drug.

Pharmacologic approaches to treating opioid addiction have been further refined by using a partial opioid agonist such as **buprenorphine.** Because of its agonist effect, buprenorphine can alleviate cravings and withdrawal symptoms. On the other hand, because it is not a full agonist, buprenorphine carries a low risk of overdose, and it can antagonize the euphorigenic effects of a full agonist (such as heroin) should the patient "slip." In addition, the withdrawal effects of buprenorphine are mild compared to those of full opioid agonists. Thus, buprenorphine functions pharmacologically similar to a combination of naltrexone and methadone. Access to buprenorphine has been limited by legislation that requires prescribers to be trained and certified in its use and permits physicians to prescribe buprenorphine to only thirty patients at a time. To further minimize abuse, buprenorphine is usually administered as a sublingual preparation (**Suboxone®**) that also contains the opiate antagonist naloxone. If Suboxone® is abused and administered parenterally, the naloxone antagonizes the agonist effects of buprenorphine; when administered sublingually, the naloxone is inactivated and the full effects of buprenorphine are experienced.

A fourth approach is to utilize medications to prevent the

long-term dysphoria and brain dysfunction (allostasis) that is common in addicts who are newly abstinent. For example, one of the consequences of long-term alcohol consumption is a hyperactive glutamate system that persists even after alcohol consumption ceases. A medication such as **acamprosate**, which modulates glutamate hyperactivity to re-establish a more normal state, has been shown to be efficacious in preventing relapse to alcohol drinking and has been approved for the treatment of alcohol dependence.

The antiepileptic medication **topiramate**, which inhibits the AMPA/kainate class of glutamate receptors, was shown to significantly reduce alcohol drinking in a double-blind placebo controlled study. It is being studied in larger clinical trials, but is not currently approved for the treatment of alcoholism.

Depressed mood and anxious affect are often observed in abstinent patients, and some clinicians treat these symptoms with anxiolytics and antidepressants. However, a recent meta-analysis of antidepressant use in addicted patients found that these medications are not effective unless patients are diagnosed with a co-occurring major depression. In fact, there is some evidence that selective serotonin reuptake inhibitors (SSRIs) may cause Type B (early onset, antisocial) alcoholics to become worse and drink more alcohol than those receiving a placebo.

In contrast to the various pharmacologic treatments available for alcohol and opioid addiction, there is a paucity of current treatments for cocaine and amphetamine abuse, and none are formally approved by the FDA. Several trials have attempted to use antidepressants, such as the tricyclic antidepressant **desipramine** or the selective serotonin reuptake inhibitor **fluoxetine.** Desipramine acts by blocking monoamine reuptake (especially norepinephrine reuptake), whereas fluoxetine inhibits serotonin reuptake. Both agents have been shown to reduce drug craving but, unfortunately, neither has been shown to prevent cocaine use. There is recent evidence that disulfiram, used to treat alcohol dependence, may have some effectiveness in the treatment of cocaine dependence. In addition to its inhibition of aldehyde dehydrogenase, disulfiram also blocks dopamine beta-hydroxylase and can increase brain dopamine levels, possibly counteracting the dopamine-depleting effects of chronic cocaine use. Because cocaine sensitization involves glutamate, antiepileptics such as topiramate are also being studied for efficacy in the treatment of cocaine dependence.

Conclusion and Future Directions

This chapter has discussed the major causes of drug dependence and addiction. Drug dependence is caused by a homeostatic adaptation to the presence of the drug. Dependence can lead to addiction, which is defined as a maladaptive pattern of use of the drug associated with context-induced craving, especially under situations of stress, that leads to clinically significant impairment or distress. Although each drug has its own molecular and cellular mechanism of action, many abused drugs affect the brain reward pathway. This chapter has also discussed the major treatments for dependence and addiction, including the pharmacologic prevention and treatment of withdrawal symptoms,

the long-term social treatments of addiction, and newer pharmacologic treatments that promote long-lasting sobriety.

As research into its mechanisms continues to support the notion that addiction is a long-term, chronic illness, akin to atherosclerosis or diabetes, new treatments for addiction will help in the long-term management of the disease. New directions in addiction research are exemplified by two very different attempts to treat cocaine abuse. First, drugs that interact with specific dopamine receptor subtypes have been explored, investigating the hypotheses that a D1-specific agonist or D4-specific antagonist could suppress drug cravings, and a D2-specific antagonist could prevent the euphorigenic effects of cocaine. These hypotheses were generated based on experiments in mice, in which priming with a D1 agonist suppressed cocaine-seeking behavior.

Second, a novel vaccine approach has been investigated. Researchers injected a protein-conjugated analogue of cocaine into rats, and the rats produced antibodies directed against cocaine. Later, when the immunized rats were injected with cocaine, their brain cocaine levels were lower than those of unimmunized rats who were similarly injected. Based on these promising animal studies, researchers have initiated large-scale clinical trials of a cocaine vaccine, under the theory that cocaine will be less euphorigenic in vaccinated persons who are exposed to the drug. Trials of an analogous anti-nicotine vaccine are forthcoming. If successful, this approach could be extended to other drugs of abuse.

Suggested Reading

American Psychiatric Association. Diagnostic and Statistical Manual of Mental Disorders. 4th ed. Text Revision (DSM-IV-TR). Washington, DC: American Psychiatric Association; 2000.

Camí J, Farré M. Mechanisms of disease: drug addiction. *N Engl J Med* 2003;349:975–986. (*Current understanding of neural mechanisms leading to addiction.*)

Hyman S. Addiction to cocaine and amphetamine. *Neuron* 1996; 17:901–904. (*Reviews how the psychostimulants interface with the brain reward pathway and how neuronal adaptations to the drugs lead to addiction.*)

Hyman S. Why does the brain prefer opium to broccoli? *Harv Rev Psychiatry* 1994;2:43–46. (*Excellent introductory article explains the basics of addiction and dependence, covering both brain reward pathways and adaptations made by cells in response to long-term drug abuse.*)

Institute of Medicine. *Improving the quality of health care for mental and substance-use conditions: quality chasm series.* Washington, DC: American Academy Press; 2006. (*Landmark study spells out how quality can be achieved in substance abuse and mental health treatment. Good review of treatment research, with important policy implications.*)

Nestler E. Under siege, the brain on opiates. *Neuron* 1996;17: 897–900. (*Explains how opioids cause addiction, focusing on psychological dependence rather than the better studied physical dependence. Also explains cellular changes in the cAMP pathway in response to opioids.*)

Nestler E, Aghajanian G. Molecular and cellular basis of addiction. *Science* 1997;278:58–63. (*Describes addiction on a molecular and cellular basis, emphasizing changes in the cAMP pathway and the cytoskeleton.*)

O'Brien CP. A range of research-based pharmacotherapies for addiction. *Science* 1997;278:66–70. (*Reviews the principal long-term pharmacologic treatments for addiction, including the administration of antagonists, agonists, and partial agonists.*)

Sofuoglu M, Kosten TR. Emerging pharmacological strategies in the fight against cocaine addiction. *Expert Opin Emerg Drugs* 2006;11:91–98. (*Reviews research in cocaine addiction and potential novel treatment strategies, including research into a possible cocaine vaccine.*)

www.aa.org. (*Offers excellent information on Alcoholics Anonymous.*)

www.niaaa.nih.gov. National Institute on Alcohol Abuse and Alcoholism. (*Links to epidemiology and clinical information as well as research summaries on prevention, treatment, and alcohol policy.*)

www.nida.nih.gov. National Institute on Drug Abuse. (*Detailed information on drugs of abuse as well as research materials for health professionals and communities.*)

www.samhsa.gov. Substance Abuse and Mental Health Services Administration. (*Contains a wealth of information about prevention and treatment and co-occurring diagnoses; also access to listings of evidence-based treatment practices.*)

Drug Summary Table	**Chapter 17 Pharmacology of Drug Dependence and Addiction**

Drug	Clinical Applications	*Serious* and **Common** Adverse Effects	Contraindications	Therapeutic Considerations
INHIBITOR OF ALCOHOL METABOLISM				
Mechanism—Ethanol is oxidized by alcohol dehydrogenase to acetaldehyde, and acetaldehyde is metabolized by aldehyde dehydrogenase. Disulfiram inhibits aldehyde dehydrogenase and thereby prevents metabolism of acetaldehyde. Accumulation of serum acetaldehyde causes a number of unpleasant symptoms.				
Disulfiram	Alcoholism	*Hepatitis, peripheral neuropathy, optic neuritis, psychotic disorder* Metallic or garlic-like aftertaste, dermatitis	Concomitant use of paraldehyde, metronidazole, ethanol, or ethanol-containing products Coronary occlusion, severe myocardial disease Psychoses	Acetaldehyde accumulation causes facial flushing, headache, nausea, vomiting, weakness, orthostatic hypotension, and respiratory difficulty; these symptoms last from 30 minutes to several hours Disulfiram's effectiveness is limited by failures in compliance Coadministration with isoniazid may result in adverse CNS effects Disulfiram increases anticoagulant effects of warfarin
OPIOID ANTAGONISTS				
Mechanism—Competitively block binding of opioids to the μ-opioid receptor				
Naloxone	Opioid overdose Rapid reversal of opioid activity	*Cardiac arrhythmia, blood pressure lability, hepatotoxicity, pulmonary edema, opioid withdrawal*	Hypersensitivity to naloxone	Interacts with opioid analgesics Short half-life
Naltrexone	Opioid dependence Alcohol dependence	*Hepatotoxicity* Abdominal pain, constipation, nausea, headache, anxiety	Acute hepatitis or liver failure Concomitant opioid analgesics	Naltrexone prevents the "high" associated with opioid abuse, but it does not alleviate cravings or withdrawal effects High likelihood of non-compliance with naltrexone; only effective in motivated individuals An injectable, sustained-release naltrexone formulation is approved to reduce heavy alcohol consumption and increase alcohol abstinence
LONG-ACTING OPIOID AGONISTS				
Mechanism—A synthetic opioid agonist that binds and activates μ-opioid receptor				
Methadone	Opioid detoxification Severe pain	*Cardiac arrest, shock, respiratory arrest, depression* Constipation, nausea, asthenia, dizziness, somnolence	Hypersensitivity to methadone	Suppresses symptoms of withdrawal in opioid-dependent individuals due to slow absorption and long half-life Produces plasma opioid levels that remain fairly constant over time and thereby mitigates cravings and prevents withdrawal symptoms Produces cross-tolerance to other opioids Coadministration with phenytoin may decrease serum methadone concentration, resulting in methadone withdrawal symptoms

OPIOID PARTIAL AGONISTS

Mechanism—Partial μ-opioid receptor agonist and κ-opioid receptor antagonist

Drug	Clinical Applications	Serious and Common Adverse Effects	Contraindications	Therapeutic Considerations
Buprenorphine	Opioid dependence Moderate to severe pain	*Bradyarrhythmia, tachyarrhythmia, hypertension, hypotension, cyanosis, dyspnea, respiratory depression* Sedation, somnolence, vertigo, dizziness, nausea	Hypersensitivity to buprenorphine	Alleviates opioid cravings and withdrawal symptoms; carries low risk of overdose The withdrawal effects of buprenorphine are mild compared to those of full opioid agonists Buprenorphine is usually administered as Suboxone®, a sublingual preparation that also contains naloxone. If suboxone is abused and administered parenterally, the naloxone antagonizes the effects of buprenorphine; when administered sublingually, the naloxone is inactivated and the full effects of buprenorphine are experienced

GABA-ERGIC AGONISTS

Mechanism—Analogue of homotaurine, a GABAergic agonist. Stimulates inhibitory GABAergic neurotransmission in the brain and antagonizes the effects of glutamate; active at postsynaptic GABA-B receptors but not at GABA-A receptors in vitro.

Drug	Clinical Applications	Serious and Common Adverse Effects	Contraindications	Therapeutic Considerations
Acamprosate	Maintenance of abstinence in alcoholism	*Cardiomyopathy, heart failure, arterial and venous thrombosis, depression, anxiety, suicide attempt, acute renal failure* Dyspepsia, somnolence, confusion, amnesia, back pain	Severe renal impairment	Modulates glutamate hyperactivity to re-establish a more normal state for the treatment of alcohol dependence Decreases spontaneous alcohol consumption in animal studies Acamprosate has little or no abuse potential and does not induce dependence

TRICYCLIC ANTIDEPRESSANTS

Mechanism—Inhibit reuptake of 5HT and NE from the synaptic cleft

Drug	
Desipramine	See Drug Summary Table: Chapter 13 Pharmacology of Serotonergic and Central Adrenergic Neurotransmission

SELECTIVE SEROTONIN REUPTAKE INHIBITOR

Mechanism—Selectively inhibit reuptake of 5HT from the synaptic cleft

Drug	
Fluoxetine	See Drug Summary Table: Chapter 13 Pharmacology of Serotonergic and Central Adrenergic Neurotransmission

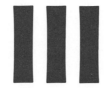

Principles of
Cardiovascular
Pharmacology

18

Pharmacology of Cardiac Rhythm

April W. Armstrong and David E. Clapham

INTRODUCTION

The human heart is both a mechanical and an electrical organ. To perfuse the body adequately with blood, the mechanical and electrical components of the heart must work in precise concert with each other. The mechanical component pumps the blood; the electrical component controls the rhythm of the pump. When the mechanical component fails despite a normal rhythm, heart failure can result (see Chapter 24, Integrative Cardiovascular Pharmacology: Hypertension, Ischemic Heart Disease, and Heart Failure). When the electrical component goes awry (called an arrhythmia), cardiac myocytes fail to contract in synchrony, and effective pumping is compromised. Changes in the membrane potential of cardiac cells directly affect cardiac rhythm, and most antiarrhythmic drugs act by modulating the activity of ion channels in the plasma membrane. This chapter discusses the ionic basis of electric rhythm formation and conduction in the heart, the pathophysiology of electric dysfunction, and the pharmacologic agents used to restore a normal cardiac rhythm.

Case

One winter morning, Dr. J, a 56-year-old professor, is lecturing on the treatment of cardiomyopathies to the second-year medical school class. He feels his heart beating irregularly and becomes nauseated. He is able to finish his lecture, but he continues to feel significantly short of breath throughout the morning. His persistent symptoms prompt him to walk down the street to the local emergency department.

Physical examination reveals an irregular heartbeat ranging from 120 to 140 beats/min. Dr. J's blood pressure is stable (132/76 mm Hg), and his oxygen saturation is 100% on room air. An electrocardiogram (ECG) confirms that Dr. J has atrial fibrillation, without any evidence of ischemia. Several intravenous boluses of diltiazem are administered, and his heart rate decreases to a range of 80–100 beats/min but his rhythm remains irregular. Further laboratory studies and a chest x-ray do not reveal an underlying cause for Dr. J's atrial fibrillation.

During observation over the next 12 hours, Dr. J remains in atrial fibrillation. Although his heart rate is under better control, he continues to experience palpitations. Under continuous ECG monitoring, a cardiologist administers an intravenous infusion of ibutilide. Twenty minutes after receiving the ibutilide, Dr. J's ECG shows a return to normal sinus rhythm. Based on his age and generally good health, Dr. J is sent home with a prescription for aspirin. He is instructed to call his doctor if he develops further symptoms of atrial fibrillation.

Dr. J feels fine at first, but he develops recurrent palpitations within 3 weeks of his initial event. After discussion with his cardiologist, he elects to start amiodarone at a maintenance dose of 200 mg/day, in addition to continuing his aspirin. Dr. J tolerates the amiodarone well and reports no difficulty breathing. He remains symptom-free during the rest of his cardiology lectures.

QUESTIONS

■ **1.** Why did diltiazem slow Dr. J's heart rate without affecting his underlying heart rhythm, atrial fibrillation?

■ **2.** Why should ibutilide be administered only under carefully monitored circumstances?

■ **3.** Why were ibutilide and amiodarone effective in converting Dr. J's heart rhythm to normal sinus rhythm?

■ **4.** What adverse effects of amiodarone could develop at higher daily doses?

ELECTRICAL PHYSIOLOGY OF THE HEART

Electrical activity in the heart, leading to rhythmic cardiac contraction, is a manifestation of the heart's exquisite control of cell depolarization and impulse conduction. Once initiated, a cardiac action potential is a spontaneous event that proceeds based on the characteristic responses of ion channels to changes in membrane voltage. At the completion of a cycle, the spontaneous depolarization of pacemaker cells ensures that the process repeats over and over, without interruption.

PACEMAKER AND NONPACEMAKER CELLS

The heart contains two types of cardiac myocytes—those that can spontaneously initiate action potentials and those that cannot. Cells possessing the ability to initiate spontaneous action potentials are termed **pacemaker cells.** All pacemaker cells possess **automaticity,** the ability to depolarize above a threshold voltage in a rhythmic fashion. Automaticity results in the generation of spontaneous action potentials. Pacemaker cells are found in the sinoatrial node (SA node), the atrioventricular node (AV node), and the ventricular conducting system (bundle of His, bundle branches, and Purkinje fibers). Together, the pacemaker cells constitute the specialized conducting system that governs the electrical activity of the heart. The second type of cardiac cells, the **nonpacemaker cells,** includes the atrial and ventricular myocytes. The nonpacemaker cells contract in response to depolarization and are responsible for the majority of cardiac contraction. In *pathologic* conditions, these nonpacemaker cells can acquire automaticity and thereby also act as pacemaker cells.

CARDIAC ACTION POTENTIALS

Ions are not distributed equally across cell membranes. Transporters (pumps) drive K^+ into cells while pumping Na^+ and Ca^{2+} out, giving rise to electrical and chemical gradients across the membrane. These gradients ultimately determine the membrane potential of a cardiac cell. The **Nernst equilibrium potential** for each ion ($E_{Na} = +70$ mV, $E_K = -94$ mV, and $E_{Ca} = +150$ mV) depends on the relative concentrations of ions inside and outside the cell. The difference between an ion's Nernst potential and the cell's membrane potential determines the driving force for ions into or out of the cell. Refer to Chapter 6, Principles of Cellular Excitability and Electrochemical Transmission, for a detailed discussion of the Nernst equilibrium potential.

When an ion-specific channel opens, the membrane potential approaches the equilibrium potential for that ion. For example, opening a K^+-selective channel drives the membrane potential towards E_K (-94 mV). The final membrane potential depends on the number of channels of each type, their conductances (i.e., the ability of each channel to pass ions), and the duration for which each channel remains open. *The resting membrane of the cardiac myocyte is relatively permeable to K^+ ions (because some types of K^+-selective channels are open) but not to Na^+ or Ca^{2+} ions;* hence, the **resting membrane potential** is close to the equilibrium potential for K^+. (The actual cardiac myocyte membrane potential is higher than the equilibrium potential for K^+, due to the contribution of other ion channels to the resting membrane potential.)

Changing the membrane potential requires the movement of relatively few ions across the membrane. Therefore, despite the opening and closing of ion channels, the ionic concentration gradients across the membrane remain relatively stable and the Nernst potential for each ion remains constant.

Cardiac action potentials are strikingly longer than those of nerve or skeletal muscle, lasting for almost half a second. Prolonged cardiac action potentials provide the sustained depolarization and contraction needed to empty the heart's chambers. Sinoatrial (SA) nodal cells pace the heart at normal resting heart rates between 60 and 100 beats/min, while ventricular muscle cells orchestrate the contraction that ejects blood from the heart (Fig. 18-1).

SA nodal cells fire spontaneously in a cycle defined by three phases, referred to as *phase 4, phase 0, and phase 3* (Fig. 18-2 and Table 18-1). **Phase 4** consists of a slow, spontaneous depolarization that is caused by an inward pacemaker current (I_f). This spontaneous depolarization accounts for the automaticity of the SA node. The channels that carry the I_f current are activated during the repolarization phase of the previous action potential. The I_f channels are nonselective cation channels, although most of the pacemaker current is carried by Na^+ ions because, at negative membrane poten-

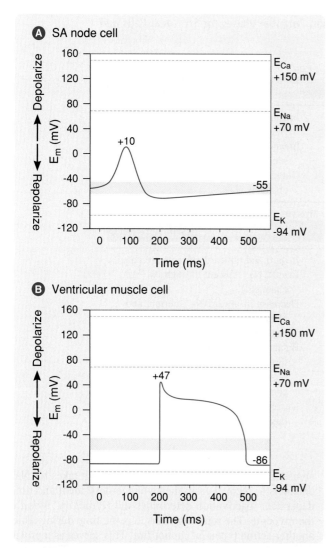

Figure 18-1. SA node and ventricular muscle cell action potentials. The resting membrane potential of a sinoatrial (SA) node cell is approximately −55 mV, while that of a ventricular muscle cell is −86 mV. The shaded areas represent the approximate depolarization required to trigger an action potential in each cell type. Together, the cardiac action potentials last for approximately half a second. SA node cells **(A)** depolarize to a peak of +10 mV, and ventricular muscle cells **(B)** depolarize to a peak of +47 mV. Note that the ventricular action potential has a much longer plateau phase. This long plateau ensures that ventricular myocytes have adequate time to contract before the onset of the next action potential. The Nernst equilibrium potentials of the major ions (E_{Ca}, E_{Na}, E_K) are shown as *dashed horizontal lines*. E_m, membrane potential.

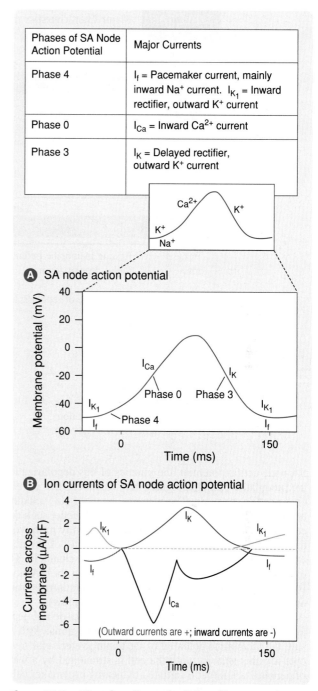

Figure 18-2. SA node action potential and ion currents. A. SA nodal cells are depolarized slowly by the pacemaker current (I_f) (phase 4), which consists of an inward flow of sodium (mostly) and calcium ions. Depolarization to the threshold potential opens highly selective voltage-gated calcium channels, which drive the membrane potential towards E_{Ca} (phase 0). As the calcium channels close and potassium channels open (phase 3), the membrane potential repolarizes. **B.** The flux of each ion species correlates roughly with each phase of the action potential. Positive currents indicate an outward flow of ions *(blue)*, while negative currents are inward *(gray)*.

tials, the driving force for Na$^+$ entry is greater than that for K$^+$ efflux. **Phase 0** consists of a more rapid depolarization mediated by highly selective voltage-gated Ca^{2+} channels that, upon opening, drive the membrane potential towards E_{Ca}. In **phase 3**, the Ca^{2+} channels slowly close and K$^+$-selective channels open, resulting in membrane repolarization. Once the membrane potential repolarizes to approximately −60 mV, the opening of I_f channels is triggered and the cycle begins again.

Although the I_f (inward pacemaker) current is responsible for the slow spontaneous depolarization in phase 4 of the

TABLE 18-1	Major Characteristics of Action Potential Phases for SA Nodal Cells and Ventricular Myocytes

SA Nodal Cells

Segment	Characteristics	Major Underlying Current
Phase 4	Slow depolarization	Inward I_f current (carried mainly by Na^+ ions)
Phase 0	Action potential upstroke	Inward Ca^{2+} current through voltage-sensitive Ca^{2+} channels (I_{Ca})
Phase 3	Repolarization	Outward K^+ current through K^+ channels (I_K)

Ventricular Myocytes

Segment	Characteristics	Major Underlying Current
Phase 4	Resting membrane potential	Inward and outward currents are equal
Phase 0	Rapid depolarization	Inward Na^+ current through Na^+ channels (I_{Na})
Phase 1	Early phase of repolarization	Decrease in inward Na^+ current and efflux of K^+ ions through K^+ channels (I_{to})
Phase 2	Plateau	Balance between inward Ca^{2+} current through Ca^{2+} channels (I_{Ca}) and outward K^+ current through K^+ channels (I_K, I_{K1})
Phase 3	Late phase of rapid repolarization	Decrease in inward Ca^{2+} current and large increase in outward K^+ current

SA node action potential, the kinetics of this depolarization are modulated by voltage-gated Na^+ channels that are also expressed in the node. There are gradients of Na^+ channel and Ca^{2+} channel expression within the SA node, such that cells at the border of the node express relatively more voltage-gated Na^+ channels and cells in the center of the node express relatively more voltage-gated Ca^{2+} channels. The expression of voltage-gated Na^+ channels in the SA node is partly responsible for the effect of certain antiarrhythmics on the automaticity of SA nodal cells (see below).

Unlike SA nodal cells, ventricular myocytes do not depolarize spontaneously under physiologic conditions. As a result, the membrane potential of the resting ventricular myocyte remains near E_K until the cell is stimulated by a wave of depolarization that is initiated by nearby pacemaker cells. The five phases of the ventricular myocyte action potential result from an intricately woven cascade of channel openings and closings; the phases are numbered from 0 to 4 (Fig. 18-3 and Table 18-1).

In **phase 0**, an action potential upstroke of very rapid depolarization is caused by a transient increase in inward Na^+ current through voltage-gated Na^+ channels. (Note that currents in phase 0 of the SA nodal and ventricular myocyte action potentials are carried by different ions—Ca^{2+} and Na^+, respectively.) The opening of Na^+ channels leads to a rapid influx of Na^+ (I_{Na}), which accounts for the depolarization and drives the membrane potential towards E_{Na} (+70 mV). Although large, the increase in Na^+ conductance during phase 0 lasts for only 1–2 milliseconds, because the Na^+ channels inactivate as a function of time and voltage. Inactivation of the fast Na^+ channels causes a dramatic de-

crease in the inward Na^+ current. The time it takes for Na^+ channels to recover from their voltage-dependent and time-dependent inactivation determines the *refractory period* of the myocyte. The refractory period is the time during which another action potential cannot fire. This serves as a protective mechanism to ensure that the heart has sufficient time to eject blood from its chambers. The refractory period lasts from the initiation of the action potential upstroke until the repolarization phase. I_{Na} is the major determinant of the velocity of impulse conduction throughout the ventricle.

The threshold-dependent activation of I_{Na} quickly depolarizes the membrane. The upstroke terminates before reaching E_{Na}, however, and is followed by an early phase of rapid repolarization to about +20 mV. This **phase 1** repolarization is a consequence of two events: (1) the rapid voltage-dependent inactivation of I_{Na}; and (2) the activation of transient K^+ currents (I_{to}; transient outward).

Phase 2, the plateau phase of the ventricular action potential, is unique to cardiac cell electrophysiology. The plateau is maintained by a finely tuned balance between an inward Ca^{2+} current through two types of Ca^{2+} channels ($I_{Ca.T}$, $I_{Ca.L}$) and an outward K^+ current through several types of K^+ channels (I_K, I_{K1}, I_{to}). Remarkably, only a few hundred channels per cell are used to maintain this fine balance. Because only a small number of channels are open, the total membrane conductance is low. The high membrane resistance during the plateau phase insulates the cardiac cells electrically, allowing rapid propagation of the action potential with little current dissipation.

During the plateau phase, two distinct Ca^{2+} cur-

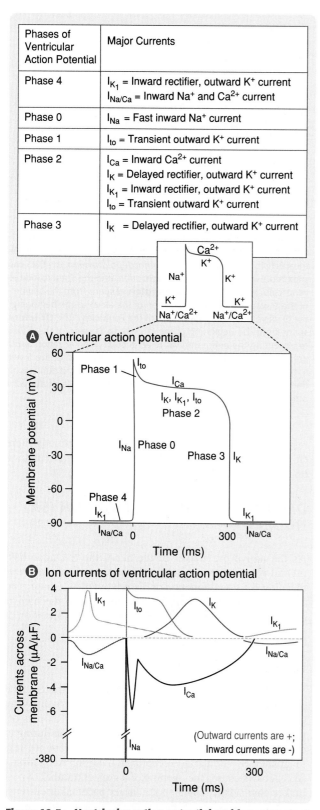

Phases of Ventricular Action Potential	Major Currents
Phase 4	I_{K_1} = Inward rectifier, outward K^+ current $I_{Na/Ca}$ = Inward Na^+ and Ca^{2+} current
Phase 0	I_{Na} = Fast inward Na^+ current
Phase 1	I_{to} = Transient outward K^+ current
Phase 2	I_{Ca} = Inward Ca^{2+} current I_K = Delayed rectifier, outward K^+ current I_{K_1} = Inward rectifier, outward K^+ current I_{to} = Transient outward K^+ current
Phase 3	I_K = Delayed rectifier, outward K^+ current

A Ventricular action potential

B Ion currents of ventricular action potential

(Outward currents are +; Inward currents are -)

Figure 18-3. Ventricular action potential and ion currents. A. At the resting membrane potential (phase 4), the inward and outward currents are equal and the membrane potential approaches the K^+ equilibrium potential (E_K). During the action potential upstroke (phase 0), a large transient increase in Na^+ conductance occurs. This event is followed by a brief period of initial repolarization (phase 1), which is mediated by a transient outward K^+ current. The plateau of the action potential (phase 2) results from the opposition of an

rents—the transient Ca^{2+} current, $I_{Ca.T}$, and the long-lasting Ca^{2+} current, $I_{Ca.L}$—mediate the influx of Ca^{2+} needed to initiate contraction. T-type Ca^{2+} channels inactivate with time and are insensitive to block by dihydropyridines such as nifedipine and nitrendipine. Current through the L-type Ca^{2+} channels ($I_{Ca.L}$) provides the dominant Ca^{2+} current in virtually all cardiac cells. $I_{Ca.L}$ is activated at -30 mV and inactivates slowly (hundreds of milliseconds). It is sensitive to block by dihydropyridines (**nifedipine**), benzothiazepines (**diltiazem**), and phenylalkylamines (**verapamil**), as discussed below. L-type Ca^{2+} channels carry inward current throughout the plateau phase; because Ca^{2+} stimulates the contraction of cardiac myocytes, these channels are crucial for coupling membrane excitability to myocardial contraction.

Opposing the inward Ca^{2+} currents are outward currents through the K^+ channels that are activated during the plateau phase. As the time-dependent inward Ca^{2+} currents inactivate, the outward K^+ currents (mostly I_K) rapidly drive the membrane potential towards E_K, thus repolarizing the cell in **phase 3.** However, these channels are unable to drive the membrane potential all the way to E_K because they deactivate at -40 mV. In **phase 4,** the resting membrane potential is reestablished by the activation of time-independent K^+ currents (I_{K_1}), which drive the membrane potential close to the K^+ equilibrium potential.

In clinical practice, the overall electrical activity of the heart is measured, rather than the ionic changes that occur at a single-cell level. This overall activity is reported in the electrocardiogram, or ECG (Box 18-1 and Fig. 18-4).

DETERMINATION OF FIRING RATE

The specialized conduction system of the heart consists of the SA node, AV node, bundle of His, and Purkinje system. These different populations of cells have different intrinsic rates of firing. Three factors determine the firing rate. First, as the rate of spontaneous depolarization in phase 4 increases, the rate of firing increases because the threshold potential (the minimum potential necessary to trigger an action potential) is reached more quickly at the end of phase 4. Second, as the threshold potential becomes more negative, the rate of firing increases because the threshold potential is reached more quickly at the end of phase 4. Third, as the maximum diastolic potential (the resting membrane potential) becomes more positive, the rate of firing increases because less time is needed to repolarize the membrane fully at the end of phase 3.

Because the various populations of pacemaker cells possess different intrinsic rates of firing, the pacemaker population with the fastest firing rate sets the heart rate. The SA

inward Ca^{2+} current and an outward K^+ current. The membrane repolarizes (phase 3) when the inward Ca^{2+} current decreases and the outward K^+ current predominates. **B.** The ion fluxes that give rise to the ventricular action potential consist of a complex pattern of changing ion permeabilities that are separated in time. Note especially that the Na^+ current in phase 0 is very large but extremely brief.

BOX 18-1. The Electrocardiogram

The electrocardiogram (ECG or EKG) is used to infer changes in cardiac impulses by recording electrical potentials at various locations on the surface of the body. An ECG recording reflects changes in the excitation of the myocardium. A basic understanding of the ECG is useful for discussions of the clinical applications of the various antiarrhythmic agents.

A normal electrocardiogram contains three electrical waveforms: the P wave, the QRS complex, and the T wave (Fig. 18-4). The **P wave** represents *atrial depolarization;* the **QRS complex** represents *ventricular depolarization;* and the **T wave** represents *ventricular repolarization.* The ECG does not show atrial repolarization explicitly, because the atrial repolarization is "drowned out" by the QRS complex. The ECG also contains two intervals and one segment: the PR interval, the QT interval, and the ST segment. The **PR interval** spans from the beginning of the P wave (initial depolarization of the atria) to the beginning of the Q wave (initial depolarization of the ventricles). Hence, the length of the PR interval varies with conduction velocity through the AV node. For example, if a patient has an electrical block in the AV node, then the conduction velocity through the AV node decreases and the PR interval increases. The **QT interval** spans from the beginning of the Q wave to the end of the T wave, representing the entire sequence of ventricular depolarization and repolarization. The **ST segment** extends from the end of the S wave to the beginning of the T wave; this segment, which represents the period during which the ventricles are depolarized, corresponds to the plateau phase of the ventricular action potential.

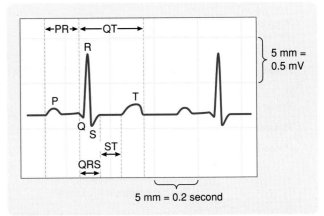

Figure 18-4. Electrocardiogram. The electrocardiogram (ECG or EKG) measures the body surface potentials induced by cardiac electrical activity. The **P wave** reflects *atrial depolarization,* the **QRS complex** represents *ventricular depolarization,* and the **T wave** indicates *ventricular repolarization.* The **PR interval** spans from the beginning of the P wave (initial depolarization of the atria) to the beginning of the Q wave (initial depolarization of the ventricles). The **QT interval** spans from the beginning of the Q wave to the end of the T wave, representing the entire interval of ventricular depolarization and repolarization. The **ST segment** extends from the end of the S wave to the beginning of the T wave, representing the period during which the ventricles are depolarized (i.e., the plateau phase of the action potential).

node possesses the fastest intrinsic firing rate—60–100 times per minute—and is the **native pacemaker** of the heart. The cells of the atrioventricular (AV) node and bundle of His fire intrinsically between 50 and 60 times per minute, and the cells of the Purkinje system have the slowest intrinsic firing rate—30–40 times per minute. The cells of the AV node, bundle of His, and Purkinje system are termed **latent pacemakers,** because their intrinsic rhythm is overridden by the faster SA-node automaticity. In a mechanism termed **overdrive suppression,** the SA node suppresses the intrinsic rhythm of the other pacemaker populations and entrains them to fire at the SA nodal firing rate.

PATHOPHYSIOLOGY OF ELECTRICAL DYSFUNCTION

Causes of electrical dysfunction in the heart can be divided into defects in impulse formation and defects in impulse conduction. In the former case, SA-node automaticity is interrupted or altered, leading to missed beats or ectopic beats,

respectively. In the latter case, impulse conduction is altered (for example, in the case of re-entrant rhythms), and sustained arrhythmias can result.

DEFECTS IN IMPULSE FORMATION (SA NODE)

As the native pacemaker of the heart, the SA node has a pivotal role in normal impulse formation. Electrical events that alter SA nodal function or disturb overdrive suppression can lead to impaired impulse formation. Two mechanisms commonly associated with defective impulse formation are altered automaticity and triggered activity.

Altered Automaticity

Some mechanisms that alter automaticity of the SA node are physiologic. In particular, the autonomic nervous system often modulates automaticity of the SA node as part of a physiologic response. In sympathetic stimulation during exercise, an increased concentration of catecholamines leads to greater β_1-adrenergic receptor activation. Activation of β_1 receptors causes the opening of a greater number of pacemaker channels (I_f channels); a larger pacemaker current is then conducted through these channels; and faster phase 4 depolarization results. Sympathetic stimulation also causes the opening of a greater number of Ca^{2+} channels, and thereby shifts the threshold to more positive potentials. Both of these mechanisms increase heart rate. The parasympathetic vagus nerve affects the SA node by a number of mechanisms that oppose the sympathetic regulation of heart rate. Vagus nerve release of acetylcholine initiates an intracellular signaling cascade that: (1) reduces the pacemaker current by decreasing the probability of pacemaker channel opening; (2) shifts the threshold to more positive potentials by reducing the probability of Ca^{2+} channel opening; and (3) makes the maximum diastolic potential (equivalent to the resting membrane potential in these spontaneously firing cells) more negative by increasing the probability of K^+ channel opening. The SA node, atria, and AV node are more sensitive than the ventricular conducting system to the effects of vagal stimulation.

In pathologic conditions, automaticity can be altered when latent pacemaker cells take over the SA node's role as the pacemaker of the heart. *When the SA nodal firing rate becomes pathologically slow* or when conduction of the SA impulse is impaired, an **escape beat** may occur as a latent pacemaker initiates an impulse. A series of escape beats, known as an **escape rhythm**, may result from prolonged SA nodal dysfunction. On the other hand, an **ectopic beat** occurs *when latent pacemaker cells develop an intrinsic rate of firing that is faster than the SA nodal rate*, in some cases despite the presence of a normally functioning SA node. A series of ectopic beats, termed an **ectopic rhythm**, can result from ischemia, electrolyte abnormalities, or heightened sympathetic tone.

Direct tissue damage (such as can occur after a myocardial infarction) also results in altered automaticity. Tissue injury can cause structural disruptions in the cell membrane. Disrupted membranes are unable to maintain ion gradients, which are critical for maintaining appropriate membrane potentials. If the resting membrane potential becomes sufficiently positive (more positive than -60 mV), nonpacemaker cells may begin to depolarize spontaneously. Another mechanism by which tissue damage leads to altered automaticity is through the loss of gap junction connectivity. Direct electrical connectivity is important for the effective delivery of overdrive suppression from the SA node to the rest of the cardiac myocytes. When connectivity is disrupted due to tissue injury, overdrive suppression is not efficiently relayed, and the unsuppressed cells can initiate their own rhythm. This abnormal rhythm can lead to cardiac arrhythmia.

Triggered Activity

Afterdepolarizations occur when a *normal* action potential triggers extra *abnormal* depolarizations. That is, the first (normal) action potential triggers additional oscillations of membrane potential, which may lead to arrhythmia. There are two types of afterdepolarizations—early afterdepolarizations and delayed afterdepolarizations.

If the afterdepolarization occurs *during the inciting action potential*, it is termed an **early afterdepolarization** (Fig. 18-5). *Conditions that prolong the action potential (e.g., drugs that prolong the QT interval, such as procainamide and ibutilide) tend to trigger early afterdepolarizations.* Specifically, an early afterdepolarization can occur during the plateau phase (phase 2) or the rapid repolarization phase (phase 3). During the plateau phase, because most of the Na^+ channels are inactivated, an inward Ca^{2+} current is responsible for the early afterdepolarization. On the other hand, during the rapid repolarization phase, partially recovered Na^+ channels can conduct an inward Na^+ current that contributes to the early afterdepolarization. If an early

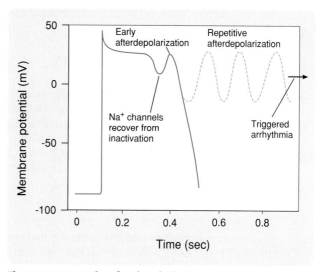

Figure 18-5. Early afterdepolarization. Early afterdepolarizations generally occur during the repolarizing phase of the action potential, although they can also occur during the plateau phase. Repetitive afterdepolarizations can trigger an arrhythmia.

afterdepolarization is sustained, it can lead to a type of ventricular arrhythmia termed **torsades de pointes.** Torsades de pointes, French for "twisting of the points," is characterized by QRS complexes of varying amplitudes as they "twist" along the baseline; this rhythm is a medical emergency that can lead to death if not treated with antiarrhythmics and/or defibrillation.

In contrast to early afterdepolarizations, **delayed afterdepolarizations** occur shortly *after the completion of repolarization* (Fig. 18-6). The mechanism of delayed afterdepolarizations is not well understood; it has been proposed that high intracellular Ca^{2+} concentrations lead to an inward Na^+

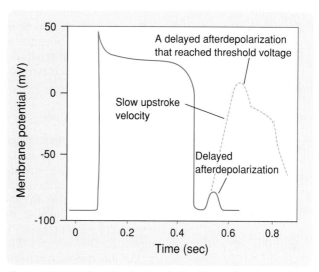

Figure 18-6. Delayed afterdepolarization. Delayed afterdepolarizations occur shortly after repolarization. Although the mechanism has not been firmly elucidated, it appears that intracellular Ca^{2+} accumulation activates the Na^+/Ca^{2+} exchanger, and the resulting electrogenic influx of 3 Na^+ for each extruded Ca^{2+} depolarizes the cell.

current, which, in turn, triggers the delayed afterdepolarization.

DEFECTS IN IMPULSE CONDUCTION

The second type of electrical disturbance of the heart involves defects in impulse conduction. Normal cardiac function requires unobstructed and timely propagation of an electrical impulse through the cardiac myocytes. In pathologic conditions, altered impulse conduction can result from one or a combination of three mechanisms: re-entry, conduction block, and accessory tract pathways.

Re-entry

Normal cardiac conduction is initiated at the SA node and propagated to the AV node, bundle of His, Purkinje system, and myocardium in an orderly fashion. The cellular refractory period ensures that stimulated regions of the myocardium depolarize only once during propagation of an impulse. Figure 18-7A depicts normal impulse conduction, in which an impulse arriving at point *a* travels synchronously down two parallel pathways, 1 and 2.

Re-entry of an electrical impulse occurs when a self-sustaining electrical circuit stimulates an area of the myocardium repeatedly and rapidly. Two conditions must be present for a re-entrant electrical circuit to occur: (1) *unidirectional block* (anterograde conduction is prohibited, but retrograde conduction is permitted); and (2) *slowed retrograde conduction velocity*. Figure 18-7B shows a re-entrant electrical circuit. As the impulse arrives at point *a*, it can travel only down pathway 1 (the left branch), because pathway 2 (the right branch) is blocked *unidirectionally* in the anterograde direction. The impulse conducts through pathway 1 and travels to point *b*. At this junction, the impulse travels in a *retrograde* fashion up pathway 2 towards point *a*. The conduction time from point *b* to point *a* is slowed because of cell damage or the presence of cells that are still in the refractory state. By the time the impulse reaches point *a*, the cells in pathway 1 have had adequate time to repolarize, and these cells are stimulated to continue conducting the action potential towards point *b*. In this manner, tachyarrhythmias result from the combination of unidirectional block and decreased conduction velocity in the abnormal pathway.

Conduction Block

Conduction block occurs when an impulse fails to propagate because of the presence of an area of inexcitable cardiac tissue. This area of inexcitable tissue could consist of normal tissue that is still refractory, or it could represent tissue that has been damaged by trauma, ischemia, or scarring. In either case, the myocardium is unable to conduct an impulse. Because conduction block removes overdrive suppression by the SA node, the cardiac myocytes are free to beat at their intrinsically slower frequency. For this reason, conduction block can be manifested clinically as bradycardia.

Accessory Tract Pathways

During the normal cardiac cycle, the SA node initiates an impulse that travels quickly through the atrial myocardium

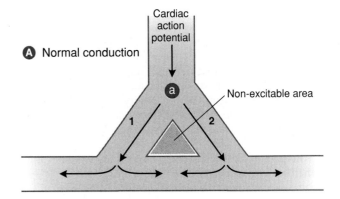

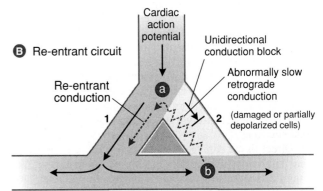

Figure 18-7. Normal and re-entrant electric pathways. A. In normal impulse conduction, an impulse traveling down a pathway arrives at point *a*, where it is able to travel down two alternate pathways, 1 and 2. In the absence of re-entry, the impulses continue on and depolarize different areas of the ventricle. **B.** A re-entrant circuit can develop if one of the branch pathways is pathologically disrupted. When the impulse arrives at point *a*, it can travel only down pathway 1 because pathway 2 is blocked *unidirectionally* (i.e., the effective refractory period of the cells in pathway 2 is prolonged to such an extent that anterograde conduction is prohibited). The impulse conducts through pathway 1 and proceeds to point *b*. At this point, the cells in pathway 2 are no longer refractory, and the impulse conducts in a retrograde fashion up pathway 2 towards point *a*. When the retrograde impulse arrives at point *a*, it can initiate re-entry. Re-entry can result in a sustained pattern of rapid depolarizations that trigger tachyarrhythmias. This mechanism can occur over small or large regions of the heart.

and arrives at the AV node. Impulse conduction then slows through the AV node, allowing sufficient time for filling of the ventricles with blood before ventricular contraction is initiated. After the impulse travels through the AV node, it again propagates quickly throughout the ventricles to trigger ventricular contraction.

Some individuals possess accessory electrical pathways that bypass the AV node. One common accessory pathway is the **bundle of Kent,** a band of myocardium that conducts impulses directly from the atria to the ventricles, bypassing the AV node (Fig. 18-8). In these individuals, an impulse originating in the SA node is conducted through the bundle of Kent to the ventricles more rapidly than the same impulse would be conducted through the AV node. Because the bundle of Kent is an *accessory* pathway, the ventricular tissue receives impulses from both the normal conduction pathway

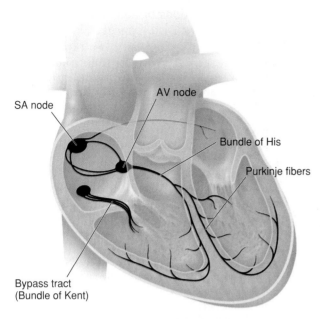

SA node

AV node

Bundle of His

Purkinje fibers

Bypass tract
(Bundle of Kent)

Figure 18-8. Bundle of Kent. The bundle of Kent is an accessory electrical pathway that conducts impulses directly from the atria to the ventricles, bypassing the AV node. Impulse conduction through this accessory tract is more rapid than conduction through the AV node, setting up the conditions for re-entrant tachyarrhythmias.

and the accessory pathway. As a result, electrocardiograms from these individuals typically exhibit a wider-than-normal QRS complex and an earlier-than-normal ventricular upstroke. More importantly, because the two conduction tracts have different conduction velocities, the presence of an accessory tract can set up the conditions for a re-entrant loop, and thereby predispose the individual to tachyarrhythmias.

PHARMACOLOGIC CLASSES AND AGENTS

Ion currents across the plasma membrane induce changes in the membrane potential of cells. Changes in the membrane potential of cardiac pacemaker cells underlie the timely contraction of cardiac myocytes. Defects in impulse formation and altered impulse conduction can lead to disturbances in cardiac rhythm. Antiarrhythmic agents are used to restore normal cardiac rhythm by targeting proarrhythmic regions of the heart.

GENERAL MECHANISMS OF ACTION OF ANTIARRHYTHMIC AGENTS

Although there are many different antiarrhythmic agents, there are surprisingly few mechanisms of antiarrhythmic action. In general, drugs that affect cardiac rhythm act by altering: (1) the maximum diastolic potential in pacemaker cells

(and/or the resting membrane potential in ventricular cells); (2) the rate of phase 4 depolarization; (3) the threshold potential; or (4) the action potential duration. The specific effect of a particular channel blocker follows directly from the role of the current carried by that channel in the cardiac action potential. For example, Na^+ and Ca^{2+} channel blockers typically alter the threshold potential, while K^+ channel blockers tend to prolong action potential duration. These drugs can access the ion channel by either traversing the pore of the channel or diffusing across the lipid bilayer within which the channel is embedded.

State-dependent ion channel block is an important concept in antiarrhythmic drug action. Ion channels are capable of switching among various conformational states, and changes in the permeability of the membrane to a particular ion are mediated by conformational changes in the channels that pass that ion. Antiarrhythmic drugs often have different affinities for different conformational states of the ion channel; that is, these drugs bind to one conformation of the channel with higher affinity than they do to other conformations of the channel. This type of binding is referred to as ''state-dependent.''

Na^+ channel blockers serve as an excellent example to illustrate the concept of state-dependent ion channel block. The Na^+ channel undergoes three major state changes (open-closed-inactivated) throughout the course of an action potential. During the upstroke, the channel is in the open conformation. The channel becomes inactivated during the plateau phase, and it changes again to the resting (closed) conformation as the membrane is repolarized to its resting potential. Most Na^+ channel blockers bind preferentially to the open and inactivated states of the Na^+ channel, not to the resting (closed) state of the channel. In this way, the drugs tend to block the channels during the action potential (cardiac systole) and to dissociate from the channels during diastole.

The unblocking rate (dissociation rate) of the various Na^+ channel blockers is an important determinant of the steady-state block of Na^+ channels. For example, when heart rate increases, the time available for unblocking (dissociation of the drug from its binding site on the channel) decreases and the degree of steady-state Na^+ channel block increases. The action of Na^+ channel blockers on ischemic tissue illustrates the therapeutic utility of state-dependent block. It has been observed that Na^+ channel blockers depress Na^+ conduction in ischemic tissue to a much greater extent than in normal tissue. In ischemic tissue, cardiac myocytes are depolarized for a longer period of time. This increase in action potential duration prolongs the inactivation state of the Na^+ channels, thereby making the inactivated Na^+ channels accessible to Na^+ channel blockers for a longer period of time. The rate of channel recovery from block is also decreased in depolarized ischemic myocytes because of the prolonged action potential. Thus, *the higher affinity of Na^+ channel blockers for open and inactivated states of the channel allows these agents to act preferentially on ischemic tissue, and thereby to block an arrhythmogenic focus at its source.* See Chapter 10, Local Anesthetic Pharmacology, for more discussion on the concept of state-dependent Na^+ channel block.

Developing and using effective antiarrhythmic treatments

is often complicated by the possibility that the antiarrhythmic agent can also cause arrhythmias. For example, many efforts have been directed at the treatment of re-entry, a mechanism responsible for a large proportion of arrhythmias. One way to treat re-entry is to block action potential propagation. If the retrograde impulse in the re-entrant circuit is *completely extinguished* by an antiarrhythmic agent, then the impulse will be unable to repeatedly depolarize the cardiac tissue in the re-entrant circuit. If the impulse is not completely extinguished, however, then the antiarrhythmic-induced slowing of conduction can actually promote re-entry arrhythmia. The ''surviving'' impulse may use the original re-entrant pathway to propagate the arrhythmia, or it may find other pathways and create new re-entrant circuits.

CLASSES OF ANTIARRHYTHMIC AGENTS

Antiarrhythmic agents have traditionally been organized into four classes based on their mechanism of action. Class I antiarrhythmics are Na^+ channel blockers; class II antiarrhythmics are β-adrenergic receptor blockers; class III antiarrhythmics are K^+ channel blockers; and class IV antiarrhythmics are Ca^{2+} channel blockers. *It is important to realize, however, that many antiarrhythmic agents are not entirely selective blockers of Na^+, K^+, or Ca^{2+} channels; rather, many of these agents block more than one channel type.* This section presents some useful definitions of common cardiac electrical disturbances (Box 18-2), and describes the mechanism of drug action for each class of antiarrhythmic agent.

Class I Antiarrhythmic Agents: Fast Na^+ Channel Blockers

Na^+ channel blockers decrease automaticity in SA nodal cells by: (1) shifting the threshold to more positive potentials, and (2) decreasing the slope of phase 4 depolarization (Fig. 18-9). The block of Na^+ channels leaves fewer channels available to open in response to membrane depolarization, thereby raising the threshold for action potential firing and slowing the rate of depolarization. Both of these effects extend the duration of phase 4, and thereby decrease heart rate. Furthermore, the shift in threshold potential means that, in patients with implanted defibrillators who are treated with Na^+ channel blockers, a higher voltage is needed to defibrillate the heart. Therefore, it is important to take into account the effect of Na^+ channel blockers when choosing appropriate settings for implanted defibrillators.

In addition to decreasing SA-node automaticity, Na^+ channel blockers act on ventricular myocytes to decrease re-entry. This is achieved mainly by decreasing the upstroke velocity of phase 0 and, for some Na^+ channel blockers, by prolonging repolarization (Fig. 18-10). By decreasing phase 0 upstroke velocity, Na^+ channel blockers decrease the conduction velocity through cardiac tissue. Ideally, conduction velocity is reduced to such an extent that the propagating wavefront is extinguished before it is able to restimulate myocytes in a re-entrant pathway. However, if conduction velocity is not sufficiently decreased, and the impulse is not extinguished, then the slowed impulse can support re-entry as it reaches cells that are no longer refractory (see above).

BOX 18-2. **Definitions of Common Cardiac Electric Disturbances**

To appreciate the clinical applications of the various antiarrhythmic agents, it is helpful to understand the basic definitions of terms that describe common electrical abnormalities of the heart.

Effective refractory period: The period during which a region of cardiac tissue cannot be excited by an electrical impulse.

Sinus tachycardia: The SA node fires between 100 and 180 times per minute, and the ECG shows normal P waves and QRS complexes. Sinus tachycardia can be a normal physiologic response (e.g., during exercise), or a pathologic condition that results from altered SA node automaticity.

Paroxysmal supraventricular tachycardia (PSVT): PSVT is characterized by atrial firing rates of 140–250 beats per minute, but it is usually transient and self-limited in nature. In 90% of cases, PSVT is caused by re-entry involving the AV node, SA node, or atrial tissue.

Atrial flutter: The atrial rate is between 280 and 300 beats per minute, and the ECG shows a rapid, ''saw-tooth'' appearance of atrial electrical activity. Because the pace of atrial firing is so rapid, some impulses from the atria reach the AV node during its refractory period. These impulses are not transmitted to the ventricles and, therefore, the ventricular rate is slower than the atrial rate. The ratio of atrial to ventricular firing rate is typically 2:1.

Atrial or ventricular fibrillation: These arrhythmias are characterized by chaotic, re-entrant impulse conduction through the atrium or ventricle. Ventricular fibrillation (VF) is invariably fatal if the arrhythmia is not converted, while atrial fibrillation (AF) can be tolerated for many years.

Ventricular tachycardia (VT): A series of three or more ventricular extrasystoles at rates between 100 and 250 beats per minute.

Torsades de pointes: This arrhythmia is often generated by afterdepolarizations in individuals with prolonged QT syndrome. The varying amplitudes of the QRS complex are often described as a ''twisting of points'' along the baseline of an ECG tracing. *Torsades* is often transient and self-limited, but can lead to more life-threatening arrhythmias.

In addition to decreasing phase 0 upstroke velocity, class IA Na^+ channel blockers prolong repolarization. Prolonged repolarization increases the effective refractory period, so that cells in a re-entrant circuit cannot be depolarized by the re-entrant action potential. In summary, *Na^+ channel blockers decrease the likelihood of re-entry, and thereby prevent arrhythmia, by: (1) decreasing conduction velocity, and (2) increasing the refractory period of ventricular myocytes.*

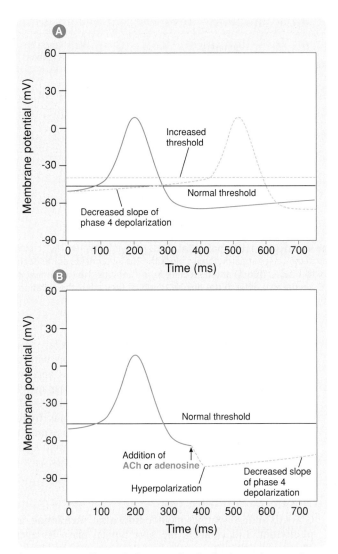

Figure 18-9. Effects of Class I Antiarrhythmics and Natural Agonists on the SA-Node Action Potential. A. The normal SA-node action potential is shown as a solid curve. Class I antiarrhythmics (Na$^+$ channel blockers) alter SA-node automaticity by affecting two aspects of the SA nodal action potential: (1) the threshold is shifted to more positive potentials; and (2) the slope of phase 4 depolarization is decreased. **B.** Acetylcholine and adenosine slow the SA nodal firing rate by activating K$^+$ channels that hyperpolarize the cell and decrease the slope of phase 4 depolarization.

Although the three subclasses of class I antiarrhythmics (class IA, IB, and IC) have similar effects on the action potential in the SA node, there are important differences in their effects on the ventricular action potential.

Class IA Antiarrhythmics

Class IA antiarrhythmics exert a moderate block on Na$^+$ channels and prolong the repolarization of both SA nodal cells and ventricular myocytes. By blocking Na$^+$ channels, these agents decrease the phase 0 upstroke velocity, which decreases conduction velocity through the myocardium. Class IA antiarrhythmics also block K$^+$ channels, and thereby reduce the outward K$^+$ current responsible for repolarization of the membrane. This prolongation of repolariza-

tion increases the effective refractory period of the cells. Together, the decreased conduction velocity and increased effective refractory period decrease re-entry.

Quinidine is often considered the prototypical drug among the class IA antiarrhythmics, but it is becoming less frequently used due to its side effects. In addition to the pharmacologic actions described above for all class IA antiarrhythmics, quinidine blocks transmitter release from the vagus nerve and thereby exerts anticholinergic (vagolytic) effects. *The anticholinergic effect is significant clinically because it can increase conduction velocity through the AV node.* Increased AV nodal conduction can have potentially detrimental effects in patients with atrial flutter. Such patients manifest an average atrial firing rate of 280–300 beats per minute. Because some of these impulses reach the AV node while it is still refractory, not all of the impulses are transmitted to the ventricles. Therefore, the atria fire much faster than the ventricles—there is typically a 2:1 or 4:1 ratio of atrial to ventricular firing rates. When quinidine is administered to patients with atrial flutter, the atrial firing rate decreases because of quinidine's pharmacologic action in slowing conduction velocity through the myocardium. At the same time, however, AV nodal conduction velocity increases because of the vagolytic effects of the drug. The increase in AV nodal conduction velocity abolishes the 2:1 or 4:1 ratio of atrial to ventricular firing rates, and a *1:1 ratio* of atrial to ventricular firing rates is often established. For example, with an atrial flutter rate of 300 and 2:1 "A–V block," the ventricles are driven at a rate of 150, which most individuals can tolerate. If the flutter rate is slowed to 200 and A–V conduction is enhanced to 1:1, however, the ventricles are driven at a rate of 200, which is usually too fast for effective ventricular pumping. For this reason, an agent that slows AV nodal conduction—such as a β-adrenergic antagonist or verapamil (a Ca$^+$ channel blocker)—should be used in conjunction with quinidine to prevent an excessively rapid ventricular response in patients with atrial flutter.

The most common adverse effects of quinidine are diarrhea, nausea, headache, and dizziness. These effects make it difficult for patients to tolerate chronic therapy with quinidine. Quinidine is contraindicated in patients with QT prolongation and in patients who are taking medications that predispose to QT prolongation, because of the increased risk of *torsades de pointes.* Relative contraindications to quinidine use include sick sinus syndrome, bundle branch block, myasthenia gravis (because of quinidine's antagonist action at muscarinic receptors), and liver failure.

Quinidine is administered orally and metabolized by cytochrome P450 enzymes in the liver. Quinidine increases plasma levels of digoxin (an inotropic agent), most likely by competing for the P450 enzymes that are responsible for digoxin metabolism. Because digoxin has a narrow therapeutic index (see Chapter 19, Pharmacology of Cardiac Contractility), quinidine-induced digoxin toxicity occurs in a significant fraction of patients. The plasma potassium level must be carefully monitored in patients treated with quinidine, because hypokalemia decreases quinidine efficacy, exacerbates QT prolongation, and, most importantly, predisposes to *torsades de pointes. It is hypothesized that torsades de pointes is the mechanism most likely responsible for quinidine-induced syncope.* Because of quinidine's numerous side effects and contraindications, this drug has largely been re-

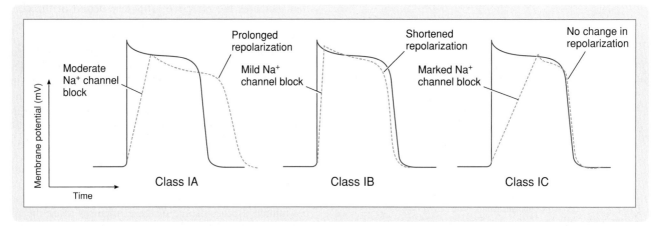

Figure 18-10. Effects of Class IA, IB, and IC antiarrhythmics on the ventricular action potential. Class I antiarrhythmics (Na$^+$ channel blockers) act on ventricular myocytes to decrease re-entry. All subclasses of the class I antiarrhythmics block the Na$^+$ channel to some degree: class IA agents exhibit moderate Na$^+$ channel block, class IB agents rapidly bind to (block) and dissociate from (unblock) Na$^+$ channels, and class IC agents produce marked Na$^+$ channel block. Class IA, IB, and IC agents also differ in the degree to which they affect the duration of the ventricular action potential.

placed by class III agents—such as ibutilide and amiodarone—for the pharmacologic conversion of atrial flutter or atrial fibrillation to normal sinus rhythm.

Procainamide is a class IA antiarrhythmic agent that is effective in the treatment of many types of supraventricular and ventricular arrhythmias. Procainamide is often used in the pharmacologic conversion of new-onset atrial fibrillation to normal sinus rhythm, although with less efficacy than intravenous ibutilide. Procainamide can be used safely to decrease the likelihood of re-entrant arrhythmias in the setting of acute myocardial infarction, even in the presence of decreased cardiac output. Procainamide can also be administered by slow intravenous infusion to treat acute ventricular tachycardia.

Unlike quinidine, procainamide has few anticholinergic effects and does not alter plasma levels of digoxin. Procainamide can cause peripheral vasodilation via inhibition of neurotransmission at sympathetic ganglia. With chronic therapy, almost all patients develop a lupus-like syndrome and positive antinuclear antibodies; the precise mechanism of this reaction is not known, but it remits if the drug is discontinued. Procainamide is acetylated in the liver to N-acetyl-procainamide (NAPA); this active metabolite produces the pure class III antiarrhythmic effects of prolonging the refractory period and lengthening the QT interval. NAPA does not appear to cause the lupus-like side effects of procainamide.

Disopyramide is similar to quinidine in its electrophysiologic and antiarrhythmic effects; the difference between the two drugs lies in their side effects. Disopyramide causes fewer gastrointestinal problems but has even more profound anticholinergic effects than quinidine, producing such side effects as urinary retention and dry mouth. It is contraindicated in patients with obstructive uropathy or glaucoma. Disopyramide is also contraindicated in patients with conduction block between the atria and ventricles and in patients with sinus-node dysfunction. Disopyramide has the prominent but unexplained effect that it depresses cardiac contractility, which has led to its use in the treatment of hypertrophic obstructive cardiomyopathy and neurocardiogenic syncope.

Because of its negative inotropic effects, disopyramide is absolutely contraindicated in patients with uncompensated heart failure. Oral disopyramide is approved only for the treatment of life-threatening ventricular arrhythmias; oral or intravenous disopyramide is sometimes used to convert supraventricular tachycardia to normal sinus rhythm. The current trend in the treatment of life-threatening arrhythmias, however, is away from class I antiarrhythmic agents and towards class III agents and electrical devices.

Class IB Antiarrhythmics

Class IB antiarrhythmics include **lidocaine**, **mexiletine**, and **phenytoin**. Lidocaine is the prototypical class IB agent. These drugs alter the ventricular action potential by blocking Na$^+$ channels and sometimes by shortening repolarization; the latter effect may be mediated by the drugs' ability to block the few Na$^+$ channels that inactivate late during phase 2 of the cardiac action potential (Fig. 18-10). In comparison to class IA antiarrhythmics, which preferentially bind to open Na$^+$ channels, *class IB drugs bind to both open and inactivated Na$^+$ channels.* Therefore, the more time Na$^+$ channels spend in the open or inactivated state, the more blockade the class IB antiarrhythmics can effect. The major distinguishing characteristic of the class IB antiarrhythmics is their *fast dissociation* from Na$^+$ channels. Because Na$^+$ channels recover quickly from class IB blockade, these drugs are most effective in blocking depolarized or rapidly driven tissues, where there is a higher likelihood of the Na$^+$ channels being in the open or inactivated state. Thus, class IB antiarrhythmics exhibit *use-dependent block* in diseased myocardium, where the cells have a tendency to fire more frequently; these antiarrhythmics have relatively little effect on normal cardiac tissue.

Myocardial ischemia provides an example of the therapeutic utility of the use-dependent block exerted by class IB antiarrhythmics. The increase in extracellular H$^+$ concentration in ischemic tissue activates membrane pumps that cause an increase in the extracellular K$^+$ concentration. This increase in extracellular K$^+$ shifts E_K to a more depolarized (more positive) value; for example, E_K may shift from -94 mV to -85 mV. The altered electrochemical K$^+$ gradient provides a *smaller* driving force for K$^+$ ions to flow out of cells, and depolarization of the membrane leads to a higher likelihood of action potential firing. Because ischemic cardiac myocytes tend to fire more frequently, the Na$^+$ channels spend more time in the open or inactivated state, serving as a better target for blockade by class IB antiarrhythmics.

Lidocaine is the antiarrhythmic agent used most commonly to treat ventricular arrhythmias in emergency situations. This drug is not effective in treating supraventricular arrhythmias. In hemodynamically stable patients, lidocaine is reserved for treatment of ventricular tachyarrhythmias or frequent premature ventricular contractions (PVCs).

Lidocaine has a short plasma half-life (approximately 20 minutes), and it is metabolically de-ethylated in the liver. Its metabolism is governed by two factors, liver blood flow and liver cytochrome P450 activity. For patients whose liver blood flow is decreased by old age or heart failure, or whose P450 enzymes are acutely inhibited, for example, by cimetidine (see Chapter 4, Drug Metabolism), a lower dose of lidocaine should be considered. For patients whose P450 enzymes are induced by drugs such as barbiturates, phenytoin, or rifampin, the dose of lidocaine should be increased.

Because lidocaine shortens repolarization, possibly by blocking the few Na$^+$ channels that inactivate late during phase 2 of the cardiac action potential, it does not prolong the QT interval. Therefore, the drug is safe for use in patients with long QT syndrome. However, because lidocaine also blocks Na$^+$ channels in the central nervous system (CNS), it can produce CNS adverse effects such as confusion, dizziness, and seizures. In addition to its use as an acute intravenous therapy for ventricular arrhythmias, lidocaine is used as a local anesthetic (see Chapter 10).

Mexiletine, an analogue of lidocaine, is available in oral formulation. While the efficacy of mexiletine is similar to that of quinidine, mexiletine does not prolong the QT interval and it lacks vagolytic side effects. In addition, little hemodynamic depression has been reported with the use of mexiletine. The primary indication for mexiletine is life-threatening ventricular arrhythmia. In practice, however, mexiletine is often used as an adjunct to other antiarrhythmic agents. For example, mexiletine is used in combination with **amiodarone** in patients with implantable cardioverter-defibrillators (ICDs) and in patients with recurrent ventricular tachycardia. Mexiletine is also used in combination with **quinidine** or **sotalol** to increase antiarrhythmic efficacy while reducing side effects. As for other class IB antiarrhythmic agents, there are no data supporting reduced mortality with the use of mexiletine. Major adverse effects of mexiletine include dose-related nausea and tremor, which can be ameliorated when the medication is taken with food. Mexiletine undergoes hepatic metabolism, and its plasma levels may be altered by inducers of hepatic enzymes such as phenytoin and rifampin.

While **phenytoin** is usually considered an antiepileptic medication, its effects on the myocardium also allow it to be classified as a class IB antiarrhythmic agent. The pharmacologic properties of phenytoin are discussed in detail in Chapter 14, Pharmacology of Abnormal Electrical Neurotransmission in the Central Nervous System. Although the use of phenytoin as an antiarrhythmic agent is limited, phenytoin has been found to be effective in ventricular tachycardia of young children. Specifically, phenytoin has been used in the treatment of congenital prolonged QT syndrome when monotherapy with β-adrenergic antagonists has failed; it is also used to treat ventricular tachycardia after congenital heart surgery. Phenytoin maintains AV conduction in digoxin-toxic arrhythmias, and it is especially useful in the rare patient who has concurrent epilepsy and cardiac arrhythmia. Phenytoin is an inducer of hepatic enzymes including P450 3A4, and thus affects serum levels of other antiarrhythmic agents such as mexiletine, lidocaine, and quinidine.

Class IC Antiarrhythmics

Class IC antiarrhythmics are the most potent Na$^+$ channel blockers, and they have little or no effect on action potential duration (Fig. 18-10). By markedly decreasing the rate of phase 0 upstroke of ventricular cells, these drugs suppress premature ventricular contractions. Class IC antiarrhythmics also prevent paroxysmal supraventricular tachycardia and atrial fibrillation. However, these drugs have marked depressive effects on cardiac function and, thus, must be used with discretion. In addition, the CAST (Cardiac Arrhythmia Suppression Trial) and other studies have brought attention to the proarrhythmic effects of these agents.

Flecainide is the prototypical class IC drug; other members of this class include **encainide**, **moricizine**, and **propafenone**. Flecainide illustrates the principle that antiarrhythmic agents can also cause arrhythmia. When flecainide is administered to patients with pre-existing ventricular tachyarrhythmias and to those with a history of myocardial infarction, it can worsen the arrhythmia even at normal doses. Currently, flecainide is approved for use only in life-threatening situations; for example, when paroxysmal supraventricular or ventricular arrhythmia is unresponsive to other measures. Flecainide is eliminated very slowly from the body; it has a plasma half-life of 12–30 hours. Because of its marked blockade of Na$^+$ channels and its suppressive effects on cardiac function, flecainide use is associated with adverse effects that include sinus-node dysfunction, a marked decrease in conduction velocity, and conduction block.

Class II Antiarrhythmic Agents: β-Adrenergic Antagonists

Class II antiarrhythmic agents are β-adrenergic antagonists (also called β-blockers). These agents act by inhibiting sympathetic input to the pacing regions of the heart. (β-Adrenergic antagonists are more extensively discussed in Chapter 9, Adrenergic Pharmacology, and Chapter 19.) Although the heart is capable of beating on its own without innervation from the autonomic nervous system, both sympathetic and parasympathetic fibers innervate the SA node and the AV node, and thereby alter the rate of automaticity. Sympathetic stimulation releases norepinephrine, which binds to β$_1$-adrenergic receptors in the nodal tissues. (β$_1$-Adrenergic receptors are the adrenergic subtype preferentially expressed in cardiac tissue.) Activation of β$_1$-adrenergic receptors in the SA node triggers an increase in the pacemaker current (I_f), which increases the rate of phase 4 depolarization and, consequently, leads to more frequent firing of the node. Stimula-

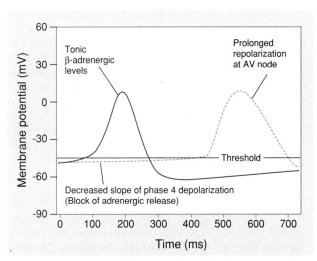

Figure 18-11. Effects of class II antiarrhythmics on pacemaker cell action potentials. Class II antiarrhythmics (β-antagonists) reverse the tonic sympathetic stimulation of cardiac β₁-adrenergic receptors. By blocking the adrenergic effects on the SA and AV nodal action potentials, these agents decrease the slope of phase 4 depolarization (especially important at the SA node) and prolong repolarization (especially important at the AV node). These agents are useful in the treatment of supraventricular and ventricular arrhythmias that are precipitated by sympathetic stimulation.

tion of β₁-adrenergic receptors in the AV node increases Ca^{2+} and K^+ currents, thereby increasing the conduction velocity and decreasing the refractory period of the node.

β₁-Antagonists block the sympathetic stimulation of β₁-adrenergic receptors in the SA and AV nodes (Fig. 18-11). The AV node is more sensitive than the SA node to the effects of β₁-antagonists. β₁-Antagonists affect the action potentials of the SA and AV nodes by: (1) decreasing the rate of phase 4 depolarization; and (2) prolonging repolarization. Decreasing the rate of phase 4 depolarization results in decreased automaticity, and this, in turn, reduces myocardial oxygen demand. Prolonged repolarization at the AV node increases the effective refractory period, which decreases the incidence of re-entry.

β₁-Antagonists are the most frequently used agents in the treatment of supraventricular and ventricular arrhythmias precipitated by sympathetic stimulation. β₁-Adrenergic antagonists have been shown to reduce mortality after myocardial infarction, even in patients with relative contraindications to this therapy such as severe diabetes mellitus or asthma. Because of their wide spectrum of clinical application and established safety record, β-adrenergic antagonists are the most useful antiarrhythmic agents currently available.

There are several generations of β-antagonists, each characterized by slightly different pharmacologic properties. First-generation β-antagonists, such as **propranolol,** are nonselective β-adrenergic antagonists that antagonize both β₁-adrenergic and β₂-adrenergic receptors. They are widely used to treat tachyarrhythmias caused by catecholamine stimulation during exercise or emotional stress. Because propranolol does not prolong repolarization in ventricular tissue, it can be used in patients with long-QT syndrome. Second-generation agents, including **atenolol, metoprolol, acebutolol,** and **bisoprolol,** are relatively selective for β₁-

adrenergic receptors when administered in low doses. Third-generation β-antagonists cause vasodilation in addition to β₁-receptor antagonism. **Labetalol** and **carvedilol** induce vasodilation by antagonizing α-adrenergic receptor-mediated vasoconstriction, while **pindolol** is a partial agonist at the β₂-adrenergic receptor.

The different generations of β-antagonists produce varying degrees of adverse effects. Three general mechanisms are responsible for the adverse effects of β-blockers. First, antagonism at β₂-adrenergic receptors causes smooth muscle spasm, leading to bronchospasm, cold extremities, and impotence. These effects are more commonly caused by the nonselective first generation β-antagonists. Second, exaggeration of the therapeutic effects of β₁-receptor antagonism can lead to excessive negative inotropic effects, heart block, and bradycardia. Third, drug penetration into the CNS can produce insomnia and depression.

Class III Antiarrhythmic Agents: Inhibitors of Repolarization

Class III antiarrhythmic agents block K^+ channels. Two types of currents determine the duration of the plateau phase of the cardiac action potential: inward, depolarizing Ca^{2+} currents and outward, hyperpolarizing K^+ currents. During a normal action potential, the hyperpolarizing K^+ currents eventually dominate, returning the membrane potential to more hyperpolarized values. Larger hyperpolarizing K^+ currents shorten plateau duration, returning the membrane potential to its resting value more rapidly, while smaller hyperpolarizing K^+ currents lengthen plateau duration and delay return of the membrane potential to its resting value.

When K^+ channels are blocked, a smaller hyperpolarizing K^+ current is generated. Therefore, K^+ channel blockers cause a longer plateau and prolong repolarization (Fig. 18-12). The ability of K^+ channel blockers to lengthen plateau

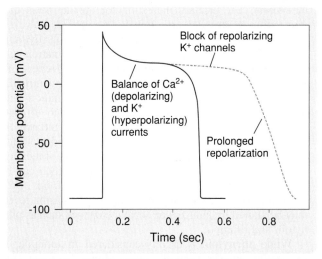

Figure 18-12. Effects of class III antiarrhythmics on the ventricular action potential. Class III antiarrhythmics (K^+ channel blockers) decrease the magnitude of the repolarizing K^+ currents during phase 2 of the action potential and, thereby, prolong action potential duration. This prolongation of the plateau phase decreases re-entry, but it can also predispose to early afterdepolarizations.

duration is responsible for both their pharmacologic uses and their adverse effects. On the beneficial side, prolongation of the plateau duration increases the effective refractory period, which, in turn, decreases the incidence of re-entry. On the toxic side, prolongation of the plateau duration increases the likelihood of developing early afterdepolarizations and *torsades de pointes.* With the exception of amiodarone, K^+ channel blockers also exhibit the undesirable property of "reverse use-dependency": action potential prolongation is most pronounced at slow rates (undesirable) and least pronounced at fast rates (desirable). K^+ channel blockers have little or no effect on the upstroke phase or conduction velocity of the impulse.

Ibutilide is a class III agent that prolongs repolarization by inhibiting the delayed rectifier K^+ current. This agent also enhances a slow inward Na^+ current that further prolongs repolarization. Ibutilide is used to terminate atrial fibrillation and flutter, as exemplified in the introductory case. The major adverse effect of ibutilide results from its prolongation of the QT interval; the serious arrhythmia *torsades de pointes* may result, requiring electrical cardioversion (delivery of an electrical shock to resynchronize the heart) in almost 2% of patients taking the drug. For this reason, Dr. J was closely monitored by a cardiologist during his ibutilide infusion. Ibutilide is generally not administered to patients with pre-existing long-QT syndrome.

Dofetilide is a class III agent that is only available orally. It inhibits exclusively the rapid component of the delayed rectifier K^+ current and has no effect on the inward Na^+ current. Dofetilide increases the action potential duration and prolongs the QT interval in a dose-dependent manner. Because dofetilide has the potential of inducing ventricular arrhythmias, it is reserved for patients with highly symptomatic atrial fibrillation and/or atrial flutter. Dofetilide is used in the cardioversion of atrial fibrillation and atrial flutter to normal sinus rhythm, and it is effective in the maintenance of sinus rhythm in such patients after cardioversion. Because dofetilide has no negative inotropic effects, it can be used in patients with depressed ejection function. Similar to ibutilide, the major adverse effect of dofetilide is *torsades de pointes,* which occurs in 1% to 3% of patients taking the drug. Because dofetilide is excreted by the kidneys, patients with renal dysfunction must have their dose of drug reduced based on their creatinine clearance.

Sotalol is a mixed class II and class III antiarrhythmic agent. This drug nonselectively antagonizes β-adrenergic receptors (class II action), and it also increases action potential duration by blocking K^+ channels (class III action). Sotalol exists in two isomeric forms, the *l*-isomer and *d*-isomer. While the two isomeric forms are equipotent in blocking K^+ channels, the *l*-form is a more potent β-antagonist. Sotalol is used to treat severe ventricular arrhythmias, especially in patients who cannot tolerate the side effects of amiodarone. Sotalol is also used to prevent recurrent atrial flutter or fibrillation, and thereby to maintain normal sinus rhythm. Like other β-antagonists, sotalol can cause fatigue and bradycardia; and like other class III antiarrhythmic agents, it can induce *torsades de pointes.*

Bretylium acts as both an antihypertensive agent and a class III antiarrhythmic agent. Like guanethidine (see Chapter 9), this drug is concentrated in the terminals of sympathetic neurons, causing an initial release of norepinephrine but then inhibiting further release of norepinephrine. In effect, bretylium performs a "chemical sympathectomy" and thereby exerts an antihypertensive effect. Bretylium also increases the action potential duration in normal and ischemic cardiac cells. Its sites of antiarrhythmic activity are mainly in the Purkinje fibers and secondarily in ventricular myocytes; it has no effect on atrial tissue. Bretylium is indicated only in patients with recurrent ventricular tachycardia or fibrillation after lidocaine and defibrillation measures have failed. Because of its sympatholytic effects, bretylium can cause marked hypotension.

Amiodarone is mainly a class III antiarrhythmic agent, but it also acts as a class I, class II, and class IV antiarrhythmic. The ability of amiodarone to exert such a diversity of effects can be explained by its mechanism of action: *alteration of the lipid membrane in which ion channels and receptors are located.* In all cardiac tissues, amiodarone lengthens the effective refractory period by blocking the K^+ channels responsible for repolarization; this prolongation of action potential duration decreases re-entry. As a potent class I agent, amiodarone blocks Na^+ channels and thereby decreases the rate of firing in pacemaker cells; it exhibits use-dependent Na^+ channel blockade by binding preferentially to channels in the inactivated conformation. Amiodarone exerts class II antiarrhythmic activity by noncompetitively antagonizing α-adrenergic and β-adrenergic receptors. Finally, as a Ca^{2+} channel blocker (class IV), amiodarone can cause significant AV nodal block and bradycardia, although fortunately its use is associated with a relatively low incidence of *torsades de pointes.*

In recent years, the results of several clinical trials have caused the popularity of amiodarone to increase from a last-resort agent to one that is frequently used to treat arrhythmias. The severity of the arrhythmia dictates the dose of amiodarone. Because high-dose amiodarone has substantial toxicity, the drug is used at full dose only in patients with hemodynamically unstable ventricular tachycardia or fibrillation after other antiarrhythmic agents have failed. At reduced doses, however, amiodarone is one of the most effective agents in preventing serious ventricular arrhythmias in patients with heart failure and/or a history of recent myocardial infarction. Amiodarone is also highly effective in the prevention of recurrent paroxysmal atrial fibrillation or flutter, as exemplified in the introductory case.

The wide spectrum of action of amiodarone is accompanied by a panoply of serious adverse effects when the drug is used for long periods or in high doses. These effects include cardiac, pulmonary, thyroid, hepatic, neurological, and idiosyncratic complications (Table 18-2). In the heart, amiodarone can decrease AV- or SA-node function by blocking Ca^{2+} channels. As an α-adrenergic antagonist, amiodarone can cause hypotension. Amiodarone can exert a negative inotropic effect by inhibiting β-adrenergic receptors, especially when the drug is used chronically. Severe pulmonary complications can occur in patients taking high doses of amiodarone (400 mg daily). Pneumonitis leading to pulmonary fibrosis is the most dreaded of all complications associated with amiodarone use. Fortunately, such complications occur rarely in patients taking prophylactic doses (200 mg daily) for prevention of ventricular or atrial arrhythmias. Because of its structural similarity to thyroxine, amiodarone affects thyroid hormone metabolism by inhibiting peripheral

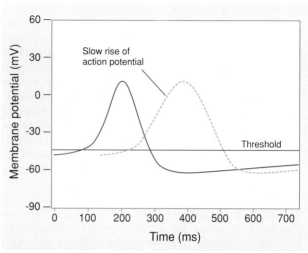

Figure 18-13. Effects of class IV antiarrhythmics on pacemaker cell action potentials. Class IV antiarrhythmics (Ca^{2+} channel blockers) decrease excitability of SA nodal cells and prolong AV nodal conduction, primarily by slowing the action potential upstroke in nodal tissue. Class IV antiarrhythmics are useful in the treatment of arrhythmias that involve re-entry through the AV node, but high doses of Ca^{2+} channel blockers can prolong AV nodal conduction to such an extent that heart block results.

conversion of thyroxine (T4) to triiodothyronine (T3). Either hyperthyroidism or hypothyroidism can occur as a consequence of this dysregulation of thyroid hormone metabolism (see Chapter 26, Pharmacology of the Thyroid Gland). Ten percent to 20% of patients taking amiodarone manifest an abnormal increase in liver enzymes, although this effect is reversible when the dose of the drug is reduced. Neurological symptoms can include peripheral neuropathy, headache, ataxia, and tremors. Patients taking amiodarone should be monitored for abnormal pulmonary, thyroid, and liver function.

Amiodarone is contraindicated in patients with cardiogenic shock, second-degree or third-degree heart block, or severe SA-node dysfunction with marked sinus bradycardia or syncope.

Class IV Antiarrhythmic Agents: Ca^{2+} Channel Blockers

Drugs that block cardiac Ca^{2+} channels act preferentially on *SA and AV nodal tissues,* because these pacemaker tissues depend on Ca^{2+} currents for the depolarization phase of the action potential (Fig. 18-2). In contrast, Ca^{2+} channel blockers have little effect on fast Na^+ channel-dependent tissues, such as Purkinje fibers and atrial and ventricular muscle. *The major therapeutic action of the class IV antiarrhythmics is to slow the action potential upstroke in AV nodal cells, leading to slowed conduction velocity through the AV node* (Fig. 18-13). This also blocks re-entrant arrhythmias in which the AV node is part of the re-entry circuit. In the introductory case, however, the re-entry circuit responsible for atrial fibrillation was isolated to the atria. This is why diltiazem, a Ca^{2+} channel blocker, slowed Dr. J's heart rate but did not change his underlying heart rhythm. (Refer to Chapter 21, Pharmacology of Vascular Tone, for a more extended discussion of Ca^{2+} channel blockers.)

Because different tissues express different subtypes of Ca^{2+} channels, and different subclasses of Ca^{2+} channel blockers interact preferentially with different Ca^{2+} channel subtypes, the various Ca^{2+} channel blockers have differen-

tial effects in different tissues. Dihydropyridines (such as **nifedipine**) have a relatively greater effect on the Ca^{2+} current in *vascular smooth muscle,* while **verapamil** and **diltiazem** are more effective in *cardiac tissues.* Verapamil and diltiazem are used to treat re-entrant paroxysmal supraventricular tachycardias, because these are often re-entrant arrhythmias that involve the AV node. Verapamil and diltiazem are *rarely* used in ventricular tachycardia. In fact, the only indications for these agents in ventricular arrhythmias are idiopathic right ventricular outflow tract tachycardia and fascicular tachycardias. Verapamil is also used to treat hypertension and vasospastic (Prinzmetal) angina. Class IV agents can cause AV nodal block by excessively reducing the conduction velocity. Administration of intravenous verapamil to patients taking β-blockers can precipitate severe heart failure and lead to irreversible electromechanical dissociation. Verapamil and diltiazem increase plasma digoxin levels by competing with digoxin for renal excretion.

Other Antiarrhythmic Agents

Adenosine and **potassium**, while not considered classical antiarrhythmic agents, have important effects on cardiac electrophysiology. Adenosine can be used to treat arrhythmias that involve aberrant AV nodal conduction. Physiologic concentrations of K^+ must be maintained to prevent arrhythmias. **Ranolazine** is a recently approved agent for the treatment of chronic stable angina; its mechanism of action appears to involve inhibition of the late Na^+ current.

Adenosine

The nucleoside **adenosine** is naturally present throughout the body. By stimulating the P1 class of purinergic receptors, adenosine opens a G protein-coupled K^+ channel (I_{KACh})

and thereby inhibits SA nodal, atrial, and AV nodal conduction. The AV node is more sensitive than the SA node to the effects of adenosine. Adenosine also inhibits the potentiation of Ca^{2+} channel activity by cAMP, and thereby suppresses Ca^{2+}-dependent action potentials. Adenosine has a plasma half-life of less than 10 seconds and is often used as the first-line agent for converting narrow-complex paroxysmal supraventricular tachycardia to normal sinus rhythm. For this indication, it is efficacious in 90% of cases. Most adverse effects of adenosine are transient, including headache, flushing, chest pain, and excessive AV or SA nodal inhibition. Adenosine can also cause bronchoconstriction lasting for up to 30 minutes in patients with asthma. In 65% of patients, a *transient* new arrhythmia occurs at the onset of adenosine administration.

Potassium

Both hypokalemia and hyperkalemia can be arrhythmogenic and, therefore, the plasma K^+ level must be carefully monitored. Hypokalemia can cause early afterdepolarizations, delayed afterdepolarizations, and ectopic beats in nonpacemaker cells. Hyperkalemia can lead to a marked slowing in conduction velocity, because increased extracellular K^+ concentrations lower E_K and thus depolarize cell membranes. The life-threatening cardiac effects of hyperkalemia are the primary impetus for initiating dialysis in patients with renal failure.

Potassium is an antiarrhythmic agent in two ways. First, serum K^+ levels outside the physiologic range (3.5–5 mM) can be an important factor in initiating and maintaining arrhythmias. Correction of hypokalemia or hyperkalemia alone can be sufficient to terminate some arrhythmias. Second, it is possible to use supraphysiologic or subphysiologic serum K^+ concentrations in an attempt to terminate arrhythmias. This is *rarely* done in clinical practice, because it is difficult to change K^+ levels reliably, and exogenously induced changes in K^+ levels are rapidly corrected by renal mechanisms.

Ranolazine

Many patients with chronic stable angina have chest pain with exertion despite mechanical revascularization and use of β-adrenergic antagonists or calcium channel blockers. **Ranolazine** is a recently approved agent that improves exercise capacity and reduces anginal events in patients with chronic stable angina. Despite extensive evaluation, the exact mechanism of action of ranolazine is uncertain. Proposed mechanisms of action include inhibition of cardiac myocyte fatty-acid β-oxidation, inhibition of the delayed rectifier K^+ current, and inhibition of the late Na^+ current. Inhibition of fatty-acid β-oxidation may improve myocardial ATP utilization, while inhibition of Na^+ channel activity may reduce the energy required for myocardial repolarization.

Ranolazine has been generally well tolerated in clinical trials; its most common adverse effects are nausea, constipation, and dizziness. Ranolazine also prolongs the QT interval. It is currently approved as a second-line treatment for patients with chronic stable angina.

Conclusion and Future Directions

Cardiac arrhythmias arise from defects in impulse formation, defects in impulse conduction, or a combination of the two mechanisms. Because derangements in ion conductance lead to arrhythmias, antiarrhythmic agents act directly or indirectly to alter the conformational states of ion channels and thereby change the membrane permeability to ions. The pharmacologic property of use-dependent ion channel blockade allows many antiarrhythmic agents to target diseased cardiac tissues preferentially, based on the altered electrophysiology of these tissues. In general, class I antiarrhythmics block Na^+ channels; class II antiarrhythmics (β-blockers) inhibit sympathetic stimulation, and thereby decrease automaticity; class III agents block K^+ channels; and class IV agents block Ca^{2+} channels. Despite continuing developments in antiarrhythmic drugs, the paradox still exists that antiarrhythmic drugs can generate arrhythmias. Nonetheless, judicious use of antiarrhythmic agents can reduce mortality in certain clinical circumstances, and careful tailoring of a drug regimen to the individual patient's clinical status can reduce the adverse effects of these agents.

The most important new directions in the pharmacology of cardiac rhythm involve identifying specific genes for ion channels in the human heart (Table 18-3). Currently, animal models are used for the majority of ion channel research; comparatively little is known about the clinical pharmacology of ion channel expression in humans. With the mouse and human genomes now completely sequenced, researchers will be able to investigate the possibility that newly identified gene products can serve as selective targets for new therapeutic agents. The identification of ion channel gene expression in the various tissues of the human heart (SA node, AV node, atrial conduction pathways, endocardium, ventricular conduction pathways, etc.), both during development and in response to injury, may provide new targets that are not now known. Many of the genes are likely to encode channels that form heteromultimers, and there are likely to be many genetic variants within the population. This enormous complexity will likely represent a boon to drug development because it will allow more tailored strategies to be employed. In parallel, the development of implantable com-

TABLE 18-3 Molecular Identity of Known Cardiac Ion Currents

ION CURRENT	CHANNEL PROTEIN
I_{Na}	$Na_V1.5$
$I_{Ca.L}$ (dihydropyridine-sensitive)	$Ca_V1.2$
$I_{Ca.T}$	$Ca_V3.1$
I_f	HCN2, HCN4
I_{to}	$K_V4.3$
$I_{Ks}*$	$K_V7.1$ (KvLQT1)
$I_{Kr}*$	K_V11, HERG
I_{K1}	Kir2.1 (inward rectifier)
I_{KACh}	Kir3.1 + Kir3.4 (G protein-gated)

*Collectively referred to as I_K.

puters, stimulators, and defibrillators will constitute an alternative strategy to prevent or terminate arrhythmias.

Suggested Reading

Ackerman MJ, Clapham DE. Chapter 18: excitability and conduction. In: Chien KR, ed. *Molecular basis of cardiovascular disease.* 2nd ed. Philadelphia: WB Saunders; 2004. (*Detailed overview of cardiac excitability and conduction.*)

Ackerman MJ, Clapham DE. Ion channels—basic science and clinical disease. *N Engl J Med* 1997;336:1575–1586. (*Broad review of ion channels.*)

Chaitman BR. Ranolazine for the treatment of chronic angina and potential use in other cardiovascular conditions. *Circulation* 2006;113:2462–2472. (*Recent review on ranolazine.*)

Delacretaz E. Clinical practice. Supraventricular tachycardia. *N Engl J Med* 2006;354:1039–1051. (*Discussion of the clinical uses of antiarrhythmic agents in treating supraventricular tachycardia.*)

Katz A. Mechanisms of disease: cardiac ion channels. *N Engl J Med* 1993;328:1244–1251. (*Molecular basis of cardiac arrhythmias.*)

Kowey PR, Marinchak RA, Rials SJ, et al. Classification and pharmacology of antiarrhythmic drugs. *Am Heart J* 2000;140:12–20. (*Synopsis of antiarrhythmic drugs.*)

Lilly L, ed. *Pathophysiology of heart disease: a collaborative project of medical students and faculty.* 3rd ed. Baltimore: Lippincott Williams & Wilkins; 2002. (*Detailed discussion of the pathophysiology of cardiac arrhythmias.*)

| Drug Summary Table | **Chapter 18 Pharmacology of Cardiac Rhythm** |

CLASS IA ANTIARRHYTHMICS

Mechanism—Moderate block of voltage-gated Na⁺ channels and block of K⁺ channels in ventricular myocytes (decreases phase 0 upstroke velocity and prolongs repolarization) and SA nodal cells (shifts threshold to more positive potentials and decreases slope of phase 4 depolarization); quinidine also blocks acetylcholine release from vagus nerve (vagolytic effect)

Drug	Clinical Applications	Serious and Common Adverse Effects	Contraindications	Therapeutic Considerations
Quinidine	Conversion of atrial flutter or fibrillation and maintenance of normal sinus rhythm Paroxysmal supraventricular tachycardia Premature atrial or ventricular contractions Paroxysmal AV junctional rhythm or atrial or ventricular tachycardia	*Torsades de pointes, complete AV block, ventricular tachycardia, agranulocytosis, thrombocytopenia, hepatotoxicity, acute asthma attack, respiratory arrest, angioedema, rare occurrence of systemic lupus* Fatigue, headache, lightheadedness, widening of QRS complex and QT and PR intervals, hypotension, PVCs, tachycardia, diarrhea, cinchonism	History of *torsades de pointes* or prolonged QT interval Concurrent use of drugs that prolong QT interval Conduction defects	Coadministration of other drugs known to prolong QT interval (such as thioridazine, ziprasidone) is contraindicated Quinidine inhibits conversion of codeine to morphine, thereby reducing codeine's analgesic effect Quinidine-induced digoxin toxicity occurs in a significant fraction of patients Amiodarone, amprenavir, azole antifungals, cimetidine, and ritonavir increase quinidine levels Coadministration of anticholinergics results in additive anticholinergic effects An agent that slows AV nodal conduction (a β-adrenergic blocker or a Ca²⁺ channel blocker) should be used in conjunction with quinidine to prevent an excessively rapid ventricular response in patients with atrial flutter
Procainamide	Symptomatic PVCs Life-threatening ventricular tachycardia Maintenance of normal sinus rhythm after conversion of atrial flutter Malignant hyperthermia	*Same as quinidine, except fewer anticholinergic effects. Additionally, lupus-like syndrome may occur after prolonged use*	Same as quinidine Additional contraindications include myasthenia gravis and systemic lupus erythematosus	Coadministration of drugs known to prolong QT interval is contraindicated Procainamide does not alter plasma levels of digoxin Ventricular rate may accelerate due to vagolytic effects on AV node; consider pretreatment with a cardiac glycoside Baseline and periodic determination of ANA, and monitor for development of lupus-like syndrome
Disopyramide	PVCs Ventricular tachycardia Conversion of atrial fibrillation, atrial flutter, and paroxysmal atrial tachycardia to normal sinus rhythm	*Same as quinidine, except more profound anticholinergic effects and fewer GI effects*	Same as quinidine	Coadministration of drugs known to prolong QT interval is contraindicated Rifampin impairs antiarrhythmic activity of disopyramide Ventricular rate may accelerate due to vagolytic effects on AV node; consider pretreatment with a cardiac glycoside Disopyramide is commonly prescribed for patients who cannot tolerate quinidine or procainamide

(Continued)

Drug Summary Table | **Chapter 18 Pharmacology of Cardiac Rhythm** (*Continued*)

Drug	Clinical Applications	Serious and Common Adverse Effects	Contraindications	Therapeutic Considerations
CLASS IB ANTIARRHYTHMICS				
Mechanism—Use-dependent block of voltage-gated Na^+ channels in ventricular myocytes (decreases phase 0 upstroke velocity); may also shorten repolarization				
Lidocaine Mexiletine (oral analogue of lidocaine)	Ventricular arrhythmias in the context of MI, cardiac manipulation, or cardiac glycosides Status epilepticus Local anesthesia of skin or mucous membranes Pain, burning, or itching Postherpetic neuralgia	*Seizures, asystole, bradycardia, cardiac arrest, new or worsened arrhythmias, respiratory depression, anaphylaxis, status asthmaticus* Restlessness, stupor, tremor, hypotension, blurred or double vision, tinnitus	Stokes-Adams syndrome Wolff-Parkinson-White syndrome Severe SA, AV, or intraventricular block Contraindications for spinal or epidural block include: inflammation or infection in puncture region, septicemia, severe hypertension, spinal deformities, neurologic disorders	Dosage of both lidocaine and mexiletine should be adjusted when co-administered with P450 inhibitors (such as cimetidine) and inducers (such as barbiturates, phenytoin, or rifampin) In severely ill patients, seizures may be the first sign of toxicity Intramuscular injection of lidocaine can cause large increase in serum creatine kinase (CK)
Phenytoin	Generalized tonic-clonic seizures, status epilepticus, non-epileptic seizures Seizures related to eclampsia Neuralgia Ventricular arrhythmias unresponsive to lidocaine or procainamide Arrhythmias induced by cardiac glycosides	*Agranulocytosis, leukopenia, pancytopenia, thrombocytopenia, hepatitis, Stevens-Johnson syndrome, toxic epidermal necrolysis* Ataxia, confusion, slurred speech, diplopia, nystagmus, gingival hyperplasia, nausea, vomiting, hirsutism	Hydantoin hypersensitivity Sinus bradycardia, SA node block, second- or third-degree AV block Stokes-Adams syndrome	Phenytoin interacts with numerous drugs due to its hepatic metabolism. Phenytoin is metabolized by P450 2C9/10 and P450 2C19. Other drugs that are metabolized by these enzymes can increase plasma concentration of phenytoin. Phenytoin can also induce various P450s, such as P450 3A4, which can lead to increased metabolism of oral contraceptives and other drugs
CLASS IC ANTIARRHYTHMICS				
Mechanism—Marked block of voltage-gated Na^+ channels in ventricular myocytes (decreases phase 0 upstroke velocity)				
Encainide Flecainide Moricizine Propafenone	Sustained ventricular tachycardia Paroxysmal supraventricular tachycardia, paroxysmal atrial fibrillation unresponsive to other measures	*Cardiac arrest, heart failure, new or worsened arrhythmia, sinus-node dysfunction, marked decrease in conduction velocity, conduction block* Dizziness, headache, syncope, visual disturbances, dyspnea	Cardiogenic shock Second- or third-degree AV block, right bundle branch block with left hemiblock Proarrhythmic effects in patients with atrial fibrillation or flutter	Associated with excessive mortality and non-fatal cardiac arrest; restrict use to patients who have failed other measures Can worsen arrhythmia in patients with pre-existing ventricular tachyarrhythmias and in those with a history of myocardial infarction May increase acute and chronic endocardial pacing threshold and suppress ventricular escape rhythms Monitor levels in patients with significant hepatic impairment

CLASS II ANTIARRHYTHMICS: β-ADRENERGIC ANTAGONISTS

Mechanism—Antagonize sympathetic stimulation of β1-adrenergic receptors in SA and AV nodal cells, thereby decreasing slope of phase 4 depolarization (important at SA node) and prolonging repolarization (important at AV node)

Propranolol Atenolol Metoprolol Acebutolol Bisoprolol	See Drug Summary Table: Chapter 9 Adrenergic Pharmacology

Labetalol
Carvedilol
Pindolol

CLASS III ANTIARRHYTHMIC AGENTS: INHIBITORS OF REPOLARIZATION

Mechanism—Block K$^+$ channels, resulting in longer action potential plateau and prolonged repolarization

Drug	Clinical uses	Serious and common adverse effects	Contraindications	Therapeutic considerations
Ibutilide	Conversion of atrial fibrillation or atrial flutter to normal sinus rhythm	*AV block, bradycardia, sustained ventricular tachycardia, 2% develop torsades de pointes requiring electrical cardioversion*	History of polymorphic ventricular tachycardia, such as *torsades de pointes*; Pre-existing long QT syndrome	Class IA and Class III antiarrhythmic agents may increase potential for prolonged refractoriness. Drugs that prolong QT interval (such as antihistamines, phenothiazines, and tricyclic antidepressants) increase the risk of arrhythmia. Monitor QT interval during ibutilide administration
Dofetilide	Conversion of atrial fibrillation or atrial flutter to normal sinus rhythm; Maintenance of normal sinus rhythm in patients with symptomatic atrial fibrillation or atrial flutter	*Same as ibutilide*	Same as ibutilide. Additional contraindications include patients with creatinine clearance less than 20 mL/min	Only available orally; Due to its potential for inducing ventricular arrhythmias, dofetilide is reserved for patients with highly symptomatic atrial fibrillation and/or atrial flutter; Reduction in dosage in patients with renal dysfunction
Sotalol	Life-threatening ventricular arrhythmias; Maintenance of normal sinus rhythm in patients with symptomatic atrial fibrillation or flutter	*Bradycardia, torsades de pointes, premature ventricular contractions, ventricular fibrillation, ventricular tachycardia, AV block, heart failure, bronchospasm*; Dyspnea, chest pain, fatigue	Severe sinus-node dysfunction, sinus bradycardia, second- or third-degree AV block; Long QT syndrome; Cardiogenic shock, uncontrolled heart failure; Asthma	Sotolol is a mixed class II and class III antiarrhythmic agent, which nonselectively antagonizes β-adrenergic receptors and prolongs action potential duration by blocking potassium channels; Used frequently in patients who cannot tolerate adverse effects of amiodarone; Use with caution in patients with impaired renal function or diabetes mellitus; Avoid coadministration with ziprasidone and sparfloxacin, which can prolong QT interval
Bretylium	Life-threatening ventricular arrhythmias	*Cardiac arrhythmia*; Marked orthostatic hypotension, bradycardia, dizziness, anxiety, increased body temperature	Digitalis-induced arrhythmias	Both an antihypertensive agent and a class III antiarrhythmic agent
Amiodarone	Recurrent ventricular fibrillation, unstable ventricular tachycardia; Atrial fibrillation; Supraventricular arrhythmias	*Arrhythmias, asystole, bradycardia, heart block, heart failure, hypotention, sinus arrest, neutropenia, pancytopenia, hepatic failure, severe pulmonary toxicity (pneumonitis, alveolitis, fibrosis), thyroid dysfunction*; Fatigue, corneal microdeposits, blue-gray skin pigmentation, photosensitivity	Patients receiving ritonavir; Severe SA-node disease; Second- or third-degree AV block; Bradycardia with syncope	IV formulation (Cordarone®) contains benzyl alcohol, which has caused gasping respiration and cardiovascular collapse (''gasping syndrome'') in neonates; Pulmonary toxicity is more common at high doses; Coadministration of beta-blockers or calcium channel blockers may increase risk of sinus bradycardia, sinus arrest, and AV block; Coadministration of cholestyramine increases amiodarone elimination; Coadministration of cyclosporine, digoxin, flecainide, lidocaine, phenytoin, procainamide, quinidine, or theophylline may lead to increased levels of these drugs

(Continued)

Drug Summary Table   Chapter 18 Pharmacology of Cardiac Rhythm (*Continued*)

Drug	Clinical Applications	Serious and Common Adverse Effects	Contraindications	Therapeutic Considerations
CLASS IV ANTIARRHYTHMIC AGENTS: CALCIUM CHANNEL BLOCKERS *Mechanism—Preferentially block cardiac Ca²⁺ channels; slow action potential upstroke in SA and AV nodal tissues*				
Verapamil Diltiazem	See Drug Summary Table, Chapter 21 Pharmacology of Vascular Tone			
OTHER ANTIARRHYTHMIC AGENTS *Mechanism—See specific drug*				
Adenosine	Conversion of paroxysmal supraventricular tachycardia to normal sinus rhythm	Facial flushing, brochoconstriction in patient with asthma, chest pressure, diaphoresis, excessive SA or AV nodal inhibition	Second- or third-degree AV block Do not use adenosine for atrial fibrillation or atrial flutter	Opens G protein-coupled K⁺ channel and suppresses Ca²⁺-dependent action potential, thereby inhibiting SA nodal, atrial, and AV nodal conduction Coadministration of carbamazepine may increase the degree of heart block Transient arrhythmia may occur at the onset of adenosine infusion
Ranolazine	Chronic angina pectoris	*Prolongs QT interval, syncope, acute renal dysfunction* Constipation, dizziness, headache	Concurrent use of drugs that prolong QT interval Pre-existing long QT syndrome Concurrent use of moderately potent P450 3A inhibitors Hepatic dysfunction	Mechanism of action unclear—may inhibit fatty-acid oxidation, delayed rectifier potassium current, or late sodium current Frequently used in combination with beta-blockers, amlodipine, or nitrates in patients who have not achieved adequate response with other anti-anginal agents Avoid concurrent use of moderately potent P450 3A inhibitors or drugs that prolong QT interval Avoid use in patients with severe renal impairment

(Top row, continued from previous page — Therapeutic Considerations column:)

Coadministration of drugs that prolong QT interval, such as disopyramide, thioridazine, phenothiazine, pimozide, quinidine, sparfloxacin, or tricyclic antidepressants, may lead to prolonged QT interval and induce *torsades de pointes*

Coadministration of phenytoin may decrease amiodarone levels

19

Pharmacology of Cardiac Contractility

Ehrin J. Armstrong and Thomas P. Rocco

INTRODUCTION

In 1785, Dr. William Withering described the cardiovascular benefits of a preparation from the foxglove plant called digitalis. He used this preparation to treat patients suffering from ''dropsy,'' a condition in which accumulation of extravascular fluid leads to dyspnea (difficulty breathing) and peripheral edema. These symptoms are now recognized as characteristic manifestations of **heart failure (HF)**, a clinical syndrome most commonly caused by systolic dysfunction of the left ventricle (LV). In this condition, the LV is unable to maintain adequate stroke volume despite normal filling volumes, and the LV end-diastolic volume increases in an effort to preserve stroke output. However, beyond a certain end-diastolic volume, LV diastolic pressures begin to increase, often precipitously. This increase in LV diastolic pressure results in increased left atrial and pulmonary capil-lary pressures which, in turn, lead to interstitial and alveolar pulmonary edema, and to increased right heart and pulmonary artery pressures. The elevated right heart pressures result in systemic venous hypertension and peripheral edema.

Dr. Withering's use of digitalis presaged the current use of **digoxin,** a member of the cardiac glycoside family of drugs, to treat conditions in which myocardial contractility is impaired. Cardiac glycosides are **positive inotropes**, defined as *agents that increase the contractile force of cardiac myocytes.* Since the advent of digitalis, elucidation of the cellular mechanism of cardiac contraction has facilitated the development of other inotropic agents. After reviewing the physiology of cardiac contraction and the cellular pathophysiology of contractile dysfunction, this chapter describes four classes of positive inotropic drugs that are either approved for use or under investigation in clinical trials. An integrated discussion of therapeutic strategies for HF can be found in Chapter 24, Integrative Cardiovascular Pharmacology: Hypertension, Ischemic Heart Disease, and Heart Failure.

▪ Case

GW, a 68-year-old man with known systolic dysfunction and heart failure, is admitted to the hospital with shortness of breath and nausea. The patient's cardiac history is notable for two prior myocardial infarctions, the more recent occurring about 2 years ago. Since the second infarction, the patient has had significant limitation of his exercise capacity. A two-dimensional echocardiogram is notable for a LV ejection fraction of 25% (normal, >55%) and moderate mitral valve regurgitation. GW has been treated with aspirin, carvedilol (a β-antagonist), captopril (an angiotensin converting enzyme inhibitor), digoxin (a cardiac glycoside), furosemide (a loop diuretic), and spironolactone (an aldosterone receptor antagonist). He has also had an automatic internal cardioverter-defibrillator (AICD) placed to prevent sustained ventricular arrhythmia and sudden cardiac death.

Physical examination in the emergency department is notable for a blood pressure of 90/50 mm Hg and an irregular heart rate of 120 beats per min. An electrocardiogram indicates that the underlying cardiac rhythm is atrial fibrillation. He is started on amiodarone (a class III anti-arrhythmic), and the heart rate decreases to approximately 80 beats/min. Laboratory tests show serum Na^+ 148 mEq/L (normal, 135–145), BUN 56 mg/dl (normal, 7–19), K^+ 2.9 mEq/L (normal, 3.5–5.1), and creatinine 4.8 mg/dL (normal, 0.6–1.2). The serum digoxin level is 3.2 ng/mL (therapeutic concentration, typically ~1 ng/mL).

Based on these findings, GW is admitted to the cardiology intensive care unit. His oral digoxin dose is held, and he is given intravenous K^+ to increase his serum potassium concentration. Based on the severity of this clinical decompensation, a pulmonary artery (PA) catheter is placed to monitor cardiac pressures. GW is also started on dobutamine and his carvedilol is held. After initiation of intravenous dobutamine, GW has increased urine output and begins to feel symptomatically improved. He is monitored for 7 days, and his digoxin level decreases to the therapeutic range.

QUESTIONS

▪ **1.** Why is GW being treated with a β-antagonist and a positive inotrope (digoxin) at the same time?
▪ **2.** What is the mechanism of action of digoxin?
▪ **3.** What is GW's major clinical manifestation of digoxin toxicity?
▪ **4.** What factors (including drug interactions) have contributed to digoxin toxicity in this patient?
▪ **5.** What is the mechanism of action of dobutamine?

PHYSIOLOGY OF CARDIAC CONTRACTION

The heart is responsible for receiving deoxygenated blood from the periphery, propelling this blood through the pulmonary circulation (where the hemoglobin is reoxygenated), and ultimately distributing this oxygenated blood to peripheral tissues. To accomplish the latter task, the left ventricle must develop sufficient tension to overcome the impedance to ejection that resides in the peripheral circulation. The relationship between the tension generated during the systolic phase of the cardiac cycle and the extent of LV filling during diastole is referred to as the **contractile state** of the myocardium. Together with **preload** (intraventricular blood volume), **afterload** (the resistance against which the left ventricle ejects), and **heart rate,** myocardial contractility is a primary determinant of cardiac output. Although cardiac pump performance at the organ level has been a central concern of cardiac physiologists for many years, the cellular and molecular mechanisms of cardiac contraction are now understood as well.

MYOCYTE ANATOMY

Like skeletal muscle, cardiac muscle contracts when action potentials depolarize the plasma membranes of cardiac muscle cells. The process of **excitation–contraction (EC) coupling,** in which the intracellular machinery transduces an electrochemical signal into mechanical force, involves the following cascade of events: voltage-gated calcium channels open, intracellular calcium increases, contractile proteins are activated, and actin–myosin interactions shorten the contractile elements.

The cellular anatomy of ventricular myocytes is well-suited to the excitation and regulation of cardiac contraction (Fig. 19-1). Specialized components of the ventricular myocyte include the sarcolemma, or myocyte plasma membrane; the sarcoplasmic reticulum (SR), a large internal membrane system that encircles the myofibrils; and the myofibrils themselves. Myofibrils are rope-like units containing precisely organized contractile proteins; the coordinated interaction of these proteins is responsible for the physical shortening of the cardiac muscle. These anatomic specializations are illustrated in Figures 19-1 and 19-2, and summarized in Table 19-1.

MYOCYTE CONTRACTION

Increased cytosolic Ca^{2+} is the link between excitation and contraction. During the ventricular action potential (see Chapter 18, Pharmacology of Cardiac Rhythm), Ca^{2+} influx through L-type Ca^{2+} channels in the sarcolemma causes an increase in the cytosolic Ca^{2+} concentration. This "trigger calcium" stimulates the ryanodine receptor in the SR membrane, causing release of stored Ca^{2+} from the SR into the cytosol. When the Ca^{2+} concentration in the cytoplasm reaches approximately 10^{-5} M, calcium binds to troponin C and induces a conformational change in tropomyosin that releases the inhibitory protein troponin I. This release of troponin I exposes an interaction site for myosin on the actin filament, and the binding of myosin to actin initiates the contraction cycle.

Figure 19-2 illustrates the cycle by which actin–myosin interactions physically shorten the sarcomere. Each myosin filament is studded with protruding flexible heads that form reversible cross-bridges with actin filaments. Formation of actin–myosin cross-bridges, bending of the myosin heads at

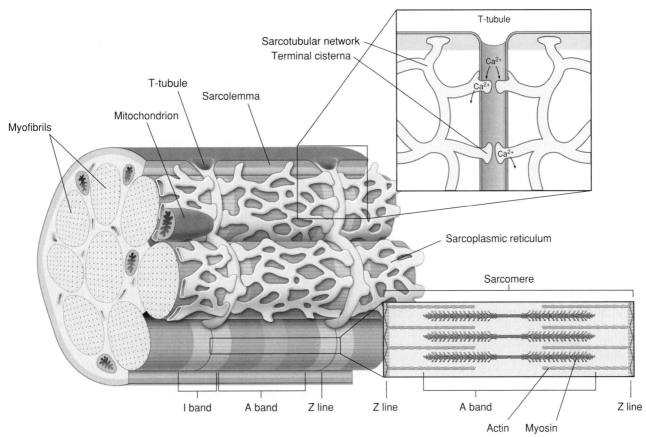

Figure 19-1. Cardiac myocyte structure. Each cardiac myocyte contains myofibrils and mitochondria surrounded by a specialized plasma membrane termed *the sarcolemma*. Invaginations of the sarcolemma, called T-tubules, provide conduits for Ca^{2+} influx. Within the cell, an extensive sarcoplasmic reticulum stores Ca^{2+} for use in contraction. Extracellular Ca^{2+} enters through the sarcolemma and its T-tubules during phase 2 of the action potential. This trigger Ca^{2+} binds to channels on the sarcoplasmic reticulum membrane, causing release into the cytosol of a large pool of so-called activation Ca^{2+}. Increased cytosolic Ca^{2+} initiates myofibril contraction. The *sarcomere* is the functional unit of the myofibril. Each sarcomere consists of interdigitating bands of actin and myosin. These bands form distinctive structures under the electron microscope. The *A* bands correspond to regions of overlapping actin and myosin. The *Z* lines demarcate the borders of each sarcomere. The *I* bands span neighboring sarcomeres and correspond to regions of actin without overlapping myosin. During cardiac myocyte contraction, the *I* bands become shorter (i.e., the *Z* lines approach one another), but the *A* bands maintain a constant length.

their flexible hinges, and detachment of the cross-bridges together allow the myosin filament to "walk up" the actin filament in both directions, and thereby to pull the two ends of the sarcomere together.

The normal function of the sarcomeric cross-bridge cycle is critically dependent on ATP. The ATP hydrolase (ATPase) activity of myosin provides the energy used both to drive contraction and to reset the contractile proteins, leading to relaxation. If an insufficient amount of ATP is available for cross-bridge cycling, myosin and actin remain "locked" in the associated state and the myocardium is unable to relax. This ATP-dependence explains the profound impact of ischemia on both systolic contraction (the contraction cycle cannot proceed) and diastolic relaxation (actin and myosin cannot dissociate) of the myocardium.

The organization of the sarcomere and the physical mechanism of contraction explain the fundamental relationship between muscle length and tension development. Increased stretch (length) of the muscle exposes additional sites for calcium binding and for actin–myosin interaction; increased stretch also effects greater release of calcium from the SR. These cellular events provide the mechanistic explanation

for the **Frank–Starling law**: *an increase in the end-diastolic volume of the left ventricle leads to an increase in ventricular stroke volume during systole.* Chapter 24 describes the organ-level implications of the Frank–Starling law in more detail.

REGULATION OF CONTRACTILITY

Three major control mechanisms regulate calcium cycling and myocardial contractility in cardiac myocytes. At the sarcolemma, calcium flux is mediated by interactions between the sodium pump and sodium-calcium exchanger. At the sarcoplasmic reticulum, calcium channels and pumps regulate the extent of calcium release and reuptake. Neurohumoral influences, especially the β-adrenergic signaling pathway, further modulate calcium cycling through these channels and transporters.

The Sodium Pump and Sodium–Calcium Exchange

In the sarcolemma, the three key proteins involved in calcium regulation are the Na^+/K^+-ATPase, hereafter referred

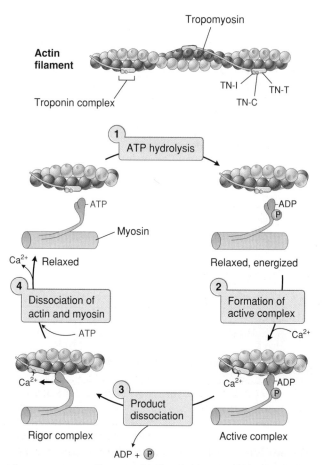

Figure 19-2. Cardiac contractile proteins and the contraction cycle. During contraction, myosin ratchets along actin filaments, resulting in an overall shortening of sarcomere length. Actin filaments **(top)** consist of two actin polymers wound around one another, three troponin proteins (TN-I, TN-C, and TN-T), and tropomyosin. In the absence of Ca^{2+}, tropomyosin is oriented on actin so that it inhibits the interaction of actin with myosin. The contraction cycle, shown in the **bottom** panel, occurs in a four-step process. 1. Cardiac myocyte contraction begins with hydrolysis of ATP to ADP by myosin; this reaction energizes the myosin head. 2. Ca^{2+} released from the sarcoplasmic reticulum binds to TN-C; this reaction causes a conformational change in tropomyosin that allows myosin to form an active complex with actin. 3. Dissociation of ADP from myosin allows the myosin head to bend; this bending pulls the *Z* lines closer together, and thus shortens the *I* band *(not shown)*. This contracted state is often referred to as a *rigor complex* because muscle will remain in a contracted state unless there is sufficient ATP available to displace the myosin heads from actin. 4. Binding of a new ATP molecule to myosin allows the actin–myosin complex to dissociate. Ca^{2+} also dissociates from TN-C, and the contraction cycle is repeated.

to as the **sodium pump,** the **sodium–calcium exchanger,** and the calcium–ATPase or **calcium pump** (Fig. 19-3). The activity of the sodium pump is crucial to maintain both the resting membrane potential and the concentration gradients of sodium and potassium across the sarcolemma ($[Na^+]_{out} = 145$ mM, $[Na^+]_{in} = 15$ mM, $[K^+]_{out} = 5$ mM, $[K^+]_{in} = 150$ mM). Sodium-pump activity is closely linked to the intracellular calcium concentration via the sodium–calcium exchanger; this antiporter exchanges sodium and calcium in both directions across the sarcolemma. Changes in the

concentration of either sodium or calcium ions inside or outside the cell affect the direction and magnitude of sodium–calcium exchange. Under normal conditions, the low intracellular sodium concentration favors sodium influx and calcium efflux. Some drugs take advantage of the functional coupling between the sodium pump and the sodium–calcium exchanger to exert their effect as positive inotropes. **Digoxin,** discussed in the introductory case and described in detail below, is the prototype of an inotropic agent that acts by inhibiting the sodium pump. A sarcolemmal calcium pump also helps to maintain calcium homeostasis by actively extruding calcium from the cytoplasm after cardiac contraction. A high concentration of ATP favors calcium removal (relaxation), both directly via the calcium pump and indirectly via the sodium pump.

Calcium Storage and Release

As described above, Ca^{2+} signaling is central to both cardiac contraction and relaxation. As such, the cardiac myocyte has well-developed systems to regulate Ca^{2+} flux during the cardiac cycle. In the SR, the calcium release channel (**ryanodine receptor**) and the calcium pump (sarcoendoplasmic reticulum calcium ATPase, **SERCA**) are critical to the regulation of contractility (Fig. 19-3). Proper contraction requires both that Ca^{2+} release into the cytoplasm is adequate to stimulate contraction and that Ca^{2+} reuptake into the SR is sufficient to permit relaxation and to replenish calcium stores. Cytoplasmic concentrations of both calcium and ATP regulate the activity of both the ryanodine receptor and SERCA.

As noted above, trigger calcium opens the ryanodine receptor. Cytoplasmic calcium concentration is directly related to the number of receptors that open. A safety mechanism also exists whereby high calcium levels lead to calcium–calmodulin complex formation: this complex inhibits calcium release by decreasing the open time of the ryanodine receptor. High concentrations of ATP favor the open channel conformation, and thereby facilitate SR calcium release into the cytosol.

In addition to opening the ryanodine receptor, cytoplasmic calcium also stimulates SERCA, which pumps calcium back into the SR. This pump provides another control mechanism to prevent a positive feedback cycle that could irreversibly deplete the SR of calcium. As calcium pumps refill the SR, the rate of Ca^{2+} reuptake slows because of the declining cytoplasmic calcium concentration. ATP also favors SERCA activity; conversely, decreased ATP impairs calcium reuptake. The latter mechanism causes the rate and extent of diastolic relaxation to decrease in ischemic myocardium.

A third mediator of SERCA activity is **phospholamban,** a SR membrane protein that inhibits SERCA. High levels of intracellular **cAMP** stimulate **protein kinase A** to phosphorylate phospholamban, which reverses its inhibition of SERCA (Fig. 19-3). Phospholamban thus controls the rate of relaxation by regulating calcium reuptake into the SR: unphosphorylated phospholamban slows relaxation, while phosphorylated phopholamban accelerates relaxation.

Adrenergic Receptor Signaling and Calcium Cycling

β_1-Adrenoceptor stimulation supports cardiac performance in several ways. First, β-receptor agonists increase β-adreno-

TABLE 19-1	Functional Anatomy of Cardiac Myocyte Contraction
Sarcolemma	
T tubules	Invaginations of sarcolemma, facilitate ion flux across the cell membrane
Voltage-gated L-type Ca^{2+} channels	Mediate influx of trigger Ca^{2+} ions when sarcolemma is depolarized
Sarcoplasmic Reticulum (SR)	
Ca^{2+} release channels	Stimulated by trigger Ca^{2+}, release internal Ca^{2+} stores
Ca^{2+}-ATPase pumps	Sequester intracellular Ca^{2+} in SR to terminate contraction
Terminal cisternae	Sacs at distal branches of SR that store Ca^{2+}
Myofibril	
Sarcomere	Basic contractile unit of the myofibril
Myosin	Thick filament, hydrolyzes ATP for energy
Actin	Thin filament, provides scaffolding for myosin binding
Tropomyosin	Coils around actin, preventing actin-myosin binding at rest
Troponin complex:	Complex of three proteins that regulate actin–myosin binding:
Troponin T	Holds troponin complex to tropomyosin
Troponin I	Inhibits actin–myosin binding at rest
Troponin C	Binds Ca^{2+}, displacing troponin I from actin–myosin binding site

ceptor-mediated increases in Ca^{2+} entry during systole; increased Ca^{2+} entry increases fractional shortening of cardiac muscle during contraction. This **positive inotropic effect** results in a greater stroke volume for any given end-diastolic volume. β-Agonists also have a **positive chronotropic effect**, increasing heart rate in a relatively linear dose-dependent manner. The net effect of these inotropic and chronotropic effects is to increase cardiac output:

$$\text{Cardiac Output (CO)} = \text{Heart Rate (HR)} \times \text{Stroke Volume (SV)} \quad \text{Equation 19-1}$$

where *CO* is cardiac output, *HR* is heart rate, and *SV* is stroke volume. A third, but less widely appreciated, mechanism by which β-agonists support cardiac performance is by enhancing the rate and extent of diastolic relaxation (sometimes called the **positive lusitropic effect**). This is a critical permissive effect of $β_1$-receptor stimulation because it facilitates maintenance of adequate LV filling (i.e., preservation of LV end-diastolic volume), despite the reduction in diastolic filling time that occurs as heart rate increases.

In the peripheral circulation, the effects of sympathetic stimulation are more complex. Activation of peripheral $β_2$-receptors dilates vascular smooth muscle, but $α_1$-receptor stimulation constricts vascular smooth muscle. Thus, *$β_2$-receptor stimulation typically decreases systemic vascular resistance (SVR) and afterload, while $α_1$-receptor stimulation increases SVR and afterload.* Dopamine receptors in the splanchnic and renal circulations also modulate the resistance vessels in these vascular beds, as discussed below.

The cardiostimulatory actions of the sympathetic nervous system are mediated by activation of several adrenergic receptor subtypes located in the heart and peripheral vasculature. Stimulation of these **G protein-coupled receptors** induces conformational changes that activate **adenylyl cyclase** and thereby elevate intracellular cAMP levels (Fig. 19-4 and Table 19-2). Higher levels of cAMP activate protein kinase A, which phosphorylates multiple targets in the cell. These targets include L-type calcium channels in the sarcolemma and phospholamban in the SR membrane. As discussed above, the phosphorylation of phospholamban releases its inhibition of SERCA, allowing calcium to be pumped from the cytosol back into the SR; this is one of the molecular mechanisms of enhanced diastolic relaxation associated with $β_1$-adrenoceptor stimulation.

Sensitivity of Contractile Proteins to Calcium

As mentioned above, the tension developed by cardiac myocytes during contraction is directly related to the pre-contraction length of the sarcomere units. Increased stretch of the sarcomeres exposes more calcium binding sites on troponin C, making more sites available for actin–myosin cross-bridge formation and thereby increasing the *sensitivity* of the contractile proteins to calcium. Several other mechanisms also regulate contractile protein sensitivity. Phosphorylation of troponin I by protein kinase A (a process that, like phospholamban phosphorylation, depends on cAMP levels) decreases contractile protein sensitivity to calcium. Expression of various isoforms of the contractile proteins, particularly troponin T, has also been linked to altered calcium sensitivity. Pharmacologic agents that sensitize contractile proteins to calcium are under active investigation.

PATHOPHYSIOLOGY

Many disease processes can lead to myocyte dysfunction or death, causing replacement of myocardium with fibrous tissue and leading to impaired contractility. The most common etiology of contractile dysfunction in the United States is coronary artery disease (CAD) resulting in myocardial in-

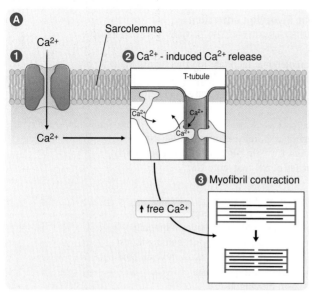

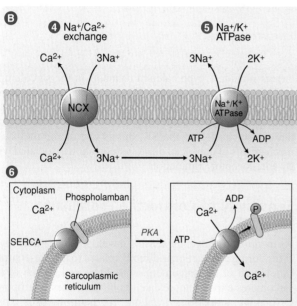

Figure 19-3. Regulation of cardiac myocyte Ca²⁺ flux. A. During contraction: 1. Extracellular Ca^{2+} enters the cardiac myocyte through Ca^{2+} channels in the sarcolemma. 2. This trigger Ca^{2+} induces release of Ca^{2+} from the sarcoplasmic reticulum into the cytosol (so-called Ca^{2+}-induced Ca^{2+} release). 3. The increased cytosolic Ca^{2+} facilitates myofibril contraction. **B.** During relaxation: 4. The Na^+/Ca^{2+} exchanger (NCX) extrudes Ca^{2+} from the cytosol, using the Na^+ gradient as a driving force. 5. The Na^+/K^+ ATPase maintains the Na^+ gradient, thus keeping the cardiac myocyte hyperpolarized. 6. The sarcoendoplasmic reticulum Ca^{2+} ATPase (SERCA) in the sarcoplasmic reticulum membrane is tonically inhibited by phospholamban. Phosphorylation of phospholamban by protein kinase A (PKA) disinhibits the Ca^{2+} ATPase, allowing sequestration of cytosolic Ca^{2+} in the sarcoplasmic reticulum.

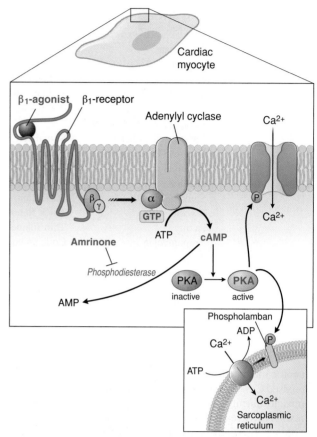

Figure 19-4. Regulation of cardiac contractility by β-adrenergic receptors. β-Adrenergic receptors increase cardiac myocyte contractility but also enhance relaxation. Binding of an endogenous or exogenous agonist to β_1-adrenergic receptors on the surface of cardiac myocytes causes Gα proteins to activate adenylyl cyclase, which in turn catalyzes the conversion of ATP to cAMP. cAMP activates multiple protein kinases, including protein kinase A (PKA). PKA phosphorylates and activates sarcolemmal Ca^{2+} channels and thereby increases cardiac myocyte contractility. PKA also phosphorylates phospholamban. The SERCA pump becomes disinhibited and pumps Ca^{2+} into the sarcoplasmic reticulum; the increased rate of Ca^{2+} sequestration enhances cardiac myocyte relaxation. cAMP is converted to AMP by phosphodiesterase, resulting in termination of β_1-adrenergic receptor-mediated actions. The phosphodiesterase is inhibited by amrinone, a drug that can be used in the treatment of heart failure.

farction; other common etiologies of contractile dysfunction include systemic hypertension and valvular heart disease. In each of the aforementioned disease states, dysfunction of the cardiac myocyte occurs as a consequence of a non-myocardial disease process. A less common cause of LV dys-

function is idiopathic cardiomyopathy, in which the principal abnormality occurs at the level of the cardiac myocyte.

Irrespective of underlying etiology, progressive contractile dysfunction of the myocardium leads ultimately to the syndrome of **systolic HF.** It is important to note, however, that HF can occur in the absence of contractile dysfunction. For example, several common cardiovascular disease states—such as acute myocardial ischemia and restrictive cardiomyopathy—are associated with abnormalities of LV relaxation and/or filling, leading to decreased chamber compliance and elevated LV diastolic pressure. This abnormal elevation of intraventricular pressure can occur even in the presence of normal systolic function, leading to a syndrome referred to as **diastolic heart failure.** The organ-level pathology and treatment of HF are discussed in detail in Chap-

TABLE 19-2	Effects of Increased Intracellular cAMP in Cardiac Cells
Sarcolemma	↑ Phosphorylation of voltage-gated Ca^{2+} channel → ↑ contractility, heart rate, and AV conduction ↑ Phosphorylation of Na^+ pump → ↑ Ca^{2+} influx into cytoplasm via Na^+/Ca^{2+} exchange
Sarcoplasmic reticulum	↑ Phosphorylation of phospholamban → ↑ Ca^{2+} uptake and release
Contractile proteins	↑ Phosphorylation of troponin I → ↓ Ca^{2+} sensitivity
Energy production	↑ Glycogenolysis → ↑ ATP availability

ter 24. Here, we focus on the salient cellular and molecular aspects of normal and abnormal contractile function.

The clinical expression of HF often reflects the impact of neurohumoral systems that are activated by inadequate forward cardiac output. In advanced stages of the disease, it may be difficult to determine whether the cellular abnormalities observed in failing cardiac myocytes reflect primary cellular defects or secondary responses to extracardiac stimuli (such as circulating cytokines and neuroendocrine peptides). Nonetheless, the cellular and molecular alterations in the failing myocardium can be contrasted with the events of normal contraction in an effort to obtain mechanistic insight, and many of these changes are active areas of investigation. Study of these alterations also promises to identify potential new molecular targets for pharmacologic intervention.

CELLULAR PATHOPHYSIOLOGY OF CONTRACTILE DYSFUNCTION

At the cellular level, changes associated with decreased cardiac contractility include dysregulation of calcium homeostasis, changes in the regulation and expression pattern of contractile proteins, and alterations in β-adrenoceptor signal transduction pathways (Fig. 19-5). As noted above, some of these alterations may result from local myocardial pathology, whereas others likely represent responses to circulating hormonal and inflammatory signals.

Altered calcium homeostasis results in prolongation of the action potential and the Ca^{2+} transient associated with each contraction in failing cardiac myocytes. Mechanisms that increase the cytosolic concentration of Ca^{2+} and deplete SR Ca^{2+} stores include reduced SR Ca^{2+} reuptake and an increased number of sodium–calcium exchangers in the sarcolemma. As described above, efficient sequestration of calcium by the SR is essential for the termination of contraction. Thus, the inability of the myocyte to regulate intracellular calcium impairs both systolic contraction and diastolic relaxation.

Dysfunctional contractile proteins are produced by changes in the transcription of various genes in failing car-

diac myocytes. The available data suggest that the myocytes enter a maladaptive growth phase, reverting to production of the fetal isoforms of some proteins. For example, failing myocytes increase expression of the fetal isoform of troponin T, which is potentially a more efficient contractile protein. Other contractile protein alterations identified in heart failure include a reduction in phosphorylation of troponin and diminished ATP hydrolysis by myosin; each of these changes results in a slower rate of cross-bridge cycling. In addition, activation of collagenase and matrix metalloproteinases may disrupt the stromal framework that maintains the structural and functional integrity of the myocardium.

Desensitization of the β-adrenergic receptor–G protein–adenylyl cyclase signaling pathway is the third major abnormal finding in cardiac myocytes of patients with systolic HF. Failing myocytes down-regulate the number of β-adrenergic receptors expressed at the cell surface, possibly as an adaptive response to the presence of increased neurohormonal stimulation. Sympathetic stimulation of the remaining receptors results in a smaller increase in cAMP than would occur in the presence of a normal number of receptors. The reduction in β-adrenergic signaling may also reflect increased expression of both **β-adrenergic receptor kinase** (which phosphorylates and thereby inhibits β-adrenoceptors) and the **inhibitory G protein ($G\alpha_i$)**. Another contributor to the reduction of β-adrenergic signaling may be **inducible nitric oxide synthase (iNOS)**, the expression of which is increased in HF. The diminished response of the failing myocytes to adrenergic stimulation causes decreased phosphorylation of phospholamban, which impairs SR Ca^{2+} uptake capacity. Decreased cAMP levels also result in a decreased ability to produce and use ATP. Together, the impaired calcium regulation and decreased cAMP levels attenuate many of the steps of cardiac myocyte contraction and relaxation.

PHARMACOLOGIC CLASSES AND AGENTS

The central roles of intracellular calcium and cAMP in cardiac myocyte contraction provide a basis for the classification of inotropic agents. The **cardiac glycosides** raise intracellular Ca^{2+} concentration via inhibition of the sarcolemmal Na^+/K^+-ATPase (sodium pump), while **β-agonists** and **phosphodiesterase inhibitors** increase intracellular levels of cAMP. **Calcium-sensitizing agents**, a class of agents under active investigation, are also discussed briefly.

CARDIAC GLYCOSIDES

The cardiac glycosides include the digitalis derivatives **digoxin** and **digitoxin** and non-digitalis agents such as **ouabain**. Glycosides are defined by a common chemical scaffold that includes a steroid nucleus, an unsaturated lactone ring, and one or more sugar residues. This common structural substrate underlies the common mechanism of action of these agents. In clinical practice, digoxin is both the most

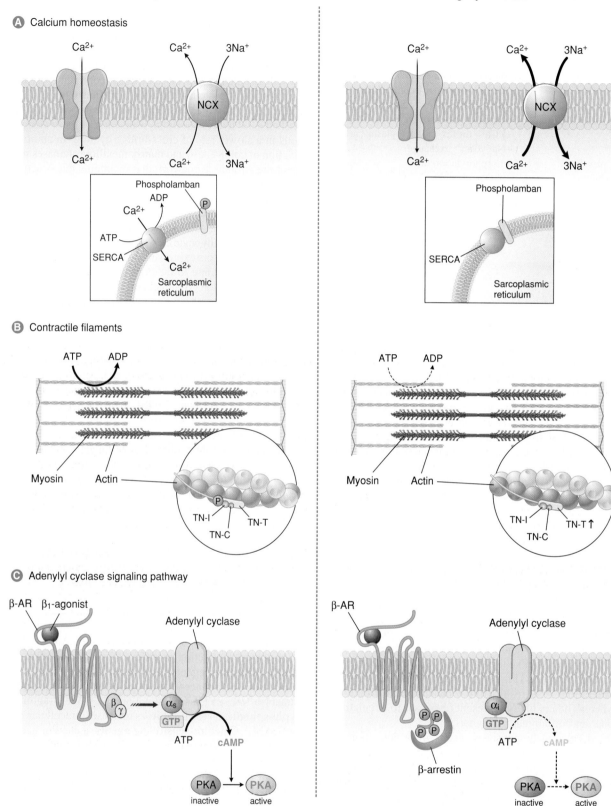

Figure 19-5. Cellular mechanisms of contractile pathophysiology. In the failing myocardium, there are derangements in Ca^{2+} homeostasis, the contractile elements, and the adenylyl cyclase signaling pathway. In each panel (*A, B,* and *C*), normal myocardium is shown on the **left** and failing myocardium on the **right. A.** In the normal myocardium, Ca^{2+} homeostasis is tightly controlled by Ca^{2+} channels, including the Na^+/Ca^{2+} exchanger (NCX) and the Ca^{2+} ATPase (SERCA). Operation of these pathways allows the myocardium to relax during diastole. In the failing myocardium, diastolic Ca^{2+} remains elevated because phospholamban is not phosphorylated and it therefore tonically inhibits SERCA. Also, the expression of NCX increases (*large arrows*), so that cytosolic Ca^{2+} is extruded from the cardiac myocyte rather than stored in the sarcoplasmic reticulum. **B.** In the normal myocardium, phosphorylation of troponin-I (TN-I) exposes the actin–myosin interaction site,

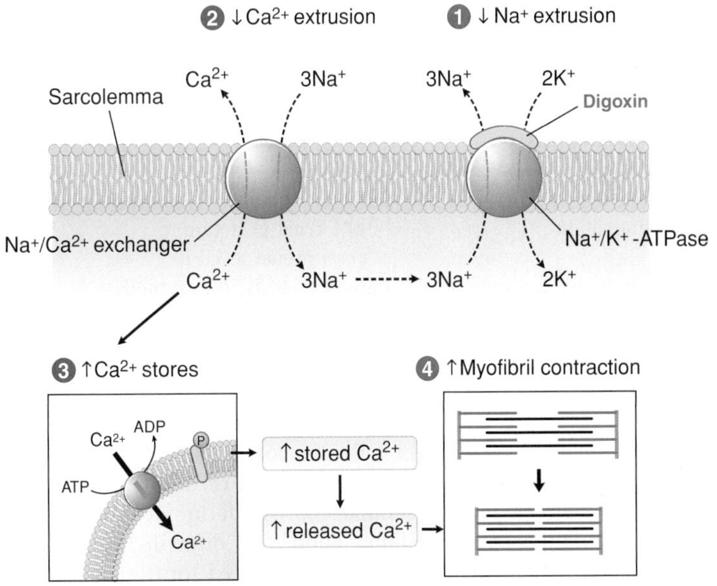

Figure 19-6. Positive inotropic mechanism of digoxin. 1. Digoxin selectively binds to and inhibits the Na^+/K^+-ATPase. Decreased Na^+ extrusion *(dashed arrows)* leads to an increased concentration of cytosolic Na^+. 2. The increased intracellular Na^+ decreases the driving force for the Na^+/Ca^{2+} exchanger *(dashed arrows)*, leading to decreased extrusion of Ca^{2+} from the cardiac myocyte into the extracellular space and to increased cytosolic Ca^{2+}. 3. An increased amount of Ca^{2+} is then pumped by the SERCA Ca^{2+}-ATPase *(large arrow)* into the sarcoplasmic reticulum, creating a net increase in Ca^{2+} that is available for release during subsequent contractions. 4. During each contraction, the increased Ca^{2+} release from the sarcoplasmic reticulum leads to increased myofibril contraction, and therefore increased cardiac inotropy.

frequently used cardiac glycoside and the most widely used inotropic agent.

Digoxin

Digoxin is a selective inhibitor of the plasma membrane sodium pump (Fig. 19-6). Cardiac myocytes exposed to digoxin extrude less sodium, leading to a rise in intracellular sodium concentration. In turn, the increase in intracellular sodium concentration alters the equilibrium of the sodium–calcium exchanger: calcium efflux is decreased because the gradient for sodium entry is decreased, while calcium influx is increased because the gradient for sodium efflux is increased. The net result is a rise in the intracellular calcium concentration. In response to this rise, the SR of the digoxin-treated cell sequesters more calcium. When the digoxin-treated cell depolarizes in response to an action potential, there is more Ca^{2+} available to bind troponin C, and tension development during contraction is facilitated.

In addition to its effects on myocardial contractility, digoxin exerts autonomic effects through its binding to sodium pumps in the plasma membranes of neurons in the central and peripheral nervous systems. These effects include inhibition of sympathetic nervous outflow, sensitization of baroreceptors, and increased parasympathetic (vagal) tone. Digoxin also alters the electrophysiologic properties of the heart by a direct action on the cardiac conduction system. At therapeutic doses, digoxin decreases automaticity at the AV node, prolonging the effective refractory period of AV nodal tissue and slowing conduction velocity through the node. These combined vagotonic and electrophysiologic

properties underlie the use of digoxin in the treatment of patients with atrial fibrillation and rapid ventricular response rates; both the decreased automaticity of AV nodal tissue and the decreased conduction velocity through the node increase the degree of AV block, and thereby decrease the ventricular response rate.

In contrast to its effects at the AV node, digoxin enhances automaticity of the infranodal (His–Purkinje) conduction system. These divergent effects at the AV node and His–Purkinje system explain the characteristic electrophysiologic disturbance of complete heart block with accelerated junctional or accelerated idioventricular escape rhythm (referred to as "regularized" atrial fibrillation) in patients with digoxin toxicity.

Digoxin has a *narrow therapeutic window,* and prevention of digoxin toxicity depends on a complete understanding of the pharmacokinetics of this agent (Table 19-3). Orally administered digoxin has a bioavailability of approximately 75%. A minority of patients harbor gut flora that metabolize digoxin to the inactive metabolite dihydrodigoxin. In these patients, it is sometimes necessary to coadminister antibiotics in order to decontaminate the gut and thereby facilitate oral absorption of digoxin. Digoxin has a large volume of distribution; the primary binding reservoir consists of Na^+/K^+-ATPase molecules in skeletal muscle. Approximately 70% of the drug is excreted unchanged by the kidney; the rest is excreted in the gut or via hepatic metabolism.

Several specific aspects of digoxin pharmacokinetics merit emphasis. *Chronic kidney disease* reduces both the volume of distribution and the clearance of digoxin, obligating a reduction in both the loading dose and the maintenance

and myosin effectively hydrolyzes ATP during each contraction cycle. In the failing myocardium, there is decreased phosphorylation of TN-I, resulting in less efficient actin–myosin crosslinking. Myosin does not hydrolyze ATP as efficiently *(dashed arrow)*, further reducing the effectiveness of each contraction cycle. There is also increased expression of the fetal isoform of TN-T in the failing myocardium; the significance of this alteration is uncertain. **C.** In the normal myocardium, β-agonists stimulate cAMP formation and subsequent activation of protein kinase A (PKA). In the failing myocardium, β-arrestin binds to and inhibits the activity of β-adrenergic receptors (β-AR), leading to decreased stimulation of adenylyl cyclase *(dashed arrows)*. Expression of the inhibitory Gα isoform Gα$_i$ is also induced in the failing myocardium.

TABLE 19-3	**Pharmacokinetics of Digoxin**
Oral bioavailability	~75%
Onset of action (intravenous)	~30 minutes
Peak effect (intravenous)	1–5 hours
Half-life	36 hours
Elimination	~90% renal excretion, proportional to GFR
Volume of distribution	Large (~640 L/70 kg): binds to skeletal muscle

dose of the drug (see Chapter 3, Pharmacokinetics). *Hypoka-lemia* increases the myocardial localization of digoxin because reductions in extracellular K^+ result in increased phosphorylation of the sodium pump, and digoxin has a higher binding affinity for the phosphorylated form of the pump than for the dephosphorylated form. (Conversely, increasing plasma K^+ can help to relieve symptoms of digoxin toxicity by promoting dephosphorylation of the sodium pump.)

Digoxin also *interacts* with many drugs. These interactions can be divided into pharmacodynamic and pharmacokinetic interactions. Pharmacodynamic interactions include those with β-adrenergic antagonists, Ca^{2+} channel blockers, and K^+-wasting diuretics. β-Adrenergic antagonists decrease AV nodal conduction, and the combined use of β-antagonists and digoxin can increase the risk of developing high grade AV block. Both β-antagonists and Ca^{2+} channel blockers can decrease cardiac contractility and potentially attenuate the effects of digoxin. K^+-wasting diuretics (e.g., furosemide) can decrease plasma potassium concentration, which can increase the affinity of digoxin for the Na^+/K^+-ATPase and thereby predispose to digoxin toxicity (see above).

Pharmacokinetic interactions can result from changes in the absorption, volume of distribution, or renal clearance of digoxin (Table 19-3). Many antibiotics, such as erythromycin, can increase digoxin absorption by killing the enteric bacteria that would ordinarily metabolize a significant fraction of orally administered digoxin before its absorption. Co-administration of digoxin with verapamil (a calcium channel blocker), quinidine (a class IA antiarrhythmic), or amiodarone (a class III antiarrhythmic) can increase digoxin levels because of the impact of these drugs on the volume of distribution and/or renal clearance of digoxin.

In the introductory case, multiple factors likely contributed to the marked increase in the patient's serum digoxin level. The glomerular filtration rate (GFR) was reduced (indicated by the elevated creatinine), resulting in decreased digoxin clearance. Administration of a loop diuretic likely contributed to the reduction in GFR. This reduction of GFR could have been exacerbated by coadministration of an angiotensin converting enzyme inhibitor via interference with angiotensin-II-mediated autoregulation of glomerular hydrostatic pressure. Together, these factors likely contributed to the elevated serum digoxin concentration (3.2 ng/mL). To put this value into perspective, toxic effects, such as ventric-

ular ectopy, begin to appear at digoxin concentrations of 2–3 ng/mL.

Treatment of digoxin toxicity relies on normalizing plasma K^+ levels and minimizing the potential for ventricular arrhythmias. In addition, life-threatening digoxin toxicity can be treated with **antidigoxin antibodies.** These polyclonal antibodies form 1:1 complexes with digoxin that are rapidly cleared from the body. Fab fragments of these antibodies (i.e., the portion of the antibody that interacts with antigen) have been shown to be less immunogenic than antidigoxin IgG, and to have a larger volume of distribution, more rapid onset of action, and increased clearance compared to the intact IgG.

It may seem counterintuitive to administer digoxin (a positive inotrope) and the β-antagonist carvedilol (a negative inotrope) simultaneously. However, both agents have been shown to provide benefit in patients with HF. β-Antagonists are known to reduce mortality by 30% or more in patients with HF. (It is postulated that these receptor antagonists counteract the cardiotoxic effects of the chronic sympathetic stimulation that can occur in patients with contractile dysfunction. β-Antagonists have been shown to effect changes in cellular morphology and chamber remodeling.) The mechanism underlying the benefit of digoxin in HF is not fully understood. It is thought to be related both to its positive effect on contractile function and its neurohumoral effects. This issue is discussed in greater detail in Chapter 24.

Several large randomized trials provide a consistent picture of the clinical efficacy and limitations of digoxin. These trials indicate that withdrawal of digoxin in patients with HF leads to a decline in clinical status compared to patients who continue digoxin therapy. For example, withdrawal of digoxin is associated with deterioration in exercise capacity and increased frequency of hospitalization for worsening heart failure. However, the use of digoxin in patients with heart failure does not have a significant impact on survival. In short, while digoxin has not been shown to improve survival, it does palliate symptoms, improve functional status, and reduce hospitalization rates. These clinical benefits can provide significant improvement in quality of life for patients with HF.

Digoxin is also frequently used to control ventricular rate in patients with long-standing atrial fibrillation. The combined bradycardic and inotropic effects of digoxin make it an especially useful agent for patients with both HF and atrial fibrillation.

Digitoxin

Digitoxin is a less frequently used digitalis preparation that may be preferable to digoxin in selected clinical circumstances. Digitoxin is structurally identical to digoxin except for the presence (digoxin) or absence (digitoxin) of a hydroxyl group at position 12 of the steroid nucleus. This structural modification renders digitoxin less hydrophilic than digoxin and significantly alters the pharmacokinetics of the drug. In particular, digitoxin is metabolized and excreted primarily by the liver; the fact that its clearance does not depend on renal excretion makes digitoxin a suitable alternative to digoxin for the treatment of patients with HF and chronic kidney disease. However, digitoxin has a very long half-life (approximately 7 days) compared even to the long half-life of digoxin (approximately 36 hours).

β-ADRENERGIC RECEPTOR AGONISTS

β-Adrenoceptor agonists are a heterogeneous group of drugs that have differential specificity for adrenergic subtypes. Inhaled formulations of these medications are also used frequently in the treatment of asthma, as discussed in Chapter 46, Integrative Inflammation Pharmacology: Asthma. For all these agents, it merits emphasis that *the differential activation of receptor subtypes is influenced both by the agent selected and the dose at which that agent is administered.* For example, dopamine administered at low infusion rates (2–5 µg/kg/min) has an overall cardiostimulatory effect (caused by increased contractility and decreased SVR), while the same drug infused at higher rates (>10 µg/kg/min) has an overall impact that is largely related to α_1-receptor activation. Thus, the pharmacodynamic effects of the agent (see Table 19-4) must be considered in the context of the patient's overall hemodynamic profile; this often requires placement of hemodynamic monitoring catheters to quantify intracardiac filling pressures, systemic vascular resistance, and cardiac output. This is the reason that, in the introductory case, GW's doctors placed a PA catheter prior to starting the dobutamine infusion.

Clinical use of the sympathomimetic inotropes is generally reserved for short-term support of the failing circulation. This is attributable to the adverse effect profile of these agents and to their pharmacodynamic and pharmacokinetic properties. In general, sympathomimetic agents that stimulate myocardial β-adrenergic receptors share the adverse effect profile of tachycardia, arrhythmia, and increased myocardial oxygen consumption. These agents also induce tolerance via rapid down-regulation of adrenergic receptors at the surface of cells in target organs. In addition, the sympathomimetic amines have low oral bioavailability, and are typically administered by continuous intravenous infusion.

Dopamine

Dopamine (DA) is an endogenous sympathomimetic amine that functions as a neurotransmitter; it is also a biosynthetic precursor of norepinephrine and epinephrine (see Chapter 9, Adrenergic Pharmacology). At low doses, dopamine has a vasodilatory effect in the periphery by stimulating dopaminergic D1 receptors in the renal and mesenteric vascular beds. This regional vascular dilation reduces the impedance to left ventricular ejection (afterload). At intermediate doses, DA causes more widespread vasodilation and a greater reduction in systemic vascular resistance, although the preferential dilation of renal and mesenteric beds is lost at this midrange dose. At these intermediate doses, DA also activates β_1-receptors, thereby increasing contractility and heart rate. At higher doses, activation of α_1-receptors predominates in the periphery, leading to generalized vasoconstriction and an increase in afterload.

Dopamine must be administered intravenously in a closely monitored setting. It is metabolized rapidly by monoamine oxidase (MAO) and dopamine β-hydroxylase to inactive metabolites that are excreted by the kidney. Patients receiving dopamine and MAO inhibitors concomitantly have decreased metabolism of dopamine; in these patients, dopamine can cause significant tachycardia, arrhythmia, and increased myocardial oxygen consumption.

Despite its complex pharmacology, DA finds wide clinical application in patients with sepsis and anaphylaxis, syndromes in which peripheral vasodilation is a major contributor to circulatory failure. At low and intermediate doses, DA is used occasionally in patients with cardiogenic shock or HF. However, its use in cardiogenic circulatory failure has largely been supplanted by alternative agents (such as dobutamine and the phosphodiesterase inhibitors) that have a more predictable vasodilator effect in the periphery and/or are less likely to induce tachycardia and ventricular arrhythmia.

Dobutamine

Dobutamine is a synthetic sympathomimetic amine that was developed in an attempt to optimize the overall hemodynamic benefits of β-adrenergic receptor activation for patients with acute cardiogenic circulatory failure. Overall, dobutamine approximates the desirable hemodynamic profile of a "pure" β_1 agonist. However, this profile is *not* the result of selective activation of β_1-receptors, but rather derives from the fact that the clinically available formulation is a racemic mixture of enantiomers that have differential

---

TABLE 19-4 Receptor Selectivity of Sympathomimetics

AGENT	RECEPTOR TYPE				
	α_1 VASOCONSTRICTS PERIPHERAL VESSELS	α_2 PRESYNAPTIC INHIBITION AT NE SYNAPSE	β_1 INCREASES HEART RATE, CONTRACTILITY, DIASTOLIC RELAXATION	β_2 VASODILATES PERIPHERAL VESSELS	D1 LOW DOSES VASODILATE RENAL VESSELS
Dopamine	+		+ +	+ +	+ +
Dobutamine	+/−		+ +	+	
Epinephrine	+ +	+ +	+ +	+ +	
Norepinephrine	+ +	+ +	+ +		

effects on adrenergic receptor subtypes. Both the (+) and (−) enantiomers stimulate β₁-receptors and, to a lesser degree, β₂-receptors, but the (+) enantiomer acts as an α₁ antagonist, whereas the (−) enantiomer is an α₁ agonist. Because the clinical formulation includes both enantiomers, the opposing hemodynamic responses produced by these enantiomers at the α₁-receptor effectively negate one another. The predominant overall effect is that of an agonist at cardiac β₁-receptors, with modest peripheral vasodilation via agonist action at peripheral β₂-receptors.

Dobutamine is administered by continuous intravenous infusion, and titrated to achieve the desired clinical effect. Catechol-O-methyl transferase rapidly metabolizes dobutamine, so that the circulating half-life is only about 2.5 minutes. As with all sympathomimetic amines with β-agonist effects, dobutamine has the potential to induce cardiac arrhythmias. In clinical practice, supraventricular tachycardia and high-grade ventricular arrhythmia occur less frequently with dobutamine than with dopamine. On the basis of this constellation of clinical effects, dobutamine has become the sympathomimetic inotrope of choice for patients with acute cardiogenic circulatory failure.

Epinephrine

Epinephrine (Epi) is a nonselective adrenergic agonist that is endogenously released by the adrenal glands to support the circulation. Exogenously administered Epi stimulates β₁, β₂, α₁, and α₂ receptors; the net effect depends on the dose. At all dose levels, Epi is a potent β₁ agonist with positive inotropic, chronotropic, and lusitropic effects. Low-dose Epi predominantly stimulates peripheral β₂-receptors, causing vasodilation. At higher Epi doses, however, stimulation of α₁-receptors causes vasoconstriction and increased afterload. These effects make high-dose Epi a suboptimal agent for patients with HF.

As with other adrenergic agonists, epinephrine is primarily administered intravenously, although it can also be administered as an inhaled agent (for treatment of asthma) or subcutaneously (for treatment of anaphylaxis). Epinephrine is rapidly metabolized to metabolites that are excreted by the kidney. At high doses, epinephrine can cause tachycardia and life-threatening ventricular arrhythmias.

The primary clinical application of Epi is in the setting of resuscitation from cardiac arrest, a situation in which rapid restoration of spontaneous circulatory function is the immediate treatment goal. In this clinical setting, the potent inotropic and chronotropic effects of Epi supersede concerns related to its adverse peripheral vasomotor effects. Noncardiovascular indications for Epi include relief of bronchospasm (via β₂-mediated bronchial relaxation), potentiation of the effect of local anesthetics (via local α₁-mediated vasoconstriction), and treatment of allergic hypersensitivity reactions.

Norepinephrine

Norepinephrine (NE) is the endogenous neurotransmitter released at sympathetic nerve terminals. NE is a potent β₁-receptor agonist and, therefore, it supports both systolic and diastolic cardiac performance. NE is also a potent α₁-receptor agonist in the peripheral vessels and, thus, it increases systemic vascular resistance. During exercise, NE release increases heart rate and contractility, enhances diastolic relaxation, and supports redistribution of the cardiac output away from non-critical circulatory beds via its α₁ agonist-mediated vasoconstriction.

Intravenous NE is rapidly metabolized by the liver to inactive metabolites. At therapeutic doses, NE may precipitate tachycardia, arrhythmia, and increased myocardial oxygen consumption. When administered to patients with contractile dysfunction, NE has a tendency to cause tachycardias involving both the SA node and ectopic sites in the atria and ventricles. Furthermore, the peripheral vasoconstriction induced by NE increases afterload, and thereby limits the inotropic benefit of this agent. The increase in afterload occurs most frequently in patients who have already recruited compensatory vasoconstrictive responses (via sympathoadrenal and renin-angiotensin–aldosterone system activation). NE is, however, frequently used for acute hemodynamic support in patients with distributive shock (e.g., gram-negative bacterial sepsis) in the absence of underlying heart disease.

Isoproterenol

Isoproterenol is a synthetic β-adrenergic agonist with relative selectivity for β₁ receptors. The hemodynamic effects of isoproterenol are dominated by a significant chronotropic response. The β₂ effects of isoproterenol can cause peripheral vasodilation and hypotension. Isoproterenol should not be administered to patients with active coronary artery disease, as it can worsen ischemia. Isoproterenol is used infrequently, but it may be indicated in patients with refractory bradycardia not responsive to atropine. It may also be administered in the treatment of β-antagonist overdose.

PHOSPHODIESTERASE (PDE) INHIBITORS

Like the β-adrenergic receptor agonists, the phosphodiesterase (PDE) inhibitors increase cardiac contractility by raising intracellular cAMP levels (Fig. 19-4). PDE inhibitors inhibit the enzyme that hydrolyzes cAMP, thereby increasing intracellular cAMP and indirectly increasing intracellular calcium concentration. There are multiple isoforms of PDE, each of which is linked to a distinct signal transduction pathway. Nonspecific PDE inhibitors, such as **theophylline**, have been studied since the 1960s. Theophylline was first used to treat obstructive airways disease (see Chapter 46), but was later observed to have possible inotropic benefits.

Although cardiac muscle expresses multiple PDE isoenzymes, selective inhibition of PDE3 has been shown to have beneficial cardiovascular effects. The relatively selective PDE3 inhibitors **inamrinone** and **milrinone** increase contractility and enhance the rate and extent of diastolic relaxation. PDE3 inhibitors also have important vasoactive effects in the peripheral circulation. These peripheral actions occur through cAMP-mediated effects on intracellular calcium handling in vascular smooth muscle, and result in decreased arterial and venous tone. In the systemic arterial circulation, vasodilation leads to a decrease in systemic vascular resistance (decreased afterload); in the systemic venous circulation, an increase in venous capacitance results in a decrease in venous return to the heart (decreased preload). The combination of positive inotropy and mixed arterial and venous dilation has led to the designation of PDE inhibitors as "inodilators."

Similar to the β-agonists, PDE inhibitors have found clinical utility in short-term support of the severely failing circulation. Widespread application of inamrinone has been limited by the adverse effect of clinically significant thrombocytopenia in about 10% of patients. The development of oral formulations of milrinone induced tremendous excitement in the cardiovascular community. Unfortunately, clinical trials of milrinone demonstrated a statistically significant *increase* in mortality in heart failure patients; the increase exceeded 50% in patients with the most severe symptoms (NYHA Class IV: symptoms at rest). Although the early data from clinical trials of a third PDE inhibitor, **vesnarinone,** suggested that this drug could have a favorable impact on survival in patients with advanced HF, detailed review of the complete trial data also demonstrated an increase in mortality in the treatment group.

CALCIUM-SENSITIZING AGENTS

Calcium-sensitizing drugs, such as **levosimendan,** are a novel class of positive inotropes that are under investigation as possible therapeutic agents. The calcium sensitizers, which have the same "ino-dilator" actions as the PDE inhibitors, augment myocardial contractility by enhancing the sensitivity of troponin C to calcium. This potentiating effect increases the extent of actin–myosin interactions at any given concentration of intracellular calcium, without a substantial increase in myocardial oxygen consumption. In the peripheral circulation, levosimendan activates ATP-sensitive K^+ channels, leading to peripheral vasodilation. Preliminary clinical trial data suggest that levosimendan improves cardiac hemodynamics in severe systolic HF and may reduce short-term mortality. Levosimendan is available in many countries, but is not currently approved for use in the United States.

■ *Conclusion and Future Directions*

Knowledge of the cellular and molecular bases for myocardial contraction has provided several pharmacologic strategies designed to increase myocardial contractility in patients with heart failure attributable to left ventricular systolic dysfunction. By inhibiting the sodium pump, *digoxin* raises intracellular calcium levels and thereby increases contractile force. This drug is the only oral inotropic agent in wide clinical use today. Although digoxin has no demonstrable impact on the mortality of patients with heart failure, it helps alleviate symptoms and improves functional capacity. Digoxin also slows AV nodal conduction, an effect that is useful in treating patients with atrial fibrillation and rapid ventricular response rates. The *β-adrenergic receptor agonists*—including the endogenous amines *dopamine, norepinephrine,* and *epinephrine* and the synthetic agents *dobutamine* and *isoproterenol*—act through G protein-mediated elevation of intracellular cAMP to enhance both myocardial

contractility and diastolic relaxation. The latter effect allows the left ventricle to fill adequately during diastole, despite the increase in heart rate that is stimulated by these agents. β-Agonists are administered intravenously, and they provide short-term hemodynamic support to patients with cardiogenic circulatory failure. The longer-term utility of these agents has been limited both by the lack of an oral formulation with acceptable bioavailability and by the adverse-effect profile of these drugs. *PDE inhibitors*, including *inamrinone* and *milrinone*, act as positive inotropes and as mixed arterial and venous dilators by increasing the levels of cyclic AMP in the heart and vascular smooth muscle. The increased mortality associated with longer-term use of these agents has similarly restricted their role to the short-term management of severe HF.

New classes of pharmacologic agents for the augmentation of myocardial contractility are under active investigation. These agents are directed at a variety of biochemical targets, including the signaling systems that regulate water resorption (e.g., vasopressin receptor antagonists) and the synthesis of contractile proteins (e.g., **cardiac neuregulins**). Alternative strategies attempt to preserve myocardial contractility by inhibiting the effects of proinflammatory cytokines associated with HF. For example, **endothelin receptor antagonists** such as **tezosentan** attenuate the progression of LV dysfunction and increase survival in animal models of HF. The PDE inhibitor vesnarinone, a positive inotrope that has been associated with increased mortality in clinical trials, is now being examined for its anticytokine potential. Finally, **gene therapy** methods to increase contractility include the delivery of genes with cardiac–specific promoters that alter the production of contractile proteins, channels, and regulators in the heart. At the present time, the most promising candidates for gene therapy include the SR calcium pump, phospholamban, and cardiac troponin I.

■ *Suggested Reading*

Gheorghiade M, Adams KF, Colucci WS. Digoxin in the management of cardiovascular disorders. *Circulation* 2004;109: 2959–2964. *(Reviews the clinical pharmacology of digoxin.)*

Gheorghiade M, Teerlink JR, Mebazaa A. Pharmacology of new agents for acute heart failure syndromes. *Am J Cardiol* 2005; 96:68G–73G. *(Describes properties of many investigational agents for acute heart failure.)*

Lilly LS, ed. *Pathophysiology of heart disease.* 3rd ed. Baltimore: Lippincott Williams & Wilkins; 2002. *[Excellent introduction to cardiovascular medicine: Chapters 1 (Basic Cardiac Structure and Function), 9 (Heart Failure), and 17 (Cardiovascular Drugs) relate to the physiology, pathophysiology, and pharmacology of contractile function.]*

Stevenson, LW. Clinical use of inotropic agents for heart failure: looking backward or forward. Part I: inotropic infusions during hospitalization. *Circulation* 2003;108:367–372. *(Clinical use of inotropic agents for acute decompensated heart failure.)*

Wehrens XH, Lehnart SE, Marks AR. Intracellular calcium release and cardiac disease. *Ann Rev Physiol* 2005;67:69–98. *(Reviews current understanding of the cellular pathophysiology of heart failure.)*

Zipes D, ed. *Braunwald's heart disease: a textbook of cardiovascular medicine.* 7th ed. Philadelphia: WB Saunders; 2004. *(Encyclopedic reference that includes a good survey of pharmacologic agents, trials, and new approaches.)*

Drug Summary Table	Chapter 19 Pharmacology of Cardiac Contractility

CARDIAC GLYCOSIDES

Mechanism—1) In myocardium, inhibit plasma membrane Na^+/K^+-ATPase, leading to increased cytoplasmic Ca^{2+} concentration, which results in positive inotropy; 2) in autonomic nervous system, inhibit sympathetic outflow and increase parasympathetic (vagal) tone; 3) at AV node, prolong effective refractory period and slow conduction velocity
Digoxin immune Fab is an antibody fragment that binds to and inhibits digoxin

Drug	Clinical Applications	Serious and Common Adverse Effects	Contraindications	Therapeutic Considerations
Digoxin Digitoxin	Systolic heart failure Supraventricular arrhythmias including atrial fibrillation, atrial flutter, and paroxysmal atrial tachycardia	*Arrhythmias (especially conduction disturbances with or without AV block, PVCs, and supraventricular tachycardias)* Agitation, fatigue, muscle weakness, blurred vision, yellow-green halo around visual images, anorexia, nausea, vomiting	Ventricular fibrillation. Ventricular tachycardia	Digoxin has numerous significant drug interactions. Coadministration with beta-blockers increases the risk of developing high-grade AV block. Beta-blockers and calcium channel blockers counteract positive inotropic effects of digoxin. Potassium-wasting diuretics and hypokalemia predispose to digoxin toxicity. Some antibiotics, such as erythromycin, increase digoxin absorption. Coadministration with verapamil, quinidine, or amiodarone can increase digoxin levels Treat digoxin toxicity by normalizing plasma potassium level or using digoxin antibodies in severe cases Chronic kidney disease requires reduction in loading dose and maintenance dose of digoxin Digoxin has not been shown to improve survival; it palliates symptoms and improves functional status Digitoxin undergoes hepatic metabolism and biliary excretion
Digoxin Immune Fab	Potentially life-threatening digitalis toxicity Acute digoxin toxicity in which ingested amount or serum digoxin level is unknown	*Heart failure, anaphylaxis*	No known contraindications Use with caution in patients allergic to ovine proteins	Keep resuscitation equipment available during administration of digoxin immune Fab

BETA-ADRENERGIC AGONISTS

Mechanism—Increase cAMP by activating G protein-coupled adrenergic receptors; acting at cardiac β1 adrenergic receptors, agonists have positive inotropic, chronotropic, and lusitropic effects

Drug	Clinical Applications	Serious and Common Adverse Effects	Contraindications	Therapeutic Considerations
Dopamine	In distributive or cardiogenic shock, use as adjunct to increase cardiac output, blood pressure, and urine flow Short-term treatment of severe, refractory, chronic heart failure	*Bradycardia, asthma attacks, widening of QRS complex, cardiac arrhythmias* Hypotension, hypertension, palpitations, tachycardia	Pheochromocytoma Uncorrected tachyarrhythmias Ventricular fibrillation	Low doses cause vasodilation in the periphery by stimulating dopaminergic D1 receptors in renal and mesenteric vascular beds Intermediate doses cause widespread vasodilation via stimulation of D1 receptors, and increased contractility and heart rate via activation of β1 receptors High doses cause generalized vasoconstriction via stimulation of α1 receptors Coadministration with MAO inhibitors results in decreased metabolism of dopamine, which can lead to significant tachycardia and arrhythmia

Drug	Clinical Applications	Adverse Effects	Notes / Contraindications
Dobutamine	Short-term treatment of cardiac decompensation secondary to depressed contractility (cardiogenic shock)	*Same as dopamine, except cardiac arrhythmias occur less frequently*	Idiopathic hypertrophic subaortic stenosis	A racemic mixture of enantiomers that have differential effects on adrenergic receptor subtypes; overall effect is predominantly β1 and modest β2 • Sympathomimetic inotrope of choice for patients with acute cardiogenic circulatory failure • Dobutamine induces less supraventricular tachycardia and high-grade ventricular arrhythmia than dopamine
Epinephrine	Bronchospasm • Hypersensitivity reaction, anaphylactic shock • Cardiac resuscitation • Hemostasis (topical use) • Prolong local anesthetic effect (local use) • Open-angle glaucoma • Nasal congestion	*Arrhythmias including ventricular fibrillation, cerebral hemorrhage, severe hypertension* • Headache, nervousness, tremor, hypertension, palpitations, tachycardia	Active labor • Angle-closure glaucoma • Shock (other than anaphylaxis) • Organic brain damage • Cardiac arrhythmias • Coronary insufficiency • Severe hypertension • Cerebral atherosclerosis	Nonselective agonist at β1, β2, α1, and α2 receptors • High doses can cause tachycardia and life-threatening ventricular arrhythmias
Norepinephrine	Blood pressure support in acute hypotensive states (shock) • Limit GI bleeding via intraperitoneal or nasogastric administration	*Same as epinephrine*	Peripheral vascular thrombosis • Profound hypoxia • Hypercapnia • Hypotension from loss of blood volume	Nonselective agonist at β1, α1, and α2 receptors • May cause tachycardias involving the SA node or ectopic atrial or ventricular sites in patients with contractile dysfunction • Avoid coadministration with MAO inhibitors or amitriptyline or imipramine-type antidepressants due to risk of severe hypertension
Isoproterenol	Emergency treatment of arrhythmias (IV) • Atropine-resistant hemodynamically significant bradycardia (IV) • Heart block and shock (IV) • Bronchospasm (inhalation)	*Same as epinephrine*	Tachycardia caused by digitalis intoxication • Angina pectoris	Nonselective β-agonist at β1 and β2 receptors • Isoproterenol may be useful in treating patients with refractory bradycardia not responsive to atropine, and in treating patients with β-antagonist overdose • Do not administer to patients with active coronary artery disease

PHOSPHODIESTERASE (PDE) INHIBITORS

Mechanism—Increase cAMP by inhibiting the PDE enzymes that hydrolyze it; in cardiac myocytes, PDE inhibitors have positive inotropic and lusitropic effects; PDE inhibitors also relax vascular smooth muscle and thereby decrease preload (venodilation) and afterload (arteriodilation)

Drug	Clinical Applications	Adverse Effects	Contraindications	Notes
Theophylline **Inamrinone** **Milrinone** **Vesnarinone**	See Drug Summary Table: Chapter 46 Integrative Inflammation Pharmacology: Asthma • Short-term treatment of severely failing circulation in patients refractory to conventional therapy	*Ventricular arrhythmias* • *Thrombocytopenia (greater incidence with inamrinone than with milrinone)* • *Reversible neutropenia and agranulocytosis (vesnarinone)*	Do not use these agents in place of surgical intervention in patients with stenotic valvular disease • Acute phase of myocardial infarction	Coadministration with disopyramide may cause severe hypotension • Use of inamrinone is limited by 10% occurrence of thrombocytopenia • Oral formulation of milrinone is available; milrinone use is associated with statistically significant increase in mortality in heart failure patients • Survival benefit of vesnarinone is controversial

CALCIUM-SENSITIZING AGENT

Mechanism—Enhances the sensitivity of troponin C to calcium, which increases the extent of actin–myosin interactions without a substantial increase in myocardial oxygen consumption

Drug	Clinical Applications	Adverse Effects	Contraindications	Notes
Levosimendan	Not approved for use in the US	*Dose-related hypotension and reflex tachycardia* • Nausea, headache	Hypersensitivity to levosimendan or racemic simendan	Preliminary data suggest that levosimendan improves cardiac hemodynamics in severe systolic HF and may reduce short-term mortality

20

Pharmacology of Volume Regulation

Mallar Bhattacharya and Seth L. Alper

INTRODUCTION

Coordinated regulation of volume homeostasis and vascular tone maintains adequate tissue perfusion in response to varying environmental stimuli. This chapter discusses the pharmacologically relevant physiology of volume regulation, with emphasis on the hormonal pathways and renal mechanisms that modulate systemic volume. (Control of vascular tone is discussed in Chapter 21, Pharmacology of Vascular Tone.) Dysregulation of volume homeostasis can result in edema, the pathologic accumulation of fluid in the extravascular space. Pharmacologic modulation of volume is targeted at reducing volume excess; this is an effective treatment for hypertension and heart failure (HF), as well as cirrhosis and the nephrotic syndrome. The two broad classes of pharmacologic agents used to modify volume status are modulators of neurohormonal regulators (e.g., angiotensin converting enzyme [ACE] inhibitors) and diuretics, agents that increase

renal Na$^+$ excretion. Drugs that modify volume regulation also have many other clinically important effects on the body, because these volume regulators act as diverse hormonal modulators in a number of physiologic pathways. Many of the clinical applications of these agents are discussed further in Chapter 24, Integrative Cardiovascular Pharmacology: Hypertension, Ischemic Heart Disease, and Heart Failure.

 Case

70-year old Mr. R is taken by ambulance to the emergency department at 1 AM after waking up with shortness of breath for the fourth night in a row. Each time he "felt tight in the chest" and "couldn't get a breath;" this discomfort was relieved somewhat by sitting up in bed. He also recalls previous episodes of shortness of breath while climbing stairs.

Physical exam reveals tachycardia, mild hypertension, pedal edema (edema of the feet and lower legs), and bilateral pulmonary crackles on inspiration. Serum chemistries show no elevation of troponin T (a marker of cardiomyocte injury) but mildly elevated creatinine and blood urea nitrogen (BUN). The electrocardiogram shows evidence of an old myocardial infarction. Echocardiography reveals diminished left ventricular ejection fraction (the fraction of blood in the ventricle at the end of diastole that is ejected when the ventricle contracts) without ventricular dilatation.

Based on the clinical findings of decreased cardiac output, pulmonary congestion, and peripheral edema, Mr. R is diagnosed with acute heart failure. His increased creatinine and BUN also indicate an element of renal insufficiency. Pharmacologic therapy is started, including a positive inotrope, a coronary vasodilator, an antihypertensive ACE inhibitor, and a loop diuretic. After Mr. R's condition stabilizes over the course of 3 days, the dose of the loop diuretic is decreased and then discontinued. Elective coronary angiography reveals significant stenosis of the left anterior descending coronary artery. Mr. R undergoes balloon angioplasty and stent placement and remains stable as an outpatient. His discharge drug regimen is accompanied by a low-salt, low-fat diet.

QUESTIONS

■ **1.** What mechanisms led to Mr. R's pulmonary congestion and pedal edema?
■ **2.** Why was Mr. R given a loop diuretic?
■ **3.** How do ACE inhibitors improve cardiovascular hemodynamics?
■ **4.** What other kinds of diuretics are available, and why were they not chosen in this acute setting?

PHYSIOLOGY OF VOLUME REGULATION

An intricate set of mechanisms sense, signal, and modulate changes in plasma volume. Volume sensors are located throughout the vascular tree, including in the atria and in the kidneys. Many of the volume regulators activated by these sensors include systemic and autocrine hormones, while others involve neural circuits. The integrated result of these signaling mechanisms is to alter vascular tone and to regulate renal Na^+ reabsorption and excretion. Vascular tone maintains end-organ tissue perfusion; changes in renal Na^+ excretion alter total volume status.

DETERMINANTS OF INTRAVASCULAR VOLUME

Intravascular volume is a small proportion of total body water, but the amount of fluid in the vascular compartment critically determines the extent of tissue perfusion. Approximately 2/3 of total body water is intracellular, while 1/3 is extracellular. Of the extracellular fluid (ECF), approximately 3/4 resides in the interstitial space, while 1/4 of ECF is plasma.

Fluid exchange between plasma and interstitial fluid occurs as a result of changes in capillary permeability, oncotic pressure, and hydrostatic pressure. Capillary permeability is largely determined by the junctions between individual endothelial cells lining a vascular space. The capillary beds of some organs are more permeable than others and, as a result, allow greater intercompartmental fluid shifts. In the context of inflammation and other pathologic conditions (see below), increased capillary permeability allows proteins and other osmotically active agents to shift between intravascular and perivascular compartments. Oncotic pressure is determined by the molecular solute components of a fluid space that are differentially partitioned between adjacent compartments (such constituents are said to be osmotically active). Because albumin, globulins, and other large plasma proteins are normally confined to the plasma space, these proteins act as osmotically active agents to retain water in the vascular space. The hydrostatic pressure gradient across the capillary barrier between compartments is another force for water movement. An elevated intracapillary pressure favors increased transudation of fluid from plasma into the interstitial space.

The relationship between fluid filtration and capillary permeability, oncotic pressure, and hydrostatic pressure is represented by the following equation:

$$\text{Fluid Filtration} = K_f\,(P_c - P_{if}) - (\Pi_c - \Pi_{if}) \quad \text{Equation 20-1}$$

where K_f = capillary permeability, P_c = capillary hydrostatic pressure, P_{if} = interstitial fluid hydrostatic pressure, Π_c = capillary oncotic pressure, and Π_{if} = interstitial fluid oncotic pressure. This equation emphasizes that transcapillary fluid movement is governed by intercompartmental gradients, rather than by the absolute value of each compartmental pressure. Note that *the hydrostatic and oncotic gradient terms have opposing vectors,* and therefore favor fluid movement in opposing directions. ΔP_c normally favors transudation from the capillary lumen to the interstitium, whereas $\Delta \Pi_c$ normally favors fluid retention within the capillary lumen.

The extent of fluid filtration that occurs along the length of the capillary differs for each tissue's capillary bed and is determined by cellular and junctional permeability properties of tissue-specific capillary endothelial cells. In the example shown in Figure 20-1, liver capillaries filter fluid into the interstitium along their entire length. At the arterial end of the capillary bed, $(P_c + \Pi_{if})$ exceeds $(P_{if} + \Pi_c)$, thus favoring plasma filtration from the capillary into the interstitial space. P_c gradually decreases along the length of the capillary, and the rate of fluid filtration into the interstitium decreases. At the venous end of the capillary, hydrostatic fluid filtration and oncotic fluid absorption are almost balanced. Liver sinusoids, which transfer fluid into the interstitial space during perfusion, return this fluid to the circulation via lymphatic flow. In capillary beds of other tissues, the integrated oncotic pressure gradient favoring fluid flow into the capillary balances the integrated hydrostatic pressure gradient, resulting in no net volume change between the vascular and interstitial spaces. Thus, the physiologic steady state of extracellular fluid represents a balance of driving forces between fluids of the intravascular and interstitial compartments. Pathologic alterations in the determinants of transcapillary fluid shifts, coupled with changes in renal

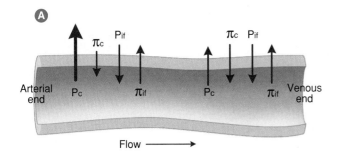

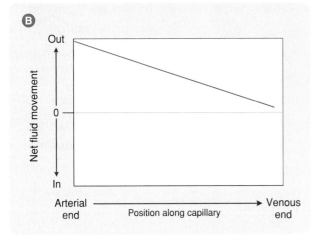

Figure 20-1. Capillary fluid filtration. The balance of hydrostatic pressure and oncotic pressure determines fluid filtration along the capillary. The example shown here is for a hypothetical capillary where fluid filtration exceeds fluid reabsorption. **A.** At the arterial end of the capillary, the capillary hydrostatic pressure (P_c) is large *(long arrow)*, and the sum of P_c and interstitial oncotic pressure (π_{if}) exceeds the sum of interstitial hydrostatic pressure (P_{if}) and capillary oncotic pressure (π_c). Therefore, fluid moves out of the capillary into the interstitial space. As fluid continues to filter along the length of the capillary, the increased fluid filtration results in decreased P_c and increased π_c, thus decreasing the driving force for fluid filtration from the capillary to the interstitium. Throughout the length of the capillary, P_{if} and Π_{if} remain relatively constant. **B.** A graphic representation of net fluid movement along the capillary length shows the decreasing driving force for fluid filtration into the interstitium. In the hypothetical capillary shown here, fluid is filtered into the interstitium along the entire capillary length; lymphatic vessels eventually return the excess interstitial fluid to the systemic circulation *(not shown)*.

Na^+ handling, can result in the formation of edema, as discussed below.

VOLUME SENSORS

Vascular volume sensors can be divided into low-pressure and high-pressure feedback systems. The low-pressure system consists of the atria and pulmonary vasculature. In response to decreased wall stress (e.g., caused by decreased intravascular volume), peripheral nervous system cells lining the atria and pulmonary vasculature transmit a signal to noradrenergic neurons in the medulla of the central nervous system (CNS). This signal is relayed to the hypothalamus, resulting in increased secretion of **antidiuretic hormone (ADH)** from the posterior pituitary gland. Together with

increased peripheral sympathetic tone, ADH maintains distal tissue perfusion. In response to increased wall stress (e.g., caused by increased intravascular volume), cells of the atria produce and secrete natriuretic peptide, promoting vasodilation and **natriuresis** (increased renal Na^+ excretion).

The high-pressure system consists of specialized baroreceptors in the aortic arch, carotid sinus, and juxtaglomerular apparatus. These sensors modulate hypothalamic control of ADH secretion and sympathetic outflow from the brainstem. In addition, sympathetic input stimulates the juxtaglomerular apparatus to secrete **renin**, a proteolytic enzyme that activates the renin-angiotensin–aldosterone system (see below).

VOLUME REGULATORS

Together, the low-pressure and high-pressure feedback systems integrate neurohumoral volume signals to maintain volume homeostasis in the face of volume perturbations. The neurohormonal response to a change in volume status is controlled by at least four main systems: the renin-angiotensin–aldosterone system (RAAS), natriuretic peptides, ADH, and renal sympathetic nerves. The RAAS, ADH, and renal sympathetic nerves are active in situations of intravascular volume depletion, while natriuretic peptides are released in response to intravascular volume overload.

Renin-Angiotensin–Aldosterone System

Renin is an aspartyl protease produced and secreted by the **juxtaglomerular apparatus,** a specialized set of smooth muscle cells that line the afferent and efferent arterioles of the renal glomerulus. The ultimate result of renin secretion is *vasoconstriction and Na^+ retention, actions that maintain tissue perfusion and increase extracellular fluid volume* (Fig. 20-2).

Three mechanisms control juxtaglomerular-cell renin release (Fig. 20-3). First, a direct pressure-sensing mechanism of the afferent arteriole increases juxtaglomerular-cell release of renin in response to decreased tension. The molecular mechanism of this release is unknown, but may involve prostaglandin signaling. Second, sympathetic innervation of juxtaglomerular cells promotes renin release via β_1-adrenoceptor signaling. Third, an autoregulatory mechanism known as **tubuloglomerular feedback** senses distal nephron sodium (or chloride) delivery and modulates renin release. Nephron anatomy is organized such that the distal end of the cortical thick ascending limb (TAL) of each nephron is closely apposed to the juxtaglomerular mesangium of that same nephron. This spatial proximity allows rapid regulation of afferent arteriolar and glomerular mesangial activity by distal nephron electrolyte concentration and/or salt load. **Macula densa** cells of the cortical thick ascending limb respond to increased luminal NaCl delivery by increasing extracellular adenosine in the juxtoglomerular interstitium and thereby activating A_1 receptors on the juxtaglomerular mesangial cells. Conversely, decreased luminal NaCl delivery activates a prostaglandin signaling cascade that culminates in increased juxtaglomerular-cell renin release. The mechanism by which the macula densa cells sense luminal NaCl delivery is thought to involve both luminal NaCl concentration and luminal fluid flow rate.

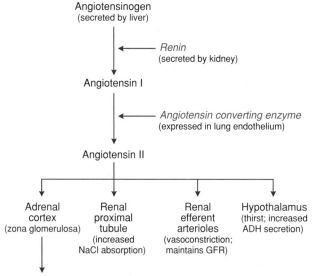

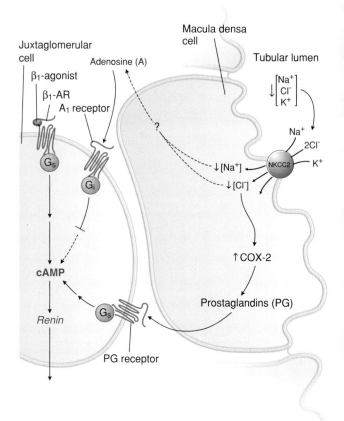

Figure 20-2. The renin–angiotensin–aldosterone axis. Angiotensinogen is a prohormone secreted into the circulation by hepatocytes. Renin, an aspartyl protease secreted by juxtaglomerular cells of the kidney, cleaves angiotensinogen to angiotensin I. Angiotensin converting enzyme (ACE), a protease expressed on pulmonary capillary endothelium (and elsewhere), cleaves angiotensin I to angiotensin II. Angiotensin II has four actions that increase intravascular volume and maintain tissue perfusion. First, angiotensin II stimulates zona glomerulosa cells of the adrenal cortex to secrete aldosterone, a hormone that increases renal NaCl reabsorption at multiple segments along the nephron. Second, angiotensin II directly stimulates renal proximal tubule reabsorption of NaCl. Third, angiotensin II causes efferent arteriolar vasoconstriction, an action that increases intraglomerular pressure and thereby increases GFR. Fourth, angiotensin II stimulates hypothalamic thirst centers and promotes ADH secretion.

Figure 20-3. Modulation of renin release. Renin is released by juxtaglomerular cells in response to diverse stimuli that signal volume depletion. First, decreased pressure in the afferent arteriole *(not shown)* stimulates increased renin release, possibly by releasing prostaglandins. Second, juxtaglomerular cells express β_1-adrenergic receptors (β_1-AR) coupled to G_s, which stimulates adenylyl cyclase to increase the intracellular level of cAMP, which is a stimulus for renin release. Third, cells lining the diluting segments of the nephron modulate renin release based on the extent of luminal NaCl flux. In cases of decreased NaCl flux, decreased Cl^- entry through the $Na^+/2Cl^-/K^+$ transporter (NKCC2) on the apical membrane of macula densa cells in the distal convoluted tubule stimulates cyclooxygenase-2 (COX-2) activity, which increases prostaglandin production. The prostaglandins diffuse to and activate juxtaglomerular-cell prostaglandin (PG) receptors, which stimulate release of renin by increasing cAMP production. In contrast, increased cortical TAL NaCl delivery leads, through still-debated mechanisms, to increased generation of adenosine in the juxtaglomerular mesangial interstitium. Activation of G_i-coupled juxtaglomerular-cell A_1 receptors decreases intracellular cAMP, which leads to decreased renin release.

Plasma renin cleaves the circulating 14-amino-acid hepatic prohormone **angiotensinogen** to the decapeptide **angiotensin I.** In turn, angiotensin I is cleaved to the active octapeptide **angiotensin II** (AT II) by the carboxypeptidase angiotensin converting enzyme (ACE) located on the endothelial cell surface. ACE is highly expressed in the pulmonary vascular endothelium, but is also present on the surface of other endothelial cells, including those lining the coronary arteries. ACE activity regulates the local production of AT II in all vascular beds. Indeed, an incompletely understood ''local'' renin–angiotensin system is also expressed in the vasculature, producing these substances as autocrine factors independently of the kidney and liver. ACE has a broad proteolytic substrate specificity that includes bradykinin and other kinins, venodilatory autacoids released in response to inflammation. For this reason, ACE is also known as **kininase II.** Kininase activity has important pharmacologic consequences, as discussed below.

AT II has at least four physiologic actions: (1) stimulation of aldosterone secretion by zona glomerulosa cells of the adrenal glands; (2) increased reabsorption of NaCl at the proximal tubule and other nephron segments; (3) stimulation of thirst and ADH secretion; and (4) arteriolar vasoconstriction. All four of these actions increase intravascular volume

and therefore help to maintain perfusion pressure: aldosterone secretion increases distal-tubule Na^+ reabsorption; proximal-tubule NaCl reabsorption increases the fraction of filtered Na^+ that is reabsorbed; stimulation of thirst increases the free water absorbed into the vasculature; secretion of ADH increases collecting-duct free water absorption; and arteriolar vasoconstriction maintains blood pressure.

All of these actions of AT II are mediated by its binding to the **AT II receptor subtype 1 (AT_1 receptor),** a G protein-coupled receptor. The actions of AT II are best understood in vascular smooth muscle cells, where AT_1 activates phospholipase C, leading to the release of Ca^{2+} from intracellular stores and activation of protein kinase C. Inhibition of AT_1 can lead to vascular smooth muscle cell relaxation, and hence decrease systemic vascular resistance and blood pressure (see below). A second G protein-coupled AT II receptor, termed AT_2, is expressed more prominently in fetal than in adult tissue. The AT_2 receptor appears to have a vasodilatory role.

Natriuretic Peptides

Natriuretic peptides are hormones released by atria, ventricles, and vascular endothelium in response to volume overload. Three natriuretic peptides have been identified: A-type, B-type, and C-type natriuretic peptides. A-type natriuretic peptide (**ANP**) is released primarily by the atria, while B-type natriuretic peptide (**BNP**) is released mainly by the ventricles. C-type natriuretic peptide (**CNP**) is released by vascular endothelial cells.

Natriuretic peptides are released in response to increased intravascular volume, an effect that may be signaled by increased stretch of natriuretic peptide-secreting cells. Circulating natriuretic peptides bind to one of three receptors, termed **NPR-A**, **NPR-B**, and **NPR-C**. NPR-A and NPR-B are transmembrane proteins with intrinsic **guanylyl cyclase** activity (see Chapter 1, Drug–Receptor Interactions); activation of these receptors increases intracellular cGMP levels. NPR-C lacks an intracellular guanylyl cyclase domain and may serve as a ''decoy'' or ''buffer'' receptor to reduce the level of circulating natriuretic peptide available to bind to the two signaling receptors. Both ANP and BNP bind with high affinity to NPR-A, while only CNP binds to NPR-B. All three natriuretic peptides bind to NPR-C (Fig. 20-4A).

Natriuretic peptides affect the cardiovascular system, the kidney, and the central nervous system. Integration of natriuretic peptide-derived signals serves to decrease volume overload and its sequelae. ANP relaxes vascular smooth muscle by increasing intracellular cGMP, which causes dephosphorylation of myosin light chain and subsequent vasorelaxation (see Chapter 21). ANP also increases capillary endothelial permeability; this effect reduces blood pressure by favoring fluid filtration from the plasma into the interstitium (see Equation 20-1).

In the kidney, natriuretic peptides promote both increased glomerular filtration rate (GFR) and natriuresis. GFR is increased because of constriction of the efferent arteriole and dilation of the afferent arteriole, resulting in higher intraglo-

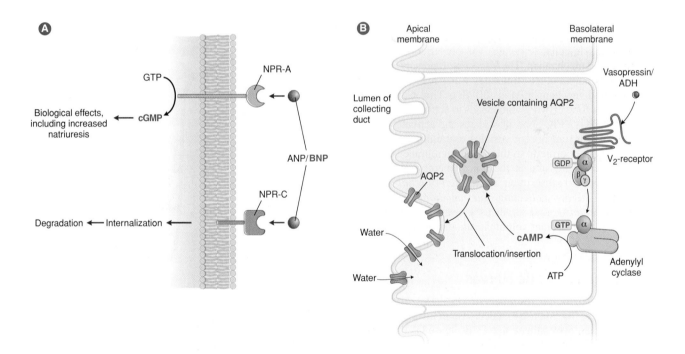

Figure 20-4. Natriuretic peptide and antidiuretic hormone signaling pathways. A. A-type and B-type natriuretic peptides (ANP and BNP) are hormones secreted in response to volume overload. These peptides bind to natriuretic peptide receptor-A (NPR-A) and natriuretic peptide receptor-C (NPR-C). NPR-A is a transmembrane receptor with intrinsic guanylyl cyclase activity. Increased intracellular cGMP levels mediate the effects of natriuretic peptides, including increased natriuresis. NPR-C is believed to be a "decoy receptor," because the protein has no identified intracellular domain. Binding of natriuretic peptide to NPR-C may result in receptor internalization and in degradation of the internalized receptor together with the bound natriuretic peptide. A third natriuretic peptide, CNP, is expressed by vascular endothelial cells and binds to NPR-B *(not shown).* **B.** Antidiuretic hormone (ADH), also known as vasopressin, is secreted by the hypothalamus in response to increased osmolality and volume depletion. ADH mediates renal collecting-duct water reabsorption by activating the G_s-coupled V_2-receptor. Activation of G_s leads to increased adenylyl cyclase activity and increased cAMP levels. cAMP increases collecting-duct water reabsorption by promoting the translocation and insertion of aquaporin water channel (AQP2)-containing vesicles into the collecting duct apical membrane. The increased apical membrane AQP2 results in increased water flux across the collecting duct, and therefore greater reabsorption of filtered water. Hydrolysis of cAMP by phosphodiesterase leads to removal of AQP2 from the luminal membrane by endocytosis of AQP2-containing vesicles *(not shown).*

merular pressure and therefore increased plasma filtration. The natriuretic effects on the kidney result from antagonism of ADH action in the collecting ducts and antagonism of Na$^+$ reabsorption in multiple segments of the distal nephron.

The central effects of natriuretic peptides are less well understood, but they include decreased perception of thirst (and therefore decreased fluid intake), decreased release of antidiuretic hormone, and decreased sympathetic tone. The signaling mechanisms mediating these actions are uncertain, but may be via CNP, as this natriuretic peptide is expressed at high levels in the brain.

Although many of the effects of natriuretic peptides are still not understood completely, these hormones appear to play an important role in regulating the pathophysiology of volume excess. Much interest has recently focused on the relationship between natriuretic peptides and heart failure, and the physiology and pharmacology of natriuretic peptides and their receptors continue to be refined.

Antidiuretic Hormone

Antidiuretic hormone (**ADH,** also referred to as **vasopressin**) is a nonapeptide hormone secreted by the posterior pituitary gland in response to increased plasma osmolality or severe hypovolemia. ADH constricts the peripheral vasculature and promotes water reabsorption in the renal collecting duct. Its actions are mediated by two distinct G protein-coupled receptors. The V$_1$ receptor, present in vascular smooth muscle cells, stimulates vasoconstriction through a G_q-mediated mechanism. The V$_2$ receptor, present in collecting-duct principal cells, stimulates water reabsorption by a G_s-mediated mechanism (Fig. 20-4B). This G_s signal increases cytosolic cAMP, which leads to activation of protein kinase A (PKA). PKA phosphorylates and activates proteins responsible for transport of vesicles containing aquaporin 2, a water channel protein, to the apical membrane. Increased aquaporin 2 expression at the apical membrane promotes increased water reabsorption. *Regulation of renal water reabsorption in the collecting duct modulates urine and plasma osmolality,* and serves as a reserve mechanism for increasing intravascular volume in situations of severe dehydration.

Renal Sympathetic Nerves

Renal sympathetic nerves innervate both afferent and efferent arterioles. In response to a decrease in intravascular volume, the renal sympathetic nerves decrease GFR by stimulating constriction of the afferent arteriole to a greater degree than the efferent arteriole. The decreased GFR resulting from preferential constriction of the afferent arteriole ultimately leads to decreased natriuresis. Renal sympathetic nerves also increase renin production by stimulation of β$_1$-adrenergic receptors on juxtaglomerular mesangial cells, and increase proximal-tubule NaCl reabsorption.

RENAL CONTROL OF NA$^+$ EXCRETION

Over the course of 24 hours, the kidneys filter approximately 180 L of fluid. To increase or decrease body fluid volume, the kidneys must increase or decrease renal Na$^+$ reabsorp-

tion from the large daily volume of glomerular filtrate. For this reason, the neurohormonal mechanisms controlling extracellular volume status have important actions on the kidney. An understanding of the renal control of Na$^+$ excretion is crucial to understanding the role of the kidney in regulation of body fluid volume.

The renal glomerulus produces an ultrafiltrate of plasma that flows through and is processed by the nephron, the functional unit of the kidney (Fig. 20-5). The postglomerular nephron is responsible for solute and water reabsorption from the filtrate, as well as for excretion of metabolic waste products and xenobiotics, including drugs. The renal tubular

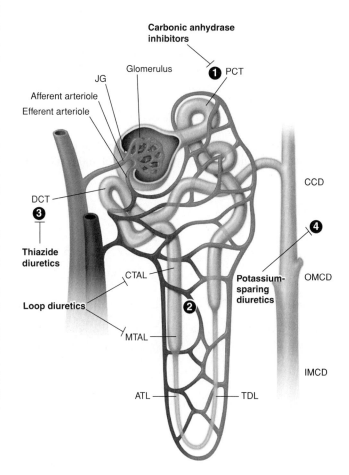

Figure 20-5. Nephron anatomy and sites of action of diuretics. Nephron fluid filtration begins at the glomerulus, where an ultrafiltrate of the plasma enters the renal epithelial (urinary) space. This ultrafiltrate then flows through four sequential segments of the nephron *(1–4)*. From the glomerulus, ultrafiltrate travels to the proximal convoluted tubule *(PCT)* (1), then to the loop of Henle (2), which includes the thin descending limb *(TDL)*, ascending thin limb *(ATL)*, medullary thick ascending limb *(MTAL)* and cortical thick ascending limb *(CTAL)* of Henle. The distal convoluted tubule *(DCT)* (3) includes the macula densa and juxtaglomerular *(JG)* apparatus. The collecting duct (4) consists of the cortical collecting duct *(CCD)*, outer medullary collecting duct *(OMCD)*, and inner medullary collecting duct *(IMCD)*. Pharmacologic agents inhibit specific solute transporters within each segment of the nephron. Carbonic anhydrase inhibitors act at the proximal convoluted tubule; loop diuretics act at the medullary and cortical thick ascending limbs; thiazide diuretics inhibit solute transport in the distal convoluted tubule; and potassium-sparing diuretics inhibit collecting-duct Na$^+$ reabsorption.

epithelial cells of the postglomerular nephron encircle a lengthy tubular lumen, the "urinary space," which leads to the ureters, urinary bladder, and urethra. The concentrations of filtered solutes in the glomerular ultrafiltrate are initially identical to those in the plasma. As the ultrafiltrate passes through the nephron, substrate-specific channels and transporters in the luminal (or apical) membrane of polarized renal tubular epithelial cells sequentially alter the filtrate solute concentrations. The function of these channels, in turn, is influenced by changes in solute concentrations in the cells themselves, as regulated in part by channels and transporters on the contraluminal (or basolateral) side of the cells. Systemic volume regulation by the kidney is accomplished by the integrated action of apical and basolateral ion channels and ion transporters, and by the accompanying reabsorption of water.

The nephron beyond the glomerulus exhibits remarkable heterogeneity along its length. Four segments of the nephron are especially relevant to the pharmacology of body volume regulation (Fig. 20-5). These are the **proximal tubule**, the **TAL** of the loop of Henle, the **distal convoluted tubule** (DCT), and the **cortical collecting duct** (CCD). In each tubular segment, a complex but tightly choreographed interplay of segment-specific ion transporters and/or channels collaborate in the reabsorption of NaCl from the lumen across the cellular monolayer of tubular epithelium into the interstitial space. NaCl reabsorption is key for systemic water retention. Solute and water transport across each segment requires coordination of transporter function in the luminal and basolateral membranes. In addition, paracellular transport of ions across the tight junctions between cells requires regulation of cell-to-cell communication. Integration of the transcellular and paracellular components of transepithelial transport requires integration of signals transmitted by sensors of extracellular and intracellular ion concentrations and of intracellular, local extracellular, and systemic volume. Alteration of ion transport by drugs in any nephron segment can induce compensatory regulation in more distal nephron segments.

Proximal Tubule

The proximal tubule (PT) is the first reabsorptive site in the nephron. It is responsible for approximately two-thirds of sodium reabsorption, 85% to 90% of bicarbonate reabsorption, and ~60% of chloride reabsorption (Fig. 20-6). Specific sodium-coupled symporters in the proximal tubule apical membrane drive renal reabsorption of glucose, amino acids, phosphate, and sulfate. The proximal tubule also mediates secretion and reabsorption of weak organic acids and bases coupled to sodium or proton symport or antiport, or to anion exchange mechanisms. Among these weak acids and bases are many of the drugs used to regulate systemic volume (see below).

Bicarbonate reabsorption requires the coordinated action of apical and basolateral ion transporters together with apical and intracellular enzymatic activities (Fig. 20-6). At the luminal surface of the proximal tubule, filtered bicarbonate encounters active proton secretion across the proximal tubule brush-border microvilli. Two-thirds of the proton efflux is in exchange for influx of Na^+ via the **NHE3 Na^+/H^+ exchanger.** The remaining third of proton efflux is mediated by the vacuolar **H^+-ATPase (vH$^+$ ATPase).**

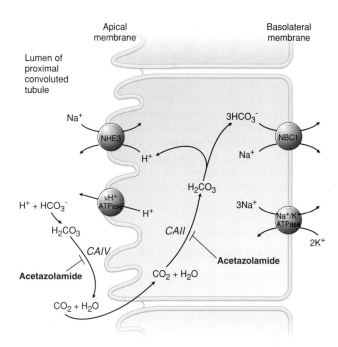

Figure 20-6. Proximal convoluted tubule cell. A significant percentage of proximal convoluted tubule Na^+ is reabsorbed via the NHE3 Na^+/H^+ antiporter. The action of this antiporter, together with that of an apical membrane vacuolar ATPase (vH$^+$ ATPase), results in significant H^+ extrusion into the proximal convoluted tubule urinary space. H^+ extrusion is coupled to HCO_3^- reabsorption by the action of an apical membrane carbonic anhydrase IV (CAIV) that catalyzes the cleavage of HCO_3^- into OH^- and CO_2. OH^- combines with H^+ to form water, while CO_2 diffuses into the cytoplasm of the epithelial cell. The cytoplasmic enzyme carbonic anhydrase II (CAII) catalyzes the formation of HCO_3^- from CO_2 and OH^-; the HCO_3^- is then transported into the interstitium together with Na^+. The net result of this process is reabsorption of HCO_3^- and Na^+ by the basolateral cotransporter NBC1. Acetazolamide inhibits both isoforms of carbonic anhydrase; the decreased carbonic anhydrase activity results in decreased Na^+ and HCO_3^- absorption.

The HCO_3^- permeability of the luminal membrane of the proximal tubular cell is low. However, the outer leaflet of the luminal membrane harbors the glycosylphosphatidylinositol-linked exo-enzyme **carbonic anhydrase IV (CAIV).** CAIV converts luminal HCO_3^- to CO_2 and OH^-. The OH^- is rapidly hydrated to water by the abundance of local protons, and the CO_2 freely diffuses into the cytoplasm of the proximal tubular epithelial cell. The intracellular CO_2 is rapidly rehydrated to HCO_3^- by cytoplasmic **carbonic anhydrase II (CAII)**; this reaction consumes the intracellular OH^- accumulated as a result of the H^+-extruding activities of apical NHE3 and vH$^+$ ATPase. The HCO_3^- produced by the CAII reaction is then cotransported with Na^+ across the basolateral membrane of the epithelial cell, accounting for the net reabsorption of sodium and bicarbonate. The Na^+/HCO_3^- cotransporter **NBC1** mediates electrogenic basolateral efflux of 3 HCO_3^- ions with each cotransported Na^+ ion. Basolateral K^+ channels maintain an inside-negative membrane potential to enhance the driving force for net efflux of two negative charges per NBC1 transport cycle. Emerging evidence also suggests the presence of several distinct forms of carbonic anhydrase at the extracellular surface of the basolateral membrane that help dissipate local accumulation of bicarbonate within the small interstitial space between the epithelial cells and peritubular capillaries.

Solute absorption in the proximal tubule is iso-osmotic—water accompanies reabsorbed ions to maintain osmotic balance. In the past, water flow was assumed to be largely paracellular. However, data from mice genetically modified to lack the **aquaporin** water channel AQP1 (and from rare cases of humans lacking AQP1) demonstrate that most proximal tubular water reabsorption is transcellular. The important role of aquaporins in transepithelial water permeability seems to hold true for all water-permeable nephron segments.

Thick Ascending Limb of the Loop of Henle

The tubular fluid emerging from the thin ascending limb is hypertonic and has an elevated NaCl concentration. The TAL reabsorbs NaCl without accompanying water, diluting the tubular fluid (Fig. 20-7). Together with urea reabsorption, NaCl reabsorption also provides the interstitial solute required for the countercurrent concentrating mechanism that generates and maintains the corticomedullary osmotic gradient of the kidney. The TAL reabsorbs between 25% and 35% of the filtered Na^+ load by means of the luminal

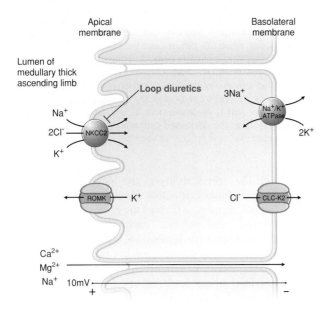

Figure 20-7. Medullary thick ascending limb cell. The medullary thick ascending limb of the loop of Henle absorbs Na^+ through an apical membrane $Na^+/K^+/2Cl^-$ (NKCC2) transporter. The Na^+/K^+-ATPase pumps sodium from the cytoplasm into the interstitium, and a basolateral Cl^- channel (CLC-K2) transports Cl^- into the interstitium. K^+ is primarily recycled into the urinary space via a luminal K^+ channel (ROMK). The combined activities of apical ROMK and basolateral CLC-K2 result in a lumen-positive transepithelial potential difference (approximately 10 mV) that drives paracellular absorption of cations, including Ca^{2+} and Mg^{2+}. Loop diuretics inhibit NKCC2, resulting in significantly increased renal sodium excretion. Disruption of the positive transepithelial potential by loop diuretics also increases the excretion of Ca^{2+} and Mg^{2+}.

membrane Na^+-K^+-$2Cl^-$ cotransporter, **NKCC2.** The Cl^- imported by NKCC2 exits the basolateral side of the cell via **ClC-K2** chloride channels. The Na^+ imported from the lumen via NKCC2 leaves the basolateral side of the cell via the Na^+/K^+-ATPase. Because Cl^- carries a negative charge, exit of Cl^- through ClC-K2 depolarizes the cell. The stoichiometry of the Na^+/K^+ ATPase, $3Na^+$ out per $2 K^+$ in, partly counters this depolarization; additional repolarization of the cell is accomplished by the apical K^+ channel **ROMK,** which recycles back into the lumen the K^+ imported into the cell via NKCC2. The coordinated operation of these apical and basolateral transporters and channels generates a lumen-positive electrical potential across the TAL. This transepithelial potential difference drives the paracellular reabsorption of additional Na^+ from lumen to interstitium. The paracellular component of Na^+ reabsorption, ~50% of the Na^+ reabsorbed by the TAL, effectively reduces by 50% the energetic cost to the TAL (measured as ATP consumption), because Na^+/K^+ transport consumes most of the TAL cell's ATP. Even with the energy conserved by the paracellular Na^+ absorptive pathway, the TAL, working at maximal capacity, can consume up to 25% of the body's total ATP production, ~65 moles per day at rest. The lumen-positive transepithelial potential of the TAL also drives paracellular reabsorption of luminal calcium and magnesium ions.

Distal Convoluted Tubule

This continuation of the diluting segment actively reabsorbs between 2% and 10% of the filtered NaCl load, while remaining impermeable to luminal water (Fig. 20-8). Luminal Na^+ enters the epithelial cells of the distal convoluted tubule via the electroneutral, K^+-independent **NCC1** Na^+-Cl^- cotransporter. Basolateral exit of Na^+ is mediated by Na^+/K^+-ATPase, while the imported Cl^- exits by basolateral anion pathways that include both electrogenic Cl^- channels and (at least in the mouse) electroneutral K^+-Cl^- cotransport. The distal convoluted tubule (DCT) also mediates transepithelial reabsorption of luminal calcium and magnesium ions via ion-specific, regulated TRPV5 calcium channels and TRPM6 magnesium channels in the apical membrane. The reabsorbed calcium crosses the DCT cell basolateral membrane via specific NCX Na^+/Ca^{2+} exchangers and Ca^{2+}-ATPases. The magnesium is believed to follow mechanistically similar pathways selective for Mg^{2+}.

Collecting Duct

This terminal portion of the nephron is divided into **cortical, outer medullary,** and **inner medullary** collecting duct segments (Fig. 20-9). The more proximal portions of the collecting duct (CD) consist of two cell types, **principal cells** and **intercalated cells.** Principal cells reabsorb between 1% and 5% of the filtered sodium load, depending on plasma aldosterone levels (aldosterone increases sodium reabsorption and water retention, see below). Luminal Na^+ enters the principal cells of the cortical collecting duct via heterotrimeric epithelial Na^+ channels, **ENaC,** in the apical membrane. Intracellular Na^+ exits the basolateral side of the cell via the Na^+/K^+-ATPase. Principal cells also secrete K^+ into the lumen to maintain tight control of plasma $[K^+]$, as well

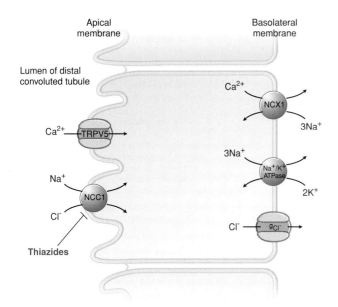

Figure 20-8. Distal convoluted tubule cell. Distal convoluted tubule cells absorb Na$^+$ via an apical membrane NaCl cotransporter (NCC1). Na$^+$ is then transported across the basolateral membrane into the interstitium via the Na$^+$/K$^+$-ATPase, and Cl$^-$ is transported from the cytosol into the interstitium via Cl$^-$ channels (g$_{Cl}^-$) and perhaps by K$^+$-Cl$^-$ cotransport *(not shown)*. Renal epithelial cells of the distal convoluted tubule also absorb Ca^{2+} via apical membrane Ca^{2+} channels (TRPV5), and Ca^{2+} is transported across the basolateral membrane into the interstitium by the Na$^+$/Ca^{2+} exchanger NCX1 and by the Ca^{2+} channel PMCA *(not shown)*. Thiazides inhibit NCC1, resulting in increased Na$^+$ excretion. Thiazides also increase epithelial cell absorption of Ca^{2+} by an unknown mechanism *(not shown)*.

as to minimize the transepithelial potential difference resulting from Na$^+$ reabsorption. In addition, cortical and outer medullary principal cells, as well as cells of the inner medullary collecting duct, express vasopressin (ADH)-responsive water channels. ADH activates water reabsorption by stimulating a G$_s$ protein-coupled V$_2$ receptor in the basolateral membrane; in turn, G$_s$ protein signaling promotes the reversible insertion of intracellular vesicles containing aquaporin 2 (AQP2) water channels into the apical membrane (Fig. 20-4B). At least two subtypes of intercalated cells contribute to systemic acid-base balance by secreting either bicarbonate or protons. Intercalated cells may also regulate Cl$^-$ absorption via anion exchangers, K$^+$ absorption by electroneutral luminal H$^+$/K$^+$-ATPases, and NH$_4^+$ secretion by proteins related to the erythroid Rhesus (Rh) antigens.

PATHOPHYSIOLOGY OF EDEMA FORMATION

Edema is defined as the *accumulation of fluid in the interstitial space*. Edema can be either exudative (having a high protein content) or transudative (having a low protein content, essentially a plasma ultrafiltrate). Exudative edema occurs as part of the acute inflammatory response (see Chapter

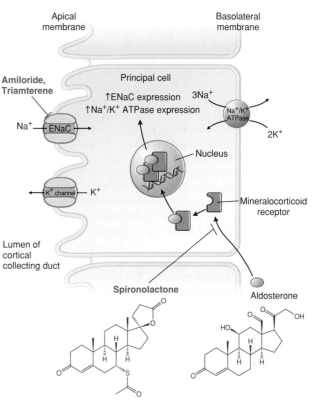

Figure 20-9. Cortical collecting duct principal cell. Cortical collecting duct principal cells absorb Na$^+$ via an apical membrane Na$^+$ channel (ENaC). Cytoplasmic Na$^+$ is then transported across the basolateral membrane via the Na$^+$/K$^+$-ATPase. In addition, collecting duct cells express apical membrane K$^+$ channels that allow K$^+$ to exit into the urinary space. ENaC expression and apical surface localization is modulated by aldosterone. Aldosterone binds to the mineralocorticoid receptor, which then increases transcription of the gene encoding ENaC as well as genes encoding other proteins involved in Na$^+$ reabsorption (such as Na$^+$/K$^+$-ATPase). The collecting duct principal cell is the site of action of the two classes of potassium-sparing diuretics. Mineralocorticoid receptor antagonists such as spironolactone competitively inhibit the interaction of aldosterone with the mineralocorticoid receptor, and thereby decrease expression of ENaC. Direct inhibitors of ENaC, such as amiloride and triamterene, inhibit Na$^+$ influx through the ENaC channel.

40, Principles of Inflammation and the Immune System). The type of edema considered here is **transudative edema,** which can result from pathologic renal retention of Na$^+$.

Under physiologic conditions, any increased fluid filtration across the capillary membrane is quickly counterbalanced by homeostatic mechanisms. This return to a physiologic set-point is mediated by three factors: osmotic forces, lymphatic drainage, and long-term modulation of volume by physiologic sensors and signals. Osmotic forces play an immediate role in fluid shifts between compartments. For example, increased fluid shift to the interstitial space will result in increased interstitial hydrostatic pressure and increased plasma oncotic pressure. Both of these variables favor fluid shift back into the intravascular space (Fig. 20-1). The lymphatic system can also increase return of filtered fluid dramatically, thereby decreasing the amount of filtered fluid that remains in the interstitial space. Over a period of days to weeks, volume sensors and signals respond to changes in volume by altering the extent of natriuresis or sodium reabsorption necessary to maintain a constant intravascular volume. These combined systems closely monitor and regulate intravascular volume. Therefore, *the pathophysiology of transudative edema formation almost always requires an element of pathologic renal Na$^+$ retention.*

The three most common clinical situations resulting in edema formation are HF, cirrhosis, and nephrotic syndrome. All of these diseases manifest deranged Na$^+$ reabsorption caused by pathologic alterations in volume regulation. Understanding the pathophysiology of edema formation in these diseases provides a rationale for the therapeutic use of natriuretic agents.

HEART FAILURE

Heart failure is defined by the inability of the heart to perfuse tissues and organs adequately. The inadequate cardiac output leads to a decreased forward flow of blood, with consequent congestion in the venous "capacitance" vessels. The "congestive" aspect of heart failure describes the edema formation, especially pulmonary edema, that occurs in situations where the increased venous pressure creates a dramatically increased capillary hydrostatic pressure favoring fluid transudation into the interstitial space. In the introductory case, Mr. R's compromised cardiac function led to pulmonary venous congestion and peripheral edema; the pulmonary congestion was responsible for his sensation of dyspnea. The pathophysiology of heart failure is discussed in further detail in Chapter 24; the current discussion is restricted to the pathophysiology of edema formation.

The fundamental cause of Na$^+$ retention in HF is *perceived volume depletion* (Fig. 20-10). The inadequate arterial blood flow is perceived by high-pressure volume receptors, including the juxtaglomerular apparatus, as a decrease in intravascular volume. The kidney therefore increases renin production, leading to increased angiotensin II (AT II) production and secretion of aldosterone by the adrenal cortex. AT II and aldosterone both increase renal Na$^+$ absorption. Other important mediators of increased renal Na$^+$ reabsorption may include endothelin, prostaglandins, and renal sympathetic nerves; these pathways act to maintain renal perfusion pressure and glomerular filtration fraction in the presence of perceived volume depletion.

Under physiologic conditions, low-pressure systems such as neural responses and natriuretic peptides sense the increased pressure resulting from venous congestion and therefore promote natriuresis. This response limits the extent of renal Na$^+$ reabsorption and prevents pathologic extracellular fluid volume expansion. However, both neural and natriuretic peptide signaling pathways are disrupted in HF. HF activates excessive sympathetic responses, in part to increase norepinephrine-induced ventricular inotropy and thereby to augment ejection fraction and maintain cardiac output. Plasma natriuretic peptide is significantly increased in HF, but co-existing end-organ resistance may blunt the natriuretic response to the increased concentration of circulating hormone.

Diuretics and ACE inhibitors have found significant application in the interruption of HF pathophysiology. As discussed below, diuretics decrease renal Na$^+$ reabsorption and

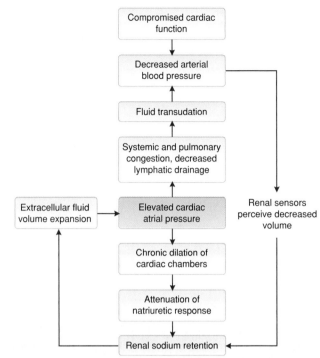

Figure 20-10. Mechanisms of Na$^+$ retention in HF. In HF, compromised cardiac function leads to decreased arterial blood pressure and subsequent activation of renal volume sensors. These sensors activate renal sodium retention to expand extracellular volume and thereby correct the decreased arterial blood pressure. The expansion of extracellular volume increases cardiac atrial pressure. In the failing heart, the increased atrial pressure leads to increased hydrostatic pressure in the pulmonary and systemic circuits, leading to fluid transudation and edema. In addition, evidence suggests that chronic dilation of the cardiac chambers leads to local resistance to stimulation by natriuretic peptide; in the absence of an appropriate natriuretic response, the kidney continues reabsorbing Na$^+$ despite the increased extracellular volume.

thereby reduce the extracellular volume expansion that provides a stimulus for edema formation. As demonstrated in the introductory case, diuretics can be used in an acute setting to reduce the extent of pulmonary edema. Over the long term, decreased Na$^+$ retention also affects afterload by reducing intravascular volume and hence systemic blood pressure and ventricular systolic pressure. ACE inhibitors may interrupt pathologic paracrine signaling pathways that otherwise lead to deterioration of cardiac tissue and worsening of HF (see below).

CIRRHOSIS

Cirrhosis is caused by hepatic parenchymal fibrosis resulting from chronic inflammation or hepatotoxic insult. The fibrotic changes alter hepatic hemodynamics by obstructing venous outflow from the liver and increasing hydrostatic pressure in the portal vein. The obstruction to flow causes portosystemic shunting of blood away from the liver and into the systemic circulation. Hepatocellular injury disrupts the synthetic and metabolic functions of the liver, leading to decreased production of albumin and other important con-

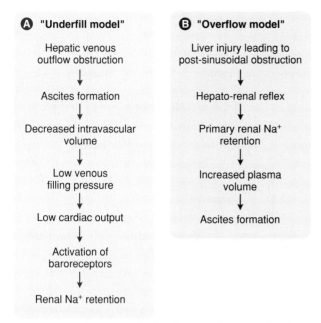

Figure 20-11. Proposed mechanisms of Na⁺ retention in cirrhosis. The post-sinusoidal obstruction in cirrhosis is associated with renal Na⁺ retention as well as the accumulation of ascites fluid. Two models have been proposed to explain the mechanisms of these effects. **A.** Hepatic venous outflow obstruction causes increased hydrostatic pressure, which initiates ascites formation. The accumulation of ascites fluid decreases intravascular volume, leading to low venous filling pressure, decreased cardiac output, and subsequent activation of arterial baroreceptors that initiate renal Na⁺ retention. **B.** Post-sinusoidal obstruction activates the hepato-renal reflex, an autonomic response involving the liver and kidney that initiates renal Na⁺ reabsorption by a poorly understood mechanism. The renal Na⁺ retention leads to an expansion of plasma volume, increased hydrostatic pressure in the portal circuit, and the formation of ascites.

tributors to plasma oncotic pressure, as well as decreased production of coagulation factors and peptide hormones.

The mechanism of renal Na⁺ retention in cirrhosis is unknown, but two models have been proposed (Fig. 20-11). The **underfill model** (Fig. 20-11A) proposes that obstruction of hepatic venous outflow leads to an increase in intrahepatic hydrostatic pressure. The increased hydrostatic pressure causes increased fluid transudation across the hepatic sinusoids, and therefore increased lymphatic flow through the thoracic duct. Under physiologic conditions, the lymphatic system is able to increase its flow dramatically and thereby limit the extent of interstitial fluid accumulation. In cirrhosis, however, lymphatic flow can exceed 20 L/day, overwhelming the ability of the lymphatic system to return transudate to the systemic circulation and leading to the formation of **ascites** (an accumulation of serous fluid in the abdominal cavity). Ascites formation decreases intravascular volume, because fluid is shunted from the plasma into the abdominal cavity. The decreased intravascular volume leads to a decrease in cardiac output, with subsequent activation of baroreceptors that increase renal Na⁺ retention. Thus, the underfill model is conceptually similar to the mechanism of edema formation in HF, in that the kidney initiates Na⁺ reabsorption in response to a *perceived* decrease in intravascular volume.

The **overflow model** postulates that ascites formation involves an element of *primary* renal Na⁺ retention (Fig. 20-11B). In this model, post-sinusoidal obstruction activates the **hepato–renal reflex,** an incompletely characterized autonomic response that results in increased renal Na⁺ retention. Pathologic retention of Na⁺ leads to intravascular volume expansion, increased portal hydrostatic pressure, and formation of ascites. Although not well understood, this mechanism is consistent with a number of experimental model systems demonstrating that renal Na⁺ retention in cirrhosis occurs before the development of ascites.

The formation of ascites may well involve elements of both the underfill and overflow models. Both models begin with the observation that cirrhosis leads to significant hepatic outflow obstruction, and both must consider compromised portal hemodynamics, decreased hepatic synthetic and secretory functions leading to decreased plasma oncotic pressure, and poorly characterized neural or hormonal interactions between the liver and the kidney. Elucidation of the mechanism of the hepato-renal reflex may lead in the future to more effective pharmacologic interventions to manage the development of ascites in cirrhosis.

NEPHROTIC SYNDROME

Nephrotic syndrome is characterized by massive proteinuria (>3.5 g/day), edema, hypoalbuminemia, and often hypercholesterolemia. The primary cause of nephrotic syndrome is *glomerular dysfunction*, which may be due to immune complex disease, diabetes, lupus, amyloidosis, or other conditions affecting glomerular function.

A classical explanation of edema formation in nephrotic syndrome follows this sequence. First, massive proteinuria leads to decreased plasma oncotic pressure, reducing the forces favoring fluid retention in the capillary and leading to fluid transudation into the interstitium. The increased net fluid transudation decreases intravascular volume, activating volume sensors to enhance renal Na⁺ retention. The resulting expansion in fluid volume, in the absence of adequate compensatory albumin synthesis, maintains low plasma oncotic pressure and continued edema formation. In this view, renal Na⁺ retention is secondary to decreased renal arterial perfusion. However, the edema of nephrotic syndrome may also be caused by an element of primary renal Na⁺ retention. The postulated primary Na⁺ retention of nephrotic syndrome may be localized to the distal nephron, arising from resistance to natriuretic peptides or from increased sympathetic nervous system activity.

Although treatment of nephrotic syndrome can include diuretics to counter renal Na⁺ retention, correction of edema typically requires correction of the underlying glomerular disorder, eventually leading to decreased proteinuria and correction of the edema. Diuretics are used in the short term to minimize edema formation.

PHARMACOLOGIC CLASSES AND AGENTS

Pharmacologic modulators of extracellular fluid volume can be divided into agents that modify neurohormonal volume regulators and agents that act directly on the nephron segments to alter renal Na$^+$ handling. The former category includes agents that interrupt the renin–angiotensin axis, alter circulating levels of natriuretic peptides, or interrupt ADH signaling. The latter category includes the various classes of diuretics, which directly target renal ion transporter or channel function or expression to increase renal Na$^+$ excretion, and thereby decrease extracellular fluid volume. Neurohormonal volume regulators may also act directly on Na$^+$ reabsorption through mechanisms less well understood than those of the diuretics.

AGENTS THAT MODIFY VOLUME REGULATORS

Inhibitors of the Renin–Angiotensin System

There are three pharmacologic strategies for interruption of the renin-angiotensin–aldosterone system. First, ACE inhibitors interrupt the conversion of angiotensin I to angiotensin II. Second, angiotensin receptor antagonists are competitive antagonists of the AT$_1$ receptor, and thus inhibit the target-organ effects of angiotensin II. Third, antagonists of the mineralocorticoid receptor block aldosterone action at the nephron collecting duct. The first two classes of agents are discussed here; because antagonists of aldosterone action are considered diuretics, these agents are addressed below (see ''Potassium-Sparing Diuretics'').

Angiotensin Converting Enzyme Inhibitors

Most commonly, pharmacologic interruption of the renin–angiotensin axis is achieved via inhibition of angiotensin converting enzyme (ACE). Because angiotensin II (AT II) is the primary mediator of the activity of the renin-angiotensin–aldosterone system, decreased conversion of AT I to AT II inhibits arteriolar vasoconstriction, decreases aldosterone synthesis, inhibits renal proximal tubule NaCl reabsorption, and decreases ADH release. All of these actions result in decreased blood pressure and increased natriuresis. In addition, because ACE proteolytically cleaves bradykinin (among other substrates), ACE inhibitors also increase bradykinin levels. Bradykinin causes vascular smooth muscle relaxation by binding to bradykinin receptors on endothelial cell surfaces, leading to Ca^{2+} mobilization, eNOS activation, and increased NO production (see Chapter 21). Thus, ACE inhibitors decrease blood pressure both by decreasing AT II levels and by increasing bradykinin levels (Fig. 20-12).

The contribution of reduced plasma aldosterone levels to the antihypertensive effects of ACE inhibitors remains unclear. This uncertainty is related to the observation that the renal vasoconstrictive effects of angiotensin II occur primarily at the efferent arteriole of the glomerulus. A preferential decrease in efferent relative to afferent arteriolar tone reduces intraglomerular pressure, resulting in decreased GFR. This reduction in GFR may counterbalance the anticipated reduction in Na$^+$/H$_2$O retention that should occur as a result of the reduced aldosterone levels.

ACE inhibitors exhibit three patterns of metabolism. The prototypical ACE inhibitor, **captopril**, represents the first

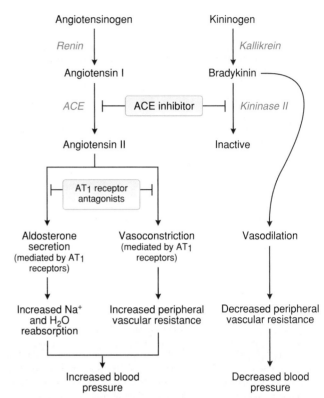

Figure 20-12. Effects of renin–angiotensin system inhibitors on blood pressure. ACE inhibitors prevent the conversion of angiotensin I to angiotensin II (both in the lung and locally in blood vessels and tissues) and inhibit the inactivation of bradykinin. Both actions of ACE inhibitors lead to vasodilation. The inhibition of angiotensin I conversion decreases AT$_1$-mediated vasoconstriction and decreases aldosterone secretion; both of these effects act to decrease blood pressure. The inhibition of kininase II activity results in higher bradykinin levels, which promote vasodilation. The increased vasodilation decreases peripheral vascular resistance, which decreases blood pressure. In contrast, AT$_1$ antagonists (also known as *angiotensin receptor blockers,* or *ARBs*) decrease aldosterone synthesis and interrupt AT$_1$-mediated vasoconstriction, but do not alter bradykinin levels. Note that bradykinin-induced cough is a major side effect of ACE inhibitors, but not of AT$_1$ antagonists.

pattern: it is active as administered, but is also processed to an active metabolite. The second and most common pattern, exemplified by **enalapril** and **ramipril,** is that of an ester prodrug converted in the plasma to an active metabolite. The active forms of each of these drugs are denoted by the letters ''-at'' added to the drug name; thus, enalaprilat and ramiprilat are the active forms of enalapril and ramipril, respectively. **Lisinopril** is the sole example of the third pattern, in which the drug is administered in active form and excreted unchanged by the kidneys. Captopril, enalapril, ramipril, and lisinopril have all been studied in large-scale clinical trials.

Although ACE inhibitors are generally well tolerated, important adverse effects of these agents include **cough** and **angioedema** caused by potentiation of bradykinin action. The cough, occurring in up to 20% of patients taking captopril, is usually dry and nonproductive. While not causing any serious physiologic effects, the cough may cause discomfort, impair voice quality, and limit patient compliance. Angioedema, which can occur in 0.1% to 0.2% of patients, is a potentially life-threatening cause of airway obstruction. This adverse effect almost always occurs within the first week of initiating therapy and may require emergent intervention.

ACE inhibitors can precipitate first-dose **hypotension** and/or **acute renal failure,** and thus are administered at a low initial dose. These adverse effects are more common in patients with bilateral renal artery stenosis. In such patients, renal function can be dependent on increased angiotensin II activity, because elevated angiotensin II maintains GFR by preferential constriction of the efferent arteriole. For this reason, bilateral renal artery stenosis is a contraindication to ACE inhibitor therapy. ACE inhibitors interrupt aldosterone synthesis, and so can produce **hyperkalemia.** Hyperkalemia is more commonly observed when ACE inhibitors are used in conjunction with potassium-sparing diuretics (see below) such as spironolactone, amiloride, and triamterene.

ACE inhibitors are widely used to treat hypertension, HF, acute myocardial infarction, and chronic kidney disease. In many cases, ACE inhibitors are increasingly considered first-line agents for hypertension, especially when a patient has concomitant left ventricular wall dysfunction or diabetes (see Chapter 24). ACE inhibitors have broad applicability to all forms of hypertension, including hypertension where there is no clear increase in plasma renin levels. Long-term use of ACE inhibitors retards progression of the cardiac contractile dysfunction observed in HF and after myocardial infarction, by little understood mechanisms that may involve inhibition of paracrine growth factors and hormones that stimulate pathologic tissue hypertrophy and fibrosis. ACE inhibitors can also delay progression of diabetic nephropathy, likely through attenuation of renal paracrine signaling pathways, with consequent improvement in renal hemodynamics. However, because the use of ACE inhibitors is associated with an increased risk of major fetal malformations, their use is contraindicated in pregnancy (including the treatment of pregnancy-associated hypertension).

Angiotensin Receptor Antagonists

AT_1 receptor antagonists, such as **losartan** and **valsartan,** inhibit the action of AT II at its receptor. Compared to ACE inhibitors, AT_1 receptor antagonists may allow more complete inhibition of AT II's actions, because ACE is not the only enzyme that can generate AT II. In addition, because AT_1 receptor antagonists have no effect on bradykinin metabolism, their use may minimize the incidence of drug-induced cough and angioedema. However, the inability of AT_1 receptor antagonists to potentiate the vasodilatory effects of bradykinin may result in less effective vasodilation. Unlike ACE inhibitors, AT_1 receptor antagonists may indirectly increase vasorelaxant AT_2 receptor activity. Both ACE inhibitors and AT_1 antagonists increase renin release as a compensatory mechanism; in the case of AT_1 blockade, the increased AT II that results could lead to increased interaction of AT II with AT_2 receptors.

AT_1 receptor antagonists are approved for the treatment of hypertension. Although these agents were initially prescribed only for patients with intolerable adverse reactions to ACE inhibitors, they are now considered potential first-line treatments for hypertension. AT_1 receptor antagonists are under study for the treatment of heart failure. Recent trials have suggested that the combination of an AT_1 receptor antagonist and an ACE inhibitor may provide survival benefit in severe heart failure, and studies testing such combinations in the treatment of chronic kidney disease and cardiac disease progression are currently underway. AT_1 receptor antagonists may also protect against stroke, not only by controlling hypertension but also by beneficial secondary effects on platelet aggregation (anti-aggregatory), uric acid metabolism (hypouricemic), diabetes (anti-diabetic), and atrial fibrillation (antiarrhythmic). The mechanisms of these secondary effects remain to be elucidated.

B-Type Natriuretic Peptide

Nesiritide, a recombinant human-sequence B-type natriuretic peptide (BNP), has recently been approved for short-term management of decompensated HF. Because nesiritide is a peptide, it is ineffective when given orally. In clinical trials of nesiritide in acute HF, the drug decreased pulmonary capillary wedge pressure (a measure of hydrostatic pressure in the pulmonary system), decreased systemic vascular resistance, and improved cardiac hemodynamic parameters such as stroke volume. Although nesiritide was not more efficacious than dobutamine in these trials (dobutamine is one of the agents commonly used in the treatment of decompensated HF; see Chapter 24), nesiritide may be associated with a lower incidence of arrhythmias than dobutamine. At low doses, nesiritide appears to promote water excretion more than sodium excretion.

Hypotension is a major adverse effect of nesiritide, reflecting the vasorelaxant properties of the natriuretic peptides. The risk of hypotension is increased by coadministration of nesiritide with an ACE inhibitor. Nesiritide treatment is also associated with an increased risk of renal dysfunction. These adverse effects have not been reported in preliminary clinical trials of an investigational peptide related to ANP, which exhibits powerful natriuretic as well as diuretic properties.

Antidiuretic Hormone (ADH) Antagonists

The tetracycline analogue **demeclocycline** is an ADH antagonist that has long been used in the treatment of syndromes of inappropriate ADH secretion (SIADH), when dietary water restriction is not feasible or sufficient. **Conivaptan** is the first specific non-peptide vasopressin receptor antagonist approved for treatment of euvolemic hyponatremias (SIADH). Its disadvantages include a requirement for intravenous administration and some V_1 receptor antagonist activity. However, approval of **tolvaptan** and **lixivaptan**—which are both V_2-selective receptor antagonists that are orally bioavailable—is anticipated soon. In clinical trials, V_2 receptor antagonists have also shown benefit in the treatment of other conditions associated with inappropriate ADH-induced water retention, including HF and cirrhotic ascites. V_2 receptor antagonists are also under evaluation as agents to retard vasopressin-driven renal cyst growth in autosomal dominant polycystic kidney disease.

Congenital nephrogenic diabetes insipidus may result from mutations in either the V_2 receptor or the collecting-duct principal-cell aquaporin AQP2. Some V_2 receptor mutations are associated with trapping of newly synthesized receptor polypeptides inside the principal cell. Vasopressin receptor antagonists may act as molecular chaperones for a subset of these mutant receptors; in these cases, antagonist binding presumably promotes a receptor conformation that allows insertion of the mutant protein into the apical membrane of the cell.

AGENTS THAT DECREASE RENAL Na$^+$ REABSORPTION

As discussed above, the kidney modifies the ionic composition of the glomerular filtrate by the concerted action of ion transporters and channels in both apical and basolateral membranes of renal tubular epithelial cells. This transepithelial ion transport can be modulated pharmacologically by the actions of diuretic drugs to regulate urinary volume and composition. Pharmacologic inhibition of ion reabsorption leads to reduction of the osmotic driving force that favors water reabsorption in the water-permeable segments of the nephron. Diuretics target sodium reabsorption along four segments of the nephron: the proximal tubule, medullary thick ascending limb, distal convoluted tubule, and collecting duct. The kidney concentrates and secretes these drugs into the tubule lumen, allowing diuretics to reach higher concentrations in the tubule than in the blood. Because of this concentrating effect, therapeutic concentrations of diuretics in the blood are often low and non-renal adverse effects are often mild.

Carbonic Anhydrase Inhibitors

Carbonic anhydrase inhibitors, exemplified by **acetazolamide,** inhibit sodium reabsorption by noncompetitively and reversibly inhibiting proximal-tubule cytoplasmic carbonic anhydrase II and luminal carbonic anhydrase IV (Fig. 20-6). Inhibition of carbonic anhydrase leads to increased delivery of sodium bicarbonate to more distal segments of the nephron. Much of this sodium bicarbonate is initially excreted, resulting in an acute decrease in plasma volume (diuresis). However, over the course of several days of therapy, the diuretic effect of the drug is diminished by compensatory up-regulation of $NaHCO_3$ reabsorption and by increased NaCl reabsorption across more distal nephron segments (by incompletely understood mechanisms).

Use of carbonic anhydrase inhibitors is often associated with mild-to-moderate metabolic acidosis, arising not only from inhibition of proximal tubular H$^+$ secretion, but also from inhibition of carbonic anhydrase in acid-secreting intercalated cells of the collecting duct. The alkalinized urine resulting from carbonic anhydrase inhibition increases the urinary excretion of organic acid anions, including aspirin.

The clinical use of carbonic anhydrase inhibitors is primarily restricted to several carbonic anhydrase-dependent conditions (see below). In addition, carbonic anhydrase inhibitors are occasionally used to restore acid-base balance in HF patients with metabolic alkalosis due to treatment with loop diuretics.

Carbonic anhydrase inhibitors also have ophthalmologic applications. The ciliary process epithelium of the anterior chamber of the eye secretes sodium chloride into the aqueous humor. This NaCl secretion requires carbonic anhydrase activity, because a portion of the basolateral Cl$^-$ uptake by the ciliary epithelium requires coupled Cl$^-$-HCO_3^- and

Na$^+$-H$^+$ exchange as well as Na$^+$-HCO_3^- symport. The basolateral membrane Na$^+$-K$^+$-2Cl$^-$ cotransporter NKCC1 mediates most remaining Cl$^-$ uptake by ciliary epithelial cells. **Glaucoma** is characterized by increased pressure in the anterior chamber of the eye. This is usually attributed to partially obstructed outflow of aqueous humor, but in some cases overproduction of aqueous humor may also contribute. Inhibition of carbonic anhydrase in the ciliary process epithelium reduces secretion of aqueous humor and may thereby reduce elevated intraocular pressure. Topical, lipophilic carbonic anhydrase inhibitors are often used in concert with topical β-adrenergic antagonists in the treatment of glaucoma (see Chapter 9, Adrenergic Pharmacology).

Ascent to altitudes greater than 3,000 m above sea level predisposes several body organs, including the brain, to edema and ionic disequilibria. Symptoms of **acute mountain sickness** can include nausea, headache, dizziness, insomnia, pulmonary edema, and confusion. Carbonic anhydrase is involved in the secretion of chloride and bicarbonate into the cerebrospinal fluid by the choroid plexus of the cerebral ventricles, and inhibition of carbonic anhydrase can be used prophylactically against acute mountain sickness. The still-controversial mechanism(s) of action include effects on the choroid plexus and ependyma, on the respiratory control centers of the brain, and on the blood–brain barrier.

The treatment of hyperuricemia or **gout** (see Chapter 47, Integrative Inflammation Pharmacology: Gout) may involve alkalinization of the urine to increase the urinary solubility of uric acid. Increased uric acid solubility prevents uric acid precipitation in the urine, with consequent uric acid nephropathy and nephrolithiasis (kidney stones). Urinary alkalinization can be achieved by oral bicarbonate, supplemented as needed by a carbonic anhydrase inhibitor to reduce renal reabsorption of the filtered bicarbonate.

Osmotic Diuresis

Osmotic diuretics, such as **mannitol**, are small molecules that are filtered at the glomerulus but not subsequently reabsorbed in the nephron. Thus, they constitute an intraluminal osmotic force limiting reabsorption of water across water-permeable nephron segments. The effect of osmotic agents is greatest in the proximal tubule, where most iso-osmotic reabsorption of water takes place. Water loss in excess of sodium excretion can sometimes lead to unintended hypernatremia. Alternatively, the increased urine volume associated with osmotic diuresis can promote vigorous natriuresis. Therefore, careful monitoring of clinical volume status and serum electrolytes is warranted. Mannitol is used primarily for rapid (emergent) treatment of **increased intracranial pressure**. In the setting of head trauma, brain hemorrhage, or a symptomatic cerebral mass, the increased intracranial pressure can be relieved, at least transiently, by the acute reduction in cerebral intravascular volume that follows the mannitol-induced reduction in systemic vascular volume.

Osmotic diuresis can also occur as a result of pathologic states. Two common examples of this phenomenon are hyperglycemia and the use of radiocontrast dyes. In diabetic hyperglycemia, the filtered glucose load exceeds the reabsorptive capacity of the proximal tubule for glucose. As a result, significant quantities of glucose remain in the lumen of the nephron and act as an osmotic agent to increase fluid retention in the tubular lumen, thereby decreasing fluid reabsorption. Radiocontrast agents, which are used in radiologic imaging studies, are filtered at the glomerulus but not reabsorbed by the tubular epithelium. Thus, the dyes constitute an osmotic load and can produce osmotic diuresis. In patients with borderline cardiovascular status, the consequent reduction in intravascular volume can lead to hypotension or to renal and/or cardiac insufficiency secondary to reduced organ perfusion.

Loop Diuretics

The so-called loop diuretics act at the TAL of the loop of Henle. These agents reversibly and competitively inhibit the Na^+-K^+-$2Cl^-$ cotransporter NKCC2 in the apical (luminal) membrane of TAL epithelial cells (Fig. 20-7). In addition to the primary effect of inhibiting Na^+ reabsorption across the TAL, inhibition of transcellular NaCl transport also reduces or abolishes the lumen-positive transepithelial potential difference across the TAL. Consequently, paracellular reabsorption of divalent cations, particularly calcium and magnesium, is also inhibited. This results in increased delivery of luminal calcium and magnesium to downstream reabsorptive sites in the distal convoluted tubule and can lead to increased excretion of calcium and magnesium. Hypocalcemia and especially hypomagnesemia can be clinically significant in some patients who require prolonged administration of loop agents. Furthermore, increased downstream delivery of sodium increases the Na^+ load presented to principal cells of the collecting duct. The increased Na^+ load stimulates increased secretion of K^+ and protons, predisposing to hypokalemia and metabolic alkalosis. Together, the clinical consequences of loop diuretic treatment are often described as **volume-contraction alkalosis.** Diuretic-associated hypokalemia can predispose to cardiac arrhythmias in the setting of coronary or cardiac insufficiency.

The prototypical loop diuretic is **furosemide.** Other drugs in this class include **bumetanide, torsemide,** and **ethacrynic acid.** All these agents are generally well tolerated. Apart from their effects on renal electrolyte handling, loop diuretics are associated with dose-related **ototoxicity,** presumably because of altered electrolyte handling in the endolymph. For this reason, coadministration of loop diuretics with aminoglycosides (which are also ototoxic; see Chapter 32, Pharmacology of Bacterial Infections: DNA Replication, Transcription, and Translation) should be avoided. The major differences among the loop diuretics are in potency and incidence of allergies. Bumetanide is approximately 40 times more potent than the other loop diuretics. Furosemide, bumetanide, and torsemide are all **sulfonamide derivatives,** while ethacrynic acid is not. Therefore, ethacrynic acid is a therapeutic option for patients who are allergic to ''sulfa'' drugs.

The high sodium reabsorption capacity of the TAL makes loop diuretics a front-line therapy for acute relief of pulmonary and peripheral edema in the context of heart failure. Loop diuretics are capable of reducing intravascular volume to the extent that filling pressures are decreased below the threshold for pulmonary and peripheral edema. This was the rationale for the intravenous furosemide used to treat Mr. R's pulmonary edema and peripheral edema in the introduc-

tory case. Hypoalbuminemia, resulting from decreased synthesis of albumin (liver disease) or increased clearance of the protein (nephrotic proteinuria), can diminish intravascular oncotic pressure and cause edema. These **edematous states** can be treated with low-dose loop diuretics.

Loop agents can be used therapeutically to increase calcium diuresis, and thereby provide acute relief of **hypercalcemia,** in states such as hyperparathyroidism or malignancy-associated hypercalcemia caused by tumor secretion of parathyroid hormone-related protein or other calciotropic hormones (see Chapter 30, Pharmacology of Bone Mineral Homeostasis). Loop agents are also used to counteract **hyperkalemia** caused by potassium-retaining adverse effects of other drugs, or by renal insufficiency with impaired urinary K^+ excretion in the context of normal or elevated dietary K^+ intake.

In **acute renal failure,** the increase in urine flow brought about by loop diuretics can facilitate clinical management of fluid balance in the face of decreased glomerular filtration. However, there is no evidence to support the oft-repeated claim that increased urine output itself intrinsically enhances renal tubular epithelial cell recovery from the ischemic or toxic event that precipitated the acute renal failure.

Thiazides

Thiazide diuretics inhibit sodium chloride reabsorption in the distal convoluted tubule (Fig. 20-8). These agents act from the apical (luminal) side as competitive antagonists of the NCC1 Na^+-Cl^- cotransporter in the luminal membrane of distal convoluted tubule cells. The modest natriuresis produced by thiazides stems from the fact that 90% of sodium reabsorption occurs upstream of their site of action in the nephron; nonetheless, thiazides do cause a modest reduction in intravascular volume. The decrease in intravascular volume, possibly combined with a poorly understood direct vasodilatory effect, decreases systemic blood pressure.

The distal tubule is also a site of parathyroid hormone-regulated reabsorption of calcium via voltage-independent TRPV5 Ca^{2+} channels. Thiazides promote increased transcellular calcium reabsorption in the distal convoluted tubule. Thiazides have been used to decrease urinary Ca^{2+} wasting in **osteoporosis** (although this is no longer common practice in the absence of hypercalciuria) and to diminish hypercalciuria in patients at risk for **nephrolithiasis.** The mechanism by which inhibition of NaCl uptake enhances apical Ca^{2+} entry remains incompletely understood, but part of the response is mediated by increased expression of the apical membrane TRPV5 Ca^{2+} channel and the basolateral membrane Na^+/Ca^{2+} exchanger. Additionally (and more speculatively), the decreased intracellular Cl^- concentration that results from thiazide inhibition of apical Na^+-Cl^- cotransport may favor Cl^- entry via basolateral Cl^- channels, and the consequent membrane hyperpolarization may favor apical Ca^{2+} entry.

Hydrochlorothiazide is the prototypical thiazide diuretic. In addition to its effects on renal electrolyte handling, hydrochlorothiazide decreases glucose tolerance and may unmask diabetes in patients at risk for impaired glucose metabolism. The mechanism of this effect is unknown, but may be attributable to drug-induced impairment of insulin secretion and/or decreased peripheral insulin sensitivity. Thiazide diuretics should not be administered concurrently with antiarrhythmic agents that prolong the QT interval (e.g., quinidine, sotalol), as coadministration of these drugs predisposes patients to *torsades de pointes* (polymorphic ventricular tachycardia, see Chapter 18, Pharmacology of Cardiac Rhythm). The mechanism of this adverse effect may be related to thiazide-induced hypokalemia, which increases the potential for cardiac arrhythmias (see Chapter 18).

Thiazide diuretics are first-line agents for treatment of hypertension (see Chapter 24). In numerous randomized clinical trials, these drugs have been shown to reduce both cardiovascular-related and total mortality. In addition, thiazide diuretics are often used together with loop agents for their synergistic diuretic effects in HF. This synergism arises because the increased Na^+ load, delivered from the loop diuretic-blocked TAL to the thiazide diuretic-blocked DCT, must now proceed to the collecting duct, which has only a limited ability to up-regulate compensatory Na^+ reabsorption. The dose of thiazide must be carefully considered in this setting, for as with loop diuretics, thiazides can increase K^+ and H^+ secretion by increasing Na^+ presentation to the collecting duct, thus leading to hypokalemic metabolic alkalosis.

Patients with impaired secretion of vasopressin by the posterior pituitary gland, or with impaired signaling by the V_2 vasopressin receptor of the collecting duct principal cells, fail to reabsorb water in the terminal nephron. These patients generate large volumes of hypotonic urine. **Central diabetes insipidus** (defective pituitary secretion of vasopressin) can be treated with the exogenous vasopressin agonist **desmopressin** (see Chapter 25, Pharmacology of the Hypothalamus and Pituitary Gland). Patients with **nephrogenic diabetes insipidus** do not respond to desmopressin; paradoxically, however, thiazide diuretics can produce a modest *decrease* in urine flow in this setting. It is thought that, by reducing intravascular volume and decreasing glomerular filtration rate, thiazides reduce the volume of tubular fluid delivered to the collecting duct and thereby decrease urine volume.

Collecting Duct (Potassium-Sparing) Diuretics

In contrast to all other diuretic classes, potassium-sparing diuretics increase nephron reabsorption of potassium. Agents in this class interrupt collecting-duct principal-cell Na^+ reabsorption by one of two mechanisms. Agents such as spironolactone inhibit the biosynthesis of new Na^+ channels in the principal cells, while agents such as amiloride and triamterene block the activity of Na^+ channels in the luminal membranes of these cells (Fig. 20-9).

The epithelial sodium channel (ENaC) of collecting duct principal cells comprises α, β, and γ subunits assembled in a complex with a (still-debated) stoichiometry of $α_2βγ$. Control of sodium channel expression is regulated primarily by aldosterone, which is secreted by the adrenal cortical zona glomerulosa under the regulation of angiotensin II and plasma potassium. Circulating aldosterone diffuses into collecting duct principal cells and binds to an intracellular mineralocorticoid receptor. Activation of the mineralocorticoid receptor increases transcription of mRNAs that encode proteins involved in Na^+ handling, including ENaC expressed in the apical membrane and Na^+/K^+-ATPase expressed in the basolateral membrane. The increased ENaC expression increases Na^+ flux across the luminal membrane, while increased Na^+/K^+-ATPase activity increases Na^+ flux from the cytoplasm across the basolateral membrane into the interstitium. These two actions of aldosterone increase Na^+ reabsorption and hence increase intravascular volume.

Spironolactone and **eplerenone** inhibit aldosterone action by binding to and preventing nuclear translocation of the mineralocorticoid receptor. **Amiloride** and **triamterene** are competitive inhibitors of the principal cell apical membrane ENaC Na^+ channel. Both types of potassium-sparing diuretics can cause **hyperkalemia**, because inhibition of electrogenic Na^+ uptake by either mechanism decreases the normal transepithelial lumen-negative potential and thus decreases the driving force for potassium secretion from collecting duct cells. Decreased Na^+ uptake through ENaC may also diminish H^+ secretion, leading to **metabolic acidosis**. Spironolactone inhibits the androgen receptor as well as the mineralocorticoid receptor; this cross-reactivity can cause adverse effects of impotence and gynecomastia in men. The more selective eplerenone minimizes the incidence of these adverse effects.

Potassium-sparing diuretics are mild diuretics when used in isolation because the collecting duct reabsorbs only 1% to 5% of filtered sodium. However, they can be used to potentiate the action of more proximally acting diuretics, including loop diuretics. Potassium-sparing diuretics are occasionally used in combination with thiazides to counteract the potassium-wasting effects of the thiazides. Amiloride and triamterene are the drugs of choice for treatment of Liddle syndrome, a rare, Mendelian form of hypertension resulting from gain-of-function mutations in the β or γ subunit of the ENaC Na^+ channel.

Potassium-sparing diuretics are used clinically to treat hypokalemic alkalosis secondary to the mineralocorticoid excess that can accompany HF, hepatic failure, and other disease processes associated with diminished aldosterone metabolism. The mild diuretic action of spironolactone or eplerenone minimizes the risk of cardiovascular compromise from excessively rapid or extensive diuresis when diminished oncotic pressure impairs the mobilization of extravascular fluid into the vasculature. Therefore, mineralocorticoid receptor antagonists are the diuretics of choice for treatment of ascites and edema associated with impaired plasma protein biosynthesis secondary to hepatic failure.

Studies have suggested that mineralocorticoid receptor antagonists preserve cardiac function in the setting of coronary ischemia, and that these agents retard the development of HF. Both spironolactone and eplerenone reduce mortality in patients with HF and in patients with significant cardiac dysfunction (ejection fraction less than 40%) after myocardial infarction. The mechanism of this effect may be related to inhibition of cardiac fibrosis resulting from a paracrine aldosterone-signaling pathway.

◼ *Conclusion and Future Directions*

This chapter has reviewed the physiology and pathophysiology of extracellular volume regulation. Control of intravascular volume maintains adequate perfusion pressure to organs and ensures that the kidney is able to filter waste products from the plasma. Regulation of extracellular volume is accomplished by integrated neurohormonal mechanisms that respond to changes in arterial and atrial wall stress. These hormones modulate numerous steps in renal Na^+ handling, and thereby maintain a homeostatic balance between dietary Na^+ intake and Na^+ excretion. Edema can develop when the capillary hydrostatic pressure gradient favoring fluid filtration exceeds the opposing oncotic forces favoring fluid entry into the intravascular space. Pharmacologic treatment of dysregulated extracellular volume involves modification of neurohormonal signaling and direct inhibition of renal Na^+ reabsorption. ACE inhibitors prevent the conversion of angiotensin I to angiotensin II; drugs in this class have important vasodilatory actions. Angiotensin receptor antagonists are also useful in interrupting the angiotensin–aldosterone axis. Both ACE inhibitors and angiotensin receptor antagonists have beneficial effects in slowing the progression of hypertrophy and fibrosis in the heart, the kidney, and the vasculature. B-type natriuretic peptide (nesiritide) is now used in the treatment of decompensated HF.

Diuretics are agents that alter nephron Na^+ reabsorption and secondarily alter the reabsorption and secretion of other ions. Essential to understanding diuretic mechanisms is an appreciation of the functional organization of the nephron. With the exception of osmotic diuretics, which increase urinary flow by osmotic retention of water throughout the nephron, a specific class of diuretic drugs targets each of the four segments of the nephron. Carbonic anhydrase inhibitors such as acetazolamide decrease sodium and bicarbonate reabsorption in the proximal tubule; loop agents such as furosemide decrease sodium and chloride reabsorption by the apical Na^+-K^+-$2Cl^-$ pump in the thick ascending loop of Henle; thiazides such as hydrochlorothiazide inhibit the apical Na^+-Cl^- cotransporter in the distal convoluted tubule; and potassium-sparing diuretics such as spironolactone and amiloride inhibit, respectively, the aldosterone receptor and the ENaC apical Na^+ channel in the collecting duct. The most important use of

diuretics is in the treatment of hypertension; the second most important use is to treat edema of any cause.

Future developments in the pharmacology of extracellular volume regulation will likely focus on interrupting the hormonal pathways implicated in the disruption of volume homeostasis. This research will focus on new drugs that interrupt the renin-angiotensin–aldosterone axis, including renin inhibitors, neutral endopeptidase inhibitors, additional AT_1 receptor antagonists, and selective aldosterone receptor antagonists. As agents with higher natriuretic potency are approved, natriuretic peptide mimetics will likely play an increasingly important role in the management of decompensated HF. Specific V2 vasopressin receptor antagonists will also be used increasingly in hypervolemic conditions accompanied by elevated ADH levels or action. Drugs interrupting these hormonal pathways have the potential to modify the pathophysiology of these disease processes, and thereby to interrupt disease progression while concomitantly regulating renal Na^+ reabsorption.

Suggested Reading

Ellison DH. Core curriculum in nephrology: disorders of sodium and water. *Am J Kidney Dis* 2005;46:356–361. *(A concise outline of salt and water homeostasis and pharmacology.)*

Greenberg A, Verbalis JG. Vasopressin receptor antagonists. *Kidney Int* 2006;69:2124–2130. *(Introduction to the physiology and clinical indications of this new drug class.)*

Koeppen BM, Stanton BA, Koeppen BH. *Renal Physiology.* 4th ed. St. Louis: Mosby; 2006. *(Concise but complete monograph on renal physiology.)*

Okusa MD, Ellison DH. Physiology and pathophysiology of diuretic action. In: Seldin DW, Giebisch G, eds. *The kidney: physiology and pathophysiology.* 3rd ed. Philadelphia: Lippincott Williams & Wilkins; 2000. *(Full discussion of the physiology and pathophysiology of diuretic action.)*

Silver MA. The natriuretic peptide system: kidney and cardiovascular effects. *Curr Opin Nephrol Hypertens* 2006;15:14–21. *(Overview of natriuretic peptide physiology in volume regulation.)*

Drug Summary Table | Chapter 20 Pharmacology of Volume Regulation

ANGIOTENSIN CONVERTING ENZYME (ACE) INHIBITORS

Mechanism—By inhibiting ACE, decrease conversion of angiotensin (AT) I to AT II, and thereby decrease arteriolar vasoconstriction, aldosterone synthesis, renal proximal tubule NaCl reabsorption, and ADH release. ACE inhibitors also inhibit the degradation of bradykinin, and thereby increase vasodilation.

Drug	Clinical Applications	Serious and Common Adverse Effects	Contraindications	Therapeutic Considerations
Captopril Enalapril Ramipril Benazepril Fosinopril Moexipril Perindopril Quinapril Trandolapril Lisinopril	Hypertension Heart failure Diabetic nephropathy Myocardial infarction	Angioedema (more frequent in Black patients), agranulocytosis, neutropenia Cough, edema, hypotension, rash, gynecomastia, hyperkalemia, proteinuria	History of angioedema Bilateral renal artery stenosis Renal failure Pregnancy	ACE inhibitors exhibit three patterns of metabolism: (1) administered as active drug and processed to active metabolite (e.g., captopril), (2) ester prodrugs converted to active metabolites in plasma (e.g., enalapril and ramipril), (3) administered as active drug and excreted unchanged (lisinopril) Cough and angioedema are caused by bradykinin action; angioedema occurs within the first week of therapy in 0.1%–0.2% of patients and can be potentially life-threatening First-dose hypotension and/or acute renal failure are more common in patients with bilateral renal artery stenosis; hyperkalemia is more common when ACE inhibitors are used in combination with potassium-sparing diuretics ACE inhibitors delay progression of cardiac contractile dysfunction in heart failure and after myocardial infarction, and delay progression of diabetic nephropathy A few case reports suggest that coadministration with allopurinol may predispose to hypersensitivity reactions including Stevens-Johnson syndrome and anaphylaxis

ANGIOTENSIN II RECEPTOR ANTAGONISTS

Mechanism—Antagonize action of angiotensin II at AT1 receptor, may also indirectly increase vasorelaxant AT2 receptor activity

| Candesartan
Irbesartan
Losartan
Telmisartan
Valsartan | Hypertension
Diabetic nephropathy
Heart failure
Myocardial infarction
Prevention of stroke | Rare thrombocytopenia, rhabdomyolysis, rare angioedema
Hypotension, diarrhea, asthenia, dizziness | Bilateral renal artery stenosis
Pregnancy | Also called angiotensin receptor blockers (ARBs)
Do not cause cough and angioedema, but may be less effective vasodilators compared to ACE inhibitors
In combination with ACE inhibitors, may provide survival benefit in severe heart failure; AT1 receptor antagonists may also protect against stroke
Initially prescribed only for patients with intolerable reactions to ACE inhibitors, but are now considered potential first-line treatments for hypertension |

B-TYPE NATRIURETIC PEPTIDE (BNP)

Mechanism—Increases intracellular concentrations of cGMP by binding to the particulate guanylyl cyclase receptor of vascular smooth muscle and endothelial cells, resulting in smooth muscle relaxation

Drug	Clinical Applications	Adverse Effects	Contraindications	Therapeutic Considerations
Nesiritide	Acutely decompensated heart failure	*Hypotension, cardiac arrhythmia, renal dysfunction* Headache, confusion, somnolence, tremor, pruritus, nausea	Cardiogenic shock Systolic blood pressure less than 90	Nesiritide decreases pulmonary capillary wedge pressure, decreases systemic vascular resistance, and improves cardiac hemodynamic parameters such as stroke volume Nesiritide may be associated with a lower incidence of arrhythmias than dobutamine The risk of hypotension is increased by co-administration with ACE inhibitors; nesiritide treatment is also associated with an increased risk of renal dysfunction

VASOPRESSIN RECEPTOR 2 (V2) ANTAGONISTS

Mechanism—Potent antagonist activity at vasopressin receptor 2 and weaker antagonist activity at V1, preventing vasopressin-stimulated water reabsorption via V2-coupled aquaporin channels in apical membrane of collecting duct cells

Drug	Clinical Applications	Adverse Effects	Contraindications	Therapeutic Considerations
Conivaptan Lixivaptan Tolvaptan	Euvolemic hyponatremia SIADH Heart failure Cirrhotic ascites Autosomal dominant polycystic kidney disease	*Atrial fibrillation* Orthostatic hypotension, hypertension, peripheral edema, injection-site reaction, hypokalemia, thirst, dyspepsia, headache, polyuria	Concurrent use of potent P450 3A4 inhibitors Hypovolemic hyponatremia	Conivaptan is relatively nonselective for V2 and V1 receptors and must be administered IV Approval of the orally bioavailable, V2-selective agents tolvaptan and lixivaptan is anticipated at the time of this writing V2 receptor antagonists are under evaluation as agents to retard vasopressin-driven renal cyst growth in autosomal dominant polycystic kidney disease

CARBONIC ANHYDRASE INHIBITORS

Mechanism—Inhibit sodium and bicarbonate reabsorption by noncompetitively and reversibly inhibiting proximal-tubule cytoplasmic carbonic anhydrase II and luminal carbonic anhydrase IV, leading to increased delivery of sodium bicarbonate to more distal segments of the nephron

Drug	Clinical Applications	Adverse Effects	Contraindications	Therapeutic Considerations
Acetazolamide	High-altitude sickness Heart failure Epilepsy Glaucoma	*Metabolic acidosis, sulfonamide adverse reactions (including anaphylaxis, blood dyscrasias, erythema multiforme, fulminant hepatic necrosis, Stevens-Johnson syndrome, toxic epidermal necrolysis)* Diarrhea, weight and appetite loss, tinnitus, nausea, vomiting, paresthesia, somnolence, polyuria	Adrenal gland failure Chronic angle-closure glaucoma Cirrhosis Hyponatremia/hypokalemia Hyperchloremic acidosis Severe hepatic or renal disease	Clinical use is associated with mild-to-moderate metabolic acidosis Used occasionally in heart failure to restore acid-base balance Carbonic anhydrase inhibition in ciliary process of the eye reduces secretion of aqueous humor and may thereby reduce elevated intraocular pressure in glaucoma Can be used prophylactically against acute mountain sickness, presumably owing to the drug's effects on choroid plexus and ependyma, respiratory control centers of brain, and blood–brain barrier Carbonic anhydrase inhibitors alkalinize urine and increase urinary excretion of endogenous (uric acid) and exogenous (aspirin) organic acid anions; can be used in the treatment of hyperuricemia or gout Aspirin increases plasma concentration of acetazolamide, potentially leading to CNS toxicity

(Continued)

Drug Summary Table   Chapter 20 Pharmacology of Volume Regulation (Continued)

Drug	Clinical Applications	Serious and Common Adverse Effects	Contraindications	Therapeutic Considerations
OSMOTIC DIURETICS				
Mechanism—Act as an osmole, filtered at the glomerulus but not subsequently reabsorbed in the nephron; exert an intraluminal osmotic force and limit reabsorption of water across water-permeable nephron segments				
Mannitol	Cerebral edema Increased intraocular pressure Prophylaxis of oliguria in acute renal failure	*Thrombophlebitis, acidosis, seizure, urinary retention, pulmonary edema* Hypotension, palpitations, fluid and/or electrolyte imbalance, diarrhea, nausea, rhinitis	Anuria Severe dehydration Heart failure, pulmonary congestion, or renal dysfunction after initiation of mannitol	Promotes vigorous natriuresis; requires careful monitoring of volume status Water loss in excess of sodium excretion can lead to unintended hypernatremia Used primarily for rapid (emergent) reduction of intracranial pressure in the setting of head trauma, brain hemorrhage, or symptomatic cerebral mass; also used rarely in treatment of compartment syndrome
LOOP DIURETICS				
Mechanism—Inhibit sodium reabsorption by reversibly and competitively inhibiting sodium-potassium-chloride cotransporter NKCC2 in apical (luminal) membrane of cells in thick ascending limb of loop of Henle; also reduce or abolish the lumen-positive transepithelial potential difference				
Furosemide Bumetanide Torsemide Ethacrynic acid	Hypertension Acute pulmonary edema Edema associated with congestive heart failure, hepatic cirrhosis, or renal dysfunction Hypercalcemia Hyperkalemia	*Hypotension, erythema multiforme, Stevens-Johnson syndrome, pancreatitis, aplastic or hemolytic anemia, leukopenia, thrombocytopenia* Volume contraction, alkalosis, ototoxicity (dose-related), hypokalemia, hyperuricemia, hypomagnesemia, hyperglycemia, rash, cramps, spasticity, headache, blurred vision, dyspepsia, glycosuria	Hypersensitivity to sulfonamides (contraindication for furosemide, bumetanide, and torsemide) Anuria Coadministration with aminoglycosides increases ototoxicity and nephrotoxicity	Bumetanide is approximately forty times more potent than the other loop diuretics; furosemide, bumetanide, and torsemide are all sulfonamide derivatives, while ethacrynic acid is not Front-line therapy for acute relief of pulmonary and peripheral edema in heart failure; edematous states secondary to diminished oncotic pressure of hypoalbuminemia (as in nephrotic proteinuria or liver disease) can be treated with low-dose loop diuretics Also used to counteract hypercalcemic and hyperkalemic states
THIAZIDE DIURETICS				
Mechanism—Inhibit sodium chloride reabsorption by acting as competitive antagonists at NCC1 sodium-chloride cotransporter in apical (luminal) membrane of distal convoluted tubule cells; promote increased transcellular calcium reabsorption in distal convoluted tubule				
Hydrochlorothiazide Bendroflumethiazide Hydroflumethiazide Polythiazide Chlorthalidone Metolazone Indapamide	Hypertension Adjunct in edema states associated with congestive heart failure, hepatic cirrhosis, renal dysfunction, corticosteroid and estrogen therapy	*Cardiac arrhythmia, Stevens-Johnson syndrome, toxic epidermal necrolysis, pancreatitis, hepatotoxicity, systemic lupus erythematosus* Hypotension, vasculitis, photosensitivity, electrolyte abnormalities, hypokalemic metabolic alkalosis, hyperglycemia, hyperuricemia, dyspepsia, headache, blurred vision, impotence, restlessness	Anuria Hypersensitivity to sulfonamides Coadministration with agents that prolong QT interval	First-line agents for treatment of hypertension; also used in combination with loop agents for synergistic diuretic effect in heart failure Used to diminish hypercalciuria in patients at risk for nephrolithiasis and (rarely) to decrease urinary calcium wasting in osteoporosis Hydrochlorothiazide decreases glucose tolerance and may unmask diabetes in patients at risk for impaired glucose metabolism Should not be administered concurrently with antiarrhythmic agents that prolong the QT interval In patients with nephrogenic diabetes insipidus, thiazide diuretics can paradoxically produce a modest decrease in urine flow

COLLECTING DUCT (POTASSIUM-SPARING) DIURETICS

Mechanism—Spironolactone and eplerenone inhibit aldosterone action by binding to and preventing nuclear translocation of the mineralocorticoid receptor. Amiloride and triamterene are competitive inhibitors of the principal cell apical membrane ENaC sodium channel.

Drug	Therapeutic uses	Adverse effects	Contraindications	Notes
Spironolactone Eplerenone	Hypertension Edema associated with congestive heart failure, liver cirrhosis (with or without ascites), or nephrotic syndrome Hypokalemia Primary aldosteronism Acne vulgaris (spironolactone) Female hirsutism (spironolactone)	*Hyperkalemic metabolic acidosis, gastrointestinal hemorrhage, agranulocytosis, systemic lupus erythematosus, breast cancer (not established)* Gynecomastia, dyspepsia, lethargy, abnormal menstruation, impotence, rash	Anuria Hyperkalemia Acute renal insuffiency	Potassium-sparing diuretics are mild diuretics when used in isolation, but can potentiate the action of more proximally acting loop diuretics Occasionally used in combination with thiazides to counteract potassium-wasting effect of thiazide Spironolactone also antagonizes the androgen receptor; this cross-reactivity can cause impotence and gynecomastia in men but confers therapeutic advantage in women with acne and hirsutism; eplerenone has less anti-androgenic activity Used to treat hypokalemic alkalotic states secondary to mineralocorticoid excess in heart failure, hepatic failure, and other disease states associated with diminished aldosterone metabolism Both spironolactone and eplerenone reduce mortality in patients with heart failure; the mechanism may be related to inhibition of cardiac fibrosis resulting from a paracrine aldosterone-signaling pathway
Amiloride Triamterene	Hypertension Liddle syndrome	*Diseases of the hematopoietic system, nephrotoxicity (triamterene), hyperkalemic metabolic acidosis* Orthostatic hypotension, hyperkalemia, dyspepsia, headache	Same as spironolactone	Amiloride and triamterene are drugs of choice for treatment of Liddle syndrome, a rare, Mendelian form of hypertension resulting from gain-of-function mutations in the β or γ subunit of the ENaC sodium channel

21

Pharmacology of Vascular Tone

Deborah Yeh Chong and Thomas Michel

INTRODUCTION

In combination with cardiac output, **vascular tone** (i.e., the degree of contraction of vascular smooth muscle) determines the adequacy of perfusion of the tissues of the body. The importance of vascular tone is underscored by the wide spectrum of disease states—ranging from angina pectoris to hypertension to Raynaud's phenomenon to migraine headaches—that are associated with dysregulated vascular tone. As the major factors that govern the regulation of blood vessel diameter have become understood at the molecular level, it has become apparent that a complex array of mechanisms is required to maintain proper vascular tone in the face of diverse stimuli. Pharmacologic strategies for intervention in these regulatory pathways have already yielded many successful therapies for disorders of vascular tone, and provide hope that, in the future, even better therapies will be available to manage the multiple types of vascular disorders.

Case

GF, a 63-year-old man with a history of hypertension, diabetes, and hypercholesterolemia, begins to develop episodes of chest pain on exertion. One week after his first episode, a bout of chest pain occurs while he is mowing the lawn. Twenty minutes after the onset of this pain, GF takes two of his wife's sublingual nitroglycerin tablets. Within a few minutes, he feels much better. GF feels so well that he decides to take one of the sildenafil (Viagra®) pills that a friend had previously offered to him. A few minutes after taking sildenafil, he feels flushed, develops a throbbing headache, and feels his heart racing. Upon standing, GF feels lightheaded and faints. He is taken immediately to the emergency department, where he is found to have severe hypotension. He is quickly placed in a supine position with his legs raised, and monitored until he regains consciousness. The physician considers administering an α-adrenergic agonist, such as phenylephrine, but the rapid amelioration of GF's hypotension after he is placed in a supine position suggests that pharmacologic intervention is unnecessary. After GF recovers, his physician discusses with him the dangers of taking medications without a prescription and, specifically, the risk of concurrent administration of organic nitrates and sildenafil.

QUESTIONS

■ **1.** What is the mechanism by which sublingual nitroglycerin acts so quickly to relieve chest pain?

■ **2.** What are the common adverse effects of nitroglycerin?

■ **3.** How can sildenafil and organic nitrates interact to precipitate severe hypotension?

■ **4.** Are nonnitrate antihypertensives, such as calcium channel blockers, also contraindicated for men taking sildenafil? How can the mechanisms of action of drugs be used to predict possible drug-drug interactions or lack of interactions?

PHYSIOLOGY OF VASCULAR SMOOTH MUSCLE CONTRACTION AND RELAXATION

Vascular tone is a key regulator of tissue perfusion, which determines whether tissues receive sufficient O_2 and nutrients to meet their demands. The delicate balance between O_2 supply and demand is critical for the function of all tissues, especially for the myocardium. Vascular tone is an important determinant of both myocardial O_2 supply and demand. Myocardial O_2 supply depends on the tone of the coronary arteries, while myocardial O_2 demand depends on the tone of both the systemic arterioles (resistance vessels) and veins (capacitance vessels).

VASCULAR RESISTANCE AND CAPACITANCE

The tone of the arterial portion of the circulation and the tone of the venous portion of the circulation play important yet distinctive roles in modulating the balance of myocardial O_2 demand. The major determinants of myocardial O_2 demand are heart rate, contractility, and ventricular wall stress. Wall stress can be expressed as:

$$\sigma = (P \times r)/2h \qquad \text{Equation 21-1}$$

where σ is wall stress, P is ventricular pressure, r is ventricular chamber radius, and h is ventricular wall thickness. Systolic and diastolic ventricular wall stresses are influenced by systemic arteriolar and venous tone, respectively. Arteriolar tone directly controls **systemic vascular resistance** and, thus, arterial blood pressure:

$$MAP = SVR \times CO \qquad \text{Equation 21-2}$$

where *MAP* is mean arterial pressure, *SVR* is systemic vascular resistance, and *CO* is cardiac output. During systole, the intraventricular pressure must exceed the arterial pressure in order for blood to be ejected. **Afterload**—defined as systolic ventricular wall stress—is equivalent to the resistance that the ventricle must overcome to eject its contents. Assuming that there is no obstruction between the ventricle and the aorta, systolic arterial blood pressure thus approximates systolic ventricular wall stress (i.e., afterload).

Although the *resistance* of the arterial circulation is the most important parameter determined by arteriolar tone, the *capacitance* of the venous circulation is the most important parameter determined by venous tone. **Venous capacitance,** in turn, regulates the volume of blood returning to the heart, which is a major determinant of the end-diastolic volume of the heart. **Preload**—defined as end-diastolic ventricular wall stress—is equivalent to the stretch on the ventricular fibers just before contraction, which is approximated by end-diastolic volume or pressure. Venous tone, thus, determines the end-diastolic ventricular wall stress (i.e., preload). Figure 21-1 and Table 21-1 summarize the dependence of myocardial O_2 supply and demand on the tone of the coronary arteries, systemic arterioles, and capacitance veins, and provide a simplified view of how modulating the tone of these different types of vessels could alter important parameters of cardiovascular physiology. (See Chapter 24, Integrative Cardiovascular Pharmacology: Hypertension, Ischemic Heart Disease, and Heart Failure, for a diagram of the overall determinants of myocardial O_2 supply and demand.)

Myocardial O_2 supply and demand must be balanced carefully to ensure adequate tissue perfusion. **Ischemia** occurs when decreased perfusion leads to an O_2 deficit. (In contrast, **hypoxia** occurs when there is O_2 deprivation despite adequate perfusion.) **Myocardial ischemia** occurs when myocardial O_2 supply and demand are imbalanced, such that coronary blood flow cannot fully meet the O_2 needs of the heart. Although there are many potential causes of O_2 supply:demand imbalance, most causes of myocardial ischemia—especially coronary artery disease—involve some aspect of abnormal vascular tone. For further discussion of the pathophysiology of myocardial ischemia and other diseases of abnormal vascular tone, see Chapter 24.

Chest pain, termed **angina pectoris,** is a common, although not always present, symptom of myocardial ischemia. Given GF's risk factors for coronary artery disease (i.e., diabetes, hypertension, hypercholesterolemia, age, and male gender) and his symptoms of exertional chest pain when mowing the lawn, it is likely that his chest pain was a manifestation of angina pectoris. A common treatment for angina pectoris is **nitroglycerin,** an agent that decreases vascular tone (see below) and thereby ameliorates the mismatch between myocardial O_2 supply and demand. Indeed, GF did experience relief of his chest pain after taking his wife's nitroglycerin. To understand better how nitroglycerin and other modulators of vascular tone act, it is essential to appreciate the molecular mechanisms that regulate vascular smooth muscle contraction and relaxation.

VASCULAR SMOOTH MUSCLE CONTRACTION AND RELAXATION

Regulators of vascular tone act by influencing the actin–myosin contractile apparatus of vascular smooth muscle cells. As in other muscle cells, the actin–myosin interaction

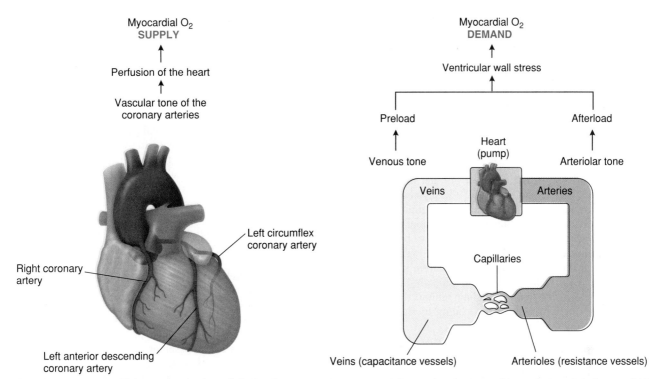

Figure 21-1. Myocardial oxygen supply and demand. Myocardial O₂ supply **(left panel)** is determined by perfusion of the heart, which is determined by the vascular tone of the coronary arteries (among other factors). The major coronary arteries are depicted on the epicardial surface of the heart. Myocardial O₂ demand **(right panel)** is determined by ventricular wall stress, which is a function of both preload (venous tone) and afterload (arteriolar tone). Venous tone determines myocardial O₂ demand by regulating the amount of blood returning to the heart, which, in turn, determines the end-diastolic ventricular wall stress. Arteriolar tone determines myocardial O₂ demand by regulating systemic vascular resistance (SVR), the pressure against which the heart must contract. Arteriolar tone, therefore, determines systolic ventricular wall stress.

leads to contraction and is regulated by the intracellular calcium (Ca^{2+}) concentration (Fig. 21-2). A steep transmembrane gradient of Ca^{2+} concentration ($[Ca^{2+}]_{extracellular} = 2 \times 10^{-3}$ M; $[Ca^{2+}]_{intracellular} = 10^{-7}$ M) is maintained by the relative impermeability of the plasma membrane to Ca^{2+} ions and by membrane pumps that actively remove Ca^{2+}

from the cytoplasm. Stimulation of vascular smooth muscle cells can increase the cytoplasmic Ca^{2+} concentration by two mechanisms. First, Ca^{2+} can enter the cell by way of **voltage-gated Ca^{2+}-selective channels** in the sarcolemma. Second, increases in cytoplasmic $[Ca^{2+}]$ can be elicited by the release of intracellular Ca^{2+} from the sarcoplasmic retic-

TABLE 21-1	Relationship Between Vascular Tone and Parameters of Cardiovascular Physiology
VESSEL TYPE	**PARAMETER OF CARDIOVASCULAR PHYSIOLOGY**
Coronary arteries	Myocardial O₂ supply
Arterioles	Afterload
	Myocardial O₂ demand
	Regional myocardial perfusion
Capacitance veins	Venous pooling
	Preload
	Myocardial O₂ demand

In a simplified model, the effects of pharmacologic agents on cardiovascular physiology can be predicted based on the vessel type on which the agents act. Coronary artery dilators increase myocardial O₂ supply. Arteriolar dilators decrease afterload, while venodilators decrease preload; both arteriolar dilators and venodilators decrease myocardial O₂ demand.

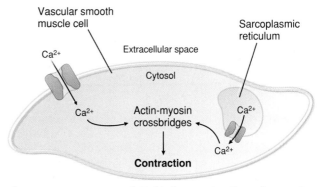

Figure 21-2. Sources of Ca^{2+} for contraction of vascular smooth muscle cells. The cytosolic concentration of Ca^{2+} is low (10^{-7} M), while the extracellular and sarcoplasmic reticulum concentrations of Ca^{2+} are high (2×10^{-3} M). Ca^{2+} can enter the vascular smooth muscle cell cytoplasm from the extracellular space or from the sarcoplasmic reticulum via Ca^{2+}-selective channels. The increased concentration of Ca^{2+} in the cytosol initiates contraction by promoting the formation of actin–myosin cross-bridges.

ulum. **Vasoconstriction** (i.e., contraction of vascular smooth muscle) is commonly initiated by the opening of **voltage-gated L-type Ca^{2+} channels** in the sarcolemma during plasma membrane depolarization. The open Ca^{2+} channels mediate Ca^{2+} flux into the cytoplasm and activation of cytoplasmic calmodulin (CaM). The Ca^{2+} − CaM complex binds to and activates **myosin light chain kinase,** which phosphorylates myosin-II light chains. When the light chain is phosphorylated, the myosin head can interact with an actin filament, leading to smooth muscle contraction (Fig. 21-3, left panel).

Vasodilation (i.e., relaxation of vascular smooth muscle) occurs upon dephosphorylation of the myosin light chain. Dephosphorylation is potentiated when **guanylyl cyclase** (discussed below) is activated inside the smooth muscle cell. Activated guanylyl cyclase increases the production of **cyclic guanosine 3′5′-monophosphate (cGMP).** The cGMP stimulates **cGMP-dependent protein kinase,** which then activates **myosin light chain phosphatase.** Dephosphorylation of the myosin light chain inhibits the interaction of the myosin head with actin, leading to smooth muscle relaxation (Fig. 21-3, right panel).

REGULATION OF VASCULAR TONE

Vascular tone is governed by a wide variety of mechanisms. Recent research has highlighted the importance of interactions between vascular endothelial cells and vascular smooth muscle cells in the control of vascular tone. The autonomic nervous system and a number of neurohormonal mediators also control vascular smooth muscle contraction and relaxation. Many of these physiologic mechanisms provide the basis for current drug discovery research.

Vascular Endothelium

Research in the past 2 decades has elucidated several signaling modes in the vascular endothelium to control vascular tone. Endothelial cells elaborate many signaling mediators and alter the expression of many genes in response to diverse stimuli. Two of the most pharmacologically relevant targets, nitric oxide and endothelin, are discussed here.

Nitric Oxide

The obligatory role of endothelial cells in regulating vascular tone was first recognized with the observation that acetylcholine causes vasoconstriction when applied directly to de-endothelialized blood vessels, but causes vasodilation when applied to normally endothelialized vessels (Fig. 21-4). It was hypothesized that muscarinic cholinergic stimulation of the endothelium induces the production of a relaxant molecule in the endothelial cell and that this molecule then diffuses to subjacent vascular smooth muscle cells to activate guanylyl cyclase. The putative vasodilatory compound was termed **endothelial-derived relaxing factor,** or **EDRF.**

Before the molecular identity of EDRF was determined to be nitric oxide (NO), **nitroglycerin**—an organic nitrate commonly prescribed for angina pectoris—was known to be metabolized in the body to form NO, and NO was known to cause relaxation of vascular smooth muscle. Based on these findings, it was hypothesized and later confirmed that the EDRF released from endothelial cells is NO, a gas that reacts with a wide range of biomolecules to elicit cellular responses.

Although acetylcholine was the first ligand to be identified that promotes endothelial-cell synthesis of NO, a number of other mediators have since been described. Shear stress, acetylcholine, histamine, bradykinin, sphingosine 1-phosphate, serotonin, substance P, and ATP can all elicit increased NO synthesis by vascular endothelial cells. NO is synthesized by a family of Ca^{2+}-CaM–activated NO synthases. The **endothelial isoform of nitric oxide synthase (eNOS)** is responsible for endothelial-cell NO synthesis; this enzyme plays a critical role in controlling vascular tone and platelet aggregation. The importance of NO in regulating

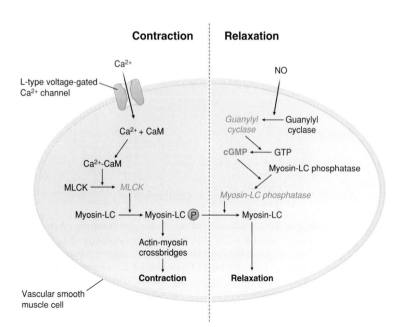

Figure 21-3. Mechanism of vascular smooth muscle cell contraction and relaxation. Vascular smooth muscle cell contraction and relaxation are controlled by the coordinated action of several intracellular signaling mediators. Ca^{2+} entry through L-type voltage-gated Ca^{2+} channels **(left panel)** is the initial stimulus for contraction. Ca^{2+} entry into the cell activates calmodulin (CaM). The Ca^{2+} − CaM complex activates myosin light chain kinase (MLCK) to phosphorylate myosin light chain (Myosin-LC). The phosphorylated myosin-LC interacts with actin to form actin–myosin cross-bridges, a process that initiates vascular smooth muscle cell contraction. Relaxation **(right panel)** is a coordinated series of steps that act to dephosphorylate (and hence inactivate) myosin-LC. Nitric oxide (NO) diffuses into the cell and activates guanylyl cyclase. The activated guanylyl cyclase catalyzes the conversion of guanosine triphosphate (GTP) to guanosine 3′,5′-cyclic monophosphate (cGMP). cGMP activates myosin-LC phosphatase, which dephosphorylates myosin light chain, preventing actin–myosin cross-bridge formation. As a result, the vascular smooth muscle cell relaxes. The active form of each enzyme is italicized and *blue*.

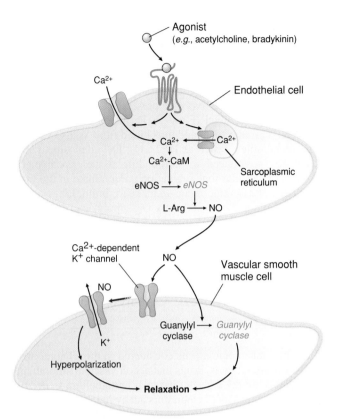

Figure 21-4. Endothelial regulation of nitric oxide-mediated vascular smooth muscle relaxation. Endothelial-cell production of nitric oxide (NO) controls the extent of vascular smooth muscle cell relaxation. Production of NO is stimulated by agonists such as acetylcholine or bradykinin. Stimulation of receptors by these agonists activates Ca^{2+} second messenger systems and promotes direct entry of Ca^{2+} into the cytosol. The increased cytosolic Ca^{2+} activates a Ca^{2+}-calmodulin complex that stimulates endothelial nitric oxide synthase (eNOS), an enzyme that catalyzes the formation of NO from L-arginine (L-Arg, an amino acid). NO diffuses from the endothelial cell into subjacent vascular smooth muscle cells, where it activates guanylyl cyclase, promoting smooth muscle cell relaxation (see Fig. 21-3). NO can also directly activate Ca^{2+}-dependent K^+ channels. This parallel signaling pathway contributes to relaxation by hyperpolarizing the smooth muscle cell. The active form of each enzyme is italicized and *blue*.

vascular tone is underscored by the observation that eNOS-deficient mice are hypertensive.

Recent evidence suggests that NO may effect vasodilation not only by activating guanylyl cyclase, but also by activating Ca^{2+}-dependent K^+ channels in vascular smooth muscle cells (Fig. 21-4). NO appears to activate these K^+ channels directly via a guanylyl cyclase-independent mechanism, leading to hyperpolarization of the cells and, subsequently, to vasodilation. (See below for a further explanation of how opening K^+ channels leads to hyperpolarization and vasodilation.)

Endothelin

Endothelin is a 21-amino acid vasoconstrictor peptide. It is the most potent endogenous vasoconstrictor yet discovered. Endothelin can be considered a functional ''mirror-image''

of NO: it is a potent endothelium-derived vasoconstrictor, while NO is a potent endothelium-derived vasodilator. In addition to its effects on the vasculature, endothelin has positive inotropic and chronotropic actions on the heart and it contributes to remodeling within the cardiovascular system. Proposed mechanisms of endothelin-induced remodeling include neointimal proliferation and increased collagen deposition leading to fibrosis. Endothelin also plays an important role in the lungs, kidneys, and brain. Three isoforms of endothelin—**ET-1, ET-2,** and **ET-3**—have been identified. ET-1—the isoform mainly involved in cardiovascular actions—is produced by endothelial cells (and vascular smooth muscle cells under inflammatory conditions) and it appears to act locally in a paracrine or autocrine fashion. The local ET-1 concentration within the vascular wall is more than 100 times greater than that in the circulation, because ET-1 is secreted chiefly on the basal side of endothelial cells (Fig. 21-5).

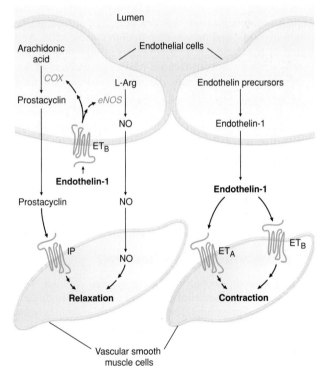

Figure 21-5. Effects of endothelin on the blood vessel wall. Endothelin mediates both contraction and relaxation of vascular smooth muscle cells. Endothelin precursors in endothelial cells are processed to endothelin-1. Endothelin-1 is secreted on the basal side of the endothelial cell, where it interacts with ET_A and ET_B receptors present on vascular smooth muscle cells. Activation of these receptors stimulates contraction by incompletely understood mechanisms. ET_B receptors are also expressed on endothelial cells. Endothelial cell ET_B activation stimulates cyclooxygenase (COX), which catalyzes the formation of prostacyclin from arachidonic acid. Prostacyclin diffuses from the endothelial cell to the vascular smooth muscle cell membrane, where it binds to and activates the isoprostanoid (IP) receptor. ET_B activation also stimulates endothelial nitric oxide synthase (eNOS), which catalyzes the formation of NO from arginine (L-Arg). Both prostacyclin and NO stimulate vascular smooth muscle cell relaxation.

Endothelin precursors are proteolytically processed in two steps to generate the mature active peptides. First, **preproendothelin** is cleaved into **big endothelin.** Second, big endothelin is cleaved by **endothelin-converting enzyme** into endothelin. There are two endothelin receptor subtypes, ET_A and ET_B. Both ET_A and ET_B are G protein-coupled receptors whose effectors likely involve phospholipase C-modulated pathways. ET-1 binds to ET_A receptors on vascular smooth muscle cells as well as ET_B receptors on both endothelial cells and vascular smooth muscle cells. ET_A receptors on vascular smooth muscle cells mediate vasoconstriction. ET_B receptors are located predominantly on vascular endothelial cells, where they mediate vasodilation via the release of prostacyclin and NO. ET_B receptors are also found on vascular smooth muscle cells, where they mediate vasoconstriction.

Autonomic Nervous System

Autonomic innervation is an important determinant of vascular tone. The sympathetic nervous system has a significant influence on vascular tone. The firing of certain sympathetic postganglionic neurons releases norepinephrine from nerve terminals that end on vascular smooth muscle cells. Activation of α_1-adrenergic receptors on vascular smooth muscle cells causes vasoconstriction, whereas activation of β_2-adrenergic receptors on vascular smooth muscle cells induces vasodilation. The effect of norepinephrine at α_1-adrenergic receptors is typically greater than its effect at β_2-adrenergic receptors, especially in organs that receive decreased blood flow during "fight or flight" responses (i.e., skin and viscera). Thus, the net effect of norepinephrine on these vascular beds is typically vasoconstrictive. In contrast, because blood vessels are not innervated by parasympathetic fibers, the parasympathetic nervous system has little influence on vascular tone.

Neurohormonal Mechanisms

Many neurohormonal mediators act on vascular smooth muscle cells, endothelial cells, and neurons to regulate vascular tone. For example, circulating catecholamines from the adrenal gland (i.e., epinephrine) can influence vascular tone via α_1-adrenergic and β_2-adrenergic receptors on vascular smooth muscle cells: as noted above, stimulation of α_1-adrenergic receptors leads to vasoconstriction, while stimulation of β_2-adrenergic receptors leads to vasodilation. Other examples of neurohormonal mediators include angiotensin II, which stimulates the angiotensin II receptor subtype 1 (AT_1) to vasoconstrict arterioles and increase intravascular volume; aldosterone, which acts via the mineralocorticoid receptor to increase intravascular volume; natriuretic peptides, which promote renal natriuresis (sodium excretion) in situations of volume overload; and antidiuretic hormone/arginine vasopressin, which stimulates arteriolar V_1 receptors to constrict arterioles and activates renal V_2 receptors to increase intravascular volume. These mediators, which also have important roles in volume regulation, are all discussed in greater detail in Chapter 20, Pharmacology of Volume Regulation.

Local Mechanisms

A panoply of local control mechanisms also modulate vascular tone. Autoregulation is a homeostatic mechanism in which vascular smooth muscle cells respond to increases or decreases in perfusion pressure by vasoconstriction or vasodilation, respectively, to preserve blood flow at a relatively constant level (Flow = Perfusion Pressure / Resistance). Vascular tone, and thus blood flow, is also governed by metabolites—such as H^+, CO_2, O_2, adenosine, lactate, and K^+—produced in surrounding tissue. Local mechanisms of vascular tone regulation predominate in the vascular beds of essential organs (e.g., heart, brain, lung, kidney), so that blood flow, and thus O_2 supply, can be adjusted quickly to meet the demands of local metabolism in these organs.

PHARMACOLOGIC CLASSES AND AGENTS

The pharmacologic agents considered in this chapter are all **vasodilators,** that is, drugs that act on vascular smooth muscle and/or on the adjacent vascular endothelium to decrease vascular tone. Most vasodilators act by reducing the contractility of actin–myosin complexes in vascular smooth muscle cells. There are a number of categories of vasodilators (Fig. 21-6). Pharmacologic donors of NO—such as the **organic nitrates** and **sodium nitroprusside**—cause vasodilation by activating guanylyl cyclase and thereby increasing the dephosphorylation of myosin light chains. Acting on the same molecular pathway, **cGMP phosphodiesterase type V (PDE5) inhibitors** prevent cGMP hydrolysis and thereby promote myosin light chain dephosphorylation, especially in smooth muscle of the corpus cavernosum. **Ca^{2+} channel blockers** cause vasodilation by reducing intracellular Ca^{2+} concentrations. **K^+ channel openers** induce vasodilation by opening ATP-sensitive K^+ channels; the resulting hyperpolarization of the cells prevents activation of the voltage-gated Ca^{2+} channels necessary for Ca^{2+} influx and vascular smooth muscle contraction. **Endothelin receptor antagonists** block endothelin-mediated vasoconstriction. **α_1-Adrenergic antagonists** inhibit the vasoconstrictive action of endogenous epinephrine and norepinephrine. **ACE inhibitors** and **angiotensin II receptor subtype 1 (AT_1) antagonists** inhibit the vasoconstrictive effects of endogenous angiotensin II, either by inhibiting angiotensin II formation (ACE inhibitors) or by blocking angiotensin II action at its cognate receptor (AT_1 antagonists). **Hydralazine** and **β-adrenergic antagonists** also modulate vascular tone. These pharmacologic classes and agents are discussed below.

ORGANIC NITRATES AND SODIUM NITROPRUSSIDE

Organic nitrates represent one of the oldest cardiac therapies still in use. Indeed, **glyceryl trinitrate**—more commonly termed **nitroglycerin (NTG)**—was first employed for relief of anginal symptoms over 100 years ago. Indications for the use of organic nitrates now include not only the classic

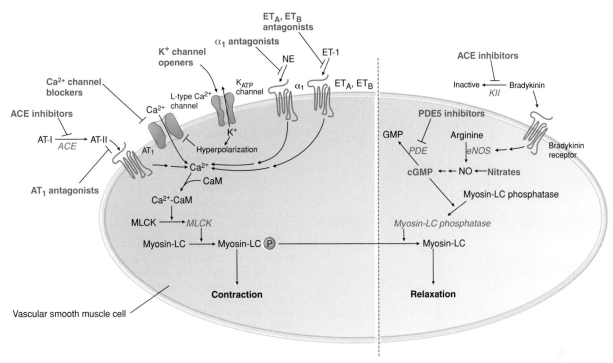

Figure 21-6. Sites of action of vasodilators. Vasodilators act at several sites in the vascular smooth muscle cell. **Left panel:** Ca²⁺ channel blockers and K⁺ channel openers inhibit the entry of Ca²⁺ into vascular smooth muscle cells by decreasing activation of L-type Ca²⁺ channels. ACE inhibitors, AT₁ antagonists, α₁-antagonists, and endothelin receptor (ETₐ, ET_B) antagonists all decrease intracellular Ca²⁺ signaling. The decreased cytosolic Ca²⁺ results in less vascular smooth muscle cell contraction, and, hence, in relaxation. **Right panel:** ACE inhibitors inhibit kininase II (KII), leading to increased levels of bradykinin. Nitrates release NO. Sildenafil inhibits phosphodiesterase (PDE). These agents all cause an increase in cGMP, an effect that promotes vascular smooth muscle relaxation. The active form of each enzyme is italicized and *blue*. α₁, α₁-adrenergic receptor. ACE, angiotensin converting enzyme. AT-I, angiotensin I. AT-II, angiotensin II. AT₁, angiotensin II receptor. CaM, calmodulin. eNOS, endothelial nitric oxide synthase. ET-1, endothelin-1. MLCK, myosin light chain kinase. Myosin-LC, myosin light chain.

indication, stable angina pectoris, but also unstable angina, acute myocardial infarction, hypertension, and acute and chronic heart failure (see Chapter 24).

Mechanism of Action

Within the body, organic nitrates are chemically reduced to release NO, a gas that can dissolve in biological fluids and in cellular membranes. NO may react directly with diverse biomolecules, including the heme moiety in guanylyl cyclase. Nitric oxide can also undergo chemical transformations to form S-nitrosothiol groups with cysteine (sulfhydryl) residues in proteins or with low-molecular–weight intracellular thiols such as glutathione. As described in detail above, NO is an endogenous signaling molecule that causes vascular smooth muscle relaxation. The various organic nitrates likely give rise to NO by different chemical and biochemical mechanisms, but the details of organic nitrate metabolism remain incompletely understood. Both extracellular and intracellular reducing agents (e.g., thiol groups) have been implicated (Fig. 21-7). The metabolism of organic nitrates to NO can apparently be catalyzed in tissues by specific enzymes such as mitochondrial aldehyde dehydrogenase; it has been hypothesized that the enzymatic release of organic nitrates allows the "targeting" of their effects to specific vascular tissues. Alternatively, some pathways for tissue-specific nitrate metabolism may be nonenzymatic (e.g., related to thiol pools). Regardless, it is clear that, *although*

NO can dilate both arteries and veins, venous dilation predominates at therapeutic doses. NO-induced venodilation increases venous capacitance, leading to a decrease in the return of blood to the right side of the heart and, consequently, to decreased right ventricular and left ventricular end-diastolic pressure and volume. This decrease in preload reduces myocardial O₂ demand. At higher concentrations of organic nitrates, arterial vasodilation may also occur. In the absence of reflex tachycardia, arterial vasodilation leads to a decrease in systemic vascular resistance, which leads to a decrease in systolic wall stress (afterload) and a decrease in myocardial O₂ demand.

In the coronary circulation, NTG dilates predominantly the large epicardial arteries (Fig. 21-8). NTG has minimal effects on the coronary resistance vessels (i.e., the coronary arterioles). This preferential dilation of the large epicardial arteries over the smaller coronary arterioles prevents the development of the **coronary steal phenomenon,** which is often encountered with agents such as **dipyridamole** (see Chapter 22, Pharmacology of Hemostasis and Thrombosis) that produce intense dilation of the coronary resistance vessels. The degree to which nitrate-mediated vasodilation of the large epicardial arteries is responsible for the beneficial effects of nitrates in patients with angina remains unclear, however. The chronic myocardial O₂ deficit in patients with coronary artery disease may, by an autoregulatory mechanism, cause maximal dilation of the coronary arteries, such that vasodilators can provide no further increase in coronary

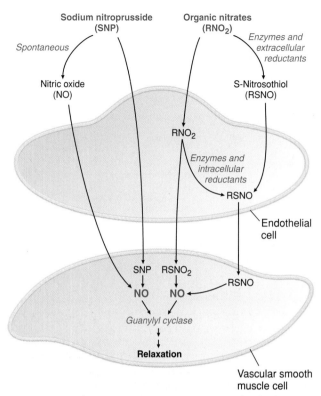

Figure 21-7. Biotransformation of organic nitrates and sodium nitroprusside. Organic nitrates and sodium nitroprusside increase local levels of NO by different mechanisms. Organic nitrates have the chemical structure RNO_2. The nitro group is reduced to form NO in the presence of specific enzymes and extracellular and/or intracellular reductants (e.g., thiols). In comparison, sodium nitroprusside releases NO spontaneously without enzymatic aid. Both agents effect relaxation via the formation of NO. However, the requirement of organic nitrates for specific cellular enzymes and/or reductants may result in tissue selectivity. Because sodium nitroprusside spontaneously converts to NO, it does not dilate vascular beds selectively.

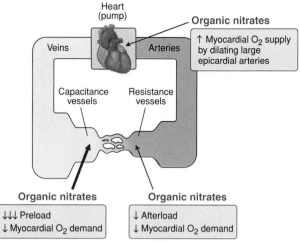

Figure 21-8. Sites of action of organic nitrates. Organic nitrates exert the majority of their vasodilator action on venous capacitance vessels. This selectivity results in greatly decreased preload, with resulting decreased myocardial O_2 demand. Organic nitrates also mildly dilate arteriolar resistance vessels, with resulting decreased afterload and decreased myocardial O_2 demand. Myocardial O_2 supply is mildly increased by dilation of large epicardial arteries.

blood flow. In addition, stiffened, calcific atherosclerotic coronary arteries may remain noncompliant, even in the face of coronary artery vasodilators.

Clinically, the administration of doses of organic nitrates sufficient to vasodilate the large epicardial arteries can be dangerous because such doses may also induce excessive peripheral arteriolar vasodilation and refractory hypotension. The excessive decrease in mean arterial pressure can be manifested as dizziness, lightheadedness, and occasionally, overt syncope, and can even lead to myocardial ischemia. Because coronary perfusion depends on the pressure gradient between the aorta and the endocardium during diastole, a marked decrease in diastolic aortic pressure can lead to an insufficient supply of O_2 to the heart. Moreover, systemic hypotension can lead to **reflex tachycardia,** which also decreases myocardial O_2 supply by shortening diastole and, thus, myocardial perfusion time. As noted above, reflex tachycardia can also harm the delicate myocardial O_2 supply: demand balance by increasing myocardial O_2 consumption. Reflex tachycardia is typically observed when baroreceptors in the aortic arch and carotid sinuses sense a decrease in blood pressure. In patients with overt heart failure, however,

reflex tachycardia is rare. Thus, nitrates can often be used to decrease pulmonary congestion in patients with heart failure (by effecting venodilation and decreasing end-diastolic pressure), without eliciting significant reflex tachycardia. Several important adverse effects of nitrates are the result of excessive vasodilation; these include flushing, caused by vasodilation of cutaneous vascular beds, and headache, caused by vasodilation of cerebral arteries.

Several different preparations of organic nitrates are currently available. The most commonly used organic nitrates include **NTG, isosorbide dinitrate,** and **isosorbide 5-mononitrate** (Fig. 21-9). Although these organic nitrates share a common mechanism of action, they differ in their routes of administration and pharmacokinetics, leading to important differences in their therapeutic utility in a variety of clinical settings.

Sodium nitroprusside is a nitrate compound that consists of a nitroso group, five cyanide groups, and an iron atom (Fig. 21-10A). As with the organic nitrates, sodium nitroprusside effects vasodilation by release of NO. Unlike the organic nitrates, however, sodium nitroprusside appears to liberate NO primarily through a nonenzymatic process (Fig. 21-7). As a result of this nonenzymatic conversion to NO, sodium nitroprusside's action does not appear to be targeted to specific types of vessels and, consequently, the drug dilates both arteries and veins.

Sodium nitroprusside is used intravenously for potent hemodynamic control in hypertensive emergencies and severe cardiac failure. Because of its rapid onset of action, short duration of action, and high efficacy, sodium nitroprusside must be infused with continuous blood pressure monitoring and careful titration of drug dose to drug effect. Sodium nitroprusside spontaneously decomposes to liberate NO and cyanide (Fig. 21-10B). The cyanide is then converted to thiocyanate in the liver, and the thiocyanate is excreted by the kidneys. Excessive cyanide accumulation can lead to acid-base disturbances, cardiac arrhythmias, and even death. Thiocyanate toxicity can also occur in patients with impaired

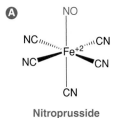

Nitroglycerin
(Glyceryl trinitrate)

Glyceryl 1,2-dinitrate   Glyceryl 1,3-dinitrate

Isosorbide dinitrate

Isosorbide 2-mononitrate   Isosorbide 5-mononitrate

Figure 21-9. Chemical structures and metabolism of nitroglycerin and isosorbide dinitrate. Nitroglycerin and isosorbide dinitrate are biologically active nitrates that are metabolized into active molecules with longer half-lives than their parent compounds. Nitroglycerin is denitrated into glyceryl 1,2-dinitrate and glyceryl 1,3-dinitrate; these active metabolites have a half-life of approximately 40 minutes. Isosorbide dinitrate is denitrated into isosorbide 2-mononitrate and isosorbide 5-mononitrate; these active metabolites have half-lives of 2 and 4 hours, respectively.

renal function, causing disorientation, psychosis, muscle spasms, and convulsions.

Nitric oxide is a gas (not to be confused with nitrous oxide, the anesthetic gas), and it can be administered by inhalation. The effects of inhaled NO are mostly restricted to the pulmonary vasculature because the free NO in the blood is rapidly inactivated, principally by binding to the heme moiety of hemoglobin. The NO gas that reaches the pulmonary vascular bed promotes vasodilation, and has been shown to ameliorate pulmonary hypertension. Inhaled NO has its clearest therapeutic application in the treatment of primary pulmonary hypertension of the newborn; the therapeutic role of inhaled NO in adults with diseases associated with pulmonary hypertension remains an active area of investigation.

Pharmacokinetics

The pharmacokinetics of the different nitrate preparations and formulations provide a basis for the preferential use of

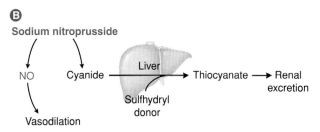

Figure 21-10. Chemical structure and metabolism of sodium nitroprusside. A. Sodium nitroprusside is a complex of iron, cyanide (CN), and a nitroso (NO) group. **B.** Sodium nitroprusside spontaneously decomposes to release NO and cyanide. NO effects vasodilation; cyanide is metabolized in the liver to thiocyanate, which undergoes renal excretion. Cyanide toxicity can result upon prolonged administration of the drug or in the presence of renal insufficiency.

specific agents and dosage forms in certain settings. For example, the rapid onset of action of sublingual nitrate preparations is desirable for rapid relief of acute anginal attacks, while longer-acting nitrates are more valuable for angina prophylaxis in the long-term management of coronary artery disease. *Orally administered* NTG and isosorbide dinitrate have low bioavailability because organic nitrate reductases in the liver rapidly metabolize these drugs. Both to circumvent the first-pass effect and to attain therapeutic blood levels within minutes, NTG or isosorbide dinitrate can be administered *sublingually. Intravenous* administration of NTG is indicated when continuous titration of drug action is necessary; for example, in the treatment of unstable angina or acute heart failure. Slow-release *transdermal* and *buccal* preparations of NTG provide therapeutic steady-state levels of NTG that can be useful for angina prevention in patients with stable coronary artery disease.

NTG has a short half-life (approximately 5 minutes), after which it is denitrated into biologically active glyceryl dinitrate metabolites that have longer half-lives (approximately 40 minutes) (Fig. 21-9). Equivalent doses of **isosorbide dinitrate** can be more effective than NTG, because isosorbide dinitrate has a longer half-life (about 1 hour). The partially denitrated metabolites of isosorbide dinitrate—isosorbide 2-mononitrate and isosorbide 5-mononitrate—have even longer half-lives (up to 2 and 4 hours, respectively) (Fig. 21-9). **Isosorbide 5-mononitrate** has itself become a popular therapeutic agent, not only because it has prolonged therapeutic effects, but also because it is well absorbed from the gastrointestinal tract and is not susceptible to extensive first-pass metabolism in the liver. The bioavailability of orally administered isosorbide 5-mononitrate is nearly 100%, allowing isosorbide 5-mononitrate to be significantly more effective than equivalent amounts of isosorbide dinitrate. After denitration, organic nitrates are typically glucuronidated in the liver and excreted renally.

Pharmacologic Tolerance

The desirable effects of nitrates can, unfortunately, be offset by compensatory sympathetic nervous system responses (e.g., a reflex increase in sympathetic vascular tone) and compensatory renal responses (e.g., increased salt and water retention). In addition to these **physiologic tolerance** mechanisms, **pharmacologic tolerance** to organic nitrates is an important and clinically relevant phenomenon that significantly limits the efficacy of this class of vasodilators. Pharmacologic tolerance was first documented in munitions workers exposed to volatile organic nitrates in the workplace. These workers suffered severe headaches at the start of the work week, but as the week progressed, the headaches tended to disappear and remain absent for the rest of the week. Upon returning to work after a weekend without nitrate exposure, however, the headaches recurred. These ''Monday morning headaches'' were initially ascribed to weekend intemperance, but it later became clear that the vasodilatory effects of NTG were responsible. Development of tolerance to NTG as the work week progressed allowed relief from the headaches, and loss of tolerance to NTG over the weekend allowed the headaches to recur upon the workers' return to work.

Although tolerance to adverse effects such as headaches can be desirable, *tolerance to the antianginal effects of nitrates diminishes their clinical efficacy.* Tolerance to NTG does not appear to depend on the route of administration. Importantly, it is possible to minimize the development of tolerance by modulating the dosing schedule to include daily ''nitrate-free intervals.'' For transdermal NTG, simple removal of the NTG patch each night can minimize the development of tolerance. In cases of severe angina that require uninterrupted nitrate therapy to manage symptoms adequately, however, patients may experience rebound angina during periods that are completely nitrate-free. The pharmacokinetic properties of oral isosorbide 5-mononitrate make this preparation an attractive solution to the dilemma of balancing nitrate tolerance and anginal rebound: its high bioavailability and long half-life produce periods of high-therapeutic plasma concentrations followed by periods of low-therapeutic (rather than zero) nitrate levels. The examples of transdermal NTG and oral isosorbide 5-mononitrate illustrate how the pharmacokinetic properties of two mechanistically similar drugs can have significant impact on their therapeutic utility.

The cellular and molecular mechanisms that underlie the development of pharmacologic tolerance to organic nitrates remain unclear. There are currently two major hypotheses. First, the so-called classic (sulfhydryl) hypothesis suggests that tolerance results mainly from intracellular depletion of sulfhydryl-containing groups, such as glutathione and/or other forms of cysteine, that are involved in the formation of NO from organic nitrates (Fig. 21-8). According to the sulfhydryl hypothesis, tolerance could be attenuated or reversed by administering reduced thiol-containing compounds such as **N-acetylcysteine.** Second, the free-radical (superoxide) hypothesis posits that cellular tolerance results from the formation of **peroxynitrite,** a highly reactive metabolite of NO that appears to inhibit guanylyl cyclase. According to the superoxide hypothesis, tolerance could be attenuated or reversed by agents that inhibit free-radical

formation. Because the specific mechanisms of nitrate tolerance remain uncertain, the most effective means of preventing tolerance is the use of a dosing strategy that includes an interval of low plasma nitrate levels every day.

Effects of Nitrates in Addition to Vasodilation

The generation of NO from organic nitrates can cause relaxation of other types of smooth muscle—such as esophageal, bronchial, biliary, intestinal, and genitourinary—in addition to vascular smooth muscle. Indeed, *the ability of NTG to relieve the angina-like chest pain of esophageal spasm can occasionally result in a misdiagnosis of coronary artery disease.* These actions of nitrates on nonvascular smooth muscle are usually of limited clinical significance, however.

NO generated from organic nitrates functions as an antiplatelet agent as well as a vascular smooth muscle relaxant. NO-mediated increases in platelet cGMP inhibit platelet aggregation; together with the vasodilatory effect of the nitrates, this antiplatelet effect may decrease the likelihood of coronary artery thrombosis. Nitrate-induced inhibition of platelet aggregation may be especially important in the treatment of **rest angina** (i.e., chest pain that occurs spontaneously at rest), because rest angina frequently results from the formation of occlusive platelet aggregates at the site of atherosclerotic coronary artery lesions. Rest angina is also known as **unstable angina** because the thrombotic occlusions that cause rest angina can evolve into complete coronary occlusion and result in myocardial infarction (see Chapter 24).

Contraindications

As discussed above, nitrates are contraindicated in patients with hypotension. Nitrates are also contraindicated in patients with elevated intracranial pressure, because NO-mediated vasodilation of cerebral arteries could further elevate intracranial pressure. Nitrates are not advised for the anginal pain associated with hypertrophic obstructive cardiomyopathy because the obstruction can be worsened by nitrate-mediated preload reduction. Nitrates should also be used with caution in patients with diastolic heart failure, who depend on an elevated ventricular preload for optimal cardiac output. A more recently discovered contraindication to nitrate use is in patients taking sildenafil or another phosphodiesterase type V inhibitor for erectile dysfunction. GF's case provides an example of the deleterious effects of concurrently administered organic nitrates and sildenafil (see below).

PHOSPHODIESTERASE INHIBITORS

Phosphodiesterase inhibitors prevent the hydrolysis of cyclic nucleotides (cAMP, cGMP) to their monophosphate forms (5'-AMP, 5'-GMP). Certain phosphodiesterase inhibitors—such as **amrinone** and **milrinone**—are selective for the isoforms of phosphodiesterase found mainly in cardiac and vascular smooth muscle, and are discussed further in Chapter 19, Pharmacology of Cardiac Contractility.

Sildenafil is the prototype phosphodiesterase inhibitor that is highly selective for **cGMP phosphodiesterase type**

V (PDE5). PDE5 is expressed mainly in the smooth muscle of the corpus cavernosum, but is also expressed in the retina and in vascular smooth muscle cells. Phosphodiesterase V inhibitors are prescribed for **erectile dysfunction (ED),** a condition that is relatively common in men, such as GF, who have vascular disease. Other PDE5 inhibitors include **vardenafil** and **tadalafil,** which are similar to sildenafil in their therapeutic efficacy and adverse-effect profiles. Tadalafil has a longer time to onset of action and a more prolonged half-life than the other PDE5 inhibitors. In normal physiology, NO released from penile nerve terminals activates guanylyl cyclase in the smooth muscle of the corpus cavernosum, leading to increased intracellular cGMP concentration, smooth muscle relaxation, inflow of blood, and penile erection. Because they inhibit the cGMP phosphodiesterase in the corpus cavernosum smooth muscle, sildenafil, vardenafil and tadalafil can potentiate the effects of endogenous NO-cGMP signaling and thereby potentiate penile erection.

Although PDE5 is expressed predominantly in erectile smooth muscle tissue, it is also expressed in small amounts in the systemic and pulmonary vasculature. Therefore, although the principal actions of PDE5 inhibitors are localized to the corpus cavernosum, the drugs can also attenuate cGMP hydrolysis in the vasculature by inhibiting the small amounts of PDE5 present in systemic and pulmonary vascular beds. Indeed, high doses of sildenafil are efficacious in the treatment of pulmonary hypertension; this observation shows that PDE5 inhibition in the pulmonary vasculature can lead to clinically significant vasorelaxation.

The adverse effects of PDE5 inhibitors probably result from drug-induced vasodilation in the systemic vasculature. Headache and flushing are likely caused by vasodilation of cerebral and cutaneous vascular beds, respectively. Sildenafil-related myocardial infarction and sudden cardiac death may also be related to its vasodilatory effects. PDE5 inhibitors have only a nominal effect on blood pressure at doses commonly used to treat erectile dysfunction, and all of the above adverse effects are relatively rare because of the small amounts of PDE5 in vascular smooth muscle. However, in the presence of excess NO (e.g., when organic nitrates are used concomitantly with PDE5 inhibitors), the inhibition of cGMP degradation can markedly amplify the vasodilatory effect. Excessive vasodilation can lead to severe refractory hypotension, as GF experienced after taking nitroglycerin and sildenafil at the same time. Therefore, *all three PDE5 inhibitors are contraindicated for patients taking organic nitrate vasodilators:* sildenafil, vardenafil, and tadalafil all have a significant and potentially dangerous drug-drug interaction with nitrates. Another adverse effect that has recently been described in case reports is a possible association of PDE5 inhibitors with transient or even permanent vision loss due to a condition termed **non-arteritic ischemic optic neuropathy.** It is unclear whether PDE5 inhibitors cause this condition or whether other factors may be involved; patients taking PDE5 inhibitors are advised to be aware of this adverse effect, with the specific caution that patients with prior episodes of vision loss may be at increased risk from drug exposure.

Given the serious consequences of combining organic nitrates and PDE5 inhibitors, one might wonder whether non-nitrate vasodilator agents are also contraindicated in patients, such as GF, who use sildenafil, vardenafil, or tadalafil.

In one preliminary study, the degree of blood pressure reduction in a cohort receiving both sildenafil and amlodipine, a vasodilatory Ca^{2+} channel blocker, did not differ significantly from that in a cohort receiving sildenafil and a placebo. Nonetheless, patients taking vasodilatory antihypertensive medications together with a PDE5 inhibitor should be regarded as *at risk* for potentially dangerous hypotension. Theoretically, the risk could be even higher for patients taking a PDE5 inhibitor in conjunction with both an antihypertensive vasodilator and a drug that inhibits degradation of the PDE5 inhibitor by hepatic P450 3A4 (see Chapter 4, Drug Metabolism).

CA^{2+} CHANNEL BLOCKERS

In contrast to organic nitrates, which have pharmacologic effects limited mostly to the vasculature, Ca^{2+} channel blockers act on both vascular smooth muscle and the myocardium. Another important difference between organic nitrates and Ca^{2+} channel blockers is that, while organic nitrates have mainly venodilatory activity, Ca^{2+} channel blockers are predominantly arteriolar dilators. Ca^{2+} channel blockers are commonly used in the treatment of hypertension, certain cardiac arrhythmias, and some forms of angina.

Mechanism of Action

Several different subtypes of voltage-gated Ca^{2+} channels have been identified (termed *L, T, N,* and *P* channels). These subtypes differ in their electrochemical and biophysical properties and in their tissue distribution patterns. Ca^{2+} influx through the L-type channel is an important determinant of vascular tone and cardiac contractility. The Ca^{2+} channel blockers in current use all act by inhibiting Ca^{2+} entry through the L-type channel, although different members of this drug class have markedly different pharmacodynamic and pharmacokinetic properties.

In smooth muscle cells, decreased Ca^{2+} entry through L-type channels keeps $[Ca^{2+}]_{intracellular}$ low, thereby reducing Ca^{2+}-CaM–mediated activation of myosin light chain kinase, actin–myosin interaction, and smooth muscle contractility (Fig. 21-3). Although Ca^{2+} channel blockers can relax many different types of smooth muscle (e.g., bronchiolar and gastrointestinal), they appear to have the greatest effect on vascular smooth muscle. Furthermore, arterial smooth muscle is more responsive than venous smooth muscle. Vasodilation of resistance arterioles reduces systemic vascular resistance and lowers arterial blood pressure, thereby decreasing ventricular systolic wall stress and myocardial O_2 demand. Drug-induced dilation of coronary arteries may also increase myocardial O_2 supply, further ameliorating the O_2 supply:demand mismatch in patients with angina. In cardiac myocytes, reduced Ca^{2+} influx through L-type channels leads to decreases in myocardial contractility, sinoatrial (SA)-node pacemaker rate, and atrioventricular (AV)-node conduction velocity. (See Chapter 18, Pharmacology of Cardiac Rhythm, for a discussion of the effects of Ca^{2+} channel blockers on cardiac impulse conduction.)

It is important to note that skeletal muscle is not significantly affected by Ca^{2+} channel blockers, because skeletal muscle depends mainly on intracellular pools of Ca^{2+} (i.e.,

Ca^{2+} from the sarcoplasmic reticulum) to support excitation–contraction coupling, and does not require as much transmembrane Ca^{2+} influx through the L-type channel. One should also distinguish between smooth muscle relaxants that block Ca^{2+} entry through the L-type Ca^{2+} channel in vascular smooth muscle cells, and skeletal muscle relaxants that block neurotransmission mediated by the nicotinic acetylcholine receptor at the neuromuscular junction (see Chapter 8, Cholinergic Pharmacology).

Chemical Classes

Three chemical classes of Ca^{2+} channel blockers—the **dihydropyridines** (exemplified by nifedipine, amlodipine and felodipine), the **benzothiazepines** (exemplified by diltiazem), and the **phenylalkylamines** (exemplified by verapamil)—are currently in clinical use. All three classes block the L-type Ca^{2+} channel, but each class has distinctive pharmacologic effects. The differences are in part attributable to different drug binding sites on the Ca^{2+} channel: nifedipine binds to the N binding site, diltiazem binds to the D binding site, and verapamil binds to the V binding site. The D and V binding sites overlap, whereas the N site is in a different region of the Ca^{2+} channel. Diltiazem and verapamil affect each other's binding in complex ways, as might be expected for two drugs with overlapping binding sites. Nifedipine and diltiazem bind synergistically, whereas nifedipine and verapamil reciprocally inhibit each other's binding. An added layer of complexity arises from the different affinities of the Ca^{2+} channel blockers for different conformational states of the channel. The drugs also have differential tissue selectivity, perhaps because different channel conformations are preferred in different tissues.

Nifedipine and **amlodipine** are representative members of the dihydropyridine class of Ca^{2+} channel blockers. Compared to the other Ca^{2+} channel blockers, the dihydropyridines cause significantly more arterial vasodilation. In contrast, the dihydropyridines have relatively little effect on cardiac tissue. Compared to diltiazem and verapamil, the dihydropyridines cause less depression of myocardial contractility and have minimal effects on SA-node automaticity and AV-node conduction velocity (Fig. 21-11).

Amlodipine (a third-generation dihydropyridine) differs from nifedipine (a first-generation dihydropyridine) principally in its pharmacokinetic properties. Because amlodipine has a pKa of 8.7, it is predominantly in a positively charged form at physiologic pH. This positive charge allows amlodipine to bind to cell membranes (which are typically negatively charged) with high affinity, and contributes to the drug's late peak plasma concentration and slow hepatic metabolism (see below).

Compared to the dihydropyridines, **diltiazem** and **verapamil** have a lower ratio of vascular-to-cardiac selectivity (Table 21-2). In the heart, both diltiazem and verapamil act as negative inotropes; verapamil has a greater suppressive effect on cardiac contractility than diltiazem. Furthermore, because diltiazem and verapamil not only reduce the transmembrane influx of Ca^{2+} but also slow the rate of Ca^{2+} channel recovery, cardiac conduction (i.e., automaticity and conduction velocity) is significantly decreased by these drugs. In contrast, as noted above, dihydropyridines do not significantly alter the rate of Ca^{2+} channel recovery, and

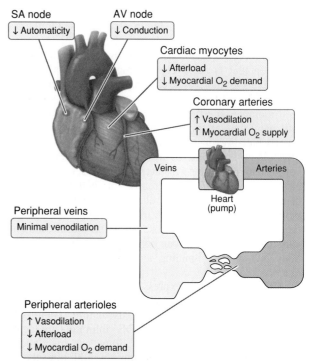

Figure 21-11. Sites of action of Ca^{2+} channel blockers. Ca^{2+} channel blockers dilate coronary arteries and peripheral arterioles, but not veins. They also decrease cardiac contractility, automaticity at the SA node, and conduction at the AV node. Dilation of the coronary arteries increases myocardial O_2 supply. Dilation of systemic (peripheral) arterioles decreases afterload and thereby decreases myocardial O_2 demand. However, some Ca^{2+} channel blockers (especially dihydropyridines) cause reflex tachycardia, which can paradoxically increase myocardial O_2 demand (not shown). Decreased cardiac contractility and decreased SA-node automaticity also decrease myocardial O_2 demand. The inhibition of AV-node conduction by some Ca^{2+} blockers makes them useful as antiarrhythmic agents. Note that the effects diagrammed here are representative effects of the class of drugs; individual agents are more or less selective for each of these effects (see Table 21-2).

thus have only minor effects on automaticity and conduction velocity.

Pharmacokinetics

Ca^{2+} channel blockers are typically used in oral dosage forms, although intravenous formulations of diltiazem and verapamil are also available. Nifedipine and verapamil are excreted by the kidney; diltiazem is excreted by the liver. Several pharmacokinetic properties of these drugs are suboptimal. First, the bioavailability of oral formulations of nifedipine, diltiazem, and verapamil is lowered by significant first-pass metabolism in the gut and liver. Furthermore, oral nifedipine has a rapid onset of action (less than 20 min) and can cause a brisk, precipitous fall in blood pressure. In turn, this drug-induced hypotension can activate severe reflex tachycardia, which can worsen myocardial ischemia by increasing myocardial O_2 demand and decreasing myocardial O_2 supply (the latter by decreasing diastolic filling time). In addition, the short half-life of oral nifedipine (about 4 h) requires that this drug be administered frequently.

Selectivity of Ca^{2+} Channel Blockers

	VASODILATION (PERIPHERAL ARTERIOLES AND CORONARY ARTERIES)	DEPRESSION OF CARDIAC CONTRACTILITY	DEPRESSION OF AUTOMATICITY (SA NODE)	DEPRESSION OF CONDUCTION (AV NODE)
Nifedipine	5	1	1	0
Diltiazem	3	2	5	4
Verapamil	4	4	5	5

The effects of the three different classes of Ca^{2+} channel blockers on vascular tone, cardiac contractility, heart rate, and AV nodal conduction are graded from 0 to 5. 0 = no effect; 5 = significant effect. Note that nifedipine is the most selective drug for peripheral vasodilation, while diltiazem and verapamil have more selective effects on the heart.

Amlodipine and nifedipine share similar pharmacodynamic profiles, but differ significantly in their pharmacokinetic profiles. Amlodipine's high bioavailability permits it to be effective at lower dosages because a greater proportion of the administered drug reaches the systemic circulation unchanged. Amlodipine's late peak plasma concentration and slow onset of action may be the reason that, as compared to nifedipine, amlodipine causes significantly less reflex tachycardia. Slow hepatic degradation of amlodipine contributes to its long plasma half-life (about 40 h) and duration of action, which enable once-daily dosing.

Toxicities and Contraindications

The toxicities of the Ca^{2+} channel blockers are mainly mechanism-based, and are therefore typically extensions of their actions. Flushing (a common adverse effect of nifedipine) and constipation (a common adverse effect of verapamil) are likely caused by excessive smooth muscle relaxation in the cutaneous vasculature and gastrointestinal tract, respectively. In excess, the negative chronotropic and negative inotropic effects of verapamil and diltiazem can lead to bradycardia, atrioventricular block, and heart failure. Patients taking β-adrenergic blockers (which are also negative inotropes) are often advised not to use diltiazem or verapamil concomitantly, because of the increased likelihood of excessive cardiac depression. Some studies have suggested that Ca^{2+} channel blockers increase the risk of mortality in patients with heart failure, and Ca^{2+} channel blockers are therefore contraindicated in the management of heart failure. Some reports also suggest that the short-acting agent nifedipine is associated with an increased risk of myocardial ischemia and infarction, by virtue of this drug's tendency to disturb the myocardial O_2 supply:demand equilibrium (see above).

K$^+$ CHANNEL OPENERS

K$^+$ channel openers cause direct arterial vasodilation by opening **ATP-modulated K$^+$ channels** (sometimes called **K$^+$ATP channels**) in the plasma membrane of vascular smooth muscle cells. Because these agents act by a mechanism that is entirely different from that of other vasodilators, K$^+$ATP channel openers represent a potent family of drugs that can be used to treat hypertension refractory to other antihypertensive therapeutics.

What is the normal function of ATP-modulated K$^+$ channels? Recall that the Nernst equilibrium potential for K$^+$ is about -90 mV, while the resting membrane potential is less negative than this value. Therefore, opening K$^+$ channels *hyperpolarizes* the membrane. If a sufficient number of K$^+$ channels are open at the same time, then normal excitatory stimuli are not able to promote membrane depolarization. In the absence of depolarization, voltage-gated Ca^{2+} channels do not open, and Ca^{2+} influx and smooth muscle contraction are inhibited (Fig. 21-3).

The K$^+$ATP channel opener drugs include **minoxidil, cromakalim, pinacidil,** and **nicorandil.** These drugs act primarily on arterial smooth muscle cells, and therefore decrease arterial blood pressure. Side effects of the K$^+$ATP channel openers include headache, caused by excessive dilation of cerebral arteries, and flushing, caused by excessive dilation of cutaneous arteries. When arterial vasodilators (e.g., Ca^{2+} channel blockers or K$^+$ATP channel openers) are used as monotherapy, the decrease in arterial pressure often elicits reflex sympathetic discharge, leading to tachycardia and increased cardiac work. As noted above in the discussion of nifedipine, reflex sympathetic discharge can offset the balance between myocardial O_2 supply and demand, precipitating myocardial ischemia; this effect is of particular concern in patients with pre-existing coronary artery disease. However, the use of β-blockers in combination with arterial vasodilators can help to block the effects of reflex sympathetic activity, and thereby preserve the therapeutic utility of the arterial vasodilators.

ENDOTHELIN RECEPTOR ANTAGONISTS

Bosentan is a competitive antagonist at ET$_A$ and ET$_B$ receptors. It is approved for use in the treatment of pulmonary hypertension. In clinical trials involving patients with severe dyspnea related to pulmonary hypertension, bosentan significantly improved 6-minute walk-test distance (i.e., the distance a patient can walk in 6 minutes) and decreased pulmonary vascular resistance relative to placebo. The major adverse effect of bosentan was an elevation in serum transaminase levels, with approximately 10% of patients having elevations exceeding three times the upper limit of normal. It is therefore necessary to monitor liver function tests monthly in patients taking bosentan. A selective ET$_A$ receptor antagonist, **sitaxsentan,** is currently under investigation.

OTHER DRUGS THAT MODULATE VASCULAR TONE

Hydralazine

Hydralazine is an orally administered arteriolar vasodilator that is sometimes used in the treatment of hypertension and, in combination with isosorbide dinitrate, in the treatment of heart failure. The mechanism of action of hydralazine remains unclear; studies have suggested that membrane hyperpolarization, K^+_{ATP} channel opening, and inhibition of IP_3-induced Ca^{2+} release from the sarcoplasmic reticulum in vascular smooth muscle cells may all be involved. Hydralazine appears to prevent the development of nitrate tolerance, perhaps by inhibiting vascular superoxide production. A combination pill containing isosorbide dinitrate and hydralazine has recently been found to reduce morbidity and mortality in Black Americans with advanced heart failure; it remains to be determined whether the benefits of this therapy extend to other patient populations. However, if the success of this hydralazine–isosorbide dinitrate combination therapy for heart failure is related to hydralazine's prevention of nitrate tolerance, then these drugs may be broadly efficacious in heart failure treatment.

The use of hydralazine has been limited because it was initially thought that the frequent dosing required for sustained blood pressure control and the rapid development of tachyphylaxis to its antihypertensive effects made chronic use of this drug impractical. As the benefits of combination therapy for hypertension and heart failure are becoming better appreciated, it may be possible for hydralazine to be used more effectively, especially in patients for whom other vasodilators (e.g., ACE inhibitors) are contraindicated.

Hydralazine typically has low bioavailability because of extensive first-pass hepatic metabolism. The rate of its metabolism depends on whether the patient is a slow or fast acetylator, however. In slow acetylators (see Chapter 4), hydralazine has a slower rate of hepatic degradation and, thus, higher bioavailability and higher plasma concentrations. A rare adverse effect of hydralazine treatment is the development of a reversible lupus erythematosus-like syndrome; this effect occurs chiefly in slow acetylators.

α_1-Adrenergic Antagonists

Epinephrine and norepinephrine stimulate **α_1-adrenergic receptors** on vascular smooth muscle, and thereby induce vasoconstriction. The α_1-adrenergic receptor is a G protein-coupled receptor that associates with the heterotrimeric G protein G_q, which activates phospholipase C to generate inositol trisphosphate and diacylglycerol. α_1-Adrenergic antagonists, such as **prazosin**, block α_1-adrenergic receptors in arterioles and venules, leading to vasodilation. The effect of these agents is greater in arterioles than in venules. The α_1-adrenergic antagonists cause a significant reduction in arterial pressure, and are thus useful in the treatment of hypertension. Initiation of therapy with α_1-adrenergic antagonists can be associated with orthostatic hypotension. Like other arterial vasodilators, the α_1-adrenergic antagonists can also cause retention of salt and water. β-Adrenergic blockers and diuretics may be used together with α_1-adrenergic antagonists to mitigate these compensatory responses. Some α_1-adrenergic antagonists, such as **terazosin,** are used principally to inhibit the contraction of nonvascular smooth muscle (e.g., prostatic smooth muscle), but these agents also have some effect on the vasculature (see Chapter 9, Adrenergic Pharmacology).

β-Adrenergic Antagonists

Activation of **β_2-adrenergic receptors** on vascular smooth muscle cells leads to vasodilation. The increased intracellular cAMP induced by β_2-receptor stimulation may cause smooth muscle relaxation by accelerating the inactivation of myosin light chain kinase and by increasing the extrusion of Ca^{2+} from the cell. Despite the beneficial vasodilatory effects of β_2-agonist action in the systemic circulation, β-adrenergic *antagonists* are of major clinical importance in the treatment of hypertension, angina, cardiac arrhythmias, and other conditions. β-Adrenergic antagonists have negative inotropic and chronotropic effects on the heart; these actions reduce cardiac output, which is an important determinant of both myocardial O_2 demand and blood pressure (see Equation 21-2). The cardiac effects of β-adrenergic antagonists are discussed in greater detail in Chapter 9. These drugs also have important effects on the vasculature: antagonism of β_2-adrenergic receptors on vascular smooth muscle cells can lead to unopposed vasoconstriction mediated by α_1-adrenergic receptors and, consequently, to an increase in systemic vascular resistance. Importantly, although some β-adrenergic antagonists may initially increase systemic vascular resistance, the net effect in most cases is a *decrease* in blood pressure. This hypotensive effect reflects the combined negative inotropic effect (leading to a decrease in cardiac output), inhibition of renin secretion, and central nervous system (CNS) effects of the β-blockers. Indeed, β-adrenergic antagonists are highly effective in the treatment of hypertension.

Renin–Angiotensin System Blockers

As discussed in Chapter 20, inhibition of the renin–angiotensin system results in significant vasorelaxation. The hypotensive effect of ACE inhibitors may be caused by decreased catabolism of bradykinin, a vasorelaxant released in response to inflammatory stimuli. Antagonists at the AT_1 receptor, which selectively inhibit angiotensin II-mediated vasoconstriction at the level of the target organ, have a more direct effect. ACE inhibitors and AT_1 receptor antagonists are considered ''balanced'' vasodilators because they affect both arterial and venous tone. Both classes of drugs are effective in the treatment of hypertension and heart failure, as discussed in Chapter 24.

Conclusion and Future Directions

Vascular tone is subject to exquisite control, as would be expected for a system that must perfuse all the tissues of the body. Vascular tone represents a balance between vascular smooth muscle contraction and relaxation. Vasoconstriction occurs when an increase in intracellular Ca^{2+} activates Ca^{2+}-CaM–dependent myosin light chain kinase (MLCK). In turn, MLCK phosphorylates myosin light chains and allows the formation of actin–myosin cross-bridges. Vascular smooth muscle relaxes when the intracellular Ca^{2+} concentration returns to basal levels and myosin light chains are dephosphorylated, terminating the formation of actin–myosin cross-bridges. Vascular tone is influenced by the state of the vascular smooth muscle cells and the overlying endothelial cells, by sympathetic innervation, and by neurohormonal and local regulators.

Diverse therapeutic agents modulate various components of this critical system, with important differences in molecular mechanisms and effects. Classes of vasodilators include nitrates, Ca^{2+} channel blockers, K^+ channel openers, α_1-adrenergic receptor antagonists, ACE inhibitors, AT_1 receptor antagonists, and endothelin receptor antagonists (Fig. 21-6). Nitrates dilate primarily veins, not arteries. These agents act by releasing NO in vascular smooth muscle cells; in turn, NO activates guanylyl cyclase, which increases intracellular cGMP, which activates cGMP-dependent protein kinase, which activates myosin light chain phosphatase, which terminates the formation of actin–myosin cross-bridges. Ca^{2+} channel blockers act mainly on arteries and resistance arterioles, and may also have direct effects on the heart. These drugs cause vasodilation by blocking L-type voltage-gated Ca^{2+} channels in the plasma membrane of vascular smooth muscle cells, and thereby inhibiting the Ca^{2+} influx through these channels that is necessary for contraction. K^+_{ATP} channel openers, as with Ca^{2+} channel blockers, are predominantly arteriodilators, not venodilators. This class of drugs opens ATP-modulated K^+ channels, thereby hyperpolarizing vascular smooth muscle cells and preventing the activation of voltage-gated Ca^{2+} channels that is necessary for Ca^{2+} influx and muscle contraction. α_1-Adrenergic receptor antagonists, AT_1 receptor antagonists, and endothelin receptor antagonists prevent vasoconstriction by inhibiting the activation of their respective receptors by endogenous agonists.

The mechanisms that control vascular tone are regulated by multiple intersecting signaling pathways. The emerging science of systems biology combines mathematical, compu-tational, and experimental approaches to understand complex signaling pathways in a wide array of tissues and organs. This integrated approach to signaling will provide novel quantitative information regarding the interplay of intracellular signaling pathways in the vasculature, and may lead to the identification of new drug targets. For example, insights into the relationships among cGMP-modulated regulatory pathways in vascular smooth muscle cells have recently led to new therapeutic applications for PDE5 inhibitors, such as sildenafil, in the treatment of pulmonary hypertension and heart failure. Continued elucidation of complex signaling pathways will likely lead to the identification of new points for pharmacologic intervention in the cellular milieu of the vascular wall, and will help to integrate the pharmacology of vascular tone across the spectrum of cardiovascular disease.

■ *Suggested Reading*

Abrams J. Chronic stable angina. *N Engl J Med* 2005;352: 2524–2533. (*An informative case vignette and review of the pathophysiology and pharmacotherapy of angina pectoris.*)

Channick RN, Sitbon O, Barst RJ, et al. Endothelin receptor antagonists in pulmonary arterial hypertension. *J Am Coll Cardiol* 2004; 43:62S–67S. (*Reviews developments in the use of endothelin receptor antagonists.*)

deLemos JA, McGuire DK, Drazner MH. B-type natriuretic peptide in cardiovascular disease. *Lancet* 2003;362:316–322. (*Concise review of the physiology and pharmacology of natriuretic peptides.*)

Mark JD, Griffiths M, Evans TW. Drug therapy: inhaled nitric oxide therapy in adults. *N Engl J Med* 2005;353:2683–2695. (*Reviews the history of inhaled NO and current indications for this therapy.*)

Opie L, Gersh BJ. *Drugs for the heart.* 6th ed. Philadelphia: WB Saunders; 2005. (*A "pocket-sized" clinician's guide with diagrams.*)

Parker JD, Parker JO. Nitrate therapy for stable angina pectoris. *N Engl J Med* 1998;338:520–531. (*Excellent reference on the pharmacokinetics and tolerance mechanisms of the organic nitrates.*)

Drug Summary Table | Chapter 21 Pharmacology of Vascular Tone

ORGANIC NITRATES AND SODIUM NITROPRUSSIDE

Mechanism—Donate NO, which activates guanylyl cyclase and increases dephosphorylation of myosin light chain in vascular smooth muscle, causing vasodilation

Drug	Clinical Applications	Serious and Common Adverse Effects	Contraindications	Therapeutic Considerations
Isosorbide dinitrate	*Short-acting (sublingual):* Prophylaxis and treatment of acute anginal attacks *Long-acting (oral, extended-release):* Prophylaxis of angina Treatment of chronic ischemic heart disease Diffuse esophageal spasm	*Refractory hypotension, angina from reflex tachycardia, palpitations, syncope* Flushing, headache	Severe hypotension, shock, or acute MI with low left ventricular filling pressure Increased intracranial pressure, angle-closure glaucoma, anginal pain associated with hypertrophic obstructive cardiomyopathy, severe anemia Coadministration with phosphodiesterase type V inhibitors (sildenafil, vardenafil, tadalafil)	Venous dilation > arteriolar dilation Continuous therapy leads to tolerance; tolerance can be avoided by providing nitrate-free interval
Isosorbide 5-mononitrate	Prophylaxis of angina Treatment of chronic ischemic heart disease	*Same as isosorbide dinitrate*	Same as isosorbide dinitrate	Same therapeutic considerations as isosorbide dinitrate Additionally, isosorbide 5-mononitrate is preferred over isosorbide dinitrate due to longer half-life, better absorption from the GI tract, non-susceptibility to extensive first-pass metabolism in the liver, less rebound angina, and greater efficacy at equivalent doses
Nitroglycerin	*Short-acting (sublingual, spray):* Short-term treatment of acute anginal attacks *Long-acting (oral, buccal, transdermal patch):* Prophylaxis of angina Treatment of chronic ischemic heart disease *Intravenous:* Unstable angina Acute heart failure	*Same as isosorbide dinitrate*	Same as isosorbide dinitrate Additionally, transdermal form is contraindicated in patients with allergy to skin tape IV form is contraindicated in patients with cardiac tamponade, restrictive cardiomyopathy, or constrictive pericarditis	Same therapeutic considerations as isosorbide dinitrate Additionally, equivalent doses of nitroglycerin may be less effective than isosorbide dinitrate due to shorter half-life of nitroglycerin Ergotamine may oppose coronary vasodilation of nitrates
Sodium nitroprusside	Hypertensive emergencies Severe cardiac failure Ergot alkaloid toxicity	*Cyanide toxicity, cardiac arrhythmia, excessive bleeding, excessive hypotension, metabolic acidosis, bowel obstruction, methemoglobinemia, increased intracranial pressure* Flushing, headache, renal azotemia	Preexisting hypotension, obstructive valvular disease, heart failure associated with reduced peripheral vascular resistance Hepatic or renal failure Optic atrophy Surgery patients with inadequate cerebral circulation Tobacco amblyopia	Venous dilation = arteriolar dilation Thiocyanate toxicity becomes life-threatening at serum concentrations of 200 mg/L Coadministration of sodium thiosulfate may reduce the risk of cyanide toxicity, but this interaction is not well-studied

PHOSPHODIESTERASE TYPE V INHIBITORS

Mechanism—Inhibit PDE5, an enzyme that converts cGMP to GMP, leading to cGMP accumulation in target tissues

Drug	Clinical Applications	Adverse Effects	Contraindications	Therapeutic Considerations
Sildenafil Vardenafil Tadalafil	Erectile dysfunction Pulmonary hypertension (sildenafil)	*Myocardial infarction, non-arteritic ischemic optic neuropathy; priapism* Headache, flushing, rash, diarrhea, dyspepsia	Concomitant use of organic nitrate vasodilators	PDE5 inhibitors promote systemic vasodilation at doses much higher than those used to treat erectile dysfunction High doses of sildenafil are efficacious in treatment of pulmonary hypertension PDE5 inhibitors are contraindicated in patients taking organic nitrate vasodilators Patients with prior episodes of vision loss may be at increased risk for non-arteritic ischemic optic neuropathy Tadalafil has longer elimination half-life than sildenafil and vardenafil

CALCIUM CHANNEL BLOCKERS

Mechanism—Block voltage-gated L-type calcium channels and prevent the influx of calcium that promotes actin-myosin cross-bridge formation. Different classes of calcium channel blockers have unique binding sites on the calcium channel and different affinities for the various conformational states of the channel.

Drug	Clinical Applications	Adverse Effects	Contraindications	Therapeutic Considerations
Dihydropyridines: Nifedipine Amlodipine Felodipine	Exertional angina Unstable angina Coronary spasm Hypertension Hypertrophic cardiomyopathy Raynaud's phenomenon Pre-eclampsia	*Increased angina, rare myocardial infarction* Palpitations, peripheral edema, flushing, constipation, heartburn, dizziness	Preexisting hypotension	Arteriolar dilation > venous dilation High vascular-to-cardiac selectivity; compared to diltiazem and verapamil, less depression of myocardial contractility and minimal effects on SA-node automaticity and AV-node conduction velocity Oral nifedipine has a rapid onset of action and can cause a brisk, precipitous fall in blood pressure, which can trigger severe reflex tachycardia Compared to nifedipine, amlodipine has higher bioavailability, longer time to peak plasma concentration, and slower hepatic metabolism Co-administration with nafcillin results in large decrease in plasma nifedipine level
Benzothiazepine: Diltiazem	Prinzmetal's or variant angina or chronic stable angina Hypertension Atrial fibrillation or flutter, paroxysmal supraventricular tachycardia	*Rare cardiac arrhythmia, atrioventricular block, bradyarrhythmia, exacerbation of heart failure* Peripheral edema, syncope, gingival hyperplasia, dizziness	Sick sinus syndrome or second- or third-degree AV block Supraventricular tachycardia associated with a bypass tract (see Fig. 18-8) Left ventricular failure Hypotension (systolic blood pressure <90 mm Hg) Acute MI with X-ray-documented pulmonary congestion	Low ratio of vascular-to-cardiac selectivity Depresses both SA-node automaticity and AV-node conduction velocity Raises serum carbamazepine levels, which may result in carbamazepine toxicity Avoid concomitant use of beta-adrenergic blockers

(Continued)

Drug Summary Table **Chapter 21 Pharmacology of Vascular Tone** (*Continued*)

Drug	Clinical Applications	*Serious* and Common Adverse Effects	Contraindications	Therapeutic Considerations
Phenylalkylamine: Verapamil	Same as diltiazem	*Same as diltiazem*	Same as diltiazem Additionally, IV verapamil is contraindicated in patients with ventricular tachycardia and patients receiving IV beta-blockers	Same therapeutic considerations as diltiazem Additionally, verapamil has a greater suppressive effect on cardiac contractility than diltiazem Alcohol consumption with chronic verapamil therapy may result in higher serum alcohol concentrations Coadministration with pimozide may result in higher pimozide concentrations and cardiac arrhythmias Coadministration with simvastatin markedly increases simvastatin concentrations

POTASSIUM CHANNEL OPENERS

Mechanism—Open ATP-modulated potassium channels and hyperpolarize plasma membrane, thereby inhibiting influx of calcium through voltage-gated calcium channels

Drug	Clinical Applications	*Serious* and Common Adverse Effects	Contraindications	Therapeutic Considerations
Minoxidil Pinacidil Nicorandil Cromakalim	Severe or refractory hypertension Male pattern alopecia (topical minoxidil)	*Angina, pericardial effusion, reflex tachycardia, Stevens-Johnson syndrome, leukopenia, thrombocytopenia* Headache, flushing, hypotension, hirsutism, hypertrichosis, fluid retention, hypernatremia	Pheochromocytoma	Arteriolar dilation > venous dilation Typically used in combination with a beta-blocker and a diuretic Use with caution in patients with impaired renal function or dissecting aortic aneurysm or after acute MI

ENDOTHELIN RECEPTOR ANTAGONIST

Mechanism—Blocks activation of endothelin receptors ET_A and ET_B by endogenous endothelin

Drug	Clinical Applications	*Serious* and Common Adverse Effects	Contraindications	Therapeutic Considerations
Bosentan	Severe pulmonary hypertension	*Hepatotoxicity, anemia, hypotension, fluid retention* Headache, flushing	Pregnancy Concomitant use of cyclosporine A or glyburide	Do not use in pregnant women Monitor liver function tests monthly in patients taking bosentan Generally avoid use in patients with moderate to severe hepatic impairment Use with caution in patients with hypovolemia, hypotension, heart failure, or anemia Potential for interactions with other drugs metabolized by P450 2C9 or P450 3A4 (e.g., hormonal contraceptives, simvastatin, warfarin, ketoconazole)

HYDRALAZINE

Mechanism—Arteriolar vasodilator. Mechanism of action is unclear; proposed mechanisms include membrane hyperpolarization, potassium channel activation, and inhibition of IP₃-induced calcium release from sarcoplasmic reticulum in vascular smooth muscle cells.

| Hydralazine | Moderate to severe hypertension
Severe heart failure | *Agranulocytosis, leukopenia, hepatotoxicity, systemic lupus erythematosus*
Headache, palpitations, tachycardia, anorexia, diarrhea | Dissecting aortic aneurysm
Coronary artery disease
Mitral valvular rheumatic heart disease | Arteriolar dilation > venous dilation
Typically used in combination with a beta-blocker and a diuretic in the treatment of hypertension
Used in combination with isosorbide dinitrate for heart failure; combination formulation with isosorbide dinitrate may have morbidity and mortality benefits in black Americans with advanced heart failure
Concomitant use of diazoxide and MAO inhibitor may cause severe hypotension |

α1-ADRENERGIC ANTAGONISTS

Mechanism—Block activation of α1-adrenergic receptors by endogenous receptor agonists

| Prazosin
Doxazosin
Terazosin | See Drug Summary Table: Chapter 9 Adrenergic Pharmacology |

β-ADRENERGIC ANTAGONISTS

Mechanism—Block activation of β-adrenergic receptors by endogenous receptor agonists

| Propranolol (nonselective)
Atenolol, metoprolol (beta 1-selective) | See Drug Summary Table: Chapter 9 Adrenergic Pharmacology |

ACE INHIBITORS

Mechanism—Inhibit cleavage of AT-I to AT-II by angiotensin converting enzyme (ACE); inhibit degradation of bradykinin by ACE

| Captopril
Enalapril
Lisinopril | See Drug Summary Table: Chapter 20 Volume Regulation |

AT1 RECEPTOR ANTAGONISTS

Mechanism—Block activation of AT1 angiotensin II (AT-II) receptors by endogenous AT-II

| Losartan
Valsartan | See Drug Summary Table: Chapter 20 Volume Regulation |

22

Pharmacology of Hemostasis and Thrombosis

April W. Armstrong and David E. Golan

INTRODUCTION

Blood carries oxygen and nutrients to tissues and takes metabolic waste products away from tissues. Humans have developed a well-regulated system of **hemostasis** to keep the blood fluid and clot-free in normal vessels and to form a localized plug rapidly in injured vessels. **Thrombosis** describes a pathologic state in which normal hemostatic processes are activated inappropriately. For example, a blood clot (thrombus) may form as the result of a relatively minor vessel injury and occlude a section of the vascular tree. This chapter presents the normal physiology of hemostasis, the pathophysiology of thrombosis, and the pharmacology of drugs that can be used to prevent or reverse a thrombotic state. Drugs introduced in this chapter are used to treat a variety of cardiovascular diseases, such as deep vein thrombosis and myocardial infarction.

 Case

Mr. S, a 55-year-old man with a history of hypertension and cigarette smoking, is awakened in the middle of the night with substernal chest pressure, sweating, and shortness of breath. He calls 911 and is taken to the emergency department. An electrocardiogram shows deep T-wave inversions in leads V2 to V5. A cardiac biomarker panel shows a creatine kinase level of 800 IU/L (normal, 60-400 IU/L) with 10% MB fraction (the heart-specific isoform), suggesting myocardial infarction. He is treated with intravenous nitroglycerin, aspirin, unfractionated heparin, and eptifibatide, but his chest pain persists. He is taken to the cardiac catheterization laboratory, where he is found to have a 90% mid-LAD (left anterior descending artery) thrombus with sluggish distal flow. He undergoes successful angioplasty and stent placement. At the time of stent placement, an intravenous loading dose of clopidogrel is administered. The heparin is stopped, eptifibatide is continued for 18 more hours, and he is transferred to the telemetry ward. Six hours later, Mr. S is noted to have an expanding hematoma (an area of localized hemorrhage) in his right thigh below the arterial access site. The eptifibatide is stopped and pressure is applied to the access site, and the hematoma ceases to expand. He is discharged two days later with prescriptions for clopidogrel and aspirin, which are administered to prevent subacute thrombosis of the stent.

QUESTIONS

■ **1.** How did a blood clot arise in Mr. S's coronary artery?
■ **2.** If low molecular weight heparin had been used instead of unfractionated heparin, how would the monitoring of the patient's coagulation status during the procedure have been affected?
■ **3.** What accounts for the efficacy of eptifibatide (a platelet GPIIb–IIIa antagonist) in inhibiting platelet aggregation?
■ **4.** When the expanding hematoma was observed, could any measure other than stopping the eptifibatide have been used to reverse the effect of this agent?
■ **5.** How do aspirin, heparin, clopidogrel, and eptifibatide act in the attempt to treat Mr. S's blood clot and to prevent recurrent thrombus formation?

PHYSIOLOGY OF HEMOSTASIS

An injured blood vessel must induce the formation of a blood clot to prevent blood loss and to allow healing. Clot formation must also remain localized to prevent widespread clotting within intact vessels. The formation of a localized clot at the site of vessel injury is accomplished in four temporally overlapping stages (Fig. 22-1). First, **localized vasoconstriction** occurs as a response to a reflex neurogenic mechanism and to the secretion of endothelium-derived vasoconstrictors such as endothelin. Immediately following vasoconstriction, **primary hemostasis** occurs. During this stage, platelets are activated and adhere to the exposed subendothelial matrix. **Platelet activation** involves both a change in shape of the platelet and the release of secretory granule contents from the platelet. The secreted granule substances recruit other platelets, causing more platelets to adhere to the subendothelial matrix and to aggregate with one another at the site of vascular injury. Primary hemostasis ultimately results in the formation of a **primary hemostatic plug.**

The goal of the final two stages of hemostasis is to form a stable, permanent plug. During **secondary hemostasis,** also known as the **coagulation cascade,** the activated endothelium and other nearby cells (see below) express a membrane-bound procoagulant factor called **tissue factor,** which complexes with coagulation factor VII to initiate the coagulation cascade. The end result of this cascade is the activation of thrombin, a critical enzyme. Thrombin serves two pivotal functions in hemostasis: (1) it converts soluble fibrinogen to an insoluble fibrin polymer that forms the matrix of the clot; and (2) it induces more platelet recruitment and activation. Recent evidence indicates that fibrin clot formation (secondary hemostasis) overlaps temporally with platelet plug formation (primary hemostasis), and that each process reinforces the other. During the final stage, platelet aggregation and fibrin polymerization lead to the formation of a stable, **permanent plug.** In addition, **antithrombotic mechanisms** restrict the permanent plug to the site of vessel injury, ensuring that the permanent plug does not inappropriately extend to occlude the vascular tree.

VASOCONSTRICTION

Transient arteriolar vasoconstriction occurs immediately after vascular injury. This vasoconstriction is mediated by a poorly understood reflex neurogenic mechanism. Local endothelial secretion of **endothelin,** a potent vasoconstrictor, potentiates the reflex vasoconstriction. Because the vasoconstriction is transient, bleeding would resume if primary hemostasis were not activated.

PRIMARY HEMOSTASIS

The goal of primary hemostasis is to form a platelet plug that rapidly stabilizes vascular injury. Platelets play a pivotal role in primary hemostasis. **Platelets** are cell fragments that arise by budding from megakaryocytes in the bone marrow; these small, membrane-bound discs contain cytoplasm but lack nuclei. Glycoprotein receptors in the platelet plasma membrane are the primary mediators by which platelets are activated. Primary hemostasis involves the transformation of platelets into a hemostatic plug through three reactions: (1) adhesion; (2) the granule release reaction; and (3) aggregation and consolidation.

Platelet Adhesion

In the first reaction, platelets adhere to subendothelial collagen that is exposed after vascular injury (Fig. 22-2). This adhesion is mediated by **von Willebrand factor (vWF),** a large multimeric protein that is secreted by both activated platelets and the injured endothelium. vWF binds both to surface receptors (especially glycoprotein Ib [GPIb]) on the platelet membrane and to the exposed collagen; this "bridging" action mediates adhesion of platelets to the collagen. The GPIb:vWF:collagen interaction is critical for initiation of primary hemostasis, because it is the only known molecular mechanism by which platelets can adhere to the injured vessel wall.

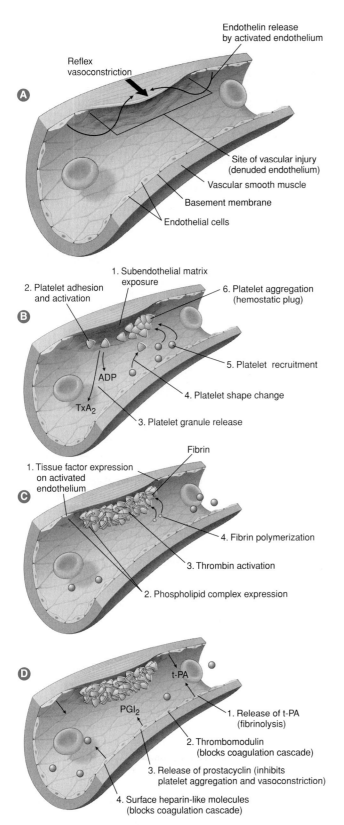

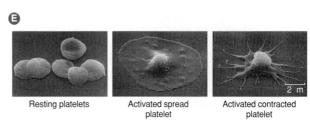

Resting platelets   Activated spread platelet   Activated contracted platelet

Figure 22-1. Sequence of events in hemostasis. The hemostatic process can be divided conceptually into four stages—vasoconstriction, primary hemostasis, secondary hemostasis, and resolution—although recent evidence suggests that these stages are temporally overlapping and may be nearly simultaneous. **A.** Vascular injury causes endothelial denudation. Endothelin, released by activated endothelium, and neurohumoral factor(s) induce transient vasoconstriction. **B.** Injury-induced exposure of the subendothelial matrix *(1)* provides a substrate for platelet adhesion and activation *(2)*. In the granule release reaction, activated platelets secrete thromboxane A_2 (TxA_2) and ADP *(3)*. TxA_2 and ADP released by activated platelets cause nearby platelets to become activated; these newly activated platelets undergo shape change *(4)* and are recruited to the site of injury *(5)*. The aggregation of activated platelets at the site of injury forms a primary hemostatic plug *(6)*. **C.** Tissue factor expressed on activated endothelial cells *(1)* and leukocyte microparticles *(not shown)*, together with acidic phospholipids expressed on activated platelets and activated endothelial cells *(2)*, initiate the steps of the coagulation cascade, culminating in the activation of thrombin *(3)*. Thrombin proteolytically activates fibrinogen to form fibrin, which polymerizes around the site of injury, resulting in the formation of a definitive (secondary) hemostatic plug *(4)*. **D.** Natural anticoagulant and thrombolytic factors limit the hemostatic process to the site of vascular injury. These factors include tissue plasminogen activator (t-PA), which activates the fibrinolytic system *(1)*; thrombomodulin, which activates inhibitors of the coagulation cascade *(2)*; prostacyclin, which inhibits both platelet activation and vasoconstriction *(3)*; and surface heparin-like molecules, which catalyze the inactivation of coagulation factors *(4)*. **E.** Scanning electron micrographs of resting platelets *(1)*, a platelet undergoing cell spreading shortly after cell activation *(2)*, and a fully activated platelet after actin filament bundling and crosslinking and myosin contraction *(3)*.

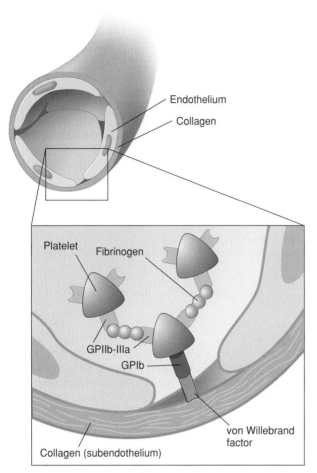

Figure 22-2.   Platelet adhesion and aggregation. von Willebrand factor mediates platelet adhesion to the subendothelium by binding both to the platelet membrane glycoprotein GPIb and to exposed subendothelial collagen. During platelet aggregation, fibrinogen crosslinks platelets to one another by binding to GPIIb–IIIa receptors on platelet membranes.

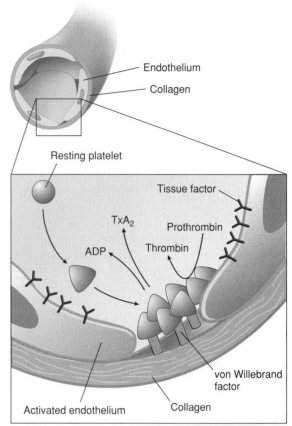

Figure 22-3.   Platelet activation. Platelet activation is initiated at the site of vascular injury when circulating platelets adhere to exposed subendothelial collagen and are activated by locally generated mediators. Activated platelets undergo shape change and granule release, and platelet aggregates are formed as additional platelets are recruited and activated. Platelet recruitment is mediated by the release of soluble platelet factors, including ADP and thromboxane A$_2$ (TxA$_2$). Tissue factor, expressed on activated endothelium, is a critical initiating component in the coagulation cascade. The membranes of activated platelets provide a surface for a number of critical reactions in the coagulation cascade, including the conversion of prothrombin to thrombin.

Platelet Granule Release Reaction

Adherent platelets undergo a process of activation (Fig. 22-3) during which the cells' granule contents are released. The release reaction is initiated by agonist binding to cell-surface receptors, which activates intracellular protein phosphorylation cascades and ultimately causes release of granule contents. Specifically, stimulation by ADP, epinephrine, and collagen leads to activation of platelet membrane phospholipase A$_2$ (PLA$_2$). PLA$_2$ cleaves membrane phospholipids and liberates **arachidonic acid,** which is converted into a **cyclic endoperoxide** by platelet cyclooxygenase. Thromboxane synthase subsequently converts the cyclic endoperoxide into **thromboxane A$_2$ (TxA$_2$).** TxA$_2$, via a G protein-coupled receptor, causes vasoconstriction at the site of vascular injury by inducing a decrease in cAMP levels within vascular smooth muscle cells. TxA$_2$ also stimulates the granule **release reaction** within platelets, thereby propagating the cascade of platelet activation and vasoconstriction.

During the release reaction, large amounts of ADP, Ca^{2+}, ATP, serotonin, vWF, and platelet factor 4 are *actively se-*

creted from platelet granules. *ADP is particularly important in mediating platelet aggregation,* causing platelets to become "sticky" and adhere to one another (see below). Although strong agonists (such as thrombin and collagen) can trigger granule secretion even when aggregation is prevented, ADP can trigger granule secretion only in the presence of platelet aggregation. Presumably, this difference is caused by the set of intracellular effectors that are coupled to the various agonist receptors. Release of Ca^{2+} ions is also important for the coagulation cascade, as discussed below.

Platelet Aggregation and Consolidation

TxA$_2$, ADP, and fibrous collagen are all potent mediators of platelet aggregation. TxA$_2$ promotes platelet aggregation through stimulation of G protein-coupled TxA$_2$ receptors in the platelet membrane (Fig. 22-4). Binding of TxA$_2$ to platelet TxA$_2$ receptors leads to activation of phospholipase C

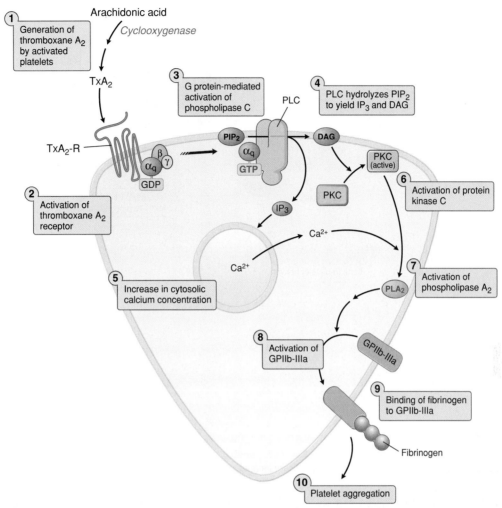

Figure 22-4. Platelet activation by thromboxane A₂. 1. Thromboxane A₂ (TxA₂) is generated from arachidonic acid in activated platelets; cyclooxygenase catalyzes the committed step in this process. 2. Secreted TxA₂ binds to the cell-surface TxA₂ receptor (TxA₂-R), a G protein-coupled receptor. 3. The Gα isoform Gα$_q$ activates phospholipase C (PLC). 4. PLC hydrolyzes phosphatidylinositol 4,5-bisphosphate (PIP₂) to yield inositol 1,4,5-trisphosphate (IP₃) and diacylglycerol (DAG). 5. IP₃ raises the cytosolic Ca²⁺ concentration by promoting vesicular release of Ca²⁺ into the cytosol. 6. DAG activates protein kinase C (PKC). 7. PKC activates phospholipase A₂ (PLA₂). 8. Through a poorly understood mechanism, activation of PLA₂ leads to the activation of GPIIb–IIIa. 9. Activated GPIIb–IIIa binds to fibrinogen. 10. Fibrinogen crosslinks platelets by binding to GPIIb–IIIa receptors on other platelets. This crosslinking leads to platelet aggregation and formation of a primary hemostatic plug.

(PLC), which hydrolyzes phosphatidylinositol 4,5-bisphosphate (PI[4,5]P₂) to yield inositol 1,4,5-trisphosphate (IP₃) and diacylglycerol (DAG). IP₃ raises the cytosolic Ca²⁺ concentration and DAG activates protein kinase C (PKC), which in turn promotes the activation of PLA₂. Through a poorly understood mechanism, PLA₂ activation induces the expression of functional GPIIb–IIIa, the membrane integrin that mediates platelet aggregation. ADP triggers platelet activation by binding to G protein-coupled ADP receptors on the platelet surface (Fig. 22-5). The two subtypes of G protein-coupled platelet ADP receptors are termed **P2Y1 receptors** and **P2Y(ADP) receptors.** P2Y1, a G$_q$-coupled receptor, releases intracellular calcium stores through activation of phospholipase C. P2Y(ADP), a G$_i$-coupled receptor, inhibits adenylyl cyclase. The P2Y(ADP) receptor is the target of the antiplatelet agents **ticlopidine** and **clopidogrel** (see below).

Activation of ADP receptors mediates platelet shape change and expression of functional GPIIb–IIIa. Fibrous collagen activates platelets by binding directly to platelet glycoprotein VI (GPVI). Ligation of GPVI by collagen leads to phospholipase C activation and platelet activation, as described above.

Platelets aggregate with one another through a bridging molecule, **fibrinogen,** which has multiple binding sites for functional GPIIb–IIIa (Fig. 22-2). *Just as the vWF:GPIb interaction is important for platelet adhesion to exposed subendothelial collagen, the fibrinogen:GPIIb–IIIa interaction is critical for platelet aggregation.* Platelet aggregation ultimately leads to the formation of a reversible clot, or a **primary hemostatic plug.**

Activation of the **coagulation cascade** proceeds nearly simultaneously with the formation of the primary hemostatic plug, as described below. Activation of the coagulation cascade leads to the generation of fibrin, initially at the periph-

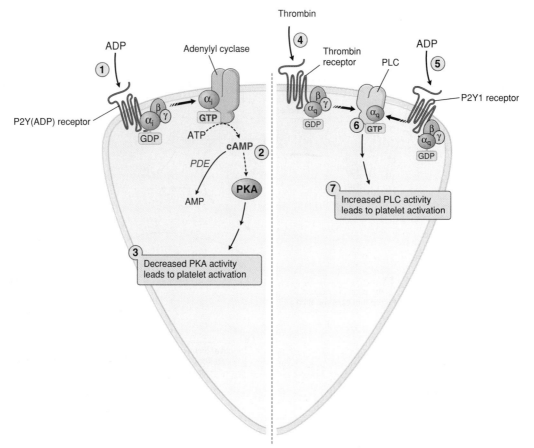

Figure 22-5. Platelet activation by ADP and thrombin. Left panel: 1. Binding of ADP to the P2Y(ADP) receptor activates a G_i protein, which inhibits adenylyl cyclase. 2. Inhibition of adenylyl cyclase decreases the synthesis of cAMP, and hence decreases protein kinase A (PKA) activation *(dashed arrow)*. cAMP is metabolized to AMP by phosphodiesterase (PDE). 3. PKA inhibits platelet activation through a series of poorly understood steps. Therefore, the decreased PKA activation that results from ADP binding to the P2Y(ADP) receptor causes platelet activation. **Right panel:** 4. Thrombin proteolytically cleaves the extracellular domain of its receptor. This cleavage creates a new N-terminus, which binds to an activation site on the thrombin receptor to activate a G_q protein. 5. ADP also activates G_q by binding to the P2Y1 receptor. 6. G_q activation (by either thrombin or ADP) activates phospholipase C (PLC). 7. PLC activity leads to platelet activation, as shown in Figure 22-4. Note that ADP can activate platelets by binding to either the P2Y(ADP) receptor or the P2Y1 receptor, although recent evidence suggests that full platelet activation requires the participation of both receptors.

ery of the primary hemostatic plug. Platelet pseudopods attach to the fibrin strands at the periphery of the plug and *contract.* Platelet contraction yields a compact, solid, irreversible clot, or a **secondary hemostatic plug.**

SECONDARY HEMOSTASIS: THE COAGULATION CASCADE

Secondary hemostasis is also termed the **coagulation cascade.** The goal of this cascade is to form a stable fibrin clot at the site of vascular injury. Details of the coagulation cascade are presented schematically in Figure 22-6. Several general principles should be noted.

First, the coagulation cascade is a sequence of enzymatic events. Most plasma coagulation factors circulate as inactive *proenzymes,* which are synthesized by the liver. These proenzymes are proteolytically cleaved, and thereby activated, by the activated factors that precede them in the cascade.

The activation reaction is catalytic and not stoichiometric. For example, one ''unit'' of activated factor X can potentially generate 40 ''units'' of thrombin. This robust amplification process rapidly generates large amounts of fibrin at a site of vascular injury.

Second, the major activation reactions in the cascade occur at sites where a *phospholipid-based protein–protein complex* has formed (Fig. 22-7). This complex is composed of a membrane surface (provided by activated platelets, activated endothelial cells, and possibly activated leukocyte microparticles [see below]), an enzyme (an activated coagulation factor), a substrate (the proenzyme form of the downstream coagulation factor), and a cofactor. The presence of negatively charged phospholipids, especially phosphatidylserine, is critical for assembly of the complex. Phosphatidylserine, which is normally sequestered in the inner leaflet of the plasma membrane, translocates to the outer leaflet of the membrane in response to agonist stimulation of platelets, endothelial cells, or leukocytes. Calcium is required for the enzyme, substrate, and cofactor to adopt the

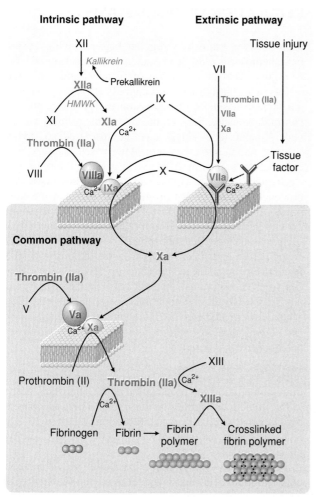

Figure 22-6. Coagulation cascade. The coagulation cascade is arbitrarily divided into the intrinsic pathway, the extrinsic pathway, and the common pathway. The intrinsic and extrinsic pathways converge at the level of factor X activation. The intrinsic pathway is largely an in vitro pathway, while the extrinsic pathway accounts for the majority of in vivo coagulation. The extrinsic pathway is initiated at sites of vascular injury by the expression of tissue factor on several different cell types, including activated endothelial cells, activated leukocytes (and leukocyte microparticles), subendothelial vascular smooth muscle cells, and subendothelial fibroblasts. Note that Ca^{2+} is a cofactor in many of the steps, and that a number of the steps occur on phospholipid surfaces provided by activated platelets, activated endothelial cells, and activated leukocytes (and leukocyte microparticles). Activated coagulation factors are shown in *blue* and indicated with a lower case "a." HMWK, high-molecular–weight kininogen.

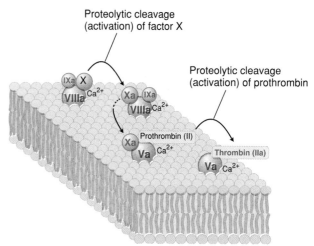

Figure 22-7. Coagulation factor activation on phospholipid surfaces. Surface catalysis is critical for a number of the activation reactions in the coagulation cascade. Each activation reaction consists of an enzyme (e.g., factor IXa), a substrate (e.g., factor X), and a cofactor or reaction accelerator (e.g., factor VIIIa), all of which are assembled on the phospholipid surface of activated platelets, endothelial cells, and leukocytes. Ca^{2+} allows the enzyme and substrate to adopt the proper conformation in each activation reaction. In the example shown, factor VIIIa and Ca^{2+} act as cofactors in the factor IXa-mediated cleavage of factor X to factor Xa. Factor Va and Ca^{2+} then act as cofactors in the factor Xa-mediated cleavage of prothrombin to thrombin.

proper conformation for the proteolytic cleavage of a coagulation factor proenzyme to its activated form.

Third, the coagulation cascade has been divided traditionally into the **intrinsic** and **extrinsic pathways** (Fig. 22-6). This division is a result of in vitro testing and is essentially arbitrary. The intrinsic pathway is activated in vitro by factor XII (Hageman factor), while the extrinsic pathway is initiated in vivo by **tissue factor,** a lipoprotein expressed by activated leukocytes (and microparticles derived from activated leukocytes; see below), activated endothelial cells, subendothelial smooth muscle cells, and subendothelial fibro-

blasts at the site of vascular injury. Although these two pathways converge at the activation of factor X, there also exists much interconnection between the two pathways. Because factor VII (activated by the extrinsic pathway) can proteolytically activate factor IX (a key factor in the intrinsic pathway), the extrinsic pathway is regarded as the primary pathway for the initiation of coagulation in vivo.

Fourth, both the intrinsic and extrinsic coagulation pathways lead to the activation of factor X. In an important reaction that requires factor V, activated factor X proteolytically cleaves prothrombin (factor II) to **thrombin** (factor IIa) (Fig. 22-8). Thrombin is a multifunctional enzyme that acts in the coagulation cascade in four important ways: (1) it converts the soluble plasma protein fibrinogen into fibrin, which then forms long, insoluble polymer fibers; (2) it activates factor XIII, which crosslinks the fibrin polymers into a highly stable meshwork or clot; (3) it amplifies the clotting cascade by catalyzing the feedback activation of factors VIII and V; and (4) it strongly activates platelets, causing granule release, platelet aggregation, and platelet-derived microparticle generation. In addition to its procoagulant properties, thrombin acts to modulate the coagulation response. Thrombin binds to thrombin receptors on the *intact* vascular endothelial cells adjacent to the area of vascular injury, and stimulates these cells to release the platelet inhibitors prostacyclin (PGI_2) and nitric oxide (NO), the profibrinolytic protein tissue plasminogen activator (t-PA), and the endogenous t-PA modulator plasminogen activator inhibitor 1 (PAI-1) (see below).

The thrombin receptor, a protease-activated G protein-coupled receptor, is expressed in the plasma membrane of

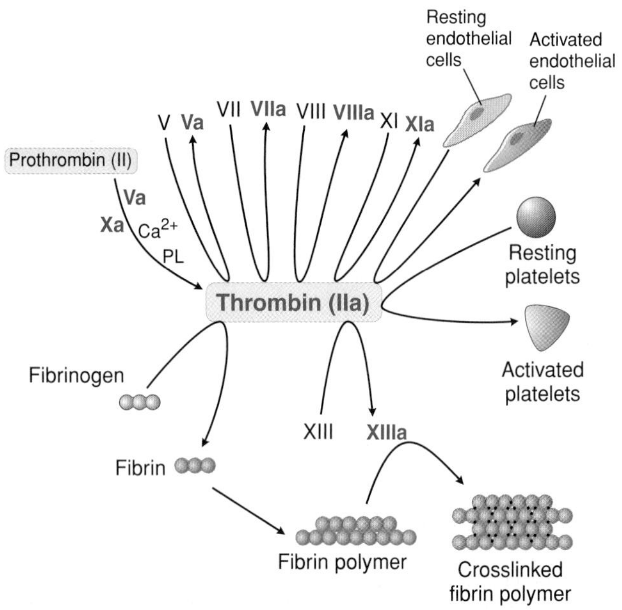

Figure 22-8. Central role of thrombin in the coagulation cascade. In the coagulation cascade, prothrombin is cleaved to thrombin by factor Xa; factor Va and Ca^{2+} act as cofactors in this reaction, and the reaction takes place on an activated (phosphatidylserine-expressing) phospholipid surface (PL). Thrombin converts the soluble plasma protein fibrinogen to fibrin, which spontaneously polymerizes. Thrombin also activates factor XIII, a transglutaminase that crosslinks the fibrin polymers into a highly stable meshwork or clot. Thrombin also activates co-factors V and VIII, as well as coagulation factors VII and XI. In addition, thrombin activates both platelets and endothelial cells. Finally, thrombin stimulates the release of several antithrombotic factors—including PGI_2, NO, and t-PA—from resting (intact) endothelial cells near the site of vascular injury; these factors limit primary and secondary hemostasis to the injured site (*not shown*).

platelets, vascular endothelial cells, smooth muscle cells, and fibroblasts. Activation of the thrombin receptor involves proteolytic *cleavage* of an extracellular domain of the receptor by thrombin. The new NH_2-terminal-tethered ligand binds intramolecularly to a discrete site within the receptor and initiates intracellular signaling. Activation of the thrombin receptor results in G protein-mediated activation of PLC (Fig. 22-5) and inhibition of adenylyl cyclase.

Finally, recent evidence from intravital (in vivo) microscopy experiments suggests that leukocyte-derived microparticles have an important role in coupling platelet plug formation (primary hemostasis) to fibrin clot formation (secondary hemostasis). A subpopulation of these microparticles, released from monocytes that are activated in the context of tissue injury and inflammation, appears to express both tissue factor and PSGL-1, a protein that binds to the P-selectin adhesion receptor expressed on activated platelets. By recruiting tissue factor-bearing microparticles throughout the developing platelet plug (primary hemostasis), thrombin generation and fibrin clot formation (secondary hemostasis) could be greatly accelerated within the plug itself. Indeed, it appears that vessel-wall tissue factor (expressed by activated endothelial cells and subendothelial fibroblasts and smooth muscle cells) and microparticle tissue factor are both important for formation of a stable clot.

REGULATION OF HEMOSTASIS

Hemostasis is exquisitely regulated for two major reasons. First, hemostasis must be restricted to the local site of vascular injury. That is, activation of platelets and coagulation factors in the plasma should occur only at the site of endothelial damage, tissue factor expression, and procoagulant phospholipid exposure. Second, the size of the primary and secondary hemostatic plugs must be restricted so that the vascular lumen remains patent. After vascular injury, intact endothelium in the immediate vicinity of the injury becomes ''activated.'' This activated endothelium presents a set of procoagulant factors that promote hemostasis at the site of injury, and anticoagulant factors that restrict propagation of the clot beyond the site of injury. The procoagulant factors, such as tissue factor and phosphatidylserine, tend to be *membrane-bound* and *localized* to the site of injury — these factors provide a surface on which the coagulation cascade can proceed. In contrast, the anticoagulant factors are generally *secreted* by the endothelium and are *soluble* in the blood. Thus, *the activated endothelium maintains a balance of procoagulant and anticoagulant factors to limit hemostasis to the site of vascular injury.*

After vascular injury, the endothelium surrounding the injured area participates in five separate mechanisms that limit the initiation and propagation of the hemostatic process to the immediate vicinity of the injury. These mechanisms involve prostacyclin (PGI_2), antithrombin III, proteins C and S, tissue factor pathway inhibitor (TFPI), and tissue-type plasminogen activator (t-PA).

Prostacyclin (PGI_2) is an eicosanoid (i.e., a metabolite of arachidonic acid) that is synthesized and secreted by the endothelium. By acting through G_s protein-coupled platelet-surface PGI_2 receptors, this metabolite increases cAMP levels within platelets and thereby inhibits platelet aggregation and platelet granule release. PGI_2 also has potent vasodilatory effects; this mediator induces vascular smooth muscle relaxation by increasing cAMP levels within the vascular smooth muscle cells. (Note that these mechanisms are physiologically antagonistic to those of TxA_2, which induces platelet activation and vasoconstriction by decreasing intracellular cAMP levels.) Therefore, PGI_2 both prevents platelets from adhering to the intact endothelium that surrounds the site of vascular injury and maintains vascular patency around the site of injury.

Antithrombin III inactivates thrombin and other coagulation factors (IXa, Xa, XIa, and XIIa, where ''a'' denotes an ''activated'' factor) by forming a stoichiometric complex with the coagulation factor (Fig. 22-9). These interactions are enhanced by a heparin-like molecule that is expressed at the surface of intact endothelial cells, ensuring that this mechanism is operative at all locations in the vascular tree *except* where endothelium is denuded at the site of vascular injury. (These endothelial cell surface proteoglycans are referred to as ''heparin-like'' because they are the physiologic equivalent of the pharmacologic agent heparin, discussed below.) Heparin-like molecules on the endothelial cells bind to and activate antithrombin III, which is then primed to complex with (and thereby inactivate) the activated coagulation factors.

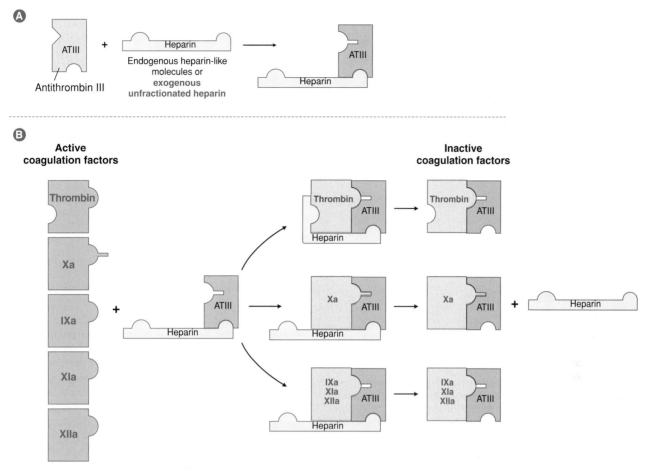

Figure 22-9.   Antithrombin III action. Antithrombin III (ATIII) inactivates thrombin and factors IXa, Xa, XIa, and XIIa by forming a stoichiometric complex with these coagulation factors. These reactions are catalyzed physiologically by heparin-like molecules expressed on healthy endothelial cells; sites of vascular injury do not express heparin-like molecules because the endothelium is denuded or damaged. Pharmacologically, these reactions are catalyzed by exogenously administered heparin. In more detail, the binding of heparin to ATIII induces a conformational change in ATIII **(A)** that allows the ATIII to bind thrombin or coagulation factors IXa, Xa, XIa or XIIa. The stoichiometric complex between ATIII and the coagulation factor is highly stable, allowing heparin to dissociate without breaking up the complex **(B)**.

Protein C and **protein S** are vitamin K-dependent proteins that slow the coagulation cascade by inactivating coagulation factors Va and VIIIa. Protein C and protein S are part of a feedback control mechanism, in which excess thrombin generation leads to activation of protein C which, in turn, helps to prevent the enlarging fibrin clot from occluding the vascular lumen. Specifically, the endothelial cell-surface protein **thrombomodulin** is a receptor for both thrombin and protein C in the plasma. Thrombomodulin binds these proteins in such a way that thrombomodulin-bound thrombin cleaves protein C to activated protein C (also known as *protein Ca*). In a reaction that requires the cofactor protein S, activated protein C then inhibits clotting by cleaving (and thereby inactivating) factors Va and VIIIa.

Tissue factor pathway inhibitor (TFPI), as its name indicates, limits the action of tissue factor (TF). The coagulation cascade is initiated when factor VIIa complexes with TF at the site of vascular injury (Fig. 22-6). The resulting VIIa:TF complex catalyzes the activation of factors IX and X. After limited quantities of factors IXa and Xa are generated, the VIIa:TF complex becomes feedback inhibited by

TFPI in a two-step reaction. First, TFPI binds to factor Xa and neutralizes its activity in a Ca^{2+}-independent reaction. Subsequently, the TFPI:Xa complex interacts with the VIIa: TF complex via a second domain on TFPI, so that a quaternary Xa:TFPI:VIIa:TF complex is formed. The molecular "knots" of the TFPI molecule hold the quaternary complex tightly together and thereby inactivate the VIIa:TF complex. In this manner, TFPI prevents excessive TF-mediated activation of factors IX and X.

Plasmin exerts its anticoagulant effect by proteolytically cleaving fibrin into fibrin degradation products. Because plasmin has powerful antithrombotic effects, the *formation* of plasmin has intrigued researchers for many years, and a number of pharmacologic agents have been developed to target the plasmin formation pathway (Fig. 22-10). Plasmin is generated by the proteolytic cleavage of plasminogen, a plasma protein that is synthesized in the liver. The proteolytic cleavage is catalyzed by **tissue plasminogen activator (t-PA),** which is synthesized and secreted by the endothelium. Plasmin activity is carefully modulated by three regulatory mechanisms in order to restrict plasmin action to the

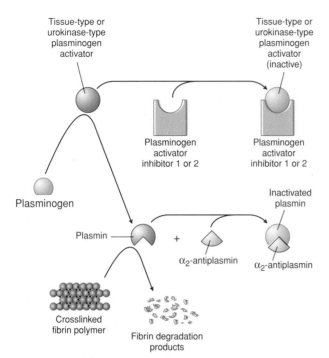

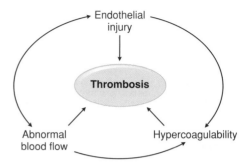

Figure 22-11. Virchow's triad. Endothelial injury, abnormal blood flow, and hypercoagulability are three factors that predispose to thrombus formation. These three factors are interrelated; endothelial injury predisposes to abnormal blood flow and hypercoagulability, while abnormal blood flow can cause both endothelial injury and hypercoagulability.

Figure 22-10. The Fibrinolytic System. Plasmin is formed by the proteolytic cleavage of plasminogen by tissue-type or urokinase-type plasminogen activator. Plasmin formation can be inhibited by plasminogen activator inhibitor 1 or 2, which binds to and inactivates plasminogen activators. In the fibrinolytic reaction, plasmin cleaves crosslinked fibrin polymers into fibrin degradation products. α_2-Antiplasmin, which circulates in the bloodstream, neutralizes free plasmin in the circulation.

ENDOTHELIAL INJURY

Endothelial injury is the dominant influence on thrombus formation in the *heart* and the *arterial circulation.* There are many possible causes of endothelial injury, including changes in shear stress associated with hypertension or turbulent flow, hyperlipidemia, elevated blood glucose in diabetes mellitus, traumatic vascular injury, and some infections. (Recall that Mr. S developed coronary artery thrombosis, which was probably attributable to endothelial injury secondary to hypertension and cigarette smoking.)

Endothelial injury predisposes the vascular lumen to thrombus formation through three mechanisms. First, platelet activators, such as exposed subendothelial collagen, promote platelet adhesion to the injured site. Second, exposure of tissue factor on injured endothelium initiates the coagulation cascade. Third, natural antithrombotics, such as t-PA and PGI_2, become depleted at the site of vascular injury because these mechanisms rely on the functioning of an intact endothelial cell layer.

ABNORMAL BLOOD FLOW

Abnormal blood flow refers to a state of **turbulence** or **stasis** rather than laminar flow. Atherosclerotic plaques commonly predispose to turbulent blood flow in the vicinity of the plaque. Bifurcations of blood vessels can also create areas of turbulent flow. Turbulent blood flow causes endothelial injury, forms countercurrents, and creates local pockets of stasis. Local stasis can also result from formation of an aneurysm (a focal out-pouching of a vessel or a cardiac chamber) and from myocardial infarction. In the latter condition, a region of noncontractile (infarcted) myocardium serves as a favored site for stasis. Cardiac arrhythmias, such as atrial fibrillation, can also generate areas of local stasis. Stasis is the major cause for the formation of *venous* thrombi.

Disruption of normal blood flow by turbulence or stasis promotes thrombosis by three major mechanisms. First, the absence of laminar blood flow allows platelets to come into close proximity to the vessel wall. Second, stasis inhibits the flow of fresh blood into the vascular bed, so that activated coagulation factors in the region are not removed or diluted.

site of clot formation. First, t-PA is most effective when it is bound to a fibrin meshwork. Second, t-PA activity can be inhibited by **plasminogen activator inhibitor (PAI).** When local concentrations of thrombin and inflammatory cytokines (such as IL-1 and TNF-α) are *high,* endothelial cells *increase* the release of PAI, preventing t-PA from activating plasmin. This ensures that a stable fibrin clot forms at the site of vascular injury. Third, α_2-antiplasmin is a plasma protein that neutralizes free plasmin in the circulation and thereby prevents random degradation of plasma fibrinogen. Plasma fibrinogen is important for platelet aggregation in primary hemostasis (see above), and it is also the precursor for the fibrin polymer that is required to form a stable clot.

PATHOGENESIS OF THROMBOSIS

Thrombosis is the pathologic extension of hemostasis. In thrombosis, coagulation reactions are inappropriately regulated so that a clot uncontrollably enlarges and occludes the lumen of a blood vessel. The pathologic clot is now termed a **thrombus.** Three major factors predispose to thrombus formation—endothelial injury, abnormal blood flow, and hypercoagulability. These three factors influence one another, and are collectively known as **Virchow's triad** (Fig. 22-11).

Third, abnormal blood flow promotes endothelial cell activation, which leads to a prothrombotic state.

HYPERCOAGULABILITY

Hypercoagulability is generally less important than endothelial injury and abnormal blood flow in predisposing to thrombosis, but this condition can be an important factor in some patients. Hypercoagulability refers to an abnormally heightened coagulation response to vascular injury, resulting from either: (1) **primary (genetic) disorders**; or (2) **secondary (acquired) disorders** (see Table 22-1). (Hypocoagulable states, or **hemorrhagic disorders,** can also result from primary or secondary causes; see Box 22-1 for an example.)

Among the genetic causes of hypercoagulability, the most prevalent known mutation resides in the gene for coagulation factor V. It is estimated that 6% of the Caucasian population in the U.S. carries mutations in the factor V gene. The most common mutation is the Leiden mutation, in which glutamine is substituted for arginine at position 506. This position is important because it is part of a site in factor Va that is marked for proteolytic cleavage by activated protein C. The mutant **factor V Leiden** protein is resistant to proteolytic cleavage by activated protein C. As a result of the Leiden mutation, factor Va is allowed to accumulate and thereby to promote coagulation.

A second common mutation (2% incidence) is the **prothrombin G20210A mutation**, in which adenine (A) is substituted for guanine (G) in the 3′-untranslated region of the prothrombin gene. This mutation leads to a 30% increase in plasma prothrombin levels. Both the factor V Leiden mutation and the prothrombin G20210A mutation are associated with a significantly increased risk of venous thrombosis and a modestly increased risk of arterial thrombosis. Other genetic disorders that predispose some individuals to thrombosis include mutations in the fibrinogen, protein C, protein S, and antithrombin III genes. Although the latter disorders are relatively uncommon (less than 1% incidence), patients with a genetic deficiency of protein C, protein S, or antithrombin III often present with spontaneous venous thrombosis.

Hypercoagulability can sometimes be acquired (secondary) rather than genetic. An example of acquired hypercoagulability is the **heparin-induced thrombocytopenia** syndrome. In some patients, administration of the anticoagulant heparin stimulates the immune system to generate circulating antibodies directed against a complex consisting of heparin and platelet factor 4. Because platelet factor 4 is present on platelet and endothelial cell surfaces, antibody binding to the heparin:platelet factor 4 complex results in antibody-mediated removal of platelets from the circulation; that is, in thrombocytopenia. In some patients, however, antibody binding also causes platelet activation, endothelial injury, and a prothrombotic state. Although both unfractionated and low molecular weight heparin (see below) can cause thrombocytopenia, it appears that low molecular weight heparin is associated with a lower incidence of thrombocytopenia than unfractionated heparin.

| TABLE 22-1 | Major Causes of Hypercoagulability |

CONDITION	MECHANISM OF HYPERCOAGULABILITY
Primary (Genetic)	
Factor V Leiden mutation (factor V R506Q) (common)	Resistance to activated protein C → excess factor Va
Hyperhomocysteinemia (common)	Endothelial damage due to accumulation of homocysteine
Prothrombin G20210A mutation (common)	Increased prothrombin level and activity
Antithrombin III deficiency (less common)	Decreased inactivation of factors IIa, IXa, and Xa
Protein C or S deficiency (less common)	Decreased proteolytic inactivation of factors VIIIa and Va
Secondary (Acquired)	
Antiphospholipid syndrome	Autoantibodies to negatively charged phospholipids → ↑ platelet adhesion
Heparin-induced thrombocytopenia	Antibodies to platelet factor 4 → platelet activation
Malignancy	Tumor cell induction of tissue factor expression
Myeloproliferative syndromes	Elevated blood viscosity, altered platelets
Nephrotic syndrome	Loss of antithrombin III in urine, ↑ fibrinogen, ↑ platelet activation
Oral contraceptive use, estrogen replacement therapy	↑ Hepatic synthesis of coagulation factors and/or effects of estrogen on endothelium (effect may be more prominent in patients with underlying primary hypercoagulability)
Paroxysmal nocturnal hemoglobinuria	Unknown, possibly "leaky" platelets
Postpartum period	Venous stasis, increased coagulation factors, tissue trauma
Surgery/trauma	Venous stasis, immobilization, tissue injury

BOX 22-1. Hemorrhagic Disorders

When the vascular endothelium is injured, the hemostatic process ensures localized, stable clot formation without obstruction of the vascular lumen. Just as thrombosis constitutes a pathologic variation on this otherwise orchestrated physiologic process, disorders involving insufficient levels of functional platelets or coagulation factors can lead to a hypocoagulable state characterized clinically by episodes of uncontrolled hemorrhage. Hemorrhagic disorders result from a multitude of causes, including disorders of the vasculature, vitamin K deficiency, and disorders or deficiencies of platelets, coagulation factors, and von Willebrand factor. Hemophilia A serves as an example of a hemorrhagic disorder in which hypocoagulability is the underlying pathology.

Hemophilia A is the most common genetic disorder of serious bleeding. The hallmark of the disorder is a reduction in the amount or activity of coagulation factor VIII. The syndrome has an X-linked mode of transmission, and the majority of patients are males or homozygous females. Thirty percent of patients have no family history of hemophilia A and presumably represent spontaneous mutations. The severity of the disease depends on the type of mutation in the factor VIII gene. Patients with 6% to 50% of normal factor VIII activity manifest a mild form of the disease; those with 2% to 5% activity manifest moderate disease; patients with less than 1% activity develop severe disease. All symptomatic patients demonstrate easy bruisability and can develop massive hemorrhage after trauma or surgery. Spontaneous hemorrhage can occur in body areas that are normally subjected to minor trauma, including joint spaces, where spontaneous hemorrhage leads to the formation of hemarthroses. Petechiae (microhemorrhages involving capillaries and small vessels, especially in mucocutaneous areas), which are usually an indication of platelet disorders, are absent in patients with hemophilia.

Patients with hemophilia A are currently treated with infusions of factor VIII that is either recombinant or derived from human plasma. Factor VIII infusion therapy is sometimes complicated in patients who develop antibodies against factor VIII. HIV infection was a serious complication of infusion therapy in patients who received factor VIII products before the institution of routine screening of blood for HIV infection (before the mid-1980s). Some sources suggest that the entire cohort of hemophiliacs who received factor VIII concentrates (factor VIII concentrated from the blood of many individuals) between 1981 and 1985 has been infected with HIV. With current blood screening practices and the development of recombinant factor VIII, the risk of contracting HIV through factor VIII infusions is now virtually zero.

PHARMACOLOGIC CLASSES AND AGENTS

Drugs have been developed to prevent and/or reverse thrombus formation. These drugs fall into three classes: antiplatelet agents, anticoagulants, and thrombolytic agents. Hemostatic agents, discussed at the end of the chapter, are occasionally used to reverse the effects of anticoagulants or to inhibit endogenous fibrinolysis.

ANTIPLATELET AGENTS

As described above, formation of a localized platelet plug in response to endothelial injury is the initial step in arterial thrombosis. Therefore, inhibition of platelet function is a useful prophylactic and therapeutic strategy against myocardial infarction and stroke caused by thrombosis in coronary and cerebral arteries, respectively. The classes of antiplatelet agents in current clinical use include cyclooxygenase (COX) inhibitors, phosphodiesterase inhibitors, ADP receptor pathway inhibitors, and GPIIb–IIIa antagonists.

Cyclooxygenase Inhibitors

Aspirin inhibits the synthesis of prostaglandins, thereby inhibiting the platelet release reaction and interfering with normal platelet aggregation.

The biochemistry of prostaglandin synthesis in platelets and endothelial cells provides a basis for understanding the mechanism of action of aspirin as an antiplatelet agent. Figure 22-12 depicts the prostaglandin synthesis pathway, which is discussed in more detail in Chapter 41, Pharmacology of Eicosanoids. Briefly, activation of both platelets and endothelial cells induces phospholipase A_2 (PLA_2) to cleave membrane phospholipids and release arachidonic acid. Arachidonic acid is then transformed into a cyclic endoperoxide (also known as **prostaglandin G_2** or **PGG_2**) by the enzyme COX. In platelets, the cyclic endoperoxide is converted into thromboxane A_2 (TxA_2). Acting through cell-surface TxA_2 receptors, TxA_2 causes localized vasoconstriction and is a potent inducer of platelet aggregation and the platelet granule release reaction. In endothelial cells, the cyclic endoperoxide is converted into prostacyclin (PGI_2). PGI_2, in turn, causes localized vasodilation and inhibits platelet aggregation and the platelet granule release reaction.

Aspirin acts by *covalently* acetylating a serine residue near the active site of the COX enzyme, thereby inhibiting the synthesis of the cyclic endoperoxide and the various metabolites of the cyclic endoperoxide. In the absence of TxA_2, there is a marked decrease in platelet aggregation and the platelet granule release reaction (Fig. 22-13A). *Because platelets do not contain DNA or RNA, these cells cannot regenerate new COX enzyme once aspirin has permanently inactivated all of the available COX enzyme.* That is, the platelets become irreversibly "poisoned" for the lifetime of these cells (7–10 days). Although aspirin also inhibits the COX enzyme in endothelial cells, its action is not permanent in endothelial cells because these cells are able to synthesize new COX molecules. Thus, the endothelial cell production

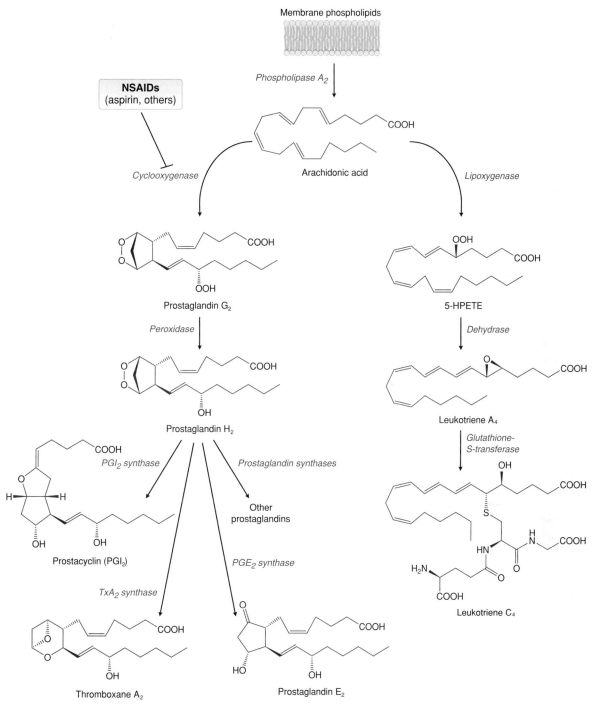

Figure 22-12. Overview of Prostaglandin Synthesis. Membrane phospholipids are cleaved by phospholipase A$_2$ to release free arachidonic acid. Arachidonic acid can be metabolized through either of two major pathways, the cyclooxygenase pathway or the lipoxygenase pathway. The cyclooxygenase pathway, which is inhibited by aspirin and other nonsteroidal anti-inflammatory drugs (NSAIDs), converts arachidonic acid into prostaglandins and thromboxanes. Platelets express TxA$_2$ synthase and synthesize the pro-aggregatory mediator thromboxane A$_2$; endothelial cells express PGI$_2$ synthase and synthesize the anti-aggregatory mediator prostacyclin. The lipoxygenase pathway converts arachidonic acid into leukotrienes, which are potent inflammatory mediators. (See Chapter 41, Pharmacology of Eicosanoids, for a detailed discussion of the lipoxygenase and cyclooxygenase pathways.) Aspirin inhibits cyclooxygenase by covalent acetylation of the enzyme near its active site. Because platelets lack the capability to synthesize new proteins, aspirin inhibits thromboxane synthesis for the life of the platelet.

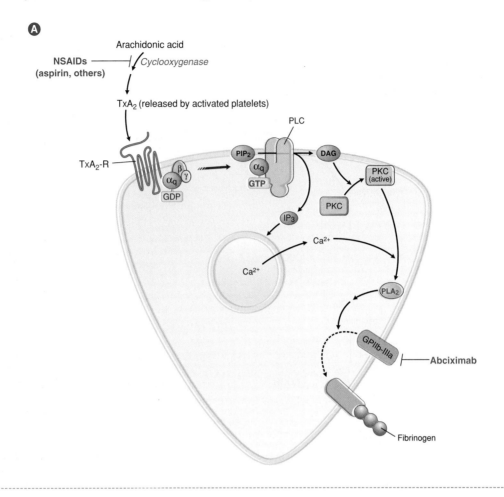

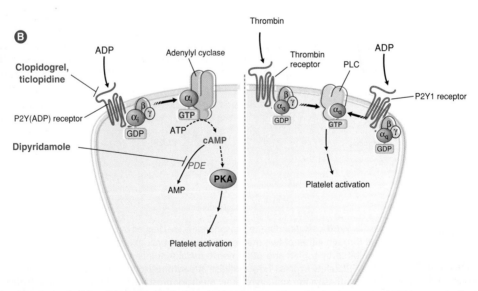

Figure 22-13. Mechanism of action of antiplatelet agents. A. NSAIDs and GPIIb-IIIa antagonists inhibit steps in thromboxane A_2 (TxA_2)-mediated platelet activation. Aspirin inhibits cyclooxygenase by covalent acetylation of the enzyme near its active site, leading to decreased TxA_2 production. The effect is profound because platelets lack the ability to synthesize new enzyme molecules. GPIIb–IIIa antagonists, such as the monoclonal antibody abciximab and the small-molecule antagonists eptifibatide and tirofiban *(not shown)*, inhibit platelet aggregation by preventing activation of GpIIb–IIIa *(dashed line)*, leading to decreased platelet crosslinking by fibrinogen. **B.** Clopidogrel, ticlopidine, and dipyridamole inhibit steps in ADP-mediated platelet activation. Clopidogrel and ticlopidine are antagonists of the P2Y(ADP) receptor. Dipyridamole inhibits phosphodiesterase (PDE), thereby preventing the breakdown of cAMP and increasing cytoplasmic cAMP concentration.

of prostacyclin is relatively unaffected by aspirin at pharmacologically low doses (see below).

Aspirin is most often used as an antiplatelet agent to prevent arterial thrombosis leading to stroke, transient ischemic attack, and myocardial infarction. Because the action of aspirin on platelets is permanent, it is most effective as a selective antiplatelet agent when taken *in low doses and/or at infrequent intervals*. For example, aspirin is often used as an antiplatelet agent at a dose of 81 mg once daily, while a typical anti-inflammatory dose of this agent could be 650 mg three to four times daily. Taken at high doses, aspirin can inhibit prostacyclin production without increasing the effectiveness of the drug as an antiplatelet agent. A more extended discussion of the uses and toxicities of aspirin is found in Chapter 41. Compared with aspirin, other nonsteroidal anti-inflammatory drugs (NSAIDs) are not as widely used in the prevention of arterial thrombosis because the inhibitory action of these drugs on cyclooxygenase is not permanent.

COX-1 is the predominant COX isoform in platelets, but endothelial cells appear to express both COX-1 and COX-2 under physiologic conditions. Because aspirin inhibits COX-1 and COX-2 nonselectively, this drug serves as an effective antiplatelet agent. In contrast, the newer selective COX-2 inhibitors cannot be used as antiplatelet agents because they are poor inhibitors of COX-1. Furthermore, use of the selective COX-2 inhibitors appears to be associated with increased cardiovascular risk, most likely because these agents inhibit endothelial production of PGI_2 without inhibiting platelet generation of TxA_2. The adverse impact of the selective COX-2 inhibitors on cardiovascular risk has resulted in the recent withdrawal of most of these agents from the market (see Chapter 41).

Phosphodiesterase Inhibitors

In platelets, an *increase* in the concentration of intracellular cAMP leads to a *decrease* in platelet aggregability. Platelet cAMP levels are regulated physiologically by TxA_2 and PGI_2, among other mediators (see above). The mechanism by which increased intracellular cAMP concentration leads to decreased platelet aggregability is not well understood. cAMP activates protein kinase A, which, through incompletely elucidated mechanisms, decreases availability of the intracellular Ca^{2+} necessary for platelet aggregation (Fig. 22-13B). Inhibitors of platelet phosphodiesterase decrease platelet aggregability by inhibiting cAMP degradation, while activators of platelet adenylyl cyclase decrease platelet aggregability by increasing cAMP synthesis. (There are currently no direct adenylyl cyclase activators in clinical use.)

Dipyridamole is an inhibitor of platelet phosphodiesterase that decreases platelet aggregability (Fig. 22-13B). Dipyridamole by itself has only weak antiplatelet effects, and is therefore usually administered in combination with warfarin or aspirin. The combination of dipyridamole and warfarin can be used to inhibit thrombus formation on prosthetic heart valves, while the combination of dipyridamole and aspirin can be used to reduce the likelihood of thrombosis in patients with a thrombotic diathesis. Dipyridamole also has vasodilatory properties. It may paradoxically induce angina in patients with coronary artery disease by causing the coronary

steal phenomenon, which involves intense dilation of coronary arterioles (see Chapter 21, Pharmacology of Vascular Tone).

ADP Receptor Pathway Inhibitors

Both **ticlopidine** and **clopidogrel** are derivatives of thienopyridine. These agents, which irreversibly inhibit the ADP-dependent pathway of platelet activation, have antiplatelet effects in vitro and in vivo. Ticlopidine and clopidogrel are thought to act by covalently modifying and inactivating the platelet P2Y(ADP) receptor (also called $P2Y_{12}$), which is physiologically coupled to the inhibition of adenylyl cyclase (Fig. 22-13B). Ticlopidine is a prodrug that requires conversion to active thiol metabolites in the liver. Maximal platelet inhibition is observed 8 to 11 days after initiating therapy with the drug; used in combination with aspirin, 4 to 7 days are needed to achieve maximal platelet inhibition. Administration of a loading dose can produce a more rapid antiplatelet response. Ticlopidine is approved in the U.S. for two indications: (1) secondary prevention of thrombotic strokes in patients intolerant of aspirin, and (2) in combination with aspirin, prevention of stent thrombosis for up to 30 days after placement of coronary artery stents. In general, ticlopidine is considered to be less safe than clopidogrel. The use of ticlopidine has occasionally been associated with neutropenia, thrombocytopenia, and thrombotic thrombocytopenic purpura (TTP); for this reason, blood counts must be monitored frequently when using ticlopidine.

Clopidogrel, a thienopyridine closely related to ticlopidine, has been used widely in combination with aspirin for improved platelet inhibition during and after elective percutaneous coronary intervention. Clopidogrel is a prodrug that must undergo oxidation by hepatic P450 3A4 to the active drug form; it may therefore interact with statins and other drugs metabolized by this P450 enzyme. Clopidogrel is approved for secondary prevention in patients with recent myocardial infarction, stroke, or peripheral vascular disease. It is also approved for use in acute coronary syndromes that are treated with either percutaneous coronary intervention or coronary artery bypass grafting. Like ticlopidine, clopidogrel requires a loading dose to achieve a maximal antiplatelet effect rapidly. For this reason, Mr. S was given an intravenous loading dose of clopidogrel in the context of his myocardial infarction. The adverse-effect profile of clopidogrel is more acceptable than that of ticlopidine: the gastrointestinal effects of clopidogrel are similar to those of aspirin, and clopidogrel lacks the significant bone marrow toxicity associated with ticlopidine.

GPIIb–IIIa Antagonists

As noted above, platelet membrane GPIIb–IIIa receptors are important because they constitute the final common pathway of platelet aggregation, serving to bind fibrinogen molecules that bridge platelets to one another. A variety of stimuli (e.g., TxA_2, ADP, epinephrine, collagen, and thrombin), acting through diverse signaling molecules, are capable of inducing the expression of functional GPIIb–IIIa on the platelet surface. It could therefore be predicted that antagonists of GPIIb–IIIa would prevent fibrinogen binding to the GPIIb–IIIa receptor and thus serve as powerful inhibitors of platelet aggregation. **Eptifibatide,** the GPIIb–IIIa receptor antagonist used in the opening case, is a highly efficacious inhibitor of platelet aggregation. A synthetic peptide, eptifibatide antagonizes the platelet GPIIb–IIIa receptor with high affinity. This drug has been used to reduce ischemic events in patients undergoing percutaneous coronary intervention and to treat unstable angina and non-ST elevation myocardial infarction.

Abciximab is a chimeric mouse–human monoclonal antibody directed against the human GPIIb–IIIa receptor. Experiments in vitro have shown that occupation of 50% of platelet GPIIb–IIIa receptors by abciximab significantly reduces platelet aggregation. The binding of abciximab to GPIIb–IIIa is essentially *irreversible*, with a dissociation half-time of 18 to 24 hours. In clinical trials, adding abciximab to conventional antithrombotic therapy reduces both long-term and short-term ischemic events in patients undergoing high-risk percutaneous coronary intervention.

Tirofiban is a nonpeptide tyrosine analogue that reversibly antagonizes fibrinogen binding to the platelet GPIIb–IIIa receptor. Both in vitro and in vivo studies have demonstrated the ability of tirofiban to inhibit platelet aggregation. Tirofiban has been approved for use in patients with acute coronary syndromes.

Because of their mechanism of action as antiplatelet agents, all of the GPIIb–IIIa antagonists can cause bleeding as an adverse effect. In the opening case, Mr. S developed a hematoma in his right thigh near the arterial access site at which eptifibatide was being infused. The expanding hematoma was caused by the excessive antiplatelet effect of a very high local concentration of eptifibatide at the infusion site. Importantly, the ability to reverse the effect of GPIIb–IIIa receptor antagonists differs for the different agents. Because abciximab is an irreversible inhibitor of platelet function, and all the abciximab previously infused is already bound to platelets, infusion of fresh platelets after the drug has been stopped can reverse the antiplatelet effect. In contrast, because the two small-molecule antagonists (eptifibatide and tirofiban) bind the receptor reversibly and are infused in great stoichiometric excess of receptor number, infusion of fresh platelets simply offers new sites to which the drug can bind, and it is not practical to deliver a sufficient number of platelets to overwhelm the vast excess of drug present. Therefore, one must stop the drug infusion and wait for platelet function to return to normal as the drug is cleared. In the case of Mr. S, no other measure could have been taken to reverse the effect of eptifibatide at the time his hematoma was recognized.

ANTICOAGULANTS

As with antiplatelet agents, anticoagulants are used both to prevent and treat thrombotic disease. There are four classes of anticoagulants: warfarin, unfractionated and low molecular weight heparins, selective factor Xa inhibitors, and direct thrombin inhibitors. Anticoagulants target various factors in the coagulation cascade, thereby interrupting the cascade and preventing the formation of a stable fibrin meshwork (secondary hemostatic plug). In this section, the four classes of anticoagulants are discussed in order of selectivity, from the least selective agents (warfarin and unfractionated heparin)

to the most selective agents (selective factor Xa inhibitors and direct thrombin inhibitors). Recombinant activated protein C also has anticoagulant activity, although its clinical indication is severe sepsis. Because of the mechanisms of action of these drugs, bleeding is an adverse effect common to all anticoagulants.

Warfarin

In the early 1900s, farmers in Canada and the North Dakota plains adopted the practice of planting sweet clover instead of corn for fodder. In the winter months of 1921 to 1922, a fatal hemorrhagic disease was reported in cattle that had foraged on the sweet clover. In almost every case, it was found that the affected cattle had foraged on sweet clover that had been spoiled by the curing process. After an intensive investigation, scientist K. P. Link reported that the spoiled clover contained the natural anticoagulant 3,3'-methylene-bis-(4-hydroxycoumarin) or ''dicumarol.'' Dicumarol and **warfarin** (a potent synthetic congener) were introduced during the 1940s as rodenticides and as oral anticoagulants. Because the oral anticoagulants act by affecting vitamin K-dependent reactions, it is important to understand how vitamin K functions.

Mechanism of Action of Vitamin K

Vitamin K (''K'' is derived from the German word ''Koagulation'') is required for the normal hepatic synthesis of four coagulation factors (II, VII, IX, and X), protein C, and protein S. The coagulation factors, protein C, and protein S are biologically inactive as unmodified polypeptides following protein synthesis on ribosomes. These proteins gain biological activity by post-translational carboxylation of their 9 to 12 amino-terminal glutamic acid residues. The γ-carboxylated glutamate residues (but not the unmodified glutamate residues) are capable of binding Ca^{2+} ions. Ca^{2+} binding induces a conformational change in these proteins that is required for efficient binding of the proteins to phospholipid surfaces. The ability of the γ-carboxylated molecules to bind Ca^{2+} increases the enzymatic activity of coagulation factors IIa, VIIa, IXa, Xa, and protein Ca by approximately 1,000-fold. Thus, vitamin K-dependent carboxylation is crucial for the enzymatic activity of the four coagulation factors and protein C, and for the cofactor function of protein S.

The carboxylation reaction requires (1) a precursor form of the target protein with its 9 to 12 amino-terminal glutamic acid residues, (2) carbon dioxide, (3) molecular oxygen, and (4) *reduced* vitamin K. The carboxylation reaction is schematically presented in Figure 22-14. During this reaction, vitamin K is oxidized to the inactive 2,3-epoxide. An enzyme, epoxide reductase, is then required to convert the inactive 2,3-epoxide into the active, reduced form of vitamin K. *Thus, the regeneration of reduced vitamin K is essential for the sustained synthesis of biologically functional clotting factors II, VII, IX, and X, all of which are critical components of the coagulation cascade.*

Mechanism of Action of Warfarin

Warfarin acts on the carboxylation pathway, not by inhibiting the carboxylase directly, but by blocking the epoxide

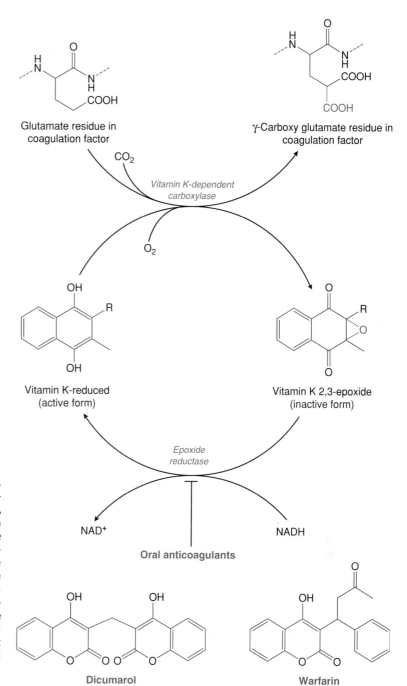

Figure 22-14. Mechanism of action of warfarin. Vitamin K is a necessary cofactor in the post-translational carboxylation of glutamate residues on factors II, VII, IX, and X. During the carboxylation reaction, vitamin K is oxidized to the inactive 2,3-epoxide. The enzyme epoxide reductase converts the inactive vitamin K 2,3-epoxide into the active, reduced form of vitamin K. The regeneration of reduced vitamin K is essential for the sustained synthesis of biologically functional coagulation factors II, VII, IX, and X. Warfarin acts on the carboxylation pathway by inhibiting the epoxide reductase that is required for the regeneration of reduced (active) vitamin K. Dicumarol is the natural anticoagulant formed in spoiled clover. Both warfarin and dicumarol are orally bioavailable, and are often termed "oral anticoagulants."

reductase that mediates the regeneration of reduced vitamin K (Fig. 22-14). Because depletion of reduced vitamin K in the liver prevents the γ-carboxylation reaction that is required for the synthesis of biologically active coagulation factors, the onset of action of the oral anticoagulants parallels the half-life of these coagulation factors in the circulation. Of the four affected clotting factors (II, VII, IX, and X), factor VII has the shortest half-life (6 hours). Thus, the pharmacologic effect of a single dose of warfarin is not manifested for approximately 18 to 24 hours (i.e., for 3 to 4 factor VII half-lives). This *delayed action* is one pharmacologic property that distinguishes the warfarin class of anticoagulants from all the other classes of anticoagulants.

Evidence from studies of long-term rodenticide use supports the hypothesis that the epoxide reductase is the molecular target of oral anticoagulant action. The use of oral anticoagulants as rodenticides has been a widespread practice in farming communities. In some areas of the United States, heavy rodenticide use has selected for a population of wild rodents that is resistant to 4-hydroxy-coumarins. In vitro studies of tissues from these rodents have demonstrated a mutation in the rodent epoxide reductase that renders the enzyme resistant to inhibition by the anticoagulant. Similarly, a small population of patients is genetically resistant to warfarin because of mutations in their epoxide reductase gene. These patients require 10

TABLE 22-2A	Examples of Drugs That Diminish Warfarin's Anticoagulant Effect
DRUG OR DRUG CLASS	**MECHANISM**
Cholestyramine	Inhibits warfarin absorption in the GI tract
Barbiturates, carbamazepine, phenytoin, rifampin	Accelerate warfarin metabolism by inducing hepatic P450 enzymes (especially P450 2C9)
Vitamin K (reduced)	Bypasses warfarin's inhibition of epoxide reductase

GI, gastrointestinal.

to 20 times the usual dose of warfarin to achieve the desired anticoagulant effect.

Clinical Uses of Warfarin

Warfarin is often administered to complete a course of anticoagulation that has been initiated with heparin (see below) and to prevent thrombosis in predisposed patients. Orally administered warfarin is nearly 100% bioavailable, and its levels in the blood peak at 0.5 to 4 hours after administration. *In the plasma, 99% of racemic warfarin is bound to plasma protein (albumin).* Warfarin has a relatively long elimination half-life (approximately 36 hours). The drug is hydroxylated by the cytochrome P450 system in the liver to inactive metabolites that are subsequently eliminated in the urine.

Drug–drug interactions must be carefully considered in patients taking warfarin. Because warfarin is highly albumin-bound in the plasma, coadministration of warfarin with other albumin-bound drugs can increase the free (unbound) plasma concentrations of both drugs. In addition, because warfarin is metabolized by P450 enzymes in the liver, coadministration of warfarin with drugs that induce and/or compete for P450 metabolism can affect the plasma concentrations of both drugs. Table 22-2A and B lists some of the major interactions between warfarin and other drugs.

Among the adverse effects of warfarin, bleeding is the most serious and predictable toxicity. Withdrawal of the drug may be recommended for patients who suffer from repeated bleeding episodes at otherwise therapeutic drug

concentrations. For severe hemorrhage, patients should promptly receive fresh frozen plasma, which contains biologically functional clotting factors II, VII, IX, and X. *Warfarin should never be administered to pregnant women* because it can cross the placenta and cause a hemorrhagic disorder in the fetus. In addition, newborns exposed to warfarin in utero may have serious congenital defects characterized by abnormal bone formation (certain bone matrix proteins are γ-carboxylated). Rarely, warfarin causes skin necrosis as a result of widespread thrombosis in the microvasculature. The fact that warfarin can cause thrombosis may seem paradoxical. Recall that, in addition to inhibiting the synthesis of biologically active coagulation factors II, VII, IX, and X, warfarin also prevents the synthesis of biologically active proteins C and S, which are natural anticoagulants. In patients who are genetically deficient in protein C or protein S (most commonly, patients who are heterozygous for protein C deficiency), an imbalance between warfarin's effects on coagulation factors and its effects on proteins C and S may lead to microvascular thrombosis and skin necrosis.

Because warfarin has a narrow therapeutic index and participates in numerous drug–drug interactions, the pharmacodynamic (functional) effect of chronic warfarin therapy must be monitored regularly (on the order of every 2 to 4 weeks). Monitoring is most easily performed using the **prothrombin time (PT)**, which is a simple test of the extrinsic and common pathways of coagulation. In this test, the patient's plasma is added to a crude preparation of tissue factor (called

TABLE 22-2B	Examples of Drugs That Enhance Warfarin's Anticoagulant Effect
DRUG OR DRUG CLASS	**MECHANISM**
Chloral hydrate	Displace warfarin from plasma albumin
Amiodarone, clopidogrel, ethanol (intoxicating dose), fluconazole, fluoxetine, metronidazole, sulfamethoxazole	Decrease warfarin metabolism by inhibiting hepatic P450 enzymes (especially P450 2C9)
Broad-spectrum antibiotics	Eliminate gut bacteria and thereby reduce availability of vitamin K in the GI tract
Anabolic steroids (testosterone)	Inhibit synthesis and increase degradation of coagulation factors

GI, gastrointestinal.

thromboplastin), and the time for formation of a fibrin clot is measured. Warfarin prolongs the PT mainly because it decreases the amount of biologically functional factor VII in the plasma. (Recall that factor VII is the vitamin K-dependent coagulation factor with the shortest half-life.) Measurement of the PT has been standardized worldwide, and is expressed as the **International Normalized Ratio (INR)** of the prothrombin time in the patient sample to that in a control sample, normalized for the international sensitivity index (ISI) of the laboratory's thromboplastin preparation compared to the World Health Organization's reference thromboplastin preparation. The formula used to calculate the INR is as follows: $\text{INR} = [\text{PT}_{\text{patient}} / \text{PT}_{\text{control}}]^{\text{ISI}}$.

Unfractionated and Low Molecular Weight Heparins

Structure of Heparin

Heparin is a sulfated mucopolysaccharide stored in the secretory granules of mast cells. It is a highly sulfated polymer of alternating uronic acid and D-glucosamine. Heparin molecules are highly negatively charged; indeed, endogenous heparin is the strongest organic acid in the human body. Commercial preparations of heparin are quite heterogeneous, with molecular weights ranging from 1 to 30 kDa. Conventionally, commercially prepared heparins have been categorized into unfractionated (standard) heparin and low molecular weight (LMW) heparin. **Unfractionated heparin,** which is often prepared from bovine lung and porcine intestinal mucosa, ranges in molecular weight from 5 to 30 kDa. **LMW heparins** are prepared from standard heparin by gel-filtration chromatography; their molecular weights range from 1 to 5 kDa.

Mechanism of Action of Heparin

Heparin's mechanism of action depends on the presence of a specific plasma protease inhibitor, antithrombin III. Antithrombin III is actually a misnomer because, in addition to inactivating thrombin, antithrombin III inactivates other serine proteases including factors IXa, Xa, XIa, and XIIa. Antithrombin III can be considered as a stoichiometric "suicide trap" for these serine proteases. When one of the proteases encounters an antithrombin III molecule, the serine residue at the active site of the protease attacks a specific Arg–Ser peptide bond in the reactive site of the antithrombin. The result of this nucleophilic attack is the formation of a covalent ester bond between the serine residue on the protease and the arginine residue on the antithrombin III. This results in a stable 1:1 complex between the protease and antithrombin molecules, which prevents the protease from further participation in the coagulation cascade.

In the absence of heparin, the binding reaction between the proteases and antithrombin III proceeds slowly. Heparin, acting as a cofactor, accelerates the reaction by 1,000-fold. Heparin has two important physiologic functions: (1) it serves as a catalytic surface to which both antithrombin III and the serine proteases bind; and (2) it induces a conformational change in antithrombin III that makes the reactive site of this molecule more accessible to the attacking protease. The first step of the reaction involves the binding of the negatively charged heparin to a lysine-rich region (a region

of positive charge) on antithrombin III. Thus, the interaction between heparin and antithrombin III is partly electrostatic. During the conjugation reaction between the protease and the antithrombin, heparin may be released from antithrombin III and become available to catalyze additional protease–antithrombin III interactions (i.e., heparin is not consumed by the conjugation reaction [Fig. 22-9]). In practice, however, heparin's high negative charge often causes this "sticky" molecule to remain electrostatically bound to protease, antithrombin or another nearby molecule in the vicinity of a thrombus.

Interestingly, heparins of different molecular weights have divergent anticoagulant activities. These divergent activities derive from the differential requirements for heparin binding exhibited by the inactivation of thrombin and factor Xa by antithrombin III (Fig. 22-15). To catalyze most efficiently the inactivation of thrombin by antithrombin III, a single molecule of heparin must bind simultaneously to both thrombin and antithrombin. This "scaffolding" function is required in addition to the heparin-induced conformational change in antithrombin III that renders the antithrombin susceptible to conjugation with thrombin. In contrast, to catalyze the inactivation of factor Xa by antithrombin III, the heparin molecule must bind only to the antithrombin, because the conformational change in antithrombin III induced by heparin binding is sufficient by itself to render the antithrombin susceptible to conjugation with factor Xa. Thus, *LMW heparins,* which have an average molecular weight of 3 to 4 kDa and contain fewer than 18 monosaccharide units, *efficiently catalyze the inactivation of factor Xa by antithrombin III but less efficiently catalyze the inactivation of thrombin by antithrombin III.* In contrast, *unfractionated heparin,* which has an average molecular weight of 20 kDa and contains more than 18 monosaccharide units, is of sufficient length to bind simultaneously to thrombin and antithrombin III, and therefore *efficiently catalyzes the inactivation of both thrombin and factor Xa by antithrombin III.* Quantitatively, LMW heparin has a threefold higher ratio of anti-Xa to anti-thrombin (anti-IIa) activity than does unfractionated heparin. LMW heparin is therefore a more selective therapeutic agent than unfractionated heparin. Both LMW heparin and unfractionated heparin use a pentasaccharide structure of high negative charge to bind antithrombin III and to induce the conformational change in antithrombin required for the conjugation reactions. This pentasaccharide has recently been approved for use as a highly selective inhibitor of factor Xa (**fondaparinux**; see below).

Clinical Uses of Heparins

Heparins are used for both prophylaxis and treatment of thromboembolic diseases. Both unfractionated and LMW heparins are used to prevent propagation of established thromboembolic disease such as deep vein thrombosis and pulmonary embolism. For prophylaxis against thrombosis, heparins are used at much lower doses than those indicated for the treatment of established thromboembolic disease. Because the enzymatic coagulation cascade functions as an amplification system (e.g., 1 unit of factor Xa generates 40 units of thrombin), the administration of relatively small amounts of circulating heparin at the first generation of factor Xa is highly effective. Heparins are highly negatively charged, and

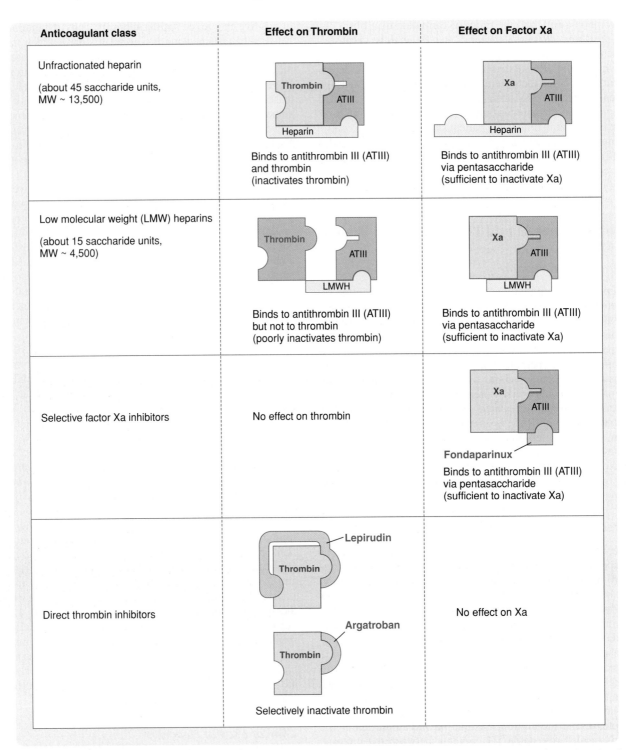

Anticoagulant class	Effect on Thrombin	Effect on Factor Xa
Unfractionated heparin (about 45 saccharide units, MW ~ 13,500)	Binds to antithrombin III (ATIII) and thrombin (inactivates thrombin)	Binds to antithrombin III (ATIII) via pentasaccharide (sufficient to inactivate Xa)
Low molecular weight (LMW) heparins (about 15 saccharide units, MW ~ 4,500)	Binds to antithrombin III (ATIII) but not to thrombin (poorly inactivates thrombin)	Binds to antithrombin III (ATIII) via pentasaccharide (sufficient to inactivate Xa)
Selective factor Xa inhibitors	No effect on thrombin	Fondaparinux Binds to antithrombin III (ATIII) via pentasaccharide (sufficient to inactivate Xa)
Direct thrombin inhibitors	Lepirudin Argatroban Selectively inactivate thrombin	No effect on Xa

Figure 22-15. **Differential effects of unfractionated heparin and low molecular weight heparin on coagulation factor inactivation.** *Effect on thrombin:* To catalyze the inactivation of thrombin, heparin must bind both to antithrombin III via a high-affinity pentasaccharide unit and to thrombin via an additional 13-saccharide unit. Low molecular weight heparin (LMWH) does not contain a sufficient number of saccharide units to bind thrombin, and therefore is a poor catalyst for thrombin inactivation. Selective factor Xa inhibitors do not inactivate thrombin, while direct thrombin inhibitors selectively inactivate thrombin. *Effect on factor Xa:* Inactivation of factor Xa requires only the binding of antithrombin III to the high-affinity pentasaccharide unit. Since unfractionated heparin, low molecular weight heparin, and fondaparinux all contain this pentasaccharide, these agents are all able to catalyze the inactivation of factor Xa. Direct thrombin inhibitors have no effect on factor Xa.

neither unfractionated heparin nor LMW heparin can cross the epithelial cell layer of the gastrointestinal tract. Hence, heparin must be administered parenterally, usually via intravenous or subcutaneous routes.

Unfractionated heparin is often used in combination with antiplatelet agents in the treatment of acute coronary syndromes. For example, Mr. S was treated with the antiplatelet agents aspirin and eptifibatide and with unfractionated heparin in an attempt to limit the extent of his myocardial infarction. Monitoring of unfractionated heparin therapy is important for maintaining the anticoagulant effect within the therapeutic range, because excessive heparin administration significantly increases the risk of bleeding. Monitoring is usually performed using the **activated partial thromboplastin time (aPTT)** assay. The aPTT is a simple test of the intrinsic and common pathways of coagulation. The patient's plasma is added to an excess of phospholipid, and fibrin forms at a normal rate only if the factors in the intrinsic and common pathways are present at normal levels. Increasing amounts of unfractionated heparin in the plasma prolong the time required for the formation of a fibrin clot.

As is true of the other anticoagulants, the major adverse effect of heparin is bleeding. Thus, it is critical to maintain the anticoagulant effect of unfractionated heparin within the therapeutic range in order to prevent the rare, devastating adverse effect of intracranial hemorrhage. In addition, a small fraction of patients taking heparin develop **heparininduced thrombocytopenia (HIT)**. In this syndrome, patients develop antibodies to a hapten created when heparin molecules bind to the platelet surface. In HIT type 1, the antibody-coated platelets are targeted for removal from the circulation, and the platelet count decreases by 50% to 75% approximately 5 days into the course of heparin therapy. The thrombocytopenia in HIT type 1 is transient and rapidly reversible upon heparin withdrawal. In HIT type 2, however, the heparin-induced antibodies not only target the platelets for destruction but also act as agonists to *activate* the platelets, leading to platelet aggregation, endothelial injury, and potentially fatal thrombosis. There is a higher incidence of HIT in patients receiving unfractionated heparin than in those receiving LMW heparin.

The LMW heparins **enoxaparin**, **dalteparin** and **tinzaparin** are each fractionated heparins of low molecular weight. As discussed above, these agents are relatively selective for anti-Xa compared to anti-IIa (anti-thrombin) activity. All LMW heparins are approved for use in the prevention and treatment of deep vein thrombosis. Additionally, enoxaparin and dalteparin have been studied in the treatment of acute myocardial infarction and as adjuncts to percutaneous coronary intervention. LMW heparins have a higher therapeutic index than unfractionated heparin, especially when used for prophylaxis. For this reason, it is generally not necessary to monitor blood activity levels of LMW heparins. Accurate measurement of the anticoagulant effect of LMW heparins requires a specialized assay for anti-factor Xa activity. Because LMW heparins are excreted via the kidneys, care should be taken to avoid excessive anticoagulation in patients with renal insufficiency.

Selective Factor Xa Inhibitors

Fondaparinux is a synthetic pentasaccharide molecule that contains the sequence of five essential carbohydrates necessary for binding to antithrombin III and inducing the conformational change in antithrombin required for conjugation to factor Xa (Fig. 22-15; see above). This agent is therefore is a specific inhibitor of Xa, with negligible anti-IIa (antithrombin) activity. Fondaparinux is approved for prevention and treatment of deep vein thrombosis, and is available as a once-daily subcutaneous injection. It is excreted via the kidneys and should not be administered to patients with renal insufficiency.

Direct Thrombin Inhibitors

As discussed above, thrombin plays a number of critical roles in the hemostatic process (Fig. 22-8). Among other effects, this clotting factor (1) proteolytically converts fibrinogen to fibrin, (2) activates factor XIII, which crosslinks fibrin polymers to form a stable clot, (3) activates platelets, and (4) induces endothelial release of PGI_2, t-PA, and PAI-1. Thus, direct thrombin inhibitors would be expected to have profound effects on coagulation. The currently approved direct thrombin inhibitors include lepirudin, desirudin, bivalirudin, and argatroban. These agents are specific inhibitors of thrombin, with negligible anti-factor Xa activity (Fig. 22-15).

Lepirudin, a recombinant 65-amino-acid polypeptide derived from the medicinal leech protein **hirudin**, is the prototypical direct thrombin inhibitor. For years, surgeons have used medicinal leeches to prevent thrombosis in the fine vessels of reattached digits. Lepirudin binds with high affinity to two sites on the thrombin molecule — the enzymatic active site and the "exosite," a region of the thrombin protein that orients substrate proteins. Lepirudin binding to thrombin prevents the thrombin-mediated activation of fibrinogen and factor XIII. Lepirudin is a highly effective anticoagulant because it can inhibit both free and *fibrin-bound* thrombin in developing clots, and because lepirudin binding to thrombin is essentially irreversible. It is approved for use in the treatment of heparin-induced thrombocytopenia. Lepirudin has a short half-life, is available parenterally, and is renally excreted. It can be administered with relative safety to patients with hepatic insufficiency. As with all direct thrombin inhibitors, bleeding is the major adverse effect of lepirudin, and clotting times must be monitored closely. A small percentage of patients may develop antihirudin antibodies, limiting the long-term effectiveness of this agent as an anticoagulant. Another recombinant formulation of hirudin, **desirudin**, has been approved for prophylaxis against deep vein thrombosis in patients undergoing hip replacement.

Bivalirudin is a synthetic 20-amino-acid peptide that, like lepirudin and desirudin, binds to both the active site and exosite of thrombin and thereby inhibits thrombin activity. Thrombin slowly cleaves an arginine–proline bond in bivalirudin, leading to reactivation of the thrombin. Bivalirudin is approved for anticoagulation in patients undergoing coronary angiography and angioplasty, and may reduce rates of bleeding relative to heparin for this indication. The drug is excreted renally and has a short half-life (25 minutes).

Argatroban is a small-molecule inhibitor of thrombin that is approved for the treatment of patients with heparin-induced thrombocytopenia. Unlike other direct thrombin inhibitors, argatroban binds only to the active site of thrombin (i.e., it does not interact with the exosite). Also unlike other direct thrombin inhibitors, argatroban is excreted by biliary secretion, and can therefore be administered with relative safety to patients with renal insufficiency.

Recombinant Activated Protein C (r-APC)

As described above, endogenously activated protein C (APC) exerts an anticoagulant effect by proteolytically cleaving factors Va and VIIIa. APC also reduces the amount of circulating plasminogen activator inhibitor 1, thereby enhancing fibrinolysis. Finally, APC reduces inflammation by inhibiting the release of tumor necrosis factor α (TNF-α) by monocytes. Because enhanced coagulability and inflammation are both hallmarks of septic shock, APC has been tested both in animal models of this disorder and in humans. **Recombinant activated protein C (r-APC)** has been found to significantly reduce mortality in patients at high risk of death from septic shock, and the U. S. Food and Drug Administration (FDA) has approved r-APC for the treatment of patients with severe sepsis who demonstrate evidence of acute organ dysfunction, shock, oliguria, acidosis, and hypoxemia. r-APC is not indicated for the treatment of patients with severe sepsis and a lower risk of death, however. As is the case with other anticoagulants, r-APC increases the risk of bleeding. This agent is therefore contraindicated in patients who have recently undergone a surgical procedure and in those with chronic liver failure, kidney failure, or thrombocytopenia.

THROMBOLYTIC AGENTS

Although warfarin, unfractionated and low molecular weight heparins, selective factor Xa inhibitors, and direct thrombin inhibitors are effective in preventing the formation and propagation of thrombi, these agents are generally ineffective against pre-existing clots. Thrombolytic agents are used to lyse already-formed clots, and thereby to restore the patency of an obstructed vessel before distal tissue necrosis occurs. Thrombolytic agents act by converting the inactive zymogen plasminogen to the active protease plasmin (Fig. 22-10). As noted above, plasmin is a relatively nonspecific protease that digests fibrin to fibrin degradation products. Unfortunately, thrombolytic therapy has the potential to dissolve not only pathologic thrombi, but also physiologically appropriate fibrin clots that have formed in response to vascular injury. Thus, the use of thrombolytic agents can lead to hemorrhage of varying severity.

Streptokinase

Streptokinase is a protein produced by β-hemolytic streptococci as a component of that organism's tissue-destroying machinery. The pharmacologic action of streptokinase involves two steps—complexation and cleavage. In the complexation reaction, streptokinase forms a stable, noncovalent 1:1 complex with plasminogen. The complexation reaction produces a conformational change in plasminogen that exposes this protein's proteolytically active site. Streptokinase-complexed plasminogen, with its active site exposed and available, can then proteolytically cleave *other* plasminogen molecules to plasmin. In fact, the thermodynamically stable streptokinase:plasminogen complex is the most catalytically efficient plasminogen activator in vitro.

Although streptokinase exerts its most dramatic and potentially beneficial effects in fresh thrombi, its use has been limited by two factors. First, streptokinase is a foreign protein that is capable of eliciting antigenic responses in humans upon repeated administration. Previous administration of streptokinase is a contraindication to its use, because of the risk of anaphylaxis. Second, the thrombolytic actions of streptokinase are relatively nonspecific and can result in systemic fibrinolysis. Currently, streptokinase is approved for treatment of ST elevation myocardial infarction and for treatment of life-threatening pulmonary embolism.

Recombinant Tissue Plasminogen Activator (t-PA)

An ideal thrombolytic agent would be nonantigenic and would cause local fibrinolysis only at the site of a pathologic thrombus. Tissue plasminogen activator (t-PA) approximates these goals. t-PA is a serine protease produced by human endothelial cells; therefore, t-PA is not antigenic. t-PA binds to newly formed (fresh) thrombi with high affinity, causing fibrinolysis at the site of a thrombus. Once bound to the fresh thrombus, t-PA undergoes a conformational change that renders it a potent activator of plasminogen. In contrast, t-PA is a poor activator of plasminogen in the absence of fibrin-binding.

Recombinant DNA technology has allowed the production of **recombinant t-PA**, generically referred to as **alteplase.** Recombinant t-PA is effective at recanalizing occluded coronary arteries, limiting cardiac dysfunction, and reducing mortality following an ST elevation myocardial infarction. At pharmacologic doses, however, recombinant t-PA can generate a systemic lytic state and (as with other thrombolytic agents) cause unwanted bleeding, including cerebral hemorrhage. Thus, its use is contraindicated in patients who have had a recent hemorrhagic stroke. Like streptokinase, t-PA is approved for use in the treatment of patients with ST elevation myocardial infarction or life-threatening pulmonary embolism. It is also approved for the treatment of acute ischemic stroke.

Tenecteplase

Tenecteplase is a genetically engineered variant of t-PA. The molecular modifications in tenecteplase increase its fibrin specificity relative to t-PA and make tenecteplase more resistant to plasminogen activator inhibitor 1. Large trials have shown that tenecteplase is identical in efficacy to t-PA, with similar (and possibly decreased) risk of bleeding. Additionally, tenecteplase has a longer half-life than t-PA. This pharmacokinetic property allows tenecteplase to be administered as a single weight-based bolus, thus simplifying administration.

Reteplase

Similar to tenecteplase, **reteplase** is a genetically engineered variant of t-PA with longer half-life and increased specificity for fibrin. Its efficacy and adverse effect profile are similar to those of streptokinase and t-PA. Because of its longer half-life, reteplase can be administered as a "double bolus" (two boluses, 30 minutes apart).

INHIBITORS OF ANTICOAGULATION AND FIBRINOLYSIS

Protamine

Protamine, a low molecular weight polycationic protein, is a chemical antagonist of heparin. This agent rapidly forms a stable complex with the negatively charged heparin molecule through multiple electrostatic interactions. Protamine is administered intravenously to reverse the effects of heparin in situations of life-threatening hemorrhage or great heparin excess (for example, at the conclusion of coronary artery bypass graft surgery). Protamine is most active against the large heparin molecules in unfractionated heparin and it can partially reverse the anticoagulant effects of low molecular weight heparins, but it is inactive against fondaparinux.

Serine-Protease Inhibitors

Aprotinin, a naturally occurring polypeptide, is an inhibitor of the serine proteases plasmin, t-PA, and thrombin. By inhibiting fibrinolysis, aprotinin promotes clot stabilization. Inhibition of thrombin may also promote platelet activity by preventing platelet hyperstimulation. At higher doses, aprotinin may also inhibit kallikrein and thereby (paradoxically) inhibit the coagulation cascade. Clinical trials have demonstrated decreased perioperative bleeding and erythrocyte transfusion requirement in patients treated with aprotinin during cardiac surgery. However, these positive findings have been tempered by recent evidence suggesting that, compared to other antifibrinolytic agents, aprotinin may increase the risk of postoperative acute renal failure.

Lysine Analogues

Aminocaproic acid and **tranexamic acid** are analogues of lysine that bind to and inhibit plasminogen and plasmin. Like aprotinin, these agents are used to reduce perioperative bleeding during coronary artery bypass grafting. Unlike aprotinin, these agents may not increase the risk of postoperative acute renal failure.

Conclusion and Future Directions

Hemostasis is a highly regulated process that maintains the fluidity of blood in normal vessels and initiates rapid formation of a stable fibrin-based clot in response to vascular injury. Pathologic thrombosis results from endothelial injury, abnormal blood flow, and hypercoagulability. Antiplatelet agents, anticoagulants, and thrombolytic agents target different stages of thrombosis and thrombolysis. Antiplatelet agents interfere with platelet adhesion, the platelet release reaction, and platelet aggregation; these agents can provide powerful prophylaxis against thrombosis in susceptible individuals. Anticoagulants primarily target plasma coagulation factors and disrupt the coagulation cascade by inhibiting crucial intermediates. After a fibrin clot has been established, thrombolytic agents mediate dissolution of the clot by promoting the conversion of plasminogen to plasmin. These classes of pharmacologic agents can be administered either individually or in combination, to prevent or disrupt thrombosis and to restore the patency of blood vessels occluded by thrombus.

Future development of new antiplatelet, anticoagulant, and thrombolytic agents will be forced to contend with two major constraints. First, for many clinical indications in this field, highly effective, orally bioavailable, and inexpensive therapeutic agents are already available: these include the antiplatelet drug aspirin and the anticoagulant warfarin. Second, virtually every antithrombotic and thrombolytic agent is associated with the mechanism-based toxicity of bleeding, and this side effect is likely to plague new agents under development. Nonetheless, opportunities remain for the development of safer and more effective therapies. It is likely that pharmacogenomic techniques (see Chapter 52, Pharmacogenomics) will be capable of identifying individuals in the population who carry an elevated genetic risk of thrombosis, and such individuals may benefit from long-term antithrombotic treatment. Combinations of antiplatelet agents, low molecular weight heparins, orally bioavailable direct thrombin inhibitors (such as the snake-venom–derived prodrug **ximelagatran,** which is not approved for use in the U.S.), and new agents that target currently unexploited components of hemostasis (such as inhibitors of the factor VIIa/tissue factor pathway) could all be useful in these settings. At the other end of the spectrum, there remains a great need for new agents that can achieve rapid, noninvasive, convenient, and selective lysis of acute thromboses associated with life-threatening emergencies such as ST elevation myocardial infarction and stroke. Carefully designed clinical trials will be critical to optimize the indications, dose, and duration of treatment for such drugs and drug combinations.

Suggested Reading

Baggish AL, Sabatine MS. Clopidogrel use in coronary artery disease. *Exp Rev Cardiovasc Ther* 2006;4:7–15. (*Reviews pharmacology and expanding clinical applications for clopidogrel.*)

Bates SM, Ginsberg JS. Treatment of deep-vein thrombosis. *N Engl J Med* 2004;351:268–277. (*Reviews treatment options for deep vein thrombosis.*)

Bauer KA. New anticoagulants: anti IIa vs anti Xa—is one better? *J Thromb Thrombolysis* 2006;21:67–72. (*Summarizes clinical trial data on selective factor Xa inhibitors and direct thrombin inhibitors.*)

Brass LF. The molecular basis for platelet activation. In: Hoffman R, Benz EJ, Shattil SJ, et al, eds. *Hematology: basic principles and practice.* 4th ed. Philadelphia: Churchill Livingstone; 2004. (*Detailed and mechanistic description of platelet activation.*)

Di Nisio M, Middeldorp S, Buller HR. Direct thrombin inhibitors. *N Engl J Med* 2005;353:1028–1040. (*Reviews mechanism of action and clinical indications for direct thrombin inhibitors.*)

Franchini M, Veneri D, Salvagno GL, et al. Inherited thrombophilia. *Crit Rev Clin Lab Sci* 2006;43:249–290. (*Reviews epidemiology, pathophysiology, and treatment of hypercoagulable states.*)

Furie B, Furie BC. Thrombus formation in vivo. *J Clin Invest* 2005; 115:3355–3362. (*Reviews molecular and cellular mechanisms of primary and secondary hemostasis in vivo.*)

Grosser T, Fries S, FitzGerald GA. Biological basis for the cardiovascular consequences of COX-2 inhibition: therapeutic challenges and opportunities. *J Clin Invest* 2006;116:4–15. (*Reviews effects of COX-2 inhibition in cellular, animal, and human studies.*)

Hirsh J, O'Donnell M, Weitz JI. New anticoagulants. *Blood* 2005; 105:453–463. (*Reviews anticoagulants in clinical development.*)

Levy JH. Hemostatic agents. *Transfusion* 2004;44:58S–62S. (*Reviews aprotinin, aminocaproic acid, and tranexamic acid.*)

Drug Summary Table	**Chapter 22 Pharmacology of Hemostasis and Thrombosis**

Drug	Clinical Applications	*Serious* and Common Adverse Effects	Contraindications	Therapeutic Considerations
ANTIPLATELET AGENTS				
Cyclooxygenase Inhibitors				
Mechanism—Inhibit platelet cyclooxygenase, thereby blocking thromboxane A2 generation and inhibiting platelet granule release reaction and platelet aggregation				
Aspirin	Prophylaxis against transient ischemic attack, myocardial infarction, and thromboembolic disorders Treatment of acute coronary syndromes Prevention of reocclusion in coronary revascularization procedures and stent implantation Arthritis, juvenile arthritis, rheumatic fever Mild pain or fever	*GI bleeding, acute renal insufficiency, thrombocytopenia, hepatitis, angioedema, asthma, Reye's syndrome* Tinitus, dyspepsia, occult bleeding, prolonged bleeding time, rash	NSAID-induced sensitivity reactions Children with chickenpox or flu-like syndromes G6PD deficiency Bleeding disorders such as hemophilia, von Willebrand's disease, or immune thrombocytopenia	Inhibits COX-1 and COX-2 nonselectively Use cautiously in patients with GI lesions, impaired renal function, hypothrombinemia, vitamin K deficiency, thrombotic thrombocytopenic purpura, or hepatic impairment Coadministration with aminoglycosides, bumetanide, capreomycin, cisplatin, erythromycin, ethacrynic acid, furosemide, or vancomycin may potentiate ototoxic effects Coadministration with ammonium chloride or other urine acidifiers may lead to aspirin toxicity Aspirin antagonizes uricosuric effects of phenylbutazone, probenecid, and sulfinpyrazone; avoid co-administration with these agents
Phosphodiesterase Inhibitors				
Mechanism—Inhibit platelet cAMP degradation and thereby decrease platelet aggregability				
Dipyridamole	Prophylaxis against thromboembolic disorders Alternative to exercise in thallium myocardial perfusion imaging	*Exacerbation of angina (IV route), rare myocardial infarction, rare ventricular arrhythmia, rare bronchospasm* Abnormal ECG, hypotension (IV route), abdominal discomfort (oral route), dizziness, headache	Hypersensitivity to dipyridamole	Weak antiplatelet effect Usually administered in combination with warfarin or aspirin Has vasodilatory properties; may paradoxically induce angina by causing the coronary steal phenomenon
ADP Receptor Pathway Inhibitors				
Mechanism—Covalently modify platelet ADP receptor, thereby preventing receptor signaling and irreversibly inhibiting ADP-dependent platelet activation pathway				
Ticlopidine	Secondary prevention of thrombotic strokes in patients intolerant of aspirin Prevention of stent thrombosis (in combination with aspirin)	*Aplastic anemia, neutropenia, thrombotic thrombocytopenic purpura* Pruritus, rash, dyspepsia, abnormal liver function tests, dizziness	Active bleeding disorder Neutropenia, thrombocytopenia Severe liver dysfunction	Use is limited by associated myelotoxicity Requires a loading dose to achieve immediate anti-platelet effect
Clopidogrel	Secondary prevention of atherosclerotic events in patients with recent myocardial infarction, stroke, or peripheral vascular disease Acute coronary syndromes Prevention of stent thrombosis (in combination with aspirin)	*Atrial fibrillation, heart failure, erythema multiforme, GI hemorrhage (in combination with aspirin), very rare anemia or neutropenia, rare intracranial hemorrhage, abnormal renal function* Chest pain, edema, hypertension, purpura, rare abnormal liver function tests, GI discomfort, arthralgia, dizziness	Active bleeding disorder	More favorable adverse effect profile than ticlopidine; significantly less myelotoxic than ticlopidine Requires a loading dose to achieve immediate anti-platelet effect

(Continued)

Drug Summary Table   Chapter 22 Pharmacology of Hemostasis and Thrombosis (Continued)

Drug	Clinical Applications	Serious and Common Adverse Effects	Contraindications	Therapeutic Considerations
GPIIb–IIIa Antagonists				
Mechanism—Bind to platelet receptor GPIIb–IIIa and thereby prevent binding of fibrinogen and other adhesive ligands				
Eptifibatide	Acute coronary syndromes Percutaneous coronary intervention	*Major bleeding, intracerebral hemorrhage, thrombocytopenia* Hypotension, bleeding	History of bleeding diathesis or recent abnormal bleeding Concomitant administration of a second glycoprotein IIb–IIIa antagonist Recent major surgery Recent stroke or history of hemorrhagic stroke Intracranial hemorrhage, mass, or arteriovenous malformation Severe uncontrolled hypertension	Avoid coadministration with a second GPIIb–IIIa antagonist Minimize use of arterial and venous punctures, urinary catheters, and nasotracheal and nasogastric tubes Eptifibatide is a synthetic peptide delivered via parenteral administration
Abciximab	Adjunct to percutaneous coronary intervention or atherectomy to prevent acute cardiac ischemic complications Unstable angina not responding to conventional therapy in patients scheduled for percutaneous coronary intervention	*Same as eptifibatide*	Same as eptifibatide	Same therapeutic considerations as eptifibatide, except abciximab is a chimeric mouse–human monoclonal antibody Adding abciximab to conventional antithrombotic therapy reduces both long-term and short-term ischemic events in patients undergoing high-risk coronary angioplasty
Tirofiban	Acute coronary syndromes in patient undergoing angioplasty or atherectomy or managed medically	*Same as eptifibatide; additionally, coronary artery dissection is rarely observed*	Same as eptifibatide	Same therapeutic considerations as eptifibatide, except tirofiban is a nonpeptide tyrosine analogue
ANTICOAGULANTS				
Warfarin				
Mechanism—Inhibit hepatic epoxide reductase that catalyzes the regeneration of reduced vitamin K, which is required for synthesis of biologically active coagulation factors II, VII, IX, and X and anticoagulant proteins C and S				
Warfarin	Prophylaxis and treatment of pulmonary embolism, deep vein thrombosis, systemic embolism after myocardial infarction, or systemic embolism associated with atrial fibrillation, rheumatic heart disease with heart valve damage, or prosthetic mechanical heart valve	*Cholesterol embolization syndrome, skin and other tissue necrosis, hemorrhage, hepatitis, hypersensitivity reaction*	Pregnancy Hemorrhagic tendency or blood dyscrasia Bleeding tendency associated with active ulceration or bleeding due to mucosal lesions, cerebrovascular hemorrhage, cerebral or aortic aneurysm, pericarditis and pericardial effusion, bacterial endocarditis Recent eye, brain, or spinal surgery Severe uncontrolled hypertension	Monitoring is required by using the prothrombin time (PT), expressed as the international normalized ratio (INR) Drug–drug interactions must be carefully considered with warfarin (refer to Table 22-2 for examples of important interactions); coadministration of warfarin with other albumin-bound drugs can increase the free (unbound) plasma concentrations of both drugs; coadministration of drugs that induce and/or compete for P450 metabolism can affect the plasma concentrations of both drugs

Drug	Clinical Applications	Serious and Common Adverse Effects	Contraindications	Therapeutic Considerations
(warfarin, continued from previous page)			Threatened abortion, eclampsia, preeclampsia Regional or lumbar block anesthesia History of warfarin-induced skin necrosis Unsupervised patients with psychosis, senility, alcoholism, or lack of cooperation, and especially those with risk of falling	Warfarin should never be given to pregnant women because it can cause a hemorrhagic disorder and/or congenital defects in the fetus Warfarin can cause skin necrosis as a result of widespread thrombosis in the microvasculature For severe hemorrhage due to warfarin, patients should promptly receive fresh frozen plasma

Unfractionated Heparin and Low Molecular Weight Heparins

Mechanism—Unfractionated heparin: combines with antithrombin III and inhibits secondary hemostasis via nonselective inactivation of thrombin (factor IIa), factor Xa, factor IXa, factor XIa, and factor XIIa. LMW heparins: combine with antithrombin III and inhibit secondary hemostasis via relatively (3-fold) selective inactivation of factor Xa.

Drug	Clinical Applications	Serious and Common Adverse Effects	Contraindications	Therapeutic Considerations
Unfractionated heparin	Prevention and treatment of pulmonary embolism, deep vein thrombosis, cerebral thrombosis, or left ventricular thrombus Prevention of systemic embolism associated with myocardial infarction Unstable angina Open-heart surgery Disseminated intravascular coagulation Maintain patency of IV catheters	*Hemorrhage, heparin-induced thrombocytopenia, hypersensitivity reactions including anaphylactoid reactions* Overly prolonged clotting time, mucosal ulceration, hematoma	Heparin-induced thrombocytopenia Active major bleeding Bleeding tendencies such as hemophilia, thrombocytopenia, or hepatic disease with hypoprothrombinemia Suspected intracranial hemorrhage Open ulcerative wounds, extensive denudation of skin Conditions that cause increased capillary permeability Bacterial endocarditis Severe hypertension	There is a higher incidence of heparin-induced thrombocytopenia in patients receiving unfractionated heparin than in those receiving LMW heparin Antihistamines, cardiac glycosides, nicotine, and tetracyclines may partially counteract anticoagulant effect Cephalosporins, penicillins, oral anticoagulants, and platelet inhibitors may increase anticoagulant effect Discourage concomitant use of herbs such as dong quai, garlic, ginger, ginkgo, motherwort, and red clover due to increased risk of bleeding
LMW heparins: Enoxaparin Dalteparin Tinzaparin	Prevention and treatment of deep vein thrombosis (all LMW heparins) Treatment of acute coronary syndromes and adjunct to percutaneous coronary intervention (enoxaparin and dalteparin)	*Hemorrhage, thrombocytopenia, abnormal liver function tests, anaphylactoid reaction, spinal hematoma* Edema, diarrhea, nausea, hematoma, normocytic hypochromic anemia, confusion, pain, dyspnea, fever, local irritation	Active major bleeding Heparin-induced thrombocytopenia Hypersensitivity to heparin or pork products Renal insufficiency (relative contraindication)	Administered as weight-based subcutaneous injection Avoid excessive anticoagulation in patients with renal insufficiency

Selective Factor Xa Inhibitors

Mechanism—Combine with antithrombin III and inhibits secondary hemostasis via highly selective inactivation of factor Xa.

Drug	Clinical Applications	Serious and Common Adverse Effects	Contraindications	Therapeutic Considerations
Fondaparinux	Prophylaxis and treatment of deep vein thrombosis Prophylaxis and treatment of pulmonary embolism	*Hemorrhage, thrombocytopenia, abnormal liver function tests, anaphylactoid reaction, spinal hematoma* Edema, diarrhea, nausea, hematoma, normocytic hypochromic anemia, confusion, pain, dyspnea, fever, local irritation	Active major bleeding Severe renal impairment Bacterial endocarditis	Fondaparinux is a pentasaccharide composed of the essential five carbohydrates necessary for binding antithrombin III; it is a specific indirect inhibitor of factor Xa, with negligible anti-thrombin (anti-IIa) activity Avoid excessive anticoagulation in patients with renal insufficiency Fondaparinux use has not been associated with heparin-induced thrombocytopenia

(Continued)

Drug Summary Table | **Chapter 22 Pharmacology of Hemostasis and Thrombosis** (*Continued*)

Drug	Clinical Applications	Serious and Common Adverse Effects	Contraindications	Therapeutic Considerations
Direct Thrombin Inhibitors *Mechanism—Bind directly to thrombin and thereby inhibit secondary hemostasis*				
Hirudin-related agents: Lepirudin Desirudin Bivalirudin	Heparin-induced thrombocytopenia (lepirudin) Prophylaxis against deep vein thrombosis (desirudin) Anticoagulation in patients undergoing coronary angiography and angioplasty (bivalirudin)	Heart failure, gastrointestinal hemorrhage, bleeding, abnormal liver function tests, anaphylaxis, hypertension, hypotension, cerebral ischemia, intracranial hemorrhage, peripheral nerve paralysis, facial nerve paralysis, hematuria, renal failure, extrinsic allergic respiratory disease, pneumonia, sepsis Cutaneous hypersensitivity, anemia, fever	Active major bleeding Pregnancy Severe uncontrolled hypertension Severe renal impairment	Recombinant polypeptides based on the medicinal leech protein hirudin; bind to both active site and exosite of thrombin Lepirudin inhibits both free and fibrin-bound thrombin After bivalirudin binds to thrombin, the thrombin slowly cleaves an arginine–proline bond in bivalirudin, leading to reactivation of thrombin Dose adjustment is required in patients with renal insufficiency because these agents are excreted via the kidneys
Argatroban	Coronary artery thrombosis Prophylaxis in percutaneous coronary intervention Heparin-induced thrombocytopenia	Cardiac arrest, cerebrovascular disorder, ventricular tachycardia, sepsis, hypotension	Active major bleeding Severe liver impairment	Binds to active site but not exosite of thrombin Dose adjustment is required in patients with liver disease because argatroban is excreted in the bile
Recombinant Activated Protein C (r-APC) *Mechanism—Proteolytically inactivates factors Va and VIIIa; may also exert anti-inflammatory effect by inhibiting tumor necrosis factor production and blocking leukocyte adhesion to selectins*				
Recombinant activated protein C (r-APC)	Severe sepsis with organ dysfunction and high risk of death	Hemorrhage	Active internal bleeding Intracranial mass Hemorrhagic stroke within 3 months Recent intracranial or intraspinal surgery or severe head trauma within 2 months Presence of an epidural catheter Major trauma with an increased risk of life-threatening bleeding	Prolongs activated partial thromboplastin time (aPTT) but has little effect on prothrombin time (PT)
THROMBOLYTIC AGENTS *Mechanism—Proteolytically activate plasminogen to form plasmin, which digests fibrin to fibrin degradation products*				
Streptokinase	ST elevation myocardial infarction Arterial thrombosis Deep vein thrombosis Pulmonary embolism Intra-arterial or intravenous catheter occlusion	Cardiac arrhythmia, cholesterol embolus syndrome, major bleeding, anaphylactoid reaction, polyneuropathy, non-cardiogenic pulmonary edema, hypotension Fever, shivering	Active internal bleeding or known bleeding diathesis Intracranial or intraspinal surgery or trauma within 2 months Cerebrovascular accident within 2 months Intracranial mass Severe uncontrolled hypertension	Streptokinase is a foreign bacterial protein that can elicit antigenic responses in humans upon repeated administration; prior administration of streptokinase is a contraindication to use due to the risk of anaphylaxis Thrombolytic actions of streptokinase are relatively nonspecific and can result in systemic fibrinolysis

Drug	Clinical Applications	Serious and Common Adverse Effects	Contraindications	Therapeutic Considerations
Recombinant tissue plasminogen activator (t-PA) (Alteplase)	Acute myocardial infarction Acute cerebrovascular thrombosis Pulmonary embolism Central venous catheter occlusion	*Cardiac arrhythmia, cholesterol embolus syndrome, gastrointestinal hemorrhage, rare allergic reaction, intracranial hemorrhage, sepsis*	Same as streptokinase	Binds to newly formed (fresh) thrombi with high affinity, causing fibrinolysis at the site of a thrombus As with other thrombolytic agents, t-PA can generate a systemic lytic state and cause unwanted bleeding
Tenecteplase Reteplase	Acute myocardial infarction	*Cardiac arrhythmia, cholesterol embolus syndrome, major bleeding, allergic reaction, anaphylaxis, cerebrovascular accident, intracranial hemorrhage*	Same as streptokinase	Genetically engineered variants of t-PA with increased specificity for fibrin Longer half-life than t-PA; tenecteplase is administered as a single weight-based bolus; reteplase is administered as a double bolus

INHIBITORS OF ANTICOAGULATION AND FIBRINOLYSIS
Protamine
Mechanism—Inactivates heparin by forming a stable 1:1 protamine:heparin complex

Drug	Clinical Applications	Serious and Common Adverse Effects	Contraindications	Therapeutic Considerations
Protamine	Heparin overdose	*Bradyarrhythmia, hypotension, anaphylactoid reaction, circulatory collapse, capillary leak, noncardiogenic pulmonary edema* Flushing, nausea, vomiting, dyspepsia	Hypersensitivity to protamine	Protamine can also partially reverse the anticoagulant effect of low molecular weight heparin, but it cannot reverse the anticoagulant effect of fondaparinux

Serine-Protease Inhibitor
Mechanism—Inhibits serine proteases, including plasmin, t-PA, and thrombin

Drug	Clinical Applications	Serious and Common Adverse Effects	Contraindications	Therapeutic Considerations
Aprotinin	Reduce perioperative bleeding during coronary artery bypass graft surgery	*Heart failure, myocardial infarction, shock, thrombotic disorder, anaphylaxis with reexposure, cerebral artery occlusion, renal failure*	Hypersensitivity to aprotinin	At higher doses, aprotinin may also inhibit kallikrein and thereby paradoxically inhibit the coagulation cascade Aprotinin may increase the risk of postoperative acute renal failure relative to other antifibrinolytic agents

Lysine Analogues
Mechanism—Analogues of lysine that bind to and inhibit plasminogen and plasmin

Drug	Clinical Applications	Serious and Common Adverse Effects	Contraindications	Therapeutic Considerations
Aminocaproic acid Tranexamic acid	Disorder involving the fibrinolytic system Hemorrhage from increased fibrinolysis	*Bradyarrhythmia, hypotension, thrombotic disorder, drug-induced myopathy (aminocaproic acid), rare renal failure*	Disseminated intravascular coagulation Hypersensitivity to aminocaproic acid	May cause less acute renal failure relative to aprotinin

23

Pharmacology of Cholesterol and Lipoprotein Metabolism

David E. Cohen and Ehrin J. Armstrong

INTRODUCTION

Lipids are insoluble or sparingly soluble molecules that are essential for membrane biogenesis and maintenance of membrane integrity. They also serve as energy sources, hormone precursors, and signaling molecules. In order to facilitate transport through the relatively aqueous blood, non-polar lipids, such as cholesteryl esters or triglycerides, are packaged within lipoproteins.

Increased concentrations of certain lipoproteins in the circulation are associated strongly with atherosclerosis. Much of the prevalence of cardiovascular disease (CVD), the leading cause of death in the US and most Western countries, can be attributed to elevated concentrations in blood of cho-

lesterol-rich low-density lipoprotein (LDL) particles as well as lipoproteins that are rich in triglycerides. Epidemiologically, decreased concentrations of high-density lipoproteins (HDL) also predispose to atherosclerotic disease. The major contributors to lipoprotein abnormalities appear to be Western diets combined with sedentary lifestyles, but a limited number of genetic causes of hyperlipidemia have also been identified. The role of genetics in the common forms of hyperlipidemia remains to be elucidated. Nevertheless, it is clear that genes modify the sensitivity of individuals to adverse dietary habits and lifestyles. This chapter highlights the biochemistry and physiology of cholesterol and lipoproteins, with an emphasis on the role of lipoproteins in atherogenesis, and the pharmacologic interventions that can ameliorate hyperlipidemia. Abundant clinical outcomes data have proven definitively that morbidity and mortality from cardiovascular disease can be reduced by the use of lipid-lowering drugs.

Case

In June 1998 Jake P, a 29-year-old construction worker, makes an appointment to see Dr. Cush. Jake complains of hard, elevated swellings around his Achilles tendon that seem to rub constantly against his construction boots. Jake had been hesitant to see the doctor (his last appointment was 10 years ago), but he remembers that his dad, who died at age 42 of a heart attack, had similar swellings. On examination, Dr. Cush recognizes the Achilles swellings as xanthomas (lipid deposits); the physical exam is otherwise within normal limits. Jake comments that his daily diet is quite "fatty," including three to four donuts each day and frequent hamburgers. Dr. Cush explains that the xanthomas on Jake's feet are the result of cholesteryl ester deposition, probably from high cholesterol levels in his blood. Dr. Cush orders a fasting plasma cholesterol level, and recommends that Jake reduce his intake of foods high in saturated fat and cholesterol, and increase his intake of poultry, fish, whole cereal grains, fruits, and vegetables. Jake has gained about 15 pounds since he was 19, and has a small paunch. Dr. Cush recommends regular exercise and weight loss.

Results of the blood test reveal a total plasma cholesterol concentration of 300 mg/dL (normal, <200), with elevated LDL cholesterol of 250 mg/dL (desirable, <100), low HDL of 35 mg/dL (normal, 35 to 100), and normal concentrations of triglycerides and VLDL. Based on these test results, his age, the Achilles heel xanthomas and a positive family history for an early myocardial infarction, Dr. Cush tells Jake that he likely has an inherited disorder of cholesterol metabolism, probably heterozygous familial hypercholesterolemia. This disease puts Jake at high risk for early atherosclerosis and myocardial infarction, but aggressive lowering of cholesterol levels can ameliorate many of the disease sequelae. The low HDL cholesterol level also contributes to his increased risk of cardiovascular disease. In addition to the dietary changes, Dr. Cush prescribes a statin to help reduce Jake's cholesterol. A starting dose of a statin reduces his LDL by 30% to 175 mg/dL, while HDL slightly increases. Dr. Cush then increases the statin dose, and this produces an additional 12% reduction in LDL. Because LDL has still not reached <100 mg/dL, and HDL remains low, Dr. Cush adds the cholesterol absorption inhibitor, ezetimibe, as well as extended-release niacin. After these modifications, Jake's LDL drops below 100 and his HDL increases to 45 mg/dL. Jake experiences cutaneous flushing during the first few months of niacin treatment, but after that period, he has only occasional flushing episodes.

QUESTIONS

■ **1.** What is the etiology of familial hypercholesterolemia?

■ **2.** How do high cholesterol levels predispose to cardiovascular disease?

■ **3.** How do statins, ezetimibe, and niacin act pharmacologically?

■ **4.** What major adverse effects of concomitant statin and niacin therapy should Jake be aware of?

BIOCHEMISTRY AND PHYSIOLOGY OF CHOLESTEROL AND LIPOPROTEIN METABOLISM

Lipoproteins are macromolecular aggregates that transport triglycerides and cholesterol in the blood. Circulating lipoproteins can be differentiated on the basis of density, size, and protein content (Table 23-1). As a general rule, larger, less dense lipoproteins have a greater percentage composition of lipids; **chylomicrons** are the largest and least dense lipoprotein subclass, whereas HDL are the smallest lipopro-

TABLE 23-1	Characteristics of Plasma Lipoproteins				
	CM	**VLDL**	**IDL**	**LDL**	**HDL**
Density (g/mL)	<0.95	0.95–1.006	1.006–1.019	1.019–1.063	1.063–1.210
Diameter (nm)	75–1,200	30–80	25–35	18–25	5–12
Total lipid (% wt)	98	90	82	75	67
Composition, % dry weight					
Protein	2	10	18	25	33
Triglycerides	83	50	31	9	8
Unesterified cholesterol and cholesteryl esters	8	22	29	45	30
Phospholipids (% wt lipid)	7	18	22	21	29
Electrophoretic mobility[a]	None	Pre-β	β	β	α or Pre-β
Major apolipoproteins	B48, AI, AIV, E, CI, CII, CIII	B100, E, CI, CII, CIII	B100, E, CI, CII, CIII	B100	AI, AII, CI, CII, CIII, E

[a] Electrophoretic mobility of lipoprotein particles is designated relative to migration of plasma α- and β-globulins.

CM, chylomicron; VLDL, very-low-density lipoprotein; IDL, intermediate-density lipoprotein; LDL, low-density lipoprotein; HDL, high-density lipoprotein.

teins, containing the lowest lipid content and the highest proportion of protein.

Structurally, lipoproteins are microscopic spherical particles ranging from 7 to 100 nm in diameter. Each lipoprotein particle consists of a monolayer of polar, amphipathic lipids that surrounds a hydrophobic core. Each lipoprotein particle also contains one or more types of apolipoprotein (Fig. 23-1). The polar lipids that comprise the surface coat are unesterified cholesterol and phospholipid molecules, arranged in a monolayer. The hydrophobic core of a lipoprotein contains the cholesteryl esters (cholesterol molecules linked by an ester bond to a fatty acid) and triglycerides (three fatty acids esterified to a glycerol molecule). The apolipoproteins (also referred to as *apoproteins*) are amphipathic proteins that intercalate into the surface coat of lipoproteins. In addition to stabilizing the structure of lipoproteins, apolipoproteins engage in biological functions. They may act as ligands for lipoprotein receptors or may activate enzymatic activities in the plasma. The apolipoprotein composition determines the metabolic fate of the lipoprotein. For example, all **LDL** contain an apoB100 molecule, which is a ligand for the low-density lipoprotein receptor (discussed below) and promotes cholesterol uptake into cells.

From a metabolic perspective, lipoprotein particles can be divided into lipoproteins that participate in the delivery of triglyceride molecules to muscle and fat tissue (the apoB-containing lipoproteins, chylomicrons, and **VLDL**) and lipoproteins that are involved primarily in cholesterol transport (**HDL** and the remnants of apoB-containing lipoproteins). HDL also serves as a reservoir for exchangeable apolipoproteins in the plasma, including apoAI, apoCII and apoE. The following discussion presents each lipoprotein class in the context of its function.

METABOLISM OF ApoB-CONTAINING LIPOPROTEINS

The primary function of apoB-containing lipoproteins is to deliver fatty acids in the form of triglycerides to muscle tissue to be used for ATP biogenesis and to adipose tissue for storage. Chylomicrons are formed in the intestine and transport dietary **triglycerides**, whereas VLDL particles are formed in the liver and transport triglycerides that are synthesized endogenously. The metabolic lifespan of apoB-containing lipoproteins can be divided into three phases: assembly, intravascular metabolism, and receptor-mediated clearance. This is a convenient categorization because pharmacologic agents are available to influence each phase.

Assembly of Apolipoprotein B-Containing Lipoproteins

The cellular mechanisms by which chylomicrons and VLDL are assembled are quite similar. Regulation of the assembly process depends on the availability of **apolipoprotein B** and triglycerides, as well as the activity of **microsomal triglyceride transfer protein** (MTP).

The gene that encodes apoB is transcribed principally in the intestine and the liver. Apart from this tissue-specific expression, there is little transcriptional regulation of the apoB gene. In contrast, a key regulatory event that differentiates chylomicron from VLDL metabolism is the editing of apoB mRNA (Fig. 23-2). Within enterocytes but not hepatocytes, a protein named **apoB editing complex-1 (apobec-1)** is expressed. This protein constitutes the catalytic subunit of the apoB editing complex, which deaminates a cytosine at position 6666 of the apoB mRNA molecule. Deamination converts the cytosine to a uridine base. As a result, the codon containing this nucleotide is converted from a glutamine to a premature stop. When translated, the intestinal form **apoB48** is 48% as long as the full-length protein that is expressed in the liver and referred to as **apoB100**. As a consequence, chylomicrons, the apoB-containing lipoprotein produced by the intestine, contains apoB48. In contrast, VLDL particles produced by the liver contain apoB100.

Figure 23-3 illustrates the cellular mechanisms for the assembly and secretion of apoB-containing lipoproteins. As the apoB protein is synthesized by ribosomes, it crosses into the endoplasmic reticulum. Within the endoplasmic reticulum, triglyceride molecules are added co-translationally to the elongating apoB protein (i.e., apoB is lipidated) by the action of a cofactor protein, MTP. Once apoB has been fully synthesized, the nascent lipoprotein is enlarged in the Golgi

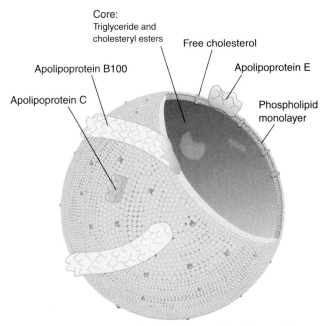

Core:
Triglyceride and cholesteryl esters

Free cholesterol

Apolipoprotein B100

Apolipoprotein E

Apolipoprotein C

Phospholipid monolayer

Figure 23-1. Structure of lipoprotein particles. Lipoproteins are spherical particles (7 to 100 nm in diameter) that transport hydrophobic molecules, principally cholesterol and triglycerides, as well as fat-soluble vitamins. The surface of the particle is composed of a monolayer of phospholipid and unesterified cholesterol molecules. These polar lipids form a coating that shields a hydrophobic core of non-polar triglyceride and cholesteryl esters from interacting with the aqueous environment of plasma. Lipoproteins contain amphipathic apolipoproteins (also called *apoproteins*) that associate with the surface lipids and hydrophobic core. Apolipoproteins provide structural stability to the lipoprotein particle and act as ligands for specific cell-surface receptors or as cofactors for enzymatic reactions. In the example shown, a very-low-density lipoprotein particle (VLDL) contains apolipoprotein E, apolipoprotein B100, and apolipoproteins CI, CII, and CIII *(shown here as apolipoprotein C).*

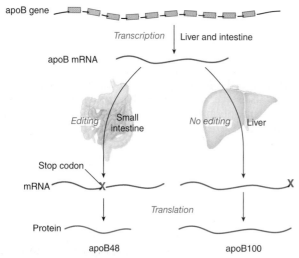

Figure 23-2. Editing of ApoB mRNA. The apoB gene, with exons represented by *rectangles* and introns by *lines,* is transcribed in both the intestine and the liver. In the intestine, but not the liver, a protein complex containing apobec-1 modifies a single nucleotide in the apoB mRNA. As a result, the codon containing this nucleotide is converted to a premature stop codon, as indicated by the "X". The protein that is synthesized in the intestine (apoB-48) is only 48% as long as the full-length protein that is synthesized in the liver (apoB-100).

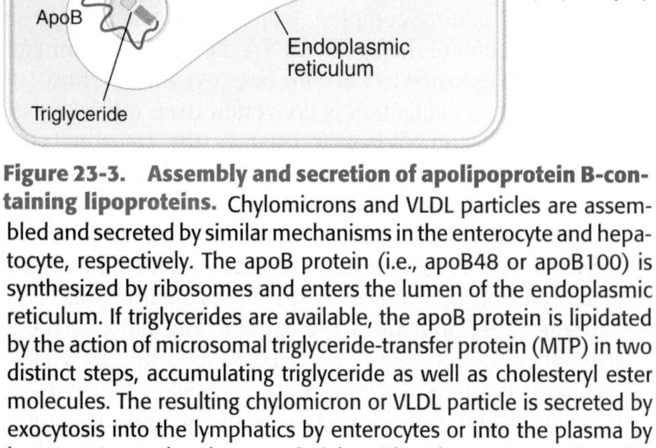

Figure 23-3. Assembly and secretion of apolipoprotein B-containing lipoproteins. Chylomicrons and VLDL particles are assembled and secreted by similar mechanisms in the enterocyte and hepatocyte, respectively. The apoB protein (i.e., apoB48 or apoB100) is synthesized by ribosomes and enters the lumen of the endoplasmic reticulum. If triglycerides are available, the apoB protein is lipidated by the action of microsomal triglyceride-transfer protein (MTP) in two distinct steps, accumulating triglyceride as well as cholesteryl ester molecules. The resulting chylomicron or VLDL particle is secreted by exocytosis into the lymphatics by enterocytes or into the plasma by hepatocytes. In the absence of triglycerides, the apoB protein is degraded *(not shown).*

apparatus; during this process, MTP adds additional triglycerides to the core of the particle. By unclear mechanisms, cholesteryl esters are also added to the core. This entire assembly process produces lipoprotein particles, each containing a single molecule of apoB.

Because the diet is the main source of triglycerides in chylomicrons (Fig. 23-4), the assembly, secretion, and metabolism of these particles are collectively referred to as the *exogenous* pathway of lipoprotein metabolism. By contrast, cholesteryl esters in chylomicrons are derived mainly from biliary cholesterol (approximately 75%), with the remainder contributed by dietary sources. During digestion, cholesteryl esters and triglycerides in food are hydrolyzed to form unesterified cholesterol, free fatty acids, and monoglycerides. Bile acids, phospholipids, and cholesterol are secreted by the liver into bile and stored in the gallbladder during fasting as micelles and vesicles, which are macromolecular lipid

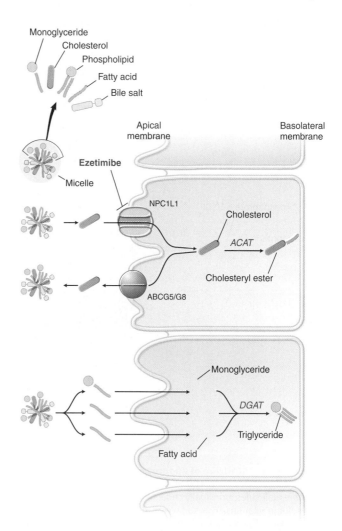

Figure 23-4. Absorption of cholesterol and triglycerides. Exogenous cholesterol and triglycerides are simultaneously absorbed from the intestinal lumen by different mechanisms. Cholesterol is taken up from micelles across a regulatory channel named **NPC1L1.** A fraction of the cholesterol is pumped back into the lumen by ABCG5/G8, a heterodimeric ATP-dependent plasma membrane protein. The remainder of the cholesterol is converted to cholesteryl esters by ACAT. Triglycerides are taken up as fatty acids and monoglycerides, which are re-esterified by DGAT.

aggregates that form due to the detergent properties of bile acid molecules. The stimulus of eating a meal promotes emptying of gallbladder bile into the small intestine, where the micelles and vesicles solubilize the digested lipids. Lipid absorption into enterocytes of the duodenum and jejunum is facilitated mainly by micelles. Long-chain fatty acids and monoglycerides are taken up separately into the enterocyte by carrier-mediated transport and then re-esterified to form triglycerides by the enzyme **diacylglycerol acyltransferase** (DGAT). By contrast, medium-chain fatty acids are absorbed directly into the portal blood and metabolized by the liver. Dietary and biliary cholesterol from micelles enter the enterocyte via a protein channel named **Niemann-Pick C1-like 1 protein (NPC1L1).** Some of this cholesterol is immediately pumped back into the intestinal lumen by the ATP-dependent action of a heterodimeric protein, ABCG5/ABCG8 (ABCG5/G8). The fraction of cholesterol that remains is esterified to a long-chain fatty acid by **acyl-CoA: cholesterol acyltransferase** (ACAT). Once triglycerides and cholesteryl esters are packaged together with apoB48, apoA1 is added as an additional structural apolipoprotein and the chylomicron particle is exocytosed into the lymphatics for transport to the circulation via the thoracic duct. The plasma concentration of triglyceride-rich chylomicrons varies in proportion to dietary fat intake.

Very-low-density lipoproteins (VLDL) comprise triglycerides that are assembled by the liver using plasma fatty acids derived from adipose tissue or synthesized *de novo*. For this reason, the assembly, secretion, and metabolism of VLDL are often referred to as the *endogenous* pathway of lipoprotein metabolism. Hepatocytes synthesize triglycerides in response to increased free fatty acid flux to the liver. This typically occurs in response to fasting, thereby ensuring a continuous supply of fatty acids for delivery to muscle in the absence of triglycerides from the diet. Interestingly, dietary saturated fats as well as carbohydrates also stimulate the synthesis of triglycerides within the liver. By cellular mechanisms that are highly similar to those that produce chylomicrons (Fig. 23-3), MTP in hepatocytes lipidates apoB100 to form nascent VLDL particles. Under the continued influence of MTP, the nascent VLDL particles coalesce with larger triglyceride droplets and are secreted directly into the circulation. VLDL particles may also acquire apoE, apoCI, apoCII, and apoCIII within the hepatocyte prior to secretion. However, these apolipoproteins may also be transferred to VLDL from HDL in the circulation.

The synthesis of apoB48 in the intestine and apoB100 in the liver is constitutive. This permits the immediate production of chylomicrons and VLDL particles when triglyceride molecules are available. In the absence of triglycerides, such as in enterocytes during fasting, apoB is degraded by a variety of cellular mechanisms.

Intravascular Metabolism of ApoB-Containing Lipoproteins

Within the circulation, chylomicrons and VLDL particles must be activated in order to target triglyceride delivery to muscle and fat tissues (Fig. 23-5). Activation requires the addition of an optimal complement of apoCII molecules, which occurs by aqueous transfer of apoCII from HDL particles. Because there is an inherent delay in the transfer of apoCII to chylomicrons and VLDL particles, there is time for widespread circulation of triglyceride-rich particles throughout the body.

Lipoprotein lipase (LPL) is a lipolytic enzyme expressed on the endothelial surface of capillaries in muscle and fat tissues. LPL is a glycoprotein that is anchored in place by electrostatic interactions with a separate glycoprotein on the endothelial cell membrane. Once chylomicrons and VLDL particles acquire apoCII, they can bind to LPL, which hydrolyzes triglycerides from the core of the lipoprotein (Fig. 23-5). LPL-mediated lipolysis liberates free fatty acids and glycerol, which are then taken up by the neighboring parenchymal cells. The expression level and intrinsic activity of LPL in muscle and fat tissue are regulated according the fed/fasting state, allowing the body to direct the delivery of fatty acids preferentially to muscle during fasting and to fat after a meal. The rate of lipolysis of chylomicron and VLDL triglycerides is also controlled by apoCIII, which is an inhibitor of LPL activity. LPL inhibition by apoCIII may be an additional mechanism promoting widespread distribution of triglyceride-rich particles in the circulation.

Receptor-Mediated Clearance of ApoB-Containing Lipoproteins

As LPL continues to hydrolyze triglycerides from chylomicrons and VLDL, the particles become progressively depleted of triglycerides and relatively enriched in cholesterol. Once approximately 50% of the triglycerides have been removed, the particles lose affinity for LPL and dissociate from the enzyme. The exchangeable apolipoproteins apoAI and apoCII (as well as apoCI and apoCIII) are then transferred to HDL in exchange for **apoE** (Fig. 23-6A), which serves as a high-affinity ligand for receptor-mediated clearance of the particles. Upon acquiring apoE, the particles are termed chylomicron or **VLDL remnants**.

Remnants of chylomicrons and VLDL are taken up by the liver in a three-step process (Fig. 23-6B). The first step is sequestration of the particles within the **Space of Disse** between the fenestrated endothelium of the liver sinusoids and the sinusoidal (basolateral) plasma membrane of the hepatocytes. Sequestration requires that the remnant particles become small enough during lipolysis to fit between the endothelial cells. Once in the Space of Disse, remnants are bound and sequestered by large heparin sulfate proteoglycans. The next step is particle remodeling within the Space of Disse by the action of **hepatic lipase**, a lipolytic enzyme that is similar to LPL but is expressed by hepatocytes. Hepatic lipase appears to optimize the triglyceride content of remnant particles so that they can be cleared efficiently by receptor-mediated mechanisms. The final phase of remnant clearance is receptor-mediated particle uptake. This is accomplished by one of four pathways. At the sinusoidal hepatocyte plasma membrane, remnant particles may be bound and taken up by the **LDL receptor**, the **LDL-receptor-related protein** (LRP) or heparin sulfate proteoglycans. A fourth pathway is mediated by the combined activities of LRP and heparin sulfate proteoglycans. These redundant mechanisms allow for efficient particle clearance, so that the half-life of remnants in the plasma is approximately 30 minutes.

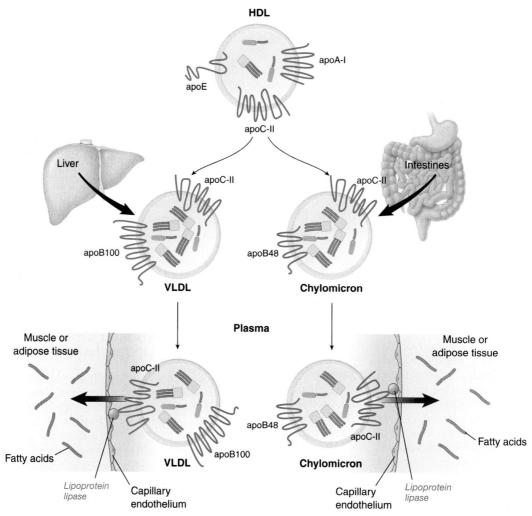

Figure 23-5. Intravascular metabolism of ApoB-containing lipoproteins. Following secretion, chylomicrons and VLDL particles are activated for lipolysis when they encounter HDL particles in the plasma and acquire the exchangeable apolipoprotein apoCII. When chylomicrons and VLDL circulate into capillaries of muscle or fat tissue, apoCII promotes binding of the particle to lipoprotein lipase, which is bound to the surface of endothelial cells. Lipoprotein lipase mediates hydrolysis of triglycerides, but not cholesteryl esters, from the core of the lipoprotein particle. The resulting fatty acids are taken up into muscle or fat tissue.

Formation and Clearance of LDL Particles

ApoB48-containing chylomicron remnants are completely cleared from the plasma. In contrast, the presence of apoB100 alters the metabolism of VLDL remnants so that only approximately 50% are cleared by the pathways for remnant particles. The difference begins with the metabolism of the remnant particles by LPL. VLDL remnants are avidly metabolized by LPL, becoming an increment smaller and relatively more deficient in triglycerides and enriched in cholesteryl esters. When converted to remnants following exchange of apolipoproteins with HDL, these more dense particles are called **intermediate-density lipoproteins** (IDL). Because IDL contains apoE, a fraction of these particles (approximately 50%) may be cleared into the liver by remnant receptor pathways (Fig. 23-6). However, the remainder are converted to LDL by hepatic lipase, which further hydrolyzes triglycerides in the core of IDL. The further reduction in size of the particle results in the transfer of apoE to HDL. As a result, *LDL is a distinct, cholesteryl ester-enriched lipoprotein with apoB100 as its only apolipoprotein* (Fig. 23-7A).

The LDL receptor is the only receptor capable of clearing significant amounts of LDL from the plasma. The LDL receptor is expressed on the surface of hepatocytes, macrophages, lymphocytes, adrenocortical cells, gonadal cells, and smooth muscle cells. Due to the lack of apoE, LDL particles are relatively weak ligands for the LDL receptor. As a result, the half-life of LDL in the circulation is markedly prolonged (2 to 4 days). This explains why LDL cholesterol accounts for approximately 65% to 75% of total plasma cholesterol.

Interaction of apoB100 with the LDL receptor facilitates receptor-mediated endocytosis of LDL particles and subsequent vesicle fusion with lysosomes (Fig. 23-7B). The LDL receptor is recycled to the cell surface, while the LDL particle is hydrolyzed to release unesterified cholesterol, which impacts three major homeostatic pathways. First, intracellular cholesterol inhibits HMG CoA reductase, the enzyme that catalyzes the rate-limiting step in *de novo* cholesterol synthesis. Second, cholesterol activates acetyl-coenzyme A:

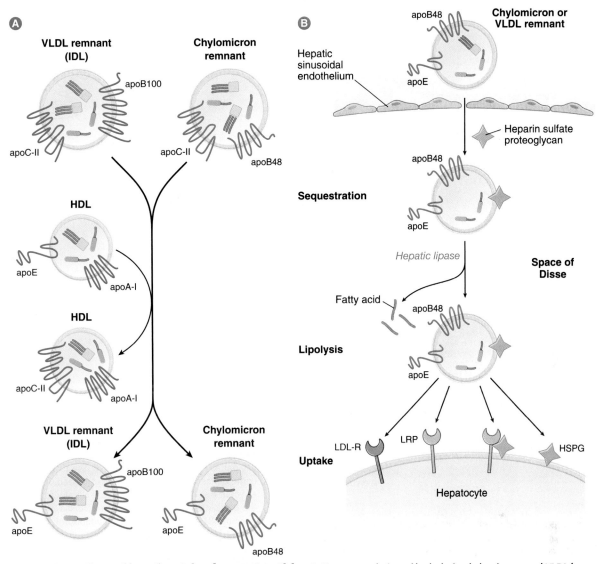

Figure 23-6. Formation and hepatic uptake of remnant particles. A. Upon completion of hydrolysis, chylomicrons and VLDL lose affinity for lipoprotein lipase. When an HDL particle is encountered, apoCII is transferred back to HDL particles in exchange for apoE. The resulting particles are chylomicron and VLDL remnants. **B.** The activity of lipoprotein lipase results in remnant lipoprotein particles that are small enough to enter the Space of Disse. Remnant lipoproteins are sequestered in the Space of Disse by binding to high-molecular-weight heparin sulfate proteoglycan (HSPG) molecules. This is followed by the action of hepatic lipase, which promotes lipolysis of some residual triglycerides in the core of the remnant lipoproteins and the release of fatty acids. Uptake of remnant lipoprotein particles into hepatocytes is mediated by the LDL receptor (LDL-R), the LDL-receptor-related protein (LRP), a complex formed between LRP and HSPG, or HSPG alone.

cholesterol acyltransferase (ACAT) to increase esterification and storage of cholesterol in the cell. Third, LDL receptor expression is down-regulated, reducing further uptake of cholesterol into the cells. The majority of LDL receptors (70%) are expressed on the surface of hepatocytes. As a result, the liver is primarily responsible for the removal of LDL particles from the circulation.

LDL particles not taken up by LDL receptor-expressing tissues may migrate into the intima of blood vessels and bind to proteoglycans (Fig. 23-8). There, they are subject to oxidization or nonenzymatic glycosylation. Oxidation of LDL results in lipid peroxidation and may create reactive aldehyde intermediates that fragment apoB100. The

modified LDL is internalized by **scavenger receptors** (e.g., SR-A), which are expressed predominantly by mononuclear phagocytic cells. Unlike the LDL receptor, scavenger receptors are not down-regulated when the phagocytic cells begin to accumulate cholesterol. As a result, the continued accumulation of oxidized LDL in macrophages can lead to **foam cell** formation (cholesterol-rich macrophages). These foam cells may undergo apoptotic or necrotic death, releasing free radicals and proteolytic enzymes. Oxidized LDL also causes up-regulation of cytokine production, impairs endothelial function, and increases expression of endothelial adhesion molecules. All of these effects increase the local inflammatory response and promote atherosclerosis. Foam cells are a

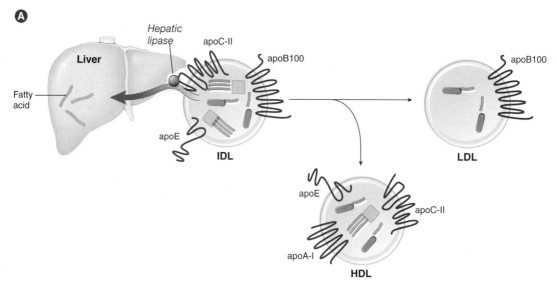

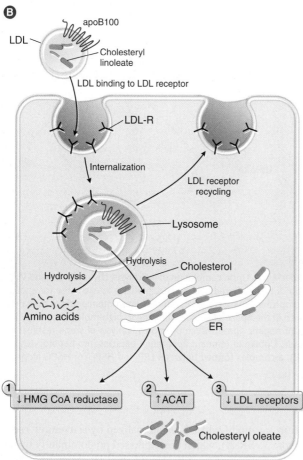

Figure 23-7. Formation and clearance of LDL particles. A. Formation of LDL occurs when IDL particles interact with hepatic lipase to become denser and cholesteryl ester-enriched. As a result, both apoE and apoCII lose affinity for the particle and are transferred to HDL, leaving only apoB100. **B.** Binding of apolipoprotein B100 to LDL receptors on hepatocytes or other cell types promotes LDL internalization into endocytic vesicles and fusion of the vesicles with lysosomes. LDL receptors are recycled to the cell surface, whereas lipoprotein particles are hydrolyzed into amino acids, releasing free cholesterol. Intracellular cholesterol has three regulatory effects on the cell. First, cholesterol decreases the activity of HMG-CoA reductase, the rate-limiting enzyme in cholesterol biosynthesis. Second, cholesterol activates acetyl CoA: cholesterol acyltransferase (ACAT), an enzyme that esterifies free cholesterol into cholesteryl esters for intracellular storage or export. Third, cholesterol inhibits the transcription of the gene encoding the LDL receptor, and, thereby, decreases further uptake of cholesterol by the cell.

major constituent of atherosclerotic lesions, and excessive foam cell death can destabilize atherosclerotic plaques. This is attributable in part to the liberation of matrix metalloproteinases. Because plaque rupture is the main cause of acute ischemic cardiovascular events, particularly heart attacks and strokes, *high plasma levels of LDL are a major risk factor for the development of atherosclerosis and subsequent cardiovascular disease.* This is why Jake's doctor became

concerned when he discovered that Jake had very high levels of circulating LDL.

HDL METABOLISM AND REVERSE CHOLESTEROL TRANSPORT

Virtually all cells in the body are capable of synthesizing all of the cholesterol they require. However, only the liver

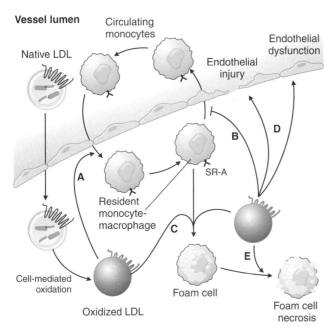

Vessel lumen
Circulating monocytes
Native LDL
Endothelial dysfunction
Endothelial injury
B
D
SR-A
A
Resident monocyte-macrophage
C
E
Cell-mediated oxidation
Foam cell
Foam cell necrosis
Oxidized LDL

Subendothelial space

Figure 23-8. LDL and atherosclerosis. Elevated LDL is a major risk factor for the development of atherosclerosis. Native LDL that migrates into the subendothelial space can undergo chemical transformation to oxidized LDL via lipid peroxidation and fragmentation of apoB100. Oxidized LDL has a number of deleterious effects on vascular function. Oxidized LDL promotes monocyte chemotaxis into the subendothelial space **(A)** and inhibits monocyte egress from that space **(B)**. Resident monocyte–macrophages bind to oxidized LDL via a scavenger receptor (SR-A), resulting in the formation of lipid-laden foam cells **(C)**. Oxidized LDL can directly injure endothelial cells and cause endothelial dysfunction **(D)**. Oxidized LDL can also cause foam cell necrosis, with release of numerous proteolytic enzymes that can damage the intima **(E)**.

has the capacity to eliminate cholesterol, and it does so by secreting unesterified cholesterol into the bile or by converting cholesterol to bile acids. As noted above, HDL serves as a reservoir for exchangeable apolipoproteins for the metabolism of apoB-containing lipoproteins. HDL also plays a key role in cholesterol homeostasis by removing excess cholesterol from cells and transporting it in plasma to the liver. This process is often referred to as **reverse cholesterol transport** (Fig. 23-9A). The major apolipoproteins of HDL are apoAI and apoAII. ApoAI, the main structural determinant of HDL, participates in the formation and interaction of the particle with its receptor, **scavenger receptor class B, type I** (SR-BI). The function of apoAII is not well understood.

HDL Formation

HDL formation occurs mainly in the liver, although a small percentage is contributed by the small intestine. The earliest events occur when lipid-poor apoAI is secreted by the liver or intestine, or dissociates from lipoprotein particles in the plasma. These amphipathic apoAI molecules interact with **ABCA1**, which is localized in the sinusoidal membrane of the hepatocyte or the basolateral membrane of the entero-

cyte. ABCA1 incorporates a small amount of membrane phospholipid and unesterified cholesterol into the apoAI molecule. The resulting small, disk-shaped particle, which consists mainly of phospholipid and apolipoprotein AI, is referred to as nascent or **pre-β-HDL**, due to its characteristic migration on agarose gels.

Intravascular Maturation of HDL

Because disk-shaped pre-β-HDL particles are relatively inefficient at removing excess cholesterol from cell membranes, these particles must mature into spherical particles in the plasma. HDL maturation occurs as a result of the activity of two distinct circulating proteins (Fig. 23-9A,B). **Lecithin:cholesterol acyltransferase** (LCAT) binds preferentially to disk-shaped HDL and converts cholesterol molecules within the particle to cholesteryl esters. This is accomplished by transesterification of a fatty acid from a phosphatidylcholine molecule on the surface of the HDL to the hydroxyl group of a cholesterol molecule. The reaction also creates a lysophosphatidylcholine molecule, which dissociates from the particle and binds to serum albumin. Because they are highly insoluble, cholesteryl esters migrate into the core of the HDL particle. The development of a hydrophobic core converts the pre-β-HDL to a spherical α-HDL particle.

The second important protein that contributes to HDL maturation in the plasma is **phospholipid transfer protein** (PLTP). PLTP transfers phospholipids from the surface coat of apoB-containing remnant particles to the surface coat of HDL. During LPL-mediated lipolysis of apoB-containing lipoproteins, the particles become smaller as triglycerides are removed from the core. This leaves a relative excess of phospholipids on the surface of the particle. Because phospholipids are highly insoluble and cannot otherwise dissociate from a particle, PLTP removes excess phospholipids and thereby maintains the appropriate surface concentration for the shrinking core. By transferring phospholipids to the surface of HDL, PLTP also replaces the molecules that are consumed by the LCAT reaction. This allows the core of HDL to continue to enlarge.

HDL-Mediated Cholesterol Efflux from Cells

Cellular cholesterol efflux is the mechanism by which excess insoluble cholesterol molecules are removed from cells. This occurs when unesterified cholesterol is transferred from the plasma membrane of cells to an HDL particle. The mechanism of cholesterol efflux varies depending on the cell type and the type of HDL particle. Lipid-poor pre-β-HDL particles can promote cholesterol efflux by interacting with ABCA1. This process is not only important in HDL formation by the liver, but is also a mechanism for removing excess cholesterol from cells within the subendothelial space and to protect macrophages from cholesterol-induced cytotoxicity. Spherical HDL very efficiently stimulates cholesterol efflux by several different mechanisms. First, the interaction of apoAI on HDL with SR-BI on the plasma membrane promotes cholesterol efflux. Second, macrophages express not only ABCA1 and SR-BI but also ABCG1, which also mediates cholesterol efflux to spherical HDL. Finally, spherical

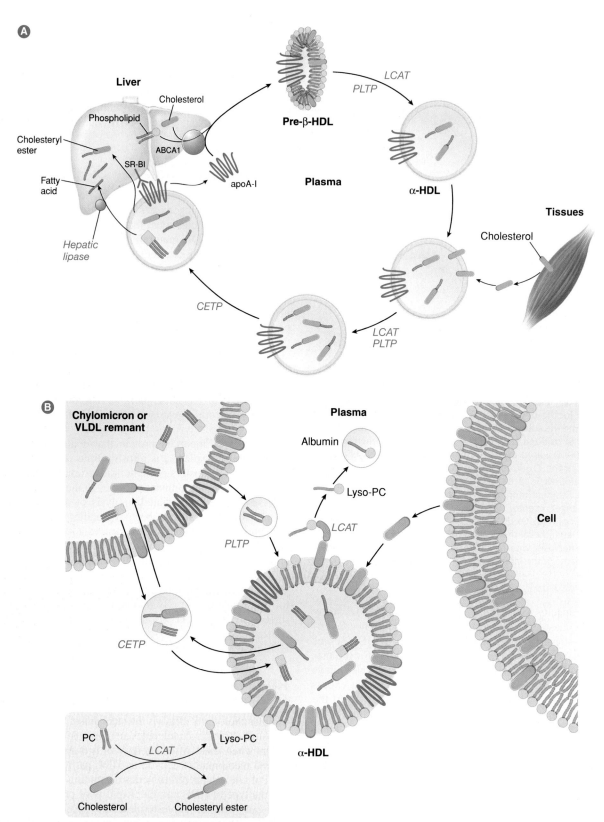

Figure 23-9. Reverse cholesterol transport. A. The process of reverse cholesterol transport begins when apoAI is secreted from the liver. ApoAI in plasma interacts with ATP binding cassette protein AI (ABCA1), which incorporates a small amount of phospholipid and unesterified cholesterol from hepatocyte plasma membranes to form a discoidal-shaped pre-β-HDL particle. Due to the activity of lecithin cholesterol: acyltransferase (LCAT) in plasma, pre-β-HDL particles mature to form spherical α-HDL. Spherical α-HDL particles function to accept excess unesterified cholesterol from the plasma membranes of cells in a wide variety of tissues. The unesterified cholesterol is transferred from the cell to nearby HDL particles by diffusion through the plasma. As explained in Panel B, LCAT and phospholipid transfer protein (PLTP) increase the capacity of HDL to accept unesterified cholesterol molecules from cells by allowing for expansion of the core and the surface coat of the particle. Cholesteryl ester transfer protein (CETP) removes cholesteryl ester molecules from HDL and replaces them with triglycerides from remnant particles. HDL particles interact with scavenger receptor, class B type I (SR-BI), which mediates selective hepatic uptake of cholesteryl esters, but not apoAI. This process is facilitated when hepatic lipase hydrolyzes triglycerides from the core of the particle. The remaining apoAI

HDL particles may promote cholesterol efflux in the absence of binding to a specific cell-surface protein. Although cholesterol has very low monomeric solubility, it can dissociate in appreciable amounts and travel short distances through the plasma to acceptor particles that are enriched with phospholipids on their surfaces. Quantitatively, *efflux to spherical HDL particles accounts for most of the removal of excess cholesterol from cells.* This capacity of HDL to remove cellular cholesterol is enhanced by the activities of LCAT and PLTP, which prevent the surface coat of the particle from becoming saturated with cholesterol.

Delivery of HDL Cholesterol to the Liver

When mature HDL particles circulate to the liver, they interact with SR-BI, the principal HDL receptor (Fig. 23-9A). SR-BI is highly expressed on the sinusoidal plasma membranes of hepatocytes. In contrast to its action on most non-hepatic cells, where SR-BI mediates *efflux* of excess cholesterol from the membrane, SR-BI in the liver promotes selective *uptake* of lipids. In this process, the cholesterol and cholesteryl esters of HDL particles are taken up into the hepatocyte in the absence of uptake of apolipoproteins. During SR-BI–mediated selective lipid uptake, apoAI is liberated to participate in pre-β-HDL formation. The ''lifespan'' of an HDL particle is 2 to 5 days, suggesting that each apoAI molecule can participate in many cycles of reverse cholesterol transport. Among the non-hepatic tissues that express high levels of SR-BI are the adrenal glands and gonads, presumably reflecting the requirement of these organs for cholesterol to support steroidogenesis.

Delivery of cholesterol from extrahepatic tissues to the liver is optimized by two additional proteins, **cholesterol ester transfer protein** (CETP) and hepatic lipase. CETP is a plasma protein that transfers cholesteryl esters from mature spherical HDL to the cores of remnant lipoproteins in exchange for a triglyceride molecule, which is inserted into the core of the HDL particle (Fig. 23-9B). This process allows the body to utilize remnant particles that have completed their function of triglyceride transport for purposes of transporting cholesterol to the liver. Removal of cholesteryl ester molecules from HDL appears to serve two functions. First, it further increases the capacity of HDL to take on additional cholesterol molecules from cells. Second, it makes the process of selective uptake by SR-BI more efficient. This is because hydrolysis of triglycerides by hepatic lipase on the hepatocyte surface facilitates the activity of SR-BI (Fig. 23-9A).

The overall process by which HDL removes cholesterol from macrophages and other extrahepatic tissues and returns it to the liver is commonly referred to as **reverse cholesterol transport**. The concept that increased plasma concentrations of HDL cholesterol may reflect increased rates of reverse cholesterol transport provides a possible explanation for the inverse relationship between plasma HDL levels and risk of cardiovascular disease. HDL particles also exert direct beneficial effects on vascular tissue, including enhancement of antioxidant enzyme activities that inhibit oxidation of LDL. HDL also inhibits the expression of inflammatory mediators (e.g., intercellular adhesion molecule (ICAM) and vascular cell adhesion molecule [VCAM]) by vascular cells. Increased understanding of HDL metabolism may lead to the development of novel biochemical targets for increasing reverse cholesterol transport in order to slow or even reverse the progression of atherosclerosis.

BILIARY LIPID SECRETION

Once cholesterol is delivered to the liver by the process of reverse cholesterol transport, it is eliminated by biliary secretion. A key essential step occurs when a fraction of the cholesterol is converted to bile acids (Fig. 23-10A). **Cholesterol 7α-hydroxylase** (CYP7A1), an enzyme expressed only in hepatocytes, catalyzes the rate-limiting step in the catabolism of cholesterol to bile acids. Bile acids, unlike cholesterol, are highly soluble in water. Moreover, bile acids are biological detergents that promote the formation of micelles (Fig. 23-10B). These macromolecular aggregates, which are rich in phospholipids derived from hepatocyte membranes, solubilize cholesterol in bile for transport from the liver to the small intestine. In this way, micelles serve as a functional counterpart to HDL particles in plasma.

Bile formation begins when bile acids are pumped into bile by the action of a canalicular membrane transport pump known as ABCB11 (Fig. 23-10B). In turn, these bile acids stimulate the biliary secretion of phospholipids and cholesterol. Phospholipid and cholesterol secretion are mediated by two additional transporters, ABCB4 for phospholipids and a heterodimer of ABCG5 and ABCG8 for cholesterol. Large amounts of bile acids, phospholipids, and cholesterol are secreted into bile at approximate rates of 24, 11, and 1.2 grams each day, respectively. Biliary lipids are stored in the gallbladder during fasting. The stimulus of a fatty meal leads to gallbladder contraction, which propels its contents into the small intestine. As described above, bile facilitates the digestion and absorption of fats, in addition to promoting the elimination of endogenous cholesterol.

---

molecules may begin the cycle of reverse cholesterol transport again. **B.** LCAT, PLTP, and CETP promote the removal of excess cholesterol from the plasma membranes of cells. LCAT removes a fatty acid from a phosphatidylcholine molecule in the surface coat of α- (or pre-β-) HDL and esterifies an unesterified cholesterol molecule on the surface of the particle. The resulting lysophosphatidylcholine (lyso-PC) becomes bound to albumin in the plasma, whereas the cholesteryl ester migrates spontaneously into the core of the lipoprotein particle. The unesterified cholesterol molecules that are consumed by LCAT are replaced by unesterified cholesterol from cells. HDL phospholipids that are consumed by LCAT action are replaced with excess phospholipids from remnant particles by the activity of PLTP. As described in Panel A, CETP increases the efficiency of cholesterol movement to the liver by transporting cholesteryl ester molecules from α-HDL to VLDL remnants in exchange for triglycerides. Unlike phospholipids, triglycerides, and cholesteryl esters, unesterified cholesterol and lyso-PC move by diffusion through the plasma.

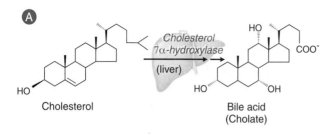

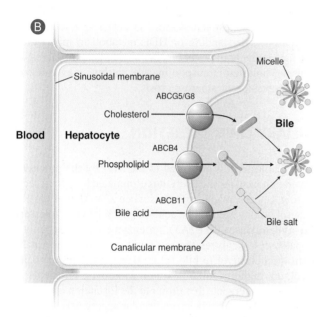

Figure 23-10. Biliary lipid secretion. A. Within hepatocytes, a portion of cholesterol is converted to bile acids. This process is rate-limited by cholesterol 7α-hydroxylase, which is expressed only in hepatocytes. Cholate is the most abundant bile salt synthesized by the human liver. **B.** Within the canalicular (apical) membranes, an ATP-dependent pump ABCB11 drives the secretion of bile acids out of the cell against a concentration gradient. Bile acids then stimulate the activities of two other proteins, ABCB4 and a heterodimer of ABCG5 and ABCG8 (ABCG5/G8), to secrete phospholipids and cholesterol, respectively, into bile. Within bile, the interactions among bile acids, phospholipids and cholesterol result in the formation of micelles.

CHOLESTEROL BALANCE

Because cholesterol is converted by the liver to bile acids and secreted unmodified into bile, overall cholesterol balance depends on the disposition of both cholesterol and bile acids. Most bile acid molecules are not lost in the feces after participating in cholesterol transport and fat digestion; instead, they are taken up and recycled by high-affinity transport proteins in the distal ileum. Bile acids enter the portal circulation and are transported back to the liver, where they are cleared from the blood by hepatocytes with high first-pass efficiency. Bile acids are then re-secreted into bile. This process of recycling bile acids between the liver and intestine is referred to as **enterohepatic circulation**.

Enterohepatic circulation is highly efficient, allowing <5% of secreted bile acids to be lost in the feces. However, because bile acids are secreted in such large amounts, the small fractional loss of bile acids amounts to about 0.4 grams

per day. Considering that cholesterol is the substrate for bile acid synthesis, fecal bile acids represent a source of cholesterol loss from the body. Sensitive nuclear hormone receptors within the liver are capable of detecting the rate of loss of bile acids into the feces. These receptors tightly regulate transcription of bile acid synthetic genes. As a result, the liver synthesizes precisely the amount of bile acids that is sufficient to replace what is lost in the feces.

In addition to the 1.2 grams of cholesterol that are secreted into bile each day, the average American diet contributes approximately 0.4 grams each day to intestinal cholesterol. Therefore, dietary cholesterol represents only a minor fraction (25%) of the total (i.e., biliary and dietary) cholesterol that passes through the intestine. The extent to which intestinal cholesterol is absorbed appears to be genetically regulated. Each individual absorbs a fixed percentage of intestinal cholesterol. In the population, percentages range from as low as 20 to more than 80. For example, when an average individual absorbs 50% of intestinal cholesterol, this will amount to half of the 1.6 grams (i.e., 1.2 grams of biliary cholesterol plus 0.4 grams of dietary cholesterol), and the other half (0.8 grams) will be lost in the feces. Combined with a loss of 0.4 grams per day of cholesterol in the form of fecal bile acids, this yields a total cholesterol loss from the body of 1.2 grams each day. Taking into account intestinal absorption of dietary cholesterol and reabsorption of biliary cholesterol, total body cholesterol synthesis is 0.8 grams per day (i.e., cholesterol synthesis = fecal loss of cholesterol plus bile acids − dietary cholesterol intake). Thus, the amount of endogenous cholesterol synthesis is about twofold greater than the amount consumed in the average diet.

PATHOPHYSIOLOGY

Numerous studies have demonstrated a definitive link between elevated plasma lipid concentrations and the risk of cardiovascular disease. Increased risk of cardiovascular mortality is most closely linked to elevated levels of LDL cholesterol and decreased levels of HDL cholesterol. In addition, hypertriglyceridemia represents an independent risk factor. The risk is further increased when hypertriglyceridemia is associated with low HDL-cholesterol concentrations, even if LDL-cholesterol concentrations are normal. From a clinical perspective, the dyslipidemias can be divided into hypercholesterolemia, hypertriglyceridemia, mixed hyperlipidemia, and disorders of HDL metabolism (Table 23-2).

Numerous causes of hyperlipidemia are appreciated. These include well-defined monogenic diseases and the contributions of genetic polymorphisms, as well as less well-defined gene–environment interactions. For many individuals, elevated cholesterol may be the consequence of a diet high in saturated fat and cholesterol superimposed on a susceptible genetic profile. The following section describes the major genetic predispositions for hyperlipidemia. This is followed by a brief overview of the secondary causes of hyperlipidemia. It is important to appreciate that the decision to treat elevated cholesterol concentrations is based on estimations of the risk of cardiovascular disease. Current clinical

TABLE 23-2	Genetic Causes of Dyslipidemia		
DISEASE	**CHARACTERISTIC LIPID PROFILE**	**ESTIMATED PREVALENCE**	**ETIOLOGY**
Primary Hypercholesterolemia			
Familial hypercholesterolemia	⇈ LDL	1:500 (heterozygote) 1:1 million (homozygote)	↓ or no functional LDL receptor expression
Autosomal recessive hypercholesterolemia	⇈ LDL	Very rare	Defective adaptor protein (ARH) that causes failure of the LDL receptor to internalize
Familial defective apoB100	↑ LDL	1:1,000	↓ Binding of apoB100 to the LDL receptor
Polygenic hypercholesterolemia	↑ Cholesterol	Common	Unknown; variants in genes for lipid metabolism increasing susceptibility to diet
Primary Hypertriglyceridemia			
Familial hypertriglyceridemia	↑ TG, ↑ VLDL, ↓ HDL	Common	Overproduction and impaired catabolism of triglyceride-rich VLDL
Familial lipoprotein lipase deficiency	⇈ TG	1:1 million	Defect in lipoprotein lipase
ApoCII deficiency	⇈ TG	1:1 million	Defect in apoCII
Mixed Hyperlipidemia			
Familial combined hyperlipidemia	↑ LDL, ↑ TG, sometimes ↓ HDL	1:100	Unknown; dominant inheritance
Familial dysbetalipoproteinemia	↑ Cholesterol, ↑ TG, ↓ LDL, ↑ remnants	1:10,000	Inheritance of apoE2 isoform
Disorders of HDL Metabolism			
Polygenic low HDL	↓ HDL	Common	Overweight, diabetes, lack of exercise, high-carbohydrate diet
Familial hypoalphalipoproteinemia	↓ HDL	1:400	Unknown; dominant inheritance
Familial apoAI deficiency	↓ HDL	Rare	ApoAI deficiency
Tangier disease	⇊ HDL	Rare	ABCA1 defect
LCAT deficiency	↓ HDL	Rare	LCAT deficiency
Fisheye disease	↓ HDL	Rare	Low activity of LCAT
CETP deficiency	↑ HDL	Rare	CETP deficiency

Dyslipidemias can be categorized by increases in plasma cholesterol, increases in triglycerides, increases in both cholesterol and triglycerides, or disturbances in HDL metabolism. The genetics of the common causes of dyslipidemia are currently largely unknown and may be ascribed to polygenic risk factors or unknown genetic susceptibilities to diet and lifestyle.

practice does not incorporate the genetic causes of hyperlipidemia into these calculations. As common genetic predispositions to dyslipidemia and the contributions of these predispositions to cardiovascular disease become better understood, lipid-lowering therapies may one day be tailored toward individual genetic susceptibilities.

HYPERCHOLESTEROLEMIA

Primary hypercholesterolemia is characterized by elevated levels of total plasma cholesterol and LDL cholesterol, with normal levels of triglyceride. The causes of primary hypercholesterolemia are familial hypercholesterolemia, familial defective apoB100 and, most commonly, polygenic hypercholesterolemia.

Familial hypercholesterolemia (FH) is an autosomal dominant disease involving defects in the LDL receptor. Mutations in the gene encoding the LDL receptor result in one of four molecular defects: lack of receptor synthesis, failure to reach the plasma membrane, defective LDL binding, and failure to internalize bound LDL particles. Heterozygous individuals (1 in 500 in the U.S.) have elevated total plasma cholesterol concentrations from birth throughout life, with adult levels averaging 275 to 500 mg/dL (normal, <200 mg/dL). Clinical features include tendon xanthomas (caused by intracellular and extracellular accumulation of cholesterol) and arcus corneae (deposition of cholesterol in the cornea). Homozygous FH is a much more severe but rare disorder (1 in 1 million in the U.S.) that is characterized by the absence of functional LDL receptors. This leads to very high plasma cholesterol concentrations (700 to 1,200 mg/dL) and cardiovascular disease that presents clinically prior to the age of 20. Heterozygotes for FH respond well to statins and other LDL-lowering drugs that up-regulate LDL receptor density on the cell surface. In the introductory case, Jake was most likely heterozygous for FH. Because homozygotes lack functional LDL receptors, the only effective treatment is plasmapheresis with immunoadsorption of LDL particles. More recently, an autosomal recessive form of hypercholesterolemia has been described in which a defective molecular adaptor protein that participates in LDL receptor internalization into the cell leads to a phenotype similar to that of FH.

Familial defective apoB100 is an autosomal dominant trait in which mutations in the apoB100 protein lead to decreased affinity of the LDL particle for LDL receptors. Due to decreased catabolism of LDL, cholesterol concentrations in familial defective apoB100 can be similar to those in patients with FH. These individuals respond well to therapy with a statin and niacin.

Polygenic hypercholesterolemia is a general term used to categorize the majority (>85%) of patients with hypercholesterolemia who have no defined genetic cause for the disorder. Polygenic hypercholesterolemia may be the result of complex gene–environment interactions and/or multiple uncharacterized genetic susceptibilities. Further research into genetic predispositions for hypercholesterolemia will be necessary in order to identify clear etiologies for the majority of patients with hypercholesterolemia.

HYPERTRIGLYCERIDEMIA

Primary hypertriglyceridemia is characterized by high plasma triglyceride concentrations (200 to 500 mg/dL; normal, <150 mg/dL), when measured following an overnight fast. Three major etiologies of hypertriglyceridemia have been identified: familial hypertriglyceridemia of unknown genetic cause, familial lipoprotein lipase (LPL) deficiency, and apoCII deficiency. Commonly, hypertriglyceridemia develops with age, weight gain, obesity, and diabetes.

Familial hypertriglyceridemia is a common autosomal dominant disorder characterized by hypertriglyceridemia with normal LDL-cholesterol concentrations. HDL-cholesterol is often reduced. Although the underlying defect in this disorder is unknown, it is hypothesized that increased hepatic triglyceride synthesis leads to accelerated production of VLDL. Decreased lipolysis of chylomicrons and VLDL by lipoprotein lipase is another cause. Fibrates are the drug of choice for familial hypertriglyceridemia, although niacin and statins may be added to this regimen.

Familial LPL deficiency is an autosomal recessive trait caused by the absence of active LPL. This condition may be diagnosed by testing the plasma for lipase activity following an infusion of heparin, which competes for binding sites on endothelial cells and dislodges LPL molecules into the plasma. Patients with LPL deficiency exhibit profound hypertriglyceridemia, which is characterized by elevated chylomicrons during infancy and impaired removal of VLDL later in life. Infants or young adults may present with pancreatitis, eruptive xanthomas, hepatomegaly, and splenomegaly attributable to the accumulation of lipid-laden foam cells. Treatment consists of a fat-free diet and avoidance of substances that increase VLDL production by the liver, such as alcohol and glucocorticoids.

ApoCII deficiency is a rare autosomal disorder with presentation and treatment similar to familial lipoprotein lipase deficiency. It may be distinguished from LPL deficiency by demonstrating that the triglyceride levels of patients are reduced following infusion of plasma that contains normal apoCII; this does not occur in patients with familial LPL deficiency.

MIXED HYPERLIPIDEMIA

Patients with mixed hyperlipidemia exhibit complex lipid profiles that may consist of elevated total cholesterol, LDL-cholesterol, and triglyceride concentrations. HDL-cholesterol is often reduced. Etiologies of mixed hyperlipidemia include **familial combined hyperlipidemia** (FCH) and **dysbetalipoproteinemia**.

FCH is a common disease associated with moderately elevated concentrations of fasting triglycerides and total cholesterol, but reduced concentrations of HDL-cholesterol. These patients often present with features of the **metabolic syndrome**, including abdominal obesity, glucose intolerance, and hypertension. The molecular defect is still under investigation. Current hypotheses focus on insulin resistance, which leads to increased lipolysis in fat tissue. Fatty acids liberated from fat tissue return to the liver, where they are reassembled into triglycerides. The increase in triglycerides increases the production of VLDL particles, which leads to an increase in apoB-containing lipoproteins in the plasma. A combination of several genetic variants is likely to be involved in the etiology of FCH, and reduced expression of LDL receptors and/or LPL may be components of the FCH phenotype. Faithful adherence to dietary modification may be an effective means of controlling FCH. However, drug treatment is often required, and statins are commonly utilized. Combination therapy that includes addition of a fibrate or niacin may be necessary to normalize triglyceride and LDL-cholesterol concentrations, as well as to increase HDL-cholesterol.

Dysbetalipoproteinemia is a disorder characterized by increased cholesterol-rich chylomicrons and IDL-like particles. These findings are the result of accumulated chylomicron and VLDL remnants, leading to both hypertriglyceridemia and hypercholesterolemia. Mutations in isoforms of apoE (E2, E3, and E4) have been implicated in the disease. Chylomicron and VLDL particles in patients with the homozygous apoE2/apoE2 phenotype have reduced affinity for their lipoprotein receptors, leading to accumulation of remnant particles in the plasma. Although the defective apoE is present at birth, symptoms generally do not present in males until age 30 and in females until menopause. The mechanism underlying this delay in expression of the phenotype is unknown, and additional metabolic factors (e.g., obesity, diabetes, or hypothyroidism) may be required to unmask the disorder. Dysbetalipoproteinemia can be managed by decreased intake of fat and cholesterol, along with weight reduction and omission of alcohol intake. In addition, niacin and fibrates are effective pharmacologic therapies.

DISORDERS OF HDL METABOLISM

Decreased HDL-cholesterol is an independent risk factor for development of atherosclerosis and cardiovascular disease.

Numerous rare genetic defects in HDL metabolism have been identified, including defects in apoAI, ABCA1, and LCAT. Each of these defects results in decreased levels of HDL, for which no effective treatments are currently available.

Variations in CETP activity have recently been characterized as a potentially more common source of interindividual variation in HDL levels. Decreased CETP activity results in increased plasma HDL concentration, attributable to a decrease in the transfer of cholesterol from HDL to remnant particles. Although it might be assumed that the increased HDL levels would be cardioprotective, this is not always observed. Decreased CETP activity may increase the risk of atherogenesis in some cases, whereas it may be cardioprotective in other cases. Additional research will be necessary before the role of CETP polymorphisms in lipid metabolism and cardiovascular disease risk can be identified.

SECONDARY HYPERLIPIDEMIA

In addition to the genetic causes of primary dyslipidemia described above, a number of secondary factors can lead to hyperlipidemia (Table 23-3). For example, alcohol intake increases the synthesis of fatty acids, which are then esterified to glycerol to form triglycerides. Therefore, excess alcohol consumption can result in increased VLDL production. Hypertriglyceridemia in type II diabetes mellitus results from increased VLDL synthesis and reduced chylomicron and VLDL catabolism by LPL. Insulin normally suppresses VLDL production by the liver, and insulin resistance in the liver causes increased VLDL production. Furthermore, apoCIII levels are increased in association with insulin resistance, and this reduces the catabolism of chylomicrons and

TABLE 23-3 Secondary Causes of Hyperlipidemia

HYPERTRIGLYCERIDEMIA	HYPERCHOLESTEROLEMIA
Diabetes mellitus	Hypothyroidism
Chronic renal failure	Nephrotic syndrome
Hypothyroidism	Anorexia nervosa
Glycogen storage disease	Acute intermittent
Stress	porphyria
Sepsis	Cholestasis
Alcohol excess	Obstructive liver disease
Lipodystrophy	Corticosteroid treatment
Pregnancy	Protease inhibitor therapy
Oral estrogen replacement therapy	
Antihypertensive drugs: beta-blockers, diuretics	
Glucocorticoid treatment	
Protease inhibitor therapy	
Acute hepatitis	
Systemic lupus erythematosus	

Numerous secondary causes of hyperlipidemia exist; screening for the presence of these underlying factors should be performed before initiating pharmacologic therapy for a dyslipidemia.

VLDL particles. Hypothyroidism is an important and common cause of secondary hyperlipidemia. Every patient with a lipid disorder should be screened for hypothyroidism.

PHARMACOLOGIC CLASSES AND AGENTS

The decision to treat dyslipidemia is largely dependent on the calculated cardiovascular risk. A number of clinical algorithms exist for determining initiation of therapy. Goals for lipid lowering were established in the 2001 National Cholesterol Education Program Adult Treatment Panel III (ATP III) guidelines, which were updated in 2004 based on the results of several additional large, randomized clinical trials. These guidelines provide target LDL levels based on 10-year risk of death from cardiovascular disease (Table 23-4). The guidelines stress that it is always important first to promote therapeutic lifestyle changes (TLC). TLC include reduction of dietary saturated fat and cholesterol intake, weight reduction, increased physical activity, and, possibly, stress reduction.

Successful dietary therapy can reduce total cholesterol by 5% to 25%, depending on adherence and the metabolic basis for elevated cholesterol concentrations. If this approach is unsuccessful or insufficient to normalize lipid levels, drug therapy is generally recommended. Five classes of agents are available for pharmacologic modification of lipid metabolism. Three of these classes (inhibitors of cholesterol synthesis, bile acid sequestrants, and cholesterol absorption inhibitors) have relatively well-defined effects on lipid metabolism. While the overall effects of the other two classes (fibrates and niacin) are clear, their molecular mechanisms of actions are diverse and remain subjects of active investigation. The inhibitors of cholesterol synthesis (i.e., HMG CoA reductase inhibitors, also known as *statins*) are the most important class due to their well-demonstrated efficacy in reducing cardiovascular morbidity and mortality. However, agents in each of the other classes act as important adjunctive therapies, and may be the agents of choice for patients with certain specific causes of dyslipidemia.

INHIBITORS OF CHOLESTEROL SYNTHESIS

HMG CoA reductase inhibitors, commonly known as statins, competitively inhibit the activity of HMG CoA reductase, the rate-limiting enzyme in cholesterol synthesis. Inhibition of this enzyme results in a transient, modest decrease in cellular cholesterol concentration (Fig. 23-11). The decrease in cholesterol concentration activates a cellular signaling cascade culminating in the activation of **sterol regulatory element binding protein 2** (SREBP2), a transcription factor that up-regulates expression of the gene encoding the LDL receptor. Increased LDL receptor expression causes increased uptake of plasma LDL, and consequently decreases plasma LDL-cholesterol concentration. Approximately 70% of LDL receptors are expressed by hepatocytes, with the remainder expressed by a variety of cell types in the body.

Statins were shown in numerous clinical trials to reduce

TABLE 23-4 Updated National Cholesterol Education Program Adult Treatment Panel III Guidelines

ATP 2004 Update: LDL-C Therapy by Risk Categories Based on Recent Clinical Trial Evidence			
RISK CATEGORY	**LDL-C GOAL**	**INITIATE THERAPEUTIC LIFESTYLE CHANGES**	**CONSIDER DRUG THERAPY**
High Risk: CHD or CHD risk equivalents (10-year risk >20%)	<100 mg/dL; *optional goal <70 mg/dL*	≥100 mg/dL	≥100 mg/dL
Moderately high risk: 2 + risk factors (10-year risk 10%–20%)	<130 mg/dL	≥130 mg/dL	≥130 mg/dL (consider drug options if 100–129 mg/dL)
Moderate risk: 2 + risk factors (10-year risk <10%)	<130 mg/dL	≥130 mg/dL	>160 mg/dL
Low risk: 0–1 risk factor	<160 mg/dL	≥160 mg/dL	≥190 mg/dL (consider drug options if 160–189 mg/dL)

Adapted with permission from Grundy SM, Cleeman JI, Merz CN, et al. Implications of recent clinical trials for the National Cholesterol Education Program Adult Treatment Panel III Guidelines. *J Am Coll Cardiol* 2004;44:720–732. (*Supplemental clinical guidelines for cholesterol lowering therapy with lower LDL cholesterol goals for high risk patients.*)

More information about lipid management guidelines and details about calculation of cardiovascular risk are available at: http://www.nhlbi.nih.gov/guidelines/cholesterol/.

mortality significantly after a myocardial infarction. This is referred to as **secondary prevention**. Recent studies have also concluded that lowering of LDL with statins can decrease mortality even in the absence of overt cardiovascular disease, which is called **primary prevention**. Despite these convincing percentage risk reductions in both secondary and primary prevention trials, it should be noted that statin use is associated with a greater absolute risk reduction in secondary prevention; the reason may be that patients in this treatment group have a greater absolute risk of death and therefore display the largest benefit from statins. It is also important to note that statins have proven to be effective in reducing cardiovascular disease risk for high-risk patients (e.g., diabetic patients) with average, or even below-average, LDL-cholesterol levels.

The magnitude of LDL-cholesterol lowering depends on the efficacy and dosage of the statin that is administered. In general, statins reduce LDL-cholesterol concentrations by 25% to 55%. Statins increase HDL-cholesterol concentrations by an average of 5%, and reduce triglyceride concentrations by 10% to 35%, depending on statin dose and degree of hypertriglyceridemia. The effect of statins on triglyceride levels is mediated by decreased VLDL production and increased clearance of remnant lipoproteins by the liver. The dose-response relationship of statins is nonlinear: the largest effect occurs with the starting dose. Each subsequent doubling of the dose produces, on average, an additional 6% LDL reduction. This is sometimes referred to as the "rule of 6's".

In addition to reducing LDL-cholesterol concentrations, statins have a number of other pharmacologic consequences. These are collectively referred to as the *pleiotropic effects of statins,* which include reversal of endothelial dysfunction, decreased coagulation, decreased inflammation, and improved stability of atherosclerotic plaques. As evidence for reversal of endothelial dysfunction, there is an improved vasodilatory response of endothelium to NO after statin administration. Improved vasodilation could help prevent ischemia. There are also decreases in prothrombin activation

and endothelial cell tissue factor production during statin therapy. Because thrombus development is at the root of most acute coronary syndromes, its reduction could contribute to the survival benefit of statins. Statin therapy is associated with a decrease in acute-phase reactants, providing evidence for diminished inflammation. Acute-phase reactants are plasma proteins that are increased during inflammatory states and may play a role in the destabilization of atherosclerotic plaques. The best characterized acute-phase reactant is **C-reactive protein**. Finally, plaque stability is enhanced during statin therapy because the fibrous cap that overlies the lipid-rich plaque becomes thicker. This effect may be attributable to decreased macrophage infiltration and inhibition of vascular smooth muscle proliferation. It is important to emphasize that many of these pleiotropic effects of statins have been demonstrated only in vitro or in animal models, and their relevance in humans is unclear. Moreover, analysis of clinical data reveals that the reductions in cardiovascular morbidity and mortality due to statins are primarily attributable to the lowering of LDL-cholesterol concentrations in the plasma.

Six statins—**lovastatin, pravastatin, simvastatin, fluvastatin, atorvastatin,** and **rosuvastatin**—are currently approved for use in hypercholesterolemia and mixed dyslipidemia. They are considered first-line therapy for increased LDL levels, and numerous trials have shown that statins decrease both cardiovascular-related and total mortality. Stroke is also reduced. All of the statins are believed to act by the same mechanism. The main differences are attributable to potency and pharmacokinetic parameters. Among the statins, fluvastatin is the least potent, and atorvastatin and rosuvastatin are the most potent. Beyond their capacity to reduce LDL-cholesterol concentrations, the clinical relevance of these potency differences has not been determined. The pharmacokinetic differences among the statins result from differential cytochrome P450 metabolism. Lovastatin, simvastatin, and atorvastatin are metabolized by P450 3A4, whereas other cytochrome P450-mediated pathways metabolize fluvastatin. Pravastatin and rosuvastatin are not me-

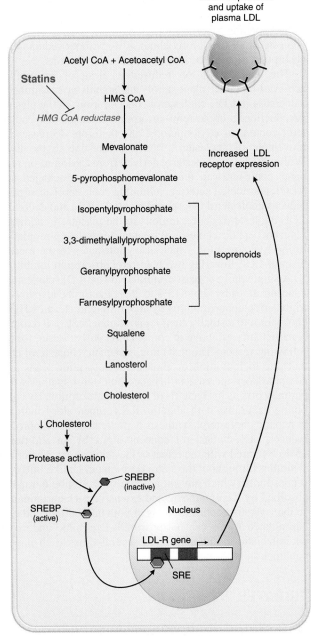

Increased
LDL-R expression
and uptake of
plasma LDL

Figure 23-11. Mechanism of LDL lowering by statins. Statins competitively inhibit HMG-CoA reductase, the enzyme that catalyzes the rate-limiting step in cholesterol biosynthesis. Decreased cellular cholesterol concentrations lead to protease activation and cleavage of the sterol regulatory element binding protein (SREBP), which is a transcription factor that normally resides in the cytoplasm. The cleaved SREBP diffuses into the nucleus, where it binds to sterol response elements (SRE), leading to up-regulation of LDL-receptor gene transcription. This leads to increased cellular LDL receptor expression. This promotes uptake of LDL particles and results in reduced LDL-cholesterol concentrations in the plasma.

tabolized via the cytochrome P450 pathway. As explained below, the pathways of statin metabolism have important implications for drug interactions.

Statins are generally well tolerated; the incidence of adverse effects is lower with statins than with any of the other lipid-lowering drug classes. The main adverse effect is myopathy and/or myositis with rhabdomyolysis. This is a very rare complication that occurs primarily at high doses of statins. At intermediate and low doses of the less potent statins (e.g., pravastatin and simvastatin), myalgia and myopathy have occurred at rates comparable to placebo in trials of about 20,000 patients. Therefore, plasma creatine kinase levels (a marker of muscle injury) are not useful for routine monitoring of statin-treated patients. High-potency statins can also cause increases in serum transaminase levels (i.e., alanine transaminase [ALT] and aspartate transaminase [AST]). These elevations are very rarely indicative of hepatotoxicity, and most likely reflect an adaptive response of the liver to changes in cholesterol homeostasis.

If a statin alone is insufficient to lower LDL to target levels, the statin can be used effectively in combination with other agents. The combination of a statin with a bile acid sequestrant or cholesterol absorption inhibitor results in additive LDL decreases, and is not associated with significant drug interactions. The combination of niacin and a statin may be most useful in patients with high levels of LDL-cholesterol and low levels of HDL-cholesterol. However, because coadministration of niacin and a statin slightly increases the risk of myopathy, this potential adverse effect should be carefully monitored. Fibrates and statins have also been reported to be efficacious in combination. However, because certain fibrates inhibit the glucuronidation of statins and thereby decrease statin clearance, these agents may raise the plasma statin concentration and increase the risk of rhabdomyolysis. This effect has been documented for **gemfibrozil** but does not occur with **fenofibrate**. Finally, in patients who require LDL lowering and are taking drugs that are metabolized by cytochrome P450—such as certain antibiotics, immunosuppressive agents, and protease inhibitors (see Chapter 4, Drug Metabolism)—a statin that is not metabolized by P450 is preferable.

INHIBITORS OF BILE ACID ABSORPTION

The bile acid sequestrants are cationic polymer resins that bind noncovalently to negatively charged bile acids in the small intestine. The resin–bile acid complex cannot be reabsorbed in the distal ileum and is excreted in the stool. Decreased bile acid reabsorption by the ileum partially interrupts enterohepatic bile acid circulation, causing hepatocytes to up-regulate 7α-hydroxylase, the rate-limiting enzyme in bile acid synthesis (Fig. 23-10A). The increase in bile acid synthesis decreases hepatocyte cholesterol concentration, leading to increased expression of the LDL receptor and enhanced LDL clearance from the circulation. The effectiveness of bile acid sequestrants in clearing LDL from plasma is partially offset by concurrent up-regulation of hepatic cholesterol and triglyceride synthesis, which stimulates the production of VLDL particles by the liver. As a result, bile acid sequestrants may also raise triglyceride levels and should be used with caution in patients with hypertriglyceridemia.

The three available bile acid sequestrants are **cholestyramine, colesevelam,** and **colestipol**. These drugs possess similar efficacy, causing 8% to 24% reductions in LDL levels at therapeutic concentrations. In order to maximize the binding of these agents to bile acids, drug administration is timed so that the drugs are present in the small intestine following a meal (i.e. after gallbladder emptying). Because bile acid sequestrants are not absorbed systemically, they have little potential for serious toxicity. However, significant bloating and dyspepsia often limit patient compliance. These adverse effects result because of increased delivery of fat and bile acids to the large intestine. Bile acid sequestrants can decrease absorption of fat-soluble vitamins, and bleeding due to vitamin K deficiency has occasionally been reported. They can also bind certain coadministered drugs, such as digoxin and warfarin, and thereby lower the bioavailability of the coadministered agents. This interaction can be eliminated by administering the bile acid sequestrant at least 1 hour after other drugs.

Because of the demonstrated clinical efficacy and tolerability of statins, bile acid sequestrants have been relegated to second-line agents for lipid reduction. Currently, bile acid sequestrants are used mainly for treatment of hypercholesterolemia in young (<25 years old) patients and in patients for whom statins alone do not provide sufficient plasma LDL reduction. Some experts prefer bile acid sequestrants for young patients (such as patients with familial hypercholesterolemia) because these agents are not absorbed and are generally considered safe for long-term use. However, other experts prefer to use a statin for initial therapy in children.

INHIBITORS OF CHOLESTEROL ABSORPTION

Cholesterol absorption inhibitors reduce cholesterol absorption by the small intestine. Although this includes reduced absorption of dietary cholesterol, the more important effect is reduced reabsorption of biliary cholesterol, which comprises the majority of intestinal cholesterol. Whereas statins and bile acid sequestrants reduce LDL-cholesterol principally by increasing LDL clearance via the LDL receptor, inhibitors of cholesterol absorption reduce LDL-cholesterol mainly by inhibiting hepatic production of VLDL.

The two available cholesterol absorption inhibitors are **plant sterols** and **ezetimibe**. Plant sterols and stanols are naturally present in vegetables and fruits, and they may be consumed in larger amounts from nutritional supplements. Plant sterols and stanols are similar in molecular structure to cholesterol, but are substantially more hydrophobic. As a result, plant sterols and stanols displace cholesterol from micelles, increasing the excretion of cholesterol in the stool. The plant sterols and stanols are themselves are poorly absorbed. Based on their mechanism of action, gram quantities of plant sterols and stanols are required to reduce plasma LDL cholesterol concentrations by approximately 15%. Because an average diet contains 200 to 400 mg of plant sterols and stanols, these molecules must be highly enriched in dietary supplements (to approximately 2 gm) in order to be effective.

Ezetimibe decreases cholesterol transport from micelles into enterocytes by selectively inhibiting cholesterol uptake through a brush border protein named NPC1L1 (Fig. 23-4A). At therapeutic concentrations, ezetimibe reduces intestinal cholesterol absorption by about 50%, without reducing the absorption of triglycerides or fat-soluble vitamins.

The end result of reduced cholesterol absorption, achieved by either plant sterols and stanols or ezetimibe, is a decrease in LDL-cholesterol concentrations in the plasma. A reduction in cholesterol absorption decreases the cholesterol content of chylomicrons, and therefore decreases the movement of cholesterol from the intestine to the liver. Within the liver, cholesterol derived from chylomicron remnants contributes to the cholesterol that is packaged into VLDL particles. Therefore, inhibiting cholesterol absorption reduces cholesterol incorporation into VLDL, and decreases LDL-cholesterol concentrations in the plasma. In addition, reduced hepatic cholesterol content leads to up-regulation of the LDL receptor, which also contributes to the mechanism of LDL lowering by cholesterol absorption inhibitors.

A single daily dose of ezetimibe lowers LDL-cholesterol concentrations by about 15% to 20%. Ezetimibe also lowers triglyceride concentrations by about 8% and elevates HDL-cholesterol to a small extent (approximately 3%). Ezetimibe is particularly effective in combination with a statin, for the following reason. The reduction in hepatic cholesterol content due to inhibition of cholesterol absorption leads to a compensatory increase in hepatic cholesterol synthesis that partially offsets the benefits of reducing absorption. By combining ezetimibe with a statin, the compensatory increase in hepatic cholesterol synthesis is prevented. This approach reduces LDL-cholesterol concentrations by an additional 15% compared with the effect of the statin alone. The effect is similar throughout the statin dose range. Unlike bile acid sequestrants (which are not absorbed), ezetimibe is rapidly absorbed by the enterocyte and extensively glucuronidated, so that systemic concentrations of both unmodified and glucuronidated forms can be measured. Ezetimibe undergoes enterohepatic circulation up to several times each day in conjunction with meals.

FIBRATES

Fibrates bind to and activate peroxisome proliferator-activated receptor α (PPARα), a nuclear receptor expressed in hepatocytes, skeletal muscle, macrophages, and the heart. Upon binding of fibrate, PPARα heterodimerizes with the retinoid X receptor (RXR). This heterodimer binds to peroxisome proliferator response elements (PPREs) in the promoter regions of specific genes, activating transcription of these genes and thereby increasing protein expression.

Activation of PPARα by fibrates results in numerous changes in lipid metabolism that act collectively to decrease plasma triglyceride levels and increase plasma HDL (Fig. 23-12). The decrease in plasma triglyceride levels is caused by increased muscle cell expression of lipoprotein lipase, decreased hepatic expression of apolipoprotein CIII, and increased hepatic oxidation of fatty acids. The increased muscle expression of lipoprotein lipase results in increased uptake of triglyceride-rich lipoproteins, with a resultant decrease in plasma triglyceride levels. Because apoCIII nor-

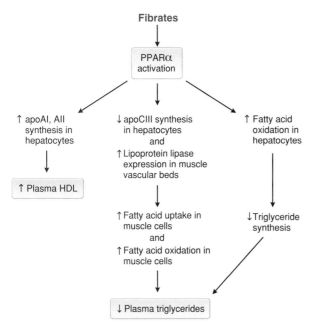

Figure 23-12. Influence of fibrates on lipid metabolism. Fibrates have several beneficial effects on lipid metabolism, all of which appear to be secondary to the activation of the transcription factor, PPARα. PPARα activation by fibrates increases hepatic synthesis of apoAI and apoAII, which lead to increased plasma HDL-cholesterol concentrations. PPARα activation also down-regulates hepatic synthesis of apoCIII, which normally inhibits lipoprotein lipase activity in muscle vascular beds, and increases lipoprotein lipase expression. Decreased apoCIII, an inhibitor of lipoprotein lipase, combined with increased lipoprotein lipase expression, leads to increased fatty acid uptake in muscle cells and increased fatty acid oxidation. PPARα also increases fatty acid oxidation in hepatocytes. The combined effects of these metabolic changes is decreased plasma triglyceride concentrations and increased plasma HDL-cholesterol. Due to decreased hepatic fatty acid and triglyceride synthesis *(not shown)*, LDL-cholesterol concentrations also decrease modestly.

mally functions to inhibit interaction of triglyceride-rich lipoproteins with their receptors, the decrease in hepatic production of apoCIII may potentiate the increased lipoprotein lipase activity.

The mechanisms by which fibrates raise plasma HDL levels are not clear. Whereas PPARα increases hepatocyte production of apolipoprotein AI in the mouse, the same has not been demonstrated convincingly in humans. Up-regulation of SR-B1 and ABCA1 in macrophages presumably promotes cholesterol efflux from these cells *in vivo*. Hepatocytes also increase expression of SR-B1 in response to PPARα, providing a pathway for increased reverse cholesterol transport, with subsequent cholesterol excretion into bile.

Fibrates also lower LDL levels modestly. The lower LDL levels result from a PPARα-mediated shift in hepatocyte metabolism toward fatty acid oxidation. PPARα increases the expression of numerous enzymes involved in fatty acid transport and oxidation. This increases fatty acid catabolism, leading to decreased triglyceride synthesis and VLDL production. PPARα activation also results in LDL particles of larger size, which appear to be taken up more efficiently by LDL receptors. Many of these effects of PPARα on lipid

metabolism remain the subject of basic and clinical investigation, which may lead to development of more selective PPARα agonists that are capable of targeting selective aspects of lipid metabolism.

Gemfibrozil and **fenofibrate** are the available fibrates in the United States. Two other fibrates, **bezafibrate** and **ciprofibrate**, are available in Europe. Fibrates are indicated for treatment of hypertriglyceridemia and hypertriglyceridemia with low HDL. In addition, fibrates are the therapy of choice for patients with type III dysbetalipoproteinemia (increased plasma levels of triglycerides and lipoprotein remnants), which results from homozygous inheritance of the apoE2 allele. The mechanism of response to fibrates in this disease is unknown, but may be related to decreased VLDL production. Because of their greater efficacy, statins are preferred over fibrates for treatment of increased LDL levels. However, fibrates can be used together with statins in cases of combined hyperlipidemia or when HDL-cholesterol is decreased.

Gastrointestinal discomfort is the most common adverse effect of fibrates. Rare adverse effects include myopathy and arrhythmias. Increases in liver transaminases occur in about 5% of patients. Gastrointestinal disturbances and myopathy are less common with fenofibrate than with gemfibrozil. Gemfibrozil-associated gallstone formation is presumably a consequence of fibrate-induced increases in biliary cholesterol excretion. Fibrates displace warfarin from albumin binding sites, resulting in increased free warfarin concentrations. Therefore, the dose of warfarin should be reduced when a fibrate is coadministered. The effect of a coadministered statin on fibrate metabolism is described above. A third important drug interaction involves fenofibrate and cyclosporine. Because fenofibrate increases the clearance of cyclosporine, plasma cyclosporine levels must be monitored in transplant patients taking both agents concurrently.

NIACIN

Niacin (nicotinic acid, vitamin B_3) is a water-soluble vitamin. At physiologic concentrations, it is a substrate in the synthesis of nicotinamide adenine dinucleotide (NAD) and nicotinamide adenine dinucleotide phosphate (NADP), which are important cofactors in intermediary metabolism.

The pharmacologic use of niacin necessitates large doses (1,500 to 3,000 mg/day), and is independent of the conversion of nicotinic acid to NAD or NADP (Fig. 23-13). Niacin decreases plasma LDL-cholesterol and triglyceride concentrations and increases HDL-cholesterol. Recent studies have identified a G protein-coupled receptor on adipocytes that appears to mediate the well documented metabolic changes associated with niacin administration. Stimulation of this receptor by niacin decreases adipocyte hormone-sensitive lipase activity, leading to reduced peripheral tissue triglyceride catabolism and therefore decreased flux of free fatty acids to the liver. This decreases the rate of hepatic triglyceride synthesis and VLDL production. Niacin also increases the half-life of apoAI, the major apolipoprotein in HDL. The increase in plasma apoAI increases plasma HDL concentrations and presumably augments reverse cholesterol transport.

Pharmacologic doses of niacin are available as oral agents

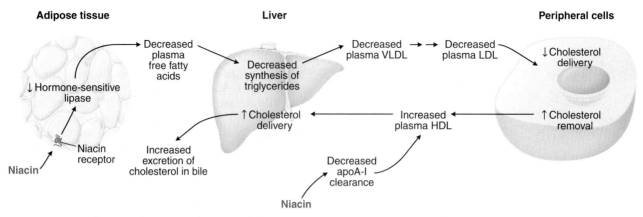

Figure 23-13. Influence of niacin on lipid metabolism. Niacin lowers triglyceride and LDL levels while increasing HDL. Activation by niacin of a G protein-coupled receptor on adipocytes results in decreased hormone-sensitive lipase activity in adipose tissue, which decreases the flux of free fatty acids to the liver. This decreased free fatty acid flux reduces hepatic triglyceride synthesis and limits VLDL synthesis. Because LDL is derived from VLDL, the decreased VLDL synthesis decreases plasma concentrations of LDL-cholesterol. Niacin also increases the half-life of apoAI, an important apolipoprotein in HDL. The increased apoAI levels directly increase levels of plasma HDL and may also augment reverse cholesterol transport, delivery of cholesterol from HDL to the liver, and excretion of cholesterol in the bile.

for daily administration. The major adverse effects of niacin are cutaneous flushing and pruritus (itching). The flushing is mediated by the G protein-coupled niacin receptor and involves the release of prostaglandins D_2 and E_2 within the skin. It can be prevented by pretreatment with aspirin or another NSAID. These adverse effects are also subject to tachyphylaxis and usually disappear after several weeks of niacin use. However, missing a single dose of niacin can lead to the resumption of adverse effects. Timed-release formulations of niacin are associated with less cutaneous flushing than the immediate-release dosage form.

In addition to flushing and pruritus, three important adverse effects of niacin are hyperuricemia, impaired insulin sensitivity, and myopathy. Hyperuricemia occurs in approximately 20% of patients, and may precipitate gout. Impaired insulin sensitivity may precipitate diabetes in patients at risk, and niacin should be used with caution in diabetic patients. Rarely, niacin may cause myopathy. Concurrent administration of niacin with a statin increases the risk of myopathy slightly.

Niacin is indicated for patients with familial combined hyperlipidemia (elevation of both triglycerides and cholesterol), usually in combination with a statin. Because niacin is currently the most effective agent available for raising HDL, it may also be the drug of choice for patients with modestly elevated LDL and decreased HDL. It is not clear whether both the LDL-lowering and HDL-raising effects of niacin contribute to improved clinical outcomes.

OMEGA-3 FATTY ACIDS

The omega-3 fatty acids **eicosapentaenoic acid** (EPA) and **docosahexaenoic acid** (DHA), also referred to as fish oils, are effective at reducing plasma triglycerides. By incompletely understood molecular mechanisms, fish oils reduce triglyceride biosynthesis and increase fatty acid oxidation in the liver. Omega-3 fatty acids are available over the counter as nutritional supplements in the form of fatty acid ethyl esters. **Omecor,** a prescription-strength form of omega-3 fatty acids, has also become available. Omecor is enriched

(84%) in EPA and DHA, whereas most dietary supplements contain 13% to 63% fish oils. The recommended dose of omecor is 4 g, once a day. Omega-3 fatty acids are generally added to therapy when plasma triglyceride concentrations exceed 500 mg/dL. The influence of omega-3 fatty acid use on clinical outcomes is uncertain.

◼ *Conclusion and Future Directions*

LDL reduction by the available lipid lowering drugs—particularly the statins—represents an important advance in reducing cardiovascular disease mortality. Future drug trials will examine the possible benefits for cardiovascular disease from raising HDL and lowering triglyceride levels. Also under development are pharmacologic therapies for new biochemical targets such as CETP and MTP. Inhibition of CETP raises HDL and lowers LDL by inhibiting the transfer of cholesterol from HDL to remnant particles, whereas inhibition of MTP reduces VLDL secretion.

◼ *Suggested Reading*

Adult Treatment Panel III. Executive summary of the National Cholesterol Education Program (NCEP) expert panel on detection, evaluation, and treatment of high blood cholesterol in adults. *JAMA* 2001;285:2486–2497. (*Clinical guidelines for cholesterol-lowering therapy.*)

Duffy D, Rader DJ. Emerging therapies targeting high-density lipoprotein metabolism and reverse cholesterol transport. *Circulation* 2006;113:1140–1150. (*Future directions in pharmacology of HDL metabolism.*)

Grundy SM, Cleeman JI, Merz CN, et al. Implications of recent clinical trials for the National Cholesterol Education Program Adult Treatment Panel III Guidelines. *J Am Coll Cardiol* 2004; 44:720–732. (*Supplemental clinical guidelines for cholesterol-lowering therapy with lower LDL-cholesterol goals for high-risk patients.*)

Tunaru S, Kero J, Schaub A, et al. PUMA-G and HM74 are receptors for nicotinic acid and mediate its anti-lipolytic effect. *Nat Med* 2003;9:352–355. (*Identification of the G protein-coupled receptor ligand for pharmacologic effects of niacin.*)

Drug Summary Table	**Chapter 23** Pharmacology of Cholesterol and Lipoprotein Metabolism

Drug	Clinical Applications	*Serious* and Common Adverse Effects	Contraindications	Therapeutic Considerations
INHIBITORS OF CHOLESTEROL SYNTHESIS *Mechanism—Inhibit HMG CoA reductase, the rate-limiting enzyme in cholesterol synthesis → LDL decreases 25% to 55%, HDL increases 5%, triglycerides decrease 10% to 25%*				
Lovastatin Pravastatin Simvastatin Fluvastatin Atorvastatin Rosuvastatin	Hypercholesterolemia Familial hypercholesterolemia Coronary atherosclerosis Prophylaxis for coronary atherosclerosis	*Myopathy, rhabdomyolysis, hepatotoxicity, dermatomyositis* Abdominal pain, constipation, diarrhea, nausea, headache	Active liver disease Pregnancy and lactation	Statins are drugs of choice for lowering LDL Atorvastatin and rosuvastatin are the most potent; fluvastatin is the least potent Lovastatin, simvastatin, and atorvastatin are metabolized by P450 3A4; inhibitors of P450 3A4 increase risk of myopathy; fluvastatin is metabolized via a different cytochrome P450-mediated pathway; pravastatin and rosuvastatin are not metabolized by cytochrome P450s; consider choosing a statin not metabolized via P450s in patients who are concurrently taking drugs that are metabolized by cytochrome P450s Combination with a bile acid sequestrant or cholesterol absorption inhibitor results in additive decrease in LDL Combination with niacin may be useful in patients with high LDL and low HDL; however, coadministration with niacin increases the risk of myopathy Coadministration with gemfibrozil decreases statin clearance and raises plasma concentration of statins, which can induce rhabdomyolysis
INHIBITORS OF BILE ACID ABSORPTION *Mechanism—Bind to bile acids, preventing enterohepatic circulation → LDL decreases 8% to 24%, HDL increases 5%*				
Cholestyramine Colesevelam Colestipol	Hypercholesterolemia Pruritus (cholestyramine only)	Increase in triglyceride levels, bloating, dyspepsia, flatulence, bleeding diathesis secondary to vitamin K deficiency	Complete biliary obstruction Hyperlipidemia types III, IV, or V (hypertriglyceridemia)	Lower LDL levels dose-dependently; increase HDL modestly Second-line agents for lipid reduction; used mainly to treat hypercholesterolemia in young patients and patients for whom statins alone do not provide sufficient LDL reduction Raise triglyceride levels Significant bloating and dyspepsia limit patient compliance Decrease absorption of fat-soluble vitamins; bleeding may result due to vitamin K deficiency; bind certain drugs, such as digoxin and warfarin

(Continued)

Drug Summary Table   **Chapter 23 Pharmacology of Cholesterol and Lipoprotein Metabolism** (*Continued*)

Drug	Clinical Applications	Serious and Common Adverse Effects	Contraindications	Therapeutic Considerations
INHIBITORS OF CHOLESTEROL ABSORPTION				
Mechanism—Decrease cholesterol transport from micelles into the enterocyte by inhibiting uptake through brush border protein NPC1L1 → LDL decreases ~19%, HDL increases ~3%, triglyceride decreases ~8%				
Ezetimibe	Primary hypercholesterolemia Familial hypercholesterolemia Sitosterolemia (very rare)	*Elevated liver function tests, myopathy* Dyspepsia, arthralgia, myalgia, headache	Active liver disease Persistently elevated liver function tests when co-administered with a statin	Modest LDL reduction; small effect on HDL and triglyceride levels Inhibition of cholesterol absorption by ezetimibe leads to a compensatory increase in hepatic cholesterol synthesis, partially offsetting the benefits of reduced cholesterol absorption; by combining a statin with ezetimibe, the compensatory increase in hepatic cholesterol synthesis is prevented Ezetimibe is rapidly absorbed by enterocytes and circulates enterohepatically Ezetimibe levels are increased by cyclosporine and fibrates
FIBRATES				
Mechanism—Agonists of peroxisome proliferator-activated receptor α (PPARα) → triglycerides decrease 35% to 70%, HDL increases 5% to 15%				
Gemfibrozil Fenofibrate	Isolated hypertriglyceridemia Hypertriglyceridemia with low HDL Type III dysbetalipoproteinemia	*Elevated liver function tests, myopathy when co-administered with a statin, arrhythmias* Dyspepsia, myalgia, gallstones, xerostomia	Concomitant gemfibrozil and cerivastatin Preexisting gallbladder disease Hepatic dysfunction Severe renal impairment	Drugs of choice for hypertriglyceridemia Bezafibrate and ciprofibrate are available in Europe Used in combination with statins for combined hyperlipidemia or when HDL cholesterol is decreased; however, there is an increased risk of myopathy when combined with statins Fenofibrate has fewer GI and myopathy adverse effects than gemfibrozil; fenofibrate increases the clearance of cyclosporine Fibrates increase warfarin levels
NIACIN				
Mechanism—Reduces free fatty acid release from adipose tissue; increases plasma residence time for apoA1				
Niacin	Isolated low HDL Low HDL with mildly elevated LDL or triglycerides Familial combined hyperlipidemia	*Hepatotoxicity; GI bleeding* Flushing, pruritus, hyperuricemia and gout, impaired insulin sensitivity, myopathy	Active liver disease Active peptic ulcer Arterial bleeding	Decreases LDL and triglyceride; increases HDL Flushing occurs during first few weeks of use and can be prevented by pretreatment with aspirin; flushing limits use Hyperuricemia occurs in 20% of patients and may precipitate gout Niacin use is associated with impaired insulin sensitivity

24

Integrative Cardiovascular Pharmacology: Hypertension, Ischemic Heart Disease, and Heart Failure

April W. Armstrong, Ehrin J. Armstrong, and Thomas P. Rocco

INTRODUCTION

In Chapters 18–23, the pharmacology of the cardiovascular system is considered in the context of individual physiologic systems. For example, diuretics are discussed in the context of volume regulation while inhibitors of angiotensin converting enzyme (ACE) are discussed in the context of vascular tone. The clinical presentation of cardiovascular diseases often involves interactions among these individual systems. As a result, pharmacologic management often necessitates the use of agents from several drug classes. This chapter presents three common cardiovascular disease states—hypertension, ischemic heart disease, and heart failure—in the context of a single, longitudinal clinical case. For each disease, an understanding of the disease pathophysiology underscores the rationale for each pharmacologic intervention, and may also highlight the potential for side effects, such as serious drug–drug interactions. This chapter aims to integrate pathophysiology with pharmacology to provide a thorough and mechanistic understanding of the contemporary management of common cardiovascular disease states.

 Case, Part I: Hypertension

Thomas N, a 45-year-old manager at a telecommunications company, presents to the cardiology clinic for evaluation of exertional shortness of breath. Mr. N had always been zealous in maintaining aerobic fitness, but about 6 months before his cardiology clinic visit, he began to note severe breathlessness as he approached the completion of his daily run, which concludes with a long but gentle uphill climb. During the intervening 6 months, the patient reports a progression in his symptoms to the point that, now, he rarely completes the first half of his daily run without resting. He denies chest discomfort at rest or with exercise. His family history is notable for hypertension and premature atherosclerosis. Mr. N has never used tobacco products.

On examination, the patient is hypertensive (blood pressure, 160/102 mm Hg), and a prominent presystolic S4 is heard at the left ventricular apex. The exam is otherwise unremarkable. The chest x-ray is reported as normal. The electrocardiogram (ECG) reveals normal sinus rhythm with voltage criteria for left ventricular hypertrophy. Mr. N is referred for noninvasive cardiac evaluation, including a treadmill exercise test and a transthoracic echocardiogram. He reaches a peak heart rate of 170 beats/min during exercise, and has to terminate the test because of severe dyspnea at a workload of 7 METS. (METS are metabolic equivalents, a measure of energy consumption; a value of 7 METS is below normal for this patient's age.) There is no evidence of myocardial ischemia by ECG criteria. The two-dimensional echocardiogram reveals concentric-pattern left ventricular hypertrophy, an enlarged left atrium, and normal aortic and mitral valves. Left ventricular diastolic filling is abnormal,

with a reduced rate of early rapid filling and a significant increase in the extent of filling during atrial systole.

QUESTIONS

■ **1.** Given the severity of hypertension in this case, Mr. N will likely require at least two drugs to achieve adequate control of his blood pressure. What are the current recommendations for initiation of antihypertensive drug therapy, and what are the therapeutic goals? When is multidrug therapy required?

■ **2.** Thiazide diuretics have been used for many years as first-line therapy in patients with hypertension. Why should diuretics be used with caution in this patient? In what clinical scenarios are thiazides appropriate first-line agents? In what context are alternative agents recommended?

PATHOPHYSIOLOGY OF HYPERTENSION

Hypertension is a widely prevalent disease and a major risk factor for adverse cardiovascular events including stroke, coronary artery disease, peripheral vascular disease, heart failure, and chronic kidney disease. In primary prevention studies, there is a continuous relationship between blood pressure and adverse cardiovascular outcomes including death. This relationship holds even within the level of blood pressure previously defined as ''normal.'' The growing appreciation of the importance of even mild hypertension has contributed to periodic revisions in the clinical approach to this disease, including criteria for the diagnosis of hypertension, stratification of hypertension severity, and indications for treatment. For example, although elevated diastolic blood pressure had been the main indication for initiating antihypertensive treatment, it is now appreciated that elevated systolic blood pressure alone (**isolated systolic hypertension**) is itself sufficient indication for treatment, particularly in elderly patients. The current criteria, which are listed in Table 24-1, are taken from the most recent consensus statement.

One of the main obstacles in the treatment of hypertension is the largely asymptomatic nature of the disease, even with marked elevation in systemic blood pressure. This disconnect between symptoms and long-term adverse consequences has earned hypertension the designation, ''silent killer.'' For example, Mr. N began to exhibit symptoms only after exercising for a prolonged period of time. Nonetheless, the severity of his hypertension puts him at major risk for developing coronary artery disease, stroke, and heart failure. Thus, effective strategies for detection and management of hypertension are critical elements in the primary and secondary prevention of cardiovascular disease.

Fortunately, the number and spectrum of agents available to treat patients with hypertension have expanded dramatically over the past 2 decades. These drugs can be administered initially as single agents (monotherapy). However, the progressive nature of hypertension characteristically leads

TABLE 24-1	Classification of Hypertension for Adults According to the JNC-VII			
	SYSTOLIC BLOOD PRESSURE (mm Hg)		**DIASTOLIC BLOOD PRESSURE (mm Hg)**	
Normal	<120	and	<80	
Prehypertension	120–139	or	80–89	
Hypertension stage 1 (moderate)	140–159	or	90–99	
Hypertension stage 2 (severe)	≥160	or	≥100	

(Seventh Report of the Joint National Committee on Prevention, Detection, Evaluation, and Treatment of High Blood Pressure; 2003.)

to the use of a multidrug regimen. Although the clinical endpoints of therapy can vary somewhat from patient to patient, the principal goal of treatment is to reduce the measured blood pressure, typically to levels in the range of 120 mm Hg systolic and less than 80 mm Hg diastolic.

Hypertension is typically categorized as either primary (essential) or secondary hypertension. **Essential hypertension**, in which the cause of the elevation in blood pressure is unknown, affects 90% to 95% of the hypertensive population. The etiology of essential hypertension is likely multifactorial, including both genetic and environmental factors such as alcohol use, obesity, and salt consumption. A more complete understanding of the pathophysiology of primary hypertension awaits the elucidation of underlying genetic predispositions and/or molecular mechanisms. **Secondary hypertension** refers to patients in whom elevated blood pressure can be attributed to a defined cause. Some examples of secondary hypertension include primary hyperaldosteronism, oral contraceptive use, primary renal disease, and renovascular disease.

The principal determinants of blood pressure are discussed in Chapter 21, Pharmacology of Vascular Tone. Briefly, *blood pressure is determined by the product of heart rate, stroke volume, and systemic vascular resistance* (Fig. 24-1). Heart rate is determined largely by sympathetic activity. Stroke volume depends on loading (preload and afterload) and contractility. Systemic vascular resistance reflects the aggregate vascular tone of the arteriolar subdivisions of the systemic circulation. A rational pharmacologic approach to the treatment of both primary and secondary hypertension requires an understanding of the physiology of normal blood pressure regulation and the mechanisms that could be responsible for hypertension in individual patients.

CARDIAC FUNCTION

One potential mechanism for persistent blood pressure elevation is a primary elevation in cardiac output ("high-output" hypertension). A "hyperkinetic" circulation can result from excessive sympathoadrenal activity and/or increased sensitivity of the heart to basal levels of neurohumoral regulators. The hemodynamic pattern of **pump-based hypertension** (i.e., *increased cardiac output [CO] with normal systemic vascular resistance [SVR]*) is most often seen in younger patients with essential hypertension; this pattern can evolve over time into a hemodynamic profile in which the

principal locus of disease appears to shift to the peripheral vasculature (see below). The underlying mechanism of high-output hypertension makes treatment with β-antagonists attractive in this population.

VASCULAR FUNCTION

Vascular resistance-based hypertension (i.e., *normal CO with increased SVR*) is a common mechanism underlying hypertension in the elderly. In individuals with this form of hypertension, it is hypothesized that the vasculature is abnormally responsive to sympathetic stimulation, circulating factors, or local regulators of vascular tone. This may be mediated in part by endothelial damage or dysfunction, which is known to disrupt the normal equilibrium between local vasodilatory (e.g., nitric oxide) and vasoconstrictive (e.g., endothelin) factors. In addition, ion channel defects in vascular smooth muscle can cause abnormal elevations in basal vasomotor tone resulting in increased systemic vascular resistance. Vascular resistance-based hypertension typically manifests as a predominant elevation of systolic blood pressure. Studies have demonstrated the effectiveness of thiazide diuretics in this population, making them the preferred initial treatment.

RENAL FUNCTION

Abnormalities of renal function can also contribute to the development of systemic hypertension. Excessive Na^+ and H_2O retention by the kidney is responsible for **volume-based hypertension**. *Renal parenchymal disease,* caused by glomerular injury with reduction of functional nephron mass and/or excessive secretion of renin, can lead to an abnormal increase in intravascular volume. Alternatively, ion channel mutations can impair normal Na^+ excretion. *Renovascular disease* (e.g., renal artery stenosis caused by atherosclerotic plaques, fibromuscular dysplasia, emboli, vasculitis, or external compression) can result in decreased renal blood flow. In response to this decrease in perfusion pressure, juxtaglomerular cells increase the secretion of renin, which in turn leads to increased production of angiotensin II and aldosterone. The latter mediators increase both vasomotor tone and Na^+/H_2O retention, leading to a hemodynamic profile in which *both CO and SVR are elevated.*

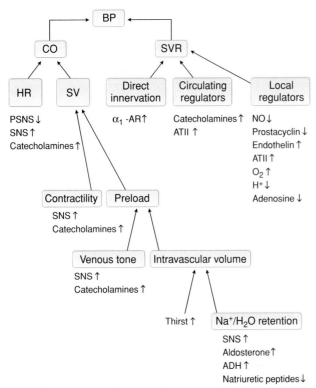

Figure 24-1. Determinants of systemic blood pressure. Blood pressure is the product of cardiac output *(CO)* and systemic vascular resistance *(SVR)*, and CO is the product of heart rate *(HR)* and stroke volume *(SV)*. These determinants are altered by a number of homeostatic mechanisms. Heart rate is increased by the sympathetic nervous system *(SNS)* and catecholamines, and decreased by the parasympathetic nervous system *(PSNS)*. Stroke volume is increased by contractility and preload, and decreased by afterload *(not shown)*; all of these determinants are important parameters for cardiac function. Preload is altered by changes in venous tone and intravascular volume. The SNS and hormones, including aldosterone, antidiuretic hormone *(ADH)*, and natriuretic peptides, are the major factors affecting intravascular volume. Systemic vascular resistance is a function of direct innervation, circulating regulators, and local regulators. Direct innervation comprises α_1-adrenergic receptors (α_1-AR), which increase SVR. Circulating regulators include catecholamines and angiotensin II (AT II), both of which increase SVR. A number of local regulators alter SVR. These include endothelial-derived signaling molecules such as nitric oxide (NO), prostacyclin, endothelin, and AT II; and local metabolic regulators such as O_2, H^+, and adenosine. SVR is the major component of afterload, which is inversely related to stroke volume. The combination of a direct effect of SVR on blood pressure and an inverse effect of afterload on stroke volume illustrates the complexity of the system. ↑ indicates a stimulatory effect; ↓ indicates an inhibitory effect on the boxed variable.

NEUROENDOCRINE FUNCTION

Dysfunction of the neuroendocrine system—including abnormal central regulation of basal sympathetic tone, atypical stress responses, and abnormal responses to signals from baroreceptors and intravascular volume receptors—can alter cardiac, vascular, and/or renal function, leading to increased systemic blood pressure. Examples of endocrine abnormalities associated with systemic hypertension include excessive secretion of catecholamines (pheochromocytoma), exces-

sive secretion of aldosterone by the adrenal cortex (primary aldosteronism), and excessive production of thyroid hormones (hyperthyroidism).

CLINICAL MANAGEMENT OF HYPERTENSION

As discussed above, hypertension presents a complex clinical challenge, as blood pressure elevation may be asymptomatic for many years even as substantial end-organ damage occurs. As a result, the effective treatment of hypertension requires strategies to identify asymptomatic patients, especially those at high risk for the adverse end-organ effects of the disease. Because antihypertensive drugs can add inconvenience to the life of a patient who is asymptomatic, long-term treatment of the hypertensive patient requires the use of drug regimens that are individualized for optimal compliance and efficacy. This requires consideration of safety profile, dosing schedule and cost.

The first line in hypertension treatment is counseling regarding the importance of lifestyle modifications. Lifestyle modifications associated with favorable results in hypertensive patients include weight loss, increased physical activity, smoking cessation, and a low-fat, low-sodium diet. Reduction or elimination of exogenous agents that can induce hypertension—such as ethanol, oral contraceptives, glucocorticoids, and stimulant drugs—can also have demonstrable clinical benefit. While nonpharmacologic therapies alone may not achieve a sufficient reduction in blood pressure, they are critical adjuncts to pharmacologic treatment.

An extensive armamentarium of drugs is used to treat systemic hypertension. Ultimately, however, these agents all exert their effects on blood pressure through a reduction in cardiac output and/or systemic vascular resistance. Strategies currently used to treat hypertension (Table 24-2 and Fig. 24-2) include reduction of intravascular volume with concomitant vasodilation (diuretics); down-regulation of sympathetic tone (β-antagonists, α₁-antagonists, central sympatholytics); modulation of vascular smooth muscle tone (calcium channel blockers, K^+ channel openers); and inhibition of the neurohumoral regulators of the circulation (ACE inhibitors, AT_1 antagonists [angiotensin II receptor antagonists]). The reduction in blood pressure caused by these agents is sensed by baroreceptors and renal juxtaglomerular cells, which can activate counter-regulatory responses that attenuate the magnitude of blood pressure reduction. These compensatory responses can be substantial, necessitating dose adjustments and/or the use of more than one agent to achieve long-term blood pressure control (Fig. 24-3).

REDUCTION OF INTRAVASCULAR VOLUME

Diuretics

Although diuretics have long been a cornerstone of antihypertensive therapy, the mechanism of action of diuretics in hypertension is incompletely understood. As discussed in Chapter 20, Pharmacology of Volume Regulation, diuretics decrease intravascular volume by increasing renal excretion

TABLE 24-2	Major Classes of Antihypertensive Agents		
DIURETICS	**SYMPATHOLYTICS**	**VASODILATORS**	**RENIN–ANGIOTENSIN SYSTEM BLOCKERS**
Thiazide diuretics	CNS sympathetic outflow blockers	Calcium channel blockers	ACE inhibitors
Loop diuretics	Ganglionic blockers	Minoxidil	AT$_1$ antagonists
K$^+$-sparing diuretics	Postganglionic adrenergic nerve terminal antagonists	Hydralazine Sodium nitroprusside	
	α_1-Adrenergic antagonists		
	β_1-Adrenergic antagonists		
	Mixed α-adrenergic/β-adrenergic antagonists		

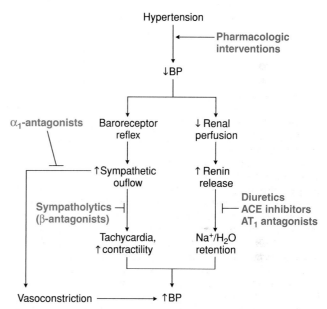

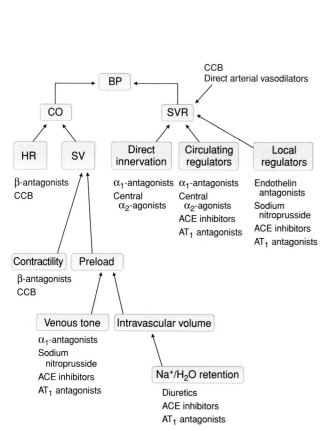

Figure 24-2. Pharmacologic effects of commonly used antihypertensive agents. Antihypertensive agents modulate blood pressure by interfering with the determinants of blood pressure. Many of these antihypertensive drugs have multiple actions. For example, renin–angiotensin system blockers, such as ACE inhibitors and AT$_1$ antagonists, alter the levels of local regulators and circulating regulators, and affect renal Na$^+$ retention and venous tone. BP, blood pressure; CO, cardiac output; SVR, systemic vascular resistance; HR, heart rate; SV, stroke volume; CCB, Ca^{2+} channel blockers; ACE, angiotensin converting enzyme.

Figure 24-3. Compensatory homeostatic responses to antihypertensive treatment. When blood pressure is lowered by pharmacologic interventions, homeostatic responses are activated to increase blood pressure. These homeostatic responses can be divided broadly into baroreceptor reflexes and renal perfusion reflexes. Baroreceptor reflexes originating in the aortic arch and carotid sinus increase sympathetic outflow, leading to tachycardia, increased contractility, and vasoconstriction; these effects all increase blood pressure. Sympatholytics, such as β-antagonists, blunt the tachycardia and contractility responses by interrupting the sympathetic nervous system. α_1-Antagonists inhibit vasoconstriction but have minimal effects on tachycardia or contractility. Decreased renal perfusion causes increased release of renin from juxtaglomerular cells of the kidney. Renin then cleaves angiotensinogen to angiotensin I, which, in turn, is activated to the potent vasoconstrictor angiotensin II *(not shown)*. Angiotensin II increases adrenal secretion of aldosterone, which acts on principal cells of the collecting duct to increase Na$^+$ (and, therefore, water) reabsorption. The increased Na$^+$ reabsorption increases intravascular volume, and thereby results in increased blood pressure. Diuretics interrupt this homeostatic response by decreasing Na$^+$ reabsorption from the nephron; angiotensin converting enzyme *(ACE)* inhibitors interrupt the formation of angiotensin II; and AT$_1$ antagonists prevent the target-organ signaling of angiotensin II.

TABLE 24-3	Diuretics Used in the Treatment of Hypertension

DRUG	DURATION OF ACTION (HOURS)
Thiazide Diuretics	
Chlorothiazide	6–12
Chlorthalidone	48–72
Hydrochlorothiazide	16–24
Indapamide	24
Metolazone	24
Loop Diuretics	
Bumetanide	4–5
Ethacrynic acid	4–5
Furosemide	4–5
Torsemide	6–8
Potassium-Sparing Diuretics	
Amiloride	6–24
Eplerenone	24
Spironolactone	72–96
Triamterene	8–12

of Na^+ and H_2O. However, volume depletion alone is unlikely to explain fully the antihypertensive effect of diuretics.

Thiazide diuretics (e.g., **hydrochlorothiazide**) are the natriuretic drugs most commonly prescribed for the treatment of hypertension (Table 24-3). The pharmacokinetic and pharmacodynamic characteristics of the thiazides make them especially useful agents in the treatment of chronic hypertension. Thiazides have high oral availability and long duration of action. The initial antihypertensive effect seems to be mediated by decreasing intravascular volume. Therefore, *thiazides are particularly effective in patients with volume-based hypertension, such as patients with primary renal disease and African-American patients.* Thiazides induce an initial decrease in intravascular volume that decreases blood pressure by lowering cardiac output. However, the decrease in cardiac output stimulates the renin–angiotensin system, which leads to volume retention and attenuation of the effect of the thiazide on volume status. It is hypothesized that a vasodilatory effect of the thiazides potentiates the compensated volume depletion, leading to a sustained decrease in blood pressure. This hypothesis is supported by the observation that the maximal antihypertensive effect of the thiazides is frequently achieved at doses lower than those needed to achieve a maximal diuretic effect. Therefore, thiazides achieve their blood pressure effect by influencing both cardiac output and systemic vascular resistance.

The Joint National Commission ''Stepped-Care'' algorithm suggests thiazide diuretics as the first-line agents of choice for the majority of patients, unless there is a specific indication for another antihypertensive drug (such as an ACE inhibitor in a patient with diabetes). This recommendation arises from the results of a large-scale trial, which found favorable outcomes and decreased cost associated with thiazide therapy.

Loop diuretics (e.g., **furosemide**) are infrequently prescribed for the treatment of mild or moderate hypertension. These agents typically have a relatively short duration of action (4–6 hr) and, despite the brisk diuresis that follows their administration, their antihypertensive efficacy is often modest. It is thought that this modest impact on blood pressure is due to the activation of compensatory responses involving the neurohumoral regulators of intravascular volume and systemic vascular resistance. *There are, however, several well-recognized clinical situations in which loop diuretics are preferable to thiazides, including malignant hypertension* (see below) *and volume-based hypertension in patients with advanced chronic kidney disease.*

K^+-sparing diuretics (e.g., **spironolactone, triamterene, amiloride**) are less efficacious than thiazide and loop diuretics, and are used primarily in combination with other diuretics to attenuate or correct drug-induced kaliuresis (K^+ excretion) and the resultant hypokalemia. *Spironolactone is an aldosterone receptor antagonist that is especially effective in the treatment of secondary hypertension caused by hyperaldosteronism.* Hypokalemia is a common metabolic side effect of the thiazide and loop diuretics, which inhibit Na^+ reabsorption in more proximal segments of the nephron and thereby increase delivery of Na^+ and water to distal segments of the nephron. Increased distal Na^+ delivery results in a compensatory increase in Na^+ reabsorption in the distal tubule, which is coupled to an increase in K^+ excretion. Because the latter effect is mediated by aldosterone (see Chapter 20), the K^+-sparing diuretics attenuate this effect and thereby help to maintain normal serum potassium levels. It should be emphasized that both ACE inhibitors (which decrease aldosterone activity and K^+ excretion) and K^+ supplements should be decreased or eliminated in patients taking K^+-sparing diuretics, because life-threatening hyperkalemia has been reported in association with clinical use of the K^+-sparing agents.

DOWN-REGULATION OF SYMPATHETIC TONE

Drugs that modulate adrenergic activity are discussed in detail in Chapter 9, Adrenergic Pharmacology; refer to that chapter for detailed descriptions of the tissue distribution of α and β receptors and the cardiovascular effects mediated by these receptors. *Sympatholytic drugs treat hypertension via two major mechanisms: reduction of systemic vascular resistance and/or reduction of cardiac output.* Clinically, these agents are broadly divided into β-adrenoceptor antagonists, α-adrenoceptor antagonists, and central sympatholytics.

β-Adrenoceptor Antagonists

β-Adrenoceptor antagonists (e.g., **propranolol, metoprolol, atenolol**) are commonly prescribed first-line agents in the treatment of hypertension. The negative chronotropic and inotropic effects of these agents (and the reductions in heart rate, stroke volume, and cardiac output that follow) account for the initial antihypertensive effect of the β-antagonists. Decreased vasomotor tone, with a consequent decrease in systemic vascular resistance, has also been reported with longer-term therapy.

The β-antagonist–induced reduction in vasomotor tone may seem paradoxical, given that β_2-adrenergic receptors in the peripheral vasculature mediate vasodilation. However, antagonism of β_1-adrenergic receptors in the kidney decreases secretion of renin and thereby decreases production of the potent vasoconstrictor, angiotensin II. The latter effect likely predominates, even when nonselective β-receptor antagonists are administered. Although β-antagonists effectively reduce blood pressure in hypertensive patients, these agents typically do not cause hypotension in individuals with normal blood pressure. Increased baseline sympathetic activity in hypertensive patients may in part explain the efficacy of β-antagonists in lowering blood pressure in these individuals. In contrast, basal activation of β-receptors in normal individuals may be sufficiently low that receptor antagonists have little hemodynamic effect. β-Antagonist therapy has been associated with both elevation of serum triglyceride levels and reduction of high-density lipoprotein (HDL) levels; the clinical significance of these potentially harmful metabolic effects remains unclear. Noncardiac side effects of β-antagonist therapy may include exacerbation of glucose intolerance (hyperglycemia), sedation, impotence, depression, and bronchoconstriction.

Mixed α–β antagonists (e.g., **labetalol**) are available in both oral and parenteral formulations. Intravenous administration of labetalol causes a substantial reduction in blood pressure, and has found wide use in the treatment of hypertensive emergencies. Oral labetalol is also used in the long-term treatment of hypertension. One potential advantage of this drug is that the decrease in blood pressure achieved by reduction of systemic vascular resistance (via antagonism of α_1-receptors) is not associated with the reflex increase in heart rate or cardiac output (because cardiac β_1-receptors are also antagonized) that can occur when pure vasodilator drugs are used as monotherapy.

α-Adrenoceptor Antagonists

α_1-Adrenergic antagonists (e.g., **prazosin, terazosin, doxazosin**) are also used in the treatment of high blood pressure. α_1-Adrenergic antagonists inhibit peripheral vasomotor tone, reducing vasoconstriction and decreasing systemic vascular resistance. The absence of adverse effects on the serum lipid profile during long-term treatment with α_1-adrenergic antagonists is often cited as a distinctive advantage of these agents relative to other antihypertensive medications. However, the long-term benefit of this advantage, if any, remains to be determined in randomized clinical trials. Furthermore, in a large trial comparing different antihypertensives, there was an increased incidence of heart failure in the group randomized to doxazosin.

Nonselective α-adrenergic antagonists (e.g., **phenoxybenzamine, phentolamine**) are not employed in the long-term treatment of hypertension, because excessive compensatory responses can result from their long-term use. For example, antagonism of central α_2-adrenergic receptors disinhibits sympathetic outflow, resulting in unopposed reflex tachycardia. However, *these agents are indicated for the treatment of pheochromocytoma.*

Central Sympatholytics

The α_2-adrenergic agonists **methyldopa, clonidine,** and **guanabenz** reduce sympathetic outflow from the medulla, leading to decreases in heart rate, contractility, and vasomotor tone. These drugs are available in oral formulations (clonidine is also available as a transdermal patch), and were widely used in the past despite their unfavorable adverse-

effect profile. The availability of multiple alternative agents, as well as the current trend towards the use of multidrug regimens at submaximal doses, have substantially diminished the clinical role of α_2-agonists in the treatment of hypertension.

Ganglionic blockers (e.g., **trimethaphan, hexamethonium**) inhibit nicotinic cholinergic activity at sympathetic ganglia. These agents are extremely effective at lowering blood pressure. However, the severe adverse effects of parasympathetic and sympathetic blockade (e.g., constipation, blurred vision, sexual dysfunction, and orthostatic hypotension) have made ganglionic blockers of historic interest only.

Some sympatholytic agents (e.g., **reserpine, guanethidine**) are taken up into the terminals of postganglionic adrenergic neurons, where they induce long-term depletion of neurotransmitter from norepinephrine-containing synaptic vesicles (see Chapter 9). These agents lower blood pressure by decreasing the activity of the sympathetic nervous system. However, reserpine and guanethidine have little role in the contemporary treatment of hypertension because of their significant adverse-effect profiles, which include severe depression (reserpine) and orthostatic hypotension and sexual dysfunction (guanethidine).

MODULATION OF VASCULAR SMOOTH MUSCLE TONE

As discussed in Chapter 21, vascular tone is dependent on the degree of vascular smooth muscle contraction. Vasodilators reduce systemic vascular resistance by acting on arteriolar smooth muscle and/or the vascular endothelium. The major mechanisms of action of the arterial vasodilators include blockade of Ca^{2+} channels and opening of metabotropic K^+ channels.

Ca^{2+} Channel Blockers

Ca^{2+} channel blockers (e.g., **verapamil, diltiazem, nifedipine, amlodipine**) are oral agents that are widely used in the long-term treatment of hypertension. Calcium channel blockers (CCBs) have a variety of hemodynamic effects, reflecting the multiple sites at which calcium is involved in the electrical and mechanical events of the cardiac cycle and in vascular regulation. These agents can act as arterial vasodilators, negative inotropes, and/or negative chronotropes. The dihydropyridine agents nifedipine and amlodipine act primarily as vasodilators. In contrast, the nondihydropyridine drugs verapamil and diltiazem act principally as negative inotropes and chronotropes, thereby decreasing myocardial contractility, heart rate, and impulse conduction. Thus, *CCBs can lower blood pressure through reduction of both systemic vascular resistance and cardiac output.* CCBs are often used in combination with other cardioactive drugs, either as components of a multidrug antihypertensive regimen or for combined antihypertensive and antianginal treatment in patients with ischemic heart disease (IHD).

Given the distinctive pharmacodynamic effects of the different CCBs, the potential adverse effects of CCB therapy (including adverse interactions with other cardiovascular therapies) are agent-specific. The nondihydropyridine agents should be used with caution in patients who have impaired

LV systolic function, as these agents can exacerbate systolic heart failure (see below). These agents should also be used with caution in patients with conduction system disease, as these drugs can potentiate functional abnormalities of the sinoatrial (SA) and atrioventricular (AV) nodes. Both of these cautions are particularly relevant in patients receiving concomitant β-antagonist therapy.

K+ Channel Openers

Minoxidil and **hydralazine** are orally available arterial vasodilators that are used in the long-term treatment of hypertension. Minoxidil is a metabotropic K+ channel opener that hyperpolarizes vascular smooth muscle cells and thereby attenuates the cellular response to depolarizing stimuli. Hydralazine is a less powerful vasodilator with an uncertain mechanism of action. Both minoxidil and hydralazine can cause compensatory retention of Na+ and H_2O as well as reflex tachycardia; these adverse effects are more frequent and more severe with minoxidil than with hydralazine. Concomitant use of a β-antagonist and a diuretic can mitigate these compensatory adverse effects. The use of hydralazine is limited by the frequent occurrence of tolerance and tachyphylaxis to the drug. In addition, increases in the total daily dose of hydralazine can be associated with a drug-induced lupus syndrome. Given the more favorable safety profile of the Ca^{2+} channel blockers, the use of minoxidil is now largely restricted to patients with severe hypertension that is refractory to other pharmacologic therapies. Of note, hydralazine (in combination with isosorbide dinitrate) has now emerged as an adjunctive therapy (i.e., in patients who are already receiving an ACE inhibitor and a β-antagonist) in the treatment of systolic heart failure in African-American patients.

MODULATION OF THE RENIN-ANGIOTENSIN–ALDOSTERONE SYSTEM

Renin–angiotensin-aldosterone system blockers include the ACE inhibitors (e.g., **captopril, enalapril, lisinopril**) and the angiotensin receptor (AT_1) antagonists (e.g., **losartan, valsartan**). These agents are being increasingly used in the treatment of hypertension.

Angiotensin Converting Enzyme Inhibitors

ACE inhibitors prevent the ACE-mediated conversion of angiotensin I to angiotensin II, leading to decreased circulating levels of angiotensin II and aldosterone. By decreasing angiotensin II levels, ACE inhibitors decrease systemic vascular resistance and thereby decrease the impedance to LV ejection. By decreasing aldosterone levels, these agents promote natriuresis and thereby reduce intravascular volume. ACE inhibitors also decrease bradykinin degradation, and the resulting increase in circulating bradykinin causes vasodilation. *ACE inhibitors are effective in patients with hyperreninemic hypertension, but these agents also reduce blood pressure in patients with low-to-normal circulating renin levels.* The antihypertensive effectiveness of ACE inhibitors in patients with low-to-normal plasma renin activity may be due to potentiation of the vasodilatory effects of bradykinin, although this hypothesis is unproven.

Therapy with ACE inhibitors is as effective as therapy with thiazide diuretics or β-antagonists in the treatment of hypertension. ACE inhibitors are attractive antihypertensive agents because these drugs seem to have unique benefits (e.g., a decrease in the loss of renal function in patients with chronic kidney disease) and relatively few adverse effects (ACE inhibitors do not increase the risk of hypokalemia or cause elevated serum glucose or lipid levels). Despite these attractive features, it merits emphasis that, in at least one large comparison trial, thiazide diuretics were more cardioprotective than ACE inhibitors.

ACE inhibitors should be administered with caution in patients with intravascular volume depletion. Such patients may have reduced renal perfusion at baseline, leading to a compensatory increase in renin and angiotensin II; this increase in angiotensin II is one of the physiologic mechanisms by which glomerular filtration rate (GFR) is maintained in the face of relative renal hypoperfusion. Administration of ACE inhibitors to such patients can disrupt this autoregulatory mechanism, leading to renal insufficiency. The same autoregulatory mechanism is the basis for the contraindication to ACE inhibitors in patients with bilateral renal artery stenosis (or unilateral stenosis in patients with a single kidney). Despite these cautionary notes, it should be emphasized that *ACE inhibitors are considered the preferred therapy in the hypertensive diabetic patient,* as these agents have been shown to delay the onset and progression of diabetic glomerular disease through favorable effects on intraglomerular pressure.

AT₁ Antagonists (Angiotensin Receptor Blockers)

Angiotensin II receptor (AT_1) antagonists (also known as **angiotensin receptor blockers** or **ARBs**) are oral antihypertensive agents that competitively antagonize the binding of angiotensin II to its cognate AT_1 receptors. In addition to their antihypertensive effect, these agents may also reduce reactive arteriolar intimal proliferation. Like ACE inhibitors, AT_1 antagonists are effective in lowering blood pressure, and are sometimes substituted for ACE inhibitors in patients with ACE inhibitor-induced cough. Cough, a common side effect of ACE inhibitor therapy, results from drug-induced increases in bradykinin levels; this side effect often leads to noncompliance or discontinuation of the drug. Because AT_1 antagonists do not affect the activity of the converting enzyme responsible for bradykinin degradation, cough is not a side effect of therapy with the ARBs.

MONOTHERAPY AND STEPPED CARE

Monotherapy (treatment with a single drug) is often sufficient to normalize blood pressure in patients with mild hypertension; this approach may improve patient compliance and avoid the risk of potential drug interactions. Controversy exists as to which antihypertensive agents are preferred as initial therapy. Thiazide diuretics, ACE inhibitors, AT_1 antagonists, β-antagonists, and calcium channel blockers (CCBs) have been shown to be similar in terms of efficacy in lowering blood pressure (each effectively lowers blood pressure in 30% to 50% of patients). Ultimately, the ideal agent is that which reduces a patient's blood pressure to the optimal range with the fewest adverse effects. Drug toxicities are often related to drug dose, and therefore the clinician must carefully consider the use of "synergistic" agents at lower doses, especially if blood pressure control is marginal or inadequate. A good example of the use of synergistic agents is the combination of a thiazide diuretic and an ACE inhibitor. By inducing a mild degree of volume depletion, thiazide diuretics activate the renin–angiotensin system. If this response is blocked by an ACE inhibitor, then the antihypertensive effect of the thiazide is potentiated. Furthermore, inhibition of the renin–angiotensin system by itself promotes natriuresis. Finally, the combination of a thiazide and an ACE inhibitor decreases systemic vascular resistance.

Certain clinical circumstances, however, favor initiating a specific class of antihypertensive medication (Table 24-4). β-Antagonists are the agents of choice in patients with a history of myocardial infarction (MI). ACE inhibitors are recommended in patients with left ventricular dysfunction, diabetes, and/or chronic kidney disease. Hypertension associated with volume retention in nephrotic syndrome responds well to diuretics. ACE inhibitors are also used in nephrotic syndrome to attenuate the degree of proteinuria.

Stepped care in the treatment of hypertension refers to the progressive, step-by-step addition of drugs to a therapeutic regimen. Combination therapy is based on the use of agents with distinct mechanisms of action; it also emphasizes the use of submaximal doses of drugs in an attempt to minimize potential adverse effects and toxicities. Although early iterations of the stepped-care approach were somewhat rigid, more recent algorithms provide far greater latitude in selecting the order of addition of the various drug classes. Current treatment algorithms recognize that any given drug will likely have effects on more than one of the interrelated systems that regulate circulatory function. For example, the initial decrease in mean arterial pressure induced by short-acting arterial vasodilators, such as hydralazine or nifedipine, activates compensatory mechanisms that can result in significant tachycardia and Na^+ and H_2O retention. The addition of a sympatholytic drug (e.g., metoprolol) and/or a diuretic (e.g., hydrochlorothiazide) can mitigate these compensatory responses. Furthermore, pharmaceutical advances have allowed for novel drug formulations that can alter the kinetics of drug metabolism and elimination. For example, the problem of compensatory tachycardia in response to short-acting CCBs of the dihydropyridine class has, to a great extent, been circumvented by the development of sustained-release formulations and of alternative drugs with more favorable pharmacokinetic profiles (see Chapter 21).

POSSIBLE DEMOGRAPHIC FACTORS

Certain classes of antihypertensive drugs have been reported to be more effective than others in special populations. Some data also suggest that distinct etiologies of hypertension may be more or less prevalent in different populations.

Elderly patients tend to respond more favorably to diuretics and dihydropyridine Ca^{2+} channel blockers than to other antihypertensive agents. β-Antagonists are more likely to cause SA or AV node dysfunction or to impair myocardial function in elderly patients; these effects are likely related to the greater prevalence of conduction system disease and LV systolic dysfunction in such patients. Elderly patients also tend to have decreased circulating levels of renin and have been reported to be less responsive to ACE inhibitors.

It has been reported that hypertension in patients of African descent is more responsive to diuretics and Ca^{2+} channel blockers than to β-antagonists and ACE inhibitors. (A nota-

TABLE 24-4	Relative Indications and Contraindications for Antihypertensive Agents	
DRUG CLASS	**INDICATIONS**	**CONTRAINDICATIONS**
Diuretics	Heart failure Systolic hypertension	Gout
β-Antagonists	Coronary artery disease Heart failure Migraine Tachyarrhythmias	Asthma Heart block
α-Antagonists	Prostatic hypertrophy	Heart failure
Calcium channel blockers	Systolic hypertension	Heart block
ACE inhibitors	Diabetic or other nephropathy Heart failure Previous myocardial infarction	Bilateral renal artery stenosis Hyperkalemia Pregnancy
AT$_1$ antagonists	ACE inhibitor-associated cough Diabetic or other nephropathy Heart failure	Bilateral renal artery stenosis Hyperkalemia Pregnancy

ble exception is the favorable response of young African-Americans to β-antagonist therapy.) Reports indicate that some African-Americans may have lower circulating renin levels, and this could account for the observation that ACE inhibitors are less effective in these patients. Recent reports have demonstrated that the prevalence of Na^+-sensitivity is substantially increased in some African-Americans, including both the hypertensive and the normotensive cohort. Although less well studied, there is some evidence of differential responsiveness to the various classes of antihypertensive agents in hypertensive Asian and Hispanic cohorts.

Despite these demographic observations, the clinical benefit of drug selection on the basis of differential responsiveness to specific drug classes has not been evaluated systematically. For example, although elderly patients are reportedly less responsive to β-antagonists, the results of the Systolic Hypertension in the Elderly Project (SHEP Trial) indicate that β-antagonists and diuretics are, in fact, associated with mortality reduction, and this favorable treatment effect is demonstrated within several years of treatment initiation. Similarly, although reports have suggested that African-Americans are less responsive to β-antagonists and ACE inhibitors, it would be difficult to apply these observations to the treatment of a hypertensive, diabetic African-American with chronic kidney disease, or to advocate for the use of a thiazide diuretic in a hypertensive African-American with a history of previous MI. Finally, it should again be emphasized that the risk of adverse events related to hypertension cannot be explained by the degree of blood pressure elevation alone. Conversely, the full spectrum of treatment benefits cannot be explained by the degree of blood pressure reduction alone. For these reasons, the empirical observation that some antihypertensive agents do not lower blood pressure as effectively in some patients does not necessarily mean that these drugs will be less effective in preventing future cardiovascular disease morbidity and mortality in these patients. Clearly, more research is needed.

HYPERTENSIVE CRISIS

The term **hypertensive crisis** refers to clinical syndromes characterized by severe (typically acute) elevations in blood pressure. This abrupt increase in blood pressure can cause acute vascular injury and derivative end-organ damage. Although most cases of severe hypertension were, at one time, designated as ''hypertensive crisis'' or ''malignant hypertension,'' current practice attempts to distinguish those patients in whom the blood pressure elevation and vascular injury are acute (**hypertensive emergency**) from the patient cohort in which the temporal course of blood pressure elevation is more gradual and the end-organ damage is chronic and slowly progressive.

A true hypertensive emergency is a life-threatening condition in which severe and acute blood pressure elevation is associated with acute vascular injury. The vascular injury can manifest clinically as retinal hemorrhages, papilledema, encephalopathy, and acute (or acute superimposed on chronic) renal insufficiency; this syndrome is often associated with acute left ventricular failure. The pathogenesis of malignant hypertension remains unclear. However, it is likely that **fibrinoid arteriolar necrosis** contributes to the

signs and symptoms of this syndrome. Fibrinoid arteriolar necrosis of specific vascular beds can result in acute vascular injury and end-organ hypoperfusion (e.g., renal failure, stroke). Fibrinoid arteriolar necrosis can also lead to microangiopathic hemolytic anemia.

The treatment of patients with hypertensive emergency necessitates rapid reduction of blood pressure to prevent end-organ damage. Drug classes used to treat this condition include parenteral vasodilators (e.g., nitroprusside), diuretics (e.g., furosemide), and/or β-antagonists (e.g., labetalol). Because of the acuteness of the syndrome and the need to titrate these powerful antihypertensive agents carefully, patients are hospitalized for treatment. After the acute episode has been controlled, subsequent lowering of the blood pressure to the normal range of the patient is then attempted more cautiously over a longer period of time (12 to 24 hours), in an effort to decrease the risk of critical-organ hypoperfusion and extension of the vascular injury.

Although malignant hypertension is a life-threatening medical emergency, it is an uncommon expression of hypertensive disease that occurs in far less than 1% of hypertensive patients. More common are cases of **hypertensive urgency,** in which the blood pressure elevation is less acute and the target organ disease has been present for some time. Conditions illustrative of hypertensive urgency include a stroke or MI that is accompanied by severe blood pressure elevation, or acute left heart failure with severe hypertension.

Case, Part II: Ischemic Heart Disease

Mr. N is treated for hypertension with a β-antagonist and an ACE inhibitor. He returns for follow-up visits at 1 month and 6 months and reports that he is doing well. He faithfully adheres to his prescribed medical regimen and notes a definite improvement in exercise capacity. His regular blood pressure measurements now show readings of 130 to 150/86 to 90 mm Hg. A serum lipid profile is notable for increased total cholesterol, with a moderately elevated LDL. Low-dose aspirin is added to his regimen. Treatment with a lipid-lowering agent is also advised, but Mr. N declines, instead requesting that his lipid profile be rechecked after a period of diet and lifestyle modifications.

An exercise tolerance test 1 year after his initial visit is notable for improved exercise capacity (10 MET workload), with blunting of the heart rate and blood pressure at peak exercise (120/min and 190/90 mm Hg, respectively); there is no evidence of myocardial ischemia by ECG criteria. A repeat LDL-cholesterol determination is within the normal range. His medications (aspirin, β-antagonist, and ACE inhibitor) are continued and routine follow-up is established.

One week later, Mr. N experiences the abrupt onset of severe retrosternal chest pressure. He is visibly diaphoretic and dyspneic. He calls 911 and is transported to the local emergency department, where an ECG shows sinus tachycardia and ST segment elevation in the inferior leads. Emergency cardiac catheterization is performed, confirming total occlusion of a dominant right coronary artery, and percutaneous transluminal coronary angioplasty (PTCA) with stent placement is performed. The procedure is successful, and he remains free of chest pain and is hemodynamically stable. ECG and serum enzyme changes (peak creatine kinase [CK], 2400 IU/L [normal, 60 to 400 IU/L]; cardiac isoform [MB] fraction, positive) are consistent with an evolving MI. A repeat echocardiogram immediately before Mr. N's discharge from the hospital demonstrates concentric left ventricular hypertrophy with a left ventricular ejection fraction of 35% (normal, >55%); the inferior wall from the base to the apex is akinetic, with thinning of the myocardium in this akinetic region.

QUESTIONS

■ **1.** What type of lipid-lowering agent is appropriate for this patient?

■ **2.** What pharmacologic interventions are appropriate during the interval between the patient's emergency department evaluation and his cardiac catheterization?

■ **3.** What are the critical drug components of a postmyocardial infarction treatment regimen in the setting of left ventricular dysfunction?

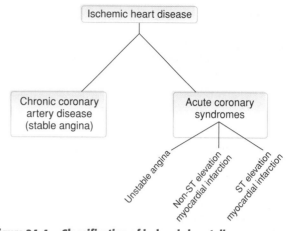

Figure 24-4. Classification of ischemic heart disease. Ischemic heart disease is divided into two broad categories: chronic coronary artery disease and acute coronary syndromes. Stable angina is the prototypical manifestation of chronic coronary artery disease. Acute coronary syndromes constitute a series (not necessarily a linear progression) of clinical presentations, including unstable angina, non-ST elevation myocardial infarction, and ST elevation myocardial infarction.

PATHOPHYSIOLOGY OF ISCHEMIC HEART DISEASE

Ischemic heart disease (IHD), the leading cause of mortality in the United States, accounts for more than 500,000 deaths each year. Since the advent of cardiac intensive care units in the early 1960's, an improved understanding of the biology of IHD has resulted in a spectrum of diagnostic and therapeutic advances. These advances, coupled with increased public awareness, healthier lifestyles, and sustained efforts to improve both primary and secondary prevention strategies, have resulted in significant mortality reduction for patients with IHD.

With respect to pharmacotherapy, IHD can be considered in two broad categories: **chronic coronary artery disease** (CAD) and **acute coronary syndromes** (ACS). Each of these clinical presentations of IHD has a distinct pathogenesis and, as a result, the pharmacologic strategies employed to treat these distinct clinical entities differ in emphasis. The therapeutic goal in patients with chronic CAD is to *maintain the balance between myocardial oxygen supply and demand*; in patients with ACS, the goal is to *restore and/or maintain patency of the coronary vascular lumen* (Fig. 24-4).

CHRONIC CORONARY ARTERY DISEASE

Chronic CAD is characterized by impaired coronary vasodilator reserve. Under conditions of hyperemic stress (i.e., stress requiring increased blood flow), this can result in an imbalance between myocardial oxygen supply and demand, leading to functional cardiac abnormalities (poor contraction of the ischemic portion of the myocardium) as well as clinical symptoms of CAD. The basic physiology of myocardial oxygen supply and demand is discussed in Chapter 21. Imbalances in myocardial oxygen supply and demand occur

mainly as a result of coronary flow reduction and endothelial dysfunction.

Coronary Flow Reduction

The coronary vasculature is composed of two types of vessels: large, proximal epicardial vessels, and small, distal endocardial vessels. The epicardial vessels are the more frequent site of atheroma formation; in disease states, total coronary artery blood flow is limited by the extent of epicardial vessel stenosis. In comparison, endocardial vessels regulate intrinsic coronary vascular resistance in response to local metabolic changes. When myocardial oxygen demand is increased, endocardial vessels dilate in response to local metabolic factors, resulting in a regional increase in myocardial blood flow and thereby providing increased oxygen to these metabolically active tissues.

Angina pectoris (Fig. 24-5) is the principal clinical manifestation of chronic CAD. This symptom is characterized by precordial pressure-like discomfort resulting from myocardial ischemia. Most patients with chronic CAD experience **stable angina**, a clinical syndrome in which *ischemic chest pain occurs at characteristic and reproducible workloads* (e.g., walking up a flight of stairs). Pathologically, chronic CAD is associated with subintimal deposition of atheroma in the epicardial coronary arteries. In general, atherosclerotic plaques in patients with chronic stable angina are characterized by an overlying fibrous cap that is thick and resistant to disruption.

The immediate cause of angina pectoris is *an imbalance between myocardial oxygen supply and demand*. Under normal physiologic conditions, coronary blood flow is modulated carefully to ensure adequate tissue perfusion in response to varying levels of myocardial oxygen demand. This ability to modulate blood flow is referred to as the **coronary flow reserve**:

$$\text{CFR} = \text{maximal CBF/resting CBF}$$

Ⓐ Normal

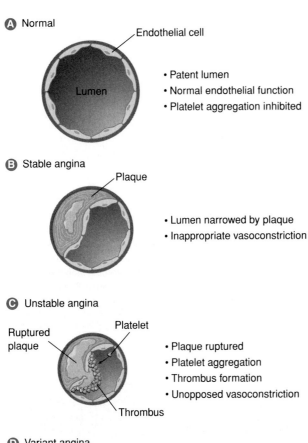

Endothelial cell

Lumen

- Patent lumen
- Normal endothelial function
- Platelet aggregation inhibited

Ⓑ Stable angina

Plaque

- Lumen narrowed by plaque
- Inappropriate vasoconstriction

Ⓒ Unstable angina

Ruptured plaque

Platelet

- Plaque ruptured
- Platelet aggregation
- Thrombus formation
- Unopposed vasoconstriction

Thrombus

Ⓓ Variant angina

- No overt plaques
- Intense vasospasm

Figure 24-5. Pathophysiology of anginal syndromes. A. Normal coronary arteries are widely patent, the endothelium functions normally, and platelet aggregation is inhibited. **B.** In stable angina, atherosclerotic plaque and inappropriate vasoconstriction (caused by endothelial damage) reduce the vessel-lumen diameter, and hence decrease coronary blood flow. **C.** In unstable angina, rupture of the plaque triggers platelet aggregation, thrombus formation, and vasoconstriction. Depending on the anatomic site of plaque rupture, this process can progress to non-Q wave (non-ST elevation) or Q wave (ST elevation) myocardial infarction. **D.** In variant angina, atherosclerotic plaques are absent, and ischemia is caused by intense vasospasm.

where CFR is coronary flow reserve, and CBF is coronary blood flow. In healthy individuals, the maximal CBF is approximately five-fold greater than the resting CBF. The overall decrease in CFR is directly related to the severity of epicardial artery stenosis. Because of this wide safety margin, the resting CBF does not decrease until an epicardial stenosis exceeds 80% of the original arterial diameter. Changes in maximal CBF can be observed more readily with exercise, as maximal CBF begins to decrease during exercise when an epicardial stenosis exceeds 50% of the original arterial diameter. In patients with chronic epicardial CAD, the coronary vasodilator reserve may be further impaired as a

consequence of endothelial dysfunction (discussed below), resulting in a further reduction in CBF. During periods in which myocardial oxygen demand exceeds CFR, demand-related ischemia occurs and the patient experiences angina pectoris.

The degree of epicardial artery stenosis and the degree of compensatory endocardial artery dilation determine the hemodynamic consequence of an atherosclerotic plaque (Fig. 24-6). If the endocardial arteries are normal, an epicardial stenosis that narrows the diameter of the arterial lumen by less than 50% does not significantly reduce maximal coronary blood flow. However, if the stenosis narrows the arterial lumen diameter by more than 80%, then the endocardial vessels must dilate to provide adequate perfusion to the myocardium, even at rest. It follows that the need for endocardial vessels to dilate at rest attenuates coronary flow reserve, in that the endocardial vessels cannot then dilate further during exercise. This reduction in coronary flow reserve leads to inadequate myocardial blood flow during hyperemic stress. Myocardial ischemia can occur at rest when the epicardial artery stenosis exceeds 90% of the lumen diameter: under these conditions, endocardial vessels cannot maintain adequate myocardial perfusion even at maximal dilation.

Endothelial Dysfunction

Endothelial dysfunction is a general term for pathologic endothelial cell regulation. Clinically, endothelial dysfunction

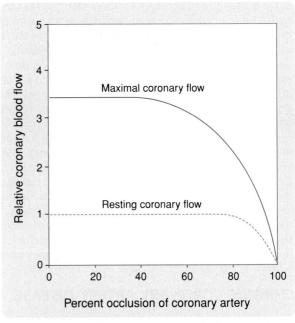

Figure 24-6. Effect of coronary artery occlusion on resting and maximal coronary blood flow. The *dotted line* depicts resting coronary blood flow, and the *solid line* represents maximal blood flow when there is full dilation of distal coronary arteries. Comparison of these two lines shows that maximal coronary blood flow is compromised when the lesion occludes more than about 50% of the arterial lumen, whereas resting coronary blood flow is relatively unaffected until the lesion exceeds about 80% of the arterial diameter. The y-axis represents coronary artery blood flow relative to the flow in a resting coronary artery with 0% occlusion.

is manifested by abnormal vascular tone and prothrombotic properties.

Abnormal vascular tone is a result of dysregulated endothelial control of smooth muscle contraction: arterial beds with endothelial dysfunction cannot dilate in response to hyperemic stimuli. For example, when mental stress or physical exertion trigger activation of the sympathetic nervous system (SNS), two opposing forces act on the coronary vascular endothelium: catecholamine-mediated vasoconstriction and nitric oxide (NO)-mediated vasodilation. Normally, endothelial release of NO is stimulated by the shear stress on the coronary vascular endothelium that results from increased blood flow. Eventually, the vasodilator effects of NO predominate over the vasoconstrictor effects of SNS activation, and the overall effect is coronary vasodilation. However, when the vascular endothelium is damaged, the production of endothelial vasodilators is decreased and catecholamine-mediated vasoconstriction predominates.

Because the endothelium also plays a crucial role in regulating platelet activation and the coagulation cascade, endothelial dysfunction can promote blood coagulation (throm-

bosis) at the site of endothelial injury. Endothelial-derived NO and prostacyclin exert significant antiplatelet effects, and molecules on the surface of healthy endothelial cells have significant anticoagulant properties (see Chapter 22, Pharmacology of Hemostasis and Thrombosis). Endothelial damage decreases these endogenous antiplatelet and anticoagulant mechanisms, leading to a local predominance of procoagulant factors and increasing the likelihood of platelet and coagulation cascade activation.

ACUTE CORONARY SYNDROMES

Acute coronary syndromes (ACS) are most often caused by the fissuring or rupture of atherosclerotic plaques. These so-called **unstable** or **vulnerable plaques** are characterized by thin fibrous caps that are prone to rupture. Plaque rupture results in the exposure of procoagulant factors, such as subendothelial collagen (Fig. 24-7), that activate platelets and the coagulation cascade. Under physiologic circumstances, hemostasis at a site of vascular injury is self-limited by endogenous anticoagulant mechanisms (see Chapter 22). How-

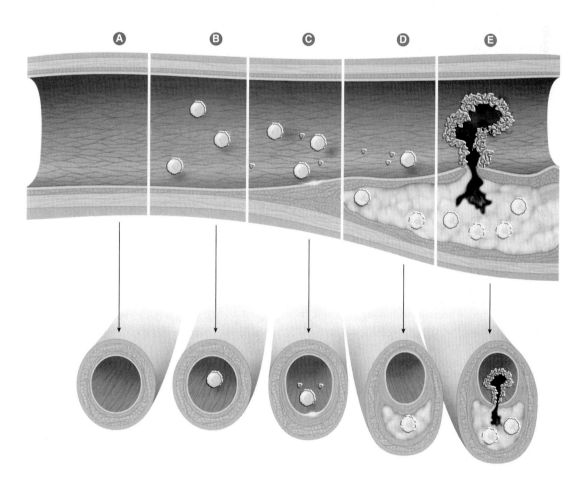

Figure 24-7. Pathogenesis of acute coronary syndromes. A. A normal coronary artery has an intact endothelium surrounded by smooth muscle cells. **B.** Endothelial cell activation or injury recruits monocytes and T lymphocytes to the site of injury, leading to development of a fatty streak. **C.** Continued oxidative stress within a fatty streak leads to development of an atherosclerotic plaque. **D.** Macrophage apoptosis and continued cholesterol deposition cause further plaque organization, and may induce the expression of additional inflammatory proteins and matrix metalloproteinases. At this stage, the cap of the fibroatheroma remains intact. **E.** Continued inflammation within an atherosclerotic plaque leads to thinning of the fibrous cap and, eventually, to plaque erosion or rupture. Exposure of plaque constituents to the bloodstream activates platelets and the coagulation cascade, with resulting coronary artery occlusion.

ever, the dysfunctional endothelium overlying the atherosclerotic plaque cannot elaborate sufficient anticoagulant factors to control the extent of clot formation. Dysregulated coagulation can then result in intraluminal thrombus formation, which leads to myocardial ischemia and potentially to irreversible myocardial damage.

The three subtypes of acute coronary syndromes are unstable angina, non-ST elevation MI, and ST elevation MI. In **unstable angina**, patients experience either acceleration in the frequency or severity of chest pain, new-onset anginal pain, or characteristic anginal chest pain that abruptly occurs at rest. Enzymatic evidence of tissue infarction (e.g., elevated troponin levels) is absent in unstable angina, but patients are at high risk for MI because of the presence of an active prothrombotic surface at the site of plaque rupture.

Non-ST elevation myocardial infarction occurs when an unstable plaque abruptly ruptures and significantly compromises (but does not completely occlude) the lumen of an epicardial coronary artery. Because the artery is partially occluded and there is a persistent prothrombotic surface at the site of plaque rupture, patients with non-ST elevation MI are at high risk for recurrence of ischemia. The pathophysiology and clinical management of unstable angina and non-ST elevation MI are very similar, and these two syndromes are often referred to by the combined acronym **unstable angina/non-ST elevation MI** (UA/NSTEMI).

If the intraluminal thrombus completely occludes the epicardial coronary artery at the site of plaque rupture, then blood flow ceases beyond the point of obstruction. Persistent, total epicardial artery occlusion provides the substrate for acute myocardial injury (**ST elevation myocardial infarction**; STEMI) that will progress inexorably to transmural infarction unless perfusion is re-established. This clinical syndrome can also present as out-of-hospital **sudden cardiac death** (~30% of patients); in these cases, death is usually caused by ischemia-induced electrical instability of the myocardium. In the absence of fatal electrical instability, ST elevation MI typically presents with unremitting chest pain that is often accompanied by dyspnea and ischemic left heart failure. *Mortality in STEMI is significantly reduced by prompt relief of the complete epicardial obstruction. Therefore, the principal management goal in STEMI is expeditious reperfusion of the occluded artery.*

The extent of myocardial necrosis following ischemic injury depends on the mass of myocardium supplied by the occluded artery, the amount of time over which the artery is totally occluded, and the degree of collateral circulation. Regions of the myocardium that are supplied directly and exclusively by the occluded artery sustain extensive ischemic injury. Cell death occurs in a "wavefront" that progresses both spatially and temporally from the subendocardial region to the epicardial surface of the myocardium. As a result, the extent of "transmurality" of an MI bears a direct relationship to the duration of coronary artery occlusion. Adjacent to the region of transmural necrosis, a border zone of myocardium receives nutrients and oxygen from collateral vessels; this collateral perfusion can maintain the viability of border-zone cells for some period of time. However, in the absence of reperfusion of the occluded (infarct-causing) artery, lethal cardiomyocyte injury eventually occurs in these border zones as well.

CLINICAL MANAGEMENT OF ISCHEMIC HEART DISEASE

As noted above, the pathophysiology as well as the clinical approach to ischemic heart disease in patients with chronic coronary disease are different than those in patients with acute coronary syndromes. Because chronic CAD results from an imbalance between myocardial oxygen supply and demand, treatment of chronic CAD focuses on modulating this balance, usually by reduction of oxygen demand. In comparison, treatment of ACS relies on re-establishing and maintaining the patency of the epicardial coronary artery as rapidly as possible. All patients with CAD, irrespective of clinical presentation, also require modification of underlying risk factors, including aggressive lipid-lowering therapy and blood pressure control.

CHRONIC CORONARY ARTERY DISEASE

The treatment goal in chronic CAD is to restore the balance between myocardial oxygen supply (coronary artery blood flow) and myocardial oxygen demand (myocardial oxygen consumption). *Pharmacologic therapies concentrate on the reduction of myocardial oxygen demand,* which is governed by heart rate, contractility, and ventricular wall stress (see Chapter 21). Antianginal drugs can be categorized on the basis of their impact on these parameters.

β-Adrenoceptor Antagonists

Activation of β_1-adrenergic receptors by the sympathoadrenal system leads to an increase in heart rate, contractility, and conduction through the AV node. It follows that antagonists acting at β_1-adrenergic receptors decrease sinus rate, reduce inotropic state, and slow AV nodal conduction.

β_1-Adrenoceptor antagonists (also referred to as "β-blockers") are the cornerstone of medical treatment regimens in patients with chronic stable angina. *β-Antagonists reduce myocardial oxygen demand by decreasing heart rate and contractility,* and the drug-induced decrease in heart rate may also increase myocardial perfusion via prolongation of the diastolic filling time. When used in chronic angina, β-antagonists decrease the peak heart rate achieved during exercise and delay the time to onset of angina. Dosing regimens for β-antagonists are drug-specific, reflecting the characteristic pharmacokinetics of each individual agent. As a general rule, the dose of drug is calibrated to maintain the resting heart rate at approximately 50 beats/minute and to maintain the peak heart rate during exertion at approximately 110 to 120 beats/minute.

β-Antagonists are frequently co-administered with organic nitrates in patients with stable angina. This combination is often more effective than either agent used alone. β-Antagonists are also frequently combined with CCBs—typically, with agents of the dihydropyridine class (see below). (In early clinical trials, short-acting formulations of the dihydropyridine CCB nifedipine were associated with reflex tachycardia when administered as monotherapy; this tachycardia was attenuated when nifedipine was co-administered with a β-antagonist. In current practice, the availability of long-acting dihydropyridine agents has effectively diminished this side effect.)

Although β-antagonists are generally well tolerated in patients with stable angina, certain clinical scenarios require caution. Combining β-antagonists with CCBs of the nondihydropyridine classes (e.g., diltiazem or verapamil) can result in synergistic suppression of SA-node automaticity (leading to extreme sinus bradycardia) and/or AV-node conduction (leading to high-grade AV conduction block). Likewise, because of their depressant effects on nodal tissues, β-antagonists may exacerbate pre-existing bradycardia and/or high-grade AV block. However, given the clear and consistent mortality benefit associated with β-antagonists in secondary prevention trials, it is currently standard clinical practice to implant a permanent transvenous pacing device if such rhythm abnormalities are the major contraindication to the use of β-antagonists. (**Secondary prevention trials** test the efficacy of pharmacologic interventions to reduce adverse cardiovascular events *in patients with known CAD*.)

β-Antagonists are now also being used in patients with clinically stable heart failure (see below). It must be emphasized that the survival benefit demonstrated in HF treatment trials occurred when these agents were initiated during periods of clinical stability. *β-Antagonists must not be administered to patients with decompensated HF.*

When used in an attempt to treat the rare patient with pure vasospastic or **variant angina** (i.e., angina in the absence of epicardial artery obstruction; see Fig. 24-5), β-antagonists can *induce coronary vasospasm* as a consequence of unopposed α-receptor–mediated vasoconstriction. β-Antagonists can also exacerbate bronchospasm in patients with asthma and chronic airway obstruction. However, in patients with chronic airway obstruction, the decision to exclude β-antagonists should be based on objective documentation of exacerbation of airflow obstruction during β-antagonist therapy. Peripheral vascular disease is another relative contraindication to β-antagonist therapy; the concern in this circumstance is the potential for antagonism of the β₂-adrenergic receptors that mediate dilation of peripheral vessels. In clinical practice, however, this concern is rarely justified. Furthermore, patients with peripheral arterial disease have an extremely high risk of concomitant CAD and are therefore likely to benefit significantly from β-antagonist therapy.

Commonly experienced side effects of β-antagonists include fatigue, lethargy, insomnia, and impotence. Although the mechanism of fatigue is unclear, decreased exercise capacity is directly related to drug-induced blunting of the physiologic tachycardia of exercise. The impotence reported by 1% of patients treated with β-antagonists is due to inhibition of β₂-adrenoceptor–mediated peripheral vasodilation.

Ca²⁺ Channel Blockers

Calcium channel blockers (CCBs) decrease the influx of calcium through voltage-gated L-type calcium channels in the plasma membrane. The resulting decrease in intracellular calcium concentration leads to reduced contraction of both cardiac myocytes and vascular smooth muscle cells (see Chapter 21).

Calcium channel blockers decrease myocardial oxygen demand and may also increase myocardial oxygen supply.

Calcium channel blockers decrease myocardial oxygen demand by decreasing systemic vascular resistance and by decreasing cardiac contractility. In the periphery, calcium entry into vascular smooth muscle cells is required for contraction of the cells and is therefore a central determinant of resting vasomotor tone. By blocking calcium entry, CCBs cause relaxation of vascular smooth muscle and thereby reduce systemic vascular resistance. Calcium channel blockers can theoretically increase myocardial oxygen supply by blocking calcium-mediated increases in coronary vasomotor tone; the resulting dilation of epicardial vessels and arteriolar resistance vessels would, in theory, increase coronary blood flow. However, the contribution of this coronary vasodilator mechanism to the clinical effects of the CCBs is controversial, because regional metabolic abnormalities that result from myocardial ischemia should effect a maximal vasodilator response in the absence of pharmacologic modulation.

The different classes of calcium channel blockers have distinctive inotropic effects on cardiac myocytes. Compared to verapamil and diltiazem, dihydropyridines (such as nifedipine) are more selective for calcium channels in the peripheral vasculature. All CCBs, however, do have the potential to impair contractile function by reducing intracellular calcium levels in cardiac myocytes. Therefore, decompensated heart failure is a contraindication to the use of certain CCBs because of their negative inotropic effects. However, newer-generation vasoselective dihydropyridines, such as amlodipine and felodipine, are typically tolerated by patients with reduced LV ejection fractions, and can therefore be administered to patients with LV dysfunction and refractory angina.

Calcium channel blockers are reported to be as effective as β-antagonists in the treatment of chronic stable angina. If the initial treatment of angina with β-antagonists alone is not successful, CCBs can be used either in combination with β-antagonists or as monotherapy. Calcium channel blockers appear to produce a greater antianginal effect when co-administered with β-antagonists than when administered alone, although combination therapy can induce bradyarrhythmias (see above). Despite this proven efficacy in reducing symptoms in patients with chronic CAD, there are no data that support a mortality benefit associated with CCB therapy as either primary or secondary prevention in patients with CAD.

Unlike the β-antagonists, *CCBs are effective in the treatment of vasospastic angina.* Calcium channel blockers relieve the vasospasm of coronary vessels by dilating both epicardial coronary arteries and arteriolar resistance vessels.

Nitrates

Organic nitrates exert their principal therapeutic effect by dilation of peripheral capacitance veins, thereby decreasing preload and reducing myocardial oxygen demand (see Chapter 21). Some investigators argue that nitrates also increase myocardial blood flow by reducing coronary vasomotor tone, although the magnitude of the incremental vasodilator effect is debated in patients with regional myocardial ischemia. Nitrates do have a coronary vasodilator effect in patients with vasospastic angina. Nitrates also have anti-aggregatory effects on platelets.

In patients with *stable exertional angina*, nitrates improve exercise tolerance when used as monotherapy and work synergistically with β-antagonists or CCBs. Sublingual nitroglycerin tablets or nitroglycerin sprays are effective for immediate relief of exertional angina. Provided that sufficient nitrate-free intervals are allowed (to attenuate the development of tolerance), long-acting nitrates (e.g., isosorbide dinitrate and mononitrate) are also effective for prophylaxis and treatment of exertional angina.

Nitrates are also effective in the treatment of both acute and chronic LV failure. This treatment effect is related to the powerful venodilator action of the nitrates, which causes peripheral redistribution of intravascular volume and marked reduction of preload. The anti-ischemic effect of nitrates may be of particular value in patients with ischemia-related diastolic dysfunction. In this clinical setting, nitrates may effect both preload reduction and restoration of normal diastolic chamber compliance and filling.

The development of tolerance is the major obstacle to long-term use of nitrates. Through uncertain mechanisms (see Chapter 21), tolerance develops to both vasodilator and antiplatelet effects of these drugs. Dosing regimens that are punctuated by sufficiently long nitrate-free intervals (8 to 12 hours) may prevent nitrate tolerance. Headache, the most common side effect of nitrate therapy, can develop as a result of cerebral vessel dilation.

Aspirin

Because platelet activation is critically important in the initiation of thrombus formation (see Chapter 22), antiplatelet agents play a central role in the treatment of patients with CAD. Aspirin irreversibly inhibits platelet cyclooxygenase, an enzyme required for generation of the pro-aggregatory compound, thromboxane A_2 (TxA_2). Therefore, the platelet inhibition that follows aspirin administration persists for the lifespan of the platelet (approximately 10 days).

Unless specific contraindications are present, aspirin is an essential therapy for patients with chronic CAD. Aspirin is used to prevent arterial thrombosis leading to stroke and transient ischemic attack as well as MI. *Aspirin is most effective as a selective antiplatelet agent when taken at low doses and/or infrequent intervals* (see Chapter 22). Clinical data have demonstrated a significant treatment benefit for aspirin in patients with unstable angina (~50% reduction in death and nonfatal MI). Aspirin is contraindicated in patients with a known allergy to the drug; in this setting, clopidogrel is indicated as an alternative. Aspirin and other antiplatelet agents should be used cautiously in patients with compromised liver function, because such patients may have a bleeding diathesis due to decreased circulating levels of hepatically-synthesized coagulation factors. Aspirin use also predisposes to gastrointestinal effects such as gastritis and peptic ulcer disease; these adverse effects can often be alleviated by coadministration of agents that decrease gastric acid production (see Chapter 45, Integrative Inflammation Pharmacology: Peptic Ulcer Disease).

Lipid-Lowering Agents

Clinical studies indicate that, in patients with known CAD, the administration of drugs that lower serum LDL-cholesterol decreases the risk of ischemic cardiovascular events. (Refer to Chapter 23, Pharmacology of Cholesterol and Li-poprotein Metabolism, for a detailed discussion of lipid-lowering agents.) The selection of a specific lipid-lowering agent is based on both clinical trial data and the patient's lipid phenotype.

HMG CoA reductase inhibitors (statins) are the most frequently used and best-studied lipid-lowering agents. Because HMG CoA reductase mediates the first committed step in sterol biosynthesis, inhibitors of HMG CoA reductase dramatically reduce the extent of hepatic cholesterol synthesis. This reduction in cholesterol synthesis results in increased hepatic LDL receptor expression, and thereby increases clearance of cholesterol-containing lipoprotein particles from the bloodstream. Clinical trials (e.g., the Scandinavian Simvastatin Survival Study and the Cholesterol and Recurrent Events Study) demonstrate that lipid-lowering therapy reduces cardiovascular event rates in patients with CAD. Dietary and other lifestyle modifications should also be included as part of a comprehensive approach to primary and secondary prevention. HMG CoA reductase inhibitors are contraindicated in women who are or may become pregnant or who are nursing.

UNSTABLE ANGINA AND NON-ST ELEVATION MYOCARDIAL INFARCTION

Unstable angina (UA) and non-ST elevation myocardial infarction (NSTEMI) may occur either as the first presentation of CAD or in patients with a history of stable CAD. (In the latter circumstance, management strategies appropriate for unstable angina take precedence over those for stable CAD.) It is estimated that patients with UA have a 15% to 20% risk of progression to acute MI over a period of 4 to 6 weeks in the absence of treatment. Aggressive treatment can reduce this risk by more than 50%. Patients with UA have no overt evidence of myocardial damage, whereas patients with NSTEMI have elevated biomarkers of cardiomyocte necrosis. Untreated UA may progress to NSTEMI, or NSTEMI may the initial result of plaque rupture with extensive inflammation and coagulation at the rupture site.

The treatment goals in UA/NSTEMI are to relieve ischemic symptoms and to prevent additional thrombus formation at the site of plaque rupture. UA/NSTEMI is typically treated with aspirin, heparin, and β-antagonists. Other antiplatelet agents (e.g., platelet GPIIb–IIIa antagonists and platelet ADP-receptor antagonists) are indicated in high-risk patients to prevent additional thrombus formation (Fig. 24-8). Although conventional antianginal drugs have no demonstrable impact on mortality in UA/NSTEMI, these "demand-based" agents are also used empirically for symptom relief.

Thrombolytic agents are contraindicated in patients with UA/NSTEMI: use of these agents in UA/NSTEMI has been associated with a significant increase in morbidity and a trend towards increased mortality. If ischemic chest discomfort recurs after initiation of treatment, urgent coronary angiography is warranted (with revascularization guided by the angiographic data).

Antianginal Drugs

Intravenous nitroglycerin is often administered for the first 24 hours after the onset of UA/NSTEMI. The intravenous

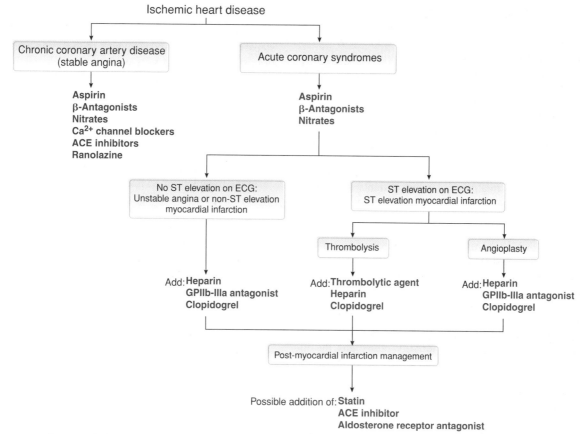

Figure 24-8. Pharmacologic management of acute coronary syndromes. All patients with chronic coronary artery disease are given aspirin unless a life-threatening contraindication is present. β-Antagonists, nitrates, calcium channel blockers, ACE inhibitors, and ranolazine are primarily used to reduce myocardial oxygen demand. All patients with symptoms that raise concerns about a possible acute coronary syndrome are given aspirin and, if tolerated, a β-antagonist. Sublingual or intravenous nitrates can also be given to relieve chest discomfort and minimize ischemia. Electrocardiographic (ECG) findings of ST elevation should prompt emergency measures to open the occluded artery, either with a thrombolytic agent (thrombolysis) or mechanical revascularization (angioplasty). Additional adjunctive pharmacologic therapies for ST elevation myocardial infarction may include aspirin, β-antagonists, nitrates, heparin, GPIIb–IIIa antagonists, and clopidogrel. For patients with acute coronary syndrome but no ST elevation on the electrocardiogram, laboratory assays of myocyte damage (e.g., troponin I or troponin T) determine whether the patient is classified as experiencing unstable angina or non-ST elevation myocardial infarction. In either case, management generally includes administration of aspirin, β-antagonists, nitrates, heparin, GPIIb–IIIa antagonists, and clopidogrel. For all patients with acute coronary syndrome, post-myocardial infarction management should include modification of risk factors, and possible addition of lipid-lowering agents (statins), ACE inhibitors, and aldosterone receptor antagonists.

formulation is used to achieve and maintain predictable blood levels of the drug. After 24 hours, the asymptomatic patient can be switched to a long-acting oral nitrate preparation. Myocardial oxygen demand should also be reduced by co-administration of a β-adrenergic antagonist. Even without symptoms of chest pain, a β-antagonist should be administered empirically because of the mortality benefit associated with β-antagonist use in the setting of MI. Although Ca^{2+} channel blockers such as verapamil and diltiazem also reduce myocardial oxygen demand, their use is purely palliative; unlike β-antagonists, these agents have not been shown to reduce the risk of recurrent MI or cardiac death in patients with UA/NSTEMI.

Heparin and Aspirin

In patients with UA/NSTEMI, heparin and aspirin reduce the risk of recurrent, life-threatening cardiovascular events by ~50%. Although these agents also increase the risk of

bleeding, the clinical benefits outweigh the potential adverse effects. The combination of heparin and aspirin appears to be more effective than either agent used alone in reducing cardiac mortality and recurrent ischemia.

Glycoprotein IIb–IIIa Antagonists

Glycoprotein IIb–IIIa (GPIIb–IIIa) antagonists are highly efficacious antiplatelet agents. During platelet aggregation, GPIIb–IIIa receptors on activated platelets bind the bridging molecule fibrinogen. GPIIb–IIIa antagonists interfere with this critical step of platelet aggregation and thereby limit the size of the platelet plug (see Chapter 22). The use of GPIIb–IIIa antagonists has increased dramatically in recent years, both in the cardiac catheterization laboratory (during percutaneous revascularization procedures) and in the pharmacologic treatment of UA/NSTEMI. GPIIb–IIIa antagonists reduce the risk of fatal and nonfatal MI in patients with UA, and these agents reduce the risk of recurrent MI and urgent revascularization in patients with NSTEMI. In UA/NSTEMI patients with ongoing ischemia or certain high-risk features, a GPIIb–IIIa antagonist should be administered in addition to aspirin and heparin; both eptifibatide and tirofiban have been approved for this use. The use of abciximab has been restricted largely to the periprocedural setting (i.e., in preparation for and immediately following percutaneous coronary intervention).

Platelet ADP-Receptor Antagonists

The platelet ADP-receptor antagonist **clopidogrel** is used increasingly in the treatment of many patients with ACS. Because it is a potent antiplatelet agent, clopidogrel is indicated in all patients with ACS who have true aspirin allergy. Clopidogrel reduces recurrent coronary events in patients with UA/NSTEMI who undergo percutaneous coronary intervention and in patients with UA/NSTEMI who are treated with a noninvasive approach (e.g., patients who do not undergo cardiac catheterization and target-vessel revascularization). Importantly, although the combination of clopidogrel, aspirin, and a GPIIb–IIIa antagonist significantly increases the risk for major bleeding, the overall reduction in cardiovascular morbidity and mortality outweighs the increased risk of bleeding in selected groups of patients.

ST ELEVATION MYOCARDIAL INFARCTION

The treatment of STEMI is aimed at expeditious reperfusion of the occluded epicardial coronary artery. As with UA/NSTEMI, aspirin and heparin are standards of care for STEMI; when used alone, however, these agents are often not sufficient to recanalize an occluded coronary artery (Fig. 24-8). There are two approaches to opening an occluded coronary artery: pharmacologic (thrombolysis) and mechanical (angioplasty or emergency coronary artery bypass). When thrombolysis is used, clopidogrel co-administration increases the likelihood that the vessel will stay open. In contrast, GPIIb–IIIa antagonists are not utilized with thrombolytics because this combination confers a significantly increased risk of bleeding, including hemorrhagic stroke. When angioplasty is performed, both clopidogrel and a GPIIb–IIIa antagonist are employed as adjunctive treatments.

Thrombolytics

The four thrombolytic agents currently used in the pharmacologic management of STEMI are streptokinase, alteplase, tenecteplase, and reteplase. (All are discussed in greater detail in Chapter 22.) One crucial factor that determines the success of thrombolytic therapy in acute MI is the timeliness of administration. *Patients who receive thrombolytic therapy within 2 hours of the onset of symptoms have a two-fold improvement in survival rate compared to patients who receive thrombolytic therapy more than 6 hours after the onset of symptoms.* This observation is consistent with the known relationship between the duration of vessel occlusion and the extent of infarction. A number of important contraindications to thrombolysis, primarily related to increased bleeding risk, may also limit use of this intervention.

Streptokinase

The pharmacologic action of streptokinase involves two steps: complexation and cleavage. In the complexation reaction, streptokinase forms a stable, noncovalent 1:1 complex with plasminogen (either free plasminogen or fibrin-bound plasminogen). The complexation reaction produces a conformational change that exposes the active site on plasminogen. Plasminogen, now with its active site exposed, can effect proteolytic cleavage of *other* plasminogen molecules (again, either free plasminogen or fibrin-bound plasminogen) to plasmin, and thereby initiate thrombolysis.

In the treatment of STEMI, streptokinase is administered as an intravenous loading dose followed by a continuous intravenous infusion. After 90 minutes of infusion, streptokinase produces reperfusion in 60% of acutely occluded vessels. However, the usefulness of streptokinase is limited by two factors. First, streptokinase is a foreign protein that is capable of eliciting antigenic reactions upon repeated administration. Patients with antibodies against streptokinase (from either a previous streptococcal infection or previous treatment with streptokinase) can develop an allergic reaction and fever. Second, because the streptokinase:plasminogen complex activates both fibrin-bound and free plasminogen molecules, its relatively nonspecific antithrombotic activity can result in systemic fibrinolysis.

Alteplase

Alteplase is the generic name for recombinant tissue plasminogen activator (t-PA). Alteplase is effective in restoring the patency of occluded coronary arteries, limiting cardiac dysfunction, and reducing mortality following STEMI. As with endogenously produced t-PA, recombinant t-PA binds to newly formed thrombi with high affinity, causing fibrinolysis at the site of a thrombus. Once bound to the nascent thrombus, t-PA undergoes a conformational change that enhances plasminogen activation. t-PA is a poor activator of plasminogen in the absence of fibrin binding.

Recombinant t-PA is typically administered intravenously at a high dose rate for 1 hour and then at a lower dose rate for the next 2 hours. Despite its high affinity for fibrin-bound plasminogen, recombinant t-PA at pharmacologic doses can (as do other thrombolytic agents) generate a systemic lytic state and cause undesirable bleeding, including cerebral hemorrhage. Thus, this agent is contraindicated in patients who have had a recent stroke or other major bleeding event.

Tenecteplase

Tenecteplase is a genetically engineered variant of t-PA. The molecular modifications in tenecteplase increase its fibrin specificity relative to t-PA and make it more resistant to plasminogen activator inhibitor-I. Large trials have shown that tenecteplase is identical in efficacy to t-PA, with similar (and possibly decreased) risk of bleeding. Additionally, tenecteplase has a longer half-life than t-PA. This pharmacokinetic property allows tenecteplase to be administered as a single, weight-based bolus, thus simplifying administration.

Reteplase

Similar to tenecteplase, **reteplase** is also a genetically engineered variant of t-PA with increased half-life and increased specificity for fibrin relative to t-PA. Its efficacy and adverse-effect profile are similar to those of t-PA. Because of its longer half-life, reteplase can be administered as a "double bolus" (two boluses, 30 minutes apart).

Primary Percutaneous Intervention

In the United States, the majority of patients with STEMI are treated with thrombolytics. Multiple studies have shown, however, that primary angioplasty, if performed within 90 minutes of presentation to the emergency room, yields a mortality benefit compared to thrombolysis. Increasingly, primary angioplasty includes placement of a **drug-eluting stent**. The two currently approved devices consist of a stainless steel stent coated with either **sirolimus** or **paclitaxel**. Each of these agents decreases early restenosis by interrupting cell cycle progression (see Chapter 44, Pharmacology of Immunosuppression). Although drug-eluting stents were originally approved for the treatment of stable coronary artery disease, these devices are now often used in the treatment of acute coronary syndromes. Recent evidence has suggested that patients with drug-eluting stents may be at increased risk for late stent thrombosis, and long-term dual antiplatelet therapy may be indicated to prevent this complication in such patients.

POST-MYOCARDIAL INFARCTION MANAGEMENT

After an MI, a patient must be carefully managed to prevent re-infarction. The goals of any post-MI medical regimen are two-fold: (1) to prevent and treat residual ischemia; and (2) to identify and treat major risk factors such as hypertension, smoking, hyperlipidemia, and diabetes mellitus. Because the extent of MI and its functional consequences vary greatly among patients, the medical regimen must be individualized. The American College of Cardiology and the American Heart Association have made the following general recommendations for the management of post-MI patients:

1. Aspirin (75 to 325 mg/d), in the absence of contraindications, or clopidogrel for patients with a contraindication to aspirin
2. β-Antagonists
3. Lipid-lowering agents (target LDL cholesterol, <100 mg/dL)
4. ACE inhibitors for patients with heart failure, left ventricular dysfunction (ejection fraction, <40%), hypertension, or diabetes
5. Spironolactone or eplerenone for patients with left ventricular dysfunction (ejection fraction, <40%)
6. Clopidogrel, in addition to aspirin, for a designated period, in patients who have undergone percutaneous coronary intervention.

In addition to designing an individualized drug regimen, the physician must also educate the patient about risk factors for the recurrence of MI. A useful mnemonic for guiding overall treatment in post-MI patients is **ABCDE**: **A**spirin, ACE inhibitors, antianginals, and aldosterone antagonists; **B**eta-antagonists and blood pressure control; **C**holesterol-lowering and cigarettes; **D**iet and diabetes control; **E**ducation and exercise.

 Case, Part III: Heart Failure

Mr. N is discharged from the hospital on a multidrug regimen that includes aspirin, clopidogrel, metoprolol, atorvastatin, captopril, and eplerenone. He does well as he increases his activity level during the first 4 to 6 weeks after the infarction. At that point, however, he once again experiences breathlessness at moderate levels of exertion. He initially attributes this to deconditioning, but he becomes concerned when he awakens from sleep with severe breathlessness in the early morning hours. He schedules an appointment with his physician for later that day.

On examination in the physician's office, Mr. N appears comfortable seated in the upright position. His heart rate is 64 beats/min, and his blood pressure is 168/100 mm Hg. The pulmonic component of S2 is prominent (representing a change from his previous exams) and the apical S4 is again noted; there is a grade III/VI apical holosystolic murmur with radiation to the left axilla. An echocardiogram reveals akinesis of the basal segment of the inferior wall of the left ventricle, with more prominent thinning and aneurysmal remodeling of the segment. The LV ejection fraction is 35%. Although the mitral valve leaflets and the supporting structures of the valve appear structurally normal, there is a degree of posterior leaflet prolapse (LV → LA) during ventricular systole. A Doppler study confirms the presence of mitral regurgitation that is at least moderate in severity. The right ventricle is dilated and hypertrophic, with relative preservation of systolic function. Repeat catheterization is performed to assess the etiology of the patient's new biventricular heart failure. Angiography shows wide patency of the right coronary artery at the site of the previous PTCA/stent intervention, and the left coronary system is free of obstruction. Hemodynamic data demonstrate increased pulmonary artery and right ventricular pressures.

QUESTIONS

■ **1.** What pharmacologic strategies are available to treat right heart failure?

■ **2.** What modifications should be made in Mr. N's medication regimen to optimize treatment of his left ventricular failure?

■ **3.** What parenteral inotropic agents are available if Mr. N's symptoms prove refractory to treatment with oral inotropes?

PATHOPHYSIOLOGY OF HEART FAILURE

Heart failure is a common clinical problem. As many as 5 million patients in the United States carry this diagnosis, with approximately 500,000 new cases diagnosed each year. The syndrome of HF has a grave prognosis: the mortality rate at 5 years approximates 50%, and in the subset of patients with the most severe clinical symptoms, the annual mortality is as high as 30% to 50%.

Because the impairment of cardiac function that underlies this syndrome is often irreversible, HF is typically a chronic illness punctuated by episodes of acute decompensation. Acute exacerbations are often multifactorial in etiology, with contributions from dietary indiscretion (excess sodium or fluid intake), nonadherence to prescribed medications, and concomitant noncardiac illness. Myocardial ischemia, progression of the proximate cause of cardiac disease, and activation of neurohumoral regulatory systems may also lead to clinical decompensation. The management of HF requires the clinician to construct, evaluate, and modify a treatment regimen that includes multiple drugs, some of which may carry significant risk for adverse interactions.

Although the discussion that follows emphasizes cardiogenic circulatory failure, it should be noted that circulatory failure can occur in the absence of contractile dysfunction (Table 24-5). Common examples include abnormalities of cardiac filling (e.g., hypovolemia), cardiac rhythm (e.g., bradycardia or tachycardia), or the peripheral circulation (e.g., distributive shock related to sepsis). As always, treatment should be tailored to the pathophysiology in each individual case.

ETIOLOGIES OF CONTRACTILE DYSFUNCTION

Left ventricular contractile dysfunction (**systolic heart failure**) is the primary cause of heart failure. Although multiple disease states can result in contractile dysfunction, the majority of cases of left HF ($\sim$70%) are attributed to CAD. Additional causes of systolic HF include chronic abnormalities of the loading conditions imposed on the heart, such as systemic arterial hypertension (pressure loading) and valvular heart disease (volume loading from mitral regurgitation or aortic insufficiency; pressure loading from aortic stenosis). The contractile performance of the myocardium is initially preserved in disease states associated with abnormal loading conditions, but cardiomyocyte injury and whole-organ contractile dysfunction supervene if the abnormal loading conditions are not corrected. The latter phase of cardiac pump

dysfunction has been referred to as cardiomyopathy of chronic overload. Systolic dysfunction can also result from diverse conditions in which the proximate pathologic abnormality is cardiomyocyte injury or dysfunction. These conditions are referred to as **dilated cardiomyopathies,** because the heart characteristically remodels to produce LV chamber dilation (with or without wall thinning) in states of primary myocyte dysfunction.

Symptomatic HF can also occur in patients with normal or near-normal LV systolic function (i.e., preserved LV ejection fraction). In such cases, the symptoms of left HF are caused by abnormalities of LV relaxation and/or filling (**diastolic heart failure**). Impaired relaxation results in an elevation of LV diastolic pressure at any given filling volume. This elevation of LV diastolic pressure causes elevation of left atrial and pulmonary capillary pressures, leading to transudation of fluid into the pulmonary interstitium (as well as secondary, or passive, elevation of pulmonary artery and right heart pressures). The most common cause of isolated diastolic HF is acute myocardial ischemia. In the setting of acute reversible ischemia (i.e., ischemia not associated with MI), LV diastolic pressures increase as a consequence of incomplete LV relaxation. (Recall from the discussion in Chapter 19, Pharmacology of Cardiac Contractility, that both contraction and relaxation of cardiomyocytes depend on adequate levels of intracellular ATP.)

Both systolic and diastolic HF can be understood by considering the determinants of cardiac performance and the pathophysiologic conditions that affect these parameters. Each of the principal factors affecting stroke volume—preload, afterload, and contractility—can be described by its effect on cardiac function curves. Figure 24-9 illustrates a normal LV pressure-volume loop. In the normal cycle, LV volume increases when the mitral valve opens during diastole. Isovolumetric contraction begins when LV pressure exceeds left atrial pressure and the mitral valve closes; during this segment of the cardiac cycle, intraventricular pressure increases while intracavitary volume remains constant. Ejection begins when the impedance to LV ejection is exceeded and the aortic valve opens; ejected blood is then transmitted to the systemic circulation by the elastic properties of the aorta. The aortic valve closes when LV pressure

TABLE 24-5	Causes of Circulatory Failure in the Absence of Cardiac Pump Dysfunction
CAUSE OF CIRCULATORY FAILURE	**MECHANISM**
Abnormal cardiac filling	Hypovolemia (e.g., hemorrhage)
	Cardiac tamponade (compression by pericardial fluid prevents normal diastolic filling)
Abnormal cardiac rhythm	Bradycardia ($\downarrow$ rate $\rightarrow$ $\downarrow$ forward output)
	Tachycardia ($\uparrow$ rate $\rightarrow$ $\downarrow$ duration of diastolic filling interval)
Abnormal peripheral circulation	Hypertensive crisis ($\uparrow$ SVR $\rightarrow$ $\uparrow$ impedance to LV ejection $\rightarrow$ $\downarrow$ stroke volume)
	Distributive shock ($\downarrow$ SVR $\rightarrow$ $\downarrow$ MAP $\rightarrow$ organ hypoperfusion)

SVR, systemic vascular resistance; MAP, mean arterial pressure.

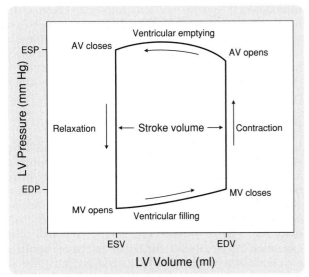

Figure 24-9.   Normal left ventricular pressure-volume loop. Mitral valve *(MV)* opening allows the left ventricular *(LV)* volume to increase as the chamber fills with blood during diastole. When ventricular pressure exceeds left atrial pressure, the mitral valve closes. During the isovolumetric phase of systolic contraction, the left ventricle generates a high pressure, which eventually forces open the aortic valve *(AV)*. Ejection of the stroke volume ensues, and the aortic valve closes when aortic pressure exceeds LV pressure. Isovolumetric relaxation returns the ventricle to its lowest pressure state, and the cycle is repeated. Stroke volume (i.e., the volume of blood ejected with each contraction cycle) is the difference between end-diastolic volume *(EDV)* and end-systolic volume *(ESV)*. EDP, end-diastolic pressure; ESP, end-systolic pressure.

falls below aortic pressure; at this point, intraventricular pressure decreases rapidly (isovolumetric relaxation), up to (and perhaps beyond) the point at which the mitral valve opens, and the cycle is repeated.

As illustrated in Figure 24-10A, the forward stroke volume ejected by the LV depends on the degree of LV filling during diastole, or **preload.** This fundamental relationship between preload and stroke volume is the **Frank–Starling law**; it derives from the relationship between muscle length and degree of muscle shortening, as described in Chapter 19. In brief, increased diastolic volume increases myocardial fiber length. As a result, a higher fraction of the actin filament length is exposed in each sarcomere and is thereby available for myosin cross-bridge formation when the cardiomyocyte is depolarized.

Impedance to LV ejection, or **afterload,** is the second determinant of stroke volume (Fig. 24-10B). As impedance to ejection (afterload) increases, the stroke output of the ventricle falls. This characteristic of the intact heart derives from the fact that increasing the resistance against which cardiac muscle must contract leads to a decrease in the extent of shortening (i.e., to reduced stroke volume). Because the sensitivity of stroke volume to outflow resistance is accentuated in the failing ventricle, agents that decrease afterload are able to increase LV stroke volume in patients with HF (see below).

A third determinant of cardiac performance is **contractility,** also described in Chapter 19. The contractile state of the LV is described by the **end-systolic pressure-volume relationship** (**ESPVR,** Fig. 24-10C). The ESPVR is, in effect, a variant of the Frank–Starling law. While the Frank–Starling law defines the relationship between LV diastolic volume (or preload) and LV stroke volume (or cardiac output), the ESPVR describes the relationship between diastolic filling volume and LV tension development during isovolumetric contraction. As shown in Figure 24-10C, an

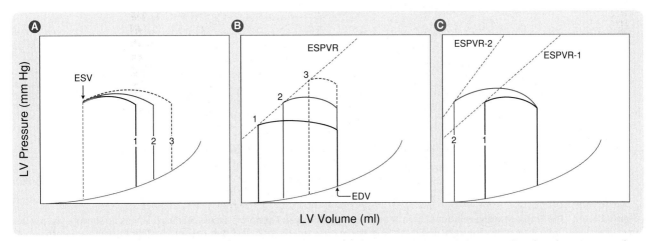

Figure 24-10.   Determinants of cardiac output. Changes in preload, afterload, and myocardial contractility alter the pressure-volume relationship of the cardiac cycle. **A.** Increases in preload (lines 1, 2, 3) result in greater stretch of ventricular myocytes, development of greater ventricular end-diastolic pressure, and ejection of greater stroke volume (the Frank–Starling mechanism). Note that the end-systolic volume *(ESV)* is the same in each case, because the contractility of the heart has not changed. **B.** Increases in afterload (points 1, 2, 3) create greater impedance to left ventricular output and result in proportionately decreased stroke volume (the difference between end-diastolic volume *(EDV)* and *ESV*). The end-systolic pressure is linearly related to ESV; this linear relationship is called the end-systolic pressure-volume relationship *(ESPVR)*. **C.** Increases in myocardial contractility (lines 1, 2), as occurs after administration of a positive inotrope, shift the ESPVR up and to the left, resulting in increased stroke volume.

increase in the contractile state of the LV, reflected by an upward shift of the ESPVR, results in a greater degree of tension development for any given end-diastolic volume. In the presence of a fixed afterload, increased contractility results in a greater degree of muscle shortening and an increase in LV stroke volume.

A final determinant of cardiac pump performance is **heart rate.** However, if LV contractile performance is preserved, then impairment of cardiac output occurs as a consequence of abnormal heart rate only at extreme rates outside the physiologic range. Heart rate can be an important determinant of cardiac output in patients with systolic contractile dysfunction.

CARDIAC COMPENSATION

As the ability of the myocardium to maintain normal forward output fails, compensatory mechanisms are activated to preserve circulatory function. The Frank–Starling mechanism increases stroke volume in direct response to increased preload. This recruitment of preload reserve is the first response of the system to hemodynamic stress. Hemodynamic stress that cannot be fully compensated by the Frank–Starling mechanism stimulates signaling systems that initiate structural changes at the cellular level, a process referred to as **remodeling** of the myocardium. Although the underlying stimuli for remodeling remain an active area of investigation, it has been noted that the specific pattern of remodeling is determined by the nature of the applied stress. If the Frank–Starling mechanism and remodeling mechanisms are unable to re-establish adequate forward cardiac output, then

neurohumoral systems are also activated. These systems modulate intravascular volume and vasomotor tone to maintain oxygen delivery to critical organs. Although each of these compensatory mechanisms contributes to the maintenance of circulatory function, each may also contribute to the development and progression of pump dysfunction and circulatory failure, as later described.

Frank–Starling Mechanism

In the intact heart, increased preload leads to increased stroke volume via the Frank–Starling mechanism. Although this mechanism remains operative in the failing heart, the relationship between end-diastolic volume and stroke volume is altered. *In patients with systolic dysfunction, the relationship between end-diastolic volume and stroke volume is characterized by a flatter plateau* (Fig. 24-11). Although volume expansion can be a useful strategy for increasing stroke volume in patients operating on the ascending limb of the Starling curve, the majority of patients with heart failure operate with *elevated* intravascular volume. This increased intravascular volume reflects the end result of neurohumoral activation (i.e., the sympathoadrenal axis and the renin-angiotensin–aldosterone system; see below). Thus, the treatment of cardiogenic circulatory failure rarely involves volume expansion. It also merits emphasis that preload expansion can result in significant LV dilation, thereby increasing LV systolic and diastolic wall stress.

Cardiac Remodeling and Hypertrophy

In the setting of increased myocardial wall stress, cardiac hypertrophy develops in order to maintain ventricular sys-

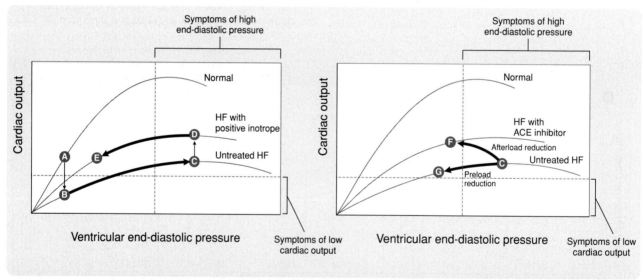

Figure 24-11. The Frank-Starling relationship in heart failure. Left panel: The normal Frank–Starling relationship shows a steep increase in cardiac output with increasing ventricular end-diastolic pressure (preload). Point *A* describes the end-diastolic pressure and cardiac output of a normal heart under resting conditions. With contractile dysfunction (untreated HF), cardiac output falls **(B)** and the Frank–Starling curve flattens, so that increasing preload translates to only a modest increase in cardiac output **(C)**. This increase in cardiac output is accompanied by symptoms of high end-diastolic pressure, such as dyspnea. Treatment with a positive inotrope, such as digitalis, shifts the Frank–Starling curve upward, and cardiac output increases **(D)**. The improvement in myocardial contractility supports a sufficient reduction in preload that the venous congestion is relieved **(E). Right panel:** Two of the principal pharmacologic treatments of HF are afterload reduction (e.g., ACE inhibitors) and preload reduction (e.g., diuretics). Afterload reduction **(F)** increases cardiac output at any given preload, and thereby elevates the Frank–Starling relationship. Preload reduction **(G)** alleviates congestive symptoms by decreasing ventricular end-diastolic pressure along the same Frank–Starling curve.

tolic performance. Because LV ejection fraction is inversely proportional to wall stress, adaptations that decrease systolic wall stress increase LV ejection fraction. **Laplace's law** states that wall stress (σ) is directly proportional to the pressure (P) and radius (R) of a chamber, and inversely proportional to wall thickness (h):

$$\sigma = P \times R/2h \qquad \text{Equation 24-1}$$

In cases of chronic pressure overload, such as aortic stenosis or systemic hypertension, the LV develops a concentric pattern of hypertrophy as contractile proteins and new sarcomeres are added in *parallel* to the existing myofilaments. **Concentric hypertrophy** simultaneously increases wall thickness (h) and decreases cavity size (R), resulting in a net reduction in systolic wall stress and thereby preserving systolic performance. The disadvantage of concentric remodeling derives from the *decrease in LV compliance* that occurs as a consequence of this pattern of hypertrophy. In a ventricle with reduced compliance, diastolic pressure in the chamber is increased at any given filling volume. This in turn leads to elevation of LA and pulmonary capillary pressures, thereby predisposing to congestive symptoms.

In conditions of chronic volume overload, such as mitral or aortic regurgitation, the LV develops an eccentric pattern of hypertrophy as contractile proteins and new sarcomeres are added in *series* to the existing myofilaments. **Eccentric hypertrophy** helps to maintain cardiac performance via modulation of diastolic wall stress. In contrast to the situation that occurs after concentric remodeling, eccentric hypertrophy is associated with *increased LV compliance*. The increase in compliance allows LV end-diastolic volume to increase without a significant elevation of left ventricular and left atrial diastolic pressures. This attenuation of the rise in chamber pressure allows the system to maintain forward cardiac output by a volume-driven increase in total stroke volume. During the compensated phase of eccentric hypertrophy, LV wall thickness increases in approximate proportion to the increase in chamber radius.

Neurohumoral Activation

Failure of the heart to provide adequate forward output activates several neurohumoral systems, often with deleterious consequences (Fig. 24-12). Decreased arterial pressure activates the baroreceptor reflex, stimulating release of catecholamines; in turn, the catecholamines produce tachycardia (via β_1-receptors) and vasoconstriction (via peripheral α_1-receptors). Stimulation of β_1-receptors on renal juxtaglomerular (JG) cells promotes the release of renin. JG cells also release renin in response to the decreased renal perfusion that accompanies decreased cardiac output. Renin cleaves circulating angiotensinogen to angiotensin I, which is subsequently converted by angiotensin converting enzyme (ACE) to angiotensin II (AT II). AT II acts through AT_1 receptors to increase arterial vasomotor tone. AT II also activates several physiologic mechanisms that increase intravascular volume, including aldosterone release from the adrenal glands (thus promoting salt and water retention), vasopressin (ADH) release from the posterior pituitary gland, and thirst center

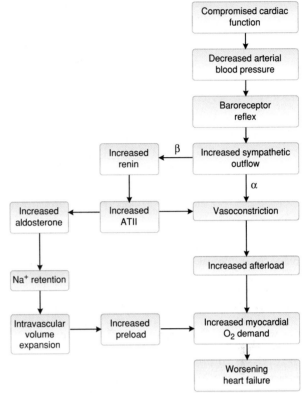

Figure 24-12. Neurohumoral effects of heart failure. Compromised cardiac function leads to decreased arterial blood pressure, which activates baroreceptors that increase sympathetic outflow. α-Adrenergic sympathetic outflow (α) causes vasoconstriction, an effect that increases afterload. The increased afterload creates a greater pressure against which the heart must contract, and thereby increases myocardial O_2 demand. β-Adrenergic sympathetic outflow (β) increases juxtaglomerular cell release of renin. Renin cleaves angiotensinogen to angiotensin I, and angiotensin I is then converted to the active hormone angiotensin II (AT II). AT II has a direct vasoconstrictor action; it also increases aldosterone synthesis and secretion. Aldosterone increases collecting duct Na^+ reabsorption, leading to intravascular volume expansion and increased preload. Together, the increased afterload and preload increase myocardial O_2 demand. In the already compromised heart, these increased stresses can lead to worsening heart failure.

activation in the hypothalamus. In addition, AT II appears to be an important mediator of vascular and myocardial hypertrophy.

The tachycardia and increased intravascular volume that accompany activation of these neurohumoral mechanisms help to maintain forward cardiac output, and the systemic vasoconstriction that occurs provides a mechanism by which central regulatory centers can override local autoregulation of blood flow. Together, these mechanisms allow the cardiovascular system to maintain perfusion of critical organs in the setting of reduced cardiac output. However, sympathetic stimulation of the heart also increases myocardial oxygen demand by increasing both afterload (arteriolar constriction) and preload (retention of sodium and water). Continued sympathetic stimulation eventually results in down-regulation of β-adrenergic receptors, further impairing the ability of the system to maintain forward output. *The central aim of the*

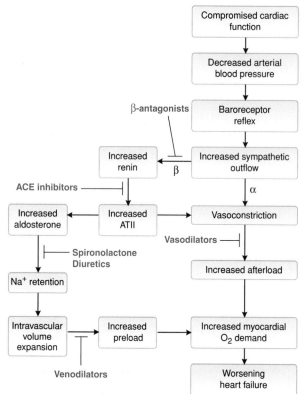

Figure 24-13. Pharmacologic modulation of the neurohumoral effects of heart failure. Many therapeutic agents used in the management of heart failure modulate the neurohumoral systems that are activated by compromised cardiac function. The renin-angiotensin–aldosterone system can be inhibited by (1) β-adrenergic antagonists, which inhibit renin release by the juxtaglomerular cells of the kidney; (2) ACE inhibitors, which prevent the conversion of angiotensin I to the active hormone angiotensin II; and (3) spironolactone, which competitively antagonizes aldosterone binding to the mineralocorticoid receptor. Diuretics promote Na^+ excretion, and thereby counteract the Na^+ retention stimulated by activation of the renin-angiotensin–aldosterone system. Venodilators counteract the effect of intravascular volume expansion by increasing peripheral venous capacitance and thereby decreasing preload. Direct arterial vasodilators alleviate the α-adrenergic receptor-mediated and angiotensin II receptor-mediated vasoconstriction induced by increased sympathetic outflow. Cardiac glycosides, β-adrenergic agonists, and cardiac phosphodiesterase inhibitors are also used in HF to increase myocardial contractility *(not shown)*.

current pharmacologic management of HF is to modulate the action of these neurohumoral effectors (Fig. 24-13).

CLINICAL MANAGEMENT OF HEART FAILURE

The pharmacologic treatment of HF has expanded dramatically over the past 3 decades. The evolution of ''load-active'' therapy has revolutionized the management of patients with HF, and numerous large-scale clinical trials have demonstrated that these therapies are associated with statistically significant reductions in morbidity and mortality. In addition, improvements in the detection and treatment of hypertension and the management of complex multivessel CAD have dramatically altered the clinical course of patients with contractile dysfunction. It is helpful to organize the treatment strategies for contractile dysfunction in patients who exhibit or are at risk to develop symptomatic heart failure according to the following physiologic goals: preload reduction, afterload reduction, and increased inotropy. Table 24-6 provides a summary of the hemodynamic effects and mechanisms of action of the drug classes that are commonly used to treat heart failure.

PRELOAD REDUCTION

Diuretics

Diuretics have long been cornerstones of the pharmacologic management of patients with LH failure and remain integral components of the treatment of patients with congestive symptoms and/or intravascular volume overload. However, despite the efficacy of these agents in reducing congestive symptoms, there is no evidence of a mortality benefit from treatment with either loop diuretics or thiazide diuretics.

The natriuretic agents most commonly used in HF are the loop diuretics, which include furosemide and bumetanide. These drugs inhibit the Na^+-K^+-$2Cl^-$ cotransporter (NKCC2) in the thick ascending limb of Henle, resulting in increased excretion of sodium, potassium, and water. Thiazide diuretics such as hydrochlorothiazide are also used to treat congestive symptoms, particularly in patients with hypertensive heart disease and LV systolic dysfunction. Thiazides inhibit sodium and chloride reabsorption via the Na^+-Cl^- cotransporter (NCC1) in the distal convoluted tubule and are less efficacious natriuretic agents than the loop diuretics. Thiazides are often ineffective as monotherapy for congestive symptoms in patients with chronic kidney disease. Thiazides are sometimes coadministered with loop diuretics in patients with reduced GFR and refractory volume overload, and in selected patients with HF in whom treatment with loop diuretics alone does not achieve adequate diuresis. (Refer to Chapter 20 for a more extended discussion of diuretics.)

Aldosterone Receptor Antagonists

Spironolactone is a potassium-sparing diuretic that acts as a competitive antagonist at the aldosterone receptor, thus decreasing sodium–potassium exchange in the distal tubule and collecting duct of the nephron. A recent clinical trial of this agent in patients with systolic HF (the RALES study) has received much attention. In this study, patients with severe HF were treated with low-dose spironolactone (25 to 50 mg daily); enrolled patients were free of significant renal impairment and were concomitantly receiving standard therapy for heart failure (ACE inhibitor, loop diuretic ± digoxin). In patients treated with spironolactone, all-cause mortality (including sudden cardiac death and death from progressive heart failure) was reduced by approximately 30%, as were hospital admissions for exacerbations of HF. Spironolactone is often administered in combination with an ACE inhibitor (see below). Because both spironolactone and ACE inhibitors decrease K^+ excretion, potassium supple-

TABLE 24-6	Pharmacologic Agents Used in the Treatment of Heart Failure		
DRUG OR DRUG CLASS	**MECHANISM OF ACTION**	**HEMODYNAMIC EFFECT**	**CLINICAL NOTES**
Drugs with Proven Mortality Reduction			
ACE inhibitors	Inhibit AT II generation → ↓ AT_1 receptor activation	Decreased afterload Decreased preload	May cause hyperkalemia
β-Antagonists	Competitive antagonists at β-adrenergic receptor → ↓ renin release	Decreased afterload Decreased preload	May be relatively contraindicated in severely decompensated heart failure
Spironolactone	Competitive antagonist at aldosterone receptor	Decreased preload	Mortality benefit may be independent of hemodynamic effects; may cause hyperkalemia
Drugs or Treatments Used for Symptomatic Improvement			
Na^+/H_2O restriction	Decrease intravascular volume	Decreased preload	May help limit edema formation
Diuretics	Inhibit renal Na^+ reabsorption	Decreased preload	Furosemide most effective for treating congestive symptoms
Digoxin	Inhibit Na^+/K^+ ATPase → ↑ intracellular Ca^{2+} → ↑ contractility	Increased contractility	Delays atrioventricular nodal conduction
Organic nitrates	Increase NO → venous smooth muscle relaxation → ↑ venous capacitance	Decreased preload	Reduces myocardial O_2 demand
Dobutamine	Stimulates β-adrenergic receptors	Increased contractility ($β_1$ effect) Decreased afterload ($β_2$ effect)	Used in the acute setting only
Amrinone, milrinone	Inhibit phosphodiesterase → ↑ β-adrenergic effect	Increased contractility Decreased afterload Decreased preload	Used in the acute setting only

mentation and plasma K^+ levels must be monitored carefully.

Venodilators

Venodilator agents are often coadministered with diuretics in patients with congestive symptoms. The prototypical venodilator is nitroglycerin (NTG). This drug increases venous capacitance and thereby decreases venous return to the heart. The decrease in venous return results in reduced LV chamber volume and reduced LV diastolic pressure. These effects of the nitrates decrease myocardial oxygen demand, which may be especially beneficial in patients with coexisting angina and LV dysfunction.

Nitrates may also be particularly effective in cases where left HF results from acute myocardial ischemia. In this condition, LV relaxation is impaired, LV compliance is decreased, and LV diastolic pressure is typically elevated. By increasing venous capacitance, nitrates reduce venous return to the heart and decrease LV diastolic volume. In turn, the decrease in diastolic volume leads to a decrease in myocardial oxygen consumption. In addition, nitrates may alleviate ischemia, thereby improving diastolic relaxation. Thus, the beneficial effects of nitrate administration in this setting include both preload reduction and improvement in LV compliance.

AFTERLOAD REDUCTION

ACE Inhibitors

ACE inhibitors reversibly inhibit angiotensin converting enzyme (ACE). The resulting decrease in angiotensin II (AT II) leads to a number of potential benefits. AT II is an important component of the neurohumoral regulation of the failing circulation. In response to renal hypoperfusion, the kidney increases renin secretion, which results in increased production of AT II, as noted above (also see Chapter 20). In turn, AT II stimulates the adrenal gland to secrete aldosterone. Overall, activation of the renin-angiotensin–aldosterone system increases vasomotor tone as well as sodium and water retention. These hemodynamic alterations result in increased intravascular volume (leading, ultimately, to increased LV diastolic filling and increased LV stroke volume) and peripheral redistribution of the cardiac output (mediated by the vasoconstrictor effects of AT II).

Administration of an ACE inhibitor reverses the vasoconstriction and volume retention that characterize renin-angiotensin–aldosterone system activation. The reduction in afterload decreases the impedance to LV ejection and thereby increases LV stroke volume. The reversal of aldosterone-related volume retention decreases preload. These effects are synergistic in patients with HF: as stroke volume increases, GFR is also increased, leading to increased delivery of sodium and water to the distal nephron, where (in the absence of renin-stimulated elevation of aldosterone levels) natriuresis and diuresis occur. ACE inhibition can also increase venous capacitance (and thereby reduce preload) by decreasing degradation of the endogenous vasodilator bradykinin. By altering the myocardial remodeling that occurs after ST elevation myocardial infarction, ACE inhibitors can provide further benefit in patients with concomitant HF and CAD.

ACE inhibitors have a statistically significant impact on survival in patients with heart failure. This mortality benefit was first demonstrated in patients with severe heart failure in the CONSENSUS trial: the mortality reduction approximated 40% at 6 months and 31% at 1 year. The mortality benefit of the ACE inhibitors was confirmed in a broader spectrum of patients in the SOLVD Treatment Trial (16% reduction in mortality) and the V-Heft II Trial (28% reduction in mortality), as well as in patients in the convalescent phase following MI (SAVE Trial, 19% reduction in mortality).

AT$_1$ antagonists (sometimes called angiotensin receptor blockers or ARBs) are a relatively new class of agents that inhibit the renin-angiotensin–aldosterone axis at the level of the angiotensin II receptor. These agents have a hemodynamic profile similar to that of the converting enzyme inhibitors. Recent clinical trials have demonstrated a mortality benefit for AT$_1$ antagonists in patients with severe systolic HF (LV ejection fraction, <40%). In some circumstances, this mortality benefit may be additive to that of a concomitantly administered ACE inhibitor (CHARM trials).

β-Adrenoceptor Antagonists

Much recent attention has been directed at the use of β-adrenoceptor antagonists in the treatment of patients with HF. Although the use of β-antagonists might seem counterintuitive, clinical trials have now established that these agents increase survival in heart failure patients. The benefits of β-antagonists in patients with heart failure have been variably attributed to (1) inhibition of renin release, (2) attenuation of the cytotoxic and signaling effects of elevated circulating catecholamines, and, more generally, (3) prevention of acute coronary syndromes. Thus, β-antagonists, like ACE inhibitors, may attenuate the adverse effects of neurohumoral regulators in patients with heart failure. Furthermore, because β-antagonists and ACE inhibitors act through distinct mechanisms and have non-overlapping toxicities, it is reasonable to coadminister these drugs to HF patients.

Vasodilators

Hydralazine is a direct-acting vasodilator that decreases systemic vascular resistance and thereby reduces afterload. The mechanism of action of hydralazine remains to be determined. The arterial vasodilation produced by hydralazine is particularly pronounced when the drug is administered intravenously. The clinical use of hydralazine has been limited by a number of factors, including the induction of reflex tachycardia during intravenous administration, the development of tachyphylaxis, and the occurrence of a drug-induced lupus syndrome during chronic administration. This agent has demonstrated a mortality benefit in HF when coadministered with organic nitrates (AHEFT Trial). The nitrate–

hydralazine combination is typically reserved for patients who cannot tolerate therapy with an ACE inhibitor.

INOTROPIC AGENTS

Cardiac Glycosides

Digitalis glycosides inhibit the sarcolemmal Na$^+$-K$^+$ ATPase in cardiac myocytes. This action increases intracellular Na$^+$, activates the Na$^+$-Ca^{2+} exchanger, and increases intracellular Ca^{2+}, including the Ca^{2+} stores in the sarcoplasmic reticulum. This, in turn, leads to increased calcium release upon myocyte stimulation, resulting in increased myocardial contractility (i.e., upward/leftward shift of the ESPVR). Although patients with HF often experience relief of congestive symptoms during treatment with the cardiac glycosides, these drugs have not been shown to decrease mortality.

Sympathomimetic Amines

Dobutamine is the parenteral sympathomimetic amine used most commonly in the treatment of systolic HF. This agent is a synthetic congener of epinephrine that stimulates β$_1$-receptors and, to a lesser extent, β$_2$-receptors and α$_1$-receptors. The stimulation of β$_1$-receptors predominates at therapeutic infusion rates, leading ultimately to an increase in the contractility of cardiac myocytes. Stimulation of vascular β$_2$-receptors causes arterial vasodilation and a reduction in afterload. The combined effects of increased contractility and decreased afterload lead to improvement in overall cardiac performance.

Phosphodiesterase Inhibitors

Phosphodiesterase inhibitors (such as **inamrinone** and **milrinone**) inhibit the degradation of cAMP in cardiac myocytes and thereby increase intracellular calcium and enhance contractility (inotropy). In the systemic vasculature, these agents cause dilation of both arteriolar resistance vessels and venous capacitance vessels, thereby decreasing afterload and preload. As a result of these aggregate effects, phosphodiesterase inhibitors have been referred to as "ino-dilators." Despite these positive actions, both phosphodiesterase inhibitors and sympathomimetic amines are reserved for short-term treatment of patients with acute decompensation of heart failure. Indeed, long-term treatment with phosphodiesterase inhibitors has been shown to *increase* mortality.

COMBINATION THERAPY

The drugs described in this chapter offer a number of approaches to the pharmacotherapy of heart failure. Some agents, most notably ACE inhibitors and β-antagonists, have demonstrated significant mortality benefit in randomized clinical trials and should probably be viewed as the new cornerstones of therapy. Others drugs, such as digoxin and diuretics, have been mainstays of symptomatic relief despite a lack of mortality benefit.

Use of combination therapies must be approached cautiously in HF patients to avoid adverse effects such as hypotension, arrhythmias, electrolyte imbalances, and renal insufficiency. Nonetheless, it is typical for these patients to require multidrug regimens to optimize their functional status.

Conclusion and Future Directions

Hypertension, ischemic heart disease, and HF are common cardiovascular diseases that occur singly and in combination. A number of therapeutic strategies target the cellular and molecular pathways that are dysfunctional in these disease states. Combination therapy with drugs from multiple classes is often required to address the complex pathophysiology of these conditions and achieve the desired therapeutic result.

Current research in cardiovascular genomics and neurohumoral pathways promises to provide new understanding of the pathophysiology of cardiovascular disease. For example, the pathophysiology of essential hypertension may, in many cases, involve mutations or polymorphisms in the genes that code for angiotensinogen, renin, the angiotensin II receptor (AT_1), endothelin, the glucocorticoid receptor, the insulin receptor, endothelial nitric oxide synthase, and the epithelial Na^+ channel (ENaC). As the genetic determinants of cardiovascular regulation are clarified, it may be possible to identify high-risk patients prospectively and to develop targeted therapies that exert their therapeutic effects on the molecular and cellular mechanisms predicted to drive the disease in these patients.

In recent years, agents targeting neurohumoral pathways—such as ACE inhibitors and β-antagonists—have become cornerstones of therapy for all cardiovascular disease. Large clinical trials have consistently demonstrated that these drugs reduce mortality in patients with hypertension, patients with coronary artery disease and prior MI, and patients with systolic HF. Over the past 25 years, increased understanding of basic disease mechanisms has improved the physician's ability to alter both the clinical expression and progression of cardiovascular diseases: examples include recent advances in the primary prevention of coronary artery disease and the positive impact of neurohumoral modulation on the progression of HF. Current research aims to identify and characterize new drug targets, including a host of signaling molecules that are abnormal in the failing heart. Elevated levels of inflammatory mediators—such as tumor necrosis factor-α (TNF-α), interleukin-6 (IL-6), and endothelin-1—and enzymes—such as inducible nitric oxide synthase, collagenases, and matrix metalloproteinases—have all been reported to contribute in some way to the detrimental structural and functional changes that occur in the failing heart.

Suggested Reading

Hypertension

ALLHAT Officers and Coordinators for the ALLHAT Collaborative Research Group. Major outcomes in high-risk hypertensive patients randomized to angiotensin-converting enzyme inhibitor or calcium channel blocker vs. diuretic: The Antihypertensive and Lipid-Lowering Treatment to Prevent Heart Attack Trial (ALLHAT). *JAMA* 2002;288:2981–2997. (*Results of a major trial comparing agents for initial treatment of hypertension.*)

August P. Initial treatment of hypertension. *N Engl J Med* 2003; 348:610–617. (*Overview of approaches to hypertension treatment.*)

Chobanian AV, Bakris GL, Black HR, et al. The seventh report of the Joint National Committee on Prevention, Detection, Evaluation, and Treatment of High Blood Pressure: the JNC 7 report. *JAMA* 2003;289:2560–2571. (*Current guidelines for classifying and treating hypertension.*)

Franse LV, Pahor M, DiBari M, et al. Hypokalemia associated with diuretic use and cardiovascular events in the SHEP trial. *Hypertension* 2000;35:1025–1030. (*Association of diuretic use with hypokalemia.*)

Vaughan CJ, Delanty N. Hypertensive emergencies. *Lancet* 2000; 356:411. (*Clinical management of hypertensive emergency.*)

Ischemic Heart Disease

Abrams J. Chronic stable angina. *N Engl J Med* 2005;352: 2524–2533. (*Clinical pharmacology of chronic coronary artery disease treatments.*)

American Heart Association 2005 guidelines for cardiopulmonary resuscitation and emergency cardiac care. Part 8: stabilization of the patient with acute coronary syndromes. *Circulation* 2005; IV(Suppl):89–110. (*Emergency management of acute coronary syndromes.*)

Armstrong EJ, Morrow DA, Sabatine MS. Inflammatory biomarkers in acute coronary syndromes. Part I: introduction and cytokines. Part II: acute-phase reactants and biomarkers of endothelial cell activation. Part III: biomarkers of oxidative stress and angiogenic growth factors; Part IV: matrix metalloproteinases and biomarkers of platelet activation. *Circulation* 2006;113: 72–75,152–155,289–292,382–385. (*Four-part series reviewing pathophysiology and clinical evidence concerning the role of inflammatory mediators in acute coronary syndromes.*)

Braunwald E, Antman EM, Beasley JW, et al. ACC/AHA 2002 guideline update for the management of patients with unstable angina and non-ST elevation myocardial infarction. Summary article: a report of the American College of Cardiology/American Heart Association Task Force on practice guidelines (Committee on the Management of Patients with Unstable Angina). *Circulation* 2002;106:1893–1900. (*Current guidelines for evaluating and treating patients with unstable angina and non-ST elevation myocardial infarction.*)

Cannon CP, Braunwald E, McCabe CH, et al. Intensive versus moderate lipid lowering with statins after acute coronary syndromes. *N Engl J Med* 2004;350:1495–1504. (*Trial demonstrating clinical benefit for aggressive statin therapy after acute coronary syndrome.*)

Davignon J, Ganz P. Role of endothelial dysfunction in atherosclerosis. *Circulation* 2004;109(Suppl 1):III27–III32. (*Molecular basis of atherosclerosis.*)

Libby P, Theroux P. Pathophysiology of coronary artery disease. *Circulation* 2005;111:3481–3488. (*Molecular basis of coronary artery disease.*)

Heart Failure

ACC/AHA 2005 guideline update for the diagnosis and management of chronic heart failure in the adult. *J Am Coll Cardiol* 2005;46:1116–1143. (*Consensus guidelines for management of heart failure.*)

Jessup M, Brozena S. Heart failure. *N Engl J Med* 2003;348: 2007–2018. (*Clinical approach to heart failure.*)

Opie LH. Cellular basis for therapeutic choices in heart failure. *Circulation* 2004;110:2559–2561. (*Molecular basis of heart failure therapeutics.*)

Stevenson LW. Clinical use of inotropic agents for heart failure: looking backward or forward. Part I: inotropic infusions during hospitalization. Part II: chronic inotropic therapy. *Circulation* 2003;108:367–372, 492–497. (*Two-part series examining use of inotropic agents in heart failure.*)

Taylor AL, Ziesche S, Yancy C, et al. Combination of isosorbide dinitrate and hydralazine in blacks with heart failure. *N Engl J Med* 2004;351:2049–2057. (*Recent trial showing mortality benefit in self-identified black patients.*)

IV

Principles of Endocrine Pharmacology

25

Pharmacology of the Hypothalamus and Pituitary Gland

Ehrin J. Armstrong and Armen H. Tashjian, Jr.

INTRODUCTION

The hypothalamus and pituitary gland function cooperatively as master regulators of the endocrine system. Together, hormones secreted by the hypothalamus and pituitary gland control important homeostatic and metabolic functions, from reproduction to control of thyroid physiology. This chapter introduces the physiology and regulation of hypothalamic and pituitary hormones through a discussion of feedback regulation and the various axes of hormonal regulation. It then discusses the pharmacologic utility of hypothalamic and pituitary factors, with emphasis on the regulation of specific endocrine pathways. Three concepts are of special importance in this chapter: (1) hypothalamic control of pituitary hormone release; (2) negative feedback inhibition; and (3) endocrine axes. A thorough understanding of these pathways and their mechanisms also provides a background for understanding all the chapters in this section.

 Case

GR is a 54 year-old hard-driving sales executive. He travels constantly, and prides himself on his high energy level and enthusiasm for surpassing his sales projections each quarter. Over the past 2 years, however, he has begun to feel increasingly fatigued, and has difficulty rushing the length of airport terminals. He has always had a muscular handshake, but lately he has also noticed that his company ring and wedding band are excessively tight. GR is also frustrated that he recently had to replace his entire dress shoe collection, because his shoe size increased from 9 ½ to 11. One afternoon while catching a flight back home, the man sitting next to GR says, "I'm sorry to bring this up, but I can't help but noticing. I'm a medical doctor, and it looks to me like you might have acromegaly."

GR scoffs at the idea that he may have any medical condition, but mentions the encounter to his wife. At her prompting, GR goes to his doctor for further evaluation. A serum insulin-like growth factor (IGF-1) level is significantly elevated after correction for GR's age, and his serum growth hormone level is 10 ng/mL (normal, <1 ng/mL) after an oral glucose load of 75 mg. A magnetic resonance imaging (MRI) of his head reveals a pituitary adenoma with maximal diameter 1.5 cm, consistent with a diagnosis of acromegaly due to a growth-hormone secreting adenoma. After referral to an endocrinologist and neurosurgeon, GR elects to undergo trans-sphenoidal pituitary surgery. GR tolerates the surgery well, but his postoperative growth hormone level remains elevated.

Based on the continued elevation in serum growth hormone levels, GR's endocrinologist recommends medical treatment with octreotide. GR tolerates the injections well, but he is annoyed by the need for injections every 8 hours, and airport security guards always make him put the needles in baggage. After 2 months of frequent injections, GR switches to a long-acting, depot form of octreotide that is injected once a month. GR is much happier with the formulation, although he continues to experience mild nausea and bloating as an adverse effect of this medication.

After 6 months of depot octreotide injections, GR's growth hormone and insulin-like growth factor levels remain elevated. GR is frustrated at the lack of improvement of his biochemical assays, but does feel that he has more energy than before treatment. GR's endocrinologist recommends treatment with pegvisomant as an alternative medical approach to treating the effects of his elevated growth hormone levels. GR begins monthly injections with pegvisomant. Six months later, GR's insulin-like growth factor level is undetectable. GR is again flying around the nation in pursuit of increased sales, and stops in town just long enough to complete his yearly head MRI and liver function tests.

QUESTIONS

■ **1.** Why are serum levels of IGF-1 an appropriate screening test for acromegaly?

■ **2.** How does somatostatin block the effects of elevated growth hormone levels?

■ **3.** Why did GR have to receive injections of octreotide and pegvisomant, rather than taking the drugs orally?

■ **4.** Why does GR have to be monitored with serial MRI and liver function tests while taking pegvisomant?

HYPOTHALAMIC AND PITUITARY PHYSIOLOGY

RELATIONSHIP BETWEEN THE HYPOTHALAMUS AND PITUITARY GLAND

From a developmental perspective, the pituitary gland consists of two closely associated organs. The **anterior pituitary** (adenohypophysis) is derived from ectodermal tissue. The **posterior pituitary** (neurohypophysis) is a neural struc-

ture derived from the ventral surface of the diencephalon. The prefixes adeno- and neuro- denote the buccal ectodermal and neural ectodermal origin of the anterior and posterior pituitary gland components, respectively. An intermediate lobe also exists in most mammals but is vestigial in humans.

Although the anterior and posterior pituitary glands derive from different embryologic origins, the hypothalamus controls the activity of both lobes. The mode of connection between hypothalamus and pituitary gland is one of the most important points of interaction between the nervous and endocrine systems. The hypothalamus acts as a neuroendocrine transducer by integrating neural signals from the brain and converting those signals into chemical messages (largely peptides) that regulate the secretion of pituitary hormones. The pituitary hormones in turn alter the activities of peripheral endocrine organs.

Hypothalamic control of the anterior pituitary gland occurs via hypothalamic secretion of hormones into the **hypothalamic–pituitary portal vascular system** (Fig. 25-1). The initial capillary bed of this portal system is formed from branches of the superior hypophyseal artery that fan around the neurons of the hypothalamus. Endothelial fenestrations in this capillary bed allow hypothalamic factors to be re-

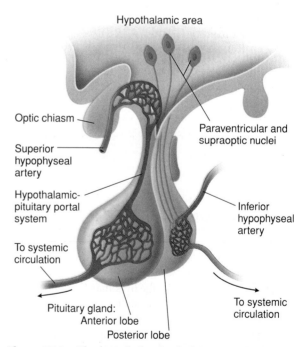

Figure 25-1. The hypothalamic-pituitary portal system. Neurons in the hypothalamus release regulatory factors that are carried by the hypothalamic–pituitary portal system to the anterior pituitary gland, where they control the release of the anterior pituitary hormones. The posterior pituitary hormones are synthesized in cell bodies of the supraoptic and paraventricular neurons in the hypothalamus, and then transported down axonal pathways to terminals in the posterior pituitary gland. These hormones are stored in the posterior pituitary gland, from which they are released into the systemic circulation. Note the separate vascular supplies to the anterior and posterior lobes of the pituitary gland.

leased into the bloodstream. These capillaries then coalesce into short veins that extend to the anterior pituitary gland. Upon arriving at the anterior pituitary, the veins branch into a second capillary bed and bathe the endocrine cells of the anterior pituitary gland with hormones secreted by the hypothalamus.

A direct neural connection exists between the hypothalamus and posterior pituitary gland. Neurons in the hypothalamus synthesize hormones, destined for storage in the posterior pituitary gland, in cell bodies of the supraoptic and paraventricular nuclei. These hormones are then transported down axons to the posterior pituitary gland, where they are stored in neuronal terminals until a release stimulus occurs. The posterior pituitary gland can, therefore, be thought of as an extension of the hypothalamus. As with the anterior pituitary gland, the endothelial cells surrounding the posterior pituitary gland are fenestrated; this facilitates release of hormones into the systemic circulation.

The anterior pituitary gland is a heterogeneous collection of numerous cell types, each of which has the capacity to respond to specific stimuli and consequently release specific hormones into the systemic circulation. There are a number of hypothalamic releasing or inhibiting factors, each of which alters the hormone secretion pattern of one or more anterior pituitary gland cell types (Table 25-1). Releasing factors also modify other cellular processes in the anterior pituitary gland, including hormone synthesis and pituitary cell growth. Interestingly, *the relationship between hypothalamic-releasing factors and pituitary gland hormones is not always 1:1, nor is the interaction always stimulatory.* Somatostatin, for example, primarily inhibits the release of growth hormone (GH), but it can also inhibit release of thyroid stimulating hormone (TSH) and prolactin. Conversely, thyrotropin-releasing hormone (TRH) primarily stimulates the release of TSH, but it can also cause release of prolactin. The overlapping activities of some releasing factors and release-inhibiting factors, together with the antagonistic actions of some stimulatory and inhibitory hypothalamic factors, provide a mechanism for the precise regulation of secretory pathways.

With the exception of dopamine, all known hypothalamic-releasing factors are peptides. The anterior pituitary gland hormones are proteins and glycoproteins. Anterior pituitary gland hormones fall into three groups. Somatotropic hormones, consisting of GH and **prolactin,** are 191 and 198 amino acids long, respectively, and exist as monomeric proteins. Glycoprotein hormones, consisting of **lutenizing hormone** (LH), **follicle-stimulating hormone** (FSH) and **thyroid-stimulating hormone** (TSH), are heterodimeric proteins with carbohydrates attached to certain residues. **Adrenocorticotropin** (ACTH) belongs to a separate class, as it is processed by proteolysis from a larger precursor protein. Of importance, intact peptides and proteins are not absorbed across the intestinal lumen; local proteases digest them into their constituent amino acids. For this reason, therapeutic administration of a peptide hormone or hormone antagonist, as in GR's case, must be accomplished by a non-oral route or by an orally available nonpeptide analogue of the natural hormone.

The anterior pituitary gland response to a hypothalamic factor is signaled through binding of the hypothalamic factor to specific G protein-coupled receptors located on the plasma membrane of the appropriate anterior pituitary cell type. Most of these receptors alter the levels of intracellular cAMP or IP_3 and calcium (see Chapter 1, Drug–Receptor Interactions). The molecular details of receptor signaling provide a basis for understanding hypothalamic factor action. For example, **growth hormone-releasing hormone** (GHRH) binding to receptors on somatotroph cells increases intracellular cAMP and Ca^{2+} levels, whereas somatostatin decreases intracellular levels of cAMP and Ca^{2+} in somatotrophs. This provides a biochemical explanation for the opposing activities of GHRH and somatostatin on somatotroph release of growth hormone.

The timing and pattern of hypothalamic factor release are important determinants of anterior pituitary cell response.

TABLE 25-1 **Anterior Pituitary Gland Cell Types, Hypothalamic Control Factors, and Hormonal Targets**

ANTERIOR PITUITARY GLAND CELL TYPE	STIMULATORY HYPOTHALAMIC FACTORS	INHIBITORY HYPOTHALAMIC FACTORS	PITUITARY HORMONES RELEASED	MAJOR TARGET ORGAN	TARGET GLAND HORMONES
Somatotroph	GHRH, Ghrelin	Somatostatin	GH	Liver	Insulin-like growth factors
Lactotroph	TRH	Dopamine, Somatostatin	Prolactin	Mammary gland	None
Gonadotroph	GnRH	None known	LH and FSH	Gonads	Estrogen, progesterone, and testosterone
Thyrotroph	TRH	Somatostatin	TSH	Thyroid gland	Thyroxine and triiodothyronine
Corticotroph	CRH	None known	ACTH	Adrenal cortex	Cortisol, adrenal androgens

Each anterior pituitary gland cell type responds to multiple hypothalamic stimulatory and inhibitory factors. Integration of these signals determines the relative extent of hormone release by the anterior pituitary gland. Each hormone has one or more specific target organs, which are, in turn, stimulated to release their own hormones. These target hormones cause feedback inhibition at the hypothalamus and anterior pituitary gland.

Most hypothalamic-releasing factors are secreted in a cyclical or pulsatile, rather than continuous, manner. For example, the hypothalamus releases pulses of gonadotropin-releasing hormone (GnRH) with a periodicity of a few hours. The frequency and magnitude of GnRH release determine the extent of pituitary gonadotropin release as well as the ratio of LH secretion to FSH secretion. Interestingly, continuous administration of GnRH suppresses rather than stimulates pituitary gonadotroph activity. These different pharmacologic effects of GnRH—depending on the frequency and pattern of administration—have important clinical consequences, as discussed below. Although not studied in as much detail, the majority of the other hypothalamic-releasing factors are also thought to be released in a pulsatile manner.

FEEDBACK INHIBITION

End-product inhibition tightly controls hypothalamic and pituitary gland hormone release. For each hypothalamic-pituitary–target organ system, an integrated picture can be constructed of how each set of hormones affects the system. Each pathway, including a hypothalamic factor(s), its pituitary gland target cell type, and the ultimate target gland(s), is referred to as an **endocrine axis**; the term *"axis"* is used to connote one of multiple homeostatic systems that the hypothalamus and pituitary gland control. A simplified model consists of five endocrine axes, with a single type of anterior pituitary gland cell at the center of each axis (Table 25-1).

Each axis regulates an important aspect of endocrine ho-

meostasis and is, therefore, subject to close regulation. Feedback inhibition is usually discussed in terms of loops, because the regulatory connection between a given hormone and its target creates a "loop" that alters the subsequent extent of hormone release. These loops, depending on the hormone and its target organ, are commonly referred to as *long loops, short loops,* and *ultrashort loops* (Fig. 25-2). The terminology is imprecise, figuratively indicating the relative distance a hormone must travel to the regulated organ. The long loop involves feedback regulation of a systemic hormone on the hypothalamus or pituitary gland. The short loop consists of pituitary hormone acting on the hypothalamus to alter release of hypothalamic factors. Ultrashort-loop feedback involves hypothalamic or pituitary hormones directly regulating the cells that secrete the hormone; ultrashort feedback is therefore synonymous with autocrine or paracrine signaling.

Just as regulatory loops are referred to based on a hormone's relationship to its target organ, many endocrine diseases are described based on whether the disease etiology is a disorder of the hypothalamus, pituitary gland, or target organ. *The disease is referred to as* primary, secondary, *or* tertiary, *depending on whether the underlying abnormality is in the target organ, pituitary gland, or hypothalamus, respectively.* Therefore, a primary endocrine disorder is caused by target organ pathology, a secondary disorder reflects pituitary disease, and a tertiary endocrine disorder results from hypothalamic pathology. Whether the underlying disease cause is primary, secondary, or tertiary can have important consequences for disease diagnosis and treatment, as discussed below.

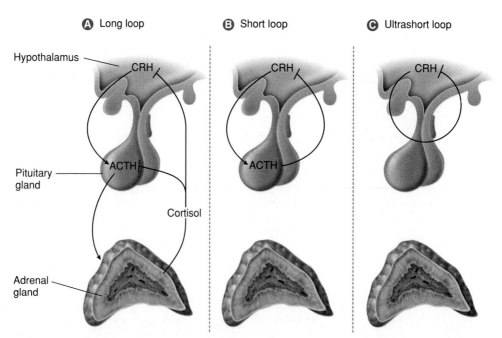

Figure 25-2. Hypothalamic-pituitary–target organ feedback. There are three general mechanisms of feedback regulation within the hypothalamic-pituitary–target organ axes, referred to as *long-loop, short-loop,* and *ultrashort-loop* feedback. Here, the hypothalamic-pituitary–adrenal axis is used to illustrate these concepts. **A.** In long-loop feedback, the target organ produces a hormone such as cortisol that, in addition to its physiologic actions on target tissues, inhibits anterior pituitary gland release of adrenocorticotropic hormone (ACTH) and hypothalamic release of corticotropin releasing hormone (CRH). **B.** In short-loop feedback, a hormone produced by the anterior pituitary gland, such as ACTH, inhibits hypothalamic release of its own releasing hormone, CRH. **C.** In ultrashort-loop feedback, the hormone produced by the hypothalamus negatively regulates itself; for example, CRH inhibits further CRH release.

PHYSIOLOGY, PATHOPHYSIOLOGY, AND PHARMACOLOGY OF INDIVIDUAL AXES

ANTERIOR PITUITARY GLAND

Hypothalamic-Pituitary–Growth Hormone Axis

The hypothalamic-pituitary–growth hormone axis regulates a number of general processes promoting growth. Growth hormone is first expressed at high concentrations during puberty; growth hormone secretion is pulsatile during this time, with the largest pulses usually occurring at night during sleep. Most of the anabolic effects of growth hormone are mediated by insulin-like growth factors, especially **insulin-like growth factor 1** (IGF-1), a hormone released by hepatocytes in response to stimulation by growth hormone.

Growth hormone secretion is enhanced by GHRH and inhibited by somatostatin. A second endogenous growth hormone-releasing peptide, **ghrelin,** promotes somatotroph secretion of growth hormone by stimulating the growth hormone secretagogue receptor (GH-S receptor), a receptor that is distinct from the GHRH receptor. Ghrelin and GHRH act synergistically on growth hormone release. The majority of ghrelin is secreted by gastric fundal cells during the fasting state, and increasing evidence suggests that ghrelin may be a key regulator of energy balance. Nonpeptide orally active ghrelin mimetics are currently under clinical investigation as growth hormone secretagogues, and antagonists are being studied for appetite control.

Pathophysiology and Pharmacology of Growth Hormone Deficiency

Failure to secrete growth hormone or to enhance IGF-1 secretion during puberty results in growth retardation (Fig. 25-3). Growth hormone deficiency most commonly results from defective hypothalamic release of GHRH (tertiary disease) or pituitary insufficiency (secondary disease). Importantly, however, failure of IGF-1 secretion in response to growth hormone (Laron dwarfism) is one etiology of short stature that is not amenable to treatment with growth hormone. **Sermorelin** (synthetic GHRH) can be administered parenterally to determine the disease etiology. If a patient possesses defective hypothalamic release of GHRH but normally functioning anterior pituitary gland somatotrophs, administration of exogenous GHRH results in increased GH release.

Most cases of growth hormone-dependent growth retardation are treated with replacement **recombinant human growth hormone**, referred to by the generic name **somatropin**. A congener of somatropin, referred to as **somatrem**, is chemically identical apart from an additional N-terminus methionine. Typical dosing schedules involve subcutaneous or intramuscular injection three times a week. To overcome this inconvenience, alternative delivery methods for growth hormone have been developed, including a slow-release depot injection of growth hormone that requires injection only once per month. Currently, however, this formulation

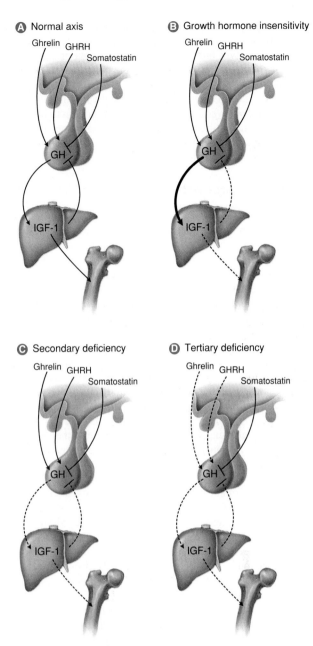

Figure 25-3. Hypothalamic-pituitary–growth hormone axis in health and disease. A. In the normal hypothalamic-pituitary–growth hormone axis, hypothalamic secretion of growth hormone-releasing hormone (GHRH) or ghrelin stimulates release of growth hormone (GH), while somatostatin inhibits release of GH. Secreted growth hormone then stimulates the liver to synthesize and secrete insulin-like growth factor I (IGF-1), which promotes bone growth. IGF-1 also inhibits GH release from the anterior pituitary gland. **B.** In growth hormone insensitivity, the anterior pituitary gland secretes growth hormone, but the liver is unresponsive to stimulation by growth hormone. As a result, IGF-1 is not secreted (indicated by dashed lines). The decreased feedback inhibition of GH release results in higher plasma levels of GH (thick line). **C.** In secondary deficiency, the pathology lies in an unresponsive anterior pituitary gland, which does not secrete growth hormone. Because GH levels are low, the liver is not stimulated to produce IGF-1. **D.** In tertiary deficiency, the hypothalamus does not secrete GHRH (dashed line); the role of ghrelin in this condition is unknown. Lack of GHRH results in lack of stimulation of GH secretion by the anterior pituitary gland and, therefore, diminished production of IGF-1.

is not being produced commercially, because it causes local reactions at the injection site. Orally bioavailable peptidomimetics of growth hormone are an active area of research.

Recombinant IGF-1, known by the generic name **mecasermin**, is an effective treatment for patients with growth hormone insensitivity (so-called Laron dwarfism). Mecasermin is also approved for use in patients with growth hormone deficiency and antibodies against growth hormone. Mecasermin administration is associated with hypoglycemia and rare intracranial hypertension.

Pathophysiology and Pharmacology of Growth Hormone Excess

Growth hormone excess usually results from a somatotroph adenoma. This entity has two differing disease presentations, depending on whether the growth hormone excess occurs before or after closure of the bone epiphyses. Gigantism occurs if growth hormone is secreted at abnormally high levels before closure of the epiphyses, because increased IGF-1 levels will promote excessive longitudinal bone growth. After the epiphyses close, abnormally high levels of growth hormone result in **acromegaly**, as illustrated in the introductory case. This condition occurs because IGF-1, although it can no longer stimulate long bone growth, can still promote growth of deep organs and cartilaginous tissue. Typical manifestations include the nonspecific symptoms that GR originally experienced, such as increased hand thickness, enlarging shoe size, and fatigue. Other frequent findings include large facial structures, macroglossia, and hepatomegaly.

Standard treatment for a somatotroph adenoma is transsphenoidal surgical removal of the tumor. As seen with the case of GR, surgical treatment has variable success, and adjuvant medical therapy is frequently required. Medical options include somatostatin analogues, dopamine agonists, and GH receptor antagonists.

Somatostatin physiologically inhibits growth hormone secretion, making it a logical therapy for somatotroph adenomas. Somatostatin itself is rarely used clinically, however, because it has a half-life of only a few minutes. **Octreotide** is a synthetic long-acting peptide analogue of somatostatin that has been shown to decrease pituitary adenoma growth in acromegalic patients. A similar synthetic analogue of somatostatin, **lanreotide**, is available in Europe. Because somatostatin and its analogues affect numerous secretory processes, octreotide can be used for several indications, including treatment of esophageal varices and certain hormone-secreting tumors. The mechanism by which octreotide ameliorates esophageal varices is unknown, but is thought to involve selective vasoconstriction of arteriolar sphincters in the splanchnic circulation. Systemic administration of octreotide can lead to adverse effects, including nausea and decreased gastrointestinal motility. A sustained-release formulation of octreotide, as exemplified in the introductory case, allows less frequent dosing but does not appear to alter the adverse effect profile.

Although dopamine stimulates GH release under physiologic conditions, patients with acromegaly have a paradoxical decrease in growth hormone secretion in response to dopamine. Based on this observation, the dopamine analogues **bromocriptine** and **cabergoline** are sometimes used

as adjunctive agents in the treatment of acromegaly. These agents are discussed below, in relation to the hypothalamic-pituitary–prolactin axis.

Pegvisomant is a GH analogue that has been modified to bind to the transmembrane GH receptor without activating subsequent intracellular signaling; it is therefore a competitive antagonist of GH activity. Pegvisomant also contains multiple polyethylene glycol (PEG) residues; this chemical modification prolongs the half-life of pegvisomant and thereby allows once-daily dosing of the drug. In clinical trials, pegvisomant significantly decreased serum IGF-1 levels. GH levels increase by one- to two-fold during pegvisomant therapy, due to decreased IGF-mediated inhibition of GH secretion. In a small percentage of patients, the underlying pituitary adenoma may increase in size during pegvisomant therapy, necessitating yearly monitoring by MRI. Liver function tests should also be monitored periodically, since some patients may have elevations in serum aminotransferase levels. Expanded applications of pegvisomant are currently being investigated, including possible use in preventing the late complications of diabetes mellitus, some of which may be mediated by GH.

Hypothalamic-Pituitary–Prolactin Axis

Lactotrophs of the anterior pituitary gland produce and secrete prolactin. Their activity is decreased in response to hypothalamic secretion of **dopamine**. TRH can enhance prolactin release. Unlike other cells of the anterior pituitary gland, lactotrophs are under tonic inhibition by the hypothalamus, presumably mediated by hypothalamic release of dopamine. *Therefore, a disease condition that interrupts the hypothalamic–pituitary portal system results in decreased secretion of most anterior pituitary gland hormones but causes increased prolactin release.* In patients taking phenothiazine antipsychotics (see Chapter 12, Pharmacology of Dopaminergic Neurotransmission), elevations of prolactin are frequently observed because these agents are dopamine receptor antagonists. Because prolactin does not stimulate secretion of hormones in its target, the mammary gland, prolactin secretion is not regulated by a negative feedback system.

The physiologic actions of prolactin involve regulation of mammary gland development and milk protein biosynthesis and secretion. Prolactin levels are normally low in men and nonpregnant women. Increased estrogen levels during pregnancy stimulate lactotroph cells of the anterior pituitary gland to secrete increasing quantities of prolactin. During pregnancy, however, estrogen antagonizes prolactin action in the breast; this prevents lactation until after parturition. Suckling provides a powerful neural stimulus for prolactin release; prolactin levels increase as much as 100-fold within 30 minutes after the initiation of breast feeding. If a mother does not breast feed, prolactin levels decrease over the course of several weeks.

Interestingly, increased prolactin levels suppress estrogen synthesis, both by antagonizing hypothalamic release of GnRH and by decreasing gonadotroph sensitivity to GnRH. This results in decreased LH and FSH release and, hence, decreased end-organ stimulation of the hypothalamic-pituitary–reproductive axis. This appears to be a physiologic mechanism to suppress ovulation while a woman is still breast-feeding. *Chronically high secretion of prolactin by a prolactinoma also suppresses the hypothalamic-pituitary–reproductive axis.* For this reason, prolactinomas are a common cause of infertility, especially in women.

Bromocriptine is a synthetic dopamine receptor agonist that inhibits lactotroph cell growth and is an established medical therapy for small prolactinomas (microadenomas). Bromocriptine is orally bioavailable. As with octreotide, many of the adverse effects of bromocriptine therapy result from systemic actions of the drug. The adverse effects include nausea and vomiting, presumably because the area postrema in the medulla, which stimulates nausea, possesses receptors for dopamine. Other members of the class of dopamine receptor agonists include **pergolide** and **cabergoline. Quinoglide** is a structurally similar agent available in Europe. Cabergoline, because it differs structurally from the other dopamine receptor agonists, may cause less nausea and vomiting than the other agents. Initial clinical studies also suggest that cabergoline may be more effective than bromocriptine at lowering prolactin levels, and that cabergoline may induce long-term remission of lactotroph adenomas.

Hypothalamic-Pituitary–Thyroid Axis

The hypothalamus secretes TRH, which stimulates thyrotrophs to produce and secrete TSH. TSH in turn promotes biosynthesis and secretion of thyroid hormone by the thyroid gland. Thyroid hormone regulates overall body energy homeostasis. Thyroid hormone negatively controls hypothalamic and pituitary release of TRH and TSH, respectively.

Because thyroid hormone replacement is an effective therapy for hypothyroidism, TRH and TSH are used mainly for diagnosis of disease etiology. If hypothyroidism is caused by an unresponsive thyroid gland, TSH levels will be high because of decreased negative feedback from thyroid hormone. If the anterior pituitary gland is unable to produce TSH in response to TRH, then pharmacologic administration of TSH should result in production and release of thyroid hormone. Finally, if the disorder is hypothalamic in origin (a tertiary endocrine disorder), addition of either exogenous TRH or exogenous TSH will stimulate increased plasma levels of thyroid hormone. Other aspects of thyroid gland pharmacology are discussed in Chapter 26, Pharmacology of the Thyroid Gland.

Hypothalamic-Pituitary–Adrenal Axis

Neurons from the paraventricular nucleus of the hypothalamus synthesize and secrete **corticotropin-releasing hormone** (CRH). After transport via the hypothalamic–pituitary portal system, CRH binds to cell surface receptors located on corticotrophs of the anterior pituitary gland. CRH binding stimulates corticotrophs to synthesize and release adrenocorticotropin-releasing hormone (ACTH). ACTH is synthesized as part of proopiomelanocortin (POMC), a precursor polypeptide that is cleaved into multiple effector molecules. In addition to ACTH, cleavage of POMC yields **melanocyte stimulating hormone** (MSH), **lipotropin,** and **β-endorphin.** MSH has effects on skin pigmentation, feeding behavior, and body weight. Because of the structural similarities between ACTH and MSH, high concentrations of ACTH can bind to and activate MSH receptors. This becomes im-

portant in primary hypoadrenalism, where increased ACTH levels result in enhanced skin pigmentation. Once secreted, ACTH binds to ACTH receptors located on cells of the adrenal cortex, especially in the zona fasciculata and zona reticularis of the cortex. ACTH stimulates the synthesis and secretion of adrenocortical steroid hormones, including glucocorticoids, androgens, and mineralocorticoids. The effect of ACTH on mineralocorticoid secretion is transient (sometimes called the "ACTH escape" phenomenon), but ACTH is required for secretion of glucocorticoids and adrenal androgens. ACTH also has a trophic effect on the zona fasciculata and zona reticularis; excessive ACTH secretion causes adrenal hyperplasia. The adrenal glucocorticoid cortisol is the main feedback inhibitor of pituitary ACTH release.

CRH is employed clinically to determine whether excessive cortisol secretion results from a pituitary adenoma or an adrenal tumor (ectopic or primary) (Fig. 25-4). If the hypercortisolism derives from a pituitary adenoma, administration of CRH will usually increase blood ACTH and cortisol levels. This response is not seen in the case of an ectopic tumor, which secretes ACTH at a constant autonomous rate. Likewise, ACTH levels will not increase after administration of CRH if a patient has a primary adrenal tumor, because the excess cortisol secretion suppresses the pituitary ACTH response to CRH.

A synthetic form of ACTH, known as **cosyntropin,** can be used to diagnose suspected cases of adrenal insufficiency; administration of cosyntropin to a patient with adrenal insufficiency will fail to increase plasma cortisol concentration. Conditions requiring physiologic replacement of glucocorticoids are usually treated with synthetic analogues of cortisol, rather than ACTH, because use of the target hormone generally allows for more precise physiologic control. Cortisol physiology and pharmacology are discussed in Chapter 27, Pharmacology of the Adrenal Cortex.

Hypothalamic-Pituitary–Reproductive Axis

Gonadotrophs are unique among anterior pituitary gland cells because they secrete two glycoprotein hormones: LH and FSH; together, these hormones are referred to as *gonadotropins.* LH and FSH are both heterodimers composed of α and β subunits. LH and FSH share the same α subunit, but possess different β subunits. Gonadotrophs regulate the secretion of FSH and LH independently. This axis is diagrammed in Figure 25-5.

Once secreted, gonadotropins control hormone production by the gonads, promoting the synthesis of androgens and estrogens. Gonadotrophs are then feedback-inhibited by testosterone and estrogen. The effects of estrogen on the anterior pituitary gland are complex. Depending on the rate of change and absolute concentration of estrogen, as well as the stage of the menstrual cycle, both inhibitory and excitatory effects can be produced. **Inhibin** and **activin** are two hormones secreted by the ovary that appear to have inhibitory and releasing effects, respectively, on FSH but not LH secretion. Endocrine control of the reproductive process is discussed in greater detail in Chapter 28, Pharmacology of Reproduction.

Peptide GnRH analogues with short half-lives can be administered in a pulsatile fashion to stimulate patterned gonadotropin release, while analogues with longer half-lives

Ⓐ Normal axis   **Ⓑ** Primary adrenal tumor

Ⓒ Pituitary adenoma   **Ⓓ** Ectopic ACTH-secreting tumor

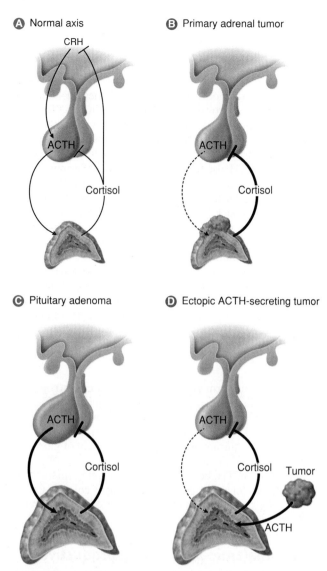

Figure 25-4. Use of CRH to determine the cause of excess cortisol secretion. A. In the normal hypothalamic-pituitary–adrenal axis, hypothalamic secretion of corticotropin releasing hormone (CRH) stimulates release of adrenocorticotropic hormone (ACTH). ACTH, in turn, stimulates synthesis and secretion of cortisol by the adrenal cortex. Cortisol then inhibits further release of CRH and ACTH. **B.** A primary adrenal tumor autonomously produces cortisol *(thick line)*, independent of regulation by ACTH. Administration of CRH will not increase ACTH and cortisol levels because the excessive cortisol produced by the tumor suppresses anterior pituitary gland responsiveness to CRH *(dashed line)*. **C.** An adenoma (tumor) in the anterior pituitary gland autonomously secretes excessive levels of ACTH *(thick line)*, which stimulate the adrenal gland to produce increased levels of cortisol *(thick line)*. Although ACTH secretion by the tumor may not be sensitive to feedback inhibition by cortisol, the pituitary adenoma may be sensitive to CRH administration. In this case, administration of CRH stimulates an acute rise in ACTH and cortisol levels. **D.** An ectopic ACTH-secreting tumor (such as a small cell carcinoma of the lung) also stimulates the adrenal gland to produce increased levels of cortisol. In this case, however, pituitary gland ACTH production is suppressed by the increased cortisol, and administration of CRH will not increase ACTH and cortisol levels.

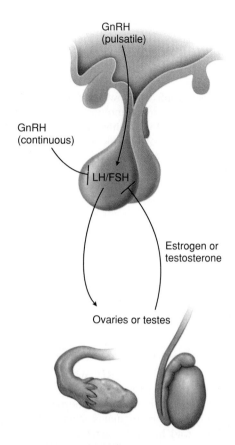

Figure 25-5. Effects of GnRH on the hypothalamic-pituitary–reproductive axis. Gonadotropin-releasing hormone (GnRH) is secreted by the hypothalamus in a pulsatile fashion, stimulating gonadotroph cells of the anterior pituitary gland to secrete luteinizing hormone (LH) and follicle-stimulating hormone (FSH). LH and FSH stimulate the ovaries or testes to produce the sex hormones estrogen or testosterone, respectively, which inhibit further release of LH and FSH. Exogenous pulsatile GnRH is used to induce ovulation in women with infertility of hypothalamic origin. Conversely, continuous administration of GnRH suppresses gonadotroph response to endogenous GnRH, and thereby causes decreased production of sex hormones. Analogues of GnRH with increased metabolic stability and prolonged half-lives take advantage of this effect, and are used to suppress sex hormone production in clinical conditions such as precocious puberty and prostate cancer.

are used to suppress production of sex hormones by desensitizing the pituitary gland to the stimulating activity of the releasing factor (Fig. 25-5). The main pharmacologic difference among the currently approved GnRH agonists is the method of administration. **Leuprolide** and **histrelin** are injected once daily; **nafarelin** is a nasal spray; **goserelin** is a depot injection administered once per month. Osmotic pump implants (see Chapter 54, Drug Delivery Modalities) are also available that deliver leuprolide acetate at a controlled rate for up to 12 months. Long-acting agonists are utilized therapeutically for treatment of several gonadotropin-dependent conditions, including endometriosis, uterine fibroids, precocious puberty, and androgen-dependent prostate cancer. Their main drawback is that gonadotroph suppression does not occur immediately; instead, there is a transient (several days) increase ("flare") in sex hormone levels, followed by a lasting suppression of hormone synthesis and secretion.

FSH is used clinically to stimulate ovulation for in vitro fertilization. Two formulations are available. **Urofollitropin** is purified FSH isolated from the urine of postmenopausal women, and **follitropin** is a recombinant form of FSH. Both agents effectively stimulate ovulation but may cause the **ovarian hyperstimulation syndrome.** Interestingly, a rare form of the ovarian hyperstimulation syndrome that occurs during pregnancy (familial gestational ovarian hyperstimulation syndrome) is caused by an inherited mutation in the FSH receptor. This mutation allows human chorionic gonadotropin (hCG), a hormone present in high concentrations during the early stages of pregnancy, to activate the FSH receptor. The resulting overstimulation of the FSH receptor is thought to cause the follicular enlargement and other sequelae characteristic of this syndrome. Whether similar mutations in the FSH receptor could be associated with cases of drug-induced ovarian hyperstimulation syndrome is an area of active investigation.

The GnRH antagonists **cetrorelix** and **ganirelix** are sometimes used during controlled ovarian stimulation. Administration of these agents in the early to mid-follicular phase of the menstrual cycle suppresses an early surge in LH, resulting in improved rates of implantation and pregnancy (see Chapter 28). A third GnRH antagonist, **abarelix**, is approved for palliation of metastatic prostate cancer in patients who have extensive metastases or tumor encroaching on the spinal cord. In this situation, a direct GnRH antagonist has the advantage of avoiding the initial surge in testosterone seen with GnRH agonists. Abarelix has been associated with cardiac QT interval prolongation, and care should be taken to avoid co-administration with other agents predisposing to QT prolongation (see Chapter 18, Pharmacology of Cardiac Rhythm).

POSTERIOR PITUITARY GLAND

In comparison to the numerous hormones of the anterior pituitary gland, the posterior lobe of the pituitary gland (neurohypophysis) secretes only two hormones, antidiuretic hormone (ADH) and oxytocin. ADH is an important regulator of plasma volume and osmolarity, whereas oxytocin has physiologic effects on uterine contraction and lactation.

Antidiuretic Hormone (ADH)

ADH is a peptide hormone produced by magnocellular cells of the hypothalamus. Cells in this region possess osmoreceptors that are able to sense changes in extracellular osmolarity. Increased osmolarity stimulates ADH secretion from nerve terminals in the posterior pituitary gland. ADH binds to two types of receptors, V_1 and V_2. V_1 receptors, located in systemic arterioles, mediate vasoconstriction. This property gives ADH its alternative name, vasopressin. V_2 receptors, located in the nephron, stimulate the cell surface expression of water channels in order to increase water reabsorption in the collecting duct, as discussed in Chapter 20, Pharmacology of Volume Regulation. These two actions of ADH combine to maintain vascular tone by: (1) increasing blood pressure; and (2) increasing water reabsorption.

Disruption of ADH homeostasis results in two important pathophysiologic conditions. Excessive secretion of ADH causes the **syndrome of inappropriate ADH** (SIADH); deficient secretion of ADH or decreased responsiveness to ADH causes diabetes insipidus. In SIADH, ADH secretion occurs irrespective of plasma volume status or osmolality. One of the most common causes of SIADH is the ectopic secretion of ADH by small cell carcinoma of the lung. This results in persistent stimulation of V_1 and V_2 receptors, causing hypertension and excessive fluid retention. The inappropriate fluid retention can result in significant edema and low extracellular sodium concentration. If the source of excess ADH cannot be removed, the only effective therapy for SIADH is restriction of fluid intake or administration of hypertonic saline. There are currently no pharmacologic agents that antagonize ADH action specifically; development of such a drug could be a potentially valuable therapy for SIADH. **Demeclocycline** (a tetracycline antibiotic: see Chapter 32, Pharmacology of Bacterial Infections) and **lithium** (possibly acting on aquaporin-2) are the two pharmacologic treatments currently used to treat SIADH. Their mechanisms of action are not well understood, however, and use of these agents is limited by their nonspecific actions and potential for adverse effects. For example, lithium has a narrow therapeutic index and may cause irreversible renal damage (see Chapter 13, Pharmacology of Central Adrenergic and Serotonergic Neurotransmission).

Both **diabetes insipidus** and diabetes mellitus are characterized by symptoms of thirst, polydipsia, and polyuria. Despite their phenotypic similarities, however, the etiologies of diabetes mellitus and diabetes insipidus are unrelated. Diabetes insipidus is a disorder of vasopressin secretion or response, whereas diabetes mellitus is caused by deficient production of insulin or target tissue insensitivity to insulin (see Chapter 29, Pharmacology of the Endocrine Pancreas). A distinction is made between two types of diabetes insipidus. **Neurogenic diabetes insipidus** results from an inability of hypothalamic neurons to synthesize or secrete ADH (Fig. 25-6). **Nephrogenic diabetes insipidus** results from an inability of renal collecting duct cells to respond to ADH. Nephrogenic diabetes insipidus is usually caused by a mutation in the V_2 receptor, such that ADH is unable to bind the receptor or stimulate receptor signaling. Neurogenic diabetes insipidus can be treated with **desmopressin,** an ADH analogue that selectively stimulates V_2 receptors. Because the drug has little cross-reactivity with V_1 receptors, it does not increase blood pressure as ADH administration could. Overdosage with desmopressin can result in hyponatremia, caused by excessive water reabsorption by the nephron. There is currently no specific pharmacologic treatment for nephrogenic diabetes insipidus; patients are typically treated by restriction of fluid intake or given diuretics to prevent excessive dilution of the urine. A hypothetical pharmacologic therapy for nephrogenic diabetes insipidus might consist of a compound that directly stimulates expression of water channels in the renal collecting duct and thereby bypasses the nonfunctional V_2 receptor.

Because heart failure is often associated with water retention, consideration is now being given to the development and use of vasopressin antagonists as adjuncts to treatment with beta-adrenergic blockers, angiotensin converting enzyme inhibitors, and aldosterone antagonists (see Chapter

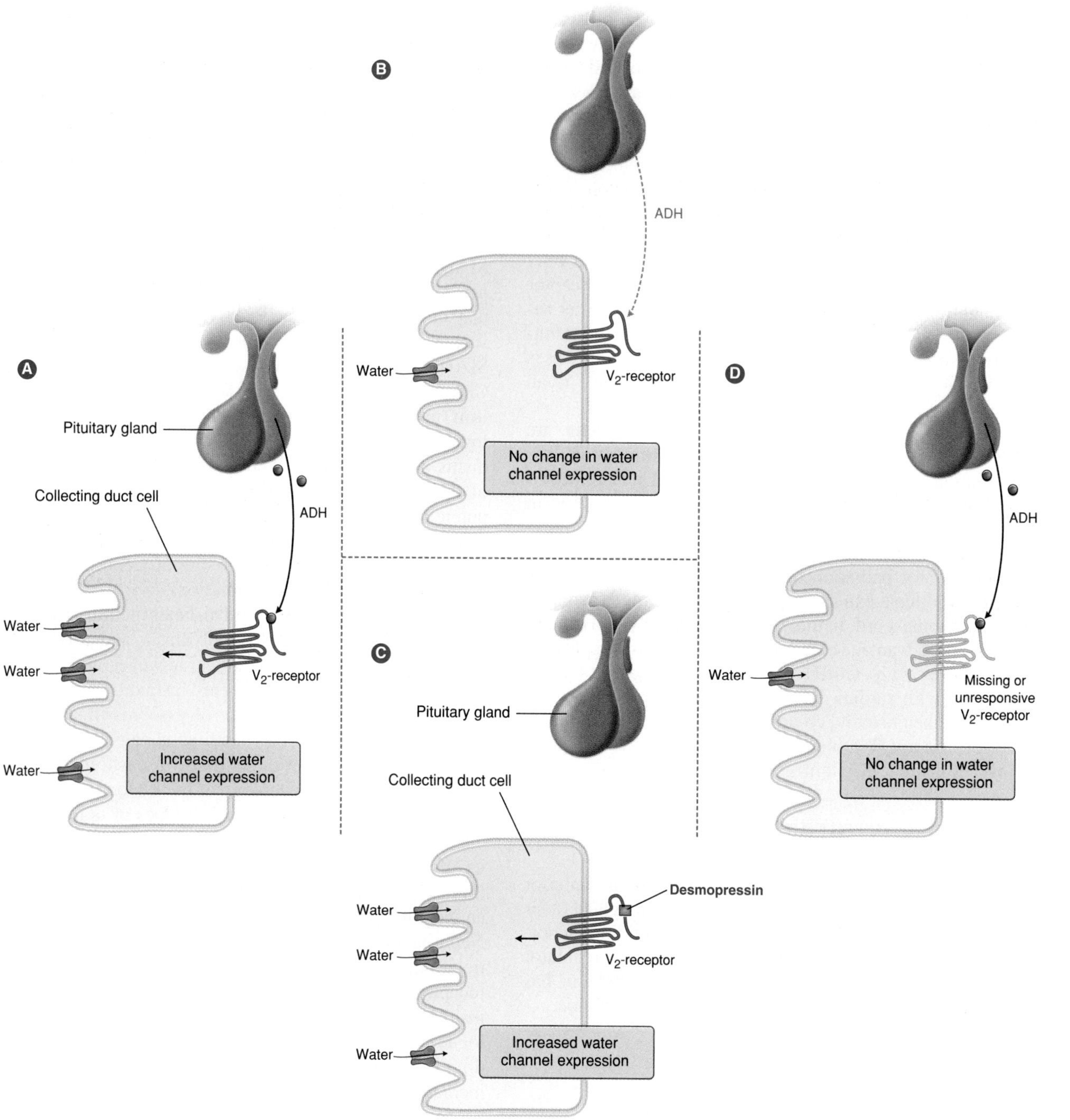

Figure 25-6. Comparison of neurogenic and nephrogenic diabetes insipidus. A. Antidiuretic hormone (ADH), released by nerve terminals in the posterior pituitary gland, stimulates V_2 receptors on renal collecting duct cells, and thereby increases expression of water channels in the apical membrane of these cells. Increased water channel expression increases the water flux through the cell, and the increased water reabsorption helps to maintain extracellular fluid volume. **B.** In neurogenic diabetes insipidus, the posterior pituitary gland is unable to secrete ADH. Consequently, there is no stimulation of renal V_2 receptors by ADH, and the collecting duct cells do not increase water channel expression. **C.** Exogenous administration of desmopressin, an ADH analogue, can replace the deficiency of posterior pituitary gland-derived ADH, and thereby treat neurogenic diabetes insipidus. **D.** In nephrogenic diabetes insipidus, the V_2 receptor gene is mutated and the V_2 receptor is either missing or unresponsive to stimulation by ADH. The lack of functional V_2 receptors prevents the cell from responding to ADH with an increase in water channel expression. There is currently no specific pharmacologic intervention for treatment of nephrogenic diabetes insipidus.

24, Integrative Cardiovascular Pharmacology). The vasopressin antagonist **conivaptan** was recently approved for the treatment of euvolemic hyponatremia, and this drug is under consideration as a treatment for hyponatremia associated with heart failure.

Oxytocin

Oxytocin is a peptide hormone produced by paraventricular cells of the hypothalamus. Many of the known physiologic roles of oxytocin involve muscular contraction; two such effects are milk release during lactation and uterine contraction. In the milk letdown response, stimuli to the hypothalamus cause oxytocin release into the blood from nerve terminals in the posterior pituitary gland. Oxytocin causes contraction of myoepithelial cells surrounding the mammary gland alveoli. This is an important physiologic action during breast feeding. In addition, it has long been known that administration of oxytocin causes uterine contraction. Oxytocin release is probably not the physiologic stimulus for initiation of labor during pregnancy; however, oxytocin is used pharmacologically to induce labor artificially.

Conclusion and Future Directions

Hormones of the hypothalamus and pituitary gland can be used as pharmacologic agents to modify the respective endocrine axes of each hormone. Hypothalamic hormones can be used to determine the causes of underlying endocrine pathology diagnostically (CRH, GHRH, TRH), or to suppress an axis (GnRH, somatostatin). Hormones of the anterior pituitary gland can be given as replacement therapy in cases of deficiency (growth hormone), or used diagnostically (ACTH, TSH). The posterior pituitary gland produces two hormones, ADH and oxytocin, which can be used for treatment of neurogenic diabetes insipidus and to induce labor, respectively. Future directions in hypothalamic and pituitary gland pharmacology will include: design of new drug delivery systems, such as nasal growth hormone secretagogue sprays; synthesis of orally active, nonpeptide analogues of hypothalamic hormones; development of ghrelin antagonists; and new pharmacologic interventions for nephrogenic diabetes insipidus. The hypothalamus is also a promising therapeutic target for new drugs to control appetite and craving disorders.

Suggested Reading

Goldsmith SR, Gheorghiade M. Vasopressin antagonism in heart failure. *J Am Coll Cardiol* 2005;46:1785–1791. (*Information regarding experimental vasopressin antagonists.*)

Kojima M, Kangawa K. Ghrelin: structure and function. *Physiol Rev* 2005;85:495–522. (*Review of recent developments in ghrelin and GHS-R research.*)

Schlechte JA. Prolactinoma. *N Engl J Med* 2003;349:2035–2041. (*Clinical information on prolactinomas.*)

Surya S, Barkan AL. GH receptor antagonist: mechanism of action and clinical utility. *Rev Endocr Metab Disord* 2005;6:5–13. (*Excellent discussion of new treatments for acromegaly.*)

Drug Summary Table   **Chapter 25 Pharmacology of the Hypothalamus and Pituitary Gland**

Drug	Clinical Applications	Serious and Common Adverse Effects	Contraindications	Therapeutic Considerations
GROWTH HORMONE AND INSULIN-LIKE GROWTH FACTOR REPLACEMENT				
Mechanism—Stimulate release of or replace growth hormone or insulin-like growth factor				
Somatropin Somatrem (GH)	Growth failure in children with GH deficiency, Turner's syndrome, Prader-Willi syndrome, and chronic kidney disease Idiopathic short stature Replacement of endogenous GH in adults with GH deficiency AIDS wasting or cachexia	*Leukemia, increased intracranial pressure, pancreatitis, rapid growth of melanocytic lesions* Hyperglycemia, peripheral edema, injection site reaction, arthralgia, headache	Patients with closed epiphyses Active underlying intracranial lesion Active malignancy Proliferative diabetic retinopathy	Caution in diabetes and in children whose GH deficiency results from an intracranial lesion Available as depot injection Glucocorticoids inhibit growth-promoting effect of somatropin
Sermorelin (GHRH)	Diagnostic evaluation of ↓ plasma growth hormone Treatment of GH deficiency GH therapy in children with tertiary (hypothalamic) deficiency	Transient flushing, chest tightness, injection site reaction, antibody development	Do not use with another drug that affects pituitary gland	Caution in children whose GH deficiency results from an intracranial lesion
Hexarelin Ghrelin	Investigational	Flushing, weight gain, drowsiness	Undetermined	Experimental agents that bind to GH-secretagogue receptor Hexarelin formulations available for intranasal use
Mecasermin	Laron dwarfism GH deficiency with neutralizing antibodies	*Hypoglycemia, slipped upper femoral epiphysis, raised intracranial pressure, seizure* Tonsillar hypertrophy, injection site reaction	Growth promotion in patients with closed epiphyses Suspected or active neoplasm	Recombinant IGF-1 Available as twice-daily and once-daily injections
AGENTS THAT DECREASE GROWTH HORMONE SECRETION OR ACTION				
Mechanism—Inhibit GHRH release, antagonize GH receptor (pegvisomant)				
Octreotide	Acromegaly Flushing and diarrhea from carcinoid tumors Carcinoid crisis Diarrhea from vasoactive intestinal peptide-secreting tumors	*Arrhythmias, bradycardia, hypoglycemia, gallstone formation* Abdominal pain, constipation, diarrhea, nausea, vomiting	Hypersensitivity to octreotide	Also used to control GI bleeding and to reduce secretory diarrhea Octreotide also available in depot formulation Decreases cyclosporine levels Lanreotide is a similar agent available in Europe
Somatostatin	VIPomas Carcinoid tumors Enterocutaneous and pancreatic fistulas Short-bowel syndrome	*Arrhythmias, erythroderma, life-threatening water retention* Glucose intolerance	Hypersensitivity to somatostatin	Upon discontinuation, may experience rebound hormonal hypersecretion Reduces analgesic effects of morphine
Pegvisomant	Acromegaly	*Increased pituitary adenoma size, elevated LFTs* Hypertension, peripheral edema, paresthesias, dizziness	Hypersensitivity to pegvisomant	Patients should have yearly MRI to exclude enlarging adenoma

AGENTS THAT DECREASE PROLACTIN LEVELS

Mechanism—Inhibit pituitary prolactin release

Bromocriptine	Amenorrhea and galactorrhea from hyperprolactinemia Acromegaly Parkinson's disease Premenstrual syndrome Cushing's syndrome Hepatic encephalopathy Neuroleptic malignant syndrome related to neuroleptic drug therapy	*Cerebral vascular accident, seizure, acute myocardial infarction* Dizziness, hypotension, abdominal cramps, nausea	Hypersensitivity to ergot derivatives Uncontrolled hypertension Toxemia of pregnancy	Ergot alkaloid; dose 2 ×/day Intravaginal administration may reduce gastrointestinal side effects Alcohol intolerance may occur First-dose phenomenon occurs in 1% of patients and may result in syncope Coadministration with amitriptyline, butyrophenones, imipramine, methyldopa, phenothiazines, or reserpine: increases prolactin levels Coadministration with antihypertensives potentiates hypotension
Pergolide Quinoglide Cabergoline	Parkinson's disease (pergolide and carbergoline) Hyperprolactinemia	*Arrhythmias, myocardial infarction, heart failure Pulmonary fibrosis and pleural effusion (cabergoline)* Nausea, dizziness, dyskinesia, dystonia, hallucinations, somnolence, orthostatic hypotension, rhinitis	Hypersensitivity to ergot derivatives Uncontrolled hypertension	Use cautiously in patients prone to arrhythmias and underlying psychiatric disorders Use cautiously in patients with history of pleuritis, pleural effusion, pleural fibrosis, pericarditis, cardiac valvulopathy, or retroperitoneal fibrosis CNS depressants have additive effects Quinoglide and cabergoline are nonergots; quinoglide is not available in U.S.; cabergoline produces less nausea than bromocriptine or pergolide

AGENTS THAT TEST THYROID FUNCTION

Mechanism—TRH stimulates TSH release from pituitary; TSH stimulates thyroid gland

Protirelin (TRH)	Diagnosis of thyroid function	*Seizure, amaurosis fugax in patients with pituitary tumors* Anxiety, diaphoresis, hyper- and hypotension		Transient changes in blood pressure can occur immediately following administration Cyproheptadine and thioridazine ↓ protirelin-mediated TSH response
Thyrotropin (TSH)	Diagnosis of malignant tumor of thyroid gland	*Anaphylactoid reaction with repeated administration* Nausea, vomiting, asthenia, headache	Adrenal insufficiency Coronary thrombosis	

AGENTS THAT TEST ADRENAL FUNCTION

Mechanism—Stimulates adrenal cortisol and androgen production

| Corticotropin (ACTH) Cosyntropin (ACTH 1-24) | Diagnosis of adrenocortical function Exacerbation of multiple sclerosis Severe allergic reactions, collagen disorders, dermatologic disorders, inflammation Infantile spasms | *Increased intracranial pressure with papilledema, pseudotumor cerebri, seizures, heart failure, necrotizing vasculitis, shock, pancreatitis, peptic ulceration with perforation, hypokalemic alkalosis, induction of latent diabetes mellitus, bronchospasm* Dizziness | Patients with peptic ulcer, scleroderma, osteoporosis, systemic fungal infections, ocular herpes simplex, heart failure, hypertension, sensitivity to pork, recent surgery, adrenocortical hyperfunction or primary insufficiency, or Cushing's syndrome | Cosyntropin (contains first 24 amino acid residues of ACTH) is less antigenic and less likely to cause allergic reactions than corticotropin (contains all 39 amino acid residues of ACTH) Patients with suspected sensitivity to porcine proteins should undergo skin testing Observe neonates of corticotropin-treated women for signs of hypoadrenalism Counteract edema by low-sodium, high-potassium intake Coadministration with NSAIDS increases risk of GI bleeding Corticotropin increases plasma level of digoxin |

(Continued)

Drug Summary Table **Chapter 25 Pharmacology of the Hypothalamus and Pituitary Gland** (*Continued*)

Drug	Clinical Applications	Serious and Common Adverse Effects	Contraindications	Therapeutic Considerations
AGENTS THAT ALTER GONADOTROPIN EXPRESSION				
Mechanism (all except GnRH receptor antagonists)—Continuous: inhibit LH and FSH release; Pulsatile: stimulate LH and FSH release				
Mechanism (ganirelix, cetrorelix, abarelix)—GnRH receptor antagonists				
Gonadorelin	Diagnosis of hypogonadism Stimulate ovulation	*Anaphylaxis with multiple administrations* Lightheadedness, flushing, headache		Normal response to gonadorelin testing indicates the presence of functional pituitary gonadotropes Pulsatile form for stimulation of ovulation
Goserelin Histrelin Leuprolide Nafarelin	All 4 agents can be used in: Breast cancer Prostate cancer Endometriosis Precocious puberty Acute intermittent porphyria	*Deep venous thrombosis (goserelin, leuprolide) Pituitary apoplexy (leuprolide)* Hot flashes, gynecomastia, osteoporosis, transient pain, sexual dysfunction	Hypersensitivity to LHRH or LHRH analogues Pregnancy	Depot formulations that result in gonadotropin suppression and consequent ↓ gonadal steroids Can initially increase testosterone and estrogen levels
Follitropin (rFSH) Urofollitropin (FSH)	Ovulation induction Male hypogonadotropic hypogonadism	*Embolism and thrombosis, acute respiratory distress syndrome, ovarian hyperstimulation syndrome* Ovarian cysts and hypertrophy, upper respiratory infection	Any endocrine disorder other than anovulation: abnormal uterine bleeding, primary gonadal failure, pituitary tumor, ovarian cyst or enlargement of unknown origin, pregnancy, sex-hormone dependent tumors, thyroid or adrenal dysfunction	May result in multiple fetuses
Ganirelix Cetrorelix Abarelix	Ovulation induction (ganirelix and cetrorelix) Prostate cancer (abarelix)	*QT interval prolongation (abarelix) Ectopic pregnancy, thrombotic disorder, spontaneous abortion (ganirelix) Anaphylaxis (cetrorelix)* Ovarian hyperstimulation syndrome	Pregnancy, lactation, ovarian cysts or enlargement not due to polycystic ovarian syndrome, primary ovarian failure, sex-hormone dependent tumors, thyroid or adrenal dysfunction, vaginal bleeding of unknown etiology	These drugs are GnRH receptor antagonists
VASOPRESSIN ANTAGONISTS				
Mechanism—Mixed V1/V2 receptor antagonists				
Conivaptan Tolvaptan	Euvolemic hyponatremia Heart failure (investigational)	Hypertension, orthostatic hypotension, injection site reaction, hypokalemia, increased thirst, polyuria	Concurrent use of potent P450 3A4 inhibitors Hypovolemic hyponatremia	Because conivaptan is a P450 3A4 substrate, it is contraindicated to use this drug concurrently with P450 3A4 inhibitors such as ketoconazole, itraconazole, ritonavir, clarithromycin, and indinavir Tolvaptan is an investigational agent specific for V2 receptor

26

Pharmacology of the Thyroid Gland

Ehrin J. Armstrong, Armen H. Tashjian, Jr., and William W. Chin

INTRODUCTION

The thyroid gland has diverse and important effects on many aspects of metabolic homeostasis. **Follicular thyroid cells** constitute the majority of thyroid tissue; these cells produce and secrete the classical thyroid hormones: thyroxine (T4), triiodothyronine (T3), and reverse triiodothyronine (rT3). Thyroid hormones regulate growth, metabolism, and energy expenditure, from oxygen consumption to cardiac contractility. **Parafollicular C cells** of the thyroid gland secrete **calcitonin,** a minor regulator of bone mineral homeostasis. Calcitonin is discussed in Chapter 30, Pharmacology of Bone Mineral Homeostasis.

The major diseases of the thyroid gland involve disruption of the normal hypothalamic-pituitary–thyroid axis (see Chapter 25, Pharmacology of the Hypothalamus and Pituitary Gland). Replacement of deficient thyroid hormone is an effective and established therapy for hypothyroidism. Treatment of hyperthyroidism is more complex, with options ranging from antithyroid drugs to surgical excision of abnormal tissue. Understanding the pathways and mechanisms of feedback regulation of thyroid hormone synthesis and thyroid hormone actions serves to explain the rationale for effective drug treatment of thyroid diseases.

Case

Over the course of a few months, Diana L, 45 years old, notices a number of disconcerting changes in the way she feels and in her general appearance. Ms. L feels nervous all the time; small events make her jumpy. She also keeps the temperature unusually cold in her house, to the point where her husband and children begin to complain. Because of these symptoms and the occasional feeling that her heart "skips a beat," Ms. L goes to see her doctor. After some questioning, he palpates her neck and notes that her thyroid gland is diffusely enlarged. He also notes that Ms. L's eyes are more prominent than normal. Tests for thyroid hormone levels reveal high serum free triiodothyronine (T3) and low thyrotropin (TSH). In addition, a test for TSH receptor antibody is positive. Ms. L is diagnosed with Graves' disease, a form of hyperthyroidism, and treated with methimazole. Although initially comforted by the fact that her doctor can explain her symptoms, she soon becomes discouraged because she does not notice any improvement for a couple of weeks. After a month, however, her symptoms begin to subside. Repeat tests confirm that her thyroid hormone levels are normalized. One year after starting treatment with methimazole, however, she begins to re-experience palpitations and feels anxious. Her doctor confirms that her thyroid hormone levels are again elevated, despite methimazole therapy. After discussion with her doctor, Ms. L elects to undergo treatment with radioactive iodide. She tolerates the treatment well, and testing over the next 3 years shows that she has normal thyroid hormone levels. However, 4 years after radioactive iodide treatment, she develops symptoms that are the opposite of her original problems: she feels tired and cold all the time, and she gains 30 pounds over the course of 6 months. Her doctor confirms that Ms. L has developed hypothyroidism. He prescribes thyroxine (T4), which she now takes once a day, and she feels well again.

QUESTIONS

■ **1.** Why was Ms. L's serum thyrotropin level low but her triiodothyronine concentration high?
■ **2.** What is the mechanism of action of methimazole? Why did methimazole eventually stop working?
■ **3.** What features of the thyroid gland make radioactive iodide a generally safe and specific therapy for hyperthyroidism?
■ **4.** Why did Ms. L develop hypothyroidism after treatment with radioactive iodide?

THYROID GLAND PHYSIOLOGY

SYNTHESIS AND SECRETION OF THYROID HORMONES

The thyroid is an endocrine gland located in the neck inferior to the larynx and spanning the ventral surface of the trachea. The main function of the thyroid gland is to produce the thyroid hormones, T3 and T4. Structurally, the thyroid hormones are built on a backbone of two tyrosine molecules that are iodinated and connected by an ether linkage (Fig. 26-1). An important structural feature of thyroid hormones is the placement of iodines on this backbone. The position and relative orientation of iodines attached to the tyrosine residues determine the specific form of thyroid hormone. **3,5,3′,5′-Tetraiodothyronine (thyroxine, T4)** has four iodines attached to the tyrosine backbones and is the major form of thyroid hormone secreted by the thyroid gland. **3,5,3′-Triiodothyronine (T3)** has three iodines. Most T3 is produced by peripheral 5′ deiodination of T4 (see below). A biologically inactive form of thyroid hormone is 3,3′,5′-triiodothyronine, also referred to as **reverse triiodothyronine (rT3)** because the single iodine is on the opposite tyrosine in the backbone relative to T3. In a normal individual, circulating thyroid hormone consists of about 90% T4, 9% T3, and 1% rT3, and most of the hormone is bound to plasma proteins (both specific binding proteins and albumin).

Iodide is a trace element that is a crucial component of thyroid hormone structure. Thyroid follicular cells, which synthesize and secrete thyroid hormones, selectively concen-

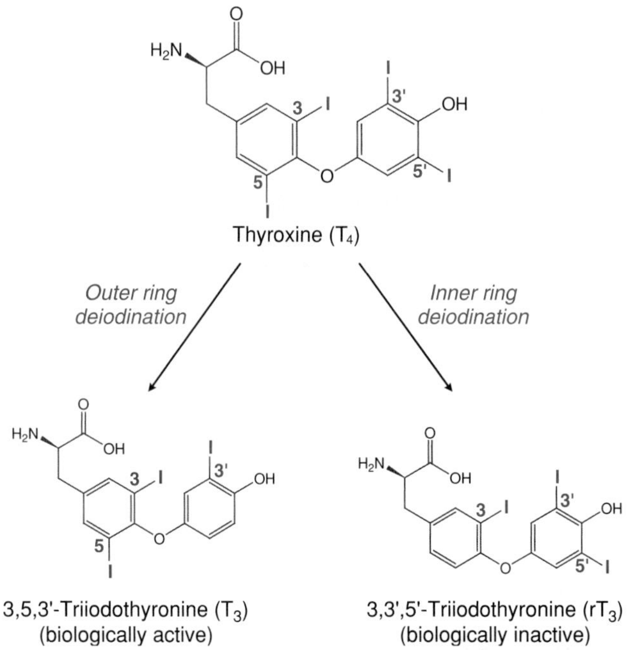

Figure 26-1.   Structure and peripheral metabolism of thyroid hormones. Thyroid hormones are synthesized from two derivatized tyrosine molecules that are attached by an ether linkage. The outer ring is hydroxylated, whereas the inner ring is linked covalently to thyroglobulin during thyroid hormone synthesis. Iodine is attached to three or four positions of the tyrosine backbone, creating several different substitution patterns. Thyroxine (T4) has four iodines attached, two on each ring. Thyroxine is the predominant thyroid hormone produced by the thyroid gland. Triiodothyronine (T3) has two iodines attached to the inner ring, but only one iodine attached to the outer ring. In contrast, reverse triiodothyronine (rT3) has two iodines on the outer ring, but only one iodine on the inner ring. During peripheral metabolism, thyroxine is deiodinated by 5′-deiodinases present in target tissues and in liver. The pattern of deiodination produces either T3 or rT3. If the iodine is removed from the outer ring, the biologically active T3 is produced. If the iodine is removed from the inner ring, the biologically inactive rT3 is produced.

trate iodide (I^-) via a Na^+/I^- symporter located on the basolateral membrane of the cell (Fig. 26-2). This active transport mechanism has the ability to concentrate iodide to intracellular concentrations up to 500 times that of plasma; most individuals have thyroid gland to plasma iodide ratios of approximately 30.

Once inside thyroid gland follicular cells, iodide is transported across the apical membrane of the cell and concurrently oxidized by the enzyme **thyroid peroxidase** (Fig. 26-2). This oxidation reaction creates a reactive iodide intermediate that couples to specific tyrosine residues on **thyroglobulin.** Thyroglobulin is a protein synthesized by thyroid follicular cells and secreted at the apical surface into the colloid space. Thyroid peroxidase is also concentrated at the apical surface, and it is thought that generation of oxidized iodide at this surface allows the iodide to react with tyrosine residues in the newly secreted thyroglobulin molecules. The process of thyroglobulin iodination is known as **organification.** Organification results in thyroglobulin molecules containing **monoiodotyrosine** (MIT) and **diiodotyrosine** (DIT) residues; these tyrosine residues have one or two covalently attached iodines, respectively.

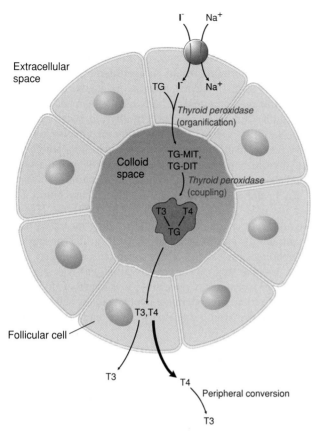

Figure 26-2. Thyroid hormone synthesis, storage, and release. Follicular cells of the thyroid gland concentrate iodide (I^-) from plasma via a basolateral membrane Na^+/I^- symporter. In a reaction (called "organification") catalyzed by thyroid peroxidase, intracellular iodide reacts covalently with tyrosine residues on thyroglobulin (TG) molecules at the apical membrane. Addition of one I^- to tyrosine results in the formation of monoiodinated tyrosine (MIT); addition of two I^- to tyrosine results in the formation of diiodinated tyrosine (DIT). MIT and DIT associate covalently on thyroglobulin via a mechanism known as "coupling," which is also catalyzed by thyroid peroxidase. The derivatized thyroglobulin is stored as colloid within follicles in the thyroid gland. Upon stimulation by TSH, thyroid follicular cells endocytose colloid into lysosomal compartments, where the thyroglobulin is degraded to yield free T4, free T3, and uncoupled MIT and DIT. T3 and T4 are secreted into the plasma, and MIT and DIT are deiodinated intracellularly to yield free iodide for use in new thyroid hormone synthesis *(not shown)*. The thyroid gland secretes more T4 than T3, although T4 is converted to T3 in peripheral tissues.

After MITs and DITs are generated within thyroglobulin, thyroid peroxidase also catalyzes **coupling** between these residues. An MIT joined to DIT generates T3, while the joining of two DITs creates T4. Note that the majority of plasma T3 is produced by metabolism of T4 in the circulation (see "Metabolism of Thyroid Hormone," below) and that nascent T3 and T4 are covalently part of the thyroglobulin protein at this point. These thyroglobulin molecules are then stored in the lumen of the follicle as **colloid.**

When thyroid-stimulating hormone (discussed below) stimulates the thyroid gland to secrete thyroid hormone, the follicular cells endocytose colloid. The ingested thyroglobulin enters lysosomes, where proteases digest the thyroglobulin. Proteolytic digestion releases free T3, T4, MIT, and

DIT. T3 and T4 are transported across the follicular cell basolateral membrane and into the blood. Free MIT and DIT are rapidly deiodinated within the cell, allowing the iodide to be recycled for new thyroid hormone synthesis.

Most endocrine organs concurrently synthesize and release new hormone when activated, rather than storing large quantities of precursor hormone. The *thyroid gland is unusual among endocrine glands in that it stores large quantities of thyroid prohormone in the form of thyroglobulin.* It is not understood why the thyroid gland maintains this elaborate pathway for hormone synthesis and release, but doing so makes it possible to maintain plasma thyroid hormone at a constant level despite fluctuations in the availability of dietary iodide.

METABOLISM OF THYROID HORMONES

Thyroid hormone circulates mostly bound to plasma proteins, notably **thyroid binding globulin (TBG)** and transthyretin. Although T4 is the predominant thyroid hormone found in the blood, T3 has four times the physiologic activity of T4 on target tissues. Some serum T4 is inactivated by deamination, decarboxylation, or conjugation and excretion by the liver. Most T4, however, is deiodinated to the more active T3 form in several locations in the body. This deiodination reaction is catalyzed by the enzyme **iodothyronine 5'-deiodinase** (Fig. 26-1).

There are three subtypes of deiodinase. **Type I 5'-deiodinase,** expressed in the liver and kidneys, is important for converting T4 to the majority of serum T3. **Type II 5'-deiodinase** is expressed primarily in the pituitary, brain, and brown fat. This enzyme is located intracellularly and converts T4 to T3 locally. **Type III 5-deiodinase** is responsible largely for conversion of T4 to the biologically inactive rT3.

The presence of T4 in the blood provides a buffer, or reservoir, for thyroid hormone effects. Most T4 to T3 conversion occurs in the liver, and many pharmacologic agents that increase hepatic cytochrome P450 enzyme activity will increase T4 to T3 conversion. In addition, T4 has a half-life in the plasma of approximately 6 days, whereas plasma T3 has a half-life of only 1 day. *Because T4 has a long plasma half-life, changes in thyroid hormone-regulated functions caused by pharmacologic intervention are generally not observed for a period of 1 to 2 weeks,* as seen with Ms. L in the introductory case.

EFFECTS OF THYROID HORMONES ON TARGET TISSUES

Thyroid hormones have effects on virtually every cell of the body. While the majority of the effects of thyroid hormones likely occur at the level of gene transcription, there is growing evidence that these hormones also act at the plasma membrane. Both modes of action are mediated by hormone binding to thyroid hormone receptors (TRs). Free hormone enters the cell by both passive diffusion and active transport, the latter mediated by hormone-specific and nonspecific carriers such as organic anion and monocarboxylate transporters.

TRs are proteins containing thyroid hormone-binding, DNA-binding, and dimerization domains. There are two classes of thyroid hormone receptor, termed **TRα** and **TRβ**. In addition, both TRα and TRβ can be expressed as multiple isoforms. TR monomers can interact in a dimerization reaction to form homodimers, or with another transcription factor, **retinoid X receptor** (RXR), to form heterodimers. These TR dimers bind to gene promoter regions and are activated by binding of thyroid hormones. Together, the multiple different combinations of TRs and the variability in their tissue distributions create tissue specificity for thyroid hormone effects.

In the absence of hormone, thyroid hormone receptor dimers associate with corepressor molecules and constitutively bind to (and thereby inactivate) thyroid hormone-stimulated genes. Binding of thyroid hormone to TR:RXR or TR:TR dimers promotes dissociation of the corepressors and recruitment of coactivators to the DNA. Thus, thyroid hormone binding to TR dimers serves as a molecular switch from inhibition to activation of gene transcription (Fig. 26-3). Thyroid hormone also acts to down-regulate gene expression by a TR-dependent mechanism, the exact nature of which is not fully understood. For example, thyroid hormone is able to down-regulate TSH gene expression, causing negative feedback of thyroid hormone on the hypothalamic-pituitary–thyroid axis (see Chapter 25). Increasing evidence suggests that thyroid hormone also has nongenomic effects on mitochondrial metabolism and that it interacts with plasma membrane receptors to stimulate intracellular signal transduction.

Thyroid hormone is important in infancy for growth and development of the nervous system. Congenital deficiency of thyroid hormone results in **cretinism,** a severe but preventable form of mental retardation. In the adult, thyroid hormone regulates general body metabolism and energy expenditure. Enzymes regulated by thyroid hormone include the Na^+/K^+ ATPase and many of the enzymes of intermediary metabolism, both anabolic and catabolic. At high levels of thyroid hormone, this effect can result in futile cycling and a consequent increase in body temperature—this is why Ms. L started turning down the heat in her home. Many of the effects of thyroid hormone resemble the effects of sympathetic neural stimulation, including increased cardiac contractility and heart rate, excitability, nervousness, and diaphoresis (sweating). These symptoms were also seen in Ms. L—she was nervous all the time and was startled by slight provocations. Conversely, low levels of thyroid hormone result in **myxedema,** a hypometabolic state characterized by lethargy, dry skin, coarse voice, and cold intolerance.

HYPOTHALAMIC-PITUITARY–THYROID AXIS

Thyroid hormone secretion follows a negative regulatory feedback scheme similar to that of the other hypothalamic-pituitary–target organ axes (Fig. 26-4). **Thyrotropin-releasing hormone (TRH)** is a tripeptide secreted by the hypothalamus that travels via the hypothalamic-pituitary portal circulation to the anterior pituitary gland (see Chapter 25). TRH binds to a G protein-coupled receptor located on the plasma membrane of anterior pituitary gland thyrotrophs, or TSH-producing cells. This stimulates a signal transduction cascade that ultimately promotes the synthesis and release of **thyroid-stimulating hormone (TSH).** TSH is the most important direct regulator of thyroid gland function. TSH stimulates every known aspect of thyroid hormone production, including iodide uptake, organification, coupling, thyroglobulin internalization, and secretion of thyroid hormone. In addition, TSH promotes increased vascularization and growth of the thyroid gland. In pathologic conditions where TSH or a TSH mimic (see below) is secreted at high levels, the thyroid gland can enlarge to several times its normal size, resulting in the characteristic diffusely hypertrophied thyroid gland referred to as a **goiter,** which Ms. L's doctor noted when he palpated her neck.

Negative feedback of the hypothalamic-pituitary–thyroid axis occurs through regulatory actions of thyroid hormone on both the hypothalamus and pituitary gland. Secreted thyroid hormone diffuses into the thyrotrophs of the anterior pituitary gland, where it binds and activates nuclear thyroid hormone receptors. These bound receptors inhibit TSH gene transcription and, hence, TSH synthesis. Thyroid hormone also has important regulatory effects on the hypothalamus; thyroid hormone binding to receptors in hypothalamic cells inhibits transcription of the gene that codes for the TRH precursor protein.

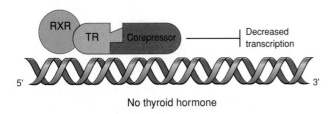

No thyroid hormone

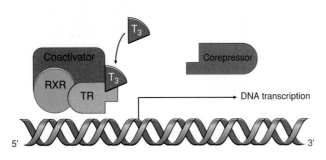

With thyroid hormone

Figure 26-3. Thyroid hormone receptor actions. In the absence of thyroid hormone, the thyroid hormone receptor (TR):retinoid X receptor (RXR) heterodimer associates with a corepressor complex, which binds to promoter regions of DNA and inhibits gene expression. In the presence of thyroid hormone (T3), the corepressor complex dissociates from the TR:RXR heterodimer, coactivators are recruited, and gene transcription occurs. This example demonstrates the action of T3 on a TR:RXR heterodimer, but similar mechanisms are probable for TR:TR homodimers. A useful strategy in the future may involve pharmacologic targeting of tissue-specific corepressors or coactivators.

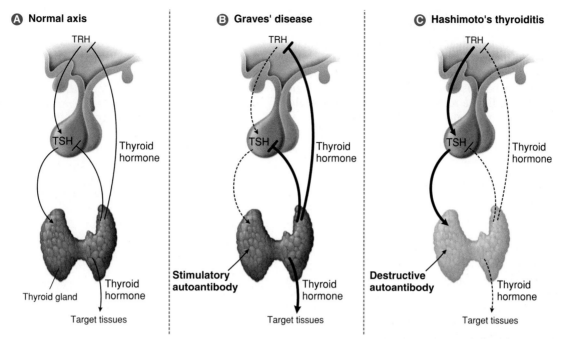

Figure 26-4. The hypothalamic-pituitary–thyroid axis in health and disease. A. In the normal axis, thyrotropin-releasing hormone (TRH) stimulates thyrotrophs of the anterior pituitary gland to release thyroid-stimulating hormone (TSH). TSH stimulates synthesis and release of thyroid hormone by the thyroid gland. Thyroid hormone, in addition to its effects on target tissues, inhibits further release of TRH and TSH by the hypothalamus and anterior pituitary gland, respectively. **B.** In Graves' disease, a stimulatory autoantibody autonomously activates the TSH receptor in the thyroid gland, resulting in sustained stimulation of the thyroid gland, increased plasma thyroid hormone *(thick lines)*, and suppression of TRH and TSH release *(dashed lines)*. **C.** In Hashimoto's thyroiditis, a destructive autoantibody attacks the thyroid gland, causing thyroid insufficiency and decreased synthesis and secretion of thyroid hormone *(dashed lines)*. Consequently, feedback inhibition on the hypothalamus and anterior pituitary gland does not occur, and plasma TSH levels rise *(thick lines)*.

PATHOPHYSIOLOGY

The pathophysiology of thyroid diseases can be understood as a disturbance of the physiologic hypothalamic-pituitary–thyroid axis. For example, a physiologic decrease in thyroid hormones normally activates TSH synthesis and release, which leads to increased release of thyroid hormones by the thyroid gland and to restoration of normal thyroid hormone levels. Thyroid gland pathology can also cause thyroid hormone insufficiency, which also reduces the negative feedback of thyroid hormone on TSH release. Although TSH levels are elevated as a consequence, there is no increase in thyroid hormone release because the thyroid gland cannot respond.

Most common thyroid diseases are best categorized as conditions that result in increased (hyperthyroid) or decreased (hypothyroid) thyroid hormone secretion. Two common thyroid diseases are **Graves' disease** and **Hashimoto's thyroiditis** (Fig. 26-4). Each is believed to be autoimmune in origin, but Graves' disease causes hyperthyroidism whereas Hashimoto's thyroiditis ultimately results in hypothyroidism.

Graves' disease demonstrates the importance of plasma thyroid hormone in regulating homeostasis of the hypothalamic-pituitary–thyroid axis. In this syndrome, an IgG autoantibody specific for the TSH receptor, known as **thyroid-stimulating immunoglobulin (TsIg),** is produced.

This antibody acts as an agonist, activating the TSH receptor and thereby stimulating thyroid follicular cells to synthesize and release thyroid hormone. *Unlike TSH, however, TsIg is not subject to negative feedback; it continues to stimulate thyroid function even when plasma thyroid hormone levels rise into the pathologic range.* Because the autoantibody in Graves' disease acts independently of the hypothalamic-pituitary–thyroid axis, thyroid hormone homeostasis is disrupted. Clinical symptoms of hyperthyroidism result, and laboratory studies show high plasma thyroid hormone levels, low or undetectable TSH levels, and high TsIg levels. In the introductory case, Ms. L's TSH levels were low because her excess plasma thyroid hormone suppressed release of TSH by her anterior pituitary gland.

Hashimoto's thyroiditis, in contrast, results in selective destruction of the thyroid gland. Antibodies specific for many thyroid gland proteins, including thyroglobulin and thyroid peroxidase, can be found in the plasma of patients with Hashimoto's thyroiditis. As with Graves' disease, the underlying etiology of this disease is thought to be autoimmune. The clinical course of Hashimoto's thyroiditis involves a gradual inflammatory destruction of the thyroid gland with resultant hypothyroidism. Early in the course of the disease, destruction of thyroid follicular cells can release excessive quantities of stored colloid, resulting in transiently increased levels of thyroid hormone. Eventually, the gland is almost completely destroyed, and clinical symptoms of hypothyroidism develop (e.g., lethargy and decreased metabolic rate). Therapy for Hashimoto's thyroiditis involves pharmacologic replacement with oral synthetic thyroid hormone.

Other causes of hypothyroidism and hyperthyroidism include developmental anomalies, subacute (DeQuervain) thyroiditis, and thyroid adenomas and carcinomas. Details of the underlying pathophysiologies differ, but pharmacologic intervention in each case rests on determining whether the patient is hypothyroid, euthyroid, or hyperthyroid.

PHARMACOLOGIC CLASSES AND AGENTS

Pharmacologic treatment of thyroid gland pathophysiology involves either replacement of deficient thyroid hormone or antagonism of excessive thyroid hormone. Replacement is self-evident, while the antagonists work at multiple steps in thyroid hormone synthesis and action (Fig. 26-5). In addition, a number of pharmacologic agents used for nonthyroid disease indications have important effects on peripheral thyroid hormone metabolism. The mechanisms of their action are discussed at the end of this section.

TREATMENT OF HYPOTHYROIDISM

Thyroid hormone is a well-established and safe therapy for long-term treatment of hypothyroidism. Therapy aims to replace missing endogenous thyroid hormone with regularly administered exogenous thyroid hormone. The exogenous thyroid hormone is structurally identical to endogenous thyroid hormone (generally T4) and is produced by chemical synthesis.

Early trials with replacement hormone debated whether it would be more efficacious to provide replacement of T3 or T4. T3 is the metabolically more active form of thyroid hormone, and one might have anticipated that replacement of deficient thyroid hormone with T3 would more effectively normalize thyroid homeostasis. However, a number of findings argue against this. First, most thyroid hormone in the blood is in the form of T4, although T4 has lower activity and is eventually metabolized to T3. Having a large reservoir of thyroid "prodrug" (T4) in the plasma may be important, perhaps as an effective buffer to normalize metabolic rates over a wide range of conditions. Second, the half-life of T4 is 6 days, as compared to the 1-day half-life of T3. The extended half-life of T4 allows a patient to take just one thyroid hormone replacement pill per day. For these reasons, **levothyroxine,** the L-isomer of T4, is the treatment of choice for hypothyroidism. (One possible exception is myxedema coma, where the faster onset of T3 may provide enhanced recovery from life-threatening hypothyroidism.) The efficacy of thyroid hormone replacement is monitored by assays of plasma TSH and thyroid hormone levels. TSH is an accurate marker of thyroid hormone activity because anterior pituitary gland release of TSH is exquisitely sensitive to feedback control by thyroid hormone in the blood.

Once a patient is taking a stable dose of levothyroxine, monitoring of TSH levels can generally be performed every 6 months to a year. Sudden alterations in TSH levels despite

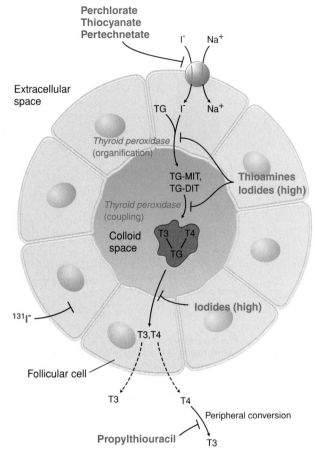

Figure 26-5. Pharmacologic interventions affecting thyroid hormone synthesis. Anions with a molecular radius approximately equal to that of the iodide anion (I^-), such as perchlorate, thiocyanate, and pertechnetate, compete with iodide for uptake by the Na^+/I^- symporter. Radioactive $^{131}I^-$, when concentrated within thyroid cells, causes selective destruction of the thyroid gland. High levels of iodide transiently depress thyroid function by inhibiting organification, coupling, and proteolysis of thyroglobulin. Thioamines, such as propylthiouracil and methimazole, inhibit organification and coupling; propylthiouracil also inhibits peripheral conversion of T4 to T3. TG-MIT, thyroglobulin-monoiodotyrosine; TG-DIT, thyroglobulin-diiodotyrosine.

constant dosing of levothyroxine may be due to drug-drug interactions affecting absorption and metabolism. For example, resins such as **sodium polystyrene sulfonate** (Kayexelate®) and **cholestyramine** may decrease absorption of T4. Drugs that increase the activity of certain hepatic P450 enzymes, including **rifampin** and **phenytoin,** increase the hepatic excretion of T4. In such cases, it may be necessary to increase the supplementary dose of T4 in order to maintain a euthyroid state.

TREATMENT OF HYPERTHYROIDISM

There are pharmacologic agents that target each step of thyroid hormone synthesis, from initial uptake of iodide, to organification, coupling, and peripheral conversion of T4 to T3. Clinically, both radioactive iodide and thioamines are available for the treatment of hyperthyroidism. β-adrenergic antagonists are also sometimes used to ameliorate some of the symptoms of hyperthyroidism.

Inhibitors of Iodide Uptake

Iodide is brought into the thyroid follicular cell via a Na$^+$/I$^-$ symporter. Certain anions with the approximate atomic radius of iodide, such as **perchlorate, thiocyanate,** and **pertechnetate,** compete with iodide for uptake into the thyroid gland follicular cell (Fig. 26-5). This results in a decreased amount of iodide available for thyroid hormone synthesis. The effects of anion uptake inhibitors are usually not immediately apparent because of the large store of preformed thyroid hormone in the colloid.

Anion uptake inhibitors can be used in the treatment of hyperthyroidism; these agents reduce the intrathyroidal supply of iodide available for thyroid hormone synthesis. However, their use is uncommon because of the potential for causing aplastic anemia, and the thioamines (see below) are generally more effective. Because many of these uptake inhibitors are also used as radiopaque contrast materials, it is important to keep this physiologic antagonism in mind whenever a patient has symptoms of hypothyroidism after extensive radiographic studies employing contrast material.

Inhibitors of Organification and Hormone Release

Iodides

Two distinct types of iodide are used in clinical practice. Both take advantage of the thyroid gland's selective uptake and concentration of iodide to levels much higher than that in the blood.

The first agent, ^{131}I$^-$, is a radioactive iodide isotope that strongly emits β-particles toxic to cells. The Na$^+$/I$^-$ channel expressed on thyroid follicular cell membranes cannot distinguish ^{131}I$^-$ from normal stable iodide (^{127}I$^-$). Therefore, ^{131}I$^-$ becomes sequestered within the thyroid gland. This makes radioactive ^{131}I$^-$ a specific and effective therapy for hyperthyroidism. The concentrated intracellular radioactive iodide continues to emit β-particles, resulting in selective local destruction of the thyroid gland. Radioactive iodide is used to treat thyrotoxicosis, and this agent serves as an alternative to surgery in the treatment of hyperthyroidism. There is a concern that patients may eventually develop hypothyroidism after treatment with radioactive iodide, because it is difficult to ascertain for a given patient the extent to which radioactive ^{131}I$^-$ will kill all or most of his or her thyroid follicular cells. *The goal is to administer enough ^{131}I$^-$ to result in a euthyroid state, without precipitating hypothyroidism.* This desired result is not always obtained; for example, Ms. L developed hypothyroidism after treatment with ^{131}I$^-$. Regardless, the development of hypothyroidism is easier to manage clinically than hyperthyroidism. Based on epidemiologic studies, it is unlikely that therapeutic doses of radioactive iodide have any effect on the incidence of thyroid cancer.

The second clinically important pharmacologic agent is, paradoxically, stable inorganic iodide. High levels of iodide inhibit thyroid hormone synthesis and release, a phenomenon known as the **Wolff–Chaikoff effect.** The negative feedback effect of high intrathyroidal iodide concentrations is reversible and transient; thyroid hormone synthesis and release returns to normal a few days after the plasma iodide concentration is increased. Therefore, inorganic iodide is not a useful long-term therapy for hyperthyroidism. This phenomenon does, however, have other important uses. For example, high iodide dosing reduces the size and vascularity of the thyroid gland. Because of this, iodide is often administered before thyroid gland surgery, resulting in technically easier excision of the gland.

Iodide can also have important preventative effects. When the nuclear accident at Chernobyl occurred, there was concern that radioactive iodide released into the air over Poland could cause population-wide thyroid gland destruction. As a preventative measure, millions of Polish children were given large doses of iodide for a number of days to suppress thyroid gland function temporarily, and thereby to avoid uptake of environmental radioactive iodide.

Thioamines

The thioamines **propylthiouracil** and **methimazole** are important and useful inhibitors of thyroid hormone production. Thioamines compete with thyroglobulin for oxidized iodide in a process that is catalyzed by the enzyme thyroid peroxidase (Fig. 26-5). This step is essential for organification and coupling of thyroid hormone precursors. *By competing for oxidized iodide, thioamine treatment causes a selective decrease in thyroid hormone production.* Iodinated thioamines may also be able to bind to thyroglobulin, further antagonizing any coupling reactions. Recall that thyroid follicular cells store a large quantity of nascent thyroid hormone in the form of colloid. This colloid can provide enough thyroid hormone for more than a week in the absence of any new synthesis. Because thioamines affect the synthesis but not the secretion of thyroid hormone, the effects of these drugs are not seen until several weeks after the initiation of treatment.

Thioamine treatment often results in goiter formation. For this reason, the drugs are commonly referred to as **goitrogens.** Inhibition of thyroid hormone production by the drug results in up-regulation of TSH release by the anterior pituitary gland in an attempt to re-establish homeostasis. The increased plasma TSH cannot raise thyroid hormone levels because of the action of the thioamine, however. In response to stimulation by the elevated TSH, the thyroid gland hypertrophies in an attempt to increase thyroid hormone synthesis. This results in the eventual formation of a goiter.

Propylthiouracil is considered the prototype thioamine; **methimazole** is another frequently used drug in this class. Propylthiouracil inhibits thyroid peroxidase as well as peripheral T4 to T3 conversion, whereas methimazole has only been shown to inhibit thyroid peroxidase. Propylthiouracil has a short half-life that necessitates dosing three times a day, while methimazole can be administered once daily.

Both propylthiouracil and methimazole are generally well tolerated. The most frequent adverse effect of these agents is a pruritic rash early in the course of treatment, which may remit spontaneously. Arthralgias are also a common reason for stopping these agents. Propylthiouracil can deplete levels of prothrombin, leading to hypoprothrombinemia and an increased bleeding tendency.

Three rare but serious complications of propylthiouracil and methimazole are agranulocytosis, hepatotoxicity, and vasculitis. Agranulocytosis occurs in <0.1% of cases, usually within the first 90 days of treatment with these agents. Because of this risk, all patients taking thioamines should have a baseline measurement of white blood cell count, and should be advised to discontinue the drug immediately if they develop fever or a sore throat. Hepatotoxicity is also a rare adverse effect of thioamines. The hepatitis is typically cholestatic in pattern, and may represent an allergic reaction to the drug. This allergic hepatitis may occur more frequently with propylthiouracil than with methimazole. Vasculitis from these agents can manifest as drug-induced lupus or an anti-neutrophil cytoplasmic antibody (ANCA)-associated vasculitis.

Because the incidence of serious adverse effects appears to be less frequent with methimazole than with propylthiouracil, methimazole is generally the preferred agent in clinical practice. Two exceptions to this rule are thyroid storm and pregnancy. In the acute management of severe hyperthyroidism (thyroid storm), the additional ability of propylthiouracil to block peripheral conversion of T4 to T3 makes this drug the more attractive agent. In pregnancy, propylthiouracil is the preferred agent because it has a more extensive safety record, and because methimazole use during pregnancy has been associated with the development of aplasia cutis.

The thioamines are generally effective at controlling hyperthyroidism. A large percentage of patients taking these agents will go into remission over the course of 6 months to a year, and may be able to maintain a euthyroid state after discontinuation of these medications. Some patients, however, will develop persistent hyperthyroisism despite treatment, as in the introductory case. Such patients require more definitive treatment of their hyperthyroidism, either by radioactive iodide therapy or surgical removal of the thyroid gland.

Inhibitors of Peripheral Thyroid Hormone Metabolism

Although the majority of thyroid hormone is synthesized in the thyroid gland as T4, thyroid hormone acts at peripheral sites principally as T3. Conversion of T4 to T3 is dependent on a peripheral 5′-deiodinase, and inhibitors of this enzyme are effective adjuncts in treating the symptoms of hyperthyroidism. As mentioned above, propylthiouracil inhibits both organification and peripheral conversion of T4 to T3. Two other agents, β-adrenergic blockers and ipodate, are discussed below.

β-Adrenergic Blockers

β-Adrenergic antagonists are useful therapies for the *symptoms* of hyperthyroidism because many of the effects of high plasma thyroid hormone levels resemble nonspecific β-adrenergic stimulation (e.g., sweating, tremor, tachycardia). In addition, it has been demonstrated that β-blockers can reduce T4/T3 conversion of thyroid hormone, but this effect is not thought to be clinically relevant. Because of its rapid onset of action and short elimination half-life (9 minutes), **esmolol** is a preferred β-adrenergic antagonist for the treatment of thyroid storm.

Ipodate

Ipodate is a radiocontrast agent formerly used for visualization of the biliary ducts in endoscopic retrograde cholangiopancreatography (ERCP) procedures. In addition to its usefulness as a radiocontrast agent, ipodate significantly inhibits conversion of T4 to T3 by inhibiting the enzyme 5′-deiodinase. Although ipodate was sometimes used in the past to treat hyperthyroidism, it is no longer commercially available.

OTHER DRUGS AFFECTING THYROID HORMONE HOMEOSTASIS

Lithium

Lithium, a drug used in the treatment of bipolar affective disorder (see Chapter 13, Pharmacology of Serotonergic and Central Adrenergic Neurotransmission), can cause hypothyroidism. Lithium is actively concentrated in the thyroid gland, and high levels of lithium have been shown to inhibit thyroid hormone release from thyroid follicular cells. There is some evidence that lithium may inhibit thyroid hormone synthesis as well. The mechanism(s) responsible for these actions is unknown.

Amiodarone

Amiodarone is an antiarrhythmic drug (see Chapter 18, Pharmacology of Cardiac Rhythm) that has both positive and negative effects on thyroid hormone function. Amiodarone structurally resembles thyroid hormone and, as a result, contains a large concentration of iodine (each 200-mg tablet of amiodarone contains 75 mg of iodine). Metabolism of amiodarone releases this iodine as iodide, resulting in increased plasma concentrations of iodide. The increased plasma iodide is concentrated in the thyroid gland; this can result in hypothyroidism by the Wolff–Chaikoff effect.

Amiodarone can also cause hyperthyroidism by two mechanisms. In type I thyrotoxicosis, the excess iodide load provided by amiodarone leads to increased thyroid hormone synthesis and release. In type II thyroiditis, an autoimmune thyroiditis is induced that leads to release of excess thyroid hormone from the colloid. Because of its close structural similarity to thyroid hormone, amiodarone may also act as a homologue of thyroid hormone at the level of the receptor.

In addition, amiodarone competitively inhibits type I 5′-deiodinase. This results in decreased T4/T3 conversion and increased plasma concentrations of rT3.

Corticosteroids

Corticosteroids, such as cortisol and glucocorticoid analogues, inhibit the 5′-deiodinase enzyme that converts T4 to the metabolically more active T3. Because T4 has less physiologic activity than T3, treatment with corticosteroids reduces net thyroid hormone activity. In addition, the decreased serum T3 results in increased release of TSH. The increased TSH stimulates greater T4 synthesis, until the amount of T4 produced generates a sufficient level of T3 to inhibit the hypothalamus. Thus, when faced with decreased peripheral T4/T3 conversion, the thyroid releases T4 at a higher rate and serum T4 and T3 levels reach a new steady-state.

Conclusion and Future Directions

Thyroid hormone synthesis consists of a complex set of synthesis and degradation steps. This pathway creates numerous points for pharmacologic intervention, from iodide uptake to peripheral conversion of T4 to T3. Thyroid hormone replacement is a safe and effective long-term therapy for thyroid hormone deficiencies. Numerous effective therapies exist for management of thyrotoxicosis. Radioactive iodide and thioamines are commonly used for this purpose, leading to selective destruction of the thyroid gland and antagonism of organification/coupling, respectively. Future potential therapies for diseases of the thyroid gland may focus on treating the etiology of autoimmune thyroid diseases, such as Graves' disease and Hashimoto's thyroiditis, and better defining the molecular targets of thyroid hormone action.

Suggested Reading

Anonymous. Drugs for hypothyroidism and hyperthyroidism. *Medical Letter* 2006;4:17–24. (*Review of therapeutic considerations, including important drug interactions.*)

Braverman L, Utiger R, eds. *Werner and Ingbar's the thyroid.* 9th ed. Baltimore: Lippincott Williams & Wilkins; 2005. (*Clinical information on the treatment of thyroid diseases.*)

Cooper DS. Antithyroid drugs. *N Engl J Med* 2005;352:905–917. (*An excellent, detailed summary of the clinical uses and adverse effects of methimazole and propylthiouracil.*)

Davis PJ, David FB, Cody V. Membrane receptors mediating thyroid hormone action. *Trends Endocrinol Metabol* 2005;16: 429–435. (*Review of recent developments in thyroid hormone signaling.*)

Weetman A. Graves' disease. *N Engl J Med* 2000;343:1236–1248. (*A very readable review of the diagnosis and treatment of Graves' disease.*)

Yen PM. Physiological and molecular basis of thyroid hormone action. *Physiol Rev* 2000;81:1097–1142. (*Excellent current review of thyroid hormone action.*)

Drug Summary Table   Chapter 26 Pharmacology of the Thyroid Gland

Drug	Clinical Applications	Serious and Common Adverse Effects	Contraindications	Therapeutic Considerations
THYROID HORMONE REPLACEMENTS *Mechanism—Replace missing endogenous thyroid hormone with exogenous thyroid hormone*				
Levothyroxine (T4) Liothyronine (T3)	Hypothyroidism Myxedema coma	*Hyperthyroidism, osteopenia, pseudotumor cerebri, seizure, myocardial infarction*	Acute myocardial infarction Uncorrected adrenal cortical insufficiency Untreated thyrotoxicosis	Cholestyramine and sodium polystyrene sulfonate decrease absorption of synthetic thyroid hormone Rifampin and phenytoin increase metabolism of synthetic thyroid hormone Because of its longer elimination half-life, T4 is usually preferred for the treatment of hypothyroidism T3 may be preferred in myxedema coma due to its faster onset of action
IODIDE UPTAKE INHIBITORS *Mechanism—Compete with iodide for uptake into the thyroid gland follicular cells via sodium-iodide symporter, thereby decreasing intrathyroidal supply of iodide available for thyroid hormone synthesis*				
Perchlorate Thiocyanate Pertechnetate	Hyperthyroidism Radiocontrast agents	Aplastic anemia GI irritation	No major contraindications	Clinical use in hyperthyroidism is limited due to the risk of developing aplastic anemia Frequently used as radiocontrast agents
INHIBITORS OF ORGANIFICATION AND THYROID HORMONE RELEASE *Mechanism—Radioactive iodide strongly emits beta-particles that are toxic to thyroid follicular cells. High-concentration iodide inhibits iodide uptake and organification via Wolff-Chaikoff effect. Propylthiouracil inhibits thyroid peroxidase and conversion of T4 to T3. Methimazole inhibits thyroid peroxidase.*				
131I (Radioactive iodide)	Hyperthyroidism	*May worsen ophthalmopathy in Graves' disease, hypothyroidism*	Pregnancy	Alternative to surgery in the treatment of hyperthyroidism Excess radiation can destroy thyroid, thereby causing hypothyroidism
Iodide (high concentrations)	Hyperthyroidism	*May worsen toxic goiter symptoms*		Used for temporary suppression of thyroid gland function Also used before thyroid gland surgery to allow technically easier excision
Propylthiouracil (PTU) Methimazole	Hyperthyroidism	*Agranulocytosis, hepatotoxicity, vasculitis, and hypoprothrombinemia (PTU)* Rash, arthralgias	Pregnancy and breast-feeding (methimazole)	Methimazole is generally preferred in the treatment of hyperthyroidism due to lower incidence of serious adverse effects PTU is the preferred agent in thyroid storm due to additional peripheral inhibition of T4-to-T3 conversion
INHIBITORS OF PERIPHERAL THYROID HORMONE METABOLISM *Mechanism—Block 5'-deiodinase, thereby inhibiting T4 to T3 conversion*				
β-blockers	See Drug Summary Table: Chapter 9 Adrenergic Pharmacology			The sympatholytic effect of beta-blockers is more important in treating the symptoms of hyperthyroidism than the minor effect of these drugs on 5'-deiodinase Esmolol is a preferred β-adrenergic antagonist for treatment of thyroid storm because of its rapid onset of action and rapid elimination half-life
Ipodate	Hyperthyroidism	Urticaria, serum sickness, may occasionally exacerbate hyperthyroid symptoms	Hypersensitivity to radiocontrast agents	Formerly used as radiocontrast agent No longer commercially available

27

Pharmacology of the Adrenal Cortex

Ehrin J. Armstrong and Robert G. Dluhy

INTRODUCTION

As with the pituitary gland, the adrenal gland consists of two organs fused together during embryologic development. The outer adrenal cortex originates from mesoderm, and the inner adrenal medulla is derived from neural crest cells. The adrenal cortex synthesizes and secretes steroid hormones essential for salt balance, intermediary metabolism, and androgenic actions in females. The adrenal medulla is important, although not essential, for maintaining sympathetic tone by means of secretion of the catecholamine epinephrine. This chapter focuses on the adrenal cortex; because of its importance in neuropharmacology, the adrenal medulla is discussed in Chapter 9, Adrenergic Pharmacology.

The pharmacologic utility of adrenocortical hormones spans almost every area of medicine. This is largely because of the usefulness of glucocorticoid analogues as efficacious

and potent anti-inflammatory agents. Unfortunately, long-term systemic glucocorticoid therapy also produces a number of predictable but undesirable adverse effects. Inhibitors of biosynthetic enzymes in the adrenal cortex can be used to treat adrenocortical hormone excess. The physiology of mineralocorticoids has been studied in the etiology of essential hypertension, and there is current interest in the use of mineralocorticoid receptor antagonists as therapies for hypertension and cardiovascular diseases. Adrenal androgens, although lacking a definitive therapeutic indication, are frequently abused for their anabolic effects at high doses.

 Case

Johnny is 8 years old when he finds that he can barely catch his breath at times, especially while exercising. His asthma comes and goes, but no therapy seems to stop the asthma attacks completely. Although his doctor is concerned that it could stunt Johnny's growth, she eventually prescribes oral prednisone (a glucocorticoid analogue), and tells Johnny's parents to make sure he takes the medication every day. After a few weeks, Johnny's asthma attacks subside, and he is able to have a fairly normal childhood. During this time, the doctor pays close attention to Johnny's linear growth. Two years later, Johnny's doctor decides that a new inhaled glucocorticoid could be a safer medication for him. Johnny switches to the inhaled glucocorticoid and discontinues oral prednisone. Three days later, he develops a respiratory infection and is brought to the emergency department with low blood pressure and a temperature of 103°F. Based on his history of prednisone use, Johnny is immediately given hydrocortisone (cortisol) intravenously, as well as a saline infusion. Johnny recovers, and for the next 6 months slowly tapers his oral prednisone dose with continued use of the inhaled glucocorticoid. Eventually, he is able to take the inhaled glucocorticoid alone as an effective therapy for his asthma.

QUESTIONS

- **1.** Why are cortisol analogues such as prednisone used for treating asthma?
- **2.** Why did the doctor monitor Johnny's linear growth?
- **3.** Why did abrupt cessation of oral prednisone precipitate Johnny's clinical presentation in the emergency department?
- **4.** Why are inhaled glucocorticoids safer than oral glucocorticoids for long-term treatment of asthma?

OVERVIEW OF THE ADRENAL CORTEX

The adrenal cortex synthesizes three classes of hormones: **mineralocorticoids, glucocorticoids,** and **androgens.** Histologically, the adrenal cortex is divided into three zones. Moving from the capsule toward the medulla, these regions are the zona glomerulosa, zona fasciculata, and zona reticularis (Fig. 27-1). The glomerulosa is responsible for mineralocorticoid production and is under the control of **angiotensin II** and plasma **potassium** concentration. The fasciculata and reticularis synthesize glucocorticoids and androgens, respectively. Both the fasciculata and reticularis are under the control of **adrenocorticotropic hormone (ACTH),** which, in turn, is regulated by corticotropin-releasing hormone (CRH) and cortisol (see Chapter 25, Pharmacology of the Hypothalamus and Pituitary Gland).

Through its mineralocorticoid, glucocorticoid, and adrenal androgen products, the adrenal cortex plays a role in diverse aspects of homeostasis. The following discussion considers the physiology, pathophysiology, and pharmacology of each class of adrenal hormones. Because of their pharmacologic importance, the glucocorticoids are discussed first, followed by the mineralocorticoids and the adrenal androgens.

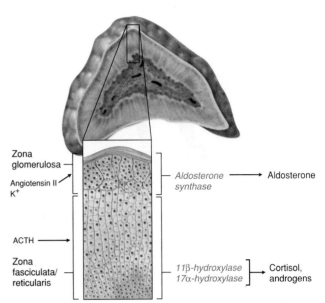

Figure 27-1. Regions of the adrenal cortex. The adrenal cortex is divided into three regions. The outermost region, the zona glomerulosa, synthesizes aldosterone and is regulated by circulating levels of angiotensin II and potassium. The zona fasciculata and zona reticularis synthesize cortisol and adrenal androgens. ACTH released from the anterior pituitary gland stimulates production of both cortisol and adrenal androgens. Tissue-specific expression of enzymes in each zone of the adrenal cortex—aldosterone synthase in the glomerulosa, steroid 11β-hydroxylase and steroid 17α-hydroxylase in the fasciculata/reticularis—determines the specificity of hormone production in that zone.

GLUCOCORTICOIDS

PHYSIOLOGY

Synthesis

Cortisol, the endogenous glucocorticoid, is synthesized from cholesterol. Its synthesis begins with the rate-limiting conversion of cholesterol to pregnenolone, a reaction catalyzed by side-chain cleavage enzyme (Fig. 27-2). This first step converts the 27-carbon cholesterol into a 21-carbon precursor common to all adrenocortical hormones. From this precursor, steroid metabolism can proceed down three different pathways to generate mineralocorticoids, glucocorticoids, or adrenal androgens.

An oxidase enzyme catalyzes each step in the pathway of adrenocortical hormone synthesis. The oxidase enzymes are mitochondrial **cytochromes,** similar to the liver cytochrome P450 oxidase system. Tissue-specific expression of particular oxidase enzymes in each zone of the adrenal cortex provides the biochemical basis for the differences among the hormonal end products of the different zones of the cortex. For example, the zona fasciculata synthesizes cortisol, but not aldosterone or androgens (Fig. 27-1). This is because enzymes required uniquely for cortisol synthesis—such as steroid 11β-hydroxylase—are expressed in the zona fasciculata, whereas enzymes required for aldosterone and androgen synthesis are not.

Figure 27-2. Hormone synthesis in the adrenal cortex. The hormones of the adrenal cortex are steroids derived from cholesterol. The rate-limiting step in adrenal hormone biosynthesis is the modification of cholesterol to pregnenolone by side-chain cleavage enzyme. From this step, pregnenolone metabolism can be directed toward the formation of aldosterone, cortisol, or androstenedione. The flux of metabolites through each of these pathways depends on the tissue-specific expression of enzymes in the different cell types of the cortex and on the relative activity of the different synthetic enzymes. Note that several enzymes are involved in more than one pathway and that defects in these enzymes can affect the synthesis of more than one hormone. For example, a defect in steroid 21-hydroxylase prevents the synthesis of both aldosterone and cortisol. This overlap of synthetic activities also contributes to the nonselective action of glucocorticoid synthesis inhibitors such as trilostane. Enzymes are shown as numbers: 17, steroid 17α-hydroxylase; 21, steroid 21-hydroxylase; 11, steroid 11β-hydroxylase. Aminoglutethimide and high levels of ketoconazole inhibit side-chain cleavage enzyme. Ketoconazole also inhibits 17, 20-lyase. Trilostane inhibits 3β-hydroxysteroid dehydrogenase. Metyrapone inhibits steroid 11β-hydroxylase.

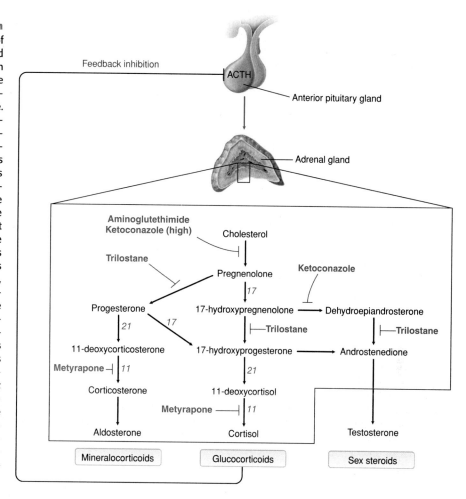

Metabolism

Approximately 90% of circulating cortisol is bound to plasma proteins, the most important of which are **corticosteroid-binding globulin** (**CBG,** also referred to as *transcortin*) and albumin. CBG has high affinity for cortisol but low overall capacity, whereas albumin has low cortisol affinity but high overall capacity. Only molecules of cortisol that are unbound to protein (the so-called *free fraction*) are bioavailable, that is, available to diffuse through plasma membranes into cells. Thus, the affinity and capacity of plasma binding proteins regulate the availability of active hormone and, consequently, hormone activity.

The liver and kidneys are the primary sites of peripheral cortisol metabolism. Through reduction and subsequent conjugation to glucuronic acid, the liver is responsible for inactivating cortisol in the plasma. The conjugation reaction makes cortisol more water soluble, thus enabling renal excretion. Importantly, the liver and kidneys express different isoforms of the enzyme **11β-hydroxysteroid dehydrogenase,** a regulator of cortisol activity. The two isoforms catalyze opposing reactions. In distal collecting duct cells of the kidney, 11β-hydroxysteroid dehydrogenase type II (11β-HSD II) converts cortisol to the biologically inactive compound **cortisone,** which (unlike cortisol) does not bind to the mineralocorticoid receptor (see below, Fig. 27-3B). In contrast,

cortisone can be converted back to cortisol (also referred to as *hydrocortisone*) in the liver by 11β-hydroxysteroid dehydrogenase type I (11β-HSDI, Fig. 27-3A). The interplay between these opposing reactions determines overall glucocorticoid activity. In addition, as discussed below, the activity of these enzymes is important in glucocorticoid pharmacology.

Physiologic Actions

As with other steroid hormones, unbound cortisol diffuses through the plasma membrane into the cytosol of target cells, where the hormone then binds to a cytosolic receptor. There are two types of glucocorticoid receptors: the **Type I (mineralocorticoid)** and **Type II glucocorticoid receptors.** The Type I receptor is expressed in the organs of excretion (kidney, colon, salivary glands, sweat glands) and the hippocampus, whereas the Type II receptor has a broader tissue distribution. *The Type I glucocorticoid receptor is synonymous with the mineralocorticoid receptor.* The nomenclature is unfortunate, and this chapter hereafter refers to the Type I receptor as the "mineralocorticoid receptor."

Once cortisol binds to its cytosolic receptor and forms a hormone–receptor complex, the complex dimerizes with another hormone–receptor complex and is transported into the nucleus. In the case of cortisol, the dimerized hormone–

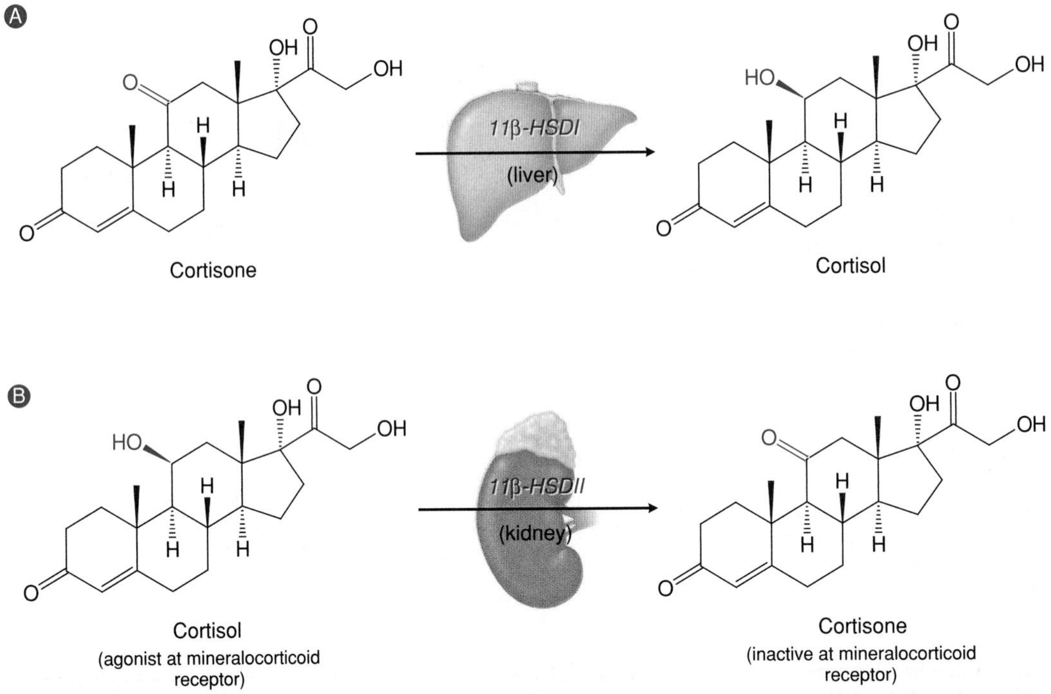

Figure 27-3. 11β-Hydroxysteroid dehydrogenase. The enzyme 11β-hydroxysteroid dehydrogenase (11β-HSD) exists in two isoforms, which catalyze opposing reactions. **A.** In the liver, 11β-hydroxysteroid dehydrogenase type I (11β-HSDI) converts 11-keto glucocorticoids such as cortisone to 11-hydroxy glucocorticoids such as cortisol. **B.** In vitro, cortisol is a potent agonist at the mineralocorticoid receptor (MR). In the kidney, however, MRs are "shielded" from cortisol by the action of the enzyme 11β-hydroxysteroid dehydrogenase type II (11β-HSD II), which converts cortisol to inactive cortisone. This mechanism ensures that, at physiologic levels, cortisol does not exert mineralocorticoid effects. At high concentrations, however, cortisol can overwhelm the activity of 11β-HSD II, leading to stimulation of renal MRs.

receptor complex binds to gene promoter elements referred to as **glucocorticoid response elements (GREs),** which may either enhance or inhibit the expression of specific genes. Cortisol has profound effects on mRNA expression; about 10% of all human genes are estimated to contain GREs. Because of the large number of genes whose expression is affected by activation of GREs, cortisol has physiologic actions in most tissues. These actions can be divided generally into metabolic effects and anti-inflammatory effects.

Metabolic effects of cortisol increase nutrient availability by raising blood glucose, amino acid, and triglyceride levels. Cortisol increases blood glucose by antagonizing insulin action and by promoting gluconeogenesis in the fasting state. Cortisol also increases muscle protein catabolism, leading to increased levels of amino acids that can be utilized by the liver as fuels for gluconeogenesis. By potentiating growth hormone action on adipocytes, cortisol increases the activity of hormone-sensitive lipase and the subsequent release of free fatty acids (lipolysis). Cortisol levels increase as a component of stress responses induced by events such as acute trauma, surgery, fear, severe infection, and pain. By elevating blood glucose, the physiologic effects of glucocorticoids maintain energy homeostasis during the stress response, thus ensuring that critical organs such as the brain continue to receive nutrients.

Cortisol also has multiple anti-inflammatory actions. Cortisol negatively regulates cytokine release from cells of the immune system; this action may be an important mechanism to limit the extent of immune responses and to regulate the inflammatory response. In turn, certain cytokines, including

IL-1, IL-2, IL-6, and TNF-α, can stimulate hypothalamic release of CRH, which stimulates ACTH and cortisol release. This series of stimulatory and inhibitory effects creates a feedback loop, in which inflammatory cytokines and cortisol are coordinately regulated to control immune and inflammatory responses (Fig. 27-4). Glucocorticoid-mediated suppression of the inflammatory response also has important pharmacologic implications for clinical conditions such as organ transplantation, rheumatoid arthritis, and asthma. Indeed, the introductory case demonstrates that glucocorticoids are an effective therapy for asthma. The exact mechanisms by which glucocorticoids act to ameliorate the symptoms of asthma are unknown but are thought to be related to the ability of glucocorticoids to reduce inflammation in the airways (see below and Chapter 46, Integrative Inflammation Pharmacology: Asthma).

Regulation

The hypothalamic–pituitary unit coordinates the production of cortisol (refer to Chapter 25 for an overview). In response to central circadian rhythms and to stress, neurons from the paraventricular nucleus of the hypothalamus synthesize and secrete **corticotropin-releasing hormone (CRH),** a peptide hormone that travels through the hypothalamic–pituitary portal system. CRH then binds to G protein-coupled receptors on the surface of corticotroph cells in the anterior pituitary gland. CRH binding stimulates the corticotrophs to synthesize **proopiomelanocortin (POMC),** a precursor polypeptide that is cleaved into multiple peptide hormones

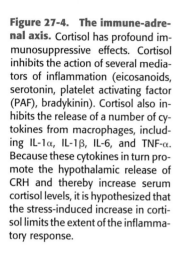
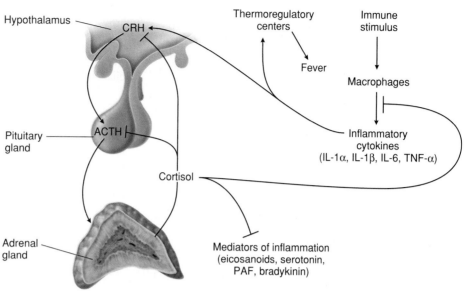

Figure 27-4. The immune-adrenal axis. Cortisol has profound immunosuppressive effects. Cortisol inhibits the action of several mediators of inflammation (eicosanoids, serotonin, platelet activating factor (PAF), bradykinin). Cortisol also inhibits the release of a number of cytokines from macrophages, including IL-1α, IL-1β, IL-6, and TNF-α. Because these cytokines in turn promote the hypothalamic release of CRH and thereby increase serum cortisol levels, it is hypothesized that the stress-induced increase in cortisol limits the extent of the inflammatory response.

including ACTH. Antidiuretic hormone, secreted by the posterior pituitary gland, synergizes with CRH to increase the release of ACTH by the anterior pituitary gland.

Proteolytic cleavage of POMC yields not only ACTH, but also γ-melanocyte–stimulating hormone (MSH), lipotropin, and β-endorphin. MSH binds to receptors on skin melanocytes, promoting melanogenesis and thereby increasing skin pigmentation. Because of the similarities between the ACTH and MSH peptide sequences, high concentrations of ACTH can also bind to and activate MSH receptors. This action becomes apparent in primary hypoadrenalism (see below), in which increased ACTH levels result in increased skin pigmentation. The role of lipotropin in human physiology is uncertain, but is thought to involve control of lipolysis. β-Endorphin is an endogenous opioid that is important for pain modulation and for regulation of reproductive physiology.

Because steroid hormones are able to diffuse freely through cell membranes, and the adrenal gland stores little cortisol, ACTH regulates cortisol production by promoting synthesis of the hormone. ACTH also has a trophic effect on the zona fasciculata and zona reticularis of the adrenal cortex, and hypertrophy of the cortex can occur in response to chronically elevated levels of ACTH.

As in other endocrine axes, there is negative feedback regulation by cortisol at the level of the hypothalamus and anterior pituitary gland. *High cortisol levels decrease both synthesis and release of CRH and ACTH.* Because ACTH has important trophic effects on the adrenal cortex, the absence of ACTH leads to atrophy of the cortisol-producing zona fasciculata and the androgen-producing zona reticularis. However, the aldosterone-producing zona glomerulosa cells continue to function in the absence of ACTH, because angiotensin II and potassium maintain production of aldosterone.

PATHOPHYSIOLOGY

Diseases affecting glucocorticoid physiology can be divided into disorders of hormone deficiency and disorders of hormone excess. Addison's disease is the classic example of adrenocortical insufficiency, whereas Cushing's syndrome exemplifies cortisol excess.

Adrenal Insufficiency

Addison's disease is an example of a *primary adrenal insufficiency* in which the adrenal cortex is selectively destroyed, most commonly by a T cell-mediated autoimmune reaction. Destruction of the cortex results in decreased synthesis of all classes of adrenocortical hormones. By comparison, *secondary adrenal insufficiency* is caused by hypothalamic or pituitary disorders or by prolonged administration of exogenous glucocorticoids. In secondary adrenal insufficiency, the decrease in ACTH levels causes decreased synthesis of sex hormones and cortisol but does not alter levels of aldosterone synthesis (see above).

Regardless of the underlying cause, adrenal insufficiency has serious consequences and can be life-threatening if left untreated in the setting of stress. If adrenal insufficiency is the result of high-dose, prolonged therapy with exogenous glucocorticoids, then the dose of glucocorticoid should be tapered slowly to allow the **hypothalamic-pituitary–adrenal (HPA) axis** to regain full activity. Importantly, it can take up to 1 year for the HPA axis to recover function following discontinuation of exogenous glucocorticoid treatment.

In the introductory case, Johnny was switched from an oral glucocorticoid to an inhaled glucocorticoid that delivered a much lower systemic concentration of glucocorticoid. His adrenal cortex had atrophied because he had been maintained for 2 years on chronically high doses of prednisone; therefore, he was unable to produce a sufficient amount of cortisol in response to the stress of a respiratory infection. As a result, he arrived at the emergency room with acute adrenal insufficiency and required intravenous therapy with saline and hydrocortisone.

Glucocorticoid Excess

Cushing's syndrome refers to a number of underlying pathophysiologies, all of which increase cortisol production. The term "Cushing's disease" is reserved for ACTH-secreting pituitary adenomas that lead to increased cortisol production (Fig. 25-4C). Other causes of Cushing's syndrome include ectopic secretion of ACTH, most commonly by small cell carcinomas of the lung (Fig. 25-4D), and (rarely) ectopic CRH production. Cushing's syndrome can also result from cortisol-secreting tumors (adenoma or carcinoma) of the adrenal cortex (Fig. 25-4B). However, iatrogenic Cushing's syndrome, secondary to pharmacologic treatment with exogenous glucocorticoids, is by far the most common cause of Cushing's syndrome.

The clinical features of Cushing's syndrome result from chronic overstimulation of target organs by endogenous or exogenous glucocorticoids. These features — which can include centripetal adipose redistribution, hypertension, proximal limb myopathy, osteoporosis, immunosuppression, and diabetes mellitus — reflect amplification of the normal physiologic actions of glucocorticoids in a variety of target tissues, and are discussed in more detail below.

PHARMACOLOGIC CLASSES AND AGENTS

Cortisol and Glucocorticoid Analogues

Drug therapy with glucocorticoids is indicated for two main purposes. First, exogenous glucocorticoids can be used as *replacement* therapy in cases of adrenal insufficiency. The goal of this therapy is to administer physiologic doses of glucocorticoids to ameliorate the effects of the adrenal insufficiency. Second, and more commonly, glucocorticoids are administered at *pharmacologic* doses to suppress inflammation and immune responses associated with disorders such as asthma, rheumatoid arthritis, and organ rejection following transplantation.

Because pharmacologic levels of systemic glucocorticoids invariably result in severe adverse effects, strategies to minimize these untoward responses to glucocorticoids have focused on local delivery of glucocorticoids to the area(s) requiring treatment. By limiting systemic exposure to the drug, HPA axis suppression and other features of iatrogenic Cushing's syndrome can be minimized or avoided. Examples of local glucocorticoid delivery include inhaled glucocorticoids for asthma, topical glucocorticoids for inflammatory skin conditions, and intra-articular glucocorticoids for arthritis.

A large number of glucocorticoid analogues have been synthesized. The following discussion highlights the differences among some commonly used cortisol analogues—including **prednisone, prednisolone, fludrocortisone,** and **dexamethasone**—by comparing the structures, potencies, and duration of action of these compounds to those of cortisol.

Structure and Potency

Glucocorticoids can be divided into two classes based on the structural moiety present at the 11-carbon position. Compounds with a hydroxyl (—OH) group at the 11 position, such as cortisol, possess intrinsic glucocorticoid activity. In contrast, compounds with a carbonyl (=O) group at the 11 carbon, such as cortisone, are inactive until the liver enzyme 11β-hydroxysteroid dehydrogenase type I (11β-HSDI) reduces the compound to its 11-hydroxyl congener (Fig. 27-3). That is, cortisone is an inactive prodrug until it is converted by the liver to the active drug cortisol. *The native activity of a glucocorticoid is especially important for topically administered drugs because the skin does not possess appreciable amounts of 11β-HSDI.* Also, whenever possible, the active drug form is preferred over the inactive prodrug form for patients with liver dysfunction, because such patients may not be able to convert the prodrug to its active form.

The basic cortisol "backbone" is essential for glucocorticoid activity, and *all synthetic glucocorticoids are analogues of the endogenous glucocorticoid cortisol* (Fig. 27-5). For example, addition of a double bond between carbons 1 and 2 of cortisol creates **prednisolone** (Fig. 27-6), which has 4–5 times the anti-inflammatory potency of cortisol. Further addition of an α-methyl group (where α is defined as the side group orientation axial to the compound, while β is the equatorial orientation) to carbon 6 of prednisolone creates **methylprednisolone,** which has an anti-inflammatory potency 5–6 times that of cortisol.

Although prednisolone and methylprednisolone have significantly greater glucocorticoid potency than cortisol, addition of an α-fluorine (F) to carbon 9 of cortisol increases both the glucocorticoid and mineralocorticoid potencies of the resulting compound, known as **fludrocortisone.** Because of its enhanced mineralocorticoid activity, fludrocortisone is useful in the treatment of conditions characterized by mineralocorticoid deficiency (see below).

Dexamethasone incorporates two of the above changes to the cortisol backbone (1,2 double bond, 9α fluorine) as well as the addition of an α-methyl group at the 16-carbon

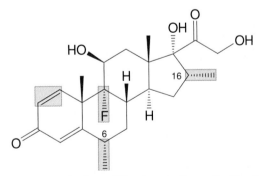

Figure 27-5. Synthetic modifications to the cortisol backbone. Four modifications to the cortisol backbone are common in synthetic glucocorticoids. Addition of a 1–2 double bond *(leftmost box),* a methyl group at carbon 6, or a methyl group at carbon 16 increases the glucocorticoid activity of the compound relative to that of cortisol. Addition of a fluorine to carbon 9 increases glucocorticoid activity and markedly increases mineralocorticoid activity; the mineralcorticoid effect is blunted if 9-fluorination is combined with 16-methylation. Simultaneous addition of the 1–2 double bond, methyl at carbon 16, and fluorine at carbon 9 creates dexamethasone, which has very potent glucocorticoid activity but essentially no mineralocorticoid activity.

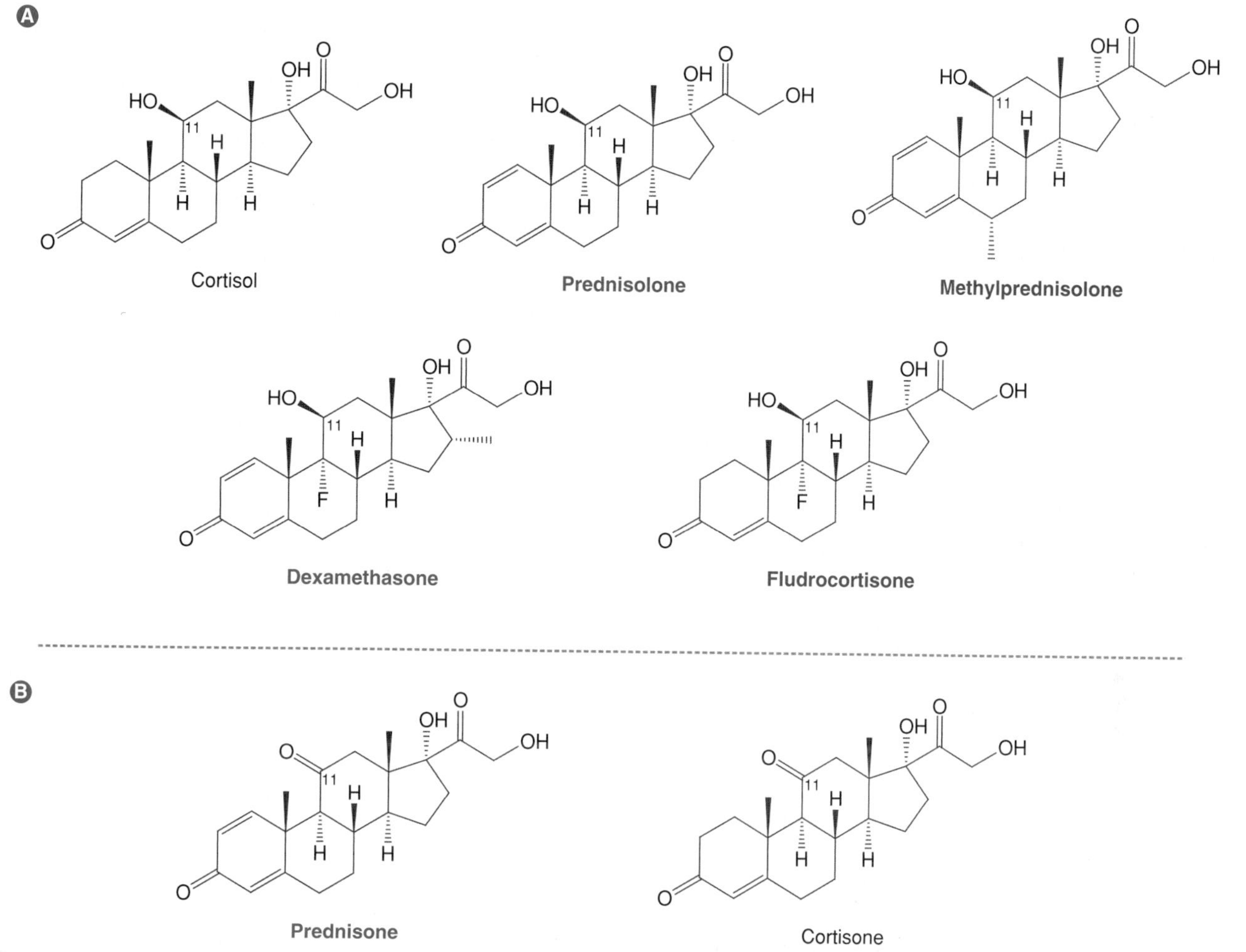

A

Cortisol

Prednisolone

Methylprednisolone

Dexamethasone

Fludrocortisone

B

Prednisone

Cortisone

Figure 27-6. Glucocorticoid analogues. Panel A shows a number of 11-hydroxy glucocorticoids, while **panel B** shows two 11-keto congeners. Note that the drugs in A are physiologically active, while the drugs in B are prodrugs that must be activated by 11β-HSDI to become active compounds. The structural class to which a glucocorticoid analogue belongs can be an important consideration in therapeutic decision-making. For example, because the skin lacks significant 11β-HSDI activity, only 11-hydroxy glucocorticoids can be used in topical glucocorticoid creams. HSD, hydroxysteroid dehydrogenase.

position. This compound has more than 18 times the gluco-corticoid potency of cortisol, but virtually no mineralocorti-coid activity.

A number of other permutations have been made to the cortisol backbone in other synthetic glucocorticoids, but the above discussion highlights the pertinent structural differ-ences among the most common synthetic glucocorticoids. *Clinically, it is most important to be aware of the potency of each agent relative to cortisol, especially when consider-ing a change from one analogue to another that has different relative glucocorticoid and mineralocorticoid activities.* Table 27-1 summarizes the relative glucocorticoid potencies

TABLE 27-1	Relative Potencies and Durations of Action of Representative Glucocorticoid Analogues		
PHARMACOLOGIC AGENT	**RELATIVE GLUCOCORTICOID POTENCY**	**RELATIVE MINERALOCORTICOID ACTIVITY**	**DURATION OF ACTION**
Hydrocortisone	1	1	Short
Prednisolone	4–5	0.25	Short
Methylprednisolone	5–6	0.25	Short
Dexamethasone	18	<0.01	Long

Short-acting agents have a tissue half-life of less than 12 hours, and long-acting agents have a half-life of greater than 48 hours.

and mineralocorticoid activities of several common glucocorticoid analogues.

Duration of Action

The duration of glucocorticoid action is a complex pharmacokinetic variable that depends on:

1. Fraction of the drug bound to plasma proteins. More than 90% of circulating cortisol is protein-bound, primarily to CBG and, to a lesser degree, to albumin. In contrast, glucocorticoid analogues generally bind to CBG with relatively low affinity. As a result, approximately 2/3 of a typical glucocorticoid analogue circulates within the plasma bound to albumin, while the rest is present as free steroid. Because only the free steroid is metabolized, the extent of binding to plasma proteins is a determinant of the drug's duration of action.
2. Affinity of the drug for 11β-HSD II. Glucocorticoids that have a lower affinity for 11β-HSD II have a longer plasma half-life because such drugs are not transformed into inactive metabolites as rapidly.
3. Lipophilicity of the drug. Increased lipophilicity promotes partitioning of the drug into adipose stores; the resulting decrease in the drug's metabolism and excretion extends its plasma half-life.
4. Affinity of the drug for the glucocorticoid receptor. Increased affinity of a glucocorticoid analogue for the glucocorticoid receptor increases the duration of action of the drug, because the fraction of drug that is bound to the receptor continues to exert its effect until the drug–receptor complex dissociates.

Together, these four variables result in a characteristic duration of action profile for each glucocorticoid analogue. Table 27-1 summarizes the duration of action of representative analogues as "short" or "long." *In general, glucocorticoid agents with higher anti-inflammatory (glucocorticoid) potency have a longer duration of action.*

Replacement Therapy

Treatment of primary adrenal insufficiency is aimed at physiologically replacing both glucocorticoids and mineralocorticoids. **Oral hydrocortisone** is the glucocorticoid of choice. Because glucocorticoid replacement therapy must continue for life, the therapeutic goal is to administer the smallest possible effective dose of glucocorticoid so as to minimize the adverse effects of chronic glucocorticoid excess. Patients with primary adrenal insufficiency also require mineralocorticoid replacement, as described below. Patients with secondary adrenal insufficiency require only glucocorticoid replacement because mineralocorticoid production is preserved by the renin–angiotensin system (see Chapter 20, Pharmacology of Volume Regulation).

Pharmacologic Dosing

Effects at Pharmacologic Levels. Glucocorticoids are important mediators of the stress response, regulating both glucose homeostasis and the immune system. Glucocorticoids have found wide clinical use as anti-inflammatory agents because of their profound effects on immune and inflammatory processes. Pharmacologic levels of glucocorticoids inhibit **cytokine release** and thereby decrease IL-1, IL-2, IL-6, and TNF-α action. Local regulation of cytokine release is crucial for leukocyte recruitment and activation, and disruption of this signaling process profoundly inhibits immune function. Glucocorticoids also block the synthesis of arachidonic acid metabolites by inhibiting the action of phospholipase A_2. As discussed in Chapter 41, Pharmacology of Eicosanoids, arachidonic acid metabolites such as thromboxanes, prostaglandins, and leukotrienes mediate many of the early steps of inflammation, including vascular permeability, platelet aggregation, and vasoconstriction. By blocking the production of these metabolites, glucocorticoids significantly down-regulate the inflammatory response.

The multiple effects described above make glucocorticoids useful drugs in the treatment of a number of inflammatory and autoimmune diseases, such as asthma, rheumatoid arthritis, Crohn's disease, polyarteritis nodosa, temporal arteritis, and immune rejection following organ transplantation. It is important to note, however, that *pharmacologic glucocorticoid therapy does not correct the underlying disease etiology, but rather limits the effects of inflammation.* For that reason, discontinuing chronic glucocorticoid therapy often results in the resumption of inflammatory symptoms, unless the disorder has gone into a spontaneous remission or been treated by other means.

Endogenous glucocorticoids affect many metabolic processes, and pharmacologic dosing with exogenous glucocorticoids amplifies those actions. Because of this, adverse effects typically accompany prolonged pharmacologic dosing. Increased *susceptibility to infection* is a potential adverse effect of long-term suppression of the inflammatory process by exogenous glucocorticoids. Glucocorticoids raise plasma *glucose levels* by antagonizing the action of insulin and promoting gluconeogenesis; pharmacologic doses of glucocorticoids amplify these effects. Insulin resistance and increased plasma glucose concentrations necessitate increased pancreatic β cell production of insulin to normalize blood glucose levels. As a result, *diabetes mellitus* is a common complication of long-term glucocorticoid administration, especially in patients with decreased pancreatic β cell reserve.

Pharmacologic dosing of glucocorticoids inhibits the vitamin D-mediated absorption of calcium. This results in *secondary hyperparathyroidism* and, therefore, an increase in bone resorption. Glucocorticoids also directly suppress osteoblast function. These two mechanisms contribute to bone loss, and long-term glucocorticoid therapy often results in *osteoporosis*. Steroid-induced bone resorption can be prevented with bisphosphonates, which inhibit osteoclast function and thus slow the progression of bone loss (see Chapter 30, Pharmacology of Bone Mineral Homeostasis). Chronic administration of glucocorticoids also slows *linear bone growth* in children, and glucocorticoid administration can cause growth retardation. Short stature can result in children who take glucocorticoids through adolescence. For this reason, Johnny's physician monitored Johnny's growth closely while he took oral prednisone.

Pharmacologic doses of glucocorticoids can cause selective atrophy of fast twitch muscle fibers, resulting in catabolism and weakness of (primarily) the proximal muscles. Glucocorticoids also cause a characteristic redistribution of fat, with peripheral wasting of adipose stores and central obesity. Excessive fat deposition occurs on the back of the neck (buffalo hump) and face (moon facies).

In considering the potential for adverse effects of glucocorticoids, it is important to understand the concept of a population at risk. Not all individuals treated with glucocorticoids develop the same adverse effects, because genetic and environmental variability place different individuals at risk for different sequelae of therapy. For example, a patient with borderline diabetes who is treated with glucocorticoids is likely to develop overt diabetes, whereas a patient with sufficient pancreatic β cell reserve may not experience this adverse effect. *By carefully defining a patient's risk factors, it is often possible to predict the patient's predisposition for adverse effects of glucocorticoids.*

Withdrawal from Glucocorticoid Treatment. A number of problems can be associated with the discontinuation of chronic glucocorticoid therapy. During long-term therapy with pharmacologic levels of glucocorticoids, high plasma glucocorticoid levels suppress the release of ACTH from the anterior pituitary gland and of CRH from the hypothalamus. Because ACTH has trophic effects on the adrenal cortex, suppression of ACTH release during glucocorticoid therapy results in atrophy of the adrenal cortex. Abrupt cessation of glucocorticoid therapy can precipitate **acute adrenal insufficiency** because a number of months are required to reactivate the hypothalamic-pituitary–adrenal axis. Even after ACTH secretion recovers, a number of additional months may be required for the adrenal cortex to begin secreting physiologic levels of cortisol. Furthermore, the underlying inflammatory disease for which therapy was initiated can worsen during this time because of disinhibition of the immune system. Thus, it is axiomatic that *chronic glucocorticoid treatment should, whenever possible, be tapered slowly with gradually decreasing doses.* This taper allows the hypothalamus, anterior pituitary gland, and adrenal cortex to resume normal function gradually, thus avoiding adrenal insufficiency and, it is hoped, avoiding exacerbation of the underlying inflammatory condition.

In the introductory case, acute adrenal insufficiency occurred because Johnny was switched acutely from oral prednisone to an inhaled glucocorticoid. On average, inhaled preparations deliver approximately 20% of the dose to the lung, while the other 80% is swallowed. However, the glucocorticoids available as inhaled formulations (see below) have significant first-pass hepatic metabolism, so that the swallowed portion is converted to inactive metabolites by the liver. Thus, Johnny's abrupt switch from an orally available glucocorticoid to an inhaled formulation caused acute adrenal insufficiency. After Johnny was placed back on oral prednisone, he was able to taper the dose slowly and, once his hypothalamic-pituitary–adrenal axis had been reactivated, use the inhaled glucocorticoid alone.

Routes of Administration

Different drug delivery methods allow selective targeting of glucocorticoid to a particular tissue. The relevant concept is that *it is possible to administer glucocorticoids locally at many times the normal plasma concentration, while minimiz-*

ing untoward systemic adverse effects. Some examples of these methods include inhaled, cutaneous, and depot preparations of glucocorticoids. The administration of glucocorticoids during pregnancy is also an example of selective targeting because the placenta can metabolically partition glucocorticoids between mother and fetus (see below).

Inhaled Glucocorticoids. Inhaled glucocorticoids are the formulation of choice in the chronic treatment of asthma. Glucocorticoids reduce asthma symptoms by inhibiting airway inflammatory responses, especially eosinophil-mediated inflammation. The exact mechanism(s) is unknown, but is thought to involve inhibition of cytokine release and subsequent inhibition of the inflammatory cascade (see Chapter 46). Because systemic therapy with glucocorticoids can lead to many serious adverse effects, efforts have been made to develop inhaled glucocorticoids with low oral bioavailability, thereby allowing high-dose delivery directly to the airway mucosa while minimizing systemic dosing. The goal of inhaled glucocorticoid therapy is to maximize the topical to systemic ratio of glucocorticoid concentration. This route of administration makes glucocorticoids safer for long-term dosing, especially when used in children.

Microcrystalline powders and metered dose inhalers of glucocorticoids such as **fluticasone, beclomethasone, flunisolide,** and **triamcinolone** (Fig. 27-7) are currently available as inhaled formulations, allowing delivery of high concentrations of these potent glucocorticoids directly to the lung epithelium. The swallowed portion is absorbed into the portal circulation and, depending on the compound, hydroxylated by the liver to inactive metabolites. The significant first-pass metabolism of fluticasone, for example, ensures that less than 1% of the swallowed glucocorticoid is systemically bioavailable. *Thus, the systemic effects can be reduced by extensive first-pass hepatic metabolism of certain agents.* Although the portion of glucocorticoid delivered to the lung is eventually absorbed into the systemic circulation, the quantity delivered to the systemic circulation is lower than that for an oral glucocorticoid such as prednisone. Because the inhaled glucocorticoid is delivered directly to the inflamed organ, rather than via the systemic circulation, less inhaled glucocorticoid than oral glucocorticoid is required to control airway inflammation.

If a patient treated chronically with systemic glucocorticoids is switched to inhaled glucocorticoids, care must be taken not to stop the systemic dosing abruptly. As noted above, it is possible to precipitate acute adrenal insufficiency by suddenly switching systemic therapy to inhaled therapy, which provides a much lower systemic dose of glucocorticoid. Acute adrenal insufficiency can be life-threatening and should be treated immediately with a large dose of intravenous glucocorticoid; for this reason, Johnny was given an intravenous infusion of hydrocortisone in the introductory case.

Oropharyngeal candidiasis is another potential complication of inhaled glucocorticoid therapy, because some glucocorticoid is delivered directly to the oral and pharyngeal mucosa. This results in local immunosuppression and allows infection with opportunistic organisms. Oropharyngeal candidiasis can be avoided by using antifungal mouthwash after each administration of aerosolized glucocorticoid.

Many patients with asthma also have symptoms of aller-

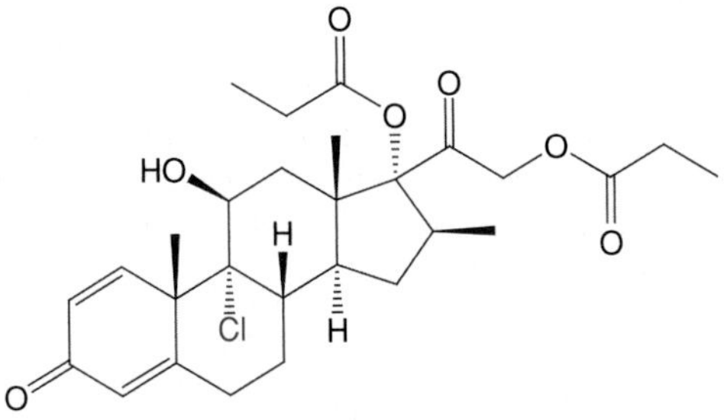

Beclomethasone dipropionate

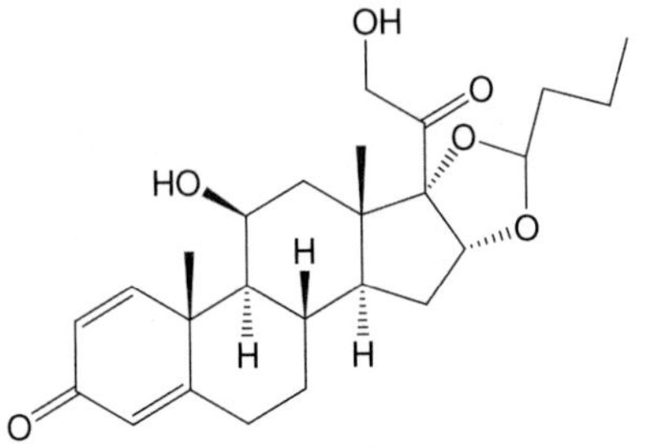

Budesonide

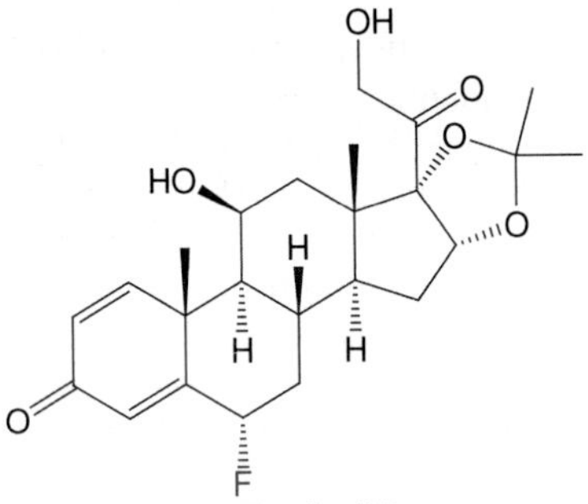

Flunisolide

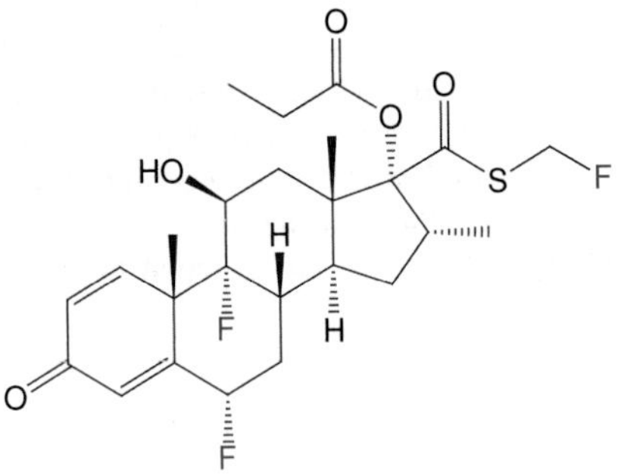

Fluticasone propionate

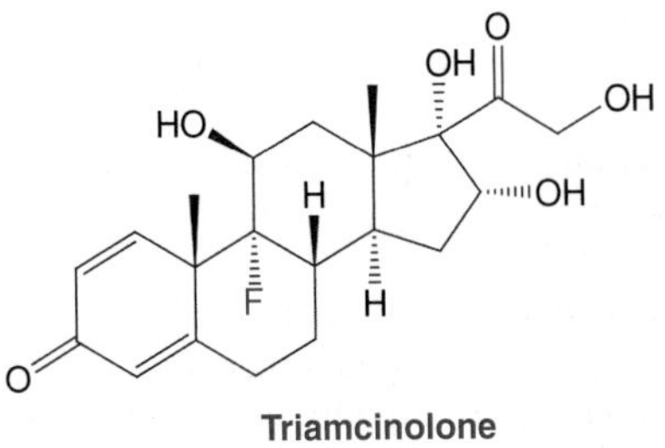

Triamcinolone

Figure 27-7. Structures of common inhaled glucocorticoids. Most of the inhaled glucocorticoids are halogenated analogues of cortisol that are highly potent glucocorticoid agonists with little mineralocorticoid activity (halogen atoms are shown in blue). Their high potency allows low doses of the inhaled glucocorticoids to inhibit

gic rhinitis. Intranasal administration of a glucocorticoid analogue is an effective therapy for these symptoms. This results in profound local suppression of the eosinophilic response and is often superior to antihistamines in the treatment of allergic rhinitis.

Cutaneous Glucocorticoids. Preparations of topical glucocorticoids are available for a number of dermatologic disorders, including psoriasis, lichen planus, and atopic dermatitis. Cutaneous administration delivers an extremely low percentage of the glucocorticoid systemically, allowing topical dosing at many-fold higher local concentrations than could be achieved safely with systemic administration. The glucocorticoid that is administered must be biologically active because the skin has little, if any, of the 11β-HSDI enzyme needed to convert glucocorticoid prodrugs to active compounds. Hydrocortisone, methylprednisolone, and dexamethasone are effective steroids for cutaneous use.

Depot Glucocorticoids. Depot intramuscular preparations of glucocorticoid analogues last for days to weeks and can be an alternative to daily or alternate-day oral glucocorticoids in the treatment of inflammatory diseases. Although depot formulations reduce the necessity for daily oral administration, these preparations are seldom used because the dose cannot be titrated on a frequent basis. Depot preparations of methylprednisolone suspended in polyethylene glycol are used, however, for **intra-articular administration.** This approach can be indicated for inflammatory processes restricted to the joints, such as rheumatoid arthritis or gout. Intra-articular glucocorticoid injection is useful in acute attacks of gout that are unresponsive to colchicine or indomethacin. Intra-articular and bursa injection requires the use of active glucocorticoid, because joint tissue lacks the 11β-HSDI enzyme required to hydroxylate and, thus, activate 11-keto glucocorticoids.

Pregnancy. The placental–maternal barrier provides another example of selective glucocorticoid targeting. During pregnancy, the placenta metabolically separates the fetus from the mother. Because of this, prednisone can be administered to the mother during pregnancy without fetal side effects. The maternal liver activates the prednisone to prednisolone, but fetal placental 11β-HSD II is capable of converting the prednisolone back to inactive prednisone. Because the liver does not function during fetal life, the fetus does not, in turn, activate prednisone. *Therefore, use of the ''prodrug'' prednisone in pregnancy does not result in delivery of an active glucocorticoid to the fetus.*

Glucocorticoids also promote lung development in the fetus. If glucocorticoid therapy is indicated to promote lung maturation in a fetus, dexamethasone is commonly adminis-

the local inflammatory response that is a critical component of asthma pathophysiology. In addition, because a number of these compounds are subject to almost complete first-pass metabolism in the liver, the fraction of inhaled glucocorticoid that is inadvertently swallowed (80% of the inhaled dose) becomes inactivated so that it is not systemically bioavailable. The fraction of inhaled glucocorticoid delivered to the lung is eventually absorbed into the systemic circulation.

tered to the mother. Dexamethasone is a poor substrate for placental 11β-HSD II, and is therefore present in active form in the fetal circulation, where it stimulates maturation of the lung. The dose must be titrated carefully because exposure to excessive glucocorticoid can have a number of deleterious effects on fetal development.

Inhibitors of Adrenocortical Hormone Synthesis

A number of compounds are available to inhibit hormone biosynthesis by the adrenal cortex. Although these drugs have some specificity for individual adrenal enzymes (Table 27-2), it is not generally possible to alter the production of a single adrenal hormone independent of other hormones. Because the enzymes necessary for adrenal hormone synthesis are P450 enzymes, use of these inhibitors is also associated with potential toxicity to hepatic P450 enzymes. In general, these agents can be divided into drugs that affect earlier versus later steps in adrenal hormone synthesis. The agents that inhibit early steps have broad effects, while those affecting later steps have more selective actions.

Mitotane, aminoglutethimide, and ketoconazole inhibit early steps in adrenal hormone synthesis. **Mitotane** is a structural analogue of DDT (a potent insecticide) that is toxic to adrenocortical mitochondria. Although used infrequently, mitotane may be indicated for medical adrenalectomy in cases of severe Cushing's disease or adrenocortical carcinoma. Patients taking mitotane commonly develop hypercholesterolemia because of the drug's concomitant inhibition of cholesterol oxidase.

Aminoglutethimide inhibits side-chain cleavage enzyme. Aminoglutethimide also inhibits the enzyme aromatase, which is important for conversion of androgens to estrogens. Because of its ability to inhibit aromatase, aminoglutethimide is under investigation as a potential therapy for breast cancer (see Chapter 28, Pharmacology of Reproduction).

Ketoconazole is an antifungal agent that acts by inhibiting the fungal P450 enzymes (see Chapter 36, Pharmacology of Fungal Infections). Because the enzymes that mediate adrenal and gonadal hormone synthesis are also members of the P450 enzyme family, high doses of ketoconazole also suppress steroid synthesis in these organs. This agent primarily inhibits 17, 20-lyase (important for adrenal androgen synthesis). High doses of ketoconazole also inhibit side-chain cleavage enzyme, the enzyme that converts cholesterol to pregnenolone. Because pregnenolone generation is required for the synthesis of all adrenal hormones, high-dose ketoconazole has broadly inhibitory effects on adrenocortical hormone synthesis.

Metyrapone and trilostane have more specific effects on adrenal hormone synthesis. **Metyrapone** inhibits 11β-hydroxylation, resulting in impaired cortisol synthesis (Fig. 27-2). Because cortisol is the adrenal steroid responsible for feedback inhibition of ACTH release, treatment with metyrapone also results in disinhibition of ACTH secretion. Thus, metyrapone can be administered as a test of ACTH reserve.

Trilostane is a reversible inhibitor of 3β-hydroxysteroid dehydrogenase. Administration of this agent leads to reduced aldosterone and cortisol production in the adrenal cortex.

Glucocorticoid Receptor Antagonists

Mifepristone (RU-486) is a progesterone receptor antagonist used to induce abortion early in pregnancy (see Chapter 28). At higher concentrations, mifepristone also blocks the glucocorticoid receptor. This action makes mifepristone potentially useful for the treatment of life-threatening elevated glucocorticoid levels, such as in ectopic ACTH syndrome, although its clinical usefulness for this purpose has not been evaluated fully.

MINERALOCORTICOIDS

PHYSIOLOGY

Synthesis

Like cortisol, **aldosterone** is a 21-carbon steroid hormone derived from cholesterol. Enzymes unique to aldosterone synthesis are expressed only in the zona glomerulosa, and

| TABLE 27-2 | Sites of Action and Pathways Affected by Inhibitors of Adrenal Hormone Synthesis |

INHIBITOR	SITE OF ACTION	ADRENAL STEROIDOGENIC PATHWAYS AFFECTED
Mitotane	Mitochondria	All
Aminoglutethimide	Side-chain cleavage enzyme	All (aromatase also inhibited in ovary)
Ketoconazole	Primarily 17, 20-lyase	Low concentrations: ↓ Androgen synthesis
		High concentrations: ↓ Synthesis of all adrenal and gonadal steroid hormones
Metyrapone	11β-hydroxylase	Cortisol synthesis
Trilostane	3β-hydroxysteroid dehydrogenase	Cortisol and aldosterone synthesis

are under the regulation of the renin–angiotensin system and potassium.

Metabolism

Circulating aldosterone binds with low affinity to transcortin, albumin, and a specific mineralocorticoid binding protein. Approximately 50% to 60% of circulating aldosterone is bound to transport proteins, resulting in a short elimination half-life (20 minutes). Orally administered aldosterone also has high first-pass hepatic metabolism, with approximately 75% of the hormone metabolized to an inactive form during each pass through the liver. As a result, orally administered aldosterone is not an effective replacement therapy in adrenal insufficiency states.

Physiologic Actions

Mineralocorticoids play important roles in regulating sodium reabsorption in sweat and salivary glands, the colon, and the kidney. In each of these organs, circulating aldosterone diffuses across the plasma membrane and binds to a cytosolic **mineralocorticoid receptor** (synonymous with the Type I glucocorticoid receptor). The aldosterone:mineralocorticoid receptor complex is then transported into the nucleus, where it binds to mineralocorticoid response elements on specific gene promoters and thus up-regulates or down-regulates gene expression. Studies have also demonstrated rapid nongenomic actions of aldosterone, which may be mediated by hormone binding to a cell surface aldosterone receptor. The physiologic role of this second signaling mechanism is currently unknown.

A major role of aldosterone is to increase **Na^+/K^+ ATPase** expression in the basolateral membrane of distal nephron cells. Enhanced Na^+/K^+ ATPase activity secondarily increases sodium reabsorption and potassium secretion across the lumenal epithelium of the nephron (see Chapter 20). As a result, sodium retention, potassium excretion, and H^+ excretion are all enhanced by aldosterone. Excess aldosterone can cause hypokalemic alkalosis, while hypoaldosteronism can cause hyperkalemic acidosis.

Although aldosterone has classically been considered important for sodium homeostasis and potassium regulation, recent data also support extrarenal actions of aldosterone in cardiovascular tissues. Animal studies have demonstrated **aldosterone-mediated cardiac fibrosis**, but only in the setting of salt loading. The fibrosis appears to be a reparative process secondary to inflammatory necrosis. Importantly, antagonists of aldosterone action at the mineralocorticoid receptor, such as spironolactone and eplerenone, may be useful pharmacologic agents for preventing these cardiac actions.

Regulation

Three systems regulate aldosterone synthesis: the renin-angiotensin–aldosterone system, plasma potassium levels, and ACTH.

The **renin-angiotensin–aldosterone system** is a central regulator of extracellular fluid volume. Decreases in extracellular fluid volume decrease perfusion pressure at the afferent arteriole of the renal glomerulus, which acts as a baro-receptor. This stimulates the juxtaglomerular cells to secrete renin, a protease that cleaves the prohormone angiotensinogen to angiotensin I. Angiotensin I is then converted to angiotensin II by angiotensin converting enzyme, which is expressed at high concentrations by the capillary endothelium of the lungs. Angiotensin II has direct arteriolar pressor effects, and it stimulates aldosterone synthesis by binding to and activating a G protein-coupled receptor in zona glomerulosa cells of the adrenal cortex.

Potassium loading increases aldosterone synthesis independent of renin activity. Because aldosterone activity at the distal nephron increases potassium excretion, this control mechanism serves a homeostatic role in regulating potassium balance.

Finally, **ACTH** acutely stimulates aldosterone synthesis in the zona glomerulosa. ACTH is believed to play only a minor physiologic role in aldosterone synthesis, however. Unlike cortisol, aldosterone does not negatively regulate ACTH secretion.

PATHOPHYSIOLOGY

Aldosterone Hypofunction

Aldosterone hypofunction (hypoaldosteronism) can result from a primary decrease in aldosterone synthesis or action, or from a secondary decrease in aldosterone regulators such as renin. Most cases of hypoaldosteronism result from decreased aldosterone synthesis. Defects in the gene coding for steroid 21-hydroxylase, an enzyme necessary for both aldosterone and glucocorticoid synthesis, lead to congenital adrenal hyperplasia (discussed under adrenal androgen pathophysiology) and cause salt wasting as a result of aldosterone deficiency. **Addison's disease,** or primary adrenal insufficiency, results in hypoaldosteronism secondary to destruction of the zona glomerulosa. Most cases of Addison's disease are caused by autoimmune adrenalitis; other causes include tuberculosis and metastatic cancer. In each case, aldosterone hypofunction can lead to salt wasting, hyperkalemia, and acidosis. Hypoaldosteronism can also result from states of decreased renin production (so-called *hyporeninemic hypoaldosteronism,* which is common in diabetic renal insufficiency), from resistance to the action of aldosterone at the level of the mineralocorticoid receptor, or from inactivating mutations of the aldosterone-regulated epithelial sodium channel (ENaC) in the cortical collecting duct of the nephron.

Aldosterone Hyperfunction

Primary hyperaldosteronism results from excess aldosterone production by the adrenal cortex. Bilateral zona glomerulosa adrenal hyperplasia and an aldosterone-producing adenoma are the two most common causes. Increased aldosterone synthesis leads to positive sodium balance, with consequent extracellular volume expansion, suppression of plasma renin activity, potassium wasting and hypokalemia, and hypertension.

PHARMACOLOGIC CLASSES AND AGENTS

Mineralocorticoid Receptor Agonists

Pathophysiologic conditions leading to hypoaldosteronism necessitate replacement with physiologic doses of a mineralocorticoid. It is not possible to administer aldosterone itself as a therapeutic agent, because the liver converts over 75% of oral aldosterone to an inactive metabolite during first-pass metabolism. Instead, the cortisol analogue **fludrocortisone,** which has minimal first-pass hepatic metabolism and a high mineralocorticoid to glucocorticoid potency ratio, is used. The adverse effects of fludrocortisone therapy are all related to the ability of this agent to mimic a state of mineralocorticoid excess, including hypertension, hypokalemia, and even cardiac failure. In order to ensure that an appropriate dose of drug is being administered, it is crucial to monitor serum potassium and blood pressure levels closely in all patients receiving fludrocortisone.

Mineralocorticoid Receptor Antagonists

Spironolactone (also discussed in Chapters 20 and 28) is a competitive antagonist at the mineralocorticoid receptor, but the drug also binds to and inhibits the androgen and progesterone receptors. The latter actions, which result in adverse effects such as gynecomastia in males, limit the usefulness of this agent in some patient subsets. **Eplerenone** is a mineralocorticoid receptor antagonist that binds selectively to the mineralocorticoid receptor; this selectivity may make eplerenone free of the unwanted adverse effects of spironolactone. Both spironolactone and eplerenone can be used as antihypertensive agents, and both are approved for use in patients with heart failure.

Antagonism of the mineralocorticoid receptor can result in significant hyperkalemia. Because many patients with heart failure are prescribed both spironolactone or eplerenone and an angiotensin converting enzyme inhibitor (which also raises plasma potassium levels), it is important to monitor potassium levels closely in these patients.

ADRENAL ANDROGENS

PHYSIOLOGY

Sex steroids produced by the adrenal cortex, primarily **dehydroepiandrosterone** (DHEA), have an uncertain role in human physiology. DHEA seems to be a prohormone that is converted to more potent androgens, primarily testosterone, in the periphery. Adrenocortical androgens are an important source of testosterone in females; these hormones are necessary for the development of female axillary and pubic hair at the time of puberty, when adrenal androgen secretion is activated (adrenarche).

PATHOPHYSIOLOGY

Congenital adrenal hyperplasia (CAH) and **polycystic ovarian syndrome** are two important diseases related to adrenocortical androgen production. *Congenital adrenal hyperplasia* is a clinical term denoting a number of inherited enzyme deficiencies in the adrenal cortex. These abnormalities cause hirsutism and virilization in females as a result of increased adrenocortical androgen production. Polycystic

ovarian syndrome, discussed in Chapter 28, may be caused by congenital adrenal hyperplasia in a subset of patients.

The most common form of congenital adrenal hyperplasia results from a deficiency of **steroid 21-hydroxylase.** Deficiency of 21-hydroxylase results in the inability of adrenocortical cells to synthesize both aldosterone and cortisol (Fig. 27-8). Because cortisol is the main negative feedback regulator of pituitary ACTH release, the decreased cortisol synthesis that results from 21-hydroxylase deficiency disinhibits ACTH release. Increased ACTH restores the level of cortisol, but there is also shunting of precursor compounds into the "unblocked" androgen pathway, resulting in greater production of DHEA and androstenedione. The liver subsequently converts these compounds into testosterone. In severe 21-hydroxylase deficiency, there may be a virilizing effect on the developing female fetus. As a result, female neonates with 21-hydroxylase deficiency typically have masculinized or ambiguous external genitalia. In the male, however, increased adrenal androgens may have little or no noticeable phenotypic effect. Instead, males with 21-hydroxylase deficiency are commonly diagnosed in infancy during an acute salt-wasting crisis, which results from the inability to synthesize aldosterone. Mild 21-hydroxylase deficiency may manifest later in life as hirsutism, acne, and oligomenorrhea in young women after menarche.

Treatment of congenital adrenal hyperplasia is aimed at glucocorticoid replacement, which suppresses excessive hypothalamic and pituitary release of CRH and ACTH, resulting in decreased production of adrenal androgens.

PHARMACOLOGIC CLASSES AND AGENTS

The androgens synthesized by the adrenal gland can be viewed as prohormones. Because no specific receptors for either DHEA or androstenedione have been described, the activity of these hormones depends on conversion of the hormones to testosterone, and subsequently to dihydrotestosterone, in peripheral target tissues. As discussed above, adrenal androgen excess can cause a variety of syndromes in women; the pharmacologic interruption of excess androgenic activity is discussed in Chapter 28.

DHEA is not regulated by the FDA and is commonly used as an "over the counter" drug. Population cross-sectional studies have shown a reciprocal relationship between an age-related decline in DHEA levels and the risk of cardiovascular disease and cancer. Replacement therapy with DHEA may be indicated for cases of Addison's disease in which there is bona fide DHEA deficiency. Some studies have reported decreased DHEA levels in chronic fatigue syndrome, but a recent large clinical trial showed no benefit of DHEA in elderly men and women with low circulating DHEA levels.

Exogenous DHEA can be converted to testosterone by the liver. As a result, DHEA is commonly abused for its anabolic effects.

Conclusion and Future Directions

Aldosterone, cortisol, and the adrenal androgens regulate many aspects of basic homeostasis. Aldosterone regulates extracellular fluid volume by promoting sodium reabsorption and fluid retention. Cortisol regulates diverse physio-

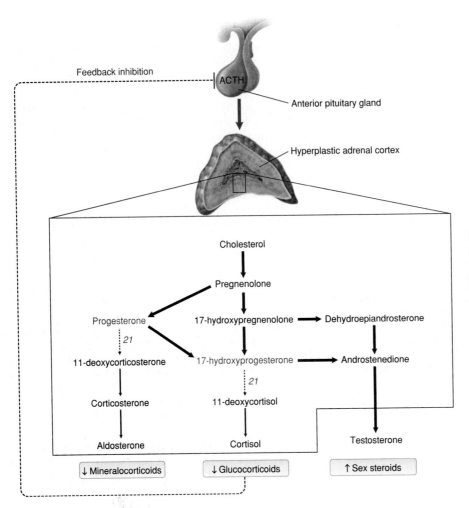

Figure 27-8. Congenital adrenal hyperplasia. Steroid 21-hydroxylase deficiency, the most common cause of congenital adrenal hyperplasia, results in impaired biosynthesis of aldosterone and cortisol *(dashed lines)*. Therefore, steroid hormone synthesis in the adrenal cortex is shunted toward increased production of sex steroids *(thick lines)*. The lack of cortisol production decreases the negative feedback on corticotroph cells of the anterior pituitary gland *(dashed line)*, causing increased ACTH release *(thick blue arrow)*. Increased levels of ACTH induce adrenal hyperplasia, and further stimulate the synthesis of sex steroids. This pathway can be interrupted by administering exogenous cortisol. The deficient enzyme is shown as a number: 21, steroid 21-hydroxylase.

logic processes, including energy homeostasis and inflammatory responses. The physiologic role of adrenal androgens is unknown, but pathophysiologic states causing increased adrenal androgen production have significant masculinizing effects in women. Antagonists of aldosterone are currently used as diuretics, and recent evidence in animal models supports an additional role for these agents in the prevention of cardiac fibrosis. To this end, antagonists specific for the aldosterone receptor may become important therapies for cardiovascular diseases. Glucocorticoid pharmacology is an immense field, primarily because glucocorticoids are used to suppress inflammation in a number of disease states. Chronic glucocorticoid use is associated with a multitude of predictable adverse effects, and future research in this area will attempt to minimize the adverse effects of glucocorticoid therapy while maintaining the anti-inflammatory actions. Such efforts could include the development of tissue-selective glucocorticoid agonists and antagonists (analogous to the selective estrogen receptor modulators), as well as further refinement of drug delivery methods. The pharmacology of adrenal androgens needs to be studied more extensively to determine the indications, if any, for DHEA therapy.

Suggested Reading

Barnes PJ. Corticosteroids: the drugs to beat. *Eur J Pharmacol* 2006;533:2–14. (*Review of glucocorticoid pharmacology, with emphasis on inhaled steroids.*)

Fuller PJ, Young MJ. Mechanisms of mineralocorticoid action. *Hypertension* 2005;46:1227–1235. (*Molecular mechanisms of mineralocorticoid action, including cardiovascular effects.*)

Nair KS, Rizza RA, O'Brien P, et al. DHEA in elderly women and DHEA or testosterone in elderly men. *N Engl J Med* 2006;355:1647–1659. (*Recent large clinical trial of DHEA.*)

Salvatori R. Adrenal insufficiency. *JAMA* 2005;294:2481–2488. (*Pathophysiology and treatment of adrenal insufficiency.*)

Sapolsky R. How do glucocorticoids influence stress responses? Integrating permissive, suppressive, stimulatory, and preparative actions. *Endocrine Rev* 2000;21:55–89. (*Thorough review discussing the numerous roles of glucocorticoids in stress responses.*)

Stellato C. Post-transcriptional and nongenomic effects of glucocorticoids. *Proc Am Thorac Soc* 2004;1:255–263. (*Details of recent advances in glucocorticoid signaling.*)

Williams JS, Williams GH. 50th anniversary of aldosterone. *J Clin Endocrinol Metab* 2003;88:2364–2372. (*Historical review of mineralocorticoids.*)

Drug Summary Table | **Chapter 27 Pharmacology of the Adrenal Gland**

Drug	Clinical Applications	Serious and Common Adverse Effects	Contraindications	Therapeutic Considerations
GLUCOCORTICOID RECEPTOR AGONISTS *Mechanism—Mimic cortisol function by acting as agonists at the glucocorticoid receptor*				
Prednisone Prednisolone Methylprednisolone Dexamethasone Hydrocortisone Fluticasone Beclomethasone Flunisolide Triamcinolone Budesonide	Inflammatory conditions in many different organs Autoimmune diseases Replacement therapy for primary and secondary adrenal insufficiency (hydrocortisone)	*Immunosuppression, cataracts, hyperglycemia, hypercortisolism, depression, euphoria, osteoporosis, growth retardation in children, muscle atrophy* Impaired wound healing, hypertension, fluid retention Inhaled glucocorticoids may also cause oropharyngeal candidiasis and dysphonia Topical glucocorticoids may also cause skin atrophy	Systemic fungal infection	See Table 27-1 for relative potency and duration of action of individual agents Pharmacologic glucocorticoid therapy does not correct the underlying disease etiology, but rather limits the effects of inflammation Chronic glucocorticoid treatment should be tapered slowly; abrupt withdrawal of systemic glucocorticoids can lead to acute adrenal insufficiency Intranasal and inhaled formulations greatly reduce systemic adverse effects; do not switch abruptly from high-dose oral to inhaled glucocorticoids The intrinsic activity of a glucocorticoid is especially important for topically administered drugs because the skin does not possess appreciable amounts of 11β-HSDI Glucocorticoid agents with higher anti-inflammatory potency typically have a longer duration of action Inhaled glucocorticoids include fluticasone, beclomethasone, flunisolide, triamcinolone, and budesonide
GLUCOCORTICOID RECEPTOR ANTAGONISTS *Mechanism—Competitive antagonist of cortisol action at the glucocorticoid receptor*				
Mifepristone (RU-486)	Abortion (through day 49 of pregnancy)	*Prolonged bleeding time, bacterial infections, sepsis* Nausea, vomiting, diarrhea, cramps, abnormal vaginal bleeding, headache	Chronic adrenal failure Ectopic pregnancy Hemorrhagic disorders Anticoagulation therapy Inherited porphyrias Intrauterine device Undiagnosed adnexal mass	Mifepristone is a progesterone receptor antagonist used to induce abortion early in pregnancy; at higher concentrations, mifepristone also blocks the glucocorticoid receptor; potentially, the latter action could make mifepristone useful for the treatment of life-threatening elevated glucocorticoid levels, such as in the ectopic ACTH syndrome
INHIBITORS OF GLUCOCORTICOID SYNTHESIS *Mechanism—Inhibit various steps in glucocorticoid hormone biosynthesis*				
Mitotane	Medical adrenalectomy in cases of severe Cushing's syndrome or adrenocortical carcinoma	*Visual disturbance, hemorrhagic cystitis* Hypercholesterolemia, somnolence, nausea, depression	Live rotavirus vaccine	Structural analogue of DDT that is toxic to adrenocortical mitochondria Hypercholesterolemia may result from inhibition of cholesterol oxidase
Aminoglutethimide	Cushing's syndrome	*Cortisol insufficiency, agranulocytosis, leukopenia, neutropenia, pancytopenia* Pruritus, nausea, hypotension, somnolence	Hypersensitivity to glutethimide or aminoglutethimide	Aminoglutethimide inhibits side-chain cleavage enzyme as well as aromatase, which is important for conversion of androgens to estrogens; therapeutic potential for breast cancer is under investigation

(Continued)

Drug Summary Table **Chapter 27 Pharmacology of the Adrenal Gland** (*Continued*)

Drug	Clinical Applications	Serious and Common Adverse Effects	Contraindications	Therapeutic Considerations
Metyrapone	Diagnostic evaluation of hypothalamic-pituitary-adrenal axis Cushing's syndrome	*Cortisol insufficiency* Hypertension	Adrenal cortical insufficiency	Inhibits 11β-hydroxylation, resulting in impaired cortisol synthesis Treatment with metyrapone also results in disinhibition of ACTH secretion; thus, metyrapone can be administered to test ACTH reserve
Trilostane	Cushing's syndrome Aldosteronism	*Addisonian crisis* Postural hypotension, hypoglycemia, diarrhea, nausea	Adrenal cortical insufficiency Renal or hepatic dysfunction	Trilostane is a reversible inhibitor of 3β-hydroxysteroid dehydrogenase, which reduces aldosterone and cortisol production in the adrenal cortex
Ketoconazole	See Drug Summary Table: Chapter 34 Pharmacology of Fungal Infections			

MINERALOCORTICOID RECEPTOR AGONISTS
Mechanism—Agonist at the mineralocorticoid receptor

Fludrocortisone	Hypoaldosteronism	*Hypertension, hypokalemia, heart failure, thrombophlebitis, secondary hypocortisolism, increased intracranial pressure* Edema, impaired wound healing, rash, myopathy, hyperglycemia, menstrual irregularities	Systemic fungal infection	The adverse effects of fludrocortisone therapy are related to its ability to mimic a state of mineralocorticoid excess, including hypertension, hypokalemia, and cardiac failure; serum potassium and blood pressure levels should be monitored closely

MINERALOCORTICOID RECEPTOR ANTAGONISTS
Mechanism—Competitive antagonists of aldosterone action at the mineralocorticoid receptor

Spironolactone Eplerenone	See Drug Summary Table: Chapter 20 Pharmacology of Volume Regulation			

ADRENAL SEX STEROID
Mechanism—DHEA is a prohormone that is converted to testosterone in the periphery

Dehydroepiandrosterone (DHEA)	Hypoaldosteronism Chronic fatigue syndrome (uncertain benefits)	Acne, hepatitis, hirsutism, androgenization	Breast, ovarian, or prostate cancer	May be used as replacement therapy for cases of Addison's disease with documented DHEA deficiency; clinical efficacy in treatment of chronic fatigue syndrome is under investigation; DHEA is commonly abused for its anabolic effects

28

Pharmacology of Reproduction

Ehrin J. Armstrong and Robert L. Barbieri

INTRODUCTION

This chapter presents endocrine pharmacology relevant to both the male and female reproductive tracts. Although men and women differ in their hormonal profiles, androgens and estrogens are both under the control of the anterior pituitary gland gonadotropins, luteinizing hormone (LH) and follicle stimulating hormone (FSH), and ultimately regulated by hypothalamic release of gonadotropin-releasing hormone (GnRH). Female hormone patterns are temporally more complex and cyclic than male patterns: hormonal control of the menstrual cycle is an illustrative example of how sex hormones are integrated into a complex physiologic system. Understanding the menstrual cycle also provides a basis for understanding the pharmacology of contraception. A number of diseases are treated pharmacologically via modification of reproductive hormone activity; these range from infertility and endometriosis to breast and prostate cancer. Key concepts in this chapter include: (1) the interactions between

estrogen and the pituitary gland; (2) the effects of GnRH release frequency on gonadotropin release; (3) the tissue selectivity of estrogen receptor agonists and antagonists; and (4) the various strategies used to antagonize the effects of endogenous sex hormones, from suppression of the hypothalamic-pituitary–reproduction axis to antagonism at the target tissue receptor. Because of its historical role in the prevention of osteoporosis, estrogen replacement therapy is discussed both here and in Chapter 30, Pharmacology of Bone Mineral Homeostasis. Androgen replacement therapy is discussed at the end of this chapter.

Case

Amy J first notices that her hair is thinning somewhat during her teenage years. Even though she loses some hair on her scalp, Ms. J notices excessive hair growth on her face; she sometimes has to shave to remove inappropriate hair growth. At age 24, she goes to her doctor complaining of both her hair problem and the fact that her periods are irregular. On further questioning, the doctor discovers that the longest interval between her menstrual cycles has been 6 months and the shortest 22 days. When Ms. J does have periods, they are heavy and last for more than her previous average of 5 days. The increased hair growth on her face, extremities, abdomen, and breasts had begun around age 15. Ms. J also reports a problem with being overweight since high school, although in middle school she had been extremely active in soccer, field hockey, and swimming. The doctor orders several tests, and finds that Ms. J has mildly elevated free and total testosterone levels and an increased ratio of plasma LH to FSH.

Based on these findings, the doctor tells Ms. J that she probably has a disorder called polycystic ovarian syndrome (PCOS). He recommends combination oral contraceptives to regularize her menstrual cycles. He also prescribes spironolactone to reduce her problems with hair growth and balding.

QUESTIONS

■ **1.** What is the pathophysiologic link between excessive hair growth and infertility in polycystic ovarian syndrome?

■ **2.** How do oral contraceptives act, and how would they help regulate Ms. J's menstrual cycles?

■ **3.** Why was spironolactone prescribed to reduce Ms. J's hair problem?

PHYSIOLOGY OF REPRODUCTIVE HORMONES

SYNTHESIS OF PROGESTINS, ANDROGENS, AND ESTROGENS

The synthesis of progestins, androgens, and estrogens is closely intertwined. All three groups are steroid hormones derived from the metabolism of cholesterol. The synthesis of these hormones is similar to that of adrenal sex hormones, which is discussed in Chapter 27, Pharmacology of the Adrenal Cortex.

The terminology *"progestins," "androgens,"* and *"estrogens"* denotes a number of related hormones, rather than a single molecule in each group (Fig. 28-1). The **progestins** consist of **progesterone,** a common precursor to testosterone and estrogen synthesis (see also Fig. 27-2), and a number of synthetically altered progesterone derivatives used for therapeutic purposes. Progestins generally exert antiproliferative effects on the female endometrium by promoting the endometrial lining to secrete rather than proliferate (see below). Progesterone is also required for the maintenance of pregnancy. **Androgens,** all of which have masculinizing properties, include dehydroepiandrosterone (DHEA), androstenedione, **testosterone,** and **dihydrotestosterone (DHT);** among the androgens, testosterone is considered the classic circulating androgen and DHT the classic intracellular androgen. Androgens are required for conversion to a male

phenotype during development and for male sexual maturation. **Estrogens** refer to a number of substances that share a common feminizing activity. **17β-Estradiol** is the most potent naturally occurring estrogen, while estrone and estriol are less potent.

Note that *all estrogens are derived from the aromatization of precursor androgens* (Fig. 28-1). The ovary and placenta most actively synthesize the **aromatase** enzyme that converts androgens to estrogens, but other non-reproductive tissues such as adipose tissue, hypothalamic neurons, and muscle can also aromatize androgens to estrogen. After menopause, the majority of circulating estrogen is derived from adipose tissue. This is also the main source of circulating estrogens in men.

HORMONE ACTION AND METABOLISM

Progestins, androgens, and estrogens are all hormones that bind to a related superfamily of nuclear hormone receptors; glucocorticoids, mineralocorticoids, vitamin D, and thyroid hormone also bind to the same superfamily of receptors. Once synthesized, these hormones diffuse into the plasma, where they bind tightly to carrier proteins such as sex-hormone binding globulin (SHBG) and albumin. Only the unbound fraction of hormone is able to diffuse into cells and bind to an intracellular receptor. Interestingly, *testosterone is essentially a prohormone.* Testosterone binds to the androgen receptor, but with only modest affinity. As a result, testosterone has only modest androgenic activity. Instead, testosterone is converted in target tissues to the more active **dihydrotestosterone** (Fig. 28-2), which binds to the androgen receptor with an affinity tenfold higher than that of testosterone. The formation of dihydrotestosterone from testosterone is catalyzed by the enzyme **5α-reductase.** There are at least two subtypes of 5α-reductase. Differential tissue expression of these enzymes provides some pharmacologic specificity for the 5α-reductase inhibitors. The importance of dihydrotestosterone as the most active androgen is highlighted in individuals with inherited deficiencies of 5α-reductase. Males lacking this enzyme are phenotypically female, because they are unable to convert testosterone to dihydrotestosterone and are thus unable to activate a program of male differentiation during development.

Although separate progesterone, androgen, and estrogen receptors exist, complete selectivity of action does not exist because of the close structural similarities among the hormones. Progesterone receptors and androgen receptors are probably derived from a single ancestral receptor. Most progestins have significant cross-reactivity with androgen receptors, and prolonged progestin administration produces an androgenic effect (**virilization,** or the development of masculine features). Most synthetic progestins used for contraception and hormone replacement therapy have been modified to minimize their androgenic effects.

The **estrogen receptor** (ER) is the best studied of the sex hormone receptors and serves as an example for all three receptor types. Because progestins, androgens, and estrogens are lipophilic steroid hormones, the fraction of hormone that remains unbound to plasma proteins can freely diffuse across the plasma membrane into the cytosol of cells. Once inside the cell, the hormone ligand binds to its specific intracellular receptor, which subsequently dimerizes. For example, asso-

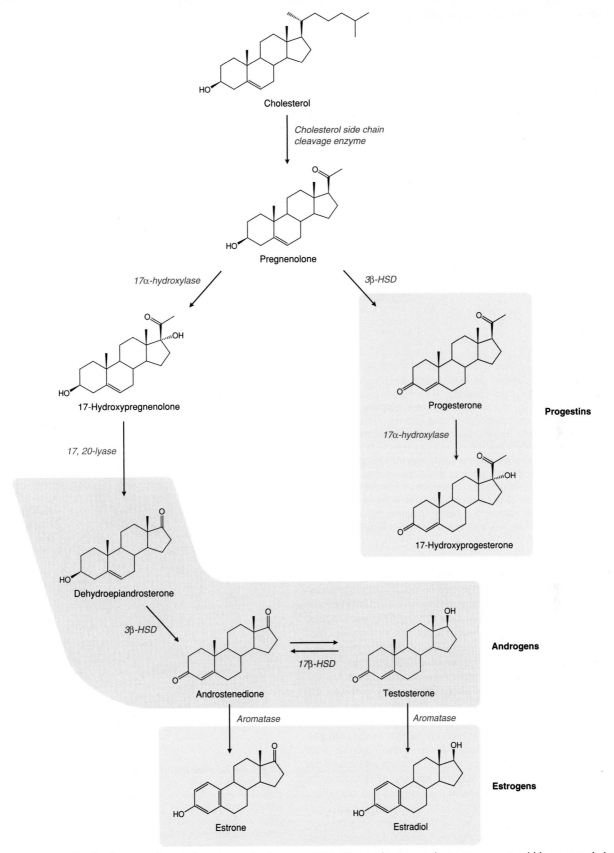

Figure 28-1. Synthesis of progestins, androgens, and estrogens. Progestins, androgens, and estrogens are steroid hormones derived from cholesterol. The major progestins include progesterone and 17α-hydroxyprogesterone. The androgens include dehydroepiandrosterone (DHEA), androstenedione, and testosterone. Estrogens include estrone and estradiol. Estrogens are aromatized forms of their conjugate androgens: androstenedione is aromatized to estrone, and testosterone is aromatized to estradiol. Estradiol and estrone are both metabolized to estriol, a weak estrogen *(not shown)*. Some of the precursor–product relationships among the hormones are omitted for clarity (see Fig. 27-2). HSD, hydroxysteroid dehydrogenase.

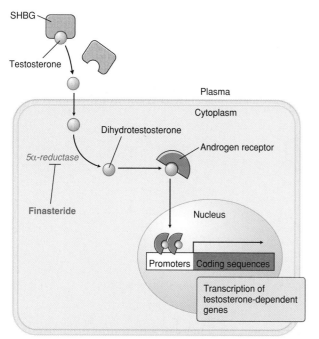

Figure 28-2. Peripheral conversion of testosterone. Testosterone circulates in the plasma bound to sex hormone binding globulin (SHBG) and/or albumin *(not shown)*. Free testosterone diffuses through the plasma membrane of cells into the cytosol. In target tissues, the enzyme 5α-reductase converts testosterone to dihydrotestosterone, which has increased androgenic activity relative to testosterone. Dihydrotestosterone binds with high affinity to the androgen receptor, forming a complex that is transported into the nucleus. Homodimers of dihydrotestosterone and androgen receptor initiate transcription of testosterone-dependent genes. Finasteride, a drug used in the treatment of benign prostatic hypertrophy and male pattern hair loss, inhibits the enzyme 5α-reductase.

ciation of estrogen with the estrogen receptor causes dimerization of two estrogen–estrogen receptor complexes, and the dimer then binds to **estrogen response elements** (EREs) in promoter regions of DNA. This binding to EREs, together with the recruitment of co-activators or co-repressors, enhances or inhibits the transcription of specific genes and thereby causes the physiologic effects of the hormone. Estrogen may also signal via membrane-bound receptors; the physiologic effects of this alternate signaling pathway are an active area of research.

There are two subtypes of estrogen receptors — ERα and ERβ. In addition, it is now recognized that many estrogen receptor actions involve association of the receptor with other transcription cofactors; that is, that dimerization of the estrogen receptor and subsequent binding of the dimer to EREs are insufficient to explain the complex and varied actions of estrogen in different tissues. *The specific transcription factors that are recruited by the estrogen receptor appear to be tissue-dependent and ligand-dependent, and probably account for some of the target specificity of estrogen action.* Although the subtypes and molecular associations of the androgen and progesterone receptors have not been studied as thoroughly as those of the estrogen receptor, it is likely that the same complexities exist for these receptors. The recognition that differential binding of modular transcription factors to ERs could alter estrogenic effects will

likely prove a burgeoning area of pharmacologic research in the near future, as pharmaceutical researchers continue to develop receptor agonists and antagonists with selective actions in specific tissues. Selective estrogen receptor modulators (SERMs, see below) are the first drugs to take advantage of the tissue selectivity of sex hormone receptor function.

HYPOTHALAMIC-PITUITARY–REPRODUCTION AXIS

A common hypothalamic-pituitary–gonadal axis regulates sex hormone synthesis. Gonadotropin-releasing hormone (GnRH) resides at the top of this three-tiered hierarchy. The hypothalamus secretes GnRH in pulses (Fig. 28-3). GnRH travels via the hypothalamic–pituitary portal system to stimulate gonadotroph cells of the anterior pituitary gland. Stim-

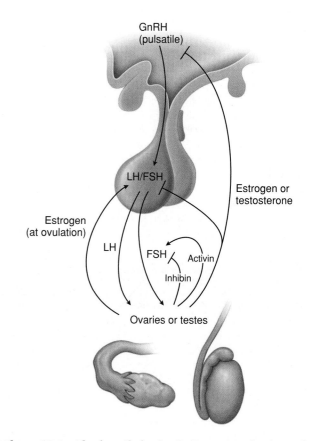

Figure 28-3. The hypothalamic-pituitary–reproduction axis. The hypothalamus secretes gonadotropin-releasing hormone (GnRH) into the hypothalamic-pituitary portal system in a pulsatile pattern. GnRH stimulates gonadotroph cells in the anterior pituitary gland to synthesize and release luteinizing hormone (LH) and follicle stimulating hormone (FSH). These two hormones, referred to as *gonadotropins,* promote ovarian and testicular synthesis of estrogen and testosterone, respectively. Estrogen and testosterone inhibit release of GnRH, LH, and FSH. Depending on the time in the menstrual cycle, the concentration of estrogen in the plasma, and the rate at which estrogen concentration increases in the plasma, estrogen can also stimulate pituitary gonadotropin release (e.g., at ovulation). Both the ovaries and testes secrete inhibin, which selectively inhibits FSH secretion, and activin, which selectively promotes FSH secretion.

ulation of gonadotroph cells via a G protein-coupled cell surface receptor increases the synthesis and secretion of LH and FSH, which are jointly referred to as the *gonadotropins.*

Although one cell type produces both LH and FSH, the synthesis and release of these two hormones are controlled independently. Current research suggests that the rate of GnRH secretion may preferentially alter the secretion patterns of LH and FSH. Pulsatile secretion of GnRH is critical for the proper functioning of the hypothalamic-pituitary–reproduction axis. *When GnRH is administered continuously, gonadotroph release of LH and FSH is suppressed rather than stimulated.* This effect has the important pharmacologic consequence that pulsatile administration of exogenous GnRH stimulates gonadotropin release, whereas continuous GnRH administration inhibits LH and FSH release and therefore blocks target cell function.

LH and FSH have analogous but somewhat different effects in males and females. The pertinent target cells in the male are the **Leydig** and **Sertoli** cells of the testis, while the **thecal** and **granulosa** cells of the ovary mediate gonadotropin function in the female (Fig. 28-4). In each case, a two-cell system is coordinated to mediate sex hormone actions. In the male, LH stimulates testicular Leydig cells to increase the synthesis of testosterone, which then diffuses into neighboring Sertoli cells. In the Sertoli cell, FSH stimulation increases the production of androgen binding protein (ABP), which is important for maintaining the high testicular concentrations of testosterone necessary for spermatogenesis. In addition, FSH stimulates the Sertoli cell to produce other proteins necessary for sperm maturation. In the female, LH stimulates the thecal cells to synthesize the androgen androstenedione, which is then aromatized to estrone and estradiol in the granulosa cells under the influence of FSH.

Both Sertoli cells and granulosa cells synthesize and secrete the regulatory proteins **inhibin A, inhibin B,** and **activin.** Inhibins secreted by the gonad act on the anterior pituitary gland to inhibit the release of FSH, while activin stimulates FSH release. Neither the inhibins nor activin has an effect on anterior pituitary gland LH release (Fig. 28-3). The role of these regulatory proteins in controlling hormone action is still not completely understood. In the male, testosterone is also an important negative regulator of pituitary gland and hypothalamic hormone release. The role of estrogen in the female is more complex, and can involve either positive or negative feedback depending on the prevailing hormonal milieu; this topic is addressed below as part of the menstrual cycle discussion. In the female, the combination of estradiol and progesterone synergistically suppresses GnRH, LH, and FSH secretion by actions at both the hypothalamus and pituitary gland.

INTEGRATION OF ENDOCRINE CONTROL: THE MENSTRUAL CYCLE

The female menstrual cycle is governed by the cycling of hormones with an approximate periodicity of 28 days (normal range, 24 to 35 days). This cycle begins at the onset of puberty and continues uninterrupted (with the exception of pregnancy) until menopause (Fig. 28-5). The start of the cycle, cycle Day 1, is arbitrarily defined as the first day of menstruation. Ovulation occurs at the midportion (about day

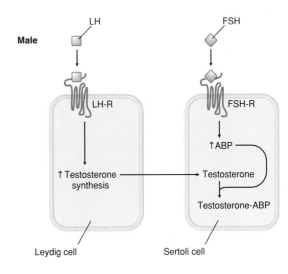

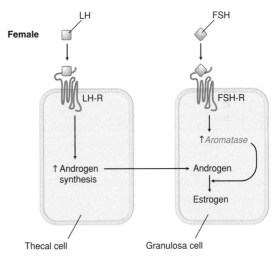

Figure 28-4. Two-cell systems for gonadal hormone action. In the **male**, the binding of luteinizing hormone (LH) to the LH receptor (LH-R) activates testosterone synthesis in Leydig cells. Testosterone then diffuses into nearby Sertoli cells, where the binding of follicle stimulating hormone (FSH) to its receptor (FSH-R) increases levels of androgen binding protein (ABP). ABP stabilizes the high concentrations of testosterone that, together with other FSH-induced proteins synthesized in Sertoli cells, promote spermatogenesis in the nearby germinal epithelium *(not shown)*. In the **female**, LH acts in an analogous manner to promote androgen (androstenedione) synthesis in thecal cells. Androgen then diffuses into nearby granulosa cells, where (after the androstenedione is converted to testosterone; *not shown*), aromatase converts testosterone to estrogen. FSH increases aromatase activity in granulosa cells, promoting the conversion of androgen to estrogen. Note that dihydrotestosterone is not a substrate for aromatase.

14) of each cycle. The portion of the menstrual cycle before ovulation is often referred to as either the **follicular** or **proliferative** phase; during this time, the developing ovarian *follicle* produces most of the gonadal hormones, which stimulate cellular *proliferation* of the endometrium. Subsequent to ovulation, the **corpus luteum** produces progesterone, and the endometrium becomes *secretory* rather than proliferative. The second half of the menstrual cycle is thus often referred to as the **luteal** or **secretory** phase, depending on

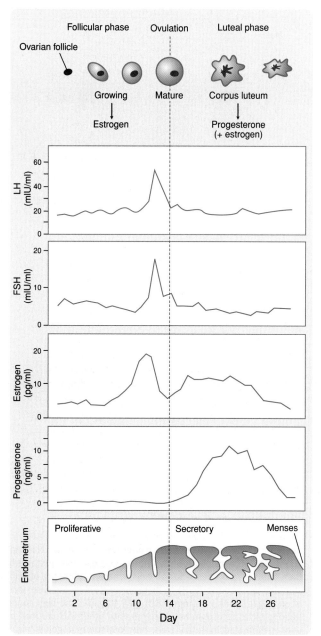

Figure 28-5. The menstrual cycle. The menstrual cycle is divided into the follicular phase and the luteal phase. Ovulation defines the transition between these two phases. During the follicular phase, gonadotroph cells of the anterior pituitary gland secrete LH and FSH in response to pulsatile GnRH stimulation. Circulating LH and FSH promote growth and maturation of ovarian follicles. Developing follicles secrete increasing amounts of estrogen. At first, the estrogen has an inhibitory effect on gonadotropin release. Just before the midpoint in the menstrual cycle, however, estrogen exerts a brief positive feedback effect on LH and FSH release. This is followed by follicular rupture and release of an egg into the fallopian tube. During the second half of the cycle, the corpus luteum secretes both estrogen and progesterone. Progesterone induces a change in the endometrium from a proliferative to a secretory type. If fertilization and implantation of a blastocyst does not occur within 14 days after ovulation, the corpus luteum involutes, secretion of estrogen and progesterone declines, menses occurs, and a new cycle begins.

whether the ovary or the endometrium is considered as the frame of reference.

At the start of the menstrual cycle, there is low production of estrogen and inhibin A. As a result, the anterior pituitary gland secretes increasing amounts of FSH and LH. These hormones stimulate the maturation of four to six follicles, each of which contains an ovum arrested in the first stage of meiosis. Maturing follicles secrete increasing concentrations of estrogen, inhibin A, and inhibin B. Estrogen causes the follicles to increase the expression of LH and FSH receptors on thecal and granulosa cells, respectively. Receptor up-regulation increases the follicular response to pituitary gland gonadotropins and allows one follicle to secrete increasing quantities of estrogen. The increased plasma estrogen and inhibin levels partially suppress pituitary gland LH and FSH release. In turn, the decreased gonadotropin levels cause other follicles to become atretic, so that usually only one follicle matures. At the same time, increased estrogen levels stimulate the uterine endometrium to proliferate rapidly in preparation for implantation of a fertilized egg.

As the dominant follicle continues to grow, it secretes high, sustained levels of estrogen. Although the mechanism is still not completely understood, the combination of high estrogen levels and the rapid rate of increase of estrogen levels causes a brief positive feedback effect on gonadotroph release of gonadotropins, stimulating rather than inhibiting release of LH and FSH. The resulting midcycle surge of LH and FSH stimulates the dominant follicle to swell and to increase the activity of its proteolytic enzymes. Approximately 40 hours after the onset of the **LH surge**, the follicle ruptures and ovulation occurs. The ovum is released into the peritoneal cavity and is then taken up by a fallopian tube, where it begins its route toward the uterus. If the oocyte becomes fertilized in the fallopian tube, it reaches the uterus approximately 4 days after ovulation and implants into the endometrium approximately 5 to 6 days after ovulation.

The cellular remains of the ruptured ovarian follicle become the corpus luteum. Cells of the corpus luteum secrete estrogen and progesterone, not just estrogen. *The presence of progesterone in the second half of the menstrual cycle causes the endometrium to switch from a proliferative to a secretory state.* The endometrium begins synthesizing proteins necessary for implantation of a fertilized egg. The blood supply to the endometrium also increases to provide increased nutrients if pregnancy ensues.

The corpus luteum has a lifespan of approximately 14 days. If fertilization and implantation of a viable blastocyst do not occur within 14 days of ovulation, the corpus luteum becomes atretic and ceases its production of estrogen and progesterone. Without the trophic effects of estrogen and progesterone, the endometrial lining sheds and menstruation begins. In the absence of estrogen and progesterone, the inhibition of gonadotrophs is removed, and production of FSH and LH increases. This stimulates the development of new ovarian follicles and the beginning of another menstrual cycle.

If fertilization does occur, however, implantation within the uterine lining causes the blastocyst to secrete **human chorionic gonadotropin** (hCG). The presence of hCG stimulates the corpus luteum to remain viable and continue secreting progesterone. Because hCG is one of the first proteins produced by the embryo that is unique to pregnancy,

pregnancy tests assay for the presence of hCG. hCG production decreases after 10 to 12 weeks of pregnancy, when the placenta begins to secrete progesterone autonomously. Special considerations attending the use of drugs in pregnancy are discussed in Box 5-1 (p. 72).

PATHOPHYSIOLOGY

Pathophysiologic processes in the reproductive tract reflect one of three general mechanisms of dysregulation (Table 28-1). The first is disruption of the hypothalamic-pituitary–reproduction axis, which causes a number of underlying disorders that can lead to infertility. The second is inappropriate growth of estrogen-dependent or testosterone-dependent tissue. This can lead to breast cancer or prostate cancer, as well as to benign but clinically important conditions such as endometriosis or endometrial hyperplasia. Finally, decreased estrogen secretion, as in menopause, or decreased androgen secretion, as in some aging men, is associated with a number of undesirable health consequences.

DISRUPTION OF THE HYPOTHALAMIC-PITUITARY–REPRODUCTION AXIS

The hypothalamic-pituitary–reproduction axis is normally tightly regulated via feedback inhibition or stimulation of hormone activity, with the goal of producing a successful menstrual cycle every month. When this axis is disrupted, infertility can result. Common causes of infertility due to disruption of sex hormone production include polycystic ovarian syndrome and prolactinomas.

Polycystic ovarian syndrome (PCOS) is a complex syndrome characterized by anovulation and by increased levels of plasma androgen. PCOS is a common problem affecting between 3% and 5% of women of reproductive age. The diagnosis is typically clinical, as in the case of Ms. J, and based on the concurrent findings of anovulation and hirsutism (excessive hair growth). Although multiple etiologies are likely to be responsible for PCOS, all of the etiologies result in increased androgen secretion and suppression of normal ovulatory cycles. The increased androgen secretion results in masculinization; as seen in Ms. J's case, male pattern baldness and inappropriate facial hair growth are common. Many women with PCOS are treated with both an estrogen–progestin contraceptive to suppress ovarian production of testosterone and an anti-androgen, such as spironolactone (see below), to abrogate the masculinizing effects of increased circulating testosterone.

Three primary hypotheses attempt to explain the development of PCOS. The first, referred to as the **LH hypothesis,** is based on the observation that many women with PCOS have an increased frequency and amplitude of pituitary LH pulses. In fact, 90% of women with PCOS have increased circulating LH. Increased LH activity stimulates thecal cells of the ovary to synthesize increased amounts of androgens, including androstenedione and testosterone. In addition, the increased LH and androgen levels prevent normal follicle growth, in turn preventing follicle secretion of large amounts of estrogen. The absence of an estrogen ''trigger'' prevents the LH surge and ovulation. As seen in the introductory case, patients with PCOS menstruate irregularly, and the menstrual periods that they do have tend to have heavy flow. The second hypothesis, referred to as the **insulin theory,** is based on the observation that many women with PCOS are obese and insulin resistant and secrete increased insulin. Increased insulin decreases the production of sex hormone binding globulin (SHBG), which results in a higher concentration of free testosterone and therefore greater androgenic effects on peripheral tissues. It has also been observed that insulin can directly synergize with LH to increase androgen production by thecal cells. Interestingly, in women with PCOS, medications that specifically treat insulin resistance, such as metformin, may result in regular ovulatory menses and normalization of testosterone levels. The third hypothesis is the **ovarian hypothesis.** This explanation posits dysregulation of sex steroid synthesis at the level of the thecal cell. For example, an abnormal increase in the activity of the oxidative enzymes responsible for androgen synthesis could lead to greater thecal cell production of androgens in response to any given stimulus. It is important to note that these hypotheses are not mutually exclusive, and that PCOS could result from a combination of two or three mechanisms. When the cellular mechanisms underlying this disease are better elucidated, new pharmacologic treatments can be de-

TABLE 28-1	General Mechanisms of Reproductive Tract Disorders for which Pharmacologic Agents are Currently Used	
MECHANISM	**EXAMPLES**
Disruption of the hypothalamic-pituitary–reproduction axis	Polycystic ovarian syndrome Prolactinoma
Inappropriate growth of hormone-dependent tissue	Breast cancer Prostatic hyperplasia, prostate cancer Endometriosis, endometrial hyperplasia Leiomyomas (uterine fibroids)
Decreased estrogen or androgen secretion	Hypogonadism Menopause

veloped that treat the etiology, rather than the effects, of the disease.

Prolactinomas are another common cause of infertility among women of reproductive age. These clonal, benign tumors of lactotrophs in the anterior pituitary gland can cause infertility through two parallel pathways. First, increased prolactin levels suppress estrogen synthesis, both by antagonizing the hypothalamic release of GnRH and by decreasing gonadotroph sensitivity to GnRH. This antagonism decreases LH and FSH release, and thereby decreases end-organ stimulation by the hypothalamic-pituitary–reproduction axis. The second mechanism, common to all pituitary gland tumors, is a crowding-out effect. Because the pituitary gland is enclosed in the bony sella turcica, lactotroph proliferation in the anterior pituitary gland leads to crowding of other cell types and thereby inhibits the function of nearby gonadotroph cells. Prolactin-secreting tumors typically remain responsive to the inhibitory effect of dopamine agonists. In most cases, chronic administration of dopamine agonists such as **cabergoline** or **bromocriptine** suppresses prolactin secretion and causes the tumor cells to shrink, thereby decreasing the size of the tumor and restoring normal gonadotroph function.

INAPPROPRIATE GROWTH OF HORMONE-DEPENDENT TISSUES

The growth of breast tissues is dependent on many hormones, including estrogen, progesterone, androgens, prolactin, and insulin-like growth factors. Many (but not all) breast cancers express the estrogen receptor (ER), and the growth of such cancers is often stimulated by endogenous levels of estrogen and inhibited by anti-estrogens. When a **breast carcinoma** is found to express the ER, an estrogen receptor antagonist (either a pure antagonist such as **fulvestrant** or a selective estrogen receptor modulator such as **tamoxifen**; see below) or an estrogen synthesis inhibitor (an aromatase inhibitor such as **anastrozole**, **letrozole**, **exemestane** or **formestane**) is commonly administered to slow tumor growth. Prostate growth is androgen-dependent and requires the local conversion of testosterone to dihydrotestosterone in stromal cells of the prostate; this conversion is mediated by the type II isoform of 5α-reductase. Both enzyme inhibition (**finasteride**) and receptor antagonist (**flutamide**) strategies are used to treat conditions in which the growth of prostate tissue is dysregulated, such as **benign prostatic hyperplasia** and metastatic **prostate cancer** (see below).

Endometriosis is the growth of endometrial tissue outside the uterus. The fact that endometriosis is usually found in areas surrounding the fallopian tube (ovaries, rectovaginal pouch, and uterine ligaments) has led to the hypothesis that endometriosis could result from retrograde migration of endometrial tissue via the fallopian tubes during menstruation. Other etiologies are possible, however, including metaplastic tissue growth from the peritoneum, or spread of endometrial cells to extra-uterine sites via lymphatic ducts. There is also evidence of increased aromatase activity in endometrial tissue from such patients. Because foci of endometriosis respond to estrogen stimulation, endometriosis grows and regresses with the menstrual cycle. This can lead to severe pain, abnormal bleeding, and the formation of ad-

hesions in the peritoneal cavity. In turn, adhesion formation can lead to infertility. Because endometriosis is usually estrogen-dependent, treatment with long half-life GnRH agonists often achieves regression of the disease (see below).

DECREASED ESTROGEN OR ANDROGEN SECRETION

The effects of decreased sex hormone production vary depending on the age of the patient at the onset of symptoms. **Hypogonadism** results if sex hormone production is impaired before adolescence. Patients with hypogonadism do not undergo sexual maturation, but proper hormone replacement can, in many cases, allow the development of secondary sexual characteristics.

Menopause is a normal physiologic response to exhaustion of the ovarian follicles. Throughout a woman's lifetime, follicles are arrested in meiosis. Only a small percentage of follicles mature during the menstrual cycle; the rest eventually become atretic. Menstrual cycles cease when all of the follicles are depleted from the ovaries. Follicle depletion leads to a decrease in estrogen and inhibins (because developing follicles are the main estrogen and inhibin source in premenopausal women) and an increase in LH and FSH (because estrogen and inhibins suppress gonadotropin release). *After menopause, androstenedione continues to be converted to estrone by aromatase in peripheral (mainly adipose) tissues. This estrone, which is a less potent estrogen than estradiol, becomes the primary estrogen in the blood.* Because of the relative lack of estrogen after menopause, many women experience hot flashes, vaginal dryness, decreased libido, and dermal atrophy, and often develop osteoporosis. The role of estrogen in the maintenance of bone mass is discussed in further detail in Chapter 30.

Men do not experience a sudden decrease in sex hormones in a manner analogous to the female menopause, but androgen secretion does decline gradually with age. Although controversy currently exists over the role of androgen therapy in normal elderly men, androgen replacement is indicated in cases of adult hypogonadism where both low testosterone levels and symptoms of hypogonadism are present.

PHARMACOLOGIC CLASSES AND AGENTS

Pharmacologic agents have been developed to target most of the steps in gonadal physiology and pathophysiology. The relevant drug classes include modulators of anterior pituitary gland gonadotroph activity and specific antagonists of peripheral hormone action. In addition, sex hormones are often used as replacement therapy or to modify gonadotropin release (Fig. 28-6).

INHIBITORS OF GONADAL HORMONES

Synthesis Inhibitors

GnRH Agonists and Antagonists

Under physiologic conditions, the hypothalamus releases GnRH in a pulsatile fashion. The frequency of GnRH pulses

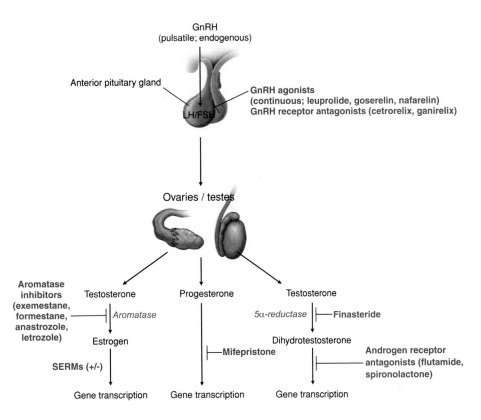

Figure 28-6. Pharmacologic modulation of gonadal hormone action. Pharmacologic modulation of gonadal hormone action can be divided into inhibitors of hormone synthesis and hormone receptor antagonists. Continuous administration of GnRH suppresses LH and FSH release from the anterior pituitary gland, thus preventing gonadal hormone synthesis. GnRH receptor antagonists (cetrorelix, ganirelix) are also used for this purpose. Finasteride inhibits the enzyme 5α-reductase, thus preventing conversion of testosterone to the more active dihydrotestosterone. Aromatase inhibitors (exemestane, formestane, anastrozole, letrozole) inhibit production of estrogens from androgens. A number of hormone receptor antagonists prevent the action of endogenous estrogens (some SERMs), androgens (flutamide, spironolactone), and progesterone (mifepristone).

controls the relative release of LH and FSH by the anterior pituitary gland. In contrast, continuous administration of GnRH suppresses, rather than stimulates, pituitary gonadotroph activity. It is possible to suppress the hypothalamic-pituitary–gonadal axis either by continuous administration of a GnRH agonist (**leuprolide, goserelin** or **nafarelin**) or by administration of a GnRH receptor antagonist (**cetrorelix** or **ganirelix**). Continuous administration of a GnRH agonist is used to treat hormone-dependent tumors such as prostate cancer and, in some cases, breast cancer. Individual agents are discussed in detail in Chapter 25, Pharmacology of the Hypothalamus and Pituitary Gland.

5α-Reductase Inhibitors

Finasteride is a selective inhibitor of type II 5α-reductase, the enzyme that converts testosterone to dihydrotestosterone. The type II reductase is highly expressed in prostate epithelial cells. Recall that dihydrotestosterone binds to the androgen receptor with higher affinity than testosterone. *Blocking the local conversion of testosterone to dihydrotestosterone effectively abrogates the local action of testosterone.* Prostate cells are dependent on androgen stimulation for survival, and administration of a reductase inhibitor slows the growth of prostate tissue. Finasteride is approved for use in benign prostatic hyperplasia, primarily to improve symptoms of decreased urine flow. The drug is a potential alternative to transurethral resection of the prostate (TURP), which is a common surgical treatment for symptomatic prostatic hyperplasia. One year of therapy with finasteride can result in up to 25% reduction in prostate size. Finasteride is most effective for patients with larger prostates, because the greatest clinical changes are observed in prostates that are already

significantly hypertrophied. Adverse effects include decreased libido and erectile dysfunction.

Aromatase Inhibitors

Because estrogens are synthesized from androgen precursors via the action of aromatase, blocking the aromatase enzyme can effectively inhibit estrogen formation. This approach is used to inhibit the growth of estrogen-dependent tumors such as breast cancer. A number of highly selective aromatase inhibitors have recently been developed. **Anastrozole** and **letrozole** are competitive inhibitors of aromatase, while **exemestane** and **formestane** bind covalently to aromatase. All of these agents are currently used in the treatment of metastatic breast cancer and in the prevention of recurrences in cancers primarily treated with surgery and radiation. Recent trials suggest that aromatase inhibitors are more effective than estrogen receptor antagonists, such as tamoxifen, for the treatment of breast cancer. However, aromatase inhibitors produce profound suppression of estrogen action, and estrogen is a major regulator of bone density. Therefore, women taking aromatase inhibitors have an increased risk of osteoporotic fractures.

Receptor Antagonists

Selective Estrogen Receptor Modulators

The term ''*Selective Estrogen Receptor Modulator*'' (SERM) is based on the observation that certain so-called antiestrogen drugs are not pure antagonists, but rather mixed agonists/antagonists (Table 28-2). These pharmacologic agents inhibit estrogenic effects in some tissues, while promoting estrogenic effects in other tissues. The basis for tissue

TABLE 28-2 **Tissue-Specific Agonist and Antagonist Activity of Selective Estrogen Receptor Modulators (SERMs)**

	BREAST	ENDOMETRIUM	BONE
Estrogen	+ + +	+ + +	+ + +
Tamoxifen	−	+	+
Raloxifene	−	−	+ +

Estrogen, the physiologic hormone, has stimulatory effects in breast, endometrium, and bone. Tamoxifen is an antagonist in breast tissue, and is therefore used in the treatment of estrogen receptor-positive breast cancer. Raloxifene, the newest SERM, is an agonist in bone but an antagonist in the breast and endometrium. Raloxifene is approved for the prevention and treatment of osteoporosis in postmenopausal women. Clomiphene (not shown in the table) is a SERM that acts as an estrogen receptor antagonist in the hypothalamus and anterior pituitary gland; it is used clinically to induce ovulation.

selectivity may include several mechanisms. First, there are two estrogen receptor subtypes, ERα and ERβ, and the expression of these receptor subtypes is tissue-specific. Second, the ability of the estrogen receptor to interact with other transcription cofactors (co-activators and co-repressors) depends on the structure of the ligand that is bound to the receptor. Figure 28-7 provides an example. Assume that the binding of 17β-estradiol (called "Estrogen" in the figure) to the estrogen receptor causes a conformational change in the receptor, so that two transcriptional cofactors, X and Y, can also bind to the receptor. This complex can then activate three genes: an X-dependent gene, a Y-dependent gene, and a gene that depends on both X and Y. In contrast, the binding of a SERM to the estrogen receptor causes a different conformational change in the receptor, so that the transcription factor X is able to bind, but the transcription factor Y is not. As a result, the SERM–receptor-X complex can activate the X-dependent gene, but not the Y-dependent gene or the (X + Y)-dependent gene.

In addition, assume that transcription factors X and Y are expressed in bone cells, but that breast cells express only transcription factor Y. In the breast, this SERM acts as an antagonist, because: (1) the inability of Y to associate with the SERM–estrogen receptor complex prevents the SERM from activating any estrogen-dependent effects; and (2) binding of the SERM to the estrogen receptor competitively inhibits the binding of endogenous estrogen to the receptor. In bone, however, this SERM acts as a partial agonist because it can activate X-dependent but not Y-dependent genes.

These tissue-specific actions of SERMs have important implications for both the desired effects and the adverse effects of pharmacologic agents. If it were possible to design a SERM that inhibits estrogen-dependent growth of breast carcinoma without causing estrogen-induced endometrial hyperplasia, then the undesirable side effects of tamoxifen (discussed below) could be reduced. Several investigational SERMs are under development, and it is likely that refined SERM specificity will, in the near future, have important implications for the treatment of osteoporosis, breast cancer, and perhaps even cardiovascular disease. The three SERMs

in current clinical use are tamoxifen, raloxifene, and clomiphene.

Tamoxifen is the only SERM currently approved for use in the treatment and prevention of breast cancer. Tamoxifen has been employed in the palliative treatment of metastatic breast cancer and as adjuvant therapy after lumpectomy. *Tamoxifen is an estrogen receptor antagonist in breast tissue, but a partial agonist in the endometrium and bone.* These pharmacodynamic effects result in inhibition of the estrogen-dependent growth of breast cancer, but also stimulation of endometrial growth. Because of the latter effect, tamoxifen administration is associated with a four-fold to six-fold increase in the incidence of endometrial cancer. Therefore, in order to minimize the risk of iatrogenic endometrial cancer, tamoxifen is typically administered for no more than 5 years.

Raloxifene is a newer SERM that possesses *estrogen receptor agonist activity in bone, but antagonist activity in both breast and endometrial tissue.* Consistent with this profile of tissue specificities, raloxifene does not appear to increase the incidence of endometrial cancer. The agonist activity of raloxifene in bone decreases bone resorption, and thus delays or prevents the progression of osteoporosis in postmenopausal women (discussed in more detail in Chapter 30). In a large clinical trial comparing raloxifene and tamoxifen for the prevention of breast cancer in women at high risk, both agents resulted in a 50% reduction in the development of invasive breast cancer. Tamoxifen treatment was associated with more cases of endometrial hyperplasia, endometrial cancer, cataracts, and deep vein thrombosis than raloxifene. However, tamoxifen prevented more cases of non-invasive breast cancer than raloxifene.

Clomiphene is a SERM used to induce ovulation. *The drug acts as an estrogen receptor antagonist in the hypothalamus and anterior pituitary gland, and as a partial agonist in the ovaries.* The antagonist activity of clomiphene in the hypothalamus and anterior pituitary gland results in relief of the negative feedback inhibition imposed by endogenous estrogen, and therefore in the increased release of GnRH and gonadotropins, respectively. The increased levels of FSH stimulate follicle growth, resulting in an estrogen trigger signal, an LH surge, and ovulation. The main adverse effect is that clomiphene can cause multiple follicles to grow, resulting in an increased ovarian size. Unlike the administration of exogenous FSH (see Chapter 25), however, clomiphene use is seldom associated with the ovarian hyperstimulation syndrome.

Androgen Receptor Antagonists

Androgen receptor antagonists competitively inhibit the binding of endogenous androgens to the androgen receptor. By this mechanism, receptor antagonists block the action of testosterone and dihydrotestosterone on their target tissues. The androgen receptor antagonists include **flutamide** and **spironolactone**. Flutamide is approved only for the treatment of metastatic prostate cancer, but the drug is also used therapeutically in the treatment of benign prostatic hyperplasia. Spironolactone, originally approved as an aldosterone receptor antagonist (see Chapter 20, Pharmacology of Volume Regulation), also has significant antagonist activity at the androgen receptor. Like flutamide, spironolactone can be used as a competitive inhibitor of testosterone action. Ms.

A Bone: both X and Y cofactors expressed

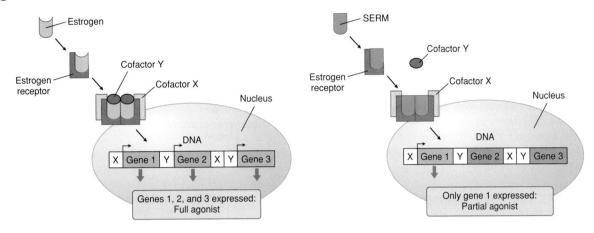

B Breast: only Y cofactor expressed

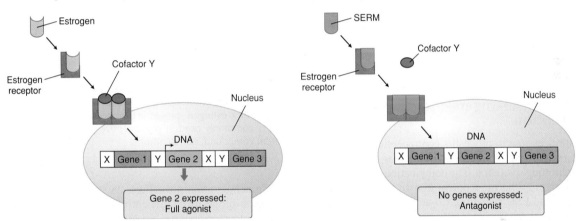

Figure 28-7. A model for the tissue specificity of action of SERMs. Selective estrogen receptor modulators (SERMs) exhibit tissue-specific estrogen receptor antagonist or partial agonist activity. This tissue specificity of action seems to be explained by the following observations: (1) transcriptional co-activators and/or co-repressors are expressed in a tissue-specific manner; (2) a SERM–estrogen receptor (ER) complex can associate with some co-activators or co-repressors, but not others; and (3) genes can be activated or inhibited by different combinations of SERM–ER and co-activators or co-repressors. In the example shown, assume that bone cells express co-activators (co-factors) X and Y, whereas breast cells express only co-activator Y. The estrogen–ER complex can associate with X and Y, whereas the SERM–ER complex can associate with only X. **A.** In bone cells, estrogen binding to ER and recruitment of co-activators X and Y induces expression of genes 1, 2, and 3. The SERM–ER complex cannot bind co-activator Y, and the SERM–ER-cofactor X complex induces expression of only gene 1. In bone, then, estrogen is a full agonist, whereas the SERM is a partial agonist. **B.** In breast cells, estrogen binding to ER and recruitment of co-activator Y induces expression of gene 2, but the SERM is unable to promote expression of any gene. In breast, then, the SERM acts as an antagonist. For simplicity, this model shows only co-activators, although co-repressors are also involved in SERM action.

J was treated with spironolactone to antagonize the excessive androgen stimulation of her hair follicles, and thus to ameliorate her hirsutism. A compound derived from spironolactone, **drospirenone,** has both progestational and anti-androgen effects. It is used as a progestin in some estrogen–progestin contraceptives.

Progesterone Receptor Antagonists

Mifepristone (also referred to as **RU-486**) is a progesterone receptor antagonist used to induce first-trimester abortion. As noted above, progesterone is crucial for maintenance of the endometrium during pregnancy; the hormone stabilizes the uterine lining and promotes vessel growth and secretory activities of the decidua. Mifepristone inhibits progesterone action by binding competitively to the progesterone receptor. Blockade of progesterone action results in decay and death of the decidua, and lack of nourishment from the decidua causes the blastocyst to die and detach from the uterus. Because the blastocyst is no longer secreting hCG, the corpus luteum involutes, and involution of the corpus luteum causes progesterone synthesis and secretion to decrease.

Mifepristone is commonly administered in conjunction with **misoprostol,** a prostaglandin analogue (see Chapter 41, Pharmacology of Eicosanoids). Misoprostol stimulates uterine contractions, and the combined effects of progesterone antagonism and uterine contractions are more than 95% effective in terminating first-trimester pregnancy.

Because mifepristone is administered as a single dose, adverse effects related to progesterone antagonism are rare.

Instead, the main potential for complication lies in the subsequent abortion, which can result in excessive vaginal bleeding. In addition, co-administration of misoprostol can cause nausea and vomiting.

Asoprisnil is a novel progesterone receptor antagonist that does not cause abortion, but inhibits the growth of tissues derived from the endometrium and myometrium. Preliminary studies indicate that asoprisnil may be effective in the treatment of endometriosis and uterine leiomyomata (fibroids). The differences in the tissue specificity of mifepristone and asoprisnil are probably due to their differences in influencing the binding of transcription cofactors to the progesterone receptor complex.

HORMONES AND HORMONE ANALOGUES: CONTRACEPTION

The development of safe, efficacious contraceptives for women has revolutionized sexual practices. The two classes of widely used oral contraceptives are **estrogen/progestin combinations** and **progestin-only contraception.** The development of male contraception is an active area of research; current approaches to this therapy are discussed briefly at the end of the section.

Combination Estrogen–Progestin Contraception

Combination estrogen–progestin contraception suppresses GnRH, LH, and FSH secretion and follicular development, thereby inhibiting ovulation. The combination of an estrogen and a progestin is the most potent known way to suppress GnRH, LH, and FSH secretion. Co-administration of estrogen and progestin may also inhibit pregnancy by a number of secondary mechanisms, including alterations in tubal peristalsis, endometrial receptivity, and cervical mucus secretions. The latter actions could together inhibit the proper transport of both egg and sperm, even if ovulation were to occur. *In combination, these mechanisms explain the >99% efficacy of combination oral contraception.*

The estrogen used in combination estrogen–progestin contraceptives is either **ethinyl estradiol** or **mestranol** (Fig. 28-8). Use of "unopposed" estrogens promotes endometrial growth, and early studies of estrogen-dominant contraceptives determined that these agents increase the risk of endometrial cancer. Because of this finding, estrogen is always co-administered with a progestin to limit the extent of endometrial growth.

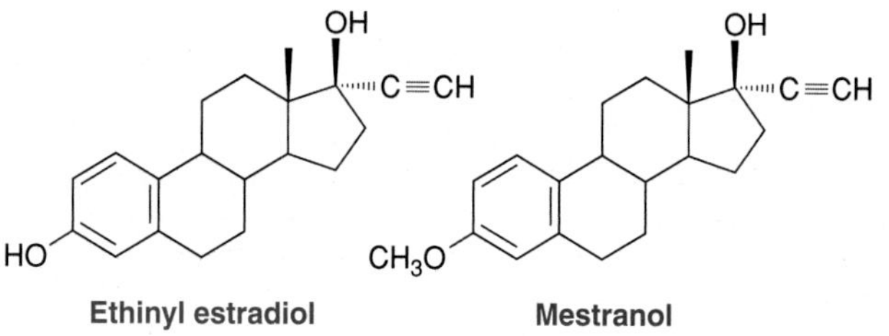

Figure 28-8. Structure of synthetic estrogens. Ethinyl estradiol and mestranol are used in combination estrogen–progestin contraceptives.

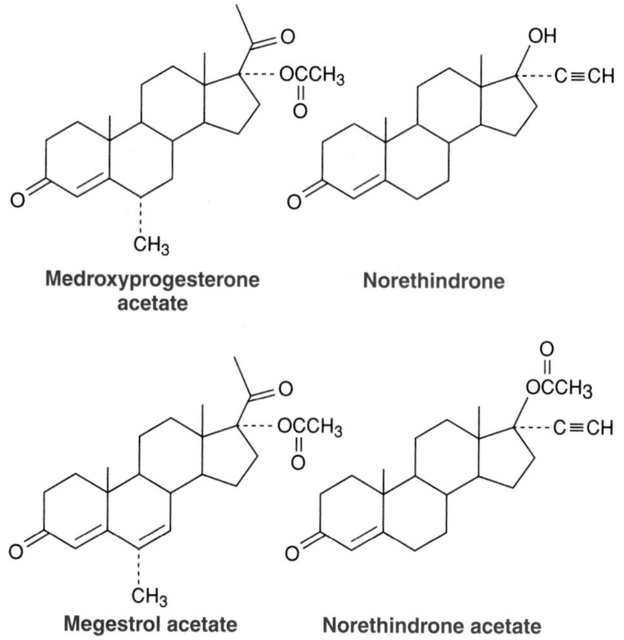

Figure 28-9. Structure of synthetic progestins. Medroxyprogesterone acetate is commonly combined with estrogen for hormone therapy in postmenopausal women. Megestrol acetate is often used as therapy for endometrial cancer. Norethindrone was the first progestin to be synthesized in quantities sufficient to mass-produce combination estrogen–progestin contraceptives. Norethindrone acetate is commonly used in contraceptives; it is metabolized to the parent compound, norethindrone.

Numerous progestins (Figs. 28-9 and 28-10) are used in estrogen–progestin contraceptives, and all are potent progesterone receptor agonists. Ideally, the progestin would possess activity only at progesterone receptors, but almost all currently available progestins also have some androgenic cross-reactivity. Progestins vary in their androgenic activity.

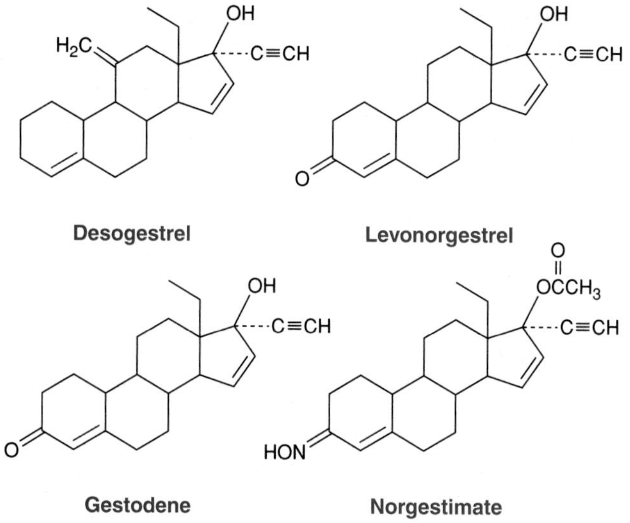

Figure 28-10. Structure of progestins commonly used in oral contraceptives. Levonorgestrel is the most androgenic of the commonly used progestins. Gestodene, norgestimate and desogestrel are less androgenic than levonorgestrel.

On a molar basis, **norgestrel** and **levonorgestrel** have the highest androgenic activity, while **norethindrone** and **norethindrone acetate** (Fig. 28-9) have lower androgenic activity. The so-called third-generation progestins — **ethynodiol, norgestimate, gestodene** and **desogestrel** (Fig. 28-10) — have even lower androgen receptor cross-reactivity. **Drospirenone** is a synthetic progestin that also has anti-androgenic activity.

Combination estrogen–progestin contraceptives are available in three delivery systems: a vaginal ring, transdermal patches, and oral tablets. The vaginal ring consists of a silastic cylinder packed with ethinyl estradiol and a progestin, **etonogestrel**. The steroids are released with zero-order kinetics (see Chapter 3, Pharmacokinetics). The ring is placed in the vagina, and remains there for 21 days. It is then removed and, 7 days later, a new ring is placed. During the 7 days following removal of the ring, menses may ensue (see below). The contraceptive transdermal patch consists of a matrix that continually releases ethinyl estradiol and a synthetic progestin, **norelgestromin**. The patch is changed weekly for 3 weeks. During the fourth week, no patch is utilized and menses may occur.

Classical regimens of combination oral contraceptive tablets consist of 21 days of drugs followed by 7 days of a placebo pill. The 7-day placebo period removes exogenous hormone stimulation, simulating the physiologic involution of the corpus luteum that occurs at the end of a normal menstrual cycle. The lack of estrogen and progestin causes the endometrium to slough, resulting in menstruation. Because the administration of progestin throughout the cycle inhibits the proliferative growth of the endometrium, most women experience lighter menstrual periods when taking combination oral contraceptives, and a woman's menstrual cycle often becomes more regular. The 21-7 cycle formulation was meant to simulate a 28-day cycle, but is relatively arbitrary. A longer cycle formulation of ethinyl estradiol and levonorgestrel is available, in which the drug combination is administered for 84 days followed by 7 days of placebo. This formulation has equal contraceptive efficacy, and reduces to four the total number of menstrual cycles each year. Formulations containing 24 daily hormone pills and 4 days of placebo are also available. An advantage of this formulation is that ovulation is not likely to occur if a woman forgets to start her new cycle for 3 or 4 days.

Combination oral contraceptive formulations consist of monophasic, biphasic, or triphasic hormone schedules. The standard formulation, used by the majority of women, is a constant (monophasic) dose of estrogen and progestin for 21 days. Biphasic preparations maintain a constant estrogen dose throughout the cycle, while the progestin is initially low but then increases during the second half of the cycle. Triphasic formulations incorporate both increased progestin in the latter half of the cycle and a midcycle increase in the estrogen dose, to prevent breakthrough bleeding. *The main advantage of biphasic or triphasic administration is that the total amount of progestin administered over each month is reduced.* Indeed, the general trend in recent years has been to decrease the quantities of administered estrogen and progestin to the smallest amount necessary for inhibition of ovulation. However, there are no clearly established differences in either the adverse effects or the clinical efficacy of monophasic compared to biphasic or triphasic therapy. In general, the lowest effective dose of ethinyl estradiol is preferred because low-dose estrogen is thought to reduce the risk of deep vein thrombosis (see below).

A number of studies have been performed to assess the adverse effects of long-term contraceptive use. These studies have shown that the incidence of **deep vein thrombosis** and the incidence of **pulmonary embolism** are increased with combination oral contraception, but that these complications occur so infrequently that the absolute number of adverse events is low. Studies have failed to demonstrate any increase (or decrease) in breast cancer. Use of oral contraceptives is associated with an increase in **gallbladder disease,** because estrogens increase the biliary concentration of cholesterol relative to that of bile salts, and the resulting decrease in cholesterol solubility promotes the formation of gallstones. *Oral contraceptives should not be administered to women over 35 who smoke, because the administration of contraceptives to this population is associated with an increase in thrombotic cardiovascular events.*

Recent studies have focused on the benefits rather than the adverse effects of oral contraception. Modern combination oral contraceptives *reduce* the incidence of endometrial cancer, probably because constant administration of a progestin inhibits endometrial growth. In addition, exogenous administration of an estrogen/progestin combination reduces the incidence of ovarian cancer, probably by lowering circulating levels of gonadotropins. *Overall, the consensus is that oral contraceptives have more beneficial than harmful medical effects.*

Progestin-Only Contraception

In situations where estrogen may be contraindicated, the use of continuous low-dose oral progestins may be warranted. The two progestin-only oral contraceptives available in the United States, commonly referred to as the ''mini-pill,'' are **norgestrel** and **norethindrone.**

Progestin-only oral contraception prevents ovulation 70% to 80% of the time, probably because progestins alter the frequency of GnRH pulsing and decrease anterior pituitary gland responsiveness to GnRH. Despite the relatively high frequency of ovulation, this form of contraception is 96% to 98% effective, suggesting that secondary mechanisms—such as alterations in cervical mucus, endometrial receptivity, and tubal peristalsis—are also at work. Because progesterone inhibits endometrial proliferation and promotes endometrial secretion, it may also be the case that an egg is unable to implant in an endometrium that is continually exposed to progestin. Patients taking these drugs do not typically menstruate, but breakthrough spotting and irregular, light menstrual periods commonly occur during the first year of administration.

Progestin-only contraceptives are also available as injectables and implants. **Medroxyprogesterone acetate** (formulated as 104 mg for subcutaneous injection or 150 mg for intramuscular injection) can be given parenterally every 3 months (Fig. 28-9). This dosage form is especially effective for women who have difficulty remembering to take a daily (pill) or weekly (patch) agent. A silastic implant that releases **etonogestrel** and is effective for 3 years is also available.

The implant is typically inserted into the dorsal side of the forearm.

Emergency (Morning-After) Contraception

Emergency contraception refers to the administration of medications to prevent pregnancy after failure of a barrier contraceptive (condom breakage) or recent unprotected intercourse (including sexual assault). Historically, estrogen–progestin tablets were given for emergency contraception. Recent clinical trials demonstrate that the most efficacious emergency contraceptive with the fewest adverse effects is oral **levonorgestrel** 0.75 mg, given as soon as possible after the exposure and repeated in 12 hours. The regimen is most effective if given within 120 hours of the exposure. Levonorgestrel is a potent progestin that can both block the LH surge, disrupting normal ovulation, and produce endometrial changes that prevent implantation.

Male Contraception

The development of an efficacious male contraceptive has been attempted for years, but has not yet met clinical success. The goal of male contraception would be to suppress endogenous production of sperm reversibly, generating a state of azoospermia (absence of sperm in the ejaculate) without suppressing libido or erectile function. Reliable inhibition of spermatogenesis is a difficult task, because even a 99% reduction in spermatogenesis would result in a sufficient number of viable sperm for fertilization. Initial studies of male contraception centered on the administration of testosterone enanthate (see below). As an end product of the hypothalamic-pituitary–gonadal axis, testosterone significantly suppresses gonadotropin release. The reduced circulating levels of LH and FSH are unable to stimulate Sertoli cell function, and decreased spermatogenesis results.

Recent clinical trials indicate that the administration of both an androgen and a progestin is superior to an androgen alone in suppressing spermatogenesis, because the combination more completely suppresses gonadotropin release. The following combinations have been demonstrated to be effective, reversible male contraceptives: parenteral **testosterone enanthate** plus daily oral levonorgestrel; and parenteral **testosterone undecanoate** plus injectable medroxyprogesterone acetate. The main difficulties with this approach have been the large population variability in the degree of spermatogenesis inhibition (on average, only 60% of men become azoospermic), and the significant adverse effects of acne, weight gain, polycythemia, and a potential increase in prostate size.

HORMONES AND HORMONE ANALOGUES: REPLACEMENT

Estrogens, progestins, and androgens are used as replacement therapies in cases of hormone deficiency.

Estrogens and Progestins

The realization that estrogen loss at menopause has many deleterious effects has led to the development of perimenopausal and postmenopausal hormone replacement therapy (for additional detail, see Chapter 30). The principal indication for such therapy is to suppress hot flashes and treat atrophy of the urogenital tissues, which may manifest as dry vagina.

For women with a uterus, estrogen therapy must be combined with progestin therapy to prevent the induction of endometrial cancer. For women without a uterus, estrogen alone is typically given for hormone therapy. The Women's Health Initiative is a large clinical trial that evaluated the health benefits and risks of hormone therapy in postmenopausal women. Separate clinical trials tested estrogen alone against a placebo in women without a uterus, and continuous estrogen–progestin against a placebo in women with a uterus. The results of the study, expressed as the relative risk for various end-points of hormone treatment versus placebo, are presented in Table 28-3. Estrogen treatment did not increase the risk of coronary heart disease or breast cancer, but it did increase the risk of stroke and thromboembolism and it decreased the risk of osteoporotic fracture. Continuous estrogen–progestin treatment increased the risk of cardiovascular events, breast cancer, and stroke, and it decreased the risk of osteoporotic fracture (see Chapter 30). Given the balance of risks and benefits, the current recommendation for postmenopausal women is to use hormone therapy only to treat bothersome symptoms such as vasomotor symptoms or vaginal dryness, and to use the lowest possible dose of hormone therapy for the shortest period of time.

Like contraceptives, hormone therapy is available as oral tablets, transdermal patches, and vaginal rings and tablets. A vaginal ring that elutes estradiol at a controlled dose rate (see Chapter 54, Drug Delivery Modalities) provides local administration of estrogen and minimal systemic absorption of the drug. The vaginal ring is an effective therapy for postmenopausal vaginal dryness and atrophy.

Androgens

Androgen replacement is an effective therapy for hypogonadism. Oral testosterone is ineffective because of its high first-pass metabolism by the liver. Two esters of testosterone, **testosterone enanthate** and **testosterone cypionate,** can be administered intramuscularly. A preparation of either of these agents, injected every 2 to 4 weeks, increases plasma testosterone to physiologic concentrations in hypogonadal men. Transdermal **testosterone patches** have also been developed; this drug delivery system has the advantages that plasma testosterone levels remain relatively constant and first-pass hepatic metabolism is bypassed. Testosterone is also available in a topical gel formulation; using this preparation on a once-a-day application schedule, plasma testosterone levels gradually increase until they reach physiologic replacement levels after 1 month of application. Testosterone can also be administered as a tablet that adheres to the buccal mucosa, resulting in rapid systemic absorption of the drug.

Aging men sometimes develop symptoms and signs of hypogonadism, such as decreased energy, decreased libido, gynecomastia, decreased muscle mass, and facial hair growth. Recent guidelines recommend that androgen replacement therapy only be offered to men with consistent

TABLE 28-3	Summary of Findings from the Women's Health Initiative	
	ESTROGEN ALONE	**CONTINUOUS ESTROGEN-PROGESTIN**
Sample size	10,739	16,608
Mean age of subjects	63 years old	63 years old
Mean duration of hormone use	6.8 years	5.2 years
Coronary heart disease	0.91 (0.75–1.12)	1.29 (1.02–1.63)
Breast cancer	0.77 (0.59–1.01)	1.26 (1.00–1.59)
Stroke	1.39 (1.10–1.77)	1.41 (1.07–1.85)
Pulmonary embolism	1.34 (0.87–2.06)	2.13 (1.39–3.25)
Osteoporotic hip fracture	0.61 (0.41–0.91)	0.67 (0.47–0.96)
Osteoporotic vertebral fracture	0.62 (0.42–0.93)	0.65 (0.46–0.92)

Data represent hazard ratios (95% confidence intervals) of various events during treatment with hormone therapy or placebo. Confidence intervals that cross the value of 1.00 are not statistically significant ($p > 0.05$).

symptoms and signs of hypogonadism and low plasma testosterone levels (< 3.0 ng/mL). Testosterone should not be administered to men with prostate cancer, because it may stimulate the growth of the tumor.

Some athletes abuse androgens by self-administration at supratherapeutic levels. Androgens have been demonstrated to increase muscle mass and fat-free mass. In one survey, approximately 5% of high school athletes reported that they had used androgen supplements. Almost every type of androgen has been abused in an attempt to enhance athletic performance, including the adrenal hormone precursors androstenedione and dehydroepiandrosterone. Covert laboratories are continuously inventing new synthetic androgens that have not yet been recognized by standard drug testing programs. These "designer" androgens are meant to enhance athletic performance and to be undetectable by sports regulatory authorities. Pharmacologic doses of androgens suppress the hypothalamic-pituitary–gonadal axis, resulting in suppression of testicular function, decreased sperm production, and impaired fertility. Because many androgens can be converted to estrogens by aromatase, pharmacologic doses of androgens can also cause an increase in plasma estrogen, resulting in gynecomastia. In addition, high plasma levels of androgens are associated with erythrocytosis, severe acne, and derangements in lipid metabolism (increased LDL and decreased HDL). Some athletes have recently started to use injections of hCG to stimulate endogenous Leydig cell testosterone production, hoping to avoid detection by sports authorities. SERMs and aromatase inhibitors have also been used by athletes in an attempt to increase endogenous LH secretion and Leydig cell testosterone production.

Conclusion and Future Directions

The male and female hormones of reproduction share significant mechanistic overlap with one another. Androgens, estrogens, and progestins are all steroid hormones that exert their physiologic action by binding to intracellular receptors, translocating to the nucleus and altering gene transcription. Recent evidence suggests that estrogens may also act on membrane receptors to mediate nongenomic effects. De-

rangements in the physiologic effects of reproductive hormones can involve disruption of the hypothalamic-pituitary–reproduction axis, inappropriate growth of hormone-dependent tissue, or decreased activity of gonadal hormones at target tissues. Currently available pharmacologic agents can modify the endocrine axis (e.g., GnRH agonists), inhibit synthesis of active hormones (e.g., 5α-reductase inhibitors, aromatase inhibitors), or inhibit end-organ effects at the receptor level (e.g., SERMs, anti-androgens, mifepristone). Oral contraceptives, such as estrogen/progestin combinations and progestin-only contraception, disrupt the exquisite chronicity of the menstrual cycle and thus suppress ovulation. The development of an effective male contraceptive has met a number of obstacles, but should represent a major pharmacologic advance in the future. Exciting progress is also being made in the design of new SERMs that possess a variety of tissue-specific activities; such research may result in new agents effective for both prevention of breast cancer and treatment of postmenopausal osteoporosis.

Suggested Reading

Anderson GL, Limacher M, Assaf AR, et al. Effects of conjugated equine estrogen in postmenopausal women with hysterectomy: the Women's Health Initiative randomized controlled trial. *JAMA* 2004;291:1701–1712. (*Reports the "Estrogen Alone" data shown in Table 28-3.*)

Bhasin S, Cunningham GR, Hayes FJ, et al. Testosterone therapy in adult men with androgen deficiency syndromes: an Endocrine Society Clinical Practice Guideline. *J Clin Endocrinol Metab* 2006;91:1995–2010. (*Aging men should have both consistent symptoms of hypogonadism and low serum testosterone in order to be treated with androgen replacement.*)

Chwalisz K, Perez MC, Demanno D, et al. Selective progesterone receptor modulator development and use in the treatment of leiomyomata and endometriosis. *Endocr Rev* 2005;26:423–438. (*Selective progesterone receptor modulators are likely to find many applications for diseases of the reproductive organs.*)

Ehrmann DA. Polycystic ovary syndrome. *N Engl J Med* 2005;352:1223–1236. (*A clinically oriented review of the polycystic ovary syndrome, the diagnosis for the patient presented in this chapter.*)

Fischer M, Bhatnagar J, Guarner J, et al. Fatal toxic shock syndrome associated with Clostridium sordellii after medical abortion. *N Engl J Med* 2005;353:2352–2360. (*Adverse effects of drugs may not become apparent until they are used by large numbers of patients.*)

Handelsman DJ. The rationale for banning human chorionic gonadotropin and estrogen blockers in sport. *J Clin Endocrinol Metab* 2006;91:1646–1653. (*Recent developments in androgen abuse by athletes.*)

Rosenfield RL. Clinical practice. Hirsutism. *N Engl J Med* 2005; 353:2578–2588. (*A clinically oriented review of the treatment of hirsutism, a chief complaint of Amy J, the patient presented in this chapter.*)

Turgeon JL, Carr MC, Maki PM, et al. Complex actions of sex steroids in adipose tissue, the cardiovascular system and brain: insights from basic science and clinical studies. *Endocr Rev* 2006;27:575–605. Epub 2006 Jun 9. (*Recent review.*)

Winer EP, Hudis C, Burstein HJ, et al. American Society of Clinical Oncology Technology Assessment on the use of aromatase inhibitors as adjuvant therapy for postmenopausal women with hormone receptor-positive breast cancer. *J Clin Oncol* 2005;23: 619–629. (*Aromatase inhibitors are replacing tamoxifen as first-line treatment of hormone receptor-positive breast cancer in postmenopausal women.*)

Writing Group for the Women's Health Initiative Investigators. Risks and benefits of estrogen plus progestin in healthy postmenopausal women: principal results from the Women's Health Initiative randomized controlled trial. *JAMA* 2002;288:321–333. (*Reports the ''Continuous Estrogen-Progestin'' data shown in Table 28-3.*)

Drug Summary Table | **Chapter 28 Pharmacology of Reproduction**

Drug	Clinical Applications	*Serious* and Common Adverse Effects	Contraindications	Therapeutic Considerations
GONADOTROPIN-RELEASING HORMONE (GnRH) AGONISTS				
Mechanism—Continuous: inhibit LH and FSH release; Pulsatile: stimulate LH and FSH release				
Gonadorelin Goserelin Histrelin Leuprolide Nafarelin	See Drug Summary Table: Chapter 25 Pharmacology of the Hypothalamus and Pituitary Gland			
GONADOTROPIN-RELEASING HORMONE (GnRH) ANTAGONISTS				
Mechanism—GnRH receptor antagonists				
Cetrorelix Ganirelix	See Drug Summary Table: Chapter 25 Pharmacology of the Hypothalamus and Pituitary Gland			
INHIBITORS OF PERIPHERAL TESTOSTERONE CONVERSION TO DHT				
Mechanism—Selectively inhibit type II 5α-reductase, the enzyme that converts testosterone to dihydrotestosterone in prostate, liver, and skin				
Finasteride	Benign prostatic hyperplasia Androgenic alopecia	*Neoplasm of male breast (rare and under investigation)* Breast tenderness, decreased libido, erectile dysfunction, ejaculatory disorder	Known or suspected pregnancy Women and children	Finasteride improves symptoms of decreased urine flow A potential alternative to transurethral resection of the prostate (TURP) One year of therapy can result in up to 25% reduction in prostate size; finasteride is most effective for patients with large prostates Women should not handle finasteride tablets
INHIBITORS OF AROMATASE				
Mechanism—Anastrozole and letrozole are competitive inhibitors of aromatase, the enzyme that catalyzes the formation of estrogens from androgen precursors. Exemestane and formestane are irreversible (covalent) inhibitors of aromatase.				
Anastrozole Letrozole Exemestane Formestane	Treatment and prevention of estrogen receptor positive early-stage, locally advanced, and metastatic breast cancer	*Osteoporotic fractures, thrombophlebitis, hypercholesterolemia, profuse vaginal bleeding* Peripheral edema, rash, nausea, arthralgia, bone pain, headache, depression, dyspnea	Hypersensitivity to anastrozole, letrozole, exemestane, or formestane	Aromatase inhibitors are used to treat estrogen-dependent tumors Aromatase inhibitors may be more effective than estrogen receptor antagonists or SERMs for the treatment of breast cancer Due to profound suppression of estrogen action, women taking aromatase inhibitors are at substantial risk for osteoporotic fractures

(Continued)

Drug Summary Table   Chapter 28 Pharmacology of Reproduction (Continued)

Drug	Clinical Applications	Serious and Common Adverse Effects	Contraindications	Therapeutic Considerations
SELECTIVE ESTROGEN RECEPTOR MODULATORS (SERMS)				
Mechanism—Estrogen antagonist in some tissues and estrogen agonist in other tissues. The basis for tissue selectivity may be related to tissue-specific expression of estrogen-receptor subtypes and the differential ability of the ligand-receptor complex to recruit transcriptional co-activators and co-repressors.				
Tamoxifen	Prevention of breast cancer	*Malignant neoplasm of*	History of deep vein thrombosis or	An estrogen receptor antagonist in breast tissue and a partial
	Palliative treatment of	*endometrium, cerebrovascular*	pulmonary embolism if used for	agonist in the endometrium and bone
	metastatic breast cancer	*accident, cataract, pulmonary*	breast cancer prevention or ductal	Because tamoxifen stimulates endometrial growth, tamoxifen
	Adjuvant therapy of breast	*embolism*	carcinoma in situ; in patients with	administration is associated with a four- to six-fold increase
	cancer after primary excision	Hot flashes, abnormal	invasive breast cancer, benefits of	in the incidence of endometrial cancer
	of the tumor (lumpectomy)	menstruation, vaginal discharge	tamoxifen outweigh risks of recurrent	Usually administered for no more than 5 years, in order to
			thromboembolic disease	minimize the risk of iatrogenic endometrial cancer
			Pregnancy	
Clomiphene	Female infertility due to	*Thromboembolism*	Pregnancy	An estrogen receptor antagonist in hypothalamus and anterior
	ovulatory disorder	Ovarian cysts, ovarian	Uncontrolled thyroid or adrenal	pituitary gland, and a partial agonist in ovaries; disinhibits
		hypertrophy, flushing,	dysfunction	GnRH release, leading to increased levels of LH and FSH;
		vasomotor symptoms,	Liver disease	the increased FSH stimulates follicle growth, resulting in an
		abdominal discomfort	Endometrial carcinoma	estrogen trigger signal, an LH surge, and ovulation
			Ovarian cysts	Unlike exogenous FSH, clomiphene use is rarely associated
			Organic intracranial lesion	with the ovarian hyperstimulation syndrome
Raloxifene	See Drug Summary Table: Chapter 30 Pharmacology of Bone Mineral Homeostasis			
ESTROGEN RECEPTOR ANTAGONISTS				
Mechanism—Competitively inhibit estrogen binding to receptor, blocking the action of estrogen on target tissues				
Fulvestrant	Treatment of estrogen receptor	Nausea, asthenia, pain,	Pregnancy	A pure estrogen receptor antagonist with no agonist activity;
	positive metastatic breast	vasodilation (hot flashes),		binds with high affinity to estrogen receptor, preventing
	cancer in postmenopausal	headache		receptor dimerization and increasing receptor degradation;
	women with disease			sometimes referred to as the first in a new class of selective
	progression following anti-			estrogen receptor down-regulators (SERDs)
	estrogen therapy			
ANDROGEN RECEPTOR ANTAGONISTS				
Mechanism—Competitively inhibit dihydrotestosterone and testosterone binding to receptor, blocking the action of testosterone and dihydrotestosterone on target tissues				
Flutamide	Metastatic prostate cancer	*Hepatotoxicity, disorders of the*	Severe hepatic impairment	Flutamide compares favorably to DES and leuprolide
	Benign prostatic hypertrophy	*hematopoietic system*		monotherapy in the treatment of prostate cancer
		Hot flash, diarrhea, nausea, rash		Flutamide is most effective when combined with medical or
				surgical castration
Spironolactone	Hirsutism	*Hyperkalemic metabolic*	Anuria	An aldosterone receptor antagonist that also has significant
	Acne vulgaris	*acidosis, gastrointestinal*	Hyperkalemia	antagonist activity at the androgen receptor
	Hypertension	*hemorrhage, agranulocytosis,*	Acute renal insufficiency	Used as a competitive inhibitor of testosterone and
	Edema associated with heart	*systemic lupus erythematosus,*		dihydrotestosterone binding to androgen receptors
	failure, cirrhosis (with or	*breast cancer (not established)*		Drospirenone (derived from spironolactone) has both
	without ascites), or nephrotic	Gynecomastia, dyspepsia,		progestational and anti-androgen effects; it is used as a
	syndrome	lethargy, abnormal		progestin in some estrogen-progestin contraceptives
	Hypokalemia	menstruation, impotence, rash		
	Primary aldosteronism			

PROGESTERONE RECEPTOR ANTAGONISTS

Mechanism—Inhibit progesterone binding to receptor; the differences in the tissue specificity of mifepristone and asoprisnil are likely due to their differences in influencing the binding of transcriptional co-activators and co-repressors to the progesterone receptor complex

Mifepristone (RU-486)	Abortion (through day 49 of pregnancy)	Chronic adrenal failure Ectopic pregnancy Hemorrhagic disorders Anticoagulation therapy Inherited porphyrias Intrauterine device Undiagnosed adnexal mass	*Prolonged bleeding time, bacterial infections, sepsis* Nausea, vomiting, diarrhea, cramps, abnormal vaginal bleeding, headache	Mifepristone (RU-486) is a progesterone receptor antagonist used to induce first-trimester abortion Blockade of progesterone action results in decay and death of the decidua, and lack of nourishment from the decidua causes the blastocyst to die and detach from the uterus Mifepristone is commonly administered in conjunction with misoprostol, a prostaglandin analogue that stimulates uterine contractions; coadministration of misoprostol can cause nausea and vomiting At higher concentrations, mifepristone also blocks the glucocorticoid receptor, which makes it potentially useful for treating conditions associated with life-threatening elevated glucocorticoid levels, such as the ectopic ACTH syndrome
Asoprisnil	Investigational agent for the treatment of endometriosis and uterine leiomyomata (fibroids)	Under investigation	Under investigation	A progesterone receptor antagonist that inhibits the growth of tissues derived from the endometrium and myometrium; preliminary studies indicate that asoprisnil may be effective in the treatment of endometriosis and uterine leiomyomata (fibroids)

COMBINATION ESTROGEN-PROGESTIN CONTRACEPTION

Mechanism—Suppress GnRH, LH, and FSH secretion and follicular development, thereby inhibiting ovulation; secondary mechanisms of pregnancy prevention include alterations in tubal peristalsis, endometrial receptivity, and cervical mucus secretions, which together prevent the proper transport of both egg and sperm

Estrogens: Ethinyl estradiol Mestranol *Progestins:* Norgestrel Levonorgestrel Norethindrone Norethindrone acetate Ethynodiol Norgestimate Gestodene Desogestrel Drospirenone	Contraception	Breast cancer Endometrial cancer or other estrogen-dependent neoplasms Cerebral vascular or coronary artery disease Cholestatic jaundice of pregnancy or jaundice with prior hormonal contraceptive use Benign or malignant liver tumors Severe hypertension Prolonged immobilization Pregnancy Female smokers over 35 years of age Thrombotic disorders	*Arterial and venous thromboembolism, pulmonary embolism, cerebral thrombosis, gallbladder disease, hypertension, hepatic neoplasm* Abnormal menstruation, break-through bleeding, breast tenderness, bloating symptoms, migraine, weight change	Because unopposed estrogen increases the risk of endometrial cancer, estrogen is always coadministered with a progestin in women with a uterus Progestins vary in their androgenic activity Norgestrel and levonorgestrel have the highest androgenic activity; norethindrone and norethindrone acetate have medium androgenic activity; ethynodiol, norgestimate, gestodene and desogestrel have low androgen receptor cross-reactivity; drospirenone is a synthetic progestin that also has anti-androgenic activity Combination estrogen-progestin contraceptives are available in oral tablets, a vaginal ring, and transdermal patches Biphasic or triphasic oral formulations have lower total amounts of progestin each month The lowest effective dose of ethinyl estradiol is preferred to reduce the risk of deep vein thrombosis Levonorgestrel is also used for emergency (morning-after) contraception

(Continued)

Drug Summary Table **Chapter 28 Pharmacology of Reproduction** (*Continued*)

Drug	Clinical Applications	Serious and Common Adverse Effects	Contraindications	Therapeutic Considerations
PROGESTIN-ONLY CONTRACEPTIVES				
Mechanism—Alter frequency of GnRH pulsing and decrease anterior pituitary gland responsiveness to GnRH. Secondary mechanisms of pregnancy prevention include alterations in tubal peristalsis, endometrial receptivity, and cervical mucus secretions, which together prevent the proper transport of both egg and sperm.				
Norgestrel Norethindrone Medroxyprogesterone acetate (injectable) Etonogestrel (silastic implant)	Contraception	Irregular periods, breast tenderness, nausea, dizziness, headache	Acute liver disease Benign or malignant liver tumors Known or suspected breast cancer Pregnancy	Breakthrough spotting and irregular, light menstrual periods commonly occur during the first year of administration Medroxyprogesterone acetate can be given parenterally every 3 months A silastic implant that releases etonogestrel is effective for 3 years Oral levonorgestrel can be used in emergency contraception
ANDROGENS USED FOR HORMONE REPLACEMENT				
Mechanism—Replacement of testosterone to produce androgenic effects, including growth and maturation of the prostate, seminal vesicles, penis, and scrotum, development of male hair distribution, laryngeal enlargement, vocal cord thickening, and alterations in body musculature and fat distribution.				
Testosterone enanthate Testosterone cypionate	Hypogonadism	*Cholestatic jaundice syndrome, liver carcinoma, benign prostatic hyperplasia, prostate cancer* Acne, gynecomastia, oral irritation with buccal delivery, skin irritation with transdermal delivery, potential transfer to female partner with topical gel formulation, headache	Breast cancer in men Prostate cancer Pregnancy when used in women	Various delivery routes have been developed for testosterone replacement therapies; testosterone replacement can be administered intramuscularly, transdermally, and via topical gel formulation; the transdermal delivery system has the advantages that plasma testosterone levels remain relatively constant and first-pass hepatic metabolism is bypassed; testosterone can also be administered as a tablet that adheres to the buccal mucosa Androgen replacement therapy should only be offered to men with consistent symptoms and signs of hypogonadism and low plasma testosterone levels (< 3.0 ng/ml); testosterone should not be administered to men with prostate cancer Some athletes abuse androgens by self-administration at supratherapeutic levels

29

Pharmacology of the Endocrine Pancreas

Aimee D. Shu, Martin G. Myers, Jr., and Steven E. Shoelson

INTRODUCTION

This chapter presents the physiology and pharmacology of the pancreatic hormones insulin, glucagon, and somatostatin. Because diabetes mellitus—caused by the absence or functional insufficiency of insulin—is clinically the most common disease of these endocrine axes, the majority of the chapter is devoted to the physiology and pharmacology of insulin. Medical students may be interested to note that Charles Best, a fourth-year medical student in Canada, had a significant role in the identification of insulin. Along with his mentor, Frederick Banting, Best isolated a pancreatic extract from dogs that could reduce blood glucose in diabetic dogs and humans. Although the 1923 Nobel Prize in Medicine or Physiology was jointly awarded to surgeon Frederick

Banting and physiologist J. J. R. MacLeod, Banting shared his award with Best.

 Case

At her annual check-up, 55-year-old Mrs. S complains of fatigue and frequent urination (polyuria), even at night. She also reports drinking large volumes of fluids (polydipsia) to quench her thirst. Although these symptoms have been "going on for a while" and are getting worse, Mrs. S has difficulty pinpointing their exact onset. She denies other urinary symptoms such as pain on urination, blood in her urine, dribbling, and incontinence. Her past medical history is remarkable for hyperlipidemia of 10 years duration. Both

529

of her parents died of coronary heart disease in their early 60s.

On physical examination, Mrs. S is moderately obese but otherwise appears normal. Glucose is detected in her urine, but proteins and ketones are not. Her blood tests are significant for elevated glucose (240 mg/dL), elevated total cholesterol (340 mg/dL), and a HbA1c level, a measure of glucose covalently bound to hemoglobin, of 9.2%. The physician explains to Mrs. S that she has Type II diabetes mellitus. In this disease, the body fails to respond normally to insulin (insulin resistance) and cannot produce a sufficient amount of insulin to overcome this resistance.

The physician discusses with Mrs. S the importance of decreasing her caloric intake and increasing her exercise to improve her metabolic state. The physician also prescribes metformin (a biguanide) for her diabetes.

QUESTIONS

1. What are the cellular and molecular actions of insulin?
2. What is the etiology of diabetes mellitus, and how is Type I diabetes mellitus different from Type II diabetes mellitus?
3. What do the blood glucose and HbA1c levels indicate about Mrs. S's diabetes? Are there circumstances under which one parameter could be elevated and the other could be normal?
4. In addition to alleviating her polyuria and polydipsia, why is it important to control Mrs. S's diabetes (i.e., what acute and chronic complications could arise)?
5. What are the mechanisms of action of the various pharmacologic agents used to treat diabetes: α-glucosidase inhibitors, sulfonylureas, meglitinides, thiazolidinediones, biguanides, and GLP-1 mimetics? Is metformin an appropriate therapy for Mrs. S?

BIOCHEMISTRY AND PHYSIOLOGY

PANCREATIC ANATOMY

The pancreas is a glandular organ that contains both exocrine and endocrine tissue. The exocrine portion—which constitutes 99% of the pancreatic mass—secretes bicarbonate and digestive enzymes into the gastrointestinal (GI) tract. Scattered within the exocrine tissue are nearly one million small islands of endocrine tissue that secrete hormones directly into the blood. These tiny endocrine glands, collectively called **Islets of Langerhans,** include several different cell types that secrete different hormones. **α cells** release **glucagon; β cells** release **insulin; δ cells** release **somatostatin** and gastrin; and PP cells release pancreatic polypeptide.

ENERGY HOMEOSTASIS

The storage of nutrients for later release into the circulation allows life to continue in the absence of continuous feeding.

Insulin and glucagon are the primary hormones involved in controlling the uptake, utilization, storage, and release of these nutrients. Insulin promotes the uptake and storage of glucose and other small, energy-containing molecules. The **"counter-regulatory" hormones** — glucagon, catecholamines (i.e., norepinephrine and epinephrine from the sympathetic nervous system and adrenal medulla), glucocorticoids (i.e., cortisol from the adrenal cortex), and growth hormone (from the pituitary gland) — oppose the action of insulin and promote the release of nutrients (see Table 29-1). Blood glucose is easily measured and provides an accurate guide to the balance of insulin and the counter-regulatory hormones. This balance normally keeps glucose levels within a narrow range (70–120 mg/dL), regardless of recent food intake. Hypoglycemia is dangerous because body organs—particularly the brain—depend on a constant supply of glucose for proper functioning. Conversely, chronic hyperglycemia is toxic to many cells and tissues.

The recently identified hormone **leptin** regulates long-term energy balance and the neuroendocrine response to energy storage. Leptin is secreted from fat cells, and its concentration in the plasma is proportional to total fat mass. Thus, leptin signals to the central nervous system the amount of energy—in the form of adipose tissue—that is stored in the body. Leptin promotes anorexia (decreased appetite) and permits the endocrine system to perform energy-expensive functions such as growth, reproduction, and maintenance of a high metabolic rate. Alternatively, the lack of leptin in states of starvation results in increased appetite and impairment of energy-expensive functions.

Fed State

After a meal, complex carbohydrates are broken down to monosaccharides (e.g., glucose, galactose, and fructose) in the lumen of the GI tract and transported into GI epithelial cells by a combination of active and passive apical membrane transporters. Sugars are then transported by basal membrane transporters from the epithelial cell cytosol to intercellular spaces, from which the sugars continue on into capillaries. When glucose in the blood is taken up by pancreatic β cells, the cells release insulin into capillaries that eventually drain into the portal vein. The liver, therefore, receives the highest concentrations of insulin concurrently with the nutrients that have been absorbed from the digestive tract. *The liver and the other energy-storing tissues, such as skeletal muscle and adipose tissue, are the primary tissue targets for insulin* (Fig. 29-1). Local actions of insulin in the Islets of Langerhans also suppress secretion of glucagon from pancreatic α cells.

Fasting State

As the plasma glucose concentration decreases, pancreatic α cells release increasing amounts of glucagon, and pancreatic β cells secrete decreasing amounts of insulin. In contrast to insulin, which promotes the cellular uptake of glucose in the fed state, glucagon mobilizes glucose from the liver by stimulating gluconeogenesis and glycogenolysis. As

TABLE 29-1	Effects of Selected Hormones on Energy Homeostasis		
HORMONE	**SOURCE**	**TARGET TISSUES**	**ACTION**
Glucagon	α Cell (pancreas)	Liver (adipose, skeletal muscle)	Promotes glycogenolysis and gluconeogenesis in liver
Insulin	β Cell (pancreas)	Liver (adipose, skeletal muscle)	Promotes uptake of glucose, amino acids, and fatty acids from blood into cells for storage as glycogen, protein, and triglyceride
Somatostatin	δ Cell (pancreas) GI tract Hypothalamus	Other islet cells, GI tract, brain and pituitary gland	Decreases release of insulin and glucagon Decreases GI tract motility and hormone release Decreases growth hormone secretion
Epinephrine	Adrenal medulla	Many	Promotes glycogenolysis in liver Lipolytic via activation of hormone-sensitive lipase
Cortisol	Adrenal cortex	Many	Antagonizes insulin action at target tissues Promotes gluconeogenesis in liver, protein breakdown in muscle
GLP-1	Ileum	Endocrine pancreas, stomach, brain, heart	Increases β cell mass and insulin secretion Delays gastric emptying Decreases food intake and glucagon secretion
Leptin	Adipocytes	CNS (basomedial hypothalamus)	Signals adequacy of body energy stores, decreases food intake, permits energy-intensive neuroendocrine functions

Physiologically, insulin and glucagon are the two most important hormones controlling glucose homeostasis. Insulin promotes energy storage in target tissues. Glucagon, epinephrine, cortisol, and growth hormone—the ''counter-regulatory'' hormones—act to raise blood glucose and thereby to counteract the effects of insulin. By acting as a ''fat sensor,'' leptin signals total body energy storage and regulates long-term energy balance. GI, gastrointestinal. GLP-1, glucagon-like peptide-1.

fasting continues, catecholamine and glucocorticoid levels also increase, promoting the release of fatty acids from adipose tissue and the breakdown of protein to amino acids in muscle.

INSULIN

Biochemistry

Insulin is a 51-amino acid protein composed of two peptide chains that are linked by two disulfide bridges. Its name comes from the Latin *insula* (meaning ''island,'' after the Islets of Langerhans). The human pancreas contains approximately 8 mg of insulin, of which 0.5 to 1.0 mg is secreted (and replenished by ongoing synthesis) daily. Insulin is initially synthesized in pancreatic β cells as preproinsulin, which is first cleaved to proinsulin and then processed to insulin and free connecting (C) peptide (Fig. 29-2).

Secretion

Resting pancreatic β cells are poised to secrete insulin, which is preformed and stored in secretory vesicles just beneath the plasma membrane. The low basal rate of insulin secretion is increased dramatically upon exposure of the cells to glucose. Glucose metabolism increases the intracellular **ATP/ADP ratio,** which stimulates insulin secretion (see below).

Plasma glucose diffuses down its concentration gradient into the β cell via a specific plasma membrane transporter,

GLUT2. In the presence of high plasma levels of glucose (e.g., in the fed state), more glucose diffuses into the cell, where it is phosphorylated to glucose-6-phosphate by hexokinase and thus started down the glycolytic pathway. Through glycolysis and the citric acid cycle, glucose metabolism generates ATP and increases the ATP/ADP ratio in the β cell. The ATP/ADP ratio modulates the activity of a membrane-spanning **ATP-sensitive K^+ channel (K^+/ATP channel).** *When open, this channel hyperpolarizes the cell by allowing an outward flux of K^+ and driving the membrane potential toward the Nernst potential for K^+; when closed, the cell depolarizes.* Because ATP inhibits the channel and ADP activates the channel, a high intracellular ATP/ADP ratio closes the K^+/ATP channel. The resulting depolarization of the cell activates voltage-gated Ca^{2+} channels, which mediate an influx of extracellular Ca^{2+}. The increase in intracellular $[Ca^{2+}]$ stimulates exocytosis of the insulin-containing vesicles. In contrast, under conditions of relatively low extracellular glucose concentrations (e.g., in the fasting state), the β cell has a low ATP/ADP ratio. In this case, the K^+/ATP channels remain open, and the β cell is maintained in a hyperpolarized state that prevents Ca^{2+} influx and insulin secretion (Fig. 29-3).

K^+/ATP channels are octameric structures containing 4 subunits of Kir6.x and 4 subunits of SURx, where ''x'' denotes one of several isoforms. The Kir6.x tetramer forms the pore of the K^+/ATP channel, while the associated SUR molecules regulate the channel's sensitivity to ADP and pharmacologic agents. Both Kir and SUR subunits must be expressed for a functional channel to be inserted into the

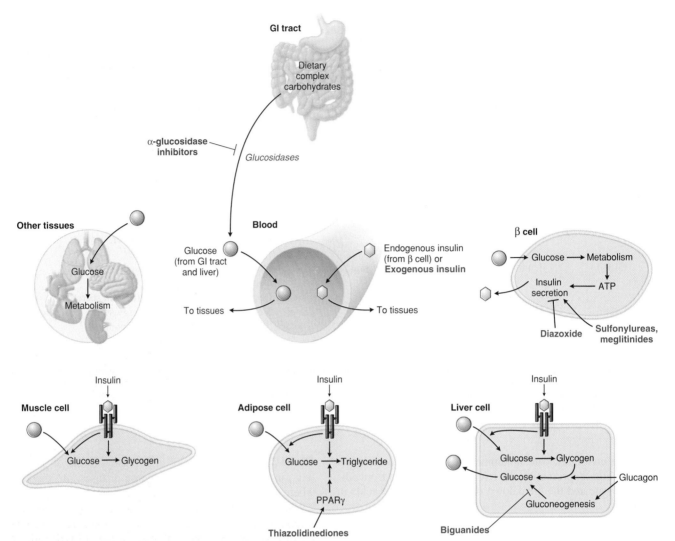

Figure 29-1. Physiologic and pharmacologic regulation of glucose homeostasis. Dietary complex carbohydrates are broken down to simple sugars in the GI tract by the action of glucosidases; simple sugars are then absorbed by GI epithelial cells and transported into the blood. Glucose in the blood is taken up by all metabolically active tissues in the body. In pancreatic β cells, glucose metabolism increases levels of cytosolic ATP, which stimulates insulin secretion. Insulin then acts on plasma membrane insulin receptors in target tissues (muscle, adipose, liver) to increase glucose uptake and storage as glycogen or triglyceride. Glucose is also taken up by other cells and tissues to fuel metabolism. In muscle cells, insulin promotes glucose storage as glycogen. In adipose cells, insulin promotes glucose conversion to triglycerides. Peroxisome proliferator-activated receptor γ (PPARγ) also promotes the conversion of glucose to triglycerides in adipose cells. In liver cells, insulin promotes glucose storage as glycogen. Glucagon promotes both gluconeogenesis and the conversion of glycogen back to glucose; glucose generated by gluconeogenesis or from glycogen is transported out of the liver cell into the blood. Note that glucose from dietary complex carbohydrates, and insulin secreted by pancreatic β cells, both enter the liver in high concentrations through the portal circulation (not shown). Pharmacologic interventions that decrease blood glucose levels include: inhibiting intestinal α-glucosidases; administering exogenous insulin; using sulfonylureas or meglitinides to augment secretion of insulin by β cells; and using biguanides or thiazolidinediones to enhance the action of insulin in liver or adipose cells, respectively. GLP-1 mimetics decrease blood glucose levels by several complementary mechanisms (not shown). Diazoxide inhibits insulin secretion from pancreatic β cells.

plasma membrane. The pancreatic β cell channel is composed of Kir6.2 and SUR1 subunits. K^+/ATP channels composed of Kir6.2 and SUR1 isoforms are also expressed in some neurons, while the channels in cardiac and smooth muscle express SUR2 isoforms. In addition, some smooth muscle cell channels contain Kir6.1 in place of Kir6.2. Mutations in Kir6.2 or SUR1 can result in hyperinsulinemic hypoglycemia, because the β cell is continually depolarized in the absence of K^+/ATP channel activity. In the future, elucidation of the mechanisms that regulate the tissue-specific

expression of the different Kir6 and SUR isoforms could lead to the development of more specific pharmacologic agents for the treatment of Type II diabetes mellitus.

Kir6.2 binds ATP directly (although the relevant nucleotide-binding motifs have not been identified), and this ATP binding inhibits the K^+ conductance of the channel. SUR1 enhances the sensitivity of the Kir6.2 channel to ATP; SUR1 also confers sensitivity of the channel to ADP and to most of the drugs that regulate the activity of the K^+/ATP channel. SUR1 contains two nucleotide-binding folds that coordi-

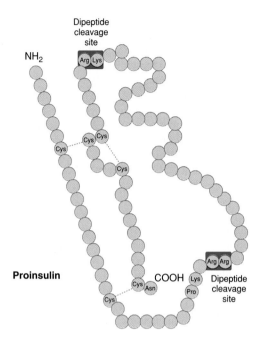

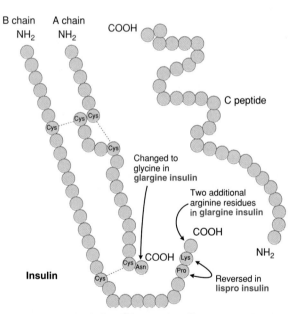

Figure 29-2. Processing of human insulin. Preproinsulin is synthesized and exported into the endoplasmic reticulum, where the signal peptide *(not shown)* is cleaved to generate proinsulin **(top panel).** Intramolecular disulfide bonds (cys–cys) aid in the proper folding of proinsulin. Proinsulin is transported to secretory vesicles, where prohormone convertases act on dipeptide cleavage sites in proinsulin *(boxes)* to generate insulin and connecting (C) peptide. Two disulfide bonds aid in holding the A-chain and B-chain of insulin together. Insulin and C-peptide are secreted together from the pancreatic β cell **(bottom panel).** In lispro, an artificial insulin designed to be absorbed more rapidly after injection, a proline and a lysine residue in the COOH-terminus of the B-chain of insulin are transposed; this minor alteration does not affect the ability of the molecule to bind the insulin receptor or to mediate insulin action. In glargine insulin, an A-chain asparagine is replaced with glycine, and two arginines are added to the COOH-terminus of the B-chain. These modifications slow the absorption of glargine insulin relative to regular insulin.

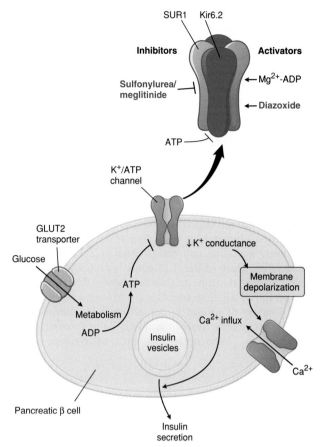

Figure 29-3. Physiologic and pharmacologic regulation of insulin release from pancreatic β cells. In the basal state, the plasma membrane of the β cell is hyperpolarized, and the rate of insulin secretion from the cell is low. When glucose is available, it enters the cell via GLUT2 transporters in the plasma membrane and is metabolized to generate intracellular ATP. ATP binds to and inhibits the plasma membrane K^+/ATP channel. Inhibition of the K^+/ATP channel decreases plasma membrane K^+ conductance; the resulting depolarization of the membrane activates voltage-gated Ca^{2+} channels and thereby stimulates an influx of Ca^{2+}. Ca^{2+} mediates fusion of insulin-containing secretory vesicles with the plasma membrane, leading to insulin secretion. The K^+/ATP channel, an octamer composed of Kir6.2 and SUR1 subunits, is the target of several physiologic and pharmacologic regulators. ATP binds to and inhibits Kir6.2, while sulfonylureas and meglitinides bind to and inhibit SUR1; all three of these agents promote insulin secretion. The GLP-1 mimetic exenatide, acting as an agonist at G protein-coupled GLP-1 receptors in the plasma membrane of the pancreatic β cell, also stimulates glucose-dependent insulin secretion. This action of exenatide appears to be mediated by an increase in intracellular cyclic AMP, and may involve an indirect effect on the K^+/ATP channel *(not shown)*. Mg^{2+}-ADP and diazoxide bind to and activate SUR1, thereby inhibiting insulin secretion. (For clarity, only four of the eight K^+/ATP channel subunits are shown.)

nate ADP complexed with Mg^{2+} (Mg^{2+}-ADP); Mg^{2+}-ADP binding to SUR1 activates the channel and thereby inhibits insulin secretion when the ATP/ADP ratio is low.

Other than plasma glucose, the stimulators of insulin release include several fuels that act to increase the intracellular ATP/ADP ratio, including some nonglucose sugars, amino acids, and fatty acids. Parasympathetic nervous system activity and the GI hormones **glucagon-like peptide-1 (GLP-1)** and glucose-dependent insulinotropic polypeptide (GIP) also decrease K⁺/ATP channel activity (and thereby stimulate insulin secretion) via G protein-mediated pathways. β Cell exposure to nutrients promotes not only insulin secretion but also insulin transcription, translation, processing, and packaging.

Action at Target Tissues

Insulin binds to receptors on the surface of target cells. Although virtually all tissues express **insulin receptors,** the energy-storing tissues (liver, muscle, and adipose) express much higher levels of insulin receptors and thus constitute the main insulin target tissues. The insulin receptor (Fig. 29-4) is a glycoprotein consisting of four disulfide-linked subunits, including two extracellular α subunits and two β subunits. Each of the β subunits is composed of a short extracellular domain, a transmembrane domain, and an intracellular tail that contains a tyrosine kinase domain. The binding of insulin to the extracellular portion of the insulin receptor activates the intracellular tyrosine kinase, resulting in "autophosphorylation" of tyrosine on the

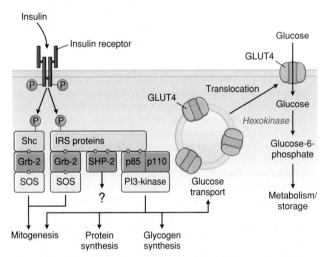

Figure 29-4. Downstream effects of insulin receptor activation. The insulin receptor is a cell surface heterotetramer composed of two α-subunits and two β-subunits. The α-subunits are entirely extracellular, while the β-subunits contain extracellular, transmembrane, and intracellular domains. Insulin binding to the extracellular portion of the receptor activates tyrosine kinase domains in the intracellular regions of the β-subunits. These tyrosine kinase domains mediate "autophosphorylation" of the receptor (actually, each β-subunit phosphorylates the other) and tyrosine-phosphorylation of cytoplasmic substrate proteins including Shc and insulin receptor substrate (IRS) proteins. Phosphorylated Shc promotes mitogenesis. Phosphorylated IRS proteins interact with many other signaling proteins (Grb-2, SHP-2, p85, and p110) to effect changes in cellular function. The IRS interaction with p85 and p110 recruits phosphatidylinositol 3′-kinase (PI3-kinase). PI3-kinase activates signaling cascades that control many aspects of cellular insulin action, including glucose transport (via the translocation of GLUT4 glucose transporters to the cell surface), protein synthesis, and glycogen synthesis. Glucose that enters the cell is rapidly phosphorylated by hexokinase, and subsequently used for metabolism or stored in the cell as glycogen or triglyceride.

nearby β subunit and in phosphorylation of several other intracellular proteins — most importantly, the **insulin receptor substrate-proteins (IRS-proteins).** Tyrosine-phosphorylated IRS-proteins recruit a variety of second messenger proteins that contain phosphotyrosine-binding src homology 2 (SH2) domains. The Type IA **phosphatidylinositol 3′-kinase (PI3-kinase)** is one of these second messenger proteins that appears to be important for many aspects of insulin action.

Although the details linking these insulin receptor second messengers to the metabolic effects of insulin remain open to investigation, the metabolic effects of insulin action are well understood: *insulin is the classic anabolic (energy-storing) hormone* (Fig. 29-1). In the liver, insulin increases glucokinase activity, thereby mediating the phosphorylation and trapping of glucose in hepatocytes. This increased supply of glucose in the hepatocyte provides fuel for glycogen synthesis, glycolysis, and fatty acid synthesis. Insulin's activation of glycogen and fatty acid synthases, and its inhibition of glycogen phosphorylase and gluconeogenic enzymes, combine to further enhance the anabolic processes.

In skeletal muscle and adipose tissue, insulin stimulates translocation of the insulin-responsive glucose transporter, GLUT4, from intracellular vesicles to the cell surface. GLUT4 translocation, in turn, facilitates the movement of glucose into the cell. In muscle, insulin also increases amino acid uptake, stimulates the ribosomal protein synthesis machinery, and promotes glycogen synthase activity and subsequent glycogen storage. In adipose tissue, insulin promotes the expression of lipoprotein lipase, which hydrolyzes triglycerides from circulating lipoproteins for uptake into fat cells. Once inside the fat cell, glucose and fatty acids are stored predominantly as triglycerides. This process is enhanced by the activation of other lipogenic enzymes, including pyruvate kinase, pyruvate dehydrogenase, acetyl-CoA carboxylase, and glycerol phosphate acyltransferase, and the deactivation of hormone-sensitive lipase, which degrades triglyceride. Insulin is degraded rapidly by insulinase enzymes in the liver and kidney; its circulating half-life is 6 minutes.

GLUCAGON

Glucagon—a single chain polypeptide of 29 amino acids—is a catabolic (energy-releasing) hormone secreted by pancreatic α cells. When plasma glucose levels are low, glucagon mobilizes glucose, fat, and protein from storage for use as sources of energy. Besides low glucose and high insulin levels, stimuli for glucagon secretion include sympathetic nervous system activity, stress, exercise, and high plasma levels of amino acids (because the latter indicates a state of starvation). Glucagon binding to its G protein-coupled receptor on the plasma membrane of target cells increases intracellular cAMP and activates protein kinase A, a serine/threonine kinase. Glucagon's main site of action is the liver, where it promotes glycogenolysis and gluconeogenesis (Fig. 29-1). Glucagon also promotes lipolysis in adipose tissue. The liver and kidneys degrade glucagon; like insulin, its circulating half-life is about 6 minutes.

SOMATOSTATIN

Somatostatin—a 14-amino acid peptide—is produced in multiple sites, including pancreatic δ cells, the gastrointestinal tract, and the hypothalamus. Somatostatin has several inhibitory effects. First, it decreases secretion of both insulin and glucagon. Second, it inhibits GI tract motility. Third, it inhibits secretion of thyroid stimulating hormone, growth hormone, and various GI hormones. The stimuli for somatostatin release are similar to those for insulin release: high plasma levels of glucose, amino acids, and fatty acids. Local somatostatin release allows the hormone to act in a paracrine fashion. The circulating half-life of somatostatin is only 2 minutes.

GLUCAGON-LIKE PEPTIDE-1

Glucagon-like peptide-1 (GLP-1) is a hormone produced primarily in enteroendocrine cells (L cells) of the distal small bowel (ileum). GLP-1 is encoded by the glucagon gene; proglucagon is alternatively processed into glucagon in pancreatic α cells or GLP-1 and other peptides in gut L cells. Bioactive forms of GLP-1 are 29 or 30 amino acids in length. GLP-1 is released from L cells during nutrient absorption in the GI tract. GLP-1 has a variety of physiologic effects in several different target tissues. In the pancreas, GLP-1 increases insulin secretion and suppresses glucagon secretion. GLP-1 acts in the stomach to delay gastric emptying, and it decreases appetite by acting in the hypothalamus. GLP-1 has a short half-life in the circulation (1–2 minutes), due to enzymatic degradation by dipeptidyl peptidase-IV (DPP-IV).

PATHOPHYSIOLOGY

DIABETES MELLITUS

As early as AD 200, the Greek physician Aretaeus observed patients who had excessive thirst and urination. He named this condition *"diabetes,"* which is Greek for "to siphon, or pass through." Later, physicians added *"mellitus"* (Latin for "honeyed, sweet") to the disease name after noticing that diabetic patients produce urine that contains sugar. The designation *diabetes mellitus* also distinguishes this disorder from *diabetes insipidus* (see Chapter 25, Pharmacology of the Hypothalamus and Pituitary Gland), in which dysregulation of the response to antidiuretic hormone (ADH) inhibits reabsorption of water in the collecting ducts of the nephron, resulting in the production of copious amounts of dilute urine.

The syndrome of diabetes mellitus results from a heterogeneous group of metabolic disorders characterized by hyperglycemia (Table 29-2). Hyperglycemia can result from an absolute lack of insulin [**Type I diabetes mellitus,** also called *insulin-dependent diabetes mellitus* (IDDM) or *juvenile-onset diabetes*] or from a relative insufficiency of insulin production in the face of insulin resistance [**Type II diabetes mellitus,** also called *noninsulin-dependent diabetes mellitus* (NIDDM) or *adult-onset diabetes*].

Type I Diabetes

Type I diabetes mellitus, which accounts for 5% to 10% of cases in the United States, results from the autoimmune

---

TABLE 29-2 Type I and Type II Diabetes Mellitus

	TYPE I	TYPE II
Etiology	Autoimmune destruction of pancreatic β cells	Insulin resistance, with inadequate β cell function to compensate
Insulin levels	Absent or negligible	Typically higher than normal
Insulin action	Absent or negligible	Decreased
Insulin resistance	Not part of syndrome but may be present (e.g., in obese patients)	Yes
Age of onset	Typically <30 years	Typically >40 years
Acute complications	Ketoacidosis Wasting	Hyperglycemia (can lead to hyperosmotic seizures and coma)
Chronic complications	Neuropathy Retinopathy Nephropathy Peripheral vascular disease Coronary artery disease	Same as Type I
Pharmacologic interventions	Insulin	A number of drug classes are available, including insulin if other therapies fail

Type I and Type II diabetes mellitus are both associated with increased blood glucose levels, but the two diseases result from distinct pathophysiologic pathways. In Type I diabetes mellitus, there is an absolute lack of insulin secondary to autoimmune destruction of pancreatic β cells. The etiology of Type II diabetes is less well understood, but seems to involve impaired insulin sensitivity and an inadequate level of compensatory insulin production by pancreatic β cells. Although Type I and Type II diabetes have different acute complications *(see text)*, they share similar chronic complications. Insulin is the primary pharmacologic intervention for Type I diabetes, while Type II diabetes can be treated with a number of different agents.

destruction of pancreatic β cells. In the absence of β cells, insulin is neither produced nor released, and circulating insulin concentrations are near zero. In the absence of insulin, insulin-responsive tissues fail to take up and store glucose, amino acids, and lipids, even when there are high circulating plasma levels of these fuels. *The unopposed action of the counter-regulatory hormones induces a starvation-like response by the cells and tissues of the body.* Thus, glycogenolysis and gluconeogenesis proceed unchecked in the liver, delivering glucose to the circulation even though the blood glucose concentrations are high. Muscle tissue breaks down protein and releases amino acids, which travel to the liver as fuel for gluconeogenesis. In adipose tissue, triglycerides are broken down and released into the circulation. In addition, the liver breaks down fatty acids for use as gluconeogenic fuels and for export as ketone bodies that could be used as fuel by the brain. These ketones equilibrate into β-hydroxybutyrate and acetoacetate. Excessively high concentrations of these acids can deplete serum bicarbonate, eventually resulting in a state of metabolic acidosis called **diabetic ketoacidosis (DKA).** DKA is a serious, potentially life-threatening medical emergency that requires immediate, aggressive treatment.

In diabetic patients, blood glucose levels exceed the kidney's capacity to reabsorb glucose from the glomerular filtrate, and the glucose that remains in the urine produces an osmotic diuresis as well as a "sweetening" of the urine. This phenomenon causes the *polyuria* and subsequent *polydipsia* experienced by many diabetic patients. Although appetite is stimulated—resulting in excessive hunger, or *polyphagia*—patients lose weight because dietary nutrients cannot be stored.

The onset of clinical disease in Type I diabetes is usually sudden, and often occurs during childhood or adolescence. The actual destruction of β cells occurs gradually, but the remaining β cells can provide a sufficient amount of insulin until approximately 85% of the total population of β cells is destroyed—resulting in the abrupt onset of symptoms. Because 15% of the β cells remain at this point in time, many patients experience a "honeymoon" phase of their illness, with intermittent periods of adequate endogenous insulin production before the eventual complete and final loss of insulin production. In many cases, a prodromal "flu-like" syndrome occurs a few weeks before the onset of symptomatic diabetes. Although some hypotheses suggest that this syndrome represents a viral illness that triggers an autoimmune reaction in genetically predisposed individuals, it is possible that these patients are instead reacting to increased levels of inflammatory mediators produced by an already-initiated autoimmune reaction.

The genetic predisposition to Type I diabetes maps most tightly to certain alleles on chromosome 6. These alleles code for human leukocyte antigens (HLA), also called *major histocompatibility complex* (MHC) proteins, which are involved in antigen presentation in the immune system. Other genetic loci may also contribute to the development of Type I diabetes. In most Type I patients, autoantibodies to β cell proteins can be detected. Environmental factors influence disease development as well; if one member of an identical twin pair is affected, the incidence of Type I diabetes in the other twin is about 50%.

Because Type I patients produce little or no endogenous insulin, therapy consists of replacement with exogenous insulin.

Type II Diabetes

Type II diabetes mellitus, which constitutes approximately 90% of cases in the United States, typically affects individuals over 40 years old. Obesity is the single most important risk factor for Type II diabetes; 80% of all Type II diabetic patients are obese. The disorder typically develops gradually, without obvious symptoms at the onset. It is frequently diagnosed either by elevated blood glucose levels in routine screening tests or, as in the introductory case, after the disease has become severe enough to cause polyuria and polydipsia.

The progression to Type II diabetes is thought to begin with a state of **insulin resistance.** Tissues that were once normally insulin-responsive become relatively refractory to insulin action and require increased insulin levels to respond appropriately. In many cases, insulin resistance is the result of obesity and a sedentary lifestyle, although the molecular predisposition in these patients is poorly characterized. Investigators have described insulin receptor defects as well as postreceptor signaling defects. However, it is unclear which, if any, of these defects could be the primary event in insulin resistance. Initially, insulin resistance is compensated for by increased production of insulin by pancreatic β cells. Indeed, many individuals with obesity and insulin resistance never progress to frank diabetes, because their β cells continue to compensate by increased secretion of insulin. In some patients like Mrs. S, however, the β cells eventually fail to keep pace with the demand for insulin.

Although patients with Type II diabetes generally have increased circulating insulin levels, these levels are insufficient to overcome insulin resistance in the target tissues. The eventual failure of β cell compensation could result from the loss of β cells through increased apoptosis (programmed cell death) or from the decreased renewal of β cells. Insulin levels that are inadequate to compensate for insulin resistance stimulate an inadequate response in target tissues, resulting in an imbalance between the actions of insulin and those of the counter-regulatory hormones. This imbalance leads to hyperglycemia and dyslipidemia, as the liver and adipose tissues inappropriately mobilize fuels from storage tissues.

The genetic basis for Type II diabetes is likely a combination of predispositions toward obesity, insulin resistance, and β cell failure. Type II diabetic patients who are lean (and insulin-sensitive) generally have a strong predisposition to β cell failure. Indeed, an early-onset form of Type II diabetes—maturity-onset diabetes in the young (MODY)—results from a predisposition to early β cell failure; in many cases, the molecular basis for this predisposition is an inherited mutation in one of the β cell-specific transcription factors. Mild or early Type II diabetes can be unmasked in predisposed individuals by states in which insulin resistance occurs suddenly, such as treatment with glucocorticoids (see Chapter 27, Pharmacology of the Adrenal Cortex) or pregnancy (gestational diabetes).

There does not seem to be an autoimmune contribution to the development of Type II diabetes, although there are rare syndromes of insulin resistance associated with autoantibodies directed against insulin or the insulin receptor. Other rare mutations in the insulin receptor can also lead to severe insulin resistance. In some cases, these individuals never progress to frank diabetes, because their β cells are able to compensate by overproducing insulin.

The ability of patients with Type II diabetes (like Mrs. S) to produce insulin suggests that such patients can be treated with orally available agents that: (1) control blood glucose levels by slowing the absorption of sugars from the GI tract; (2) increase insulin secretion by pancreatic β cells; or (3) sensitize target cells to the action of insulin. Type II diabetic patients who have lost a great deal of β cell function can come to resemble Type I diabetic patients clinically, and may require exogenous insulin therapy.

Morbidity and Mortality

Type I and Type II diabetes are associated with type-specific acute morbidities and common chronic complications. In uncontrolled Type I diabetes, the unopposed action of counter-regulatory hormones leads to ketoacidosis, which can progress rapidly to coma and death. In fact, the diagnosis of Type I diabetes is often made in the emergency room in a patient who presents for the first time with diabetic ketoacidosis. Even in the absence of severe ketoacidosis, if left untreated, the lack of insulin in Type I diabetes leads to tissue wasting and death over a period of weeks to months. Ketoacidosis does not generally occur in Type II diabetes, because these patients generally produce endogenous insulin. However, extreme hyperglycemia in Type I or Type II diabetes can cause a hyperosmotic syndrome that leads to mental status changes and can progress to seizures, coma, and death.

Both Type I and Type II diabetes are associated with long-term vascular pathology. These **chronic complications** include *premature atherosclerosis, retinopathy, nephropathy,* and *neuropathy.* Although the exact mechanisms are unclear, it appears that these complications may result from a combination of hyperglycemia, hyperlipidemia, and increases in inflammatory signaling over many years. In treating Mrs. S's diabetes, the goals are not only to improve her polydipsia and polyuria and to normalize her laboratory values as ends in themselves, but also to prevent these serious chronic complications.

Because uncontrolled diabetes has such severe complications, it is critical to assess accurately the level of control achieved with any therapy. The results of the landmark Diabetes Control and Complications Trial (DCCT), a multicenter clinical trial (1983–1996) involving Type I diabetic patients, and the United Kingdom Prospective Diabetes Study (UKPDS, 1998) involving Type II diabetics, suggest that *intensive therapy to maintain continuous normoglycemia dramatically reduces the incidence of the long-term complications of diabetes.*

Blood glucose levels are assessed in two ways: acutely, by measuring blood glucose with a glucose monitor, and chronically, by measuring **glycohemoglobin (HbA1c).** "Tight control," or the maintenance of near normal glycemia, is generally achieved by measuring acute blood glucose levels several times throughout the day, and altering diet and insulin doses to keep blood glucose levels within the normal range. To obtain an estimate of the average blood glucose level over the previous several months, physicians can measure HbA1c. Glucose in the blood nonenzymatically glycosylates blood proteins; the nonenzymatic glycosylation of hemoglobin in red blood cells generates HbA1c. Because nonenzymatic glycosylation occurs at a rate that is proportional to the level of glucose in the blood, and the lifespan of a red blood cell is approximately 120 days, the HbA1c level yields an estimate of the average blood glucose level over the preceding several months. Consequently, the HbA1c value can be elevated in a patient at the same time that the blood glucose level is normal—meaning that, although the blood glucose level is acutely normal, glucose levels have been chronically elevated over the previous several months. Mrs. S's HbA1c level of 9.2% is cause for concern, because the rate of chronic diabetic complications rises dramatically with HbA1c levels greater than 7.5%. HbA1c levels may be misleadingly low in patients with a shortened red blood cell lifespan (e.g., in patients with hemolytic anemia).

HYPERINSULINEMIA

Hyperinsulinemia is one of several conditions that can result in hypoglycemia. Hypoglycemia is a problematic condition because the brain requires a constant supply of glucose and cannot rely on alternate fuels as readily as peripheral tissues can. Hyperinsulinemia has various causes, the most common of which is iatrogenic (i.e., exogenous insulin overdose in the course of insulin therapy for Type I or Type II diabetes). A central challenge in the therapy of diabetes (Type I or Type II) is to normalize glucose levels adequately while avoiding overtreatment and causing hypoglycemia. Other rare causes of hypoglycemia include insulinomas (insulin-secreting tumors of pancreatic β cells), mutations in the β cell K^+/ATP channel (e.g., mutations in Kir6.2 or SUR1 that result in constitutive depolarization), and activating autoantibodies directed against the insulin receptor.

PHARMACOLOGIC CLASSES AND AGENTS

THERAPY FOR DIABETES

Strategies of Therapy

The major goal of pharmacologic therapy for diabetes is to normalize metabolic parameters, such as blood sugar, in order to reduce the risk of long-term complications. For Type I diabetic patients, the pharmacologic strategy is to administer a sufficient amount of exogenous insulin to achieve normoglycemia, without inducing hypoglycemia. Appropriate treatment of Type I diabetic patients not only achieves normoglycemia, but also reverses the metabolic starvation response mediated by the unopposed action of counter-regulatory hormones. For example, insulin treatment reverses amino acid breakdown in muscle and ketogenesis in the liver.

The treatment of Type II diabetes is multifaceted. First, obese patients should endeavor to reduce body weight and increase exercise in order to improve insulin sensitivity. Some Type II patients can achieve good control of their diabetes by modifying their diet and exercise habits; Mrs. S's diabetes would likely be improved dramatically by such lifestyle changes. Pharmacologically, treatments include orally available agents that act to slow glucose absorption from the gut (α-glucosidase inhibitors), to increase insulin secretion by β cells (sulfonylureas, meglitinides, and GLP-1 mimetics), or to increase insulin sensitivity at target tissues (thiazolidinediones and biguanides). These agents are generally ineffective for patients with Type I diabetes. Patients with Type II diabetes are frequently treated with combinations of these drugs and are therefore utilizing multiple strategies; nonetheless, some will eventually require exogenous insulin therapy. The various agents are discussed below in a framework that highlights their sites and mechanisms of action, by following the path of glucose metabolism from intestinal glucose absorption to insulin secretion to the metabolism and storage of glucose in target tissues (Fig. 29-1).

Inhibitors of Intestinal Glucose Absorption: α-Glucosidase Inhibitors

α-Glucosidase inhibitors—nicknamed "starch blockers"—are carbohydrate analogues that bind 1,000 times more avidly than dietary carbohydrates to intestinal brush border α-glucosidase enzymes. Glucosidases—maltase, isomaltase, sucrase, and glucoamylase—aid absorption by cleaving complex carbohydrates to yield glucose. By reversibly inhibiting these enzymes, α-glucosidase inhibitors increase the time required for absorption of carbohydrates such as starch, dextrin, and disaccharides. These drugs also increase the intestinal surface area for absorption because carbohydrates that would have been absorbed in the upper intestine are absorbed instead—in smaller quantities—throughout the length of the small intestine. Therefore, these drugs help reduce the postprandial peak in blood sugar. α-Glucosidase inhibitors are effective when taken with meals, but they are not effective at other times. Mrs. S's increased *fasting* blood glucose level suggests that, in her case, monotherapy with an α-glucosidase inhibitor would likely be ineffective.

Acarbose was introduced in the United States in 1996, and **miglitol** was introduced in 1999; these two agents are similarly effective. When used as monotherapy, these agents reduce fasting blood glucose by 25 to 30 mg/dL (1.3 to 1.7 mmol/L), postprandial blood glucose by 40 to 50 mg/dL (2.2 to 2.8 mmol/L), and HbA1c by 0.7% to 0.9%, and they pose no risk of hypoglycemia. α-Glucosidase inhibitors are also useful as adjunctive therapy. These drugs are most useful for patients with predominantly postprandial hyperglycemia, and for new-onset patients with mild hyperglycemia. Flatulence, bloating, abdominal discomfort, and diarrhea are common adverse effects, all of which result from gas released by bacteria acting on undigested carbohydrates that reach the large intestine. The gastrointestinal distress usually diminishes with continued use of an α-glucosidase inhibitor, but these agents are contraindicated for patients with inflammatory bowel disease. Serum aminotransferase levels should be monitored during therapy; these drugs are associated with a dose-dependent increase in aminotransferase levels that is reversible upon drug discontinuation. In addition, α-glucosidase inhibitors are associated with modest increases in plasma triglycerides. Use of these agents is not associated with any change in weight.

Insulin Replacement: Exogenous Insulin

Insulin is the only treatment for patients with Type I diabetes. Insulin is also used for patients with Type II diabetes if diet and other therapies are not sufficiently effective at controlling the hyperglycemia. Insulin preparations are classified according to onset of action, duration of action, and species of origin (i.e., human, pig, or cow). Recombinant DNA techniques have been employed to produce human insulin in vitro, making this form of the drug an increasingly popular choice relative to other (porcine or bovine) preparations that can violate certain religious restrictions and/or provoke an immune response.

Because insulin is a protein that is subject to rapid degradation in the GI tract, it is not effective as an oral agent. Instead, insulin is administered parenterally, typically by subcutaneous injection with a fine-gauge needle that creates a small depot of insulin at the site of injection. The rate at which this depot of insulin is absorbed depends on a variety of factors, including the solubility of the insulin preparation and the local circulation. The more quickly a particular preparation is absorbed, the faster its onset of action, and the shorter its duration of action. Person-to-person and site-to-site variability can produce great differences in the rate of absorption and, thus, the action profile of the injected insulin. Table 29-3 divides the most commonly used insulin preparations into four categories, based on their onset, peak, and duration of action.

Regular insulin, a short-acting preparation, is structurally identical to endogenous insulin, but zinc ions are added for stability. Regular insulin tends to aggregate into hexamers, and dissociation of the hexamers to monomers is the rate-limiting step for absorption. *Lispro* insulin, an ultrarapid-acting insulin, was designed to keep the molecule in a monomeric form in order to speed absorption. Lispro insulin is structurally similar to regular insulin, except that a sequence of two amino acids (lysine and proline) near the carboxy-terminus of the B-chain has been switched (see Fig. 29-2). Lispro offers flexibility and convenience for patients because it can be injected minutes before a meal, whereas the proper use of longer-acting insulins requires a time lag between insulin injection and the consumption of a meal. In *NPH (neutral protamine Hagedorn) insulin,* an intermediate-acting preparation, insulin is combined with protamine—a protein isolated from rainbow trout sperm—in a zinc suspension. Protamine prolongs the time required for absorption of insulin because it remains complexed with insulin until proteolytic enzymes cleave the protamine from the insulin. *Ultralente* insulin, a long-acting preparation, is a crystalline suspension of insulin and zinc in an acetate buffer. This formulation delays the onset of action of insulin. *Semilente* insulin is semicrystalline, or "amorphous," and is short-acting. *Lente* insulin is a combination of crystalline (i.e., ultralente) and semicrystalline (i.e., semilente) insulin and zinc suspended in an acetate buffer. This formulation is slower acting than semilente but faster acting than ultralente, and is therefore in the intermediate-acting category. *Glargine* insulin is regular insulin in which a glycine replaces an asparagine on the A-chain and two additional arginines

| TABLE 29-3 | Commonly Used Insulin Preparations |

TYPE AND PREPARATION	CONSTITUENTS	Action Profile (Hours)			USAGE
		ONSET	PEAK	DURATION	
Ultrarapid-Acting					
Lispro (human analogue)	Identical to regular human insulin, except for transposed lysine and proline in B chain	0.2–0.5	0.5–2	3–4	For meals or acute hyperglycemia
Short-Acting					
Regular (human)	Solution of unmodified zinc insulin crystals	0.5–1	2–3	6–8	For meals or acute hyperglycemia
Semilente (human)	Semicrystalline (amorphous) suspension	1–2	2–5	8–12	
Intermediate-Acting					
NPH (human)	Protamine zinc, phosphate buffer	1.5	4–10	16–24	Provide basal insulin and overnight coverage
Lente (human)	Crystalline/amorphous mix, acetate buffer	1.5–3	7–15	16–24	
Long-Acting					
Ultralente (human)	Crystalline suspension, acetate buffer	4–6	8–30	24–36	Provide basal insulin and overnight coverage
Glargine (human analogue)	Similar to regular human insulin, with glycine in place of asparagine in A chain, and 2 extra arginines in B chain	4–6	None	18–24	

Modifications to native human insulin consist of either (1) alterations in the amino acid sequence of the molecule or (2) changes in the physical form of the molecule. These changes affect the rate at which insulin is absorbed and the temporal profile of insulin action. Alterations in the amino acid sequence change the tendency for insulin to aggregate. The modification in lispro decreases aggregation, resulting in faster absorption and more rapid action. In contrast, a crystalline suspension (ultralente) delays the rate of absorption of insulin from its subcutaneous injection site, making this preparation a long-acting dosage form.

are added at the carboxy terminus of the B-chain (Fig. 29-2). These modifications make the pKa of the insulin more neutral, thus slowing its absorption into the neutral environment of the blood. Glargine has the advantages of long duration of action and steady release without a peak (mimicking so-called ''basal'' insulin secretion).

Insulin regimens—including the preparation, dose, and frequency of the insulin—are tailored for each individual patient. Furthermore, regimens are often adjusted slightly on a daily basis according to the patient's activity, meal size and composition, and blood glucose levels. For example, some patients inject short-acting insulin before meals, and long-acting insulin to provide basal insulin levels through the night. Advances in insulin therapy are still evolving. Pharmaceutical companies continue to design preparations that will more closely mimic physiologic postprandial blood insulin levels. Researchers are also attempting to make longer-lasting preparations with steadier absorption rates. In addition, new drug delivery techniques are being tested to

create alternatives to subcutaneous injection (see Chapter 54, Drug Delivery Modalities), such as intranasal and pulmonary dosage forms, as well as miniature pumps for continuous delivery.

The major danger with insulin therapy is that administration of insulin in the absence of adequate carbohydrate intake can result in hypoglycemia. Thus, patients—both Type I and Type II diabetics—must be cautioned not to take too much insulin. While tight glycemic control that aims to maintain normoglycemia does decrease the incidence of diabetic complications, it also increases the frequency of hypoglycemic attacks. Indeed, it is challenging to maintain the fine balance between insufficient and excessive insulin.

In Type II diabetic patients such as Mrs. S, insulin resistance is typically more severe in muscle and liver than in fat cells. For this reason, insulin preferentially deposits calories in adipose tissue, and insulin therapy in insulin-resistant patients (especially those who are already obese, like Mrs. S) often results in weight gain.

Insulin Secretagogues: Sulfonylureas and Meglitinides

Sulfonylureas

Since the 1950s, **sulfonylureas** have been the major oral agents available in the United States for the treatment of Type II diabetes. Sulfonylureas stimulate insulin release from pancreatic β cells, thereby increasing circulating insulin to levels sufficient to overcome the insulin resistance. *At the molecular level, sulfonylureas act by inhibiting the β cell K^+/ATP channel at the SUR1 subunit* (Fig. 29-3). (The SUR subunit was so named because it is the "*SU*lfonylurea *Receptor*.") Sulfonylureas may act by displacing endogenous Mg^{2+}-ADP, which binds to SUR1 and activates the channel. The sulfonylureas used to treat Type II diabetes bind with a higher affinity to SUR1 than to SUR2 isoforms, accounting for their relative β cell specificity. The inhibition of the K^+/ATP channel by sulfonylureas is functionally similar to the molecular events induced physiologically in the fed state, in which increased glucose metabolism causes β cell accumulation of intracellular ATP, membrane depolarization, Ca^{2+} influx, fusion of insulin-containing vesicles with the plasma membrane, and insulin secretion.

Sulfonylureas are orally available and are metabolized by the liver. These drugs are generally safe; their major adverse effect is hypoglycemia resulting from oversecretion of insulin. Thus, these medications should be used cautiously in patients who are unable to recognize or respond appropriately to hypoglycemia, such as those with impaired sympathetic function, mental status changes, or advanced age. Studies show that sulfonylurea use is associated with a marginal decrease in circulating lipids. These agents can cause weight gain secondary to increased insulin activity on adipose tissue; this adverse effect is obviously counterproductive in obese patients such as Mrs. S. Therefore, sulfonylureas are better suited for nonobese patients. Because first-generation sulfonylureas bind with lower affinity to SUR1 than second-generation agents do, first-generation agents must be administered in higher doses to achieve the same degree of glucose lowering. Sulfonylureas are generally effective, safe, and inexpensive (generically available) drugs, and are a mainstay of treatment for Type II diabetes.

Meglitinides

As with sulfonylureas, **meglitinides** stimulate insulin release by binding to SUR1 and inhibiting the β cell K^+/ATP channel. Although both sulfonylureas and meglitinides act on the SUR1 subunit, these two classes of drugs bind to distinct regions of the SUR1 molecule. The absorption, metabolism, and adverse effect profiles of meglitinides are similar to those of sulfonylureas.

Insulin Sensitizers: Thiazolidinediones and Biguanides

Thiazolidinediones

The **thiazolidinedione (TZD)** drugs are a relatively new class of oral medication for Type II diabetes; the two currently available in the United States—**rosiglitazone** and **pioglitazone**—were FDA-approved for use in 1999. The TZDs do not affect insulin secretion, but rather *enhance the action of insulin at target tissues*. TZDs are agonists for the nuclear hormone receptor **peroxisome proliferator activated receptor-γ (PPARγ)**. The identities of the endogenous ligand(s) for PPARγ remain to be elucidated. PPARγ functions as a heterodimer with the retinoid X receptor (RXR, another nuclear hormone receptor) to activate transcription of a subset of genes involved in glucose and lipid metabolism; not all of these genes have been identified. PPARγ is expressed primarily in adipose tissue and is involved in adipocyte differentiation. Studies show that cells made to overexpress PPARγ accumulate triglyceride and acquire other adipocyte markers when treated with TZDs. Although treatment with TZDs improves insulin sensitivity not only in adipose tissue but also in liver and muscle (the primary sites of insulin resistance in Type II diabetes), the mechanisms responsible for the effects of TZDs in liver and muscle are mysterious, especially because PPARγ is expressed at low levels in these tissues. In fact, the effect of TZDs on liver and muscle is likely to be indirect, because in vitro TZD treatment of these isolated tissues has little effect (except for inhibition of gluconeogenesis in hepatocytes). One theory suggests that TZD/PPARγ-mediated changes in adipocyte gene expression result in changes in fat metabolism that alter the metabolic environment of the liver and muscle cells, ultimately increasing the insulin sensitivity of these tissues.

Although our understanding of the molecular mechanisms by which TZDs act remains incomplete, it is clear that TZD treatment does increase insulin sensitivity, leading to lowering of blood glucose and insulin levels. The insulin-sensitizing effects of TZDs are beneficial in treating not only Type II diabetes, but also other insulin resistance/hyperinsulinemia-associated syndromes such as polycystic ovarian syndrome (PCOS; see Chapter 28, Pharmacology of Reproduction).

Because TZDs are a newer class of drugs, their adverse effect profile is still being defined. Effects such as weight gain and decreases in circulating triglyceride and free fatty acid levels can be explained by the stimulatory effect of TZDs on adipocytes. Unlike the insulin secretagogues, the TZDs do not increase insulin levels, and therefore do not induce hypoglycemia. The original TZD introduced in the United States (troglitazone) was associated with rare hepatotoxicity, resulting in its withdrawal from the market. Newer TZDs appear to have less hepatotoxicity.

Biguanides

Like TZDs, **biguanides** act by increasing insulin sensitivity. The molecular target of the biguanides appears to be the AMP-dependent protein kinase (AMPPK—not to be confused with protein kinase A). Biguanides activate AMPPK to block the breakdown of fatty acids and to inhibit hepatic gluconeogenesis and glycogenolysis. Secondary effects include increased insulin signaling (i.e., increased activity of the insulin receptor) as well as increased metabolic responsiveness by the liver and skeletal muscle. The most common adverse effect is mild gastrointestinal distress, which is usually transient and can be minimized by slow titration of the dose. A potentially more serious adverse effect is **lactic acidosis.** Because biguanides decrease the flux of metabolic acids through gluconeogenic pathways, lactic acid can accumulate to dangerous levels in biguanide-treated patients. With **metformin,** introduced in the United States in 1995 and the only biguanide currently available in the US, the incidence of lactic acidosis is low and predictable. Lactic acidosis is more common when metformin is taken by patients who have other conditions predisposing to metabolic acidosis. Thus, metformin should not be administered to patients with hepatic disease, heart failure, respiratory disease, hypoxemia, severe infection, alcohol abuse, a tendency to ketoacidosis, or renal disease (the latter because biguanides are excreted by the kidneys).

Like TZDs, biguanides do not directly affect insulin secretion, and their use is not associated with hypoglycemia. Furthermore, unlike insulin and insulin secretagogues, biguanides are associated with a lowering of serum lipids and a decrease in weight. Also like TZDs, biguanides are useful in the treatment of other conditions, such as PCOS, that are associated with insulin resistance and hyperinsulinemia.

GLP-1 Agonists and Mimetics

GLP-1 mimetics are the newest class of drugs developed for the treatment of diabetes. Because GLP-1 is a peptide hormone with a short circulating half-life, molecular modifications were necessary to increase its bioactivity. **Exenatide** is a long-acting analogue of GLP-1 derived from the salivary gland of the Gila monster. It acts as a full agonist at human GLP-1 receptors. Exenatide was approved for clinical use in the US in 2005. The drug must be injected, typically twice a day, and it is used in combination with metformin or a sulfonylurea to improve glucose control. As a GLP-1 mimetic, exenatide has several modes of action that benefit patients with diabetes: it increases secretion of insulin by pancreatic β cells, particularly when glucose levels are elevated; it suppresses secretion of glucagon by pancreatic α cells; it slows gastric emptying (and thereby slows the rate of nutrient entry into the circulation); and it decreases appetite.

Sitagliptin is a selective inhibitor of DPP-IV, the plasma enzyme that rapidly inactivates circulating incretin hormones such as GLP-1. In clinical trials, sitagliptin therapy increased circulating GLP-1 and insulin concentrations, decreased glucagon concentration, and increased the responsiveness of insulin release to an oral glucose load in patients with Type II diabetes. On the basis of these trials, sitagliptin was approved in 2006 as an adjunct to diet and exercise to improve glucose control in Type II diabetes. It can be used as monotherapy or in combination with a TZD or metformin (see below).

Combination Therapy

As discussed above, insulin-requiring patients with diabetes (including both Type I and Type II diabetes) benefit from individual optimization of therapy using combinations of short-acting and long-acting insulin preparations. As more oral agents have become available for the treatment of Type II diabetes, **oral combination therapy** has also become a reality for these patients. *In general, combination therapy with drugs that affect different molecular targets, and that have different mechanisms of actions, has the advantage of improving glycemic control while using a lower dose of each drug, and thus reducing adverse effects.* For example, combining an insulin sensitizer (e.g., a TZD or metformin) with insulin or an insulin secretagogue (e.g., a sulfonylurea) can both improve glycemic control in a poorly controlled Type II diabetic patient and lower the dose of each drug required to achieve a therapeutic effect. TZDs and metformin, which are both insulin sensitizers but with different mechanisms of action, can also be used together effectively. Combining two different insulin secretagogues does not improve therapeutic outcomes, however.

What, then, is the optimal treatment for Mrs. S, given that there are a number of agents from which to choose? First, it is important (as in all cases of diabetes) to promote weight loss and increased exercise. Type II diabetic patients—especially those who are older and obese—are often started on an insulin-sensitizing agent that does not predispose to either hypoglycemia or weight gain. Because Mrs. S does not appear to have renal disease or another contraindication to biguanide treatment, metformin could be a reasonable choice. A TZD would also be a reasonable starting point. If monotherapy with metformin or a TZD did not adequately decrease her blood glucose and HbA1c levels, then a combination of the two could be tried. Alternatively, adding a sulfonylurea to the insulin sensitizer could be a reasonable choice. See Table 29-4 for a comparison of adverse effects associated with the long-term use of several different therapies for Type II diabetes.

THERAPY FOR HYPERINSULINEMIA

Although surgical excision is ultimately the treatment of choice for insulinomas, **diazoxide** and **octreotide** are two

---

TABLE 29-4 Adverse Effects over 10 Years of Use: A Comparison of Several Agents Used as Monotherapy for Type II Diabetes Mellitus

AGENT	INCREASE IN WEIGHT (COMPARED TO DIET THERAPY ALONE), *kg*	SEVERE HYPOGLYCEMIA,* % OF SUBJECTS	SYMPTOMATIC HYPOGLYCEMIA,** % OF SUBJECTS
Insulin	4.0	2.3	36
Sulfonylurea	2.2	0.5	14
Biguanide	0	0	4

Because diabetes is a chronic disease, the long-term implications of therapy are an important consideration. Insulin and sulfonylureas are both capable of lowering blood glucose to dangerous levels, while biguanides lack this adverse effect. In addition, biguanide use is not associated with an increase in body weight, while patients taking insulin or a sulfonylurea tend to gain weight.
*Severe hypoglycemia is defined as hypoglycemia requiring hospitalization or other third-party intervention.
**Symptomatic hypoglycemia is defined as hypoglycemia not requiring hospitalization. (Data from the United Kingdom Prospective Diabetes Study [UKPDS] 1998.)

drugs that are often used to stabilize hypoglycemic patients preoperatively. Diazoxide binds to the SUR1 subunit of K^+/ATP channels in pancreatic β cells, and stabilizes the ATP-bound (open) state of the channel so that the β cells remain hyperpolarized. A number of K^+/ATP channel-openers of this type are known, but most are specific for SUR2 isoforms and thus are not useful to target the SUR1/Kir6.2 channel expressed by pancreatic β cells. Diazoxide binds channels containing either SUR1 or SUR2 isoforms, and is therefore used not only to decrease insulin secretion by pancreatic β cells, but also to hyperpolarize SUR2-expressing cardiac and smooth muscle cells and, by maintaining these cells in a more relaxed state, to decrease blood pressure in hypertensive emergencies. In a rare form of genetic hyperinsulinemic hypoglycemia, a mutant SUR1 isoform is relatively insensitive to Mg^{2+}-ADP but does respond to diazoxide; in most forms of this disease, however, the mutant channel is not transported to the cell surface, and diazoxide is ineffective.

Octreotide is a somatostatin analogue (see Chapter 25) that is longer acting than endogenous somatostatin. As with somatostatin, this agent blocks hormone release from endocrine-secreting tumors, such as insulinomas, glucagonomas, and thyrotropin-secreting pituitary adenomas.

GLUCAGON AS A THERAPEUTIC AGENT

Glucagon is used to treat severe hypoglycemia when oral or intravenous glucose administration is not possible. As with insulin, glucagon is administered by subcutaneous injection. The hyperglycemic action of glucagon is transient, and it requires a sufficient hepatic store of glycogen. Glucagon is also used as an intestinal relaxant before radiographic or magnetic resonance imaging (MRI) of the gastrointestinal tract. The mechanism by which glucagon mediates intestinal relaxation remains uncertain.

Conclusion and Future Directions

The pancreatic hormones insulin, glucagon, and somatostatin are involved in fuel homeostasis. When the levels of these hormones are pathologically altered, an individual can become hyperglycemic (as in diabetes mellitus) or hypoglycemic. Various pharmacologic agents act at several different cellular and molecular sites to normalize blood glucose levels. α-Glucosidase inhibitors slow the intestinal absorption of carbohydrates. Exogenous insulin, sulfonylureas, and meglitinides increase insulin levels, while diazoxide reduces insulin levels. Thiazolidinediones and biguanides increase insulin sensitivity at target tissues. Octreotide, a synthetic form of somatostatin, has wide-ranging inhibitory effects on hormone secretion. Exogenous glucagon can be used to increase plasma glucose levels. Future research on the pharmacologic treatment of diabetes will focus on better delineation of the molecular mechanisms of current treatments and better understanding of the molecular and cellular pathophysiology of Type II diabetes mellitus. This research will include, but not be limited to, elucidation of the targets of PPARγ action, optimization of GLP-1 mimetics, and inhibition of the counter-regulatory role of glucagon. In addition, clinical studies will continue to refine the role of combination oral therapy for Type II diabetes mellitus, in an attempt to maintain long-term normoglycemia without episodes of hypoglycemia.

Suggested Reading

DeWitt DE, Hirsch IB. Outpatient insulin therapy in type 1 and type 2 diabetes mellitus: scientific review. *JAMA* 2003;299:2254–2264. (*Reviews currently available insulin preparations and their pharmacodynamic and pharmacokinetic profiles.*)

Drucker DJ. The biology of incretin hormones. *Cell Metab* 2006;3:153–165. (*Reviews basic physiology of GLP-1 and related hormones.*)

Hardie DG. Minireview: the AMP-activated protein kinase cascade: the key sensor of cellular energy status. *Endocrinology* 2003;144:5179–5183. (*Reviews function and mechanism of action of probable biguanide target.*)

Krentz AJ, Bailey CJ. Oral antidiabetic agents: current role in type 2 diabetes mellitus. *Drugs* 2005;65:385–411. (*Thorough review of the pharmacology of oral agents for the treatment of diabetes, with an emphasis on therapeutics.*)

Nathan DM. Initial management of glycemia in type 2 diabetes mellitus. *N Engl J Med* 2002;347:1342–1349. (*Clinically oriented approach to treatment of type 2 diabetes, including diet, exercise, insulin, oral agents, and combination therapy.*)

| Drug Summary Table | **Chapter 29 Pharmacology of Endocrine Pancreas** |

Drug	Clinical Applications	*Serious* and Common Adverse Effects	Contraindications	Therapeutic Considerations
α-GLUCOSIDASE INHIBITORS				
Mechanism—Carbohydrate analogues that bind avidly to intestinal brush border α-glucosidase enzymes, slowing breakdown and absorption of dietary carbohydrates such as starch, dextrin, and disaccharides				
Acarbose Miglitol Voglibose	Type 2 diabetes mellitus	Abdominal pain, diarrhea, flatulence, elevated serum aminotransferase levels, elevated plasma triglycerides	Cirrhosis Diabetic ketoacidosis Severe digestive problems Inflammatory bowel disease Bowel obstruction	There is no risk of hypoglycemia with these agents Most useful for patients with predominantly postprandial hyperglycemia, and for new-onset patients with mild hyperglycemia GI distress usually diminishes with continued use of an α-glucosidase inhibitor Serum aminotransferase levels should be monitored during therapy Modest increases in plasma triglycerides may occur with therapy
EXOGENOUS INSULIN				
Mechanism—The classic anabolic hormone, insulin promotes carbohydrate metabolism and facilitates glucose, amino acid, and triglyceride uptake and storage in liver, cardiac and skeletal muscle, and adipose tissue				
Lispro ultra-rapid acting **Regular short acting** **Semilente short acting** **NPH intermediate acting** **Lente intermediate acting** **Ultralente long acting** **Glargine long acting**	Diabetes mellitus	*Hypoglycemia* Injection site reaction, lipodystrophy	Hypoglycemia	Not orally available; must be delivered parenterally; subcutaneous route is most common Lispro insulin is ultrarapid-acting; offers flexibility and convenience because it can be injected minutes before a meal Regular insulin is short-acting; recently approved for pulmonary insulin delivery NPH is intermediate-acting; contains protamine, which prolongs the time required for absorption of the insulin Ultralente insulin is long-acting; semilente insulin is short-acting; lente insulin is intermediate-acting Glargine insulin has the advantage of long-acting, steady release without a peak (mimicking "basal" insulin secretion) The major danger with insulin therapy is that hypoglycemia can result from insulin administration in the absence of adequate carbohydrate intake

(Continued)

Drug Summary Table   **Chapter 29 Pharmacology of Endocrine Pancreas** (*Continued*)

Drug	Clinical Applications	Serious and Common Adverse Effects	Contraindications	Therapeutic Considerations
INSULIN SECRETAGOGUES: SULFONYLUREAS AND MEGLITINIDES				
Mechanism—Sulfonylureas and meglitinides inhibit the β cell K+/ATP channel at the SUR1 subunit, thereby stimulating insulin release from pancreatic β cells and increasing circulating insulin to levels sufficient to overcome insulin resistance				
First-generation sulfonylureas: Acetohexamide Chlorpropamide Tolazamide Tolbutamide *Second-generation sulfonylureas:* Glimepiride Glipizide Glibenclamide (Glyburide) Gliclazide Gliquidone	Type 2 diabetes mellitus	*Hypoglycemia* Rash, diarrhea, nausea, dizziness	Diabetic ketoacidosis	Sulfonylureas are the mainstay of treatment for Type II diabetes; orally available and metabolized by the liver The major adverse effect is hypoglycemia resulting from oversecretion of insulin; therefore, should be used cautiously in patients who are unable to recognize or respond to hypoglycemia Can cause weight gain secondary to increased insulin activity in adipose tissue; therefore, are better suited for nonobese patients Because first-generation agents bind with lower affinity to SUR1 than second-generation agents do, first-generation agents must be administered in higher doses to achieve the same degree of glucose-lowering
Meglitinides: Nateglinide Repaglinide	Type 2 diabetes mellitus	*Hypoglycemia* Diarrhea, nausea, upper respiratory infection	Diabetic ketoacidosis Type 1 diabetes mellitus	Meglitinides have similar therapeutic considerations as sulfonylureas
INSULIN SENSITIZERS: THIAZOLIDINEDIONES (TZDs)				
Mechanism—Bind and stimulate the nuclear hormone receptor peroxisome proliferator activated receptor-γ (PPARγ), thereby increasing insulin sensitivity in adipose tissue, liver, and muscle				
Pioglitazone Rosiglitazone	Type 2 diabetes mellitus Polycystic ovarian syndrome	Heart failure, cholestatic hepatitis, hepatotoxicity, diabetic macular edema Edema, weight gain, increased HDL and LDL, decreased circulating triglycerides and free fatty acids	Hypersensitivity to pioglitazone or rosiglitazone	TZDs do not increase insulin levels and therefore do not induce hypoglycemia Newer TZDs appear to have less hepatotoxicity
INSULIN SENSITIZERS: BIGUANIDES				
Mechanism—Activates AMP-dependent protein kinase (AMPPK) to block breakdown of fatty acids and to inhibit hepatic gluconeogenesis and glycogenolysis; increases insulin receptor activity and metabolic responsiveness in liver and skeletal muscle				
Metformin	Type 2 diabetes mellitus Polycystic ovarian syndrome	*Lactic acidosis* Diarrhea, dyspepsia, flatulence, nausea, vomiting, cobalamin deficiency	Heart failure Septicemia Alcohol abuse Hepatic disease Respiratory disease Renal impairment Iodinated contrast media if acute alteration of renal function is suspected, as this may result in lactic acidosis Metabolic acidosis	GI distress associated with metformin use is usually transient and can be minimized by slow titration of the dose Incidence of lactic acidosis is low and predictable; lactic acidosis typically occurs with metformin use in patients who have other conditions that predispose to metabolic acidosis Does not induce hypoglycemia Lowers serum lipids and decreases weight

GLP-1 AGONISTS AND MIMETICS

Mechanism—Glucagon-like peptide-1 (GLP-1) receptor agonist that enhances glucose-dependent insulin secretion, inhibits glucagon secretion, delays gastric emptying, and decreases appetite (exenatide); dipeptidyl peptidase-IV (DPP-IV) inhibitor that slows the proteolytic inactivation of GLP-1 and other incretin hormones (sitagliptin)

Drug	Indications	Adverse Effects	Contraindications	Notes
Exenatide	Type 2 diabetes mellitus	Hypoglycemia, nausea, vomiting, diarrhea, nervousness, dizziness, headache	Type 1 diabetes mellitus Diabetic ketoacidosis	Exenatide is not orally available and must be injected Typically used in combination with metformin or a sulfonylurea to improve glucose control
Sitagliptin	Type 2 diabetes mellitus	Upper respiratory tract infection, nasopharyngitis, headache, nausea, diarrhea, mild increase in serum creatinine level	Type 1 diabetes mellitus Diabetic ketoacidosis	Dose adjustment is necessary in patients with moderate or severe kidney disease May cause hypoglycemia in combination with sulfonylureas and insulin Digoxin levels should be monitored in patients receiving digoxin and sitagliptin

DIAZOXIDE

Mechanism—Binds to SUR1 subunit of K + /ATP channels in pancreatic β cells and stabilizes the ATP-bound (open) state of the channel so that the β cells remain hyperpolarized; this decreases insulin secretion by the cells

Drug	Indications	Adverse Effects	Contraindications	Notes
Diazoxide	Hypoglycemia due to hyperinsulinism Malignant hypertension	*Heart failure, fluid retention, diabetic ketoacidosis, hypernatremia, bowel obstruction, pancreatitis, neutropenia, thrombocytopenia, extrapyramidal disease* Angina, hypotension, tachyarrhythmia, hirsutism, hyperglycemia, dyspepsia, dizziness, glucosuria	Hypersensitivity to diazoxide	Diazoxide also hyperpolarizes SUR2-containing channels in cardiac and smooth muscle cells, and can be used to decrease blood pressure in hypertensive emergencies

SOMATOSTATIN ANALOGUES

Mechanism—Inhibits GHRH release

Drug	Notes
Octreotide	See Drug Summary Table: Chapter 25 Pharmacology of the Hypothalamus and Pituitary Gland

EXOGENOUS GLUCAGON

Mechanism—A polypeptide hormone, produced by alpha cells in the islets of Langerhans in the pancreas, that stimulates gluconeogenesis and glycogenolysis in the liver, resulting in an increase in blood sugar

Drug	Indications	Adverse Effects	Contraindications	Notes
Glucagon	Hypoglycemia Intestinal relaxant before radiography of gastrointestinal tract	Rash, nausea, vomiting	Known pheochromocytoma	Used to treat severe hypoglycemia when oral or intravenous glucose administration is not possible The hyperglycemic action of glucagon is transient and depends on a sufficient hepatic store of glycogen

30

Pharmacology of Bone Mineral Homeostasis

Allen S. Liu, Ariel Weissmann, Ehrin J. Armstrong, and Armen H. Tashjian, Jr.

INTRODUCTION

The 206 bones of the human skeleton are far from the lifeless structures they are commonly imagined to be. Bones are remodeled continuously and are involved in many functions besides structural support and protection of internal organs, including hematopoiesis and mineral storage. The focus of this chapter is on the critical role of bone in mineral homeostasis, the process and regulation of bone remodeling, the diseases that can result when the delicate balances of mineral homeostasis and bone remodeling are perturbed, and the pharmacologic therapies employed to treat these conditions. A key concept regarding the pharmacologic agents discussed in this chapter is the distinction between bone antiresorptive agents, which slow bone loss, and bone anabolic agents, which have the potential to increase overall bone mass.

Case

MS is a 60-year-old Caucasian female who comes to her physician with the recent onset of low back pain that began when she unexpectedly stepped into a pothole. She is otherwise in good health.

Her menstrual periods ceased when she was 54 years old. She had little in the way of postmenopausal symptoms and never took hormone replacement therapy. Menarche was at age 11. She has one child who was born when MS was 38 years old. Her mother died at age 55 with breast cancer and her sister, age 58, was recently diagnosed with breast cancer. The patient is moderately active, playing tennis for 1 hour about once a week. Her father and maternal aunt died in their 60s with coronary artery disease.

On physical examination, she has point tenderness over lumbar vertebra L1. Her weight is 135 lb., and she is 64 inches tall but believes she has lost some height over the last year. Laboratory studies are all within normal limits.

Lateral X-ray of the spine shows a compression fracture of L1 and generalized osteopenia. Measurement of bone mineral density (BMD) at the spine and hip reveals values that are 2.6 standard deviations below the healthy peak female value.

Her physician diagnoses postmenopausal osteoporosis and a recent compression fracture of L1. MS asks her physician to discuss with her the available therapeutic options, and is particularly interested in the potential risks and benefits of each option.

QUESTIONS

■ **1.** Why is MS at particularly high risk for osteoporosis?

■ **2.** Is this patient at risk for breast cancer and/or cardiovascular disease? How does this alter the choice of pharmacologic agents that could be prescribed?

■ **3.** What are the therapeutic options available for MS? What are the advantages and disadvantages of each option?

PHYSIOLOGY OF BONE MINERAL HOMEOSTASIS

Specialized cells called osteoblasts and osteoclasts continually remodel the human skeleton in response to mechanical forces and humoral factors. Several of these humoral factors— parathyroid hormone, vitamin D, and calcitonin—control the remodeling of bone for the purpose of maintaining calcium homeostasis. Other hormones, such as glucocorticoids, thyroid hormone, and gonadal steroids, also have important effects on bone integrity. This section reviews the cellular and molecular mechanisms that mediate bone formation and bone resorption and the mechanisms by which hormones (especially parathyroid hormone and vitamin D) maintain plasma calcium levels within a narrow concentration range.

STRUCTURE OF BONE

Figure 30-1 illustrates the structure of a long bone. Note that the cortical bone forms a thick outer layer, or "cortex," around a medulla that consists of trabecular bone and bone marrow. In bones such as vertebral bodies, and in the neck and head of the femur, the cortical bone forms a thinner layer surrounding a larger core of trabecular bone. Osteoblasts and osteoclasts are found both on the outer surface of bone (beneath the periosteum) and on all inner surfaces of the bone, including the endosteum that lines the central canals in cortical bone and all of the many surfaces in trabecular bone.

Bone consists of 25% organic and 75% inorganic components. The organic component includes the cells (osteoblasts, osteoclasts, osteocytes, and bone lining cells), osteoid (a matrix consisting primarily of type I collagen fibers), and several other low-abundance proteins. The inorganic component consists of crystalline calcium phosphate salts, primarily **hy-**

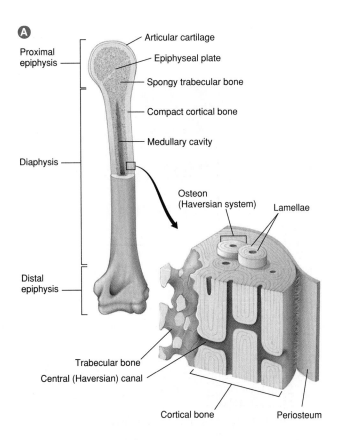

A

Proximal epiphysis — Articular cartilage — Epiphyseal plate — Spongy trabecular bone — Compact cortical bone — Medullary cavity

Diaphysis

Osteon (Haversian system) — Lamellae

Distal epiphysis

Trabecular bone
Central (Haversian) canal

Cortical bone   Periosteum

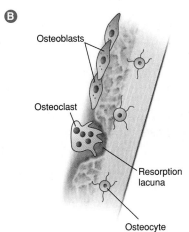

B

Osteoblasts

Osteoclast

Resorption lacuna

Osteocyte

Figure 30-1. Structure of bone. A. The upper panel depicts the structure of a long bone (exemplified by the humerus). Note that the diaphysis has a thick shell of compact cortical bone, while the epiphysis is composed predominantly of trabecular bone. The lower panel shows the detailed structure of bone. **B.** Bone remodeling is a dynamic balance between the catabolic activity of osteoclasts and the anabolic activity of osteoblasts. The majority of bone remodeling occurs in trabecular bone. Therefore, any condition that disrupts the process of mineralization and/or bone turnover preferentially affects the skeletal sites and regions of bone that have large trabecular areas. For this reason, osteoporotic fractures occur commonly in vertebral bodies and the neck of the femur.

droxyapatite. The chemical formula of hydroxyapatite is $(Ca)_5(PO_4)_3OH$. Ninety-nine percent of the calcium in the body is stored in the skeleton, mostly as hydroxyapatite.

MINERAL BALANCE

Calcium is absorbed in the small intestine by two mechanisms: facilitated transport, which occurs throughout the small intestine, and vitamin D-dependent active transport, which occurs mainly in the duodenum. Approximately 300 mg, or less than a third of the 1,000-mg average daily intake of dietary calcium, is absorbed by the intestine under normal conditions; the balance is excreted in the feces (Fig. 30-2). Calcium absorption can be increased to as much as 600 mg per day in the presence of **calcitriol** (the active form of vitamin D), as discussed below. To maintain calcium homeostasis, the absorption of calcium from the intestine is balanced by daily calcium losses through renal excretion (about 200 mg per day) and through secretions (primarily saliva and bile) that are eliminated in the feces (about 100 mg per day; Fig. 30-2). Compared with calcium homeostasis, phosphate homeostasis is not as tightly regulated.

REGULATION OF BONE REMODELING

Bone homeostasis can be viewed as a dynamic balance between anabolic (bone formation) and catabolic (bone resorption) processes. *Osteoblasts are the cells most responsible for anabolic activity, while osteoclasts are responsible for catabolic activity.* Regulation of these two cell types by hormones, mechanical factors, and cytokines determines the balance between bone formation and bone resorption (see below).

To maintain its strength over time and to respond adaptively to physical stresses, human bone is continually resorbed and reformed. This process is called **remodeling.** Partly because of its large surface area on which remodeling can take place, 25% of trabecular bone is remodeled each year in adults. In contrast, only 3% of cortical bone is remodeled each year. This difference is important because *pathologic conditions that disturb bone remodeling preferentially affect bones with a high content of trabecular bone, such as the femoral neck and vertebral bodies.*

Remodeling is carried out by the coordinated activity of millions of cellular units—**basic multicellular units** (BMU)—consisting of osteoblasts and osteoclasts. The process of resorption begins when physical or chemical signals (discussed below) recruit osteoclasts, which begin excavating small cavities on the surface of the bone (Fig. 30-3). Osteoclasts extend villus-like projections toward the bone surface. These villi secrete proteolytic enzymes, such as collagenase, that digest the organic matrix. After attaching tightly to the bone surface, the osteoclasts create an acidic microenvironment by producing various organic acids, including lactic acid, carbonic acid, and citric acid, and by using a H^+-ATPase in the villi to pump protons onto the bone surface. The dissolution of hydroxyapatite can be expressed as follows:

$$(Ca)_5(PO_4)_3OH \rightarrow 5Ca^{2+} + 3PO_4^{-3} + OH^- \quad \text{Equation 30-1}$$

The secretion of organic acids and protons by osteoclasts consumes hydroxide at the bone surface; according to Le Châtelier's principle, OH^- consumption drives the reaction to the right and results in increased dissolution of the hydroxyapatite. This is an important mechanism exploited by osteoclasts to resorb the mineral component of bone.

After a period of about 3 weeks of bone resorption, cytokines and other factors liberated from the matrix begin to stimulate osteoblast proliferation, differentiation, and activation. These osteoblasts replace the osteoclasts in the resorption cavity (lacuna), and begin to refill the cavity with concentric layers, or **lamellae,** of unmineralized organic matrix (osteoid) (Fig. 30-3). As osteoblasts continue to lay down matrix, they eventually become completely surrounded with matrix and are then called osteocytes (Fig. 30-1). Mature osteocytes may act as mechanosensors in bone. As the cavity is filled with new osteoid, various factors essential for the process of mineralization are secreted by the osteoblasts. These factors include **alkaline phosphatase** and calcium-binding proteins. Alkaline phosphatase hydrolyzes various phosphate esters; among these esters is pyrophosphate, which is an inhibitor of bone mineralization. The hydrolysis of pyrophosphate also increases the local concentration of inorganic phosphate. Together, the alkaline phosphatase-

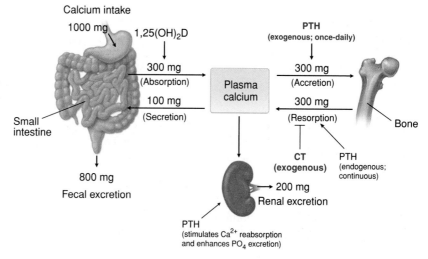

Figure 30-2. Daily whole-body calcium balance. In a state of whole-body calcium balance, the flux of calcium includes net uptake of 200 mg per day from the GI tract and excretion of 200 mg per day by the kidneys. Vitamin D [$1,25(OH)_2D_3$] enhances absorption of Ca^{2+} from the GI tract. Endogenous secretion of parathyroid hormone (PTH) modulates bone resorption and stimulates tubular reabsorption of calcium in the nephron; both effects raise plasma Ca^{2+}. PTH also enhances urinary excretion of inorganic phosphate (PO_4). In contrast, exogenous once-daily injection of PTH *(in blue)* stimulates new bone formation (accretion). Exogenous calcitonin (CT; *in blue*) inhibits bone resorption.

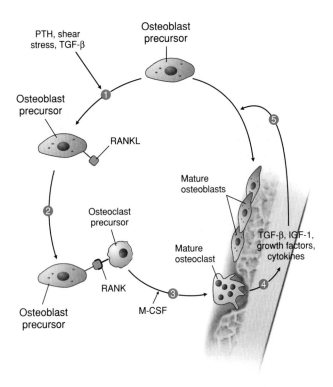

Figure 30-3. Interaction of osteoblasts and osteoclasts in bone remodeling. Bone resorption and bone formation are coupled by the interactions between osteoblasts and osteoclasts: (1) Factors such as parathyroid hormone (PTH), shear stress, and transforming growth factor β (TGF-β) cause osteoblast precursors to express the osteoclast differentiation factor RANK-ligand (RANKL). (2) RANKL binds to RANK, a receptor expressed on osteoclast precursors. (3) The RANKL–RANK binding interaction, together with other factors such as macrophage colony stimulating factor (M-CSF), cause osteoclast precursors to differentiate into mature osteoclasts. (4) As mature osteoclasts resorb bone, matrix-bound factors such as TGF-β, insulin-like growth factor 1 (IGF-1), other growth factors, and cytokines are released. (5) These liberated factors stimulate osteoblast precursors to develop into mature osteoblasts, which begin to refill the resorption cavities excavated by the osteoclasts.

catalyzed hydrolysis of pyrophosphate and liberation of inorganic phosphate promote the crystallization of calcium phosphate salts. In a complementary fashion, the secretion of calcium-binding proteins increases the local concentration of calcium, and thereby further facilitates hydroxyapatite formation.

HORMONAL CONTROL OF CALCIUM AND PHOSPHATE

Calcium is essential for many important physiologic processes, such as neurotransmitter release, muscle contraction, and blood coagulation. Even small deviations in extracellular calcium levels can have serious consequences. Therefore, calcium homeostasis is very carefully regulated. Phosphate homeostasis must also be regulated, because changes in plasma phosphate concentrations affect plasma calcium levels (see below). Three main hormones—parathyroid hormone (PTH), vitamin D, and, to a lesser extent, calcitonin—mediate calcium and phosphate homeostasis. In

addition, glucocorticoids, thyroid hormone, and gonadal steroids have lesser effects on calcium and phosphate homeostasis. Table 30-1 summarizes the mechanisms and effects of these hormones on calcium and phosphate homeostasis.

Parathyroid Hormone

The most important endocrine regulator of calcium homeostasis is **parathyroid hormone**, an 84-amino acid peptide hormone secreted by the parathyroid glands. The secretion of PTH is finely regulated in response to plasma calcium levels. Calcium-sensing receptors reside on the plasma membrane of chief cells in the parathyroid gland; when bound by extracellular calcium ions, these G protein-coupled receptors mediate increases in the level of intracellular free calcium, which, in turn, decreases secretion of preformed PTH. By this mechanism, *high plasma calcium concentration suppresses PTH secretion, while low plasma calcium stimulates PTH secretion.* (Note: In many other secretory tissues, an increase in intracellular calcium enhances secretion. Thus, the parathyroid chief cell is somewhat unique in its response to changes in intracellular calcium.)

PTH acts on three organs to raise the plasma calcium concentration: it acts directly on kidney and bone, and indirectly on the gastrointestinal (GI) tract (Fig. 30-4). The most rapid physiologic effects of PTH are to increase reabsorption of calcium and to decrease reabsorption of phosphate by the kidney. These actions decrease urinary excretion of calcium while increasing urinary excretion of phosphate. In this manner, PTH raises plasma calcium levels and decreases plasma phosphate concentrations.

Another important, although slower, effect of PTH results from its direct action on bone cells. Physiologic levels of PTH stimulate cell surface PTH receptors on osteoblasts, causing these cells to increase their expression of a number of proteins. One of these PTH-induced proteins is the osteoclast differentiation factor **RANK ligand (RANKL).** RANKL binds to **RANK,** a receptor expressed on osteoclast precursor cells in the bone marrow, promoting the differentiation of these precursors into mature osteoclasts (Fig. 30-3). The ensuing increase in osteoclastic activity results in increased bone resorption and, therefore, in liberation of calcium and phosphate into the circulation. By this mechanism, the direct action of PTH on bone raises plasma calcium concentrations.

Finally, PTH raises plasma calcium by an indirect effect on the intestine. PTH stimulates the kidney not only to increase calcium reabsorption and decrease phosphate reabsorption, as described above, but also to increase the conversion of the 25-hydroxy precursor form of vitamin D to biologically active 1,25-dihydroxy vitamin D (calcitriol). This hydroxylation takes place in cells of the proximal tubule. Calcitriol, in turn, increases calcium absorption in the small intestine (discussed below).

Although PTH has generally been considered a bone catabolic hormone, *current evidence indicates that, under certain conditions, PTH can also increase bone formation and bone mass.* Under these conditions, it appears that PTH can enhance osteoblast survival and promote differentiation of osteoblast precursors to mature osteoblasts. Specifically, intermittent, brief (1 to 2 hours) interaction of PTH with its receptor on mature osteoblasts stimulates $G\alpha_s$, which in-

TABLE 30-1	Summary of Endocrine Control of Calcium and Phosphate Homeostasis		
HORMONE	**TARGET ORGAN**	**MECHANISM**	**NET EFFECT**
PTH	GI tract	↑ Ca^{2+} absorption via vitamin D action	↑ $[Ca^{2+}]$ ↓ $[P_i]$
	Kidney	↑ Ca^{2+} reabsorption; ↓ P_i reabsorption	↑ $[Ca^{2+}]$ ↓ $[P_i]$
	Bone	↑ Osteoclast activity (continuous PTH)	↓ Bone mass
		↑ Osteoblast activity (once-daily PTH)	↑ Bone mass
Vitamin D	GI tract	↑ Ca^{2+} and P_i absorption	↑ $[Ca^{2+}]$ ↑ $[P_i]$
	Kidney	↑ Ca^{2+} and P_i reabsorption	
	Bone	↑ Osteoclast number and activity	
	Parathyroid gland	Inhibition of PTH synthesis	
Calcitonin	Bone	↓ Osteoclast activity	↓ $[Ca^{2+}]$ ↓ $[P_i]$
Glucocorticoids	GI tract	↓ Ca^{2+} absorption, leading to ↑ PTH	Osteopenia
	Kidney	↓ Ca^{2+} and P_i reabsorption	Osteoporosis
	Bone	↓ Osteoblast activity;	
		↑ osteoblast apoptosis	
Thyroid hormone	Bone	Bone resorption > formation	Osteopenia
Gonadal steroids	Bone	↓ Osteoclast activity;	↓ Bone resorption
		↑ osteoclast apoptosis	
		↓ Osteoblast apoptosis	

P_i, inorganic phosphate; GI, gastrointestinal.

creases adenylyl cyclase activity, which, in turn, increases intracellular cAMP. The transient PTH-induced increase in cAMP has an anti-apoptotic effect on the osteoblasts. In addition, the increase in cAMP promotes osteoblast release of IGF-1, which induces osteoblast precursor cells in the bone marrow to differentiate into mature osteoblasts (Fig. 30-3). Although intermittent PTH also induces the production of cytokines such as IL-6 by stromal precursor cells, and these cytokines ultimately stimulate osteoclast proliferation, this catabolic effect is dominated acutely by the PTH-induced activation of the bone formation-enhancing activity of osteoblasts.

In contrast, continuous interaction of PTH with its receptor on mature osteoblasts stimulates these cells to produce IGF-binding proteins (IGFBP). The resulting decrease in free IGF-1 levels reduces the stimulus to differentiation of osteoblast precursor cells. In addition, as described above, continuous PTH induces the expression of osteoclast differentiation factors such as RANKL on osteoblasts. The net result of continuous PTH exposure is that osteoclasts outnumber osteoblasts, and bone resorption overrides bone formation. Conceptually, the differential effects of intermittent versus continuous PTH exposure are similar to the situation with GnRH: recall that pulsatile GnRH stimulates LH and FSH secretion by the anterior pituitary gland, whereas continuous GnRH suppresses release of these gonadotropins (see Chapter 25, Pharmacology of the Hypothalamus and Pituitary Gland). Because of this differential effect of PTH, intermittent administration of PTH by once-daily injection or by some other drug delivery technology allows the use of PTH to promote osteoblast activity, and thereby to increase bone matrix production, bone mineral density, bone quality, and bone mass (see below).

Vitamin D

Despite its name, **vitamin D** is produced by the body in sufficient amounts that it is not required in the diet under normal conditions. Because it is produced endogenously and it travels in the blood to effect responses in distant target tissues, vitamin D is properly considered a hormone. The term vitamin D applies to two related compounds, **cholecalciferol** and **ergocalciferol.** Cholecalciferol, or vitamin D_3, is the form synthesized in the skin from a precursor called 7-dehydrocholesterol. This biosynthetic pathway is stimulated by exposure of the skin to the ultraviolet radiation in sunlight (Fig. 30-5). Ergocalciferol, or vitamin D_2, is the form produced by plants. (Vitamin D_2 is also the form present in many commercial preparations, as well as the form added to milk.) Vitamin D_2 and D_3 have equal biological activities, and the "D" in compounds discussed below refers to both the D_2 and D_3 forms of the hormone.

Whether from an endogenous (skin) or an exogenous (dietary) source, vitamin D travels to the liver, where it is either stored or converted to calcifediol [25-hydroxy vitamin D, or 25(OH)D] by the first of two enzymatic hydroxylation steps. The second enzymatic hydroxylation, which is PTH-dependent and takes place in the proximal tubule of the kidney, converts calcifediol to the final, active form of vitamin D called calcitriol [1α,25-hydroxy vitamin D, or 1,25(OH)₂D].

Calcitriol's primary effect on calcium balance is in the small intestine, where it increases the absorption of dietary calcium. Calcitriol enhances Ca^{2+} absorption by acting on nuclear receptors in the enterocyte to up-regulate the expression of genes coding for a number of brush border proteins. Calcitriol also promotes the transcellular transport of Ca^{2+} through the enterocyte by inducing the expression of: (1) a calcium uptake pump on the luminal surface of the enterocyte; (2) calbindin, an intracellular Ca^{2+}-binding protein; and (3) an ATP-dependent Ca^{2+} pump that extrudes Ca^{2+} from the enterocyte into the surrounding capillaries.

Calcitriol has less well understood effects on other target organs, including the parathyroid gland, bone, kidneys, and

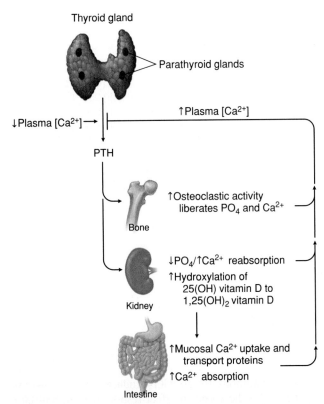

Figure 30-4. Summary of the actions of PTH on bone, kidney, and intestine. Decreased plasma [Ca²⁺] is the primary stimulus for parathyroid hormone (PTH) secretion by the parathyroid glands. PTH acts to raise plasma Ca²⁺ levels via its effects on bone, kidney, and intestine. In bone, PTH promotes increased differentiation of osteo-clast precursors into mature osteoclasts. Osteoclasts resorb bone and thereby liberate inorganic phosphate (PO₄) and Ca²⁺ into the plasma. In the kidney, PTH increases the tubular reabsorption of Ca²⁺ and decreases the distal tubular reabsorption of PO₄. In addition, PTH stimulates proximal tubule cells to hydroxylate 25(OH) vitamin D, forming 1,25(OH)₂ vitamin D. 1,25(OH)₂ vitamin D then stimu-lates intestinal absorption of Ca²⁺ by increasing the expression of mucosal Ca²⁺ uptake and transport proteins. Note that the effect of PTH on the intestine is indirect, via increased renal synthesis of the active form of vitamin D. In a tightly controlled negative feedback loop, increased plasma [Ca²⁺] inhibits further PTH secretion by the parathyroid glands.

the immune system. Calcitriol binds to nuclear receptors in parathyroid cells, and thereby inhibits PTH synthesis and release. In bone, calcitriol increases osteoclast number and activity, resulting in increased bone resorption. Some evidence suggests that calcitriol (or analogues of calcitriol) may also increase bone formation. In the distal tubule of the kidney, calcitriol increases the reabsorption of both calcium and phosphate. In the immune system, calcitriol production by macrophages may act as a local suppressant of adaptive immune cells; this observation has led to the use of vitamin D in the treatment of psoriasis, an autoimmune dermatologic disease.

Calcitonin

The third hormone involved in calcium homeostasis is **calci-tonin.** Calcitonin is a 32-amino acid peptide that is produced

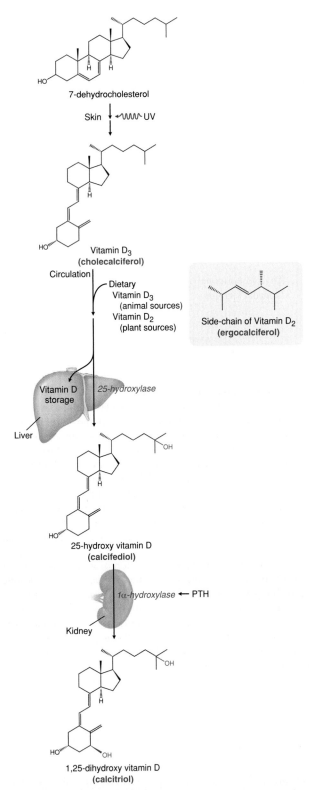

Figure 30-5. Photobiosynthesis and activation of vitamin D. Both endogenous and exogenous vitamin D are converted to 25-hy-droxy vitamin D in the liver and then to calcitriol in the kidney. Calcitriol is the active metabolite of vitamin D. Endogenous vitamin D₃ is synthe-sized in the skin from 7-dehydrocholesterol, in a reaction that is cata-lyzed by ultraviolet light. Exogenous vitamin D can be provided as D₃ (from animal sources) or as D₂ (from plant sources); D₃ and D₂ have the same biological activity. Parathyroid hormone (PTH) increases the activity of 1α-hydroxylase in the kidney and thereby stimulates the conversion of 25-hydroxy vitamin D to calcitriol.

and released by parafollicular C cells of the thyroid gland in response to hypercalcemia. *Calcitonin binds directly to receptors on osteoclasts; this binding inhibits the resorptive activity of the osteoclasts, and thereby decreases bone resorption and plasma calcium levels.* In adult humans, there is only a weak effect of endogenous calcitonin on plasma calcium levels, and the elimination of calcitonin secretion after thyroidectomy generally causes no significant changes in plasma calcium levels. Nevertheless, exogenous calcitonin has seen therapeutic use in the treatment of osteoporosis, as discussed below.

Glucocorticoids, Thyroid Hormone, and Gonadal Steroids

Although PTH, vitamin D, and, to a lesser extent, calcitonin are the primary regulators of calcium homeostasis, several other endogenous hormones have important effects on bone mineral metabolism. These hormones include glucocorticoids, thyroid hormone, estrogens, and androgens.

Pharmacologic doses of glucocorticoids decrease both intestinal absorption of calcium and renal tubular reabsorption of calcium. Although both of these effects would tend to lower plasma calcium levels, glucocorticoid use is not associated with hypocalcemia. In part, this may be explained by a compensatory increase in PTH that is stimulated by the decrease in intestinal calcium absorption and renal calcium reabsorption. In addition, glucocorticoids have direct effects on bone by inhibiting osteoblast maturation and osteoblast activity and by promoting osteoblast apoptosis. Thus, glucocorticoids preserve plasma calcium within normal limits, but at the expense of bone integrity. In fact, prolonged administration of pharmacologic doses of glucocorticoids is a common cause of iatrogenic osteoporosis. It is important, when taking the history of a patient such as MS, to determine whether she has ever taken glucocorticoids for an extended period of time, because this could represent a significant risk factor for osteoporosis.

Excess thyroid hormone also increases bone turnover. By stimulating bone resorption more than bone formation, prolonged high levels of thyroid hormone can cause osteopenia. In fact, osteopenia can be a manifestation of hyperthyroidism. The evaluation of MS's osteoporosis should, therefore, include determination of her thyroid hormone and TSH levels to rule out hyperthyroidism (see Chapter 26, Pharmacology of the Thyroid Gland).

Estrogens and androgens exert inhibitory effects on osteoclastic activity, and thereby slow the rate of bone turnover and bone loss. Specifically, the gonadal steroids inhibit the production by osteoblasts of cytokines—such as interleukin-6—that recruit and activate osteoclasts. Estrogen also has a pro-apoptotic effect on the osteoclasts themselves and an anti-apoptotic effect on osteoblasts and osteocytes. As described in more detail in Chapter 28, Pharmacology of Reproduction, estrogen exerts its actions principally by binding to the estrogen receptor (ER), which is a nuclear transcription factor. Binding of estrogen facilitates dimerization of the ER, allowing the estrogen–ER complex to recruit co-activator or co-repressor molecules and bind to promoter regions of target genes. In this way, estrogen regulates the transcription of target genes encoding, for example, the cytokines that are important in bone turnover.

PATHOPHYSIOLOGY

Bone turnover, including repeated cycles of bone resorption and bone formation, is required to maintain the integrity of the skeleton. **Osteoporosis** and **chronic kidney disease** are two common disorders of bone mineral homeostasis. In osteoporosis, bone turnover is disrupted such that bone resorption exceeds bone formation. In chronic kidney disease, the pathophysiology involves a complex interplay between decreased mineral absorption and **secondary hyperparathyroidism.** A brief summary of these and other diseases of bone mineral homeostasis, including their mechanisms, clinical features, and treatments, is provided in Table 30-2.

OSTEOPOROSIS

Osteoporosis is a common condition that results from decreased production of bone matrix and decreased BMD. The reduced bone mass predisposes to fracture after minimal trauma. Normal BMD is defined as a value that is within one standard deviation of the mean BMD in young adults (the "T score"), as determined by radiographic techniques. Values of 1.0 to 2.5 standard deviations below the mean are defined as **osteopenia**, and values more than 2.5 standard deviations below the mean are defined as **osteoporosis**.

Osteoporosis leads to an increased risk of fracture, especially in the vertebrae, femoral neck, and radius (spine, hip, and Colles' fractures, respectively). MS's presentation, with back pain from a compression fracture in a lumbar vertebra, is typical.

There are two categories of osteoporosis—**primary** and **secondary osteoporosis**—and two types of primary osteoporosis—**senile** and **postmenopausal osteoporosis.** Peak bone mass is achieved in young adulthood and is determined by several factors; these factors include dietary calcium levels, hormonal state, physical activity levels, and genetic factors such as alleles for the vitamin D receptor. *Once peak bone mass is attained, there is a gradual decline in bone mass during mid to late adult life.* This decline probably results from imperfections in the bone remodeling process: osteoblast-mediated bone formation does not completely keep pace with osteoclast-mediated bone resorption. Moreover, with age, the osteoblasts have a reduced capacity to proliferate, to synthesize organic bone matrix, and to respond to growth factors. As a result, there is an average loss of 0.7% of bone mass per year. Eventually, this rate of bone loss can lead to senile osteoporosis in old age (Fig. 30-6).

Postmenopausal osteoporosis begins in the first 3 to 5 years after menopause, when there is a rapid loss in bone mass related to the marked decline in estrogen production. MS, for example, was diagnosed with osteoporosis about 6 years after completing menopause. The decline in estrogen levels leads to an increase in osteoclast activity and bone turnover rate, which causes an imbalance between bone formation and bone resorption. The longer lifespan of osteoclasts in the absence of estrogen allows these cells to excavate deeper cavities in trabecular bone, leading to bone remodeling characterized by widely spaced and thin trabeculae with fewer interconnections. These remodeled trabeculae

TABLE 30-2	Mechanisms, Clinical Features, and Treatments for Common Diseases of Bone Mineral Homeostasis		
DISEASE	**MECHANISM**	**CLINICAL FEATURES**	**TREATMENT**

Osteoporosis
  Senile
  Postmenopausal
	Bone resorption > bone
	  formation
	↓ Estrogen
		Fragile bone
		Vulnerable to fracture
			Calcium
			Vitamin D
			Bisphosphonates
			Raloxifene (SERM)
			Calcitonin
			PTH

Chronic kidney disease	↓ Excretion of phosphate ↓ Production of 1,25(OH)$_2$D	Osteomalacia Osteitis fibrosa cystica	Phosphate restriction Active vitamin D Calcimimetics

Rickets
  Nutritional
  Vitamin D resistant
	Inadequate sunlight or dietary
	  ↓ vitamin D
	Defect in renal reabsorption of
	  phosphate and production of
	  vitamin D
		Skeletal deformities in children
		Osteomalacia in adults
			Vitamin D
			
			Oral phosphate
			Calcitriol

Type I vitamin D dependent	↓ Production of 1,25(OH)$_2$D		Oral phosphate Calcitriol

Type II vitamin D
    dependent
	Defective receptors for
	  1,25(OH)$_2$D
			Calcitriol (high dose)

Primary hyperparathyroidism	↑ PTH → ↑ bone resorption →
	  hypercalcemia
		Osteoporosis
		Nephrolithiasis
		Osteitis fibrosa cystica
		Depression
			Surgical removal
			Calcimimetic agents
			  (investigational)

Familial hypocalciuric
  hypercalcemia (FHH)
	Mutation in Ca^{2+}-sensing
	  receptor
		Hypocalciuria
		Hypercalcemia
		Hypermagnesemia
			None

Hypoparathyroidism	Decreased activity or absence
	  of parathyroid gland; →
	  hypocalcemia and
	  hyperphosphatemia
		Neuromuscular excitability
		Tetany
		Depression
			Calcium
			Vitamin D

Pseudohypoparathyroidism	Impaired response to PTH → hypocalcemia	Short stature Short metacarpals	Calcium Vitamin D
Paget's disease	↑ Local bone turnover	Bone pain Hearing loss High-output cardiac failure	Bisphosphonates Calcitonin

are structurally weaker in weight-bearing regions than the well-connected, closely spaced, thick trabeculae characteristic of bone in premenopausal women. In the cortical bone, deeper cavities coalesce to form porous spaces. The lack of estrogen also leads to increased apoptosis of osteoblasts, rendering these cells unable to keep pace with the osteoclasts, and to increased apoptosis of osteocytes, impairing the mechanosensory network that detects microdamage and stimulates bone repair. Increased bone resorption and the accumulation of microdamage lead to increased bone fragility. In summary, *the fragile bone in postmenopausal osteoporosis results from a bone turnover defect characterized by increased osteoclast activity and decreased osteoblast activity, deeper and larger resorption cavities, and impairment of the osteocyte mechanosensory network* (Fig. 30-7).

As discussed above, remodeling takes place to a greater degree in trabecular bone than in compact bone. Because appendicular bones, such as the long bones of the limbs, contain considerable amounts of compact cortical bone, while axial bones, such as the spine and pelvis, contain pre-dominantly trabecular bone, axial bones are more prone to osteoporosis than appendicular bones. Within 25 to 35 years after menopause, women may lose as much as 35% of their cortical bone mass and as much as 50% of their trabecular bone mass.

Certain systemic illnesses and medications induce **secondary osteoporosis.** Common predisposing causes include thyrotoxicosis, hyperparathyroidism, high doses of glucocorticoids, smoking, and alcohol abuse. Secondary osteoporosis is best treated through resolution of the underlying cause.

CHRONIC KIDNEY DISEASE

Chronic kidney disease affects bone mineral homeostasis mainly through **secondary hyperparathyroidism**, which enhances the resorption of bone. Under the influence of secondary hyperparathyroidism, bones develop both **osteomalacia** (decreased mineralization) and **osteitis fibrosa cystica**

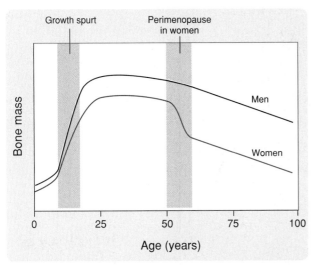

Figure 30-6. Bone mass as a function of age. In both men and women, bone mass increases with age until a peak is reached in young adulthood, after which bone mass gradually declines by approximately 0.7% per year. In women, the onset of menopause precipitates a sharp decline in bone mass as the decrease in estrogen production leads to increased bone resorption. As bone mass decreases with age, the skeleton may become sufficiently fragile that minor trauma can cause fractures. The goal of antiresorptive agents is to decrease the rate of decline of bone mass. In contrast, bone anabolic agents can be used to increase bone mass and thereby to correct situations in which significant loss of bone mass has already occurred.

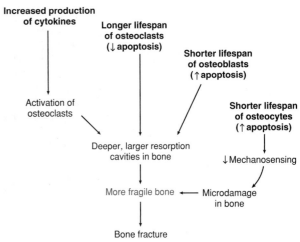

Figure 30-7. Pathophysiologic basis of osteoporosis. Several interrelated factors contribute to the development of osteoporosis. Many of these factors are activated by the decline in estrogen levels in perimenopausal women. Disinhibited production of cytokines and other regulatory molecules leads to the activation of osteoclasts. Decreased estrogen allows these osteoclasts to have a longer functional lifespan; conversely, the lack of estrogen promotes apoptosis in osteoblasts and osteocytes. The resulting imbalance between osteoclast and osteoblast activity leads to the formation of deep and large resorption cavities, which make the bone fragile and prone to fracture. The relative paucity of osteocytes impairs the mechanosensory network on which repair of microdamage in bone depends. Increased microdamage also predisposes to bone fragility and eventual fracture. Estrogen and raloxifene reverse this pathophysiologic sequence of events by suppressing cytokine production, promoting osteoclast apoptosis, and inhibiting osteoblast and osteocyte apoptosis *(not shown)*.

(increased osteoclastic resorption of bone with replacement by fibrous tissue). *Hyperparathyroidism in chronic kidney disease stems from the interplay of several factors, including decreased production of 1,25(OH)$_2$vitamin D, hypocalcemia, and hyperphosphatemia* (Figure 30-8). Each of these factors originates as a result of a decrease in renal function, manifested as an impairment in both renal synthetic ability (important for, among other processes, the 1α-hydroxylation step in 1,25(OH)$_2$ vitamin D synthesis) and renal tubular function (important for phosphate excretion).

Inadequate levels of 1,25(OH)$_2$ vitamin D (1,25(OH)$_2$D) lead to inadequate intestinal absorption of calcium. The resulting hypocalcemia stimulates PTH synthesis and secretion, and suppresses PTH degradation. The low levels of 1,25(OH)$_2$D are also thought to cause a reduction in calcium receptor synthesis in the chief cells of the parathyroid gland. The decrease in calcium receptor number raises the set-point for calcium regulation, so that a higher concentration of calcium is required to suppress PTH secretion. By this mechanism, hyperparathyroidism can persist even in the setting of hypercalcemia. In addition, evidence suggests that 1,25(OH)$_2$D normally suppresses both growth of the parathyroid gland and transcription of the PTH gene. Therefore, the deficiency of 1,25(OH)$_2$D in chronic kidney disease causes secondary hyperparathyroidism by several different mechanisms. This understanding has led to the development of several treatments for the metabolic sequelae of chronic kidney disease, including active vitamin D analogues—which bypass the requirement for 1α-hydroxylase activity in the kidney—and the calcimimetic cinacalcet—which

adjusts the sensitivity of the calcium-sensing receptor on parathyroid chief cells (see below).

Hyperphosphatemia, resulting from decreased renal excretion of phosphate, further exacerbates the hypocalcemia of chronic kidney disease. Hyperphosphatemia induces hypocalcemia by altering the equilibrium for hydroxyapatite formation and dissolution, as described in Equation 30-1. Extravascular precipitates of calcium phosphate can also damage other tissues.

PHARMACOLOGIC CLASSES AND AGENTS

Significant advances have occurred in recent years in the treatment of osteoporosis and chronic kidney disease. For osteoporosis, the relevant pharmacologic agents can be divided into two main categories: *drugs that inhibit bone resorption* and *drugs that stimulate bone formation*. Antiresorptive agents consist of hormone replacement therapy (HRT), selective estrogen receptor modulators, bisphosphonates, and calcitonin; while bone anabolic agents consist of fluoride and parathyroid hormone. For chronic kidney disease, the relevant pharmacologic agents include *drugs that lower plasma phosphate levels* (oral phosphate binders) and

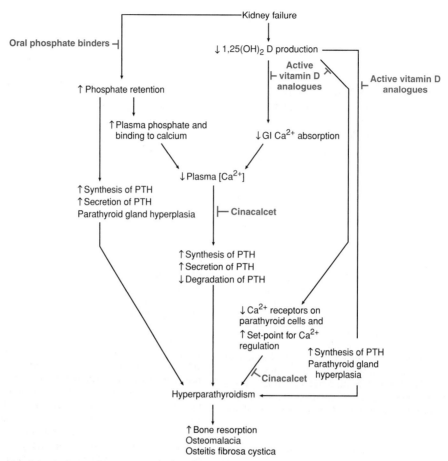

Figure 30-8. Pathophysiologic basis for osteomalacia and osteitis fibrosa cystica in chronic kidney disease. In chronic kidney disease, compromised renal function leads to decreased $1,25(OH)_2$ vitamin D synthesis and decreased phosphate excretion. The decrease in $1,25(OH)_2$ vitamin D causes decreased gastrointestinal (GI) absorption of Ca^{2+}, while the increased phosphate retention causes an increase in the levels of plasma phosphate, which complexes with Ca^{2+}. Therefore, by these two mechanisms, chronic kidney disease leads to hypocalcemia. Hypocalcemia stimulates synthesis and secretion of parathyroid hormone (PTH) and suppresses degradation of PTH. Decreased levels of $1,25(OH)_2$ vitamin D stimulate PTH synthesis and parathyroid gland hyperplasia, and lead to a decreased number of Ca^{2+} receptors on parathyroid gland chief cells and an elevated set-point for Ca^{2+} regulation. Hyperphosphatemia may also stimulate increased synthesis and secretion of PTH directly. This combination of complex regulatory events leads to hyperparathyroidism, a syndrome characterized by increased bone resorption, osteomalacia, and osteitis fibrosa cystica. Oral phosphate binders lower plasma phosphate levels by preventing dietary phosphate absorption. Active vitamin D analogues bypass the defect in renal 1α-hydroxylase activity that accompanies chronic kidney disease. Cinacalcet modulates the activity of the Ca^{2+}-sensing receptor on chief cells, such that the receptor is activated at lower plasma Ca^{2+} concentrations.

drugs that decrease parathyroid hormone synthesis and secretion (vitamin D, vitamin D analogues, and calcimimetics). Oral calcium and vitamin D also play an important role in the prevention and treatment of osteoporosis, rickets, and hypoparathyroidism.

ANTIRESORPTIVE AGENTS

Most drugs used to treat disorders of bone homeostasis are antiresorptive agents, which act by suppressing osteoclastic bone resorption. However, because bone resorption and bone formation are closely coupled processes, a decrease in one typically leads to a decrease in the other. As a result, antiresorptive drugs induce little net gain in bone mass, although they largely prevent progressive loss of skeletal mass. The increase in BMD during the initial period of antiresorptive therapy is thought to represent mineralization of resorption

cavities that had been produced during the previous period of excessive bone resorption. Subsequent increases in BMD are due to continuing mineral deposition (secondary mineralization), which occurs because resorption is inhibited.

Hormone Replacement Therapy (HRT)

Estrogen has been one of the most commonly prescribed drugs for postmenopausal osteoporosis. Estrogen acts to reduce bone resorption by suppressing the transcription of genes coding for cytokines, such as IL-6, that induce osteoclast proliferation, differentiation, and activation. Estrogen also promotes the apoptosis of osteoclasts while inhibiting the apoptosis of osteoblasts and osteocytes. Estrogen does not increase bone formation, but it does maintain bone mass or slow bone loss through its antiresorptive properties.

Estrogen is administered cyclically with a progestational agent to reduce the risk of endometrial cancer (see Chapter

28). HRT also relieves postmenopausal symptoms including hot flashes and vaginal dryness. Compliance is often a problem with HRT, because the adverse effects of estrogen, including vaginal bleeding and breast tenderness, can cause patients to discontinue treatment. HRT also increases the risk of venous thromboembolism, because estrogen promotes the hepatic synthesis of clotting factors. For many women, the greatest concern regarding HRT is the increased long-term risk of breast cancer, which is small but statistically significant. In 2002, a large government (National Institutes of Health) sponsored study concluded that the increased risks of cardiovascular disease and breast cancer outweigh the potential benefits of HRT on bone and other tissues. These findings have stimulated the use of alternative therapies for osteoporosis and the search for new and safer pharmacologic agents. Because MS has two close relatives with breast cancer, she should strongly consider an alternative to HRT for treatment of her osteoporosis.

Selective Estrogen Receptor Modulators

Selective estrogen receptor modulators (SERMs) are a group of compounds that bind to the estrogen receptor (ER) and have tissue-selective effects on the target organs of estrogen. Depending on the tissue, a SERM is capable of acting as an estrogen agonist or an estrogen antagonist. The mechanisms by which a compound can have both estrogenic and antiestrogenic effects are beginning to be understood. It appears that SERM-ER complexes: (1) bind selectively to tissue-specific hormone response elements; and/or (2) recruit tissue-selective transcriptional co-repressors and co-activators (see Chapter 28).

The goal of SERM development is to retain the beneficial effects of estrogen in one or more tissues, while eliminating the undesirable effects of estrogen in other tissues. SERMs are promising agents for the prevention and treatment of postmenopausal osteoporosis. **Raloxifene,** for example, is an estrogen agonist in bone, but an estrogen antagonist in the endometrium and breast (Fig. 30-9). This agent has been approved for the prevention and treatment of osteoporosis. Raloxifene has been demonstrated to increase both vertebral and nonvertebral bone mineral density, and to decrease vertebral fracture risk. Conclusive evidence of a beneficial effect on reducing the risk of hip fractures is lacking. The use of raloxifene is not associated with breast or endometrial cancer. In fact, there is accumulating evidence that raloxifene reduces the risk of breast cancer. Furthermore, raloxifene lowers LDL cholesterol levels, and may therefore have a role in the prevention of heart disease. However, like estrogen, raloxifene does increase the risk of venous thromboembolism.

Raloxifene may be the preferred therapy for osteoporosis in women with breast cancer, women with a past history or family history of breast or endometrial cancer, or women who wish to avoid adverse effects (such as vaginal bleeding and breast tenderness) that can be associated with HRT. Because of her family history of breast cancer, MS could potentially benefit from raloxifene.

Bisphosphonates

Bisphosphonates (BPs), currently the most widely used class of antiresorptive drugs, are analogues of pyrophosphate in

Figure 30-9. Structures of 17β-estradiol and raloxifene. Although raloxifene is not a steroid molecule, it is conformationally similar to 17β-estradiol. Raloxifene binds to the ligand binding domain on the estrogen receptor, allowing it to act as a partial estrogen agonist in some tissues (bone) and as an estrogen antagonist in other tissues (endometrium and breast). This selective action occurs because the raloxifene–estrogen receptor complex can recruit either transcriptional co-activator or co-repressor factors in a tissue-specific manner (see Chapter 28, Pharmacology of Reproduction, for further details). The benzothiophene nucleus of raloxifene is highlighted in a blue box. (See the inside front cover of this textbook for crystal structures of 17β-estradiol and raloxifene bound to the ligand-binding domain of the estrogen receptor.)

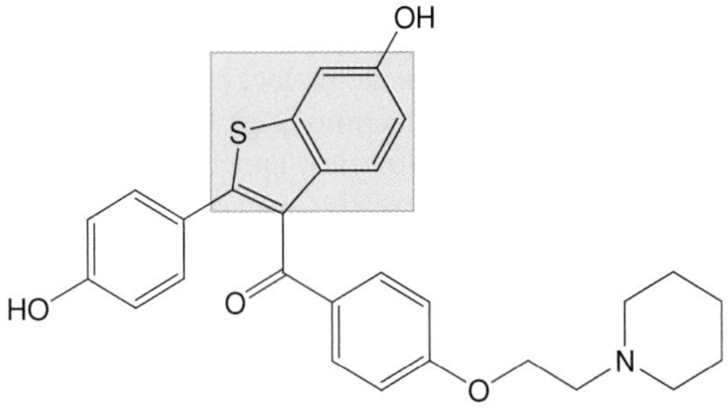

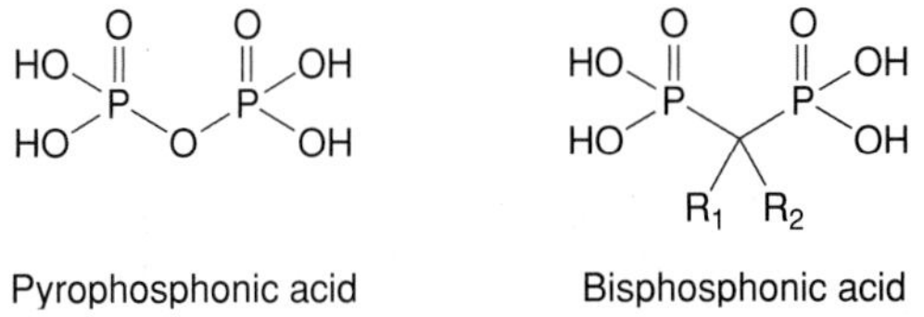

which the P-O-P bond has been replaced by a nonhydrolyzable P-C-P bond (Fig. 30-10). Four widely used bisphosphonates (the so-called amino-bisphosphonates)—**alendronate, risedronate, pamidronate,** and **ibandronate**—contain an amino moiety in one of the side chains, which greatly enhances their activity. The most recently introduced bisphosphonate, **zoledronic acid,** contains an imidazole side chain.

Because the oxygen atoms in the phosphonate groups can coordinate with divalent cations such as calcium, BPs tend to concentrate in bone, where they are incorporated into the mineralized matrix. BPs remain in the matrix until the bone

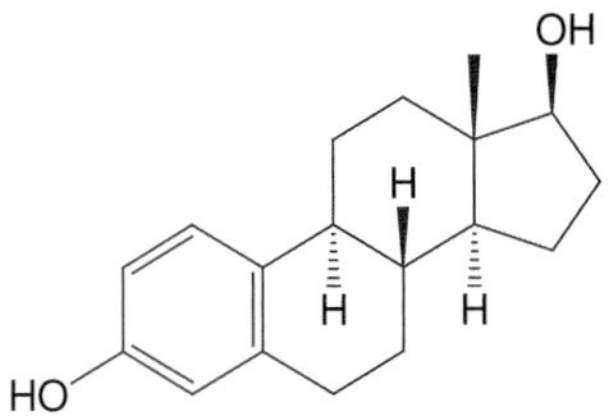

Figure 30-10. Structures of pyrophosphate and bisphosphonate. Note that the P-O-P structure of pyrophosphate (the protonated form of which is pyrophosphonic acid) is replaced with a P-C-P structure in bisphosphonate (the protonated form of which is bisphosphonic acid). This motif is conserved across all the bisphosphonates. The R-groups differ among the different bisphosphonates; those with an amine moiety have higher potency *(not shown)*.

is subsequently remodeled, at which time the acids secreted by osteoclasts dissolve the mineral matrix and release the BPs. (BPs also decrease the solubility of hydroxyapatite, rendering it more resistant to osteoclastic resorption.) Some of the released BP molecules are then internalized by the highly phagocytic osteoclasts. Within the osteoclasts, the amino-bisphosphonates inhibit a step in the **mevalonate pathway,** which is important for protein prenylation. (Prenylation, which includes farnesylation and geranylgeranylation, involves the post-translational addition of lipids to certain intracellular signaling proteins, such as GTPases.) Disruption of the mevalonate pathway leads to the loss of a number of osteoclastic functions (e.g., H^+-ATPase activity) and ultimately causes osteoclast apoptosis. Because osteoclastic bone resorption greatly increases the concentration of BP in the local vicinity of the osteoclasts, the cellular effects of mevalonate pathway inhibition appear to be limited to the osteoclasts.

The antiresorptive effects of BPs allow these agents to be used in the treatment of osteoporosis, hypercalcemia of malignancy, and Paget's disease. Alendronate, risedronate, and ibandronate are currently approved for the prevention and treatment of osteoporosis. They are all oral agents that have been shown in clinical trials to increase spine and hip BMD in postmenopausal women with osteopenia and osteoporosis. In established osteoporosis, all three agents have been shown to decrease the risk of vertebral and nonvertebral fractures. Therefore, oral BPs would be a reasonable therapeutic option for MS. Once-a-week formulations of alendronate and risedronate improve patient convenience and compliance. Ibandronate is available in a once-a-month formulation.

Hypercalcemia of malignancy occurs when certain tumors produce parathyroid hormone-related peptide (PTHrP). This peptide is structurally and functionally similar to PTH, and it can cause hypercalcemia by the same mechanism as PTH. Intravenous **pamidronate** and **zoledronate** have been approved for the treatment of this condition (Box 30-1); these agents rapidly inhibit the accelerated bone resorption that results from PTHrP-mediated osteoclastic hyperactivity.

BPs have been shown to decrease bone turnover rates in Paget's disease, and thereby to decrease the progressive deformity, pain, and fractures that are characteristic of this disease.

Because of low oral bioavailability, BPs should be administered with substantial water upon waking in the morning or on an empty stomach. Oral BPs can cause local esophagitis and esophageal erosion; for this reason, patients are advised to remain in the upright position for 30 minutes after

---

BOX 30-1. Treatment of Hypercalcemia and Hypocalcemia

HYPERCALCEMIA AND ITS TREATMENT

Hypercalcemia is most commonly treated by one or more of three different approaches: decreasing intestinal calcium absorption, increasing renal calcium excretion, and/or inhibiting bone resorption. Granulomatous diseases, such as tuberculosis and sarcoidosis, can cause hypercalcemia because of excessive ectopic calcitriol production by mononuclear cells. The resulting increase in calcium absorption by the GI tract can be blunted by the administration of **oral phosphate,** which forms insoluble complexes with dietary calcium and, thereby, decreases calcium absorption. Glucocorticoids (most commonly, prednisone) can also be administered to decrease the ectopic production of calcitriol.

The hypercalcemia of malignancy (e.g., breast cancer metastatic to bone) is often treated by increasing renal calcium excretion and inhibiting bone resorption. For acute hypercalcemia, first-line therapy consists of **saline diuresis.** In this treatment, intravenous saline is administered together with a loop diuretic that increases renal calcium excretion, such as furosemide. Saline diuresis is very effective at rapidly reducing elevated plasma calcium levels. The saline infusion also rehydrates the patient and ensures adequate renal filtration. Calcium reabsorption in the kidney is, in part, passive, driven by the electrochemical gradient associated with sodium reabsorption. By inhibiting sodium reabsorption, loop diuretics decrease calcium reabsorption and, thus, increase renal calcium excretion.

Acute hypercalcemia can also be treated with **calcitonin.** As noted in the text, this agent decreases plasma calcium levels by inhibiting osteoclastic activity. The effects of calcitonin are rapid, but limited, in duration because of the development of tachyphylaxis within several days.

Long-term management of hypercalcemia can be achieved by using **bisphosphonates.** These agents, like calcitonin, lower plasma calcium by inhibiting osteoclastic activity. Unlike calcitonin, BPs do not induce tachyphylaxis. Several BPs are effective for this purpose, but pamidronate and zoledronic acid are first-line therapies.

Severe or symptomatic acute hypercalcemia (plasma calcium >12 mg/dL) is generally treated by a combination of all three of the above approaches: saline diuresis with furosemide, calcitonin, and pamidronate. The first two agents are typically effective within the first 24 hours, whereas pamidronate is typically effective by the third day.

HYPOCALCEMIA AND ITS TREATMENT

Several possible causes for hypocalcemia are known, and treatment is best implemented after the etiology has been identified. For example, hypomagnesemia, which induces target-organ resistance to PTH and decreases PTH synthesis, is a common nutritional cause of hypocalcemia. In this case, treatment with **magnesium sulfate** will, ultimately, increase plasma calcium. In cases where the plasma magnesium concentration is within normal limits, the treatment of hypocalcemia consists principally of oral calcium and vitamin D (either calcitriol or ergocalciferol).

taking the medication, and then to have a meal before lying down.

Although bisphosphonates have been in clinical use for over 10 years and appear safe, there is a lingering concern that long-term marked inhibition of bone turnover could lead to hypermineralization and structural changes that could adversely affect bone quality and strength. It is now recognized that some patients with extensive dental disease and oral surgery may experience osteonecrosis of the jaw after taking the potent amino-bisphosphonates. This may also be a concern in patients with cancer-associated hypercalcemia who are treated with intravenous bisphosphonates.

Calcitonin

As discussed above, calcitonin binds to and activates a G protein-coupled receptor on osteoclasts, thereby decreasing the resorptive activity of these cells. Because of this action, exogenous calcitonin can be used to treat conditions characterized by high osteoclastic activity, such as Paget's disease, osteoporosis, and hypercalcemia. The clinically used preparation of calcitonin is derived from salmon, because salmon calcitonin has a higher affinity for the human calcitonin receptor and a longer half-life than human calcitonin. Calcitonin is a peptide and therefore cannot be taken orally; instead, it is administered subcutaneously or as a nasal spray. An important drawback to long-term calcitonin administration is the tachyphylaxis that can result from desensitization of the receptor-signaling pathway.

In clinical trials, intranasal calcitonin has been shown to retard vertebral bone loss and to decrease the incidence of vertebral fractures in postmenopausal women. Although the efficacy of calcitonin is lower than that of raloxifene or bisphosphonates, calcitonin can be used as an alternative to these agents in patients who are unable or unwilling to take them. Calcitonin also has weak analgesic properties, possibly because of its effects on endorphin levels. Calcitonin would be a therapeutic option for MS, but its lower efficacy relative to raloxifene would make it a second-line agent.

BONE ANABOLIC AGENTS

Antiresorptive agents slow the rate of bone loss but do not build new bone. For patients who have already lost a large amount of bone mass (BMD more than 3.0 standard deviations below normal) or who have already experienced one or more osteoporotic fragility fractures, antiresorptive agents are not optimal therapies. This need has led to the development of bone anabolic agents, which are drugs that actually increase bone mass, not just prevent its loss. The first bone anabolic agent was fluoride, and the second, more effective, agent is parathyroid hormone.

Fluoride

Fluoride is a mitogen for osteoblasts. Clinical studies have shown that fluoride, at concentrations higher than those used to fluoridate public water systems, increases trabecular bone mass. Use of fluoride, however, leads to the conversion of hydroxyapatite to fluoroapatite, which is denser but more brittle. Whether fluoride is effective in preventing osteoporosis-related fractures remains uncertain; to date, studies have shown inconsistent results.

Parathyroid Hormone

As noted above, a persistently elevated plasma concentration of PTH, such as occurs in hyperparathyroidism, leads to increased bone remodeling, with more bone resorbed than formed. As a result, bone can become weak and susceptible to fracture and osteitis fibrosa cystica. In contrast, intermittent stimulation of bone cells by PTH also increases bone remodeling, but with more new bone formed than old bone resorbed. The increase in bone formation occurs because PTH acutely promotes osteoblast differentiation and stimulates osteoblast activity; in comparison, the osteoclast-promoting activity of the hormone predominates at high or continuous exposure to PTH. Thus, *once-daily subcutaneous administration of PTH favors bone anabolism, while high continuous exposure to PTH favors bone catabolism.*

Native PTH is an 84-amino acid peptide, but N-terminal fragments containing the first 31–34 amino acids of PTH retain essentially all the important functional properties of the native protein. Thus, the 1–34 fragment has been shown in clinical trials to act as a powerful anabolic agent that builds new bone. Because **PTH(1–34)** is a peptide, the bioavailability of this agent is close to zero when administered orally. The currently available formulation is a subcutaneous injection (designed to be self-administered); whether the peptide could be formulated in an alternative dosage form (e.g., pulmonary) remains to be determined. PTH(1–34) is approved under the generic name **teriparatide** for the treatment of osteoporosis both in postmenopausal women and in men.

TREATMENT OF SECONDARY HYPERPARATHYROIDISM

There are currently three pharmacologic approaches to preventing and modifying the metabolic sequelae of chronic kidney disease—oral phosphate binders, vitamin D and analogues, and calcimimetics.

Oral Phosphate Binders

In patients with chronic kidney disease, the increased plasma phosphate can complex with circulating calcium. The resulting decrease in plasma calcium concentration can lead to hyperparathyroidism. It has increasingly been recognized that early intervention with dietary phosphate restriction and use of oral phosphate binders may limit the sequelae of chronic kidney disease.

Aluminum hydroxide was one of the first agents used to treat the hyperphosphatemia of chronic kidney disease. Aluminum precipitates with phosphate in the gastrointestinal tract, leading to the formation of nonabsorbable complexes. While effective at lowering plasma phosphate levels, this approach has the disadvantage of a significant long-term risk of aluminum toxicity. Over the course of years, chronic use of aluminum-based phosphate binders can lead to chronic anemia, osteomalacia, and neurotoxicity. For these reasons, aluminum has largely been abandoned as a treatment for hyperphosphatemia, except in cases of refractory hyperphosphatemia.

Oral preparations of **calcium carbonate** and **calcium acetate** are often used to lower plasma phosphate. These agents, when administered with meals, bind to dietary phosphate and thereby inhibit its absorption. At the doses required for phosphate binding, however, these agents can also cause iatrogenic hypercalcemia and may increase the risk of vascular calcifications.

Sevelamer is a nonabsorbable cationic ion-exchange resin that binds intestinal phosphate, thereby decreasing the absorption of dietary phosphate. Sevelamer also binds bile acids, leading to interruption of the enterohepatic circulation and to decreased cholesterol absorption.

Vitamin D and Analogues

Because impaired synthesis of 1α-vitamin D derivatives is one of the main homeostatic disturbances leading to secondary hyperparathyroidism in chronic kidney disease, vitamin D is a logical replacement therapy in this disease. Three active (i.e., 1α-hydroxylated) vitamin D congeners are approved for treatment of secondary hyperparathyroidism. *All of these agents bypass the need for 1α-hydroxylation in the kidney, and are therefore useful in the treatment of bone diseases that complicate renal failure.* Active vitamin D increases dietary absorption of calcium, and the resulting increase in plasma calcium suppresses the secretion of preformed PTH by chief cells of the parathyroid gland. In addition, these agents bind to and activate vitamin D receptors on the chief cells, and thereby suppress PTH gene transcription. Care should be taken to avoid hypercalcemia when administering any of the active vitamin D congeners.

Calcitriol [1,25(OH)$_2$D$_3$] is the dihydroxylated form of vitamin D$_3$. Calcitriol is available in oral and intravenous forms; some data suggest that the intravenous formulation may be more effective in patients on hemodialysis. Calcitriol should not be administered to patients with chronic kidney disease until hyperphosphatemia has been controlled with diet and/or pharmacologic agents, because the addition of calcitriol can cause increased plasma levels of both calcium and phosphate.

Paricalcitol [19-nor-1,25(OH)$_2$D$_2$] is a synthetic analogue of vitamin D that may lower plasma PTH levels without significantly raising plasma calcium levels. **Doxecalciferol** [1α-(OH)D$_2$] is the 1α-hydroxylated form of vitamin D$_2$; it is 25-hydroxylated to the fully active 1,25-dihydroxy form in the liver.

Calcimimetics

Although vitamin D and its analogues can be effective in the treatment of secondary hyperparathyroidism, these agents can also lead to unwanted hypercalcemia and hyperphosphatemia. The so-called calcimimetics—agents that modulate the activity of the calcium-sensing receptor on chief cells—may be effective treatments for hyperparathyroidism that do not cause these unwanted effects. **Cinacalcet**, the first FDA-approved calcimimetic, binds to the transmembrane region of the calcium-sensing receptor, and thereby modulates receptor activity by increasing its sensitivity to calcium. Because the cinacalcet-bound receptor is activated at lower calcium concentrations, PTH synthesis and secretion are also suppressed at lower calcium concentrations. As shown in Figure 30-8, these effects interrupt the pathophysiologic sequence of events leading from chronic kidney disease to secondary hyperparathyroidism. Cinacalcet is approved for the treatment of secondary hyperparathyroidism and for the treatment of hypercalcemia associated with parathyroid carcinoma.

ORAL CALCIUM

Oral calcium has both therapeutic and prophylactic utility. It is administered as a therapy for hypocalcemic states associated with disorders such as vitamin D-dependent rickets and hypoparathyroidism. In severe cases of hypocalcemia, calcium can be administered intravenously. Commonly used intravenous formulations include **calcium gluconate** and **calcium chloride**. Calcium gluconate is often the preparation of choice, because it produces less venous irritation.

As a preventative measure against osteoporosis or in cases of mild hypocalcemia, calcium is typically administered orally as a calcium salt. Commonly used oral formulations include **calcium citrate**, **calcium carbonate**, **calcium phosphate**, and **calcium lactate**. Calcium citrate is the most readily absorbed form, but calcium carbonate is the most widely used because of its low cost, wide availability (e.g., *Tums*), and antacid properties.

Dietary calcium supplementation has been shown in clinical trials to reduce vertebral bone loss modestly in postmenopausal women, although its effects on fracture prevention are less clear. Because women lose about 15% of skeletal calcium after menopause, prophylactic calcium supplementation in the premenopausal period may help to maintain bone density above the critical fracture threshold even in the face of rapid postmenopausal bone loss.

If MS had taken calcium regularly in the premenopausal and perimenopausal periods, it might have helped to reduce her risk of a spine fracture. Because she has no history of kidney stones, she should now be counseled to take daily calcium (and vitamin D) supplementation as part of her therapy for osteoporosis.

VITAMIN D

Vitamin D preparations include **cholecalciferol** (vitamin D$_3$), **ergocalciferol** (vitamin D$_2$), **calcifediol** (25(OH)D), and **calcitriol** [1,25(OH)$_2$D$_3$] (Fig. 30-5). A number of synthetic vitamin D analogues are also available, as noted above (see "Vitamin D and Analogues").

Vitamin D is used in the treatment of hypoparathyroidism, rickets, osteomalacia, osteoporosis, and chronic kidney disease. When rapidity of action is desired, calcitriol is preferred because this active form of the vitamin is capable of raising plasma calcium concentrations within 24 to 48 hours. Because vitamin D increases both plasma calcium and plasma phosphate, the plasma levels of these minerals should be monitored carefully.

In the case of *hypoparathyroidism,* large doses of vitamin D and calcium are used to restore normocalcemia and normophosphatemia. Calcitriol can be administered for more rapid onset of action, but probably does not offer an advantage over vitamin D for long-term treatment.

For *nutritional rickets,* vitamin D is used at low doses as a preventive measure and at higher doses as a treatment. In vitamin D-resistant rickets accompanied by hypophosphatemia, both oral phosphate and high doses of vitamin D are administered; calcitriol has also proved to be useful. For type I vitamin D-dependent rickets, either vitamin D or calcitriol can be used. Type II vitamin D-dependent rickets is refractory to treatment with conventional vitamin D, although high doses of calcitriol have proven to be effective for some patients with this disease.

Conclusive evidence regarding the effectiveness of vitamin D and its analogues as monotherapy in the prevention or treatment of osteoporosis has yet to be obtained. Vitamin D and dietary calcium supplements are used in combination to prevent as well as treat *osteoporosis,* possibly because many elderly individuals have poor calcium intake and are also vitamin D-deficient. The combination has been demonstrated to be modestly efficacious in preventing fracture at vertebral sites, while evidence for antifracture efficacy at nonvertebral sites is lacking.

Conclusion and Future Directions

Bone is composed of organic and inorganic components. The organic component consists of cells (osteoblasts, osteoclasts, and osteocytes) and an organic matrix called osteoid (mainly type I collagen). The inorganic component consists primarily of the calcium phosphate salt hydroxyapatite. The dynamic structure of bone depends on the relative balance between anabolic and catabolic processes, and on the physiologic regulators of calcium and phosphate homeostasis. The most important modulators of bone remodeling and bone mineral homeostasis are parathyroid hormone (PTH) and vitamin D. Through their actions on bone, kidney, and intestine, these two hormones preserve bone mineral homeostasis, sometimes at the expense of bone integrity. Bone disorders can result from abnormal levels of these hormones (e.g., high levels of PTH in hyperparathyroidism, low levels of vitamin D in rickets), increased rates of bone remodeling (e.g., increased bone resorption in osteoporosis, increased formation of disorganized bone in Paget's disease), or failure of organs that are important in maintaining mineral homeostasis (e.g., chronic kidney disease). Bone disorders usually lead to structurally weakened bone, because of either: (1) a reduction in bone mass and quality as a result of increased bone resorption; or (2) formation of architecturally unsound bone. In turn, structural weakening of the bone predisposes to bone fracture or deformity. Bone disorders can be treated by correcting the underlying hormonal or mineral imbalances (e.g.,

vitamin D, calcium), or by modulating bone remodeling (e.g., SERMs, bisphosphonates). Pharmacologic interventions directed at the physiology of bone remodeling can be divided into two main categories: antiresorptive agents and bone anabolic agents. The majority of drugs currently approved by the FDA for the treatment of osteoporosis are antiresorptive agents. These drugs act by inhibiting osteoclastic bone resorption, and thus slowing the loss of bone mass. However, these drugs do not stimulate new bone formation and *do not increase true bone mass (matrix plus mineral).* Hence, antiresorptive agents do not represent optimal therapy for individuals who have already sustained significant loss of bone mass. The only FDA-approved bone anabolic agent is once-daily PTH(1–34), which acts by increasing bone formation and is therefore the most beneficial agent for patients with very low bone mass. Clinical trials are currently underway for **denosumab**, a fully humanized antibody against RANK ligand that may inhibit bone resorption. **Strontium ranelate** has been approved in Europe for the treatment of osteoporosis. Its mechanism of action has not been elucidated, but it has been reported to inhibit bone resorption and stimulate bone formation.

Suggested Reading

Andress DL. Vitamin D treatment in chronic kidney disease. *Semin Dial* 2005;18:315–321. (*Reviews progression of chronic kidney disease and indications for vitamin D therapy.*)

Fiorelli G, Brandi ML. Skeletal effects of estrogens. *J Endocrinol Invest* 1999;22:589–593. (*Reviews the indices for bone mass and mechanisms of estrogen in controlling bone mineralization.*)

Manolagas SC. Birth and death of bone cells: basic regulatory mechanisms and implications for the pathogenesis and treatment of osteoporosis. *Endocr Rev* 2000;21:115–137. (*In-depth analysis of the signaling relationships between osteoblasts and osteoclasts.*)

Querfeld U. The therapeutic potential of novel phosphate binders. *Pediatr Nephrol* 2005;20:389–392. (*Review of agents used to lower serum phosphate levels.*)

Raisz LG. Pathogenesis of osteoporosis: concepts, conflicts, and prospects. *J Clin Invest* 2005;115:3318–3325. (*Current understanding of osteoporosis pathophysiology.*)

Rodan GA, Martin TJ. Therapeutic approaches to bone diseases. *Science* 2000;289:1508–1514. (*Discussion of future pharmacologic targets.*)

Rosen CJ. Postmenopausal osteoporosis. *N Engl J Med* 2005;353: 595–603. (*Succinct overview of the clinical management of osteoporosis.*)

Rubin MR, Bilezikian JP. The anabolic effects of parathyroid hormone therapy. *Clin Geriatr Med* 2003;19:415–432. (*Understanding of the anabolic actions of PTH.*)

Steddon SJ, Cunningham J. Calcimimetics and calcilytics—fooling the calcium receptor. *Lancet* 2005;365:2237–2239. (*New approaches to pharmacologic modulation of the calcium-sensing receptor.*)

Drug Summary Table   Chapter 30 Pharmacology of Bone Mineral Homeostasis

Drug	Clinical Applications	Serious and Common Adverse Effects	Contraindications	Therapeutic Considerations
HORMONE REPLACEMENT THERAPY *Mechanism—Promotes osteoclast apoptosis and inhibits osteoblast and osteocyte apoptosis*				
Estrogen + progestin	Osteoporosis prevention and treatment	See Drug Summary Table: Chapter 28 Pharmacology of Reproduction		
Selective Estrogen Receptor Modulators (SERMs) *Mechanism—Estrogen receptor agonist in bone and estrogen receptor antagonist in uterus and breast*				
Raloxifene	Osteoporosis prevention and treatment	*Retinal vascular occlusion, venous thromboembolism* Hot flashes, leg cramps	Pregnancy, history or presence of venous thromboembolism	Decreases risk of invasive breast cancer in postmenopausal women with osteoporosis
BISPHOSPHONATES *Mechanism—Inhibit mevalonate pathway, resulting in osteoclast apoptosis; decrease solubility of hydroxyapatite*				
Alendronate Ibandronate Pamidronate Risedronate Zoledronic acid	Osteoporosis prevention and treatment Paget's disease Hypercalcemia of malignancy (pamidronate and zoledronic acid)	*Esophageal pain and erosion, esophagitis, jaw osteonecrosis* Acid reflux, headache	Esophageal erosions Delayed gastric emptying Hypocalcemia Inability to sit up for 30 minutes after taking drug orally	Long-term effects of profound inhibition of bone turnover unknown Zoledronate is administered IV only Ibandronate is available as a monthly formulation
CALCITONIN *Mechanism—Decreases osteoclast resorptive activity*				
Salmon Calcitonin	Osteoporosis Hypercalcemia Paget's disease	Facial flushing, nausea, diarrhea, anorexia	Hypersensitivity to salmon calcitonin	Weak analgesic activity Nasal-spray formulation used most widely Plicamycin may enhance hypocalcemic effect
BONE ANABOLIC AGENTS *Mechanism—Increase osteoblast differentiation and activity*				
Once-daily PTH(1-34)	Severe osteoporosis	*Hypotension, syncope, arthralgias*	Hypersensitivity to PTH	Only approved bone formation-enhancing agent Induces osteosarcoma in long-term rat studies
Fluoride Strontium ranelate	Investigational agents			

ORAL PHOSPHATE BINDERS
Mechanism—Decrease absorption of dietary phosphate

Drug	Clinical Applications	Serious and Common Adverse Effects	Contraindications	Therapeutic Considerations
Aluminum hydroxide	Chronic kidney disease	*Confusion (chronic administration), anemia, osteomalacia* Constipation	Hypersensitivity to aluminum hydroxide	Rarely used due to adverse-effect profile
Calcium carbonate Calcium acetate	Chronic kidney disease Osteoporosis Hypocalcemia Antacid	*Milk-alkali syndrome* Constipation	Hypercalcemia Vitamin D toxicity	Calcium carbonate requires acidic environment for effective action Calcium acetate effective in acidic or alkaline environment
Sevelamer	Chronic kidney disease	*Thrombosis* Hypertenion, constipation	Hypophosphatemia Bowel obstruction	Also lowers serum cholesterol levels by binding bile acids

VITAMIN D AND ANALOGUES
Mechanism—Increase calcium absorption and decrease transcription of PTH gene

Drug	Clinical Applications	Serious and Common Adverse Effects	Contraindications	Therapeutic Considerations
Calcifediol $(25(OH)D)$ Calcitriol $[1,25(OH)_2D_3]$ Cholecalciferol (vit D_3) Doxecalciferol $[1\alpha-(OH)D_2]$ Ergocalciferol (vit D_2) Paricalcitol $[19\text{-nor-}1,25(OH)_2D_2]$	Chronic kidney disease (secondary hyperparathyroidism) Hypoparathyroidism Rickets Osteomalacia Osteoporosis	*Hypercalcemia, renal calculi, hypophosphatemia* Edema (paricalcitol)	Hypercalcemia Vitamin D toxicity	Calcitriol is the preferred agent if rapid therapeutic action is desired Calcitriol also used in treatment of Vitamin D-dependent rickets Paricalcitol may cause less hypercalcemia than calcitriol

CALCIMIMETIC
Mechanism—Increases sensitivity of calcium-sensing receptor to calcium in parathyroid gland chief cells, causing decreased secretion of PTH

Drug	Clinical Applications	Serious and Common Adverse Effects	Contraindications	Therapeutic Considerations
Cinacalcet	Chronic kidney disease Parathyroid carcinoma	Hypocalcemia, hypertension, dizziness	Hypersensitivity to cinacalcet	Sometimes used off-label in treatment of primary hyperparathyroidism

CALCIUM
Mechanism—Essential for bone mineralization

Drug	Clinical Applications	Serious and Common Adverse Effects	Contraindications	Therapeutic Considerations
Calcium gluconate Calcium carbonate	Vitamin D-dependent rickets Hypoparathyroidism Hypocalcemia Osteoporosis	Headache, GI disturbance, renal calculi	Hypersensitivity to calcium gluconate or calcium carbonate	When administered intravenously, calcium gluconate causes less venous irritation

V

Principles of Chemotherapy

31

Principles of Antimicrobial and Antineoplastic Pharmacology

Heidi Harbison, Harris S. Rose, Donald M. Coen, and David E. Golan

INTRODUCTION

Although infectious diseases and cancers have different underlying etiologies, from a pharmacologic perspective, the broad principles of treatment are similar. Both sets of diseases are among the most deadly afflictions plaguing human societies. The World Health Organization (WHO) has estimated that, in the year 2002, infectious diseases caused 10.9 million of the 57 million total deaths worldwide, and malignant neoplasms were responsible for 7.1 million deaths. Among infectious diseases, the most common causes of mortality worldwide included lower respiratory infections (3.9 million), HIV/AIDS (2.8 million), diarrheal diseases (1.8 million), tuberculosis (1.6 million), and malaria (1.3 million). In the developed world, although infectious disease mortality is increasing, cancer (along with heart disease and stroke) is a more significant cause of death. The most deadly cancers in the United States presently include lung cancer (162,000 estimated deaths in 2006), colon cancer (55,000), breast cancer (41,000), pancreas cancer (32,000), and prostate cancer (27,000). Both infectious and neoplastic patterns of disease will likely change as increasingly effective treatments are developed and distributed. The common thread in these pharmacologic strategies is the *targeting of selective differences between the microbe or cancer cell and the normal host cell*. Because both microbes and cancer cells can evolve resistance to drug therapies, the development of new treatments is also a continually evolving process.

Although antimicrobial and antineoplastic drugs are the focus of this chapter, there are many other important and effective strategies to combat microbes and cancer. These strategies include public health measures, vaccinations, and screening procedures. Most public health and vaccination programs aim to prevent infections rather than treat existing infections. Smallpox, for example, was eradicated worldwide in 1977 through aggressive vaccination programs, although concerns have recently been raised about the potential use of this virus as a bioterror agent. Similar campaigns to eradicate polio are ongoing. Cancer screening, through regular mammograms, colonoscopy, and other tests, is widely used to detect cancer in its early and more treatable stages. Early detection through the widespread use of Papanicolaou cytologic tests (Pap smears) has caused the mortality of cervical cancer to decrease by more than two thirds in the United States; cervical cancer has moved from the primary to the fifteenth leading cause of cancer deaths in women. It is hoped that widespread vaccination against the human papilloma virus, the most common causative agent of cervical cancer, will further reduce the mortality of this cancer type. Effective strategies against disease, including drug therapy, also depend on socioeconomic factors. In affluent countries, the widespread use of antimicrobial drugs and improvements in sanitation and nutrition have markedly reduced mortality from infectious diseases. This progress has not been realized in the developing world, however, where otherwise treatable infectious diseases such as pneumonia, HIV/AIDS, diarrheal disease, tuberculosis, and malaria remain the predominant causes of mortality.

Despite the importance of public health measures, vaccinations, and screening procedures, drug therapy remains a major tool in the treatment of microbial disease and cancer. The inevitable development of resistance to pharmacologic interventions suggests that the general principles and mechanisms of antimicrobial and antineoplastic pharmacology must be understood in order to prescribe existing drugs effectively and to continue to discover new drugs.

■ Case

The country is Germany and the year is 1935. Hildegard, daughter of Dr. Gerhard Domagk, is near death with a streptococcal infection from a pinprick. She has failed to respond to any treatments. In desperation, Hildegard's father injects her with prontosil, a red dye with which he has been experimenting in his laboratory. Miraculously, she makes a complete recovery.

This story actually begins 3 years earlier, when Dr. Domagk observed that prontosil protects mice and rabbits from lethal doses of staphylococci and streptococci. He discovered this by screening thousands of dyes (which are, in actuality, simply chemicals that bind to proteins) for antibacterial activity. When his daughter became ill, however, Domagk was not sure whether prontosil's antibacterial efficacy in mice would carry over to infections in humans. He kept his personal test of the drug a secret until data from other physicians indicated that the drug had been successful in curing other patients of their infections. In 1939, Gerhard Domagk was awarded the Nobel Prize in Physiology or Medicine for his discovery of the therapeutic benefit of prontosil.

QUESTIONS

■ **1.** What is the mechanism responsible for the antibacterial action of prontosil?
■ **2.** Why does prontosil kill bacteria but not human cells?
■ **3.** What has caused the utility of drugs such as prontosil to decline over the past 70 years?
■ **4.** Why are drugs of the same class as prontosil now used in combination with other antibacterial agents?

MECHANISMS OF SELECTIVE TARGETING

The goal of antimicrobial and antineoplastic drug therapy is **selective toxicity,** i.e., inhibiting pathways or targets that are critical for pathogen or cancer cell survival and replication at concentrations of drug lower than those required to affect host pathways. Selectivity can be realized by attacking: (1) targets unique to the pathogen or cancer cell that are not present in the host; (2) targets in the pathogen or cancer cell that are similar but not identical to those in the host; and (3) targets in the pathogen or cancer cell that are shared by the host but that vary in importance between pathogen and host and thus impart selectivity (Table 31-1). These selectively targeted differences can be as great as a protein that is unique to the pathogen or as slight as the difference in cell cycling

TABLE 31-1	Mechanisms of Selective Targeting by Chemotherapeutic Agents	
TYPE OF TARGETING	**MECHANISM**	**EXAMPLE**
Unique	Drug targets genetic or biochemical pathway that is unique to pathogen	Bacterial cell wall synthesis inhibitor
Selective	Drug targets protein isoform that is unique to pathogen	Dihydrofolate reductase (DHFR) inhibitor
Common	Drug targets metabolic requirement that is specific to pathogen	5-Fluorouracil

and growth rates between some cancer cells and normal cells. In principle, drugs exhibit the least toxicity to the host when they target unique differences and the most toxicity when they target common pathways. For this reason, many antineoplastic drugs are more toxic to the host than many antimicrobial drugs.

The ratio of the toxic dose to the therapeutic dose of a drug is called the **therapeutic index** or therapeutic window (see Chapter 2, Pharmacodynamics). The therapeutic index is therefore an indication of how selective the drug is in producing the desired effects. A highly selective drug, such as penicillin, can often be prescribed safely because of the large difference between its therapeutic and toxic concentrations. The margin of safety in a less selective drug, such as the anticancer drug methotrexate, is much lower because of its low therapeutic index. As more is learned about the biology of pathogens and cancer cells, drugs can be designed against more selective targets. For example, imatinib mesylate is a highly specific anticancer agent that targets the product of a novel gene rearrangement present in chronic myelogenous leukemia cells but not in normal cells (see Chapter 1, Drug-Receptor Interactions). It is important to recognize, however, that many known potential targets remain unexploited because of the unexpected adverse effects, unfavorable pharmacokinetic properties, or prohibitive cost associated with experimental drugs that have been developed to date against these targets.

UNIQUE DRUG TARGETS

Unique drug targets include metabolic pathways, enzymes, and mutated genes and gene products that are present in the pathogen or cancer cell but lacking in the host. One common target for antibacterial drugs is the bacterial peptidoglycan cell wall (see Chapter 33, Pharmacology of Bacterial Infections: Cell Wall Synthesis). This structure is both biochemically unique and essential for the survival of growing bacteria. Penicillin and other β-lactam antibiotics inhibit the transpeptidase enzymes that catalyze the final cross-linking step in peptidoglycan synthesis. Without peptidoglycans, bacterial cell wall synthesis is compromised and cell lysis ensues. Because of their unique specificity for bacterial transpeptidase proteins, the penicillins have minimal host toxicity—in fact, nonmechanism-based allergic hypersensitivity is the major adverse reaction.

Fungi lack a cell wall and are enveloped only by a lipid bilayer similar to that of human cells, making selective targeting more challenging. Ergosterol, a sterol moiety present in the fungal but not the host membrane, represents one of the few unique targets for antifungal drugs (see Chapter 34, Pharmacology of Fungal Infections). There are currently two classes of drugs that target ergosterol: one class (azoles) blocks ergosterol biosynthesis in fungal cells, and the other class (polyenes) chelates ergosterol in fungal membranes. Both types of drugs alter membrane permeability and cause fungal cell death. Some of these drugs can affect cholesterol metabolism in human cells as well as ergosterol metabolism in fungal cells; such drugs have a low therapeutic index, and their use is associated with significant adverse effects. For example, amphotericin, a polyene used to treat systemic fungal infections, commonly causes fever, rigors, and renal

toxicity. Thus, even with a unique target, selectivity can pose a significant challenge.

SELECTIVE INHIBITION OF SIMILAR TARGETS

Many organisms have metabolic pathways similar to those of humans but, because of evolutionary divergence, possess unique enzyme or receptor isoforms. Drugs can have quantitatively different binding specificities based on these biochemical differences. Because these targets are different but not unique, the resulting therapeutic windows are usually smaller than with unique targets. Examples of this strategy include inhibitors of the enzyme dihydrofolate reductase (DHFR) and inhibitors of bacterial protein synthesis. DHFR is a crucial enzyme in the synthesis of the purine and pyrimidine building blocks of DNA in many organisms (see below). Humans, bacteria, and protozoa all utilize DHFR in DNA synthesis, but the DHFR isoforms are genetically and structurally distinct and can therefore be targeted by different drugs. The anticancer drug **methotrexate** powerfully inhibits the DHFR isoforms in human as well as bacterial and protozoal cells, and this drug's low selectivity produces high toxicity in host cells. The basis for the selectivity of methotrexate in cancer treatment lies not in a difference in the isoform of the enzyme between cancer cells and normal cells, but rather in the ability of the drug to induce apoptosis in cancer cells but not in most normal cells. In contrast, **trimethoprim** selectively inhibits the bacterial DHFR and **pyrimethamine** selectively inhibits the malarial DHFR. Thus, although all of these DHFR isoforms bind the same substrate and catalyze the same reaction, biochemical differences in DHFR structure can be exploited for selective inhibition. Determining the amino acid sequence and three-dimensional structure of DHFR isoforms from different species may provide a molecular basis for the rational design of more potent and selective inhibitors in the future (Box 31-1).

Similar to protein synthesis in humans, bacterial protein synthesis is a multistep process that involves binding of mRNA to the ribosome, decoding of mRNA, synthesis of peptide bonds, translocation of the polypeptide chain, and release of the polypeptide from the ribosome. The bacterial protein synthesis machinery differs from the human machinery in that different-sized ribosomes and different ribosomal RNAs and proteins are used. Several drug classes, including the macrolides and aminoglycosides, inhibit bacterial protein synthesis (see Chapter 32, Pharmacology of Bacterial Infections: DNA Replication, Transcription, and Translation). Macrolide antibiotics such as **erythromycin** bind to the 50S bacterial ribosomal subunit and block the peptide translocation step, preventing emergence of the protein from the ribosome. Aminoglycoside antibiotics such as **streptomycin** and **gentamicin** bind to the 30S bacterial ribosomal subunit and disrupt the decoding of mRNA.

The bacterial protein synthesis inhibitors include a wide variety of individual drugs with diverse mechanisms, and the selectivity and dose-limiting toxicities of these drugs are often class- and/or drug-specific. For example, the macrolides rarely cause serious adverse effects, whereas some of the aminoglycosides have dose-limiting ototoxicity and

---

BOX 31-1. The Future of Dihydrofolate Reductase Inhibitors

Despite the effectiveness of the available DHFR inhibitors, there is much interest in developing new compounds. Drug resistance is a problem, and, for many species, no selective inhibitor is available. Recent developments have allowed researchers to determine the amino acid sequences and three-dimensional structures of DHFRs from several different organisms, including complexes of the enzyme with small-molecule inhibitors. These studies have provided a molecular basis for understanding both enzymatic catalysis and inhibition (for example, why some inhibitors, such as trimethoprim, effectively inhibit bacterial but not mammalian DHFRs). Importantly, these studies also suggest how one could design a new drug that is capable of even more potent or selective inhibition. Thus, instead of employing ''random screening'' methods (which have been successful, but inefficient, in the development of many current enzyme inhibitors), it may soon be possible to apply this powerful technology for efficient design of more selective agents. ''Rational drug design'' is currently at an early stage, but this technology holds substantial promise for the future.

---

nephrotoxicity. Some adverse effects appear to result from drug binding to human mitochondrial ribosomes in addition to bacterial ribosomes. Thus, selective inhibition of similar targets, as exemplified by DHFR inhibitors and protein synthesis inhibitors, can result in effects characterized by therapeutic indices that range from low to high, depending on the individual drug or drug class under consideration.

COMMON TARGETS

When the host and pathogen or cancer share common biochemical and physiologic pathways, a basis for selectivity may be found if the pathogen or cancer requires a metabolic activity or is affected by its inhibition to a greater degree than the host. These relatively minor differences are often exploited in cancer pharmacology, explaining the narrow therapeutic indices of many of these drugs. Tumor cells arise from normal cells that have been transformed by genetic mutations into cells with dysregulated growth. These cells utilize the same machinery for growth and replication as do normal cells. Therefore, selective inhibition of cancer cell growth is a major challenge.

Recent discoveries in cancer biology have identified a number of mutated or overexpressed proteins, inhibitors of which have entered clinical use (see Chapter 38, Pharmacology of Cancer: Signal Transduction). The basis for the selectivity of most currently used antineoplastic drugs arises not from biochemical differences, however, but from variations in cancer cell growth behavior and from increased susceptibility of cancer cells to induction of apoptosis. Cancer, as a disease of persistent proliferation, requires continued cell division. Therefore, drugs targeting processes involved in DNA synthesis, mitosis, and cell cycle progression may kill rapidly cycling cancer cells preferentially over their normal

relatives. (An important correlate to this statement is that many chemotherapeutic strategies are more successful against rapidly growing than slowly growing cancers.) Antimetabolites such as **5-fluorouracil** (5-FU) inhibit DNA synthesis in dividing cells (see Chapter 37, Pharmacology of Cancer: Genome Synthesis, Stability, and Maintenance). 5-FU inhibits thymidylate synthase, the enzyme responsible for converting dUMP to dTMP, a pyrimidine building block of DNA. As a pyrimidine analogue, 5-FU is also incorporated into growing RNA and DNA strands, thereby interrupting the synthesis of these strands. By causing DNA damage, 5-FU induces the cell to activate its apoptotic pathway, resulting in programmed cell death. 5-FU is toxic to all human cells undergoing DNA synthesis and, thus, is selectively toxic both for rapidly cycling tumor cells (therapeutic effect) and for high-turnover host tissues such as the bone marrow and gastrointestinal (GI) mucosa (adverse effect).

These examples illustrate the importance of studying the cell biology, molecular biology, and biochemistry of microbes and cancer cells to identify specific targets for selective inhibition. Clinically, an awareness of drug mechanisms and the basis of drug selectivity can help to explain the narrow or broad therapeutic windows that have an impact on drug dosing and treatment strategies. Understanding the selectivity of drugs for their targets is also important in combating drug resistance. Thus, the fundamental pharmacologic principles of drug-receptor interactions, therapeutic and adverse effects, and drug resistance form the basis for selective targeting in antimicrobial and antineoplastic drug therapy.

PATHOGENS, CANCER CELL BIOLOGY, AND DRUG CLASSES

Pharmacologic interventions target specific differences between the host and the microbial pathogen or cancer cell. This section examines some of the unique characteristics evolution has bestowed on organisms and the major drug classes that target these molecular differences among host cells, pathogens, and cancer cells.

BACTERIA

Bacteria are prokaryotic organisms that often contain unique targets for pharmacologic intervention. Some of these drug targets have been discussed previously and are illustrated in Figure 31-1. Currently available drugs act to interrupt bacterial DNA replication and repair (this chapter and Chapter 32), transcription and translation (Chapter 32), and cell wall synthesis (Chapter 33).

Depending on the role of the drug target in bacterial physiology, antibacterial drugs can produce bacteriostatic or bactericidal effects. Drugs that inhibit the growth of the pathogen without causing cell death are called **bacteriostatic.** These drugs target metabolic pathways that are necessary for bacterial growth but not for bacterial survival. Most protein synthesis inhibitors (aminoglycosides are one exception) have a bacteriostatic effect. The clinical effectiveness of these drugs relies on an intact host immune system to clear

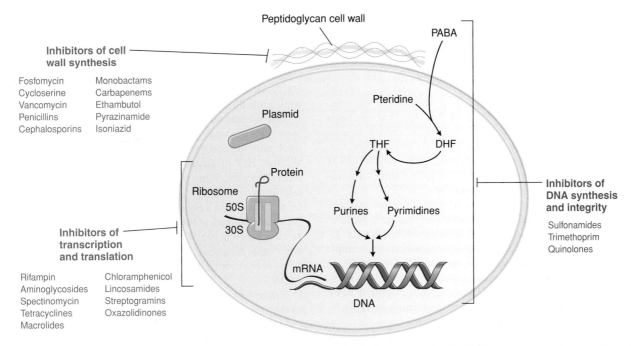

Figure 31-1. Sites of action of antibacterial drug classes. Antibacterial drug classes can be divided into three general groups. Drugs in one group inhibit specific enzymes involved in DNA synthesis and integrity: sulfonamides and trimethoprim inhibit the formation or use of folate compounds that are necessary for nucleotide synthesis; quinolones inhibit bacterial type II topoisomerases. Drugs targeting transcription and translation inhibit bacterial processes that mediate RNA and protein synthesis: rifampin inhibits bacterial DNA-dependent RNA polymerase; aminoglycosides, spectinomycin, and tetracyclines inhibit the bacterial 30S ribosomal subunit; macrolides, chloramphenicol, lincosamides, streptogramins, and oxazolidinones inhibit the bacterial 50S ribosomal subunit. A third group of drugs inhibits specific steps in bacterial cell wall synthesis: fosfomycin and cycloserine inhibit early steps in peptidoglycan monomer synthesis; vancomycin binds to peptidoglycan intermediates, inhibiting their polymerization; penicillins, cephalosporins, monobactams, and carbapenems inhibit peptidoglycan cross-linking; ethambutol, pyrazinamide, and isoniazid inhibit processes necessary for synthesis of the cell wall and outer membrane of *Mycobacterium tuberculosis.* There are several clinically useful antibacterial drugs that do not fit into one of these three groups; one recent example is daptomycin. The development of resistance is a problem for all antibacterial agents. Many bacteria carry plasmids (small, circular segments of DNA) with genes that confer resistance to an antibacterial agent or class of agents. PABA, para-aminobenzoic acid; DHF, dihydrofolate; THF, tetrahydrofolate.

the nongrowing (but viable) bacteria. In contrast, **bactericidal** drugs kill bacteria. For example, cell wall synthesis inhibitors (e.g., penicillins and cephalosporins) cause bacterial lysis when the bacteria grow in or are exposed to hypertonic or hypotonic environments. Thus, bacterial infections in immunocompetent hosts can often be treated with bacteriostatic drugs, whereas the treatment of bacterial infections in immunocompromised hosts often requires bactericidal drugs.

Bacteriostatic and bactericidal effects are also important to consider when antibiotics are used clinically in combination (see Chapter 39, Principles of Combination Chemotherapy). *The combination of a bacteriostatic drug with a bactericidal drug can result in* **antagonistic** *effects.* For example, the bacteriostatic drug tetracycline inhibits protein synthesis and thereby retards cell growth and division. The action of this drug antagonizes the effects of a cell wall synthesis inhibitor, such as penicillin, which requires bacterial growth in order to be effective. In contrast, *the combination of two bactericidal drugs can be* **synergistic;** *that is, the effect of the combination is greater than the sum of the effects of each drug alone (at the same doses of the two drugs). For example, a penicillin-aminoglycoside combination can have a synergistic effect, because inhibition of bacterial cell wall synthesis by the penicillin allows increased entry of the aminoglycoside.

FUNGI AND PARASITES

Eukaryotes, which include fungi (yeasts and molds) and parasites (protozoa and helminths) as well as all multicellular organisms, are more complex then prokaryotes. Cells in these organisms contain a nucleus and membrane-bound organelles, as well as a plasma membrane. Eukaryotic cells reproduce by mitotic division rather than binary fission. Because of the similarities among human, fungal, and parasitic cells, infections caused by fungi and parasites can be more difficult to target than bacterial infections. However, the burden of disease from these organisms is vast. Parasitic infections caused by protozoa and helminths (worms) affect more than 3 billion people worldwide, especially in less developed countries where morbidity and mortality can be devastating. In both developed and less developed parts of the world, increasing numbers of patients are immunocompromised from AIDS, cancer chemotherapy, organ transplants, and old age. Such patients are especially susceptible to fungal and parasitic infections, which are becoming more prominent and will require greater attention in the future.

The currently available antifungal drugs can be divided into three main classes. As mentioned above, polyenes (e.g., **amphotericin**, **nystatin**) and azoles (e.g., **miconazole**, **fluconazole**) selectively target ergosterol in the fungal cell membrane. Pyrimidines such as **5-fluorocytosine** inhibit

DNA synthesis. Another class of miscellaneous antifungals, mostly acids, are used only topically because of their unacceptable systemic toxicity. As with antibacterials, antifungals can be fungistatic or fungicidal; this distinction is usually determined empirically. For example, the azoles interfere with fungal cytochrome P450-mediated ergosterol metabolism. Many azoles (e.g., **itraconazole** and **fluconazole**) are fungistatic. Newer azole agents (e.g., **voriconazole** and **ravuconazole**) may have fungicidal activity against some fungal species. As compared to fungistatic drugs, fungicidal drugs are more efficacious and faster acting and allow more favorable dosing regimens. Antifungal drugs are discussed in further detail in Chapter 34.

Parasites exhibit complex and diverse life cycles and metabolic pathways, and the treatment of parasitic infections utilizes a wide array of antiparasitic drugs (see Chapter 35, Pharmacology of Parasitic Infections). Malaria is an example of a complex parasite that, while theoretically susceptible to numerous classes of drugs, is becoming resistant to many currently available therapies. Malaria is transmitted when the female *Anopheles* mosquito deposits *Plasmodia* sporozoites in the human bloodstream. The parasites leave the circulation and develop into tissue schizonts in the liver. The tissue schizonts rupture, releasing merozoites that again enter the circulation to infect red blood cells (erythrocytes). The parasites then mature to trophozoites and, finally, to mature schizonts. The mature schizonts are released into the bloodstream when the erythrocytes rupture, causing the typical cyclic fever associated with malaria. Antimalarial drugs target different stages of the protozoal life cycle; several classes of drugs can be used, depending on the local pattern of resistance. Aminoquinolines (such as the previous first-line drug, **chloroquine**) inhibit the polymerization of heme within the erythrocyte; it is thought that nonpolymerized heme is toxic to intraerythrocytic *Plasmodia*. As chloroquine resistance has increased, cinchona alkaloids (**quinine** and **quinidine**) and quinoline-methanols (**mefloquine**) have been used as first-line agents, despite their low therapeutic indices. Dihydrofolate reductase inhibitors, protein synthesis inhibitors, and other classes of drugs are also used in malaria treatment. Malaria is but one example that illustrates the complexities of both the parasitic life cycle and the use of drugs to treat parasitic infections.

VIRUSES

Viruses are noncellular organisms that typically consist of a nucleic acid core of RNA or DNA enclosed in a proteinaceous capsid. Some viruses also posses a host cell-derived lipid envelope containing viral proteins. Viruses lack the capability to synthesize proteins themselves, relying instead on the host cell machinery. Because viral replication is dependent on the normal synthetic processes of the host cell, there are fewer antiviral drug classes than antibacterial drug classes, and antiviral drugs are generally more toxic to the host than are antibacterial drugs. Most viruses also encode unique proteins not normally produced by human cells, however. Many of these proteins are involved in the viral life cycle, mediating virus attachment and entry into the host cell, viral capsid uncoating, viral genome replication, viral particle assembly and maturation, and release of viral prog-

eny from the host cell. These virus-specific processes are often targeted by antiviral drugs. A schematic diagram of the general viral life cycle is presented to illustrate the stages of viral replication that can be targeted by antiviral drugs (Fig. 31-2). Because these targets are present only during active viral replication, viruses that exhibit latency are not well controlled by antiviral drugs.

One unique viral protein is the HIV protease. This enzyme cleaves viral precursor proteins to generate the structural proteins and enzymes necessary for virus maturation. Without HIV protease, only immature and noninfective virions (individual virus particles) are produced. HIV protease inhibitors structurally mimic natural substrates of the protease, but contain a noncleavable bond. These drugs are competitive inhibitors at the active site of the enzyme (see Chapter 36, Pharmacology of Viral Infections). In combination with other classes of anti-HIV drugs, protease inhibitors have revolutionized the treatment of patients with HIV/AIDS.

Several classes of drugs target proteins that are unique to the influenza virus. **Zanamivir** and **oseltamivir** target a viral neuraminidase that is vital for virion release from host cells. **Amantadine** and **rimantadine** act on the influenza virus membrane protein M2 (a proton channel) to inhibit viral uncoating. Although these anti-influenza drugs are highly effective inhibitors of the viral neuraminidase and proton channel, respectively, they have not revolutionized influenza therapy to the extent that anti-HIV drugs have for HIV. Because most flu infections are identified clinically when the immune system has already begun to eradicate the virus, these drugs have only a limited effect on flu symptoms. This example illustrates the point that even selective inhibitors with high therapeutic indices do not necessarily become highly effective drugs in the clinic.

Currently, the most important antiviral drugs are the polymerase inhibitors. Most viruses use a viral polymerase, either an RNA or DNA polymerase, to replicate their genetic material. Polymerase inhibitors are especially effective against human herpesviruses, HIV, and hepatitis B virus. Two types of polymerase inhibitors are the nucleoside analogues and the nonnucleoside reverse transcriptase (NNRT) inhibitors. Nucleoside analogues (such as **zidovudine** [AZT] and **acyclovir**) become phosphorylated and thereby activated by viral or cellular kinases (phosphorylating enzymes), at which point they competitively inhibit the viral polymerase and, in some cases, are incorporated into the growing DNA strand. Selectivity is dependent on the relative affinities of the nucleoside analogue for the viral and cellular kinases and polymerases. Nonnucleoside reverse transcriptase inhibitors (such as **efavirenz**) inhibit viral reverse transcriptase, preventing DNA replication. Mutations in viral polymerase genes are a major mechanism of resistance to polymerase inhibitors.

Chapter 36 provides a detailed discussion of the pharmacology of antiviral drugs.

CANCER CELLS

Cancer is a disease of cell proliferation in which normal cells are transformed by genetic mutation into cells with

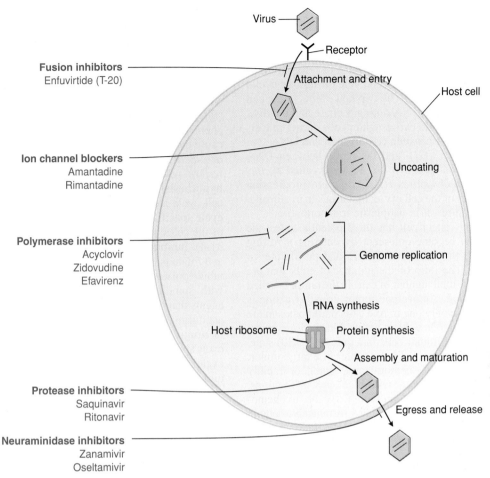

Figure 31-2. Stages of the viral life cycle targeted by antiviral drug classes. The viral life cycle begins with attachment of the virus to a host cell receptor and entry of the virus into the cell. The virus then uncoats, sometimes in an endosomal compartment. The uncoated viral nucleic acid undergoes genome replication; viral genes are transcribed (RNA synthesis); and virally coded RNA is translated into proteins on host cell ribosomes. The replicated viral genome and viral proteins are assembled into a virion (viral particle), which is then released from the host cell. The process of virion assembly and/or release is accompanied by maturation of the virus into an infective agent that is able to repeat this life cycle with a new host cell. The anti-HIV drug enfuvirtide (T-20) blocks the entry of HIV into host cells. The ion channel blockers amantadine and rimantadine inhibit influenza virus uncoating. Polymerase inhibitors are a large class of antiviral agents that include acyclovir, zidovudine, and efavirenz; these drugs inhibit viral genome replication by interfering with viral DNA polymerase (acyclovir) and reverse transcriptase (zidovudine and efavirenz). Protease inhibitors, such as the anti-HIV drugs saquinavir and ritonavir, inhibit viral maturation. Neuraminidase inhibitors block the release of influenza virus particles from the host cell.

dysregulated growth. Neoplastic cells compete with normal cells for energy and nutrition, resulting in deterioration of normal organ function. Cancers also impinge on vital organs by mass effects. Carcinogenesis, chemotherapy, and the log cell kill model of tumor regression are discussed below to provide an overview of cancer pharmacology. Chapters 37 and 38 should be read with these principles in mind, and Chapter 39 provides integrated examples of the clinical applications of combination antineoplastic chemotherapy.

Carcinogenesis and Cell Proliferation

Carcinogenesis occurs in three main steps—transformation, proliferation, and metastasis. **Transformation** denotes a change in phenotype from a cell with normal growth controls to a cell with dysregulated growth. Nonlethal genetic damage (mutations) can be inherited in the germ line, can occur spontaneously, or can be caused by environmental agents

such as chemicals, radiation, or viruses. If the DNA damage is not repaired, the mutated genes (e.g., genes involved in growth regulation and DNA repair) can express altered gene products that allow abnormal cell growth and proliferation. Mutations can activate growth-promoting genes, inactivate growth-inhibiting genes, alter apoptosis-regulating genes, confer immortalization, and inactivate DNA repair genes. Expression of altered gene products and/or loss of regulatory proteins can cause genetic instability and dysregulated growth. Most cancers are initially clonal (i.e., genetically identical to a single precursor cell), but evolve to heterogeneity as new mutations increase the genetic variation among daughter cells. When progeny cells with higher survival capacity are selected, increased cell proliferation ensues, and the tumor progresses to greater and greater heterogeneity. Thus, carcinogenesis, the progression from a normal cell to a malignant tumor, is a multistep process that requires an accumulation of multiple genetic alterations. As more is learned about the molecular basis for carcinogenesis, these genetic differences can be targeted for selective drug therapy.

The growth of transformed cells into a tumor requires **proliferation,** or an increase in the number of cells. Dividing human cells progress through a cell cycle (or mitotic cycle) consisting of distinct phases. The two key events in the cell cycle are the synthesis of DNA during S phase and the division of the parent cell into two daughter cells during mitosis or M phase. The phase between cell division and DNA synthesis is called *gap 1 (G1),* and the phase between DNA synthesis and mitosis is called *G2.* Proteins called *cyclins* and *cyclin-dependent kinases (CDKs)* govern progression through the phases of the cell cycle; mutations in cyclin and/or CDK genes can result in neoplastic transformation.

A proliferating cancer cell has three potential fates: the daughter cell can become quiescent by entering a resting phase called *G0;* the cell can enter G1 and proliferate; or the cell can die. The ratio of the number of cells that are proliferating to the total number of cells in the tumor is called the **growth fraction.** An average tumor growth fraction is about 20%, because only one in five cells participates in the cell cycle at any given time. Most antineoplastic drugs target dividing cells. Hence, tumor cells in a quiescent (G0) state, such as nutrient-starved cells in the center of a large tumor, are not easily killed by chemotherapy. Small or rapidly growing cancers (i.e., cancers with high growth fractions, such as leukemias) often respond more favorably to chemotherapy than do large bulky tumors. Unfortunately, cells in normal tissues characterized by high growth fractions, such as the bone marrow and gastrointestinal mucosa, are also killed by antineoplastic drugs, resulting in dose-limiting toxicities.

Tumor cells do not proliferate in isolation. Transformed cancer cells secrete a variety of chemical mediators to induce a specialized local environment. These chemical mediators include growth factors such as epidermal growth factor (EGF), and inhibitors of growth factor signaling have been developed for clinical use as cancer chemotherapeutic agents. Some tumors create a protective fibrous connective tissue stroma; for example, this property makes breast cancer nodules palpable. Most solid tumors also require the induction of blood vessel growth (angiogenesis) to deliver nutrients into the center of the tumor; for this reason, angiogenesis inhibitors represent a valuable new class of antineoplastic drugs.

Cancer cells may acquire the capability to invade tissues and **metastasize** throughout the body. In order to metastasize, tumor cells must acquire mutations that allow invasion into tissues and vessels, seeding of cavities, spread through lymph or blood vessels, and growth in a new environment. Aggressive, rapidly growing primary tumors are generally more likely to metastasize than are more indolent and slowly growing tumors. In the process of gaining mutations, tumor cells can also evolve differential receptor expression patterns and drug sensitivities. Often, although the primary tumor may respond well to chemotherapy, the more dedifferentiated metastatic cells respond poorly. Thus, metastatic spread often represents a poor prognostic sign.

Chemotherapy

By the time a typical solid tumor is clinically evident, it contains at least 10^9 cells, has progressed to heterogeneity,

and has developed surrounding stroma. The tumor may or may not have metastasized from its site of origin ("primary site") to one or more secondary sites. These factors can render the cancer difficult to treat pharmacologically. Currently, most chemotherapeutic agents interfere with cell proliferation and rely on rapid cell cycling and/or promotion of apoptosis for their relative selectivity against cancer cells (Fig. 31-3). As noted above, tumors are most sensitive to chemotherapy when they are growing rapidly, primarily because they are progressing through the cell cycle. *These metabolically active cells are thus susceptible to drugs that interfere with cell growth and division* (the **mitotoxicity hypothesis**). Many antineoplastic drugs interfere with the cell cycle at a particular phase; such drugs are called **cell-cycle specific.** Other antineoplastic drugs act independently of the cell cycle and are called **cell-cycle nonspecific** (Fig. 31-4). Inhibitors of DNA synthesis, such as antimetabolites and folate pathway antagonists, are S-phase specific. Microtubule poisons, such as taxanes and vinca alkaloids, interfere with spindle formation during M phase. The alkylating agents that damage DNA and other cellular macromolecules act during all phases of the cell cycle. These various classes of drugs can be administered in combination, using cell-cycle specific drugs to target mitotically active cells and cell-cycle nonspecific agents to kill both cycling and noncycling tumor cells (see Chapter 39).

The mitotoxicity hypothesis of anticancer therapy leaves some puzzles unresolved, however. Although cancer chemotherapy is often toxic to the bone marrow, gastrointestinal mucosa, and hair follicles, these tissues usually recover while (in successful treatment) cancers with similar growth kinetics are eradicated. *It has now been established that almost all chemotherapeutic drugs also cause apoptosis of cancer cells.* DNA damage is normally sensed by molecules, such as p53, that arrest the cell cycle in order to allow time for the damage to be repaired. If the damage is not repaired, a cascade of biochemical events is triggered, which results in **apoptosis** (programmed cell death). Therefore, a cancer cell that has a defective capability for DNA repair may undergo apoptosis, whereas a normal cell can repair its DNA and recover. Cancers that express wild-type p53, such as most leukemias, lymphomas, and testicular cancers, are often highly responsive to chemotherapy. In contrast, cancers that acquire a mutation in p53, including many pancreatic, lung, and colon cancers, are often minimally responsive or even resistant to DNA-damaging drugs.

Log Cell Kill Model

The **log cell kill model** is based on experimentally observed rates of tumor growth and tumor regression in response to chemotherapy. Tumor growth is typically exponential, with a doubling time (i.e., time required for the total number of cancer cells to double) that depends on the type of cancer. For example, testicular cancer often has a doubling time of less than 1 month, whereas colon cancer tends to double every 3 months. In solid tumors, the cancer may grow exponentially until a clinically observable tumor size is achieved. (Typically, a newly detected 1-cm tumor contains about 10^9 cells.) *The log cell kill model states that the cell destruction caused by cancer chemotherapy is first-order; that is, that*

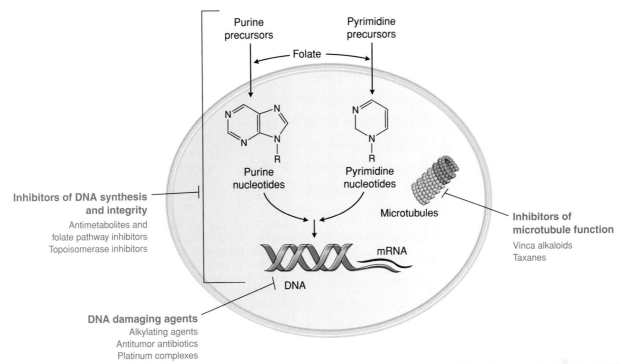

Figure 31-3. Antineoplastic drug classes. Many cancer cells divide more frequently than normal cells, and cancer cells can often be killed preferentially by targeting three critical processes in cell growth and division. DNA damaging agents alter the structure of DNA and thereby promote apoptosis of the cell. These drugs include alkylating agents (which covalently couple alkyl groups to nucleophilic sites on DNA), antitumor antibiotics (which cause free radical damage to DNA), and platinum complexes (which crosslink DNA). Inhibitors of DNA synthesis and integrity block intermediate steps in DNA synthesis; these agents include antimetabolites and folate pathway inhibitors (which inhibit purine and pyrimidine metabolism) and topoisomerase inhibitors (which induce damage to DNA during winding and unwinding). Inhibitors of microtubule function interfere with the mitotic spindle that is required for cell division. This group of drugs includes vinca alkaloids, which inhibit microtubule polymerization, and taxanes, which stabilize polymerized microtubules. Additional classes of antineoplastic agents—such as hormones, tumor-specific monoclonal antibodies, growth factor receptor antagonists, signal transduction inhibitors, proteasome inhibitors, and angiogenesis inhibitors—are not shown.

each dose of chemotherapy kills a constant fraction of cells. If the tumor starts with 10^{12} cells and 99.99% are killed, then 10^{8} malignant cells will remain. The next dose of chemotherapy will then kill 99.99% of the remaining cells, and so on. Unlike antibacterial drugs, which can often be used in a constant high dose until the bacteria are eradicated, most antineoplastic drugs must be used intermittently to reduce toxic side effects. Intermittent dosing allows partial recovery of normal cells, but also provides time for cancer cell regrowth and for evolution of drug resistance. As shown in Figure 31-5, intermittent ''cycles'' of chemotherapy are administered until all the cancer cells are killed or the tumor develops resistance. Drug-resistant cells continue to grow exponentially despite treatment, eventually resulting in death of the host. Improvements in the rates of eradication of malignant cell populations are likely to require either higher doses of chemotherapeutic agents (which are limited by toxicity and resistance) or initiation of therapy at a time when the tumor contains fewer cells (which implies earlier detection). Adjuvant therapies, such as surgery and radiation, are other important modalities used to reduce the number of tumor cells before chemotherapy is initiated. Surgery and radiation may also recruit more tumor cells into the cell cycle and thus increase the susceptibility of these cells to cell-cycle–specific agents.

MECHANISMS OF DRUG RESISTANCE

Having provided a general introduction to the pharmacology of drug targets in bacteria, fungi, parasites, viruses, and cancer, the discussion now turns to the mechanisms of drug resistance, which is a major problem in all of antimicrobial and antineoplastic pharmacology. Although resistance to current drug therapies is emerging relatively rapidly, the rate of introduction of new drugs (especially antimicrobial drugs) is relatively slow. Formerly curable diseases such as gonorrhea and typhoid fever are becoming more difficult to treat, and old killers such as tuberculosis and malaria are growing increasingly resistant worldwide. The WHO estimates that 99% of gonorrhea isolates in China are multidrug resistant. In the United States, 60% of hospital-acquired (nosocomial) infections due to Gram-positive bacteria are caused by drug-resistant microbes. Tuberculosis, the fourth leading cause of infectious disease deaths worldwide, currently has an estimated 2% overall multidrug resistance (MDR) rate, although the rate is as high as 10% to 30% in some central Asian countries such as Uzbekistan and Turkmenistan. The recent appearance of MDR tuberculosis in the United States is of special concern because of the airborne spread of this organ-

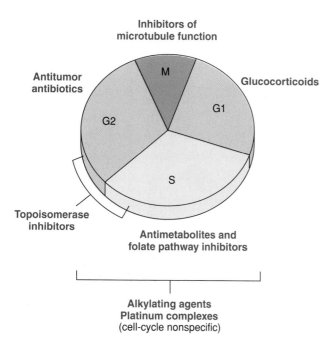

Figure 31-4. Cell-cycle specificity of antineoplastic drug classes. The cell cycle is divided into four phases. Cell division into two identical daughter cells occurs during mitosis (M phase). Cells then enter the gap 1 (G1) phase, which is characterized by active metabolism in the absence of DNA synthesis. Cells replicate their DNA during the synthesis (S) phase. After completion of S phase, the cell prepares for mitosis during the gap 2 (G2) phase. Antineoplastic drugs exhibit specificity for different phases of the cell cycle, depending on their mechanism of action. Inhibitors of microtubule function affect cells in M phase; glucocorticoids inhibit cells in G1; antimetabolites and folate pathway inhibitors inhibit cells in S phase; antitumor antibiotics inhibit cells in G2; topoisomerase inhibitors inhibit cells in S phase and G2. Alkylating agents and platinum complexes affect cell function in all phases and are therefore cell-cycle nonspecific. The differential cell-cycle specificity of the various drug classes allows them to be used in combination to target different populations of cells. For example, cell-cycle–specific drugs can be administered to target actively replicating neoplastic cells, whereas cell-cycle nonspecific agents can be used to target quiescent (non-replicating) neoplastic cells.

ism. Despite these ominous trends, only three new classes of antibiotics—oxazolidinones, streptogramins, and dapto-mycin—have been developed in the past 3 decades. The numerous examples of rapidly emerging drug-resistant organisms suggest that this problem must be addressed promptly.

Because pathogens and cancer cells are primed to evolve rapidly in response to adaptive pressure, resistance can eventually appear with the use of any antimicrobial or antineoplastic drug. In a population of microbes or transformed cells, the cells that contain random mutations promoting fitness will survive. Thus, high cell number, rapid growth rate, and high mutation rate all promote the development of a heterogeneous population of cells that can acquire resistance through mutational escape. Because the use of a drug inherently selects for organisms that can survive in the presence of high concentrations of that drug, resistance is an omnipresent consequence of drug therapy. In many cases, the emergence of drug resistance confounds effective treatment.

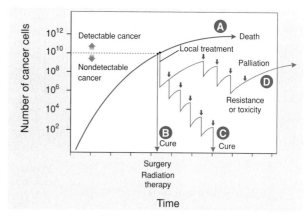

Figure 31-5. Log cell kill model of tumor growth and regression. The log cell kill model predicts that the effects of antineoplastic chemotherapy can be modeled as a first-order process. That is, a given dose of drug kills a constant *fraction* of tumor cells, and the number of cells killed depends on the total number of cells remaining. The four curves (*A–D*) represent four possible outcomes of antineoplastic therapy. *Curve A* is the growth curve of untreated cancer. The cancer continues to grow over time, eventually resulting in the death of the patient. *Curve B* represents curative local treatment (surgery and/or radiation therapy) before metastatic spread of the malignancy. *Curve C* represents local treatment of the primary tumor, followed immediately by systemic chemotherapy administered in cycles (*down arrows*) to eradicate the remaining metastatic cancer cells. Note that each cycle of chemotherapy reduces the number of cancer cells by a constant fraction (here, by about two "logs," or by about 99%), and that some cancer growth occurs as the normal tissues are given time to recover between cycles of chemotherapy. *Curve D* represents local treatment followed by systemic chemotherapy that fails when the tumor becomes resistant to the drugs or when toxic drug effects occur that are intolerable to the patient. Note that 10^9 to 10^{10} cancer cells must typically be present for a tumor to be detectable; for this reason, multiple cycles of chemotherapy are required to eradicate the cancer, even when there is no detectable tumor remaining.

GENETIC CAUSES OF DRUG RESISTANCE

The recent explosion in drug resistance has both genetic and nongenetic causes. Genetic mechanisms of resistance arise from chromosomal mutations and from exchange of genetic material. Chromosomal mutations typically occur in the gene(s) that code(s) for the drug target or in genes that code for drug transport or metabolism systems. These mutations can then be transferred to daughter cells (**vertical transmission**) to create drug-resistant organisms. Alternatively, bacteria can acquire resistance by gaining genetic material from other bacteria (**horizontal transmission**). For example, methicillin-resistant *Staphylococcus aureus* (MRSA) and vancomycin-resistant enterococcus (VRE) are able to cause highly feared nosocomial infections because these bacteria have acquired resistance genes. Bacteria acquire genetic material by three main mechanisms: conjugation, transduction, and transformation. In **conjugation,** chromosomal or plasmid DNA is transferred directly between bacteria. DNA can also be transferred from one cell to another by a bacterial virus, or bacteriophage, in a process called **transduction.** In **transformation,** naked DNA in the environment is taken up by the bacteria. Drug resistance is most often caused by the transfer of plasmids, which are extrachromosomal strands of DNA that contain drug resistance genes.

Transfer of a DNA plasmid is especially important for drug resistance because this mechanism occurs at high rates both within and between bacterial species, and because multidrug resistance genes can be transferred. Specific mechanisms of resistance for each type of organism are discussed in subsequent chapters. Table 31-2 lists the major mechanisms of genetic drug resistance that can be caused by either chromosomal mutation or genetic exchange.

Reduced Intracellular Drug Concentration

Drugs must reach their targets in order to be effective. When an insufficient amount of drug reaches the target, the growth of pathogens or tumor cells and the emergence of resistant strains are allowed. Microbes and tumor cells have evolved a number of mechanisms to *inactivate drugs* before the drugs can bind to their targets. Many bacteria are resistant to penicillins and cephalosporins because they produce a hydrolytic enzyme, **β-lactamase**, which cleaves the β-lactam ring and thereby disables the drug's active site. A single β-lactamase enzyme can hydrolyze 10^3 penicillin molecules per second, significantly reducing the intracellular concentration of active drug. As another example, tumor cells that overexpress a deaminase enzyme can rapidly inactivate purine or pyrimidine analogues (antimetabolites), making these drugs less effective.

Pathogens and cancer cells can also acquire mutations that *prevent uptake of the drug* into the cell or otherwise prevent access of the drug to the target molecule. For example, cancer cells with mutated folate-transport systems become resistant to folate analogues, such as **methotrexate**, that require active transport into cells in order to inhibit DHFR.

Finally, both bacteria and tumor cells can acquire the ability to cause active *drug efflux* from the cell. Bacteria typically possess membrane pumps to transport lipophilic or amphipathic molecules (such as antibiotics) in and out of the cells. Overproduction of these membrane proteins or their variants can mediate active pumping of a therapeutic antibiotic out of the cell faster than the drug can enter the cell.

Despite the achievement of therapeutic blood levels of the antibiotic, this active efflux mechanism can cause intrabacterial drug concentrations to be ineffectively low. Similarly, the emergence of multidrug resistant (MDR) cancers is often associated with tumor cell overexpression of a membrane-bound glycoprotein, the **P-glycoprotein** (p170 or MDR1), which actively pumps antineoplastic drugs out of the cell. These efflux pumps are especially important because they are capable of pumping out more than one type of drug, thus allowing pathogens or tumors to become resistant to multiple drugs of different classes.

Altered Target

In addition to destroying drugs chemically or pumping out drugs, cells can also reprogram or camouflage drug targets. Alteration in the target of a drug through mutation of the gene(s) that codes for that target is a common mechanism for development of drug resistance. In vancomycin-resistant enterococcus, the vanHAX genes encode a novel enzymatic pathway that reprograms the surface peptidoglycan so as to terminate in the sequence D-Ala-D-Lactate instead of the normal D-Ala-D-Ala. This substitution does not affect the peptidoglycan crosslinking process in bacterial cell wall synthesis, but it does lower the binding affinity of **vancomycin** for the dipeptide by 1,000-fold. In cancer cells, both quantitative and qualitative changes in the enzyme targets of antineoplastic drugs—such as DHFR, thymidylate synthase, and topoisomerase—can reduce drug binding (potency) and thereby confer drug resistance.

Insensitivity to Apoptosis

Drug resistance in cancer cells occurs through chromosomal mutations that are then passed to daughter cells to create a resistant tumor. Although cytotoxic anticancer drugs act at a variety of molecular targets, most, if not all, ultimately cause cell death by inducing apoptosis. In general, drug-induced **molecular lesions** can lead to cell-cycle arrest, activation of repair processes, or apoptosis. Mutations in key proteins associated with the control of apoptosis, such as p53 and Bcl-2, can result in failure to induce the apoptotic

---

TABLE 31-2 **Mechanisms of Genetic Drug Resistance**

MECHANISM	EXAMPLE: ANTIMICROBIAL	EXAMPLE: ANTINEOPLASTIC
Reduced Intracellular Concentration of Drug		
Inactivate drug	Inactivation of β-lactam antibiotics by β-lactamase	Inactivation of antimetabolites by deaminase
Prevent uptake of drug	Prevention of aminoglycoside entry by altered porins	Decreased methotrexate entry by decreased expression of reduced folate carrier
Promote efflux of drug	Efflux of multiple drugs by MDR membrane efflux pump	Efflux of multiple drugs by p170 membrane efflux pump (MDR1)
Altered Drug Target	Expression of altered peptidoglycan that no longer binds vancomycin	Expression of mutant DHFR that no longer binds methotrexate
Insensitivity to Apoptosis	Not applicable	Loss of active p53
Bypass Metabolic Requirement for Target	Inhibition of thymidylate synthase bypassed by exogenous thymidine	Loss of estrogen receptor-dependent growth results in tamoxifen resistance

response to DNA damage and can thereby reduce the sensitivity of tumor cells to anticancer drugs. As noted above, tumors with wild-type p53, such as many leukemias, lymphomas, and testicular cancers, are often highly responsive to chemotherapy. In contrast, many pancreatic, lung, and colon cancers have a high incidence of p53 mutations and are minimally responsive to chemotherapy.

Thus, the genetic causes of drug resistance include both mutations in chromosomal DNA and external acquisition of genetic material. Genetic resistance can be caused by drug inactivation, decreased drug uptake, increased drug efflux, reprogramming of the target structure or pathway, repair of drug-induced lesions, and insensitivity to apoptosis. Resistance is probably the major limiting factor in the effective treatment of both infections and cancer. Drug therapy is a dynamic balance, an ''evolutionary arms race,'' between the design of new drugs and the evolution of changes leading to drug resistance.

NONGENETIC CAUSES OF TREATMENT FAILURE

The treatment of an infection or cancer can fail for numerous reasons. One of the most important mechanisms of drug resistance is the excessive overprescription of antibiotics that are not indicated for the clinical situation. Overprescription is a problem not only in humans, but also in the treatment and prophylaxis of animal infections. Such widespread use promotes drug resistance, which is then transferred from one bacterium to another by the mechanisms described above. Other mechanisms of resistance involve pharmacologic and anatomic drug barriers, such as the wall of an abscess or the blood-brain barrier. Poor patient compliance can also promote resistance, as can the erratic drug availability found in parts of the developing world (and even in some communities in the developed world). International travel promotes a global disease community, ensuring that the multidrug-resistant tuberculosis found in Russia or Peru will eventually emerge in hospitals in the United States. Finally, demographic shifts and other trends have created large susceptible populations, such as immunocompromised cancer patients, AIDS patients, and the elderly population.

METHODS OF TREATMENT

COMBINATION CHEMOTHERAPY

The development of drug resistance depends on such factors as the number of microbial or tumor cells in the pretreatment population, the rate of replication or ''generation time'' of the pathogenic cell population, and the intrinsic rate of mutation in the population. Compared to treatment with a single agent, treatment with a combination of drugs can significantly decrease the probability that resistance will develop. Combination chemotherapy is now the standard-of-care in HIV therapy and most antineoplastic drug regimens. There are several major reasons to administer multiple drugs simultaneously in a combination chemotherapy regimen; the ra-

tionales are discussed in further detail in Chapter 39. First, the use of multiple drugs with different mechanisms of action targets multiple steps in microbial or cancer cell growth, leading to the maximum possible rate of cell killing. Second, the use of combinations of drugs that target different pathways or molecules in the pathogen or cancer cell makes it more difficult for the foreign cell to become resistant to the therapy. Even if the likelihood of development of a resistance mutation to one drug is relatively high, the concurrent emergence of separate mutations against several different drugs is less likely. Third, the use of lower doses of synergistically acting drugs in the combination can reduce drug-associated adverse effects. This is especially important in antimicrobial chemotherapy, where synergistic activity of drug combinations has been clearly demonstrated. Fourth, because many antineoplastic drugs have different dose-limiting adverse effects, it is often possible to give each drug to its maximally tolerated dose, and thereby achieve increased overall cell killing. Finally, the concept of combination chemotherapy is being redefined as new treatments become available. In the future, immunotherapies, hormone therapies, and biotherapies will become increasingly integrated into combination chemotherapy regimens (see Chapter 53, Protein-Based Therapies).

PROPHYLACTIC CHEMOTHERAPEUTICS

In most instances, antimicrobial and antineoplastic drugs are used to treat overt disease. These classes of drugs can also be used to prevent diseases from occurring (chemoprophylaxis), both before a potential exposure and after a known exposure. The potential benefit of chemoprophylaxis must always be weighed against the risk of creating drug-resistant pathogens or cancer cells and the potential for toxicity attributable to the chemoprophylactic agent. Antimicrobial chemoprophylaxis is frequently used in high-risk patients to prevent infection. Travelers to malaria-infested areas, for example, often take prophylactic antimalarial drugs such as mefloquine (see Chapter 35). Chemoprophylaxis is also used in some types of surgery to prevent wound infections. Antibiotics are commonly administered prophylactically during surgical procedures that could release bacteria into the wound site, such as colon resection. Antibiotics are also used prophylactically before dental procedures in patients at high risk for endocarditis, because such procedures can produce a transient bacteremia. In certain situations, immunocompromised patients are given antibacterial, antifungal, antiviral, and/or antiparasitic drugs prophylactically to prevent opportunistic infections. For example, **acyclovir** can protect previously infected immunocompromised patients against disease caused by reactivation of latent herpes simplex virus.

Chemoprophylaxis or pre-emptive therapy can also be used in healthy persons after exposures to certain pathogens. Prophylactic therapy after known or suspected exposure to gonorrhea, syphilis, bacterial meningitis, HIV, and other infections can often prevent disease. The risk of seroconversion after a single needle stick exposure to HIV-infected blood ranges from 0.1% to 4.5%, depending on the type of exposure. Although limited data are available regarding the reduction of risk achievable with prophylaxis, the Centers for Disease Control and Prevention (CDC) currently recommends postexposure treatment with a two- or three-drug anti-retroviral therapy regimen (e.g., **zidovudine** (AZT) and **lamivudine** (3TC) or AZT, 3TC, and **lopinavir/ritonavir**) for 4 weeks. Zidovudine has also been shown to reduce maternal transmission of HIV, representing chemoprophylaxis for the fetus (see Chapter 36).

INHIBITORS OF FOLATE METABOLISM: EXAMPLES OF SELECTIVE TARGETING AND SYNERGISTIC DRUG INTERACTIONS

Folic acid is a vitamin that participates in a number of enzymatic reactions involving the transfer of one-carbon units. These reactions are essential for the biosynthesis of DNA and RNA precursors, the amino acids glycine, methionine, and glutamic acid, the formyl-methionine initiator tRNA, and other essential metabolites. Given the importance of folate metabolism in the biochemistry of the cell, it is not surprising that inhibition of folate biosynthesis and interference with the folate cycle have been used widely in the treatment of bacterial infections, parasitic infections, and cancer.

FOLATE METABOLISM

The structure of folic acid contains three chemical moieties (Fig. 31-6A): a pteridine ring system, **para-aminobenzoic acid** (PABA), and the amino acid glutamate. (Because of its ability to absorb UV light, PABA is the active ingredient in many topical sunscreens.) For humans, folate is an essential vitamin that must be provided intact in the diet. In lower organisms, however, folate is synthesized from precursors, as shown in Figure 31-7.

Both dietary folate and folate synthesized from precursors enter the folate cycle (Fig. 31-7). In this cycle, dihydrofolate is reduced to tetrahydrofolate by dihydrofolate reductase (DHFR). Tetrahydrofolate then enters the many metabolic interconversions that involve one-carbon transfers. For example, congeners of tetrahydrofolate are essential donors of carbon atoms in the synthesis of inosine monophosphate (IMP) (leading to adenosine monophosphate [AMP] and guanosine monophosphate [GMP]) and in the conversion of deoxyuridine monophosphate (dUMP) to deoxythymidine monophosphate (dTMP) (see Fig. 37-2). In all of these reactions, tetrahydrofolate congeners donate a carbon atom and, in the process, are oxidized to dihydrofolate. For further rounds of nucleotide synthesis to occur, the dihydrofolate must be reduced to tetrahydrofolate by DHFR.

INHIBITORS OF FOLATE METABOLISM

Antimetabolites can be divided into inhibitors of folate metabolism, inhibitors of purine metabolism, inhibitors of ribonucleotide reductase, and nucleotide analogues that are incorporated into DNA. This chapter uses the **inhibitors of folate metabolism** to exemplify the basis for selective targeting of antimicrobial and antineoplastic drugs according

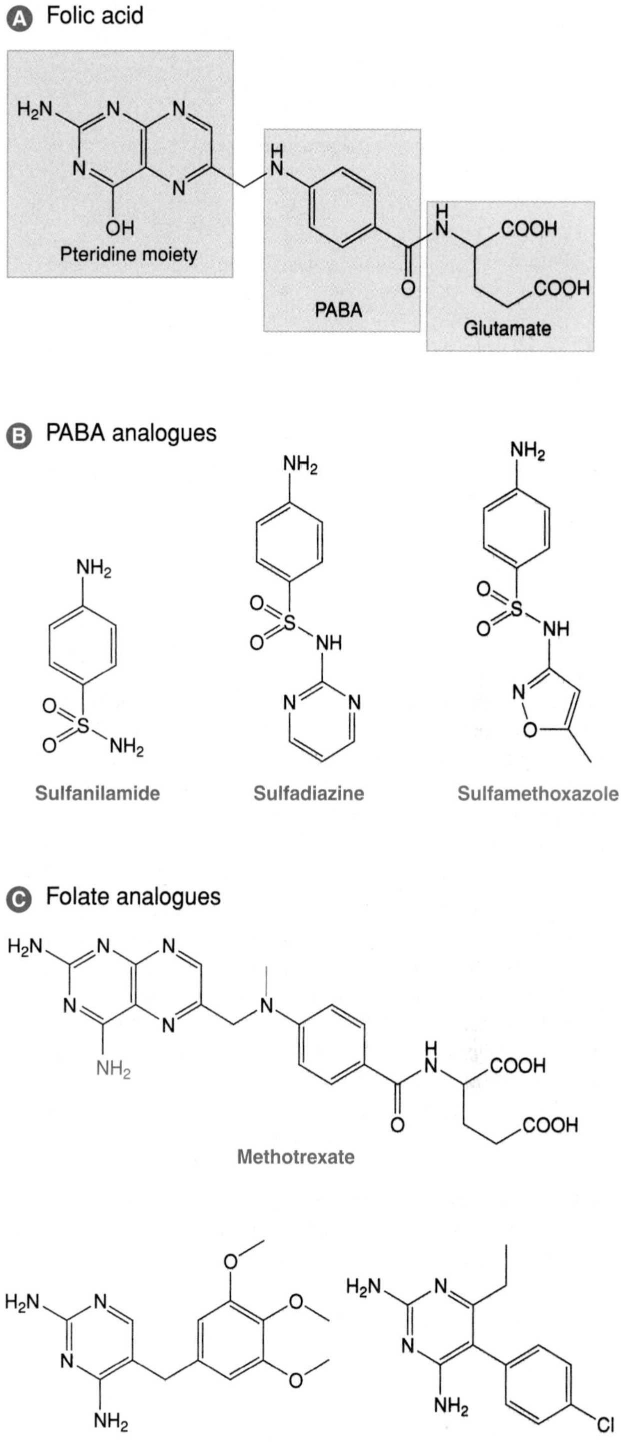

Figure 31-6. Structures of folic acid, PABA analogues (sulfonamides), and folate analogues (dihydrofolate reductase inhibitors). A. Folic acid is formed by the condensation of pteridine, para-aminobenzoic acid (PABA), and glutamate (see Fig. 31-7). Folate is the deprotonated form of folic acid. **B.** PABA analogues (sulfonamides) structurally resemble PABA. These drugs inhibit dihydropteroate synthase, the enzyme that catalyzes the formation of dihydropteroic acid from PABA and pteridine (see Fig. 31-7). **C.** Folate analogues (dihydrofolate reductase inhibitors) structurally resemble folic acid. These drugs inhibit dihydrofolate reductase, the enzyme that converts dihydrofolate to tetrahydrofolate.

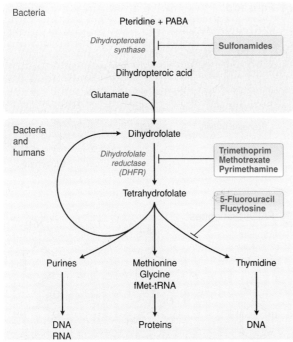

Figure 31-7. Folate synthesis and functions. Folate synthesis begins with the formation of dihydropteroic acid from pteridine and para-aminobenzoic acid (PABA); this reaction is catalyzed by dihydropteroate synthase. Glutamate and dihydropteroic acid condense to form dihydrofolate (DHF). DHF is reduced to tetrahydrofolate (THF) by dihydrofolate reductase (DHFR). THF and its congeners *(not shown)* serve as one-carbon donors in numerous reactions necessary for the formation of DNA, RNA, and proteins. In each such reaction, the reduced folate *(THF)* becomes oxidized to DHF, and the THF must then be regenerated via reduction by DHFR. Inhibitors of folate metabolism target three steps in the folate pathway. Sulfonamides inhibit dihydropteroate synthase; trimethoprim, methotrexate, and pyrimethamine inhibit DHFR; 5-fluorouracil (5-FU) and flucytosine inhibit thymidylate synthase (see Fig. 37-4). Note that bacteria synthesize folate de novo from pteridine and PABA, whereas humans require dietary folate.

to the relative uniqueness of the drug target. (The other antimetabolite drug classes are discussed in Chapter 37.) As described above, selectivity can take the form of: (1) a genetic or biochemical pathway that is unique to the pathogen or cancer cell; (2) a structure (isoform) of a protein that is unique to the pathogen or cancer cell; or (3) a metabolic requirement that is unique to the pathogen or cancer cell. Where relevant, the following discussion emphasizes the basis for selectivity of each therapeutic agent.

Inhibitors of folate metabolism include inhibitors of dihydropteroate synthase and inhibitors of dihydrofolate reductase. In each case, drugs that structurally resemble the physiologic substrate of the enzyme act as enzyme inhibitors.

Unique Drug Targets: Antimicrobial Dihydropteroate Synthase Inhibitors

Bacteria are unable to take up folic acid from the environment and therefore must synthesize the vitamin de novo from PABA, pteridine, and glutamate (Fig. 31-7). Mammalian

cells, in contrast, use folate receptors and folate carriers in the plasma membrane to scavenge the intact vitamin. This fundamental metabolic difference between pathogen and host cells makes dihydropteroate synthase an ideal target for antibacterial therapy. The **sulfa** drugs, such as **sulfamethoxazole** and **sulfadiazine,** are PABA analogues that competitively inhibit dihydropteroate synthase and thereby prevent the synthesis of folic acid in bacteria. The lack of folic acid, in turn, prevents bacterial synthesis of purines, pyrimidines, and some amino acids, and eventually results in cessation of bacterial growth. Sulfa drugs are bacteriostatic because they prevent bacterial growth but do not kill the bacteria. There are two structural classes of sulfa drugs, sulfonamides and sulfones.

Sulfonamides and Sulfones

As demonstrated in the case of Hildegard Domagk, **sulfonamides** were the first modern agents to be employed in the treatment of bacterial infections (prontosil is a sulfonamide precursor). Figure 31-6 shows the similarity in structure between PABA and the sulfonamide analogues **sulfanilamide, sulfadiazine,** and **sulfamethoxazole.** Sulfonamides are highly selective drugs, because bacterial growth requires activity of the enzyme that is inhibited by the sulfonamides, whereas mammalian cells do not even express this enzyme. Therefore, mammalian cells are essentially unaffected by the sulfonamides, and the use of these drugs is relatively free of adverse effects (except in the special case of neonates, noted below).

Despite the exquisite selectivity of the sulfonamides, the development of resistance to these drugs has resulted in their diminished use. Resistance to sulfonamides can develop because of: (1) overproduction of the endogenous substrate, PABA, by bacteria exposed to sulfonamides; (2) a mutation in the PABA binding site on dihydropteroate synthase, resulting in reduced affinity of the enzyme for sulfonamides; or (3) decreased permeability of the bacterial membrane to sulfonamides. Some resistant streptococci produce levels of PABA that are 70-fold greater than the normal value. Decreased membrane permeability to sulfonamides can be conferred by bacterial transfer of a resistance plasmid.

Because of the high incidence of sulfonamide resistance in the bacterial population, these drugs are rarely administered as single agents. Instead, they are commonly administered in combination with a synergistic drug such as **trimethoprim** or **pyrimethamine,** as discussed below.

Sulfonamides compete with bilirubin for binding sites on serum albumin and can cause kernicterus in newborns. **Kernicterus,** the condition characterized by markedly elevated concentrations of unconjugated (free) bilirubin in the blood of neonates, can lead to severe brain damage. For this reason, newborns should not be treated with sulfonamides.

Dapsone, a member of the **sulfone** class of dihydropteroate synthase inhibitors, is used in the treatment of leprosy and *Pneumocystis carinii* pneumonia. Because the mechanism of action of dapsone is the same as that of the sulfonamides, dapsone and trimethoprim or pyrimethamine can also be used as a synergistic drug combination (see discussion below). One relatively common adverse effect of dapsone is that about 5% of patients develop **methemoglobinemia** after administration of the drug. Susceptible patients are typically deficient in the erythrocyte enzyme glucose-6-phosphate dehydrogenase, which is involved in the detoxification of endogenous and exogenous oxidizing agents (such as dapsone).

Selective Inhibition of Similar Targets: Antimicrobial Dihydrofolate Reductase Inhibitors

Dihydrofolate reductase (DHFR) is the enzyme that reduces dihydrofolate (DHF) to tetrahydrofolate (THF). Several drugs, including **trimethoprim, pyrimethamine,** and **methotrexate,** are folate analogues that competitively inhibit DHFR and prevent the regeneration of THF from DHF (Figs. 31-6 and 31-7). By doing so, these drugs prevent the synthesis of purine nucleotides as well as the methylation of dUMP to dTMP (see above). Pharmacologic inhibition of DHFR is used both in the treatment of infection and in cancer chemotherapy.

Many inhibitors of DHFR have been developed. As shown in Table 31-3, **methotrexate** is a potent (subnanomolar) inhibitor of DHFR, although it exhibits little selectivity among the mammalian, bacterial, and protozoal isoforms of the enzyme. In contrast, inhibitors with structures that are more divergent from that of folate, such as **trimethoprim** and **pyrimethamine** (see Fig. 31-6), show considerable selectivity of DHFR inhibition among the various isoforms of the enzyme. Thus, trimethoprim is a potent and selective antibacterial agent, whereas pyrimethamine is a potent and selective antimalarial drug.

Why are trimethoprim and pyrimethamine each selective for one particular isoform of DHFR, while methotrexate is not? The amino acid sequences of DHFR enzymes from many species have been determined, and these sequences vary greatly among the bacteria, protozoans, and humans. In contrast, the substrates of DHFR, dihydrofolate and NADPH, have not changed at all over the course of evolution. Nonetheless, all of the various enzyme isoforms can efficiently catalyze the reduction of DHF to THF. (Similar observations have been made for many enzymes, including glycolytic enzymes.) This implies that there are many ways to encode a protein containing the binding sites and conformational flexibility required for catalysis. The basis for selectivity must therefore reside in differences in enzyme structure that are largely irrelevant for binding of the natural substrates, but that have an important role in analogue (drug) binding. Correspondingly, the very close structural resemblance between methotrexate (MTX) and the normal substrate dihydrofolate (see Fig. 31-6) may explain why MTX exhibits little selectivity for DHFR isoforms across a wide range of species, whereas the more divergent structures of trimethoprim and pyrimethamine are associated with higher selectivity of isoform binding and inhibition. Increased understanding of the molecular basis for DHFR inhibition may lead to the development of still more selective agents (see Box 31-1).

Trimethoprim

Trimethoprim is a folate analogue that selectively inhibits bacterial DHFR (Fig. 31-6C; Table 31-3) and thereby prevents the conversion of DHF to THF. As with the sulfonamides, trimethoprim is bacteriostatic. Because trimethoprim is excreted unchanged in the urine, it can be used as a single agent to treat uncomplicated urinary tract infections. For most infections, however, trimethoprim is used in combination with sulfamethoxazole. The rationale for this combination antibacterial chemotherapy is described below.

Pyrimethamine

Pyrimethamine is a folate analogue that selectively inhibits parasitic DHFR (Fig. 31-6C; Table 31-3). Pyrimethamine is currently the only effective chemotherapeutic agent against toxoplasmosis; for this indication, it is typically administered in combination with sulfadiazine. Pyrimethamine has also been used to treat malaria, although widespread resistance has limited its effectiveness in recent years. Further discussion of the therapeutic applications of pyrimethamine and sulfadiazine can be found in Chapter 35.

Common Targets: Antineoplastic Dihydrofolate Reductase Inhibitors

Methotrexate

As described above, **methotrexate (MTX)** is a folate analogue that reversibly inhibits DHFR. In mammalian cells, DHFR inhibition causes a critical shortage of intracellular supplies of tetrahydrofolate, resulting in cessation of de novo purine and thymidylate synthesis and, therefore, cessation of DNA and RNA synthesis. Because the synthesis of DNA is halted, mammalian cells treated with methotrexate are arrested in the S phase of the cell cycle.

The basis for the relative selectivity of methotrexate for cancer cells compared to normal cells is thought to be that rapidly growing cancer cells have an increased requirement for the various compounds that depend on folate intermediates, especially those (such as purines and thymidylate) required for DNA synthesis. In addition, malignant cells may be more susceptible than normal cells to the apoptosis-inducing effects of MTX (see discussion below). The use of high-dose MTX in cancer chemotherapy has been broadened by the application of **folinic acid rescue.** In this technique, folinic acid (N-5 formyltetrahydrofolate, also called **leuko-vorin**) is administered to the patient several hours after an otherwise lethal dose of methotrexate. The rationale for this

TABLE 31-3	IC$_{50}$ Values for Three Dihydrofolate Reductase Inhibitors		
	DHFR ISOFORM		
DHFR INHIBITOR	**_E. coli_ DHFR**	**MALARIAL DHFR**	**MAMMALIAN DHFR**
Trimethoprim	7	1,800	350,000
Pyrimethamine	2,500	0.5	1,800
Methotrexate	0.1	0.7	0.2

All values are reported in nM (10^{-9} M) units. Trimethoprim and pyrimethamine are selective inhibitors of the _E. coli_ and malarial isoforms of DHFR, respectively. In contrast, methotrexate is a nonselective inhibitor of all three DHFR isoforms. DHFR, dihydrofolate reductase. IC$_{50}$, concentration required for 50% enzyme inhibition.

technique is that the malignant cells are killed selectively, while the normal cells are "rescued" by the folinic acid. The molecular explanation for the effectiveness of folinic acid rescue is unclear. One hypothesis suggests that normal (nonmalignant) cells are able to concentrate the folinic acid (and, thus, to protect themselves from the effects of MTX), whereas malignant cells have a reduced rate of folinic acid transport (and, therefore, are preferentially harmed by high doses of MTX). Another hypothesis suggests that high-dose MTX induces apoptosis in malignant cells but cell-cycle arrest in normal cells; the normal cells are then able to use the folinic acid to resume cell growth and division, while the malignant cells are already committed to programmed cell death.

MTX is used to treat many tumor types, including carcinomas of the breast, lung, head and neck, acute lymphoblastic leukemia, and choriocarcinoma. MTX can also be used to treat psoriasis, certain autoimmune diseases, and early stage ectopic pregnancy. Methotrexate toxicity is manifested primarily in rapidly dividing host cells, causing damage to the gastrointestinal mucosa and the bone marrow. These effects are generally reversible after therapy is discontinued. MTX is extremely toxic to the fetus, because folic acid is essential for the proper differentiation of fetal cells and for closure of the neural tube. MTX has recently undergone clinical trials as an abortion-inducing agent, either alone or in combination with the prostaglandin analogue **misoprostol.**

Synergy of DHFR Inhibitors and Sulfonamides

Both trimethoprim and pyrimethamine can be used in combination with sulfonamides to block sequential steps in the biosynthetic pathway leading to tetrahydrofolate (Fig. 31-7). This type of combination chemotherapy, called **sequential blockade,** has been effective in the treatment of parasitic infections (pyrimethamine and sulfadiazine) and bacterial infections (trimethoprim and sulfamethoxazole). One rationale for the use of a DHFR inhibitor and a sulfa drug in combination is the marked synergistic interaction between these two classes of drugs (see Chapter 39). The sulfonamide decreases the intracellular concentration of dihydrofolate; this increases the effectiveness of the DHFR inhibitor, which competes with dihydrofolate for binding to the enzyme. The sulfa/DHFR inhibitor combination can also be effective in treating strains of bacteria and parasites that exhibit resistance to monotherapy with a DHFR inhibitor. Typically, this drug resistance phenotype is caused by the expression of a structurally altered DHFR that has a lower affinity for the inhibitor. The tradeoff for the bacteria or parasite is that the altered DHFR also has a lower affinity for the natural ligand dihydrofolate. In such strains, sulfonamide treatment can decrease the intracellular concentration of dihydrofolate to the point that the altered DHFR cannot meet the metabolic requirements of the cell.

Another important rationale for the use of a combination such as trimethoprim/sulfamethoxazole is that resistance to trimethoprim alone or sulfamethoxazole alone develops rather quickly, whereas resistance to the drug combination develops much more slowly. Because the two drugs act on different enzymes, two different mutations would have to occur simultaneously for the bacteria to develop resistance to the drug combination. Compared to the rate of development of a single mutation, the likelihood that two mutations will occur simultaneously is much lower (see Chapter 39).

Conclusion and Future Directions

Many of the principles underlying the pharmacologic treatment of microbial diseases and cancer are similar. Pharmacologic treatments of both infection and cancer rely on selective inhibition of the pathogen or cancer cell to prevent its growth or survival, with a minimum of adverse effects that could interfere with host cell function. Selective inhibition of a unique target, such as the bacterial cell wall, is ideal. Often, less selective therapies, targeting a molecule or pathway that is similar or even identical between the pathogen or cancer cell and the host, must be employed. Even highly selective drugs aimed at an entirely unique target can be rendered ineffective if the microbe or cancer cell mutates to become resistant. Both microbes and cancer cells grow rapidly, with the potential for evolving or acquiring mutations that confer resistance. Physicians attempt to circumvent the development of resistance by initiating treatment early, using maximally tolerated doses of drugs, and administering multiple drugs in combination. Despite these strategies, however, resistance has become a major impediment to successful therapy. As more is learned about the biology of microbes and cancer cells, and more unique targets are discovered, it is hoped that treatments will become more selective, less toxic, and less prone to the development of drug resistance.

Suggested Reading

American Cancer Society Statistics. Available at http://www.cancer.org/docroot/STT/stt_0.asp. (*Source of cancer statistics provided in this chapter.*)

Antimicrobial Resistance Prevention Initiative: proceedings of an expert panel on resistance. *Am J Med* 2006;119(6 Suppl 1): S1–S76. (*Series of seven articles and discussion on current status and mechanisms of antimicrobial drug resistance.*)

Mandell GL, Bennett JE, Dolin R, eds. *Principles and Practice of Infectious Diseases.* 6th ed. Philadelphia: Churchill Livingstone Inc.; 2004. (*Authoritative textbook on clinical management of infectious diseases.*)

Moscow J, Morrow CS, Cowan KH. Drug resistance and its clinical circumvention. In: Kufe DW, Bast RC Jr, Hait W, et al, eds. *Holland-Frei Cancer Medicine.* 7th ed. Hamilton (Canada): BC Decker and American Association for Cancer Research; 2005. (*Discusses mechanisms of resistance to antineoplastic agents.*)

Okeke IN, Laxminarayan R, Bhutta ZA, et al. Antimicrobial resistance in developing countries. Part I: recent trends and current status. *Lancet Infect Dis* 2005;5:481–493. (*Documents rise of antimicrobial drug resistance in developing countries.*)

Walsh CT. *Antibiotics: Actions, Origins, Resistance.* Washington, DC: ASM Press; 2003. (*Reviews structural and chemical basis for drug resistance.*)

WHO Statistical Information System. Available at http://www.who.int/whosis/. (*Source of world health statistics provided in this chapter.*)

Drug Summary Table	**Chapter 31 Principles of Antimicrobial and Antineoplastic Pharmacology**			
Drug	**Clinical Applications**	**Serious and Common Adverse Effects**	**Contraindications**	**Therapeutic Considerations**
ANTIMICROBIAL DIHYDROPTEROATE SYNTHASE INHIBITORS				
Mechanism—PABA analogues that competitively inhibit microbial dihydropteroate synthase and thereby prevent the synthesis of folic acid				
Sulfonamides: Sulfanilamide Sulfadiazine Sulfamethoxazole Sulfadoxine (See Chapter 35) Sulfalene (See Chapter 35)	Susceptible vaginal infections (sulfanilamide) Toxoplasmosis (sulfadiazine) *Pneumocystis carinii* pneumonia, shigellosis, traveler's diarrhea, urinary tract infection, granuloma inguinale, acute otitis media (sulfamethoxazole/ trimethoprim)	*Kernicterus in newborns, crystalluria, Stevens-Johnson syndrome, agranulocytosis, aplastic anemia, hepatic failure* Gastrointestinal disturbance, rash	Infants less than 2 months old Pregnant women at term Breastfeeding Megaloblastic anemia due to folate deficiency	Because of the high incidence of sulfonamide resistance, sulfonamides are commonly administered in combination with a synergistic drug such as trimethoprim or pyrimethamine Sulfonamides compete with bilirubin for binding sites on serum albumin and can cause kernicterus in newborns Avoid coadministration with PABA, which is the natural substrate for dihydropteroate synthase
Sulfones: Dapsone	Leprosy Dermatitis herpetiformis *Pneumocystis carinii* pneumonia	*Hemolytic anemia, methemoglobinemia, toxic epidermal necrolysis, erythema nodosum, pancreatitis, toxic hepatitis, peripheral neuropathy* Abdominal pain	Glucose-6-phosphate dehydrogenase (G6PD) deficiency	Dapsone and trimethoprim or pyrimethamine can be used as a synergistic drug combination Patients susceptible to hemolytic anemia and methemoglobinemia are typically deficient in the erythrocyte enzyme G6PD
ANTIMICROBIAL DIHYDROFOLATE REDUCTASE INHIBITORS				
Mechanism—Folate analogues that competitively inhibit microbial dihydrofolate reductase (DHFR) and thereby prevent the regeneration of tetrahydrofolate from dihydrofolate				
Trimethoprim	Urinary tract infection See above for applications of sulfamethoxazole/ trimethoprim combination therapy	*Stevens-Johnson syndrome, leukopenia, megaloblastic anemia* Rash, pruritus	Megaloblastic anemia due to folate deficiency	Selectively inhibits bacterial DHFR Trimethoprim is bacteriostatic and can be used as a single agent to treat uncomplicated urinary tract infection Typically used in combination with sulfamethoxazole
Pyrimethamine	Toxoplasmosis Malaria	*Stevens-Johnson syndrome, leukopenia, megaloblastic anemia* Rash	Megaloblastic anemia due to folate deficiency	Selectively inhibits parasitic DHFR Typically used in combination with sulfadiazine for treatment of toxoplasmosis Folic acid may interfere with the efficacy of pyrimethamine

(Continued)

Drug Summary Table   Chapter 31 Principles of Antimicrobial and Antineoplastic Pharmacology (Continued)

ANTINEOPLASTIC DIHYDROFOLATE REDUCTASE INHIBITOR

Mechanism—Folate analogue that competitively inhibits mammalian DHFR and thereby prevents the regeneration of tetrahydrofolate from dihydrofolate

Drug	Clinical Applications	*Serious* and Common Adverse Effects	Contraindications	Therapeutic Considerations
Methotrexate	Many tumor types, including carcinomas of the breast, lung, head and neck; acute lymphoblastic leukemia; choriocarcinoma Autoimmune diseases including psoriasis, rheumatoid arthritis Early stage ectopic pregnancy	*Myelosuppression, liver failure, gastrointestinal hemorrhage, mucous membrane inflammation, hepatic cirrhosis, kidney disease, interstitial pulmonary disease, hyperuricemia* Gastrointestinal disturbance, stomatitis, alopecia, photosensitivity, rash	Pregnancy Breastfeeding Patients with psoriasis/rheumatoid arthritis who also have alcoholism, alcoholic liver disease, chronic liver disease, preexisting blood dyscrasia, or laboratory evidence of immunodeficiency syndrome	The use of high-dose methotrexate in cancer chemotherapy has been broadened by the application of folinic acid rescue Methotrexate toxicity to the gastrointestinal mucosa and bone marrow is generally reversible after therapy is discontinued Extremely toxic to the fetus because folic acid is essential for differentiation of fetal cells and for neural tube closure Under investigation as an abortion-inducing agent, either alone or in combination with the prostaglandin analogue misoprostol Avoid coadministration of polio vaccine in immunosuppressed patients receiving methotrexate as a component of chemotherapy Avoid concurrent alcohol intake Use extreme caution with coadministration of naproxen and phenylbutazone due to sporadic case reports of deaths Coadministration with trimethoprim may result in severe methotrexate toxicity Oral absorption of methotrexate can be decreased by up to 50% in patients receiving oral antibiotic mixtures containing paromomycin, neomycin, nystatin, and vancomycin

32

Pharmacology of Bacterial Infections: DNA Replication, Transcription, and Translation

Marvin Ryou and Donald M. Coen

INTRODUCTION

Fundamental biochemical differences between bacteria and humans are exploited for the development and clinical use of antibiotics. The central dogma processes—DNA replication, transcription, and translation—share many similarities between bacteria and humans. There are, however, important differences in the biochemistry of prokaryotic (i.e., bacterial) compared with eukaryotic (i.e., human) central dogma processes. Three such differences are targeted by antibacterial chemotherapeutic drugs: (1) *topoisomerases*, which regulate supercoiling of DNA and mediate segregation of replicated strands of DNA; (2) *RNA polymerases*, which transcribe DNA into RNA; and (3) *ribosomes*, which translate messenger RNA (mRNA) into protein.

Quinolone antibiotics are broad-spectrum agents; they not only inhibit certain topoisomerases but also convert these enzymes into DNA-damaging agents. Rifamycin derivatives bind to and inhibit bacterial RNA polymerase. (One such derivative, rifampin, is a mainstay in the therapy of tuberculosis.) A number of drugs bind bacterial ribosomes to inhibit protein synthesis. Specifically, aminoglycosides, tetracyclines, and spectinomycin bind the 30S ribosomal subunit, while macrolides, chloramphenicol, lincosamides, strepto-

gramins, and oxazolidinones target the 50S ribosomal subunit. These inhibitors of protein synthesis generally act on both Gram-positive and Gram-negative organisms and are therefore in wide clinical use (see Chapter 33 for a discussion of Gram-positive and Gram-negative bacteria). This chapter briefly reviews the biochemistry of central dogma processes in prokaryotes and discusses certain relevant differences between these processes in prokaryotes and eukaryotes. With this background, the chapter discusses the mechanisms by which pharmacologic inhibitors interrupt bacterial DNA replication, transcription, and translation.

Case

It is the summer of 1976. Participants returning from an American Legion convention in Philadelphia are falling severely ill with a mysterious type of pneumonia. The outbreak centers on the Bellevue Stratford Hotel, where 150 hotel occupants and 32 passersby contract "Legionnaires' disease." Twenty-nine victims ultimately die. Conventional sputum stains, cultures, and even autopsy material show no consistent pathogens. The terror of an unknown epidemic disease sparks rumors and news reports of poison gases, tainted water supplies, terrorists, and deadly viruses.

Several months later, laboratory and field investigation teams from the Centers for Disease Control and Prevention (CDC) identify the causative aerobic Gram-negative bacterium and name it *Legionella pneumophila*. It is observed that cases treated with erythromycin and tetracycline have better outcomes than those treated with other agents. Today, erythromycin and the other macrolides, clarithromycin and azithromycin, are often used for treating Legionnaires' disease—as well as many chlamydial, streptococcal, and staphylococcal infections.

QUESTIONS

■ **1.** Which steps in translation are blocked by tetracyclines and macrolides?
■ **2.** How do bacteria develop resistance to these drugs and to other inhibitors of transcription and translation?
■ **3.** Why are macrolides bacteriostatic, while some antibiotics, such as quinolones and aminoglycosides, are bactericidal?
■ **4.** Why are macrolides an effective treatment for Legionnaires' disease?

BIOCHEMISTRY OF PROKARYOTIC DNA REPLICATION, TRANSCRIPTION, AND TRANSLATION

The central dogma of molecular biology begins with the structure of DNA, which is the macromolecule that carries genetic information. To transmit all of the genetic information in a cell to two progeny cells, the parental DNA must be copied in its entirety (replicated), and the two resulting copies must be segregated—one copy going to each progeny cell. In order to express the genes that are embedded in the DNA, these specific portions of the DNA are copied (transcribed) into RNA. Some RNAs (mRNAs) are then read (translated) by the protein synthesis machinery in order to produce proteins. Other RNAs, such as transfer RNAs (tRNAs) and ribosomal RNAs (rRNAs), perform complex functions essential to protein synthesis. It is important to note that the following discussion of these prokaryotic processes is simplified to emphasize the steps that are inhibited by antibiotics.

DNA STRUCTURE

DNA is composed of two strands of polymerized deoxyribonucleotides that wind around one another in a "double helix" conformation. The 5'-hydroxyl group of each nucleotide's deoxyribose ring is joined by a phosphate group to the 3'-hydroxyl group of the next nucleotide, thereby forming the phosphodiester backbone of each side of the double helical "ladder" (Figs. 32-1 and 32-2). The purines **adenine** *(A)* and **guanine** *(G)* and the pyrimidines **thymine** *(T)* and **cytosine** *(C)*, which are covalently linked to the deoxyribose

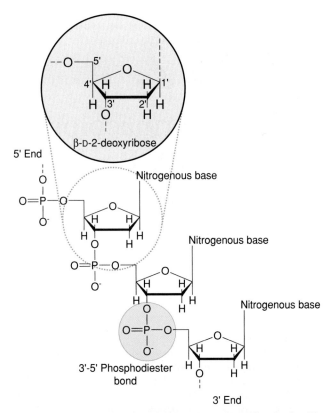

Figure 32-1. Backbone structure of DNA. DNA is a nucleotide polymer in which a phosphodiester bond connects the 2'-deoxyribose sugars of each neighboring nucleotide. The phosphodiester bond links the 3'-OH of one deoxyribose to the 5'-OH of the next deoxyribose, thus forming the backbone of the DNA strand.

ring, associate with one another (*A* with *T*, *G* with *C*) via hydrogen bonds to form the "rungs" of the ladder (Fig. 32-2). It is the linear sequence of bases that encodes the genetic information of a cell. How the nucleotide precursors to these bases are synthesized is reviewed in Chapter 37, Pharmacology of Cancer: Genome Synthesis, Stability, and Maintenance. DNA structure is essentially the same between prokaryotes and eukaryotes. However, prokaryotic chromosomes are usually circular DNAs, while eukaryotic chromosomes, including our own, are linear molecules.

DNA REPLICATION, SEGREGATION, AND TOPOISOMERASES

The faithful replication and segregation of bacterial DNA to progeny cells involve numerous steps, many of which could make good targets for antibacterial drugs. To date, the enzymes in this process that have been most successfully targeted are **topoisomerases.** These enzymes perform several functions during DNA replication and segregation.

During DNA replication, complementary strands of DNA are synthesized bidirectionally, forming two so-called replication forks. To initiate this process, the two DNA strands that comprise the double helix must unwind and separate. In so doing, the DNA strands form **"supercoils"** in which

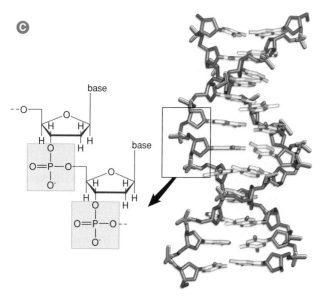

Figure 32-2. Hydrogen bonding between DNA strands. A and **B.** The *dashed lines* indicate hydrogen bonds between complementary bases on opposite DNA strands. Adenine *(A)* and thymine *(T)* form two hydrogen bonds, while guanine *(G)* and cytosine *(C)* form three hydrogen bonds. **C.** These A-T and G-C base pairs form the "rungs" of the DNA double helical "ladder." Note that the deoxyribose moieties and phosphodiester bonds are located on the outside of the DNA double helix, while the purine and pyrimidine bases stack in the center of the DNA molecule.

tate; this process would be complex and energy-consuming and could entangle the entire molecule.

When DNA replication is completed, the two progeny DNA copies are wrapped around each other. In bacteria, because the chromosomes are circular, the intertwined progeny copies form interlocking rings (catenanes). These intertwined rings must be separated (resolved) before they can be segregated to the progeny cells.

Topoisomerases perform both of these functions—removing excess DNA supercoils during DNA replication and separating intertwined progeny DNA. *Topoisomerases catalyze these activities by breaking, rotating, and religating DNA strands.* There are two types of topoisomerases. **Type I topoisomerases** form and reseal single-stranded breaks in DNA to decrease positive supercoiling (Fig. 32-3). **Type II topoisomerases** perform these nuclease and ligase operations on both strands of DNA (Fig. 32-4). Both types of topoisomerases can remove excess DNA supercoils during DNA replication. However, only type II topoisomerases can resolve intertwined copies of double-stranded DNA to permit segregation of the DNA to daughter cells. Type II enzymes are both more complex and more versatile than type I topoisomerases, and the type II enzyme serves as a more frequent molecular target for chemotherapeutic agents.

The mechanism of action of a type II topoisomerase proceeds in two steps. First, the enzyme binds a segment of DNA and forms covalent bonds with phosphates from each strand, thereby nicking both strands. Second, the enzyme causes a second stretch of DNA from the same molecule to pass through the break, relieving supercoiling (Fig. 32-4). This passage of double-stranded DNA through a double-stranded break is what permits separation of intertwined copies of DNA following replication and, thereby, segregation of DNA into progeny cells.

There are two main bacterial type II topoisomerases. The first to be identified, **DNA gyrase,** is a bacterial type II topoisomerase that is unusual in that it can introduce negative supercoils before the DNA strands separate, and thereby neutralize positive supercoils that form as the strands unwind. The second major type II topoisomerase is **topoisomerase IV.** DNA gyrase is particularly crucial for segregation in some bacteria, while topoisomerase IV is the critical enzyme in other bacteria.

Because supercoiling is important for transcription as well as segregation, topoisomerases influence this central dogma process as well. Given their multiple functions, topoisomerases are usually engaged with DNA, and this is important for their roles as drug targets. These enzymes are not only important as antibacterial drug targets, but also as targets for cancer chemotherapy (see Chapter 37).

BACTERIAL TRANSCRIPTION

the helical polymer overtwists as it rotates in the same direction as the turn of the helix. (This is similar to what happens to telephone cords during use.) Supercoils increase tension in DNA strands and thereby interfere with further unwinding. In the absence of a process to relieve the stress created by the supercoils, the entire chromosome would have to ro-

Gene expression begins with transcription, which involves the synthesis of single-stranded RNA transcripts from a DNA template. Transcription is catalyzed by the enzyme **RNA polymerase.** In bacteria, five subunits (2 α, 1 β, 1 β′, and 1 σ) associate to form the holoenzyme. As discussed below, the σ subunit is instrumental for initiating transcrip-

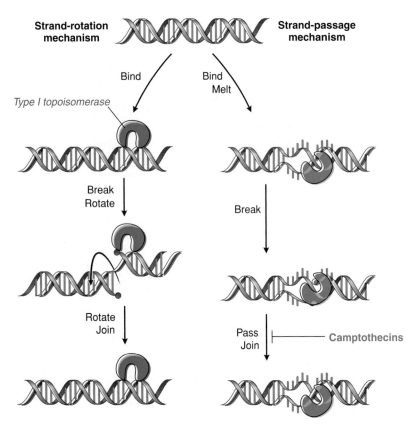

Strand-rotation mechanism

Strand-passage mechanism

Bind

Bind
Melt

Type I topoisomerase

Break
Rotate

Break

Rotate
Join

Pass
Join | Camptothecins

Figure 32-3. Regulation of DNA supercoiling by type I topoisomerases. Two mechanisms have been proposed for the action of type I topoisomerases. In the strand-rotation model, type I topoisomerase binds to opposite strands of the DNA double helix. The topoisomerase then nicks one strand and remains bound to one of the nicked ends *(filled gray circle)*. The unbound end of the nicked strand is able to unwind by one or more turns and is then joined (religated) to its parent strand. In the strand-passage model, type I topoisomerase binding to the DNA double helix results in melting (separation) of the two DNA strands. The DNA-bound topoisomerase then introduces a nick into one strand, while remaining bound to each end of the broken DNA strand *(filled blue circles)*. The broken strand is then passed through the helix and joined (religated), resulting in a net unwinding of the DNA. Camptothecins, which are used in cancer chemotherapy (see Chapter 37), inhibit the joining of the broken strand of DNA after strand passage.

tion, while the rest of the RNA polymerase enzyme—also known as the core enzyme—contains the catalytic machinery for RNA synthesis.

The process of transcription occurs in three stages: initiation, elongation, and termination (Fig. 32-5). During initiation, the RNA polymerase holoenzyme separates the strands of a short segment of double-helical DNA after its σ subunit recognizes an upstream site. Once the double helix is unwound to form a single-stranded template, RNA polymerase initiates RNA synthesis at a start site on the DNA. During elongation, RNA polymerase synthesizes a complementary RNA strand by joining together ribonucleoside triphosphates via phosphodiester bonds. In the process, the σ subunit dissociates from the holoenzyme. RNA synthesis proceeds in the $5' \rightarrow 3'$ direction, with the nascent RNA strand emerging from the enzyme, until a termination sequence is reached.

The RNA polymerase enzyme differs between bacteria and humans and thus can serve as a selective target for antibacterial drug action. In bacteria, one RNA polymerase synthesizes all of the RNA in the cell (except for the short RNA primers needed for DNA replication, which are made by **primase**). Furthermore, bacterial RNA polymerase is composed of only five subunits. In contrast, eukaryotes express three different RNA polymerases, and each enzyme is considerably more complex in its subunit structure than the bacterial counterpart. For example, the type II eukaryotic RNA polymerase, which synthesizes the precursors of mRNA, consists of 8 to 12 subunits.

BACTERIAL PROTEIN SYNTHESIS

Once the mRNA transcripts are synthesized, these transcripts are translated by the bacterial translational machinery. Al-

though the overall process of translation is similar between bacteria and higher organisms, there are a number of pharmacologically exploitable differences in the details of the mechanisms. In particular, the number and composition of the rRNA molecules differ between bacterial and human ribosomes. Thus, bacterial ribosomes can also serve as selective targets for antibiotics.

The ribosome of a representative bacterium, *Escherichia coli,* has a sedimentation coefficient of **70S** and is composed of a **30S subunit** and a **50S subunit.** The 30S subunit contains a single **16S rRNA** molecule and 21 different proteins, while the 50S subunit contains two rRNA molecules—**23S rRNA** and **5S rRNA**—and more than 30 different proteins. Importantly, it is the rRNA rather than the protein components of the ribosome that are responsible for the ribosome's key activities, namely, decoding the mRNA, linking together amino acids, and translocating the translation machine. The 70S ribosome contains two sites that bind tRNAs during translation: the **P** or **"peptidyl" site,** which contains the growing peptide chain, and the **A** or **"aminoacyl" site** (also known as the **"acceptor" site**), which binds incoming tRNA molecules carrying the various amino acids (Fig. 32-6). (There is also an E or "exit" site, which binds the tRNAs that have been used during translation before they are ejected from the ribosome.)

Translation, like transcription, can be divided into three steps (Fig. 32-7). During **initiation,** the components of the translation system assemble together. First, the mRNA joins with the 30S subunit of the bacterial ribosome and with a specific tRNA molecule linked to **formylated methionine** (fMet), the first amino acid encoded by every bacterial

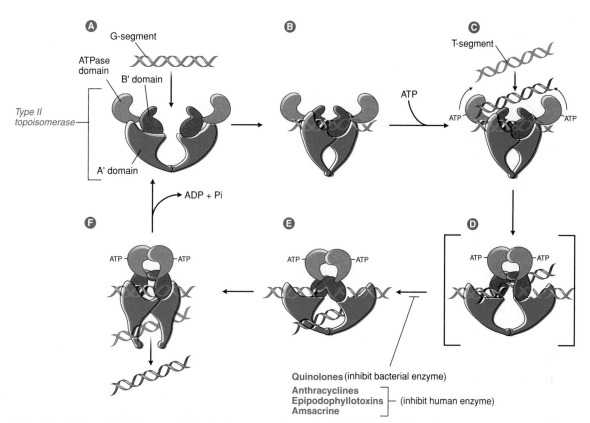

Figure 32-4. Regulation of DNA supercoiling by type II topoisomerases. A. The type II topoisomerase enzymes contain A′, B′, and ATPase domains. The A′ and B′ domains engage a segment of the DNA double helix (G-segment). **B.** Interaction with the G-segment induces a conformational change in the type II isomerase, causing it to "lock" around the DNA G-segment. **C.** ATP binds to the ATPase domains of the topoisomerase, and a second segment of the DNA double helix (T-segment) enters and is "locked" into the B′ domains. **D.** Once the enzyme is engaged with both DNA segments, the topoisomerase cuts both strands of the G-segment DNA. **E.** This double-stranded nick in the G-segment allows the T-segment to pass through the G-segment to the opposite side of the topoisomerase. **F.** The T-segment is released from the topoisomerase, and the G-segment nick is religated. ATP is hydrolyzed to ADP, ADP dissociates from the topoisomerase, and the cycle begins anew. The result of each cycle is to change the coiling number of DNA by one or, when two separate circular DNA molecules are involved, to resolve catenanes. Quinolone antibiotics inhibit passage of the T-segment and religation of the nicked G-segment by bacterial type II topoisomerases. At therapeutic concentrations, quinolones also promote topoisomerase subunit dissociation, resulting in double-stranded breaks in the DNA and killing of the bacteria. Several classes of cancer chemotherapeutic agents, including the anthracyclines, epipodophyllotoxins, and amsacrine, inhibit passage of the T-segment and religation of the nicked G-segment by human type II topoisomerases, thereby causing double-stranded DNA breaks and inducing apoptosis of the cancer cells (see Chapter 37).

mRNA. The tRNA-formylated methionine molecule (fMet-tRNA$_f$) binds to its initiation codon (AUG) on the mRNA. Next, the 50S subunit joins with the 30S subunit to form the complete 70S ribosome. The fMet-tRNA$_f$ now occupies the P site of the 70S ribosome.

Elongation involves the addition of amino acids to the carboxyl end of the growing polypeptide chain, as the ribosome moves from the 5′-end to the 3′-end of the mRNA that is being translated. tRNA molecules carrying specific amino acids (aminoacyl tRNAs) enter the ribosomal A site and base-pair to their complementary codons on the mRNA. Utilization of the correct tRNA requires not only anticodon-codon recognition between tRNA and mRNA, respectively, but also **decoding** functions provided by the 16S rRNA in the 30S ribosomal subunit. **Peptidyl transferase,** an enzyme whose activity derives from the 23S rRNA of the 50S subunit (i.e., peptidyl transferase is a ribozyme), catalyzes the formation of a peptide bond between fMet and the next amino acid. The peptide bond links fMet to the next amino acid, which, in turn, is linked to the tRNA in the A site (i.e., the

tRNA in the A site has "accepted" the fMet). After the peptide bond has been formed, the ribosome advances three nucleotides toward the 3′-end of the mRNA. In the process, the tRNA$_f$ that was originally linked to the fMet is ejected from the P site (and binds to the E site), the tRNA that is now linked to two amino acids shifts from the A site to the unoccupied P site, the A site becomes available, and the growing peptide emerges from the exit tunnel of the ribosome. This process is known as **translocation.** In this manner, polypeptide chain elongation results from multiple cycles of aminoacyl tRNA binding to the A site, peptide bond formation, and translocation.

During **termination,** proteins called **release factors** recognize the termination codon in the A site, and activate discharge of the newly synthesized protein and dissociation of the ribosome-mRNA complex. In at least some cases, this process seems to involve structural mimicry of tRNAs by the release factors.

Three general points are worth noting about bacterial translation. First, *the two ribosomal subunits demonstrate*

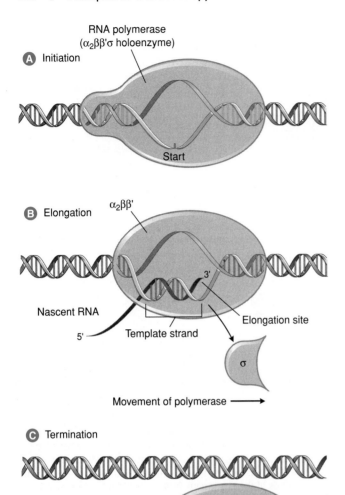

Figure 32-5. Prokaryotic transcription. A. During initiation, the RNA polymerase holoenzyme ($\alpha_2\beta\beta'\sigma$) searches for and recognizes promoter sequences on DNA. The holoenzyme then separates the strands of the double helical DNA, exposing the start site for transcription. **B.** During elongation, the core enzyme (without the σ subunit) synthesizes the new RNA strand in the $5'\rightarrow3'$ direction, using the unwound DNA strand as a template. RNA polymerase separates the strands of the DNA double helix as it moves along the template strand, extruding the $5'$ end of the transcript behind it. Rifampin blocks elongation by complexing with the β subunit of RNA polymerase *(not shown)*. **C.** Upon reaching a termination sequence, the DNA, core enzyme, and newly synthesized RNA separate from one another.

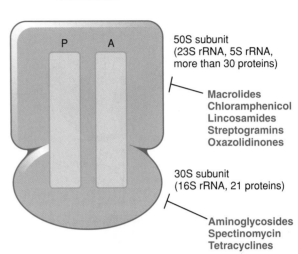

Figure 32-6. The prokaryotic 70S ribosome. The prokaryotic 70S ribosome consists of a 30S subunit and a 50S subunit. Each subunit is composed of ribosomal RNA (rRNA) and numerous proteins. The rRNAs are responsible for most of the important activities of the ribosome and are the targets of antibiotic drugs that inhibit translation. Aminoglycosides, spectinomycin, and tetracyclines bind to and inhibit the activity of 16S rRNA in the 30S subunit. Macrolides, chloramphenicol, lincosamides, streptogramins, and oxazolidinones bind to and inhibit the activity of 23S rRNA in the 50S subunit. *A,* aminoacyl site (site of binding of aminoacyl tRNA); *P,* peptidyl site (site of binding of tRNA that is covalently joined to the elongating peptide chain).

PHARMACOLOGIC CLASSES AND AGENTS

Elucidation of the mechanisms of action of the agents described below has depended crucially on the field of bacterial genetics. In particular, the molecular targets of antibiotics have been identified by the isolation of bacteria that are resistant to the particular antibiotic (e.g., rifampin), followed by showing that the target molecule (e.g., RNA polymerase) exhibits biochemical resistance to the antibiotic, and, finally, showing that the drug-resistance mutation lies within the gene encoding the target. More recent work, using nuclear magnetic resonance spectroscopy and x-ray crystallography, has further elucidated the structures of the targets as well as the molecular nature of the various drug-target interactions.

INHIBITORS OF TOPOISOMERASES: Quinolones

Quinolones are a major class of bactericidal antibiotics that act by inhibiting bacterial type II topoisomerases. One of the earliest quinolones to enter clinical use was **nalidixic acid** (Fig. 32-8), and the mechanism of action of the quinolones was elucidated largely by studying this drug. Most of the more recently introduced quinolones are fluorinated, including **ciprofloxacin, ofloxacin,** and **levofloxacin.** These and other fluorinated quinolones (**fluoroquinolones**) are

segregated functions: the 30S subunit is responsible for faithful decoding of the mRNA message, while the 50S subunit catalyzes peptide bond formation. Translocation, however, seems to involve both subunits. Second, *the catalytic machinery resides in the RNA component of the ribosome, not in the ribosomal proteins.* In other words, it is the rRNA that "does the work." Third, *inhibitors of protein synthesis block the process of translation at different steps.*

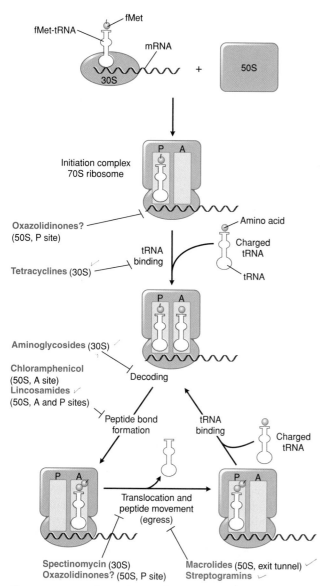

Figure 32-7. Prokaryotic translation. Prokaryotic translation begins with the assembly of a complex containing a 30S ribosomal subunit, mRNA, formyl-methionine-linked tRNA (fMet-tRNA), and a 50S ribosomal subunit. This assembly step is dependent on the binding of fMet-tRNA to an initiator codon in the mRNA. The assembled 70S ribosome contains two binding sites, referred to as the aminoacyl *(A)* and peptidyl *(P)* sites. The A site accepts incoming triplet codons of mRNA and allows the corresponding amino acid-linked tRNA (i.e., charged tRNA) to bind to its corresponding triplet. The decoding function of 16S rRNA helps ensure that the mRNA codon binds to the correct tRNA. Once a charged tRNA has entered the A site, the peptidyl transferase activity of the 23S rRNA catalyzes the formation of a peptide bond between the amino acid occupying the A site and the carboxy-terminus of the nascent peptide residing in the P site. Once the peptide bond has formed, the tRNA–mRNA complex translocates from the A site to the P site, the tRNA molecule that had occupied the P site dissociates from the P site, and the elongating polypeptide chain moves out through the exit tunnel. The A site is now empty, and introduction of the next charged tRNA molecule into the A site completes the cycle. Translation continues until a stop codon is encountered in the mRNA, at which point the newly synthesized protein is released from the ribosome.

Pharmacologic agents that inhibit translation interfere with the activities of the prokaryotic ribosome. Aminoglycosides bind to rRNA

identifiable by their generic names, which typically end in ''-floxacin'' (Fig. 32-8). The fluoroquinolones are widely used to treat common urogenital, respiratory, and gastrointestinal infections caused by Gram-negative microbes, including *E. coli, Klebsiella pneumoniae, Campylobacter jejuni, Pseudomonas aeruginosa, Neisseria gonorrhoeae,* and *Enterobacter, Salmonella,* and *Shigella* species. Bacteria typically evolve resistance to the quinolones through chromosomal mutations in the genes that encode type II topoisomerases or through alterations in the expression of membrane porins and efflux pumps that determine the concentration of drug inside the bacteria. Adverse effects are infrequent, but can include nausea, vomiting, and diarrhea.

Quinolones act by inhibiting one or both of the two prokaryotic type II topoisomerases in sensitive bacteria, **DNA gyrase** (topoisomerase II) and **topoisomerase IV.** Selectivity of action against bacterial topoisomerases results from differences in structure between the prokaryotic and eukaryotic forms of these enzymes. Quinolones primarily inhibit DNA gyrase in Gram-negative organisms, and they inhibit topoisomerase IV in Gram-positive organisms such as *Staphylococcus aureus.* Because resistant *S. aureus* is pervasive, the quinolones are less effective in treating infections caused by this bacterium. Thus, this class of drugs is used most frequently to treat Gram-negative organisms.

The mechanism of action of the quinolones involves subverting the function of prokaryotic type II topoisomerases. Ordinarily, type II topoisomerases bind to and nick both strands of a DNA molecule, allowing another stretch of the same molecule to pass through the double-stranded DNA break (Fig. 32-4). Quinolones inhibit these enzymes before the second segment of DNA can pass through, thereby stabilizing the form of the complex in which the DNA polymer is broken. At low concentrations, quinolones inhibit type II topoisomerases reversibly, and their action is bacteriostatic. At higher concentrations, however—which are readily achieved in patients—quinolones convert the topoisomerases into DNA-damaging agents by stimulating dissociation of the enzyme subunits from the broken DNA. Doubly-nicked DNA cannot be replicated, and transcription cannot proceed through such breaks. Topoisomerase dissociation from the DNA and/or the bacterial response to the double-stranded break lead ultimately to cell death. Thus, at therapeutic doses, the quinolone antibiotics are bactericidal.

INHIBITORS OF TRANSCRIPTION: Rifamycin Derivatives

Rifampin and its structural relative, **rifabutin**, are two semisynthetic derivatives of the naturally occurring antibiotic **rifamycin B** (Fig. 32-8). Although rifampin can be used for

in the 30S subunit and enable the binding of incorrect tRNAs to mRNA; tetracyclines block aminoacyl-tRNA binding to the A site; chloramphenicol and lincosamides inhibit the peptidyl transferase activity of the 50S subunit. Spectinomycin, macrolides, and streptogramins inhibit peptide translocation. The mechanism(s) of action of the oxazolidinones are uncertain, but some possible sites of action are indicated.

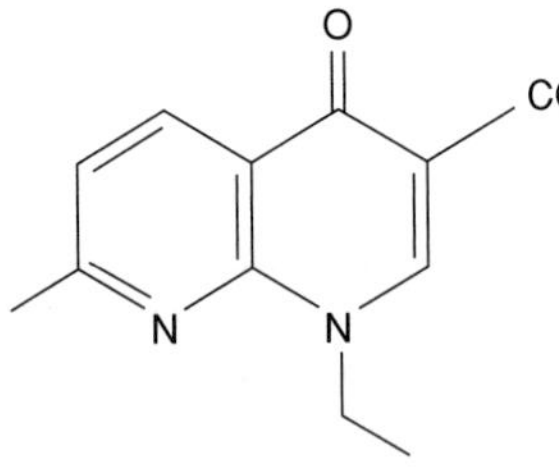

Figure 32-8. Structures of antimicrobial drugs targeting bacterial topoisomerases and transcription. Nalidixic acid and ciprofloxacin are quinolone antibiotics that inhibit bacterial type II topoisomerases. Rifampin and rifabutin inhibit bacterial DNA-dependent RNA polymerase.

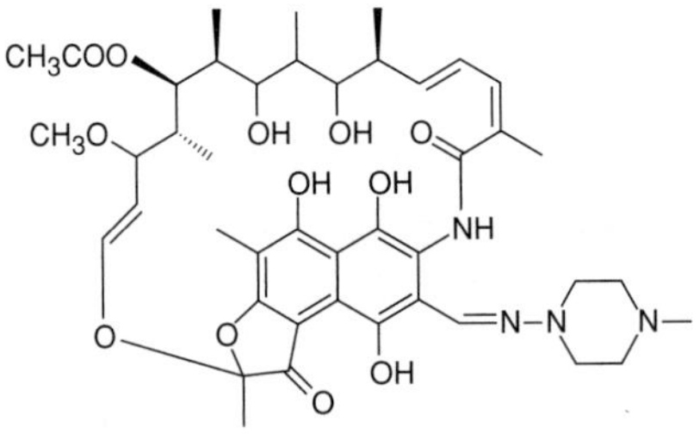

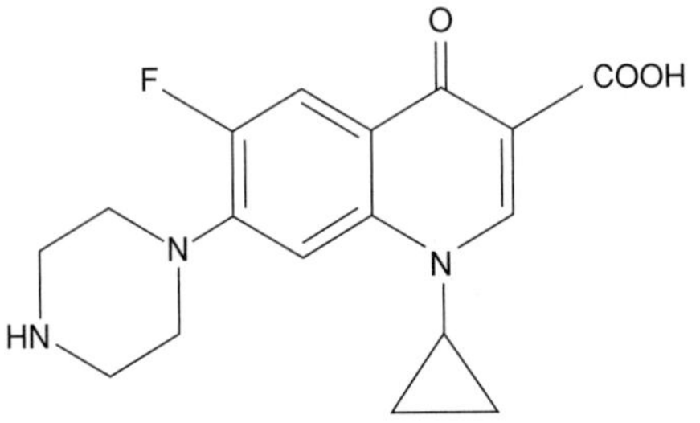

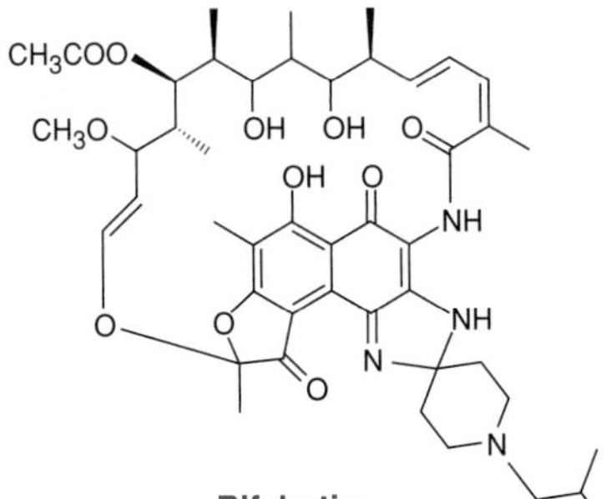

prophylaxis of meningococcal disease and for treatment of some other bacterial infections, its major use is in the treatment of tuberculosis and other mycobacterial infections. Rifampin is particularly effective against phagosome-dwelling mycobacteria because it is bactericidal for intracellular as well as extracellular bacteria. Furthermore, rifampin increases the in vitro activity of **isoniazid**, another first-line drug used in the combination therapy of tuberculosis (see Chapter 33, Pharmacology of Bacterial Infections: Cell Wall Synthesis, and Chapter 39, Principles of Combination Chemotherapy).

Rifampin exerts its bactericidal activity by forming a stable complex with bacterial DNA-dependent RNA polymerase, thereby inhibiting RNA synthesis. The drug targets the β subunit of bacterial RNA polymerase. Rifampin permits the initiation of transcription, but then blocks elongation once the length of the nascent RNA reaches 2 to 3 nucleotides. Exactly how this occurs has not been completely resolved; for certain bacterial RNA polymerases, there is evidence that rifampin occludes the path by which the nascent RNA emerges from the enzyme. Rifampin displays high selectivity for bacteria, as mammalian polymerases (even those of mitochondria, which are considered prokaryote-like) are inhibited by rifampin only at far higher concentrations. Hence, rifampin is generally well tolerated, and the incidence of adverse effects (typically, rash, fever, nausea, vomiting, and jaundice) is low.

Because the rapid emergence of resistance makes single-drug therapy of tuberculosis not only ineffective but also counterproductive, rifampin is administered in combination with other antituberculosis drugs. In vitro experiments show that 1 out of every 10^6 to 10^8 tubercle bacilli can develop resistance to rifampin via a one-step mutational process that appears to occur within the binding site of the drug on the polymerase. However, as a component of a multidrug thera-

peutic regimen, rifampin can markedly reduce the lifetime rate of reactivation of latent tuberculosis (see Chapter 39).

INHIBITORS OF TRANSLATION

Three general considerations apply to inhibitors of bacterial translation. First, *translation inhibitors target either the 30S or 50S subunit of the bacterial ribosome.* Although the details can be confusing, as in the case of the new oxazolidinone class of drugs, the following discussion of translation inhibitors is presented in terms of 30S versus 50S inhibition (Table 32-1).

The second consideration concerns selectivity. *In addition to their inhibitory effects on bacterial ribosomes, protein synthesis inhibitors can affect mammalian mitochondrial ribosomes, cytosolic ribosomes, or both.* Inhibition of host ribosomes is one common mechanism by which these drugs cause adverse effects. For some antibiotics, such as chloramphenicol, inhibition of mammalian ribosomes represents a major drawback and can lead to serious, even lethal, adverse effects. Tetracyclines can also inhibit mammalian ribosomes in vitro; fortunately, however, this class of drugs is concentrated selectively in bacterial cells. Certain other translation inhibitors exhibit little or no inhibition of mammalian ribosomes at clinically relevant concentrations; for these agents, the dose-limiting toxicities appear to be attributable to other mechanisms. As with most orally available, broad-spectrum antibiotics, gastrointestinal adverse events appear to be due to elimination of normal gut flora.

An interesting twist on the issue of selectivity emerged in the 1990s. It was discovered that certain aminoglycoside, macrolide, and lincosamide antibiotics demonstrate some efficacy against eukaryotic microorganisms (e.g., protozoan parasites) that cause opportunistic infections in patients with AIDS and in other immunocompromised individuals. In

TABLE 32-1	Sites and Mechanisms of Action of Antibacterial Translation Inhibitors	
DRUG OR DRUG CLASS	**SITE OF ACTION**	**MECHANISM OF ACTION**
Drugs targeting the 30S ribosomal subunit		
Aminoglycosides	16S rRNA	Induce misreading; halt protein synthesis at higher concentrations
Spectinomycin	16S rRNA	Inhibits translocation
Tetracyclines	16S rRNA	Block aminoacyl tRNA binding to A site
Drugs targeting the 50S ribosomal subunit		
Macrolides	23S rRNA	Inhibit translocation
Chloramphenicol	23S rRNA	Inhibits peptidyl transferase by interfering with tRNA positioning
Lincosamides	23S rRNA	Inhibit peptidyl transferase by blocking the growing polypeptide chain and by inhibiting the A site and P site
Streptogramins	23S rRNA	Inhibit peptidyl transferase; probable overlap with mechanism of action of macrolides
Oxazolidinones	23S rRNA?	Not yet known

these microorganisms, it appears that the activity of the antibiotics can be attributed to their inhibition of organellar protein synthesis in the microorganism (see Chapter 35, Pharmacology of Parasitic Infections).

The third consideration is that *complete inhibition of protein synthesis is not sufficient to kill a bacterium.* Bacteria can generate a number of responses to various growth-stifling treatments that allow them to remain dormant until the treatment is removed. One of these responses permits the bacteria to survive complete inhibition of protein synthesis. As a result, most inhibitors of protein synthesis are bacteriostatic. Aminoglycosides are the major exception to this rule.

Antimicrobial Drugs Targeting the 30S Ribosomal Subunit

Aminoglycosides

Aminoglycosides are used mainly to treat infections caused by Gram-negative bacteria. These agents are charged molecules that are not orally bioavailable, so they must be administered parenterally. The aminoglycosides include **streptomycin** (the first aminoglycoside, discovered in 1944), **neomycin, kanamycin, tobramycin, paromomycin, gentamicin, netilmicin,** and **amikacin** (Fig. 32-9). Of these, gentamicin, tobramycin, and amikacin are the most widely used agents because of their lower toxicity and broader coverage of target organisms. (Even these agents are not active against anaerobes and many Gram-positive bacteria, however.)

Aminoglycosides bind to the 16S rRNA of the 30S subunit and elicit concentration-dependent effects on protein synthesis. At low concentrations, aminoglycosides induce ribosomes to misread mRNA during elongation, leading to synthesis of proteins containing incorrect amino acids. It is logical to infer from this effect that aminoglycosides inter-

fere with the mRNA-decoding function of the 30S subunit. (Indeed, crystal structures of 30S-aminoglycoside complexes have greatly aided our understanding of the decoding process.) How aminoglycosides affect decoding is best understood for paromomycin, whose binding causes a conformational change that mimics the change caused by the correct binding of a tRNA anticodon to an mRNA codon. It is thought that this conformational change causes the 30S subunit to signal the 50S subunit to form a peptide bond, even when the incorrect tRNA is present in the A site. (Streptomycin also induces misreading, but this is thought to occur by a different mechanism.) At higher concentrations, aminoglycosides completely inhibit protein synthesis. Exactly how this occurs is not understood, but ribosomes become trapped at the AUG start codons of mRNA. Eventually, accumulation of these abnormal initiation complexes halts translation, despite the presence of ribosomes that are not bound to drug.

In contrast to other protein synthesis inhibitors, aminoglycosides are **bactericidal.** This is an important feature in the treatment of serious infections. Although the precise mechanism for bactericidal activity is not known, one appealing model, developed by the late Bernard Davis, has gained some acceptance (Fig. 32-10). The **Davis model** frames the story of cell death in terms of the concentration-dependent effects of aminoglycosides. When drug first enters the cell, it is poorly transported across bacterial membranes. At these initial low concentrations, misreading occurs, leading to synthesis of aberrant proteins. Some of these proteins insert into membranes and cause the formation of membrane pores, which allow aminoglycosides to flood the cell and halt protein synthesis completely. As a result, the damage to the membrane cannot be repaired, and leakage of ions and, later, larger molecules leads to cell death.

Another important aspect of aminoglycoside activity is that these drugs act synergistically with agents, such as β-lactams, which inhibit cell wall synthesis. Therefore, aminoglycosides and β-lactams are commonly used in combina-

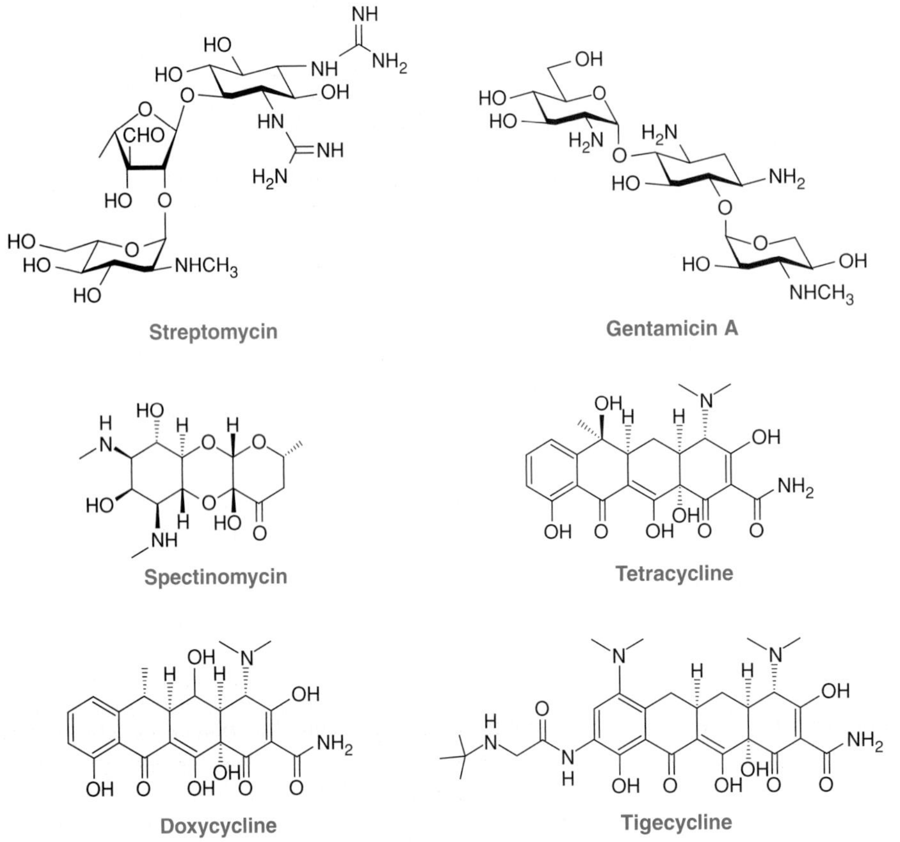

Figure 32-9. Structures of antimicrobial drugs targeting the 30S ribosomal subunit. Streptomycin and gentamicin are aminoglycosides. Spectinomycin is a structural relative of the aminoglycosides. Tetracycline and doxycycline are tetracyclines. Tigecycline is a glycylcycline.

tion (see Chapter 39). The explanation most commonly suggested for this synergy is that inhibition of cell wall synthesis increases the entry of aminoglycosides into the bacteria. The synergy between β-lactams and the aminoglycosides contrasts sharply with the antagonism between β-lactams and the bacteriostatic inhibitors of protein synthesis discussed below.

Three general mechanisms have been established for resistance to aminoglycosides. First, and clinically most common, is the plasmid-encoded production of a transferase enzyme or enzymes that inactivate aminoglycosides by adenylation, acetylation, or phosphorylation. Second, drug entry into the cell can be impaired, perhaps by alteration or elimination of porins or other proteins involved in drug transport. Third, the drug target on the 30S ribosomal subunit can become resistant to drug binding by virtue of mutation or the activity of a plasmid-encoded enzyme.

In addition to several general types of toxicity, such as hypersensitivity reactions and drug-induced fever, the aminoglycosides can cause three specific adverse effects: ototoxicity, nephrotoxicity, and neuromuscular blockade. Of these, **ototoxicity** (manifesting as either auditory or vestibular damage) is the single most important factor restricting aminoglycoside use. There is excellent evidence that ototoxicity is caused by aminoglycoside inhibition of host mitochondrial ribosomes. The aminoglycosides are known to accumulate in the perilymph and endolymph of the inner ear and, at high concentrations, to damage highly sensitive hair cells. Aminoglycosides can also cause **acute renal failure,** apparently as a result of drug accumulation in proximal tubular cells. The biochemistry involved in this toxicity is poorly

understood, although both mitochondrial poisoning and perturbation of the plasma membrane are suspected. At very high concentrations, aminoglycosides can produce nondepolarizing neuromuscular blockade, potentially causing respiratory paralysis. This effect is thought to result from drug competition with calcium at presynaptic sites, leading to reduction in acetylcholine release, failure of the postsynaptic end-plate to depolarize, and muscle paralysis.

Spectinomycin

Spectinomycin is a structural relative of the aminoglycosides that also binds to the 16S rRNA of the 30S ribosomal subunit (albeit at a location different from the aminoglycoside binding site). Spectinomycin permits formation of the 70S complex but inhibits translocation. Unlike the aminoglycosides, spectinomycin does not induce codon misreading and is not bactericidal. Spectinomycin is administered parenterally and is used clinically only as an alternative therapy for gonorrheal infections.

Tetracyclines and Glycylcyclines

Tetracyclines have been used clinically for many years. There are seven **tetracyclines** available in the United States: **chlortetracycline, oxytetracycline, tetracycline, demeclocycline, methacycline, doxycycline,** and **minocycline.** All are close structural relatives and can be considered as a group. Differences in clinical efficacy are minor and relate largely to the pharmacokinetics of absorption, distribution, and excretion of the individual drugs. Tetracyclines are

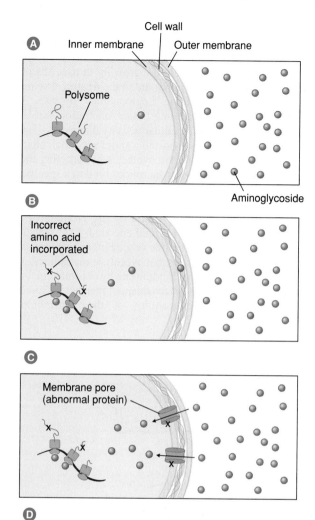

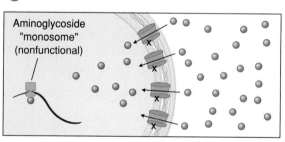

Figure 32-10. The Davis model explains the bactericidal activity of aminoglycosides. The Davis model of aminoglycoside action proposes that low concentrations of aminoglycosides induce protein misreading and that the misread (abnormal) proteins allow higher concentrations of aminoglycosides to enter the cell and halt protein synthesis. **A.** Initially, aminoglycosides are present at low concentrations inside the bacterial cell, despite therapeutic (high) extracellular concentrations of drug, because the drug molecules have poor uptake across the bacterial membranes. **B.** Low intracellular concentrations of aminoglycoside bind to bacterial ribosomes and cause incorporation of incorrect amino acids (misreading) into nascent polypeptides. **C.** The abnormal proteins insert into the bacterial membranes, forming pores and causing membrane damage. **D.** The damaged membranes allow additional aminoglycoside molecules to flood into the cell, causing complete inhibition of ribosome activity. The effect is irreversible, perhaps because of trapping of drug inside the cell ("caging"). The membrane damage cannot be repaired because new proteins cannot be synthesized, and cell death ensues.

broad-spectrum, bacteriostatic antibiotics that are used widely.

Tetracyclines bind reversibly to the 16S rRNA of the 30S subunit and inhibit protein synthesis by blocking the binding of aminoacyl tRNA to the A site on the mRNA-ribosome complex. This action prevents the addition of further amino acids to the nascent peptide. However, inhibition of protein synthesis does not account entirely for the high bacterial selectivity of tetracyclines, because these drugs can also halt eukaryotic protein synthesis in vitro at not much higher concentrations. *Rather, the high selectivity of tetracyclines derives from the active accumulation of these drugs in bacteria but not in mammalian cells.* Tetracyclines enter Gram-negative bacteria by passive diffusion through porin proteins in the outer membrane, followed by active (energy-dependent) transport across the inner cytoplasmic membrane. Uptake into Gram-positive bacteria, such as *Bacillus anthracis* (the causative agent of anthrax), occurs similarly via an energy-dependent transport system. In contrast, mammalian cells lack the active transport system found in susceptible bacteria.

Since the bacterial selectivity of tetracyclines results from drug-concentrating mechanisms, it follows that resistance can occur through increased drug efflux or decreased drug influx. In fact, plasmid-encoded **efflux pumps** represent the most widespread mechanism employed by tetracycline-resistant microbes. A second form of resistance arises through the production of proteins that interfere with the binding of tetracyclines to the ribosome. Yet a third mechanism is the enzymatic inactivation of tetracyclines.

An important pharmacokinetic feature of the tetracyclines is the interaction of these drugs with foods high in calcium, such as dairy products, and with medicines that contain divalent and trivalent cations, such as antacids. Because these products and medicines impair the absorption of tetracyclines, the tetracyclines are generally taken on an empty stomach. Once tetracyclines are in the circulation, however, the same interaction with cations—in particular, with calcium—can cause sequestration of the drug in bone and teeth, potentially leading to developmental abnormalities in pediatric patients. Teeth can also become discolored because of the ultraviolet (UV)-absorbing properties of tetracyclines, and these drugs can cause significant cutaneous photosensitivity.

Kidney toxicity and gastrointestinal distress are the two most problematic adverse effects of the tetracyclines, and nausea and vomiting are the most common reasons for premature discontinuation of a course of tetracycline. All tetracyclines are excreted in both urine and bile, with the urine being the primary route for most drugs in this class. Compared to the other tetracyclines, a lower fraction of **doxycycline** is eliminated via the kidney, making this drug safer for use in patients with renal failure. Also, doxycycline is excreted in the feces largely in an inactive form, so this agent has the added advantage of minimally altering intestinal flora. Hence, doxycycline use is associated with a lower incidence of nausea, vomiting, and superinfection with pathogenic organisms than the other tetracyclines, especially in immunocompromised patients.

Tigecycline (Fig. 32-9) is the first member of a new class of antibiotics—**glycylcyclines**. This antibiotic was approved in 2005. The four-ring structure of tigecycline resembles that of the tetracyclines. Tigecycline has a broad spectrum of activity and has been approved for intravenous administration in the treatment of serious skin and abdominal infections.

Antimicrobial Drugs Targeting the 50S Ribosomal Subunit

The best understood of the antibiotics that target the 50S subunit (i.e., the macrolides, chloramphenicol, and lincosamides) bind to a small region of 23S rRNA near the peptidyl transferase active center. Small differences in their binding sites may be responsible for differences in their detailed mechanisms of action.

Macrolides and Ketolides

Macrolides are named for their large lactone rings. Attached to these rings are one or more deoxy sugars (Fig. 32-11).

Erythromycin is the best-known member of this group. Two semisynthetic derivatives of erythromycin, **azithromycin** and **clarithromycin,** are broader in spectrum than erythromycin and are therefore growing in use. Macrolides have proven especially important in the treatment of pulmonary infections, including Legionnaires' disease. These agents display excellent lung tissue penetration and, as important, they have intracellular activity against *Legionella.*

Macrolides are bacteriostatic antibiotics that block the translocation step of protein synthesis by targeting the 23S rRNA of the 50S subunit. Macrolides bind to a specific segment of 23S rRNA and block the exit tunnel from which nascent peptides emerge.

Macrolide use is complicated by the problem of resistance, which is usually plasmid-encoded. One mechanism employed by resistant strains (e.g., *Enterobacteriaceae*) is the production of esterases that hydrolyze macrolides. Modification of the ribosomal binding site by chromosomal mutation represents a second mechanism of resistance. Some bacteria reduce the permeability of their membrane to

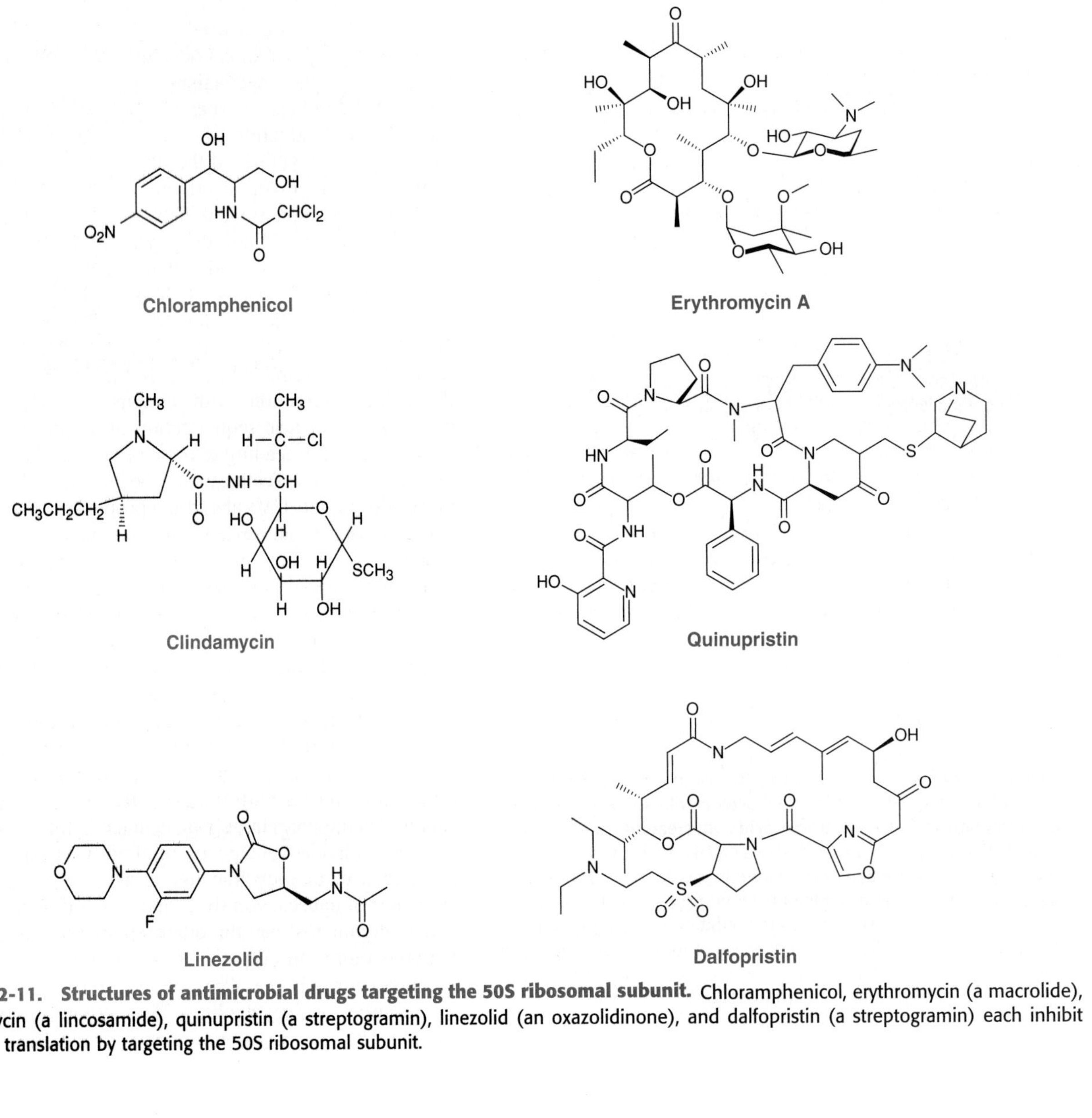

Figure 32-11.   Structures of antimicrobial drugs targeting the 50S ribosomal subunit. Chloramphenicol, erythromycin (a macrolide), clindamycin (a lincosamide), quinupristin (a streptogramin), linezolid (an oxazolidinone), and dalfopristin (a streptogramin) each inhibit bacterial translation by targeting the 50S ribosomal subunit.

macrolides, or (more commonly) increase active drug efflux. Methylase production accounts for the vast majority of resistance to macrolides in Gram-positive organisms. Methylase modifies the ribosomal target of the macrolides, leading to decreased drug binding. Constitutive production of methylase also confers resistance to structurally unrelated but mechanistically similar compounds, such as **clindamycin** and **streptogramin B** (see discussion below).

Adverse reactions to erythromycin typically involve the gastrointestinal tract or the liver. Gastrointestinal intolerance represents the most frequent reason for discontinuing erythromycin, as the drug can directly stimulate gut motility and cause nausea, vomiting, diarrhea, and sometimes anorexia. Erythromycin can also produce acute cholestatic hepatitis (with fever, jaundice, and impaired liver function), probably as a hypersensitivity reaction. Metabolites of erythromycin can inhibit certain cytochrome P450 isozymes in the liver, and thus increase the plasma concentration of numerous drugs that are also metabolized by these liver enzymes. Azithromycin and clarithromycin are generally well tolerated, although these drugs can also cause liver impairment.

Telithromycin, a third semisynthetic derivative of erythromycin, was approved by the FDA in 2004. Formally known as a **ketolide** rather than a macrolide, telithromycin has a mechanism of action similar to that of the macrolides, but with a higher affinity for the 50S ribosomal subunit due to its ability to bind an additional site on 23S rRNA. This higher affinity allows the use of telithromycin in treating infections due to certain bacterial strains that are resistant to macrolides. Like erythromycin, telithromycin can be involved in numerous drug-drug interactions, and rare cases of fulminant hepatic necrosis have been reported.

Chloramphenicol

Chloramphenicol is a bacteriostatic broad-spectrum antibiotic that is active against both aerobic and anaerobic Gram-positive and Gram-negative organisms. The most highly susceptible organisms include *Haemophilus influenzae, Neisseria meningitidis,* and some strains of *Bacteroides.* However, the potential for serious toxicity has limited the systemic use of chloramphenicol. The drug is still used occasionally in the treatment of typhoid fever, bacterial meningitis, and rickettsial diseases, but only when safer alternatives are not available, as in the case of resistance or serious drug allergy.

Chloramphenicol binds to 23S rRNA and inhibits peptide bond formation, apparently by occupying a site that interferes with proper positioning of the aminoacyl moiety of tRNA in the A site.

Microbes have developed resistance to chloramphenicol by two major mechanisms. Low-level resistance has emerged in large chloramphenicol-susceptible populations by the selection of mutants with decreased permeability to the drug. The more clinically significant type of chloramphenicol resistance has arisen from the spread of specific plasmid-encoded **acetyltransferases** (at least three types of which have been characterized) that inactivate the drug.

The fundamental mechanism underlying the toxicity of chloramphenicol appears to involve inhibition of mitochondrial protein synthesis. One manifestation of this toxicity is the **gray baby syndrome,** which can occur when chloramphenicol is administered at high doses to newborn infants.

Because newborns lack an effective glucuronic acid conjugation mechanism for the degradation and detoxification of chloramphenicol, the drug can accumulate to toxic levels and cause vomiting, flaccidity, hypothermia, gray color, respiratory distress, and metabolic acidosis. More frequently, chloramphenicol causes dose-related, reversible depression of erythropoiesis and gastrointestinal distress (nausea, vomiting, and diarrhea). **Aplastic anemia,** a rare but potentially fatal toxicity, occurs via an idiopathic mechanism that is unrelated to dose.

Of special interest are the adverse effects that chloramphenicol can cause in tandem with other drugs. Like the macrolides, chloramphenicol increases the half-lives of certain drugs, such as phenytoin and warfarin, by inhibiting the cytochrome P450 enzymes that metabolize these drugs. Chloramphenicol also antagonizes the bactericidal effects of penicillins and aminoglycosides, as do other bacteriostatic inhibitors of microbial protein synthesis.

Lincosamides

The major **lincosamide** in clinical use is **clindamycin** (Fig. 32-11). Clindamycin blocks peptide bond formation, apparently through interactions with both the A site (like chloramphenicol) and the P site.

The most important indications for clindamycin are the treatment of serious anaerobic infections caused by *Bacteroides* and the treatment of mixed infections involving other anaerobes. Clindamycin has been implicated as a potential cause of **pseudomembranous colitis** caused by *Clostridium difficile* superinfection. An infrequent member of the normal fecal flora, *C. difficile* is selected for during the administration of clindamycin or other broad-spectrum oral antibiotics. *C. difficile* elaborates a cytotoxin that can cause colitis characterized by mucosal ulcerations, severe diarrhea, and fever. This serious adverse effect is a major concern in the use of clindamycin.

Streptogramins

In 1999 the FDA approved the first drug in the **streptogramin** class of protein synthesis inhibitors. This drug was approved for the treatment of serious or life-threatening infections caused by vancomycin-resistant *Enterococcus faecium* or *Streptococcus pyogenes.* The drug is a mixture of two distinct chemicals: **dalfopristin,** a group A streptogramin, and **quinupristin,** a group B streptogramin (Fig. 32-11). The streptogramins inhibit protein synthesis by binding to the peptidyl transferase center of bacterial 23S rRNA. Mutations and modifications affecting this region can confer resistance. The binding site for the B component overlaps with that of the macrolides, and it is thought that, like the macrolides, the streptogramins block emergence of nascent peptides from the ribosome. The A component can inhibit peptidyl transferase in vitro, but whether the mechanism is the same in vivo remains uncertain.

Streptogramins are unusual among the 50S antibiotics in that they are bactericidal against many, but not all, susceptible bacterial species. A clear explanation for this phenomenon remains elusive; the current hypothesis is that, unlike the other 50S antibiotics, the streptogramins induce a conformational change in the ribosome that is reversible only after subunit dissociation.

Oxazolidinones

In 2000 the FDA approved **linezolid** (Fig. 32-11), the first drug in the **oxazolidinone** class of antibacterial agents. Linezolid demonstrates excellent activity against drug-resistant Gram-positive bacteria, including methicillin-resistant *S. aureus* (MRSA), penicillin-resistant streptococcus, and vancomycin-resistant enterococcus (VRE). Although the precise mechanism of action of linezolid remains uncertain, the drug appears to act at the 50S ribosomal subunit because mutations in 23S rRNA can confer drug resistance.

■ Conclusion and Future Directions

A number of classes of antibiotics target the prokaryotic machinery responsible for the central dogma processes, disrupting bacterial gene expression at multiple steps. Most of these drugs demonstrate selective binding to prokaryotic enzymes or RNAs and have relatively few adverse effects. All are associated with some degree of toxicity, however, and some (e.g., chloramphenicol) have limited clinical use because of their potential to cause life-threatening adverse effects. Several of these antibiotic classes—the quinolones, rifamycin derivatives, and several of the protein synthesis inhibitors—are bactericidal, but most protein synthesis inhibitors are bacteriostatic. Drug resistance is a persistent and serious problem for all of these agents. Although the emergence of resistance is an expected consequence of antibiotic use, judicious drug administration, multidrug therapies, and the continued development of new antibacterial agents can combat the emergence of resistance. The development of the new glycylcycline, streptogramin, and oxazolidinone classes of bacterial ribosome inhibitors represents an important advance in the search for drugs that are effective against resistant bacteria. Further elucidation of the mechanism of action of these drugs will both inform the basic biology of translation and define new biochemical targets for pharmacologic intervention.

■ Suggested Reading

Campbell EA, Korzheva N, Mustaev A, et al. Structural mechanism for rifampicin inhibition of bacterial RNA polymerase. *Cell* 2001;104:901–912. (*Mechanism of rifampin action.*)

Ogle JM, Murphy FV, Tarry MJ, et al. Selection of tRNA by the ribosome requires a transition from an open to a closed form. *Cell* 2002;111:721–732. (*Structural basis for the mechanism of aminoglycoside-induced codon misreading.*)

Sabria M, Pedro-Botet ML, Gomez J, et al. Fluoroquinolones vs. macrolides in the treatment of Legionnaires' disease. *Chest* 2005; 128:1401–1405. (*A prospective study suggesting that fluoroquinolones may be the drug class of choice for treatment of Legionella infection.*)

Steitz TA, Moore PB. RNA, the first macromolecular catalyst: the ribosome is a ribozyme. *Trends Biochem Sci* 2003;28:411–418. (*Reviews function of RNA as a target of antibiotic action in the 50S subunit.*)

Walsh CT. *Antibiotics: Actions, Origins, Resistance.* Washington, DC: ASM Press; 2003. (*Reviews antibiotic synthesis, action, and mechanisms of resistance.*)

Drug Summary Table | **Chapter 32 Pharmacology of Bacterial Infections: DNA Replication, Transcription, and Translation**

Drug	Clinical Applications	Serious and Common Adverse Effects	Contraindications	Therapeutic Considerations
INHIBITORS OF TOPOISOMERASES: QUINOLONES *Mechanism—Inhibit prokaryotic type II topoisomerases. At therapeutic concentrations, quinolones have a bactericidal effect by causing dissociation of the topoisomerase from nicked DNA, leading to double-stranded DNA breaks and cell death.*				
Ciprofloxacin Gatifloxacin Levofloxacin Moxifloxacin Norfloxacin Ofloxacin	Gram-negative infections	Cartilage damage, tendon rupture, peripheral neuropathy, increased intracranial pressure, seizure, severe hypersensitivity reaction Rash, gastrointestinal disturbance	Concomitant tizanidine administration (ciprofloxacin) Hypersensitivity reactions to quinolones	Bacteria evolve resistance through chromosomal mutations in the genes that encode type II topoisomerases, or through alterations in the expression of membrane porins and efflux pumps that determine drug levels inside the bacteria Avoid coadministration of thioridazine due to increased risk of cardiotoxicity (QT prolongation, torsades de pointes, cardiac arrest)
INHIBITORS OF TRANSCRIPTION *Mechanism—Form a stable complex with bacterial DNA-dependent RNA polymerase, thereby inhibiting RNA synthesis*				
Rifabutin Rifampin	Prophylaxis of meningococcal disease (rifampin) Mycobacterial infections, including tuberculosis	Thrombocytopenia, hepatotoxicity Saliva, tear, sweat, and urine discoloration, influenza-like illness, elevated liver function tests, gastrointestinal disturbance	Active *Neisseria meningitidis* infection	Rifampin is not used as a single agent because of rapid development of resistance Rifampin may reduce cyclosporine concentration and efficacy Avoid concurrent administration of clarithromycin with rifampin, because clarithromycin increases plasma concentration of rifabutin and rifabutin reduces plasma concentration of clarithromycin
ANTIMICROBIAL DRUGS TARGETING THE 30S RIBOSOMAL SUBUNIT *Mechunism—Bind to 16S rRNA of the 30S ribosomal subunit and elicit concentration-dependent effects on protein synthesis. Most drugs are bacteriostatic. Aminoglycosides are bactericidal due to induction of mRNA misreading; misread mRNA causes synthesis of aberrant proteins that insert into membrane, forming pores that eventually lead to cell death.*				
Aminoglycosides: Amikacin Gentamicin Kanamycin Neomycin Netilmicin Paromomycin Streptomycin Tobramycin	Serious Gram-negative infections	Ototoxicity, acute renal failure, neuromuscular blockade, respiratory paralysis	Hypersensitivity to aminoglycosides	Act synergistically with β-lactam antibiotics Resistance can occur by three mechanisms: 1. Plasmid-encoded production of a transferase enzyme or enzymes that inactivate aminoglycosides 2. Impaired drug entry, possibly by alteration or elimination of porins or other proteins involved in drug transport 3. Mutation of the drug target on the 30S ribosomal subunit
Spectinomycin	Gonorrhea (alternative therapy)	Injection site pain, nausea, dizziness, insomnia	Hypersensitivity to spectinomycin	Permits formation of the 70S complex but inhibits translocation
Tetracyclines: Chlortetracycline Demeclocycline Doxycycline Methacycline Minocycline Oxytetracycline Tetracycline	Used to treat a variety of infections, notably those due to *Corynebacterium acnes, Haemophilus influenzae, Vibrio cholerae,* spirochetes, *Mycoplasma pneumoniae, Chlamydia* species, and rickettsial species Malaria prophylaxis (doxycycline)	Bulging fontanelle, discoloration and hypoplasia of teeth and temporary stunting of growth, hepatotoxicity, pseudotumor cerebri Photosensitivity, rash, gastrointestinal disturbance, vestibular disturbance (minocycline), candidal infection	Last half of pregnancy Infancy Childhood up to 8 years of age Patients with severe renal impairment should not be treated with any of the tetracyclines except doxycycline	Tetracyclines are actively transported into bacterial cells Resistance occurs by plasmid-encoded efflux pumps, production of proteins that interfere with binding of tetracyclines to the ribosome, or enzymatic inactivation of tetracyclines Tetracyclines should be taken on an empty stomach, because calcium products interfere with absorption

(Continued)

Drug Summary Table **Chapter 32 Pharmacology of Bacterial Infections: DNA Replication, Transcription, and Translation (Continued)**

ANTIMICROBIAL DRUGS TARGETING THE 50S RIBOSOMAL SUBUNIT

Mechanism—Bind to a small region of 23S rRNA of the 50S ribosomal subunit near the peptidyl transferase active center. All drugs are bacteriostatic except for streptogramins, which are bactericidal.

Drug	Clinical Applications	Serious and Common Adverse Effects	Contraindications	Therapeutic Considerations
Glycylcyclines: Tigecycline	Skin or subcutaneous infection Complicated abdominal infection	Gastrointestinal disturbance	Hypersensitivity to tigecycline	Avoid coadministration with acitretin due to increased risk of elevated intracranial pressure Structure is similar to tetracyclines
Macrolides and Ketolides: Azithromycin Clarithromycin Erythromycin Telithromycin	Erythromycin is used to treat a variety of infections, notably those due to *Corynebacterium acnes*, *Legionella pneumophila*, *Treponema pallidum* (syphilis), *Mycoplasma pneumoniae*, and *Chlamydia* species Clarithromycin has increased activity against *H. influenzae* Azithromycin has increased activity against *H. influenzae* and *Moraxella catarrhalis*	*Acute cholestatic hepatitis, ototoxicity, fulminant hepatic necrosis (rare, telithromycin)* Gastrointestinal disturbance	Hepatic dysfunction	Resistance can be conferred by chromosomal mutations leading to alteration of the 50S ribosomal binding site, production of methylases that alter the 50S binding site, or production of esterases that degrade macrolides Macrolides and ketolides inhibit hepatic metabolism of cyclosporine, carbamazepine, warfarin, and theophylline, and can lead to toxic levels of these drugs Macrolides eliminate certain species of intestinal flora that inactivate digoxin, thereby leading to greater oral absorption of digoxin in some patients
Chloramphenicol	Broad-spectrum antibiotic active against bacteria (especially anaerobes) and rickettsiae	*Hemolytic anemia in patients with low levels of G6PD, aplastic anemia, gray baby syndrome*	Hypersensitivity to chloramphenicol	Chloramphenicol antagonizes the bactericidal effects of penicillins and aminoglycosides Most adverse effects are due to inhibition of mitochondrial function Inhibits hepatic metabolism of warfarin, phenytoin, tolbutamide, and chlorpropamide, and thereby potentiates their effects
Lincosamides: Clindamycin	Bacterial infections due to anaerobic organisms	*Pseudomembranous colitis, increased liver function tests, jaundice* Gastrointestinal disturbance, rash	Hypersensitivity to clindamycin	Clindamycin is associated with overgrowth of *C. difficile*, which can result in pseudomembranous colitis
Streptogramins: Dalfopristin/ quinupristin	Vancomycin-resistant enterococcus (VRE) infection Skin and subcutaneous infection caused by staphylococcal or streptococcal species	Injection site inflammation, gastrointestinal disturbance, hyperbilirubinemia, arthralgia, myalgia, headache	Hypersensitivity to dalfopristin/ quinupristin	Should not be coadministered with SSRIs, due to risk of serotonin syndrome Coadministration with pimozide should be avoided due to increased risk of cardiotoxicity (QT prolongation, torsades de pointes, cardiac arrest)
Oxazolidinones: Linezolid	Gram-positive bacterial infections, especially VRE, methicillin-resistant *S. aureus* (MRSA), *S. agalactiae*, *S. pneumoniae* (including multi-drug resistant strains) and *S. pyogenes* Nosocomial pneumonia Complicated diabetic foot infections	*Myelosuppression, peripheral neuropathy, optic neuropathy* Gastrointestinal disturbance, headache	Hypersensitivity to linezolid	The precise mechanism of action of linezolid remains uncertain Linezolid is available in both oral and IV formulations

33

Pharmacology of Bacterial Infections: Cell Wall Synthesis

Anne G. Kasmar and David Hooper

INTRODUCTION

In 1928, Alexander Fleming made a chance discovery that would revolutionize the treatment of bacterial infections. That discovery was **penicillin,** the first of a long line of antibiotics that act by inhibiting synthesis of the bacterial **cell wall.** The cell wall's unique chemical and structural properties make it an attractive and prominent target for antibacterial chemotherapy. The emergence and spread of antibiotic resistance increasingly complicates the clinical use of cell wall synthesis inhibitors, however. This chapter reviews the biochemistry of bacterial cell wall synthesis and describes the mechanisms of action, uses, and limitations (which include resistance, toxicity, and drug-drug interactions) of the antibiotics that interfere with this process.

Case

It is April 1953. The Korean War has reached an uneasy stalemate. In the general hospital in Tokyo, Dr. Alan Pierce's ward has just received a new casualty from the front. Three days earlier, 22-year-old Private (Pvt.) Morgan H had been caught by sniper fire while on reconnaissance and had been hit just above the left knee. At the MASH unit, the wound had been debrided and dressed, and Pvt. H had been started immediately on a course of high-dose penicillin. Nevertheless, by the time he reaches Tokyo, Pvt. H has grown faint and delirious and has developed a fever to 103°F. On initial inspection, Dr. Pierce notices a sickly sweet odor about Pvt. H's leg. When he removes the dressing, he finds the leg bloated below the knee and the wound soaked in putrid, bloody pus. His diagnosis is gangrene, an infection caused by the Gram-positive bacterium *Clostridium perfringens.* Dr. Pierce orders immediate amputation in hopes of saving the young private's life.

Dr. Pierce is troubled by the case. In the past year, he has seen any number of wounds worse than that of Pvt. H, but they have always responded well to aggressive treatment with penicillin. As he is thinking this over, he receives word of more incoming patients—eight men, rumored to be suffering from tuberculosis, who have just been released as part of the Operation Little Switch prisoner exchange. Dr. Pierce knows he has streptomycin on hand but decides to see what he can do about getting a 6-month supply of the new antituberculosis drug, isoniazid, from the United States.

QUESTIONS

■ **1.** What is penicillin, and what is its mechanism of action?

■ **2.** Why did penicillin fail for Pvt. H when this drug had worked for others before him?

■ **3.** Why did Dr. Pierce request a supply of isoniazid from the United States?

BIOCHEMISTRY OF BACTERIAL CELL WALL SYNTHESIS

CELL WALL STRUCTURE AND FUNCTION

The bacterial cell wall is a three-dimensional meshwork of peptide-crosslinked sugar polymers that surrounds the cell just outside its cytoplasmic membrane (Fig. 33-1). Chemically, the cell wall is known interchangeably as **peptidoglycan,** after its peptide and sugar composition, or **murein,** after the Latin *murus,* meaning "wall." The cell wall is a feature of nearly all clinically important bacteria. The major exceptions are *Mycoplasma pneumoniae,* which can cause atypical pneumonia, and the intracellular form (or "reticulate body") of *Chlamydia trachomatis,* which can cause a sexually transmitted disease. The cell wall is critically important for bacteria because of its tensile strength. This strength allows the cell to maintain its intracellular **osmotic pressure** in environments of variable tonicity. The tensile strength of the bacterial cell wall resides in its peptide crosslinks, making inhibition of peptide crosslinking an attractive target for antibacterial therapy. In fact, the largest and most widely used class of bacterial cell wall synthesis inhibitors, the **beta-lactam (β-lactam) antibiotics,** acts by inhibiting **transpeptidase** enzymes that mediate peptide crosslinking.

Bacteria are conventionally divided into two groups, **Gram-positive** and **Gram-negative,** based on the relative ability of these bacteria to retain the purple color of the gentian violet component of the **Gram stain** after being washed with an organic solvent such as acetone. Gram-positive bacteria retain the stain and appear purple, whereas Gram-negative bacteria lose the stain and appear pink from the subsequently applied safranin stain. Gram staining is frequently used to help identify the bacteria present in a specimen of body fluid such as urine, sputum, or pus. The Gram stain is one way Dr. Pierce confirmed the diagnosis of *C. perfringens* back in 1953, and the technique is still standard practice today. The ability to retain Gram stain results from two distinguishing characteristics of cell wall architecture (Fig. 33-1). First, the cell wall of Gram-positive bacteria is simply a coat of murein, whereas Gram-negative bacteria possess a second lipid bilayer, called the outer membrane, outside the murein coat. The second difference is that the murein layer of Gram-positive bacteria is generally much thicker than that of Gram-negative bacteria.

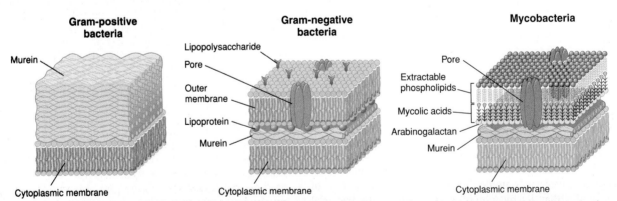

Figure 33-1. Bacterial cell wall architecture. In Gram-positive bacteria **(left),** the cell wall is composed of a thick layer of murein, through which nutrients, waste products, and antibiotics can diffuse. Lipoteichoic acids in the outer leaflet of the cytoplasmic membrane intercalate through the cell wall to the outer surface of Gram-positive bacteria *(not shown)*; the hydrophilic side chains of these molecules are involved in bacterial adherence, feeding, and evasion of the host immune system. In Gram-negative bacteria **(center),** the murein layer is thinner and is surrounded by a second, outer lipid bilayer membrane. Hydrophilic molecules cross this outer membrane through channels, which are formed by a cylindrical arrangement of pore proteins (porins). Gram-negative bacteria also have lipopolysaccharide (LPS) in the outer membrane; LPS is a major antigen for the immune response to Gram-negative organisms. The cell wall of mycobacteria **(right),** which include the causative agents of tuberculosis (*M. tuberculosis*) and leprosy (*M. leprae*), is analogous to that of Gram-negative bacteria. The main difference between the surface architecture of mycobacteria and that of Gram-negative bacteria is that, in mycobacteria, the two leaflets of the outer membrane are asymmetric in size and composition; the inner leaflet of the outer membrane is composed of arabinogalactan and mycolic acids, whereas the outer leaflet is composed of extractable phospholipids.

Because it is composed of lipid, the outer membrane of Gram-negative bacteria hinders transport of hydrophilic substances such as nutrients and waste products. (The murein layer, by contrast, is sufficiently porous to allow diffusion of many hydrophilic molecules.) To enhance uptake of hydrophilic nutrients and excretion of hydrophilic waste products, Gram-negative bacteria have **pores**—composed of proteins called **porins**—that traverse the outer membrane (see Fig. 33-1). Porins are important pharmacologically because it is through these pores that most hydrophilic antibiotics gain access to the murein layer and to the structures beneath this layer. Also important pharmacologically are the **lipopolysaccharides** in the outer leaflet of the outer membrane of Gram-negative bacteria; these amphipathic molecules protect the bacteria from disruption by hydrophilic host molecules such as bile salts, and are important for bacterial adherence to host cells and evasion of the host immune response. Hence, the relative hydrophilicity and hydrophobicity of the various classes of antibacterial drugs help to determine the cell wall architecture against which these antibiotics are most effective, as discussed below.

CELL WALL BIOSYNTHESIS

Cell wall biosynthesis takes place in three major phases. First is the synthesis of murein monomers from amino acids and sugar building blocks; second is the polymerization of the murein monomers into linear peptidoglycan polymers; and third is the crosslinking of the polymers into two-dimensional lattices and three-dimensional mats (Fig. 33-2). The first phase is intracellular and takes place in the cytoplasm; the second is lipid-mediated and takes place at the cytoplasmic membrane; and the third is extracellular and takes place in the **periplasmic space** between the cytoplasmic membrane and the murein layer. (If a bacterium had no cell wall, no periplasmic space would exist. In practice, most bacterial cell wall synthesis consists of remodeling. That is, bacteria add new cell wall components to a previously existing cell wall.) In principle, any of the biochemical steps in any of the three phases of bacterial cell wall synthesis could be a target for inhibition by an antibacterial drug; however, only a few of the biochemical steps are blocked by existing drugs (see discussion below). The details of bacterial cell wall synthesis can be daunting; therefore, it is important to keep in mind these three phases—*monomer synthesis, monomer polymerization,* and *polymer crosslinking*—during the discussion that follows.

Synthesis of Murein Monomers

Murein (peptidoglycan) is synthesized from amino acids and sugars. Murein monomer synthesis begins with the conversion of glucose into two derivatives, *N*-acetylglucosamine (*N*-acetyl-β-D-glucosamine [NAG]) and *N*-acetylmuramic acid (NAM; see Fig. 33-2). NAG is synthesized from the closed-chain glucose β-D-glucopyranose by amidation and phosphorylation to glucosamine-1-phosphate, which is then acetylated and activated by the addition of **uridine diphosphate (UDP)** to form UDP-NAG. NAM is itself a NAG derivative and is formed from UDP-NAG in two reactions. First, **phosphoenolpyruvate** is added to UDP-NAG to form

UDP-NAG pyruvate enol ether, a step catalyzed by the enzyme **MurA** (also known as **enol pyruvate transferase;** Box 33-1); second, **MurB** (also known as **UDP-NAG-enol pyruvate reductase**) reduces this molecule to UDP-NAM. This completes the synthesis of the sugar components.

Next, the peptide component is added. This is performed by a series of peptide transferases (**MurC, MurD,** and **MurE**), which sequentially add the amino acids L-alanine, D-glutamate, and a diamino acid—either L-lysine or **diamino pimelic acid (DAP)**—to UDP-NAM. DAP differs from lysine only in having an additional carboxyl group. Most Gram-positive bacteria use L-lysine, whereas a minority of Gram-positive and all known Gram-negative bacteria use DAP. This is noteworthy because DAP is not found in humans and it therefore offers a unique target for future drug development.

Peptide formation continues with the addition of a D-alanyl-D-alanine dipeptide (D-Ala-D-Ala) to the diamino acid. The dipeptide is synthesized from two molecules of L-alanine in two reactions. Because amino acids are usually available in the environment in the L-conformation—which is the conformation found in most mammalian proteins—the first reaction requires the transformation of two molecules of L-alanine into D-alanine. This reaction is catalyzed by the enzyme **alanine racemase.** In the second reaction, an enzyme called D-Ala-D-Ala synthetase (or **D-Ala-D-Ala ligase**) joins the two D-alanines together; this reaction requires ATP. The resulting D-Ala-D-Ala dipeptide is added by the enzyme **MurF** to the peptide-substituted UDP-NAM to form UDP-NAM-L-Ala-D-Glu-L-Lys-(or DAP-)D-Ala-D-Ala, a molecule referred to as the **Park peptide** (Fig. 33-2A).

Two more reactions complete the synthesis of a murein monomer. These reactions take place at the inner surface of the cytoplasmic membrane in association with a lipid carrier molecule, **bactoprenol.** Bactoprenol is also used to ferry the completed monomer to the outer surface of the cytoplasmic membrane, where polymerization occurs (Fig. 33-2B). These reactions begin with the **MraY**-mediated transfer of the Park peptide to phosphorylated bactoprenol. This transfer liberates UMP, resulting in a pyrophosphate bond between bactoprenol and the Park peptide. In a reaction catalyzed by the enzyme **MurG,** this new molecule then reacts with a molecule of UDP-NAG, liberating UDP and resulting in the formation of a bond between the NAM of the Park peptide and NAG. Finally, in Gram-positive bacteria, a linker polypeptide, typically composed of five glycine residues, is usually added at the lysine (or DAP) position; as discussed below, this **interbridge** allows polymer crosslinking in Gram-positive bacteria. In Gram-negative bacteria, the murein monomers are usually crosslinked to one another directly, without the use of a linker polypeptide. These steps complete the synthesis of a **murein monomer.**

Polymerization

The last two phases in cell wall biosynthesis—polymerization (transglycosylation) and crosslinking (transpeptidation)—take place outside the cytoplasm in the periplasmic space. For murein monomers to reach the periplasmic space, they must cross the lipid bilayer of the cytoplasmic membrane. As noted previously, this "ferrying" requires bactoprenol. A long, lipophilic molecule, bactoprenol is thought to wrap around the murein monomer, rendering it sufficiently

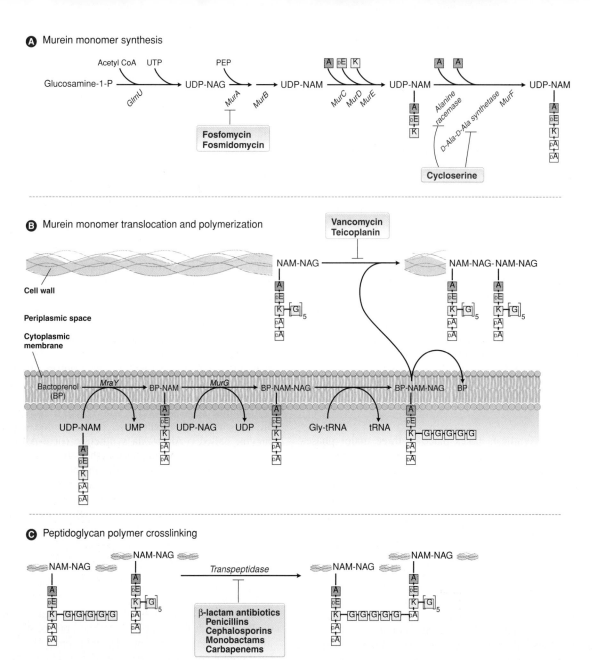

Figure 33-2. Bacterial cell wall biosynthesis and its inhibition by pharmacologic agents. Bacterial cell wall biosynthesis can be divided into three steps. **A.** In murein monomer synthesis, glucose is amidated and phosphorylated to glucosamine-1-phosphate *(not shown)*, which is acetylated and conjugated to a uridine diphosphate (UDP) nucleotide by the enzyme GlmU to form UDP-*N*-acetylglucosamine (UDP-NAG). Addition of phosphoenolpyruvate (PEP) by enol pyruvate transferase (MurA), and reduction of the resulting product by MurB, forms UDP-*N*-acetylmuramic acid (UDP-NAM). Fosfomycin and fosmidomycin are selective inhibitors of enol pyruvate transferase. NAG and NAM are the two sugar building blocks for subsequent cell wall synthesis. MurC, MurD, and MurE sequentially add the amino acids L-alanine *(A)*, D-glutamate *(DE)*, and L-lysine *(K)* to UDP-NAM. In some bacteria, diamino pimelic acid (DAP) is added instead of L-lysine. Alanine racemase converts L-alanine to D-alanine *(DA)*, and D-Ala-D-Ala synthetase forms the dipeptide D-Ala-D-Ala. This dipeptide is then added to the A-DE-K (or A-DE-DAP) tripeptide by MurF, resulting in a UDP-NAM molecule linked to five amino acids (Park peptide). Cycloserine inhibits both alanine racemase and D-Ala-D-Ala synthetase, thereby preventing the addition of alanine residues to the growing peptide chain. **B.** The NAM-penta-peptide complex is transferred from UDP to the lipid carrier bactoprenol (BP) by the enzyme MraY, and NAG is added from UDP-NAG by MurG. In some bacteria, one to five amino acids can then be added to K or DAP to form a branched peptidoglycan; the amino acids are added from amino acyl tRNA. (Here, as an example, five glycine [G] residues are added from glycyl-tRNA.) In the murein monomer translocation and polymerization step, the BP-peptidoglycan complex is transported from the bacterial inner membrane to the periplasmic space, where transglycosylases join the murein monomer to the growing peptidoglycan chain. Simultaneously, the BP is liberated to catalyze another round of murein monomer translocation. Completion of this set of reactions depends on serial phosphorylation and dephosphorylation of the bactoprenol molecule *(not shown)*. Bacitracin inhibits bactoprenol dephosphorylation and thereby interrupts murein monomer translocation *(not shown)*. Vancomycin and teicoplanin bind the D-Ala-D-Ala terminus of the BP-conjugated murein monomer unit and thereby prevent the transglycosidase-mediated addition of the murein monomer to the growing peptidoglycan chain. **C.** In the final step of cell wall biosynthesis, adjacent glycopeptide polymers are crosslinked in a reaction catalyzed by bacterial transpeptidases. In the example shown, a transpeptidase crosslinks a glycine (G) pentapeptide on one peptidoglycan chain to a D-Ala residue on an adjacent peptidoglycan chain; as shown in detail in Figure 33-3, the terminal D-Ala residue is displaced in this reaction. The β-lactam antibiotics (penicillins, cephalosporins, monobactams, and carbapenems) inhibit the transpeptidase enzymes that crosslink adjacent peptidoglycan polymers.

604

Like most enzymes, the enzymes of cell wall biosynthesis are known by multiple names. The Mur naming convention used here is the emerging standard, but the enzymes are also still known by the following descriptive names (among others):

GlmU   Diamine N-acetyltransferase
MurA   Enol pyruvate transferase
MurB   UDP–NAG-enol pyruvate reductase
MurC   UDP–NAM-L-Ala synthetase
MurD   UDP–NAM-L-Ala-D-Glu synthetase
MurE   UDP–NAM-L-Ala-D-Glu-2,6-diaminopimelate synthetase
MurF   UDP–NAM-tripeptide-D-Ala-D-Ala synthetase
MraY   UDP–NAM-pentapeptide:undecaprenyl-phosphate transferase
MurG   Undecaprenyldiphospho-NAM-pentapeptide: NAG transferase

Note: Undecaprenol is another name for bactoprenol.

lipophilic to cross the bilayer. Once in the periplasmic space, the monomer is attached to a growing murein chain via bonds between the NAM of the murein monomer and the NAG of the growing peptidoglycan polymer. This transfer, which is catalyzed by transglycosylases, frees bactoprenol pyrophosphate. Bactoprenol pyrophosphate then returns to the inner surface of the cytoplasmic membrane. There, it loses a phosphate group to form bactoprenol phosphate; this step is catalyzed by a **dephosphorylase.** Bactoprenol phosphate is now ready to accept another Park peptide (Fig. 33-2B).

Crosslinking

In the third and final phase of cell wall synthesis, murein chains are crosslinked to one another by enzymes called **transpeptidases.** Because transpeptidases were first identified as the molecular targets of penicillin binding, they are also called **penicillin-binding proteins** (**PBPs**). The transpeptidase enzyme displaces the terminal D-Ala residue on one peptide chain to form an enzyme-peptidoglycan intermediate; the free amino group on the terminal amino acid of the interbridge peptide (glycine for most Gram-positive bacteria) or on DAP (Gram-negative bacteria) then attacks this intermediate, resulting in formation of the crosslink (Figs. 33-2C and 33-3). Differences in chain length and in the number and type of crosslink give each bacterial species its characteristic shape and size and the cell wall of each species its characteristic thickness.

Bacteria typically have several transpeptidases of different but overlapping specificities. These different enzyme isoforms are used to build different parts of the wall. *Escherichia coli,* for example, has six transpeptidases, some of which build the cylindrical middle of this rod-shaped bacteria, whereas others build its hemispherical ends. Also, the suite of transpeptidases differs from species to species, and

especially between rods such as *E. coli* and *C. perfringens* and spherical cocci such as streptococci and staphylococci.

MYCOBACTERIAL CELL WALL

The cell wall structures described above apply to the vast majority of clinically relevant bacteria, including Gram-positive cocci such as streptococci and staphylococci, Gram-negative rods such as *E. coli* and *Pseudomonas aeruginosa,* and Gram-positive rods such as *C. perfringens.* However, the cell wall of one group of bacteria, the **mycobacteria,** differs in several important respects. Because of the resurgent clinical impact of *Mycobacterium tuberculosis,* the bacterium that causes tuberculosis, it is important to examine the mycobacterial cell wall in some detail.

As with the cell wall of Gram-negative bacteria, the cell wall of mycobacteria consists of a relatively thin layer of murein just outside the cytoplasmic membrane. However, dissimilar to Gram-negative bacteria, the NAM residues of the cell wall in mycobacteria are modified by the addition of a long, branched chain consisting of a NAG-**arabinogalactan** linker topped with **mycolic acid.** Structurally, the lipophilic mycolic acid layer acts as the inner half of an asymmetric outer membrane; the outer half of this membrane is composed of secreted phospholipids, called **extractable lipids,** that are analogous to the lipids that form the outer half of the cytoplasmic membrane (see Fig. 33-1). Overall, then, an analogy can be drawn between the mycobacterial and the Gram-negative cell wall and associated structures. Both mycobacteria and Gram-negative bacteria are enclosed by an inner (cytoplasmic) membrane, a murein (cell wall) layer, and an outer membrane; the main structural difference is that the outer membrane of mycobacteria is thick, asymmetric, and highly impermeable to both hydrophilic and hydrophobic substances.

The synthesis of NAG-arabinogalactan begins with the transfer of a molecule of NAG phosphate from UDP-NAG to mycobacterial bactoprenol phosphate. Next, a molecule of the sugar rhamnose is added, followed by the addition of the several galactose and arabinose units that make up arabinogalactan. Addition of the arabinose units is catalyzed by the enzyme **arabinosyl transferase.**

Mycolic acid is a long, complex, branched fatty acid. The starting materials for its synthesis include a number of long, saturated hydrocarbon chains that are synthesized from two-carbon units carried by acetyl CoA. The enzyme **fatty acid synthetase 1 (FAS1)** catalyzes the formation of these saturated hydrocarbon chains, whereas the enzyme **fatty acid synthetase 2 (FAS2)** catalyzes the linkage of these chains. The linked product then undergoes several enzymatic transformations to become mycolic acid. Mycolic acid is eventually added to NAG-arabinogalactan, which, in turn, is attached to NAM to form the complete inner half of the mycobacterial outer membrane (Figs. 33-1 and 33-4).

In principle, any step in this process is susceptible to pharmacologic intervention. As discussed below, standard antimycobacterial treatment regimens include antibiotics that target both the synthesis of NAG-arabinogalactan and the early reactions of mycolic acid synthesis.

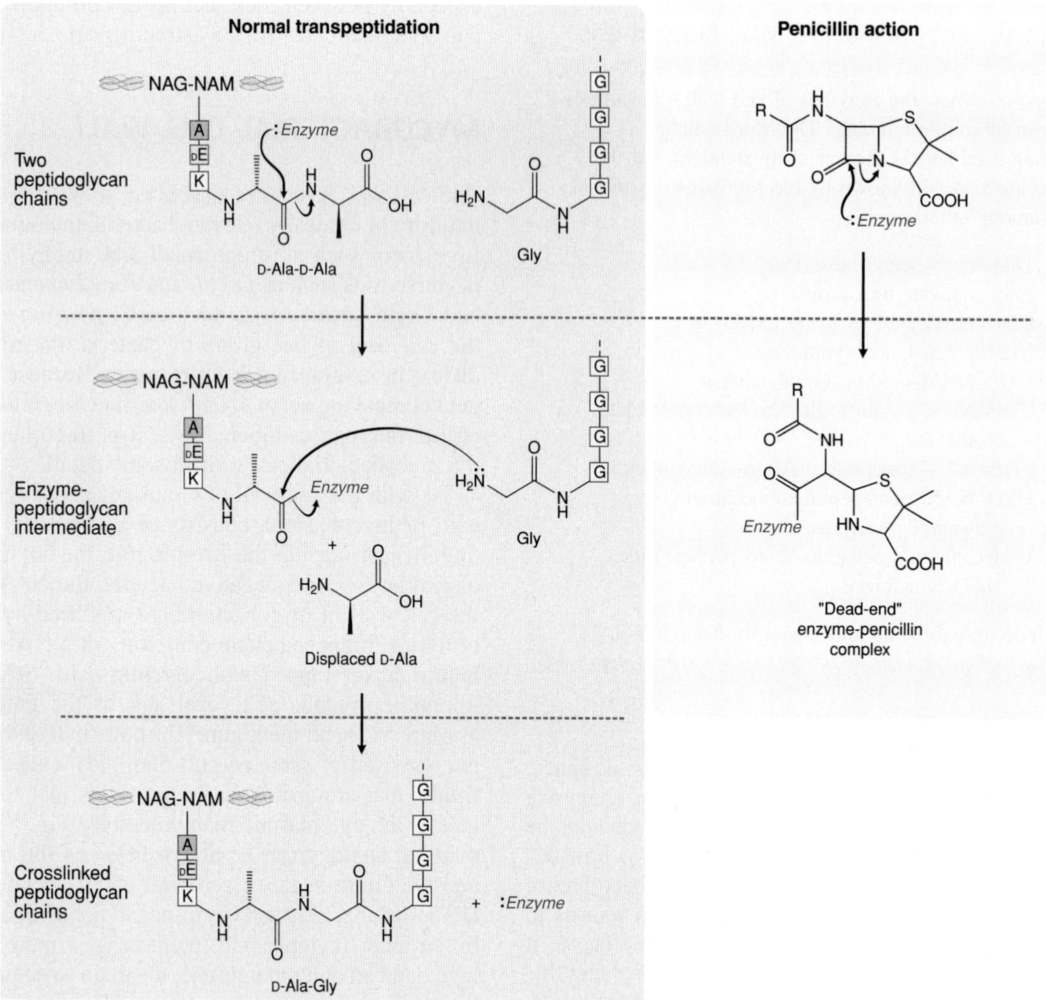

Figure 33-3. Transpeptidase action and its inhibition by penicillin. The left side of the figure shows the mechanism by which transpeptidases catalyze transpeptidation, a reaction that occurs in bacteria but not in mammalian cells. A nucleophilic group on the transpeptidase (Enzyme) attacks the peptide bond between the two D-Ala residues at the terminus of a pentapeptide moiety on one peptidoglycan chain **(top panel).** The terminal D-alanine residue is displaced from the peptidoglycan chain, and an enzyme-D-alanine-peptidoglycan intermediate is formed. This intermediate is then attacked by the amino terminus of a polyglycine pentapeptide linked at its carboxy terminus to L-lysine or diaminopimelic acid on an adjacent peptidoglycan chain (see Fig. 33-2) **(middle panel).** As the enzyme is liberated from the intermediate, a new peptide bond (crosslink) is formed between the terminal glycine residue on one peptidoglycan chain and the enzyme-activated D-alanine residue on the adjacent peptidoglycan chain. The free enzyme can then catalyze another transpeptidation reaction **(bottom panel).** The right side of the figure shows the mechanism by which penicillin interferes with transpeptidation, leading to the formation of a penicilloyl-enzyme "dead-end complex." In this form, the enzyme is incapable of catalyzing further transpeptidation (crosslinking) reactions.

AUTOLYSINS AND CELL WALL DEGRADATION

For bacteria to grow, bacterial cell walls must expand; for expansion to occur, new murein units must be incorporated into the existing cell wall. This is difficult to accomplish in a "finished" cell wall, where the murein polymer chains are already of the desired length and the desired type and degree of polymer crosslinking already exist. In addition, for a bacterium to divide into two daughter cells, its cell wall must at some point be broken. Bacteria address these issues by using **autolysins.** These enzymes (**NAM-L-ala-nine amidase,** for example) punch small holes in the cell wall that allow for cell wall remodeling and expansion.

Clearly, new murein synthesis and autolysin-mediated destruction must be carefully balanced for the bacteria to survive. Indeed, studies have shown that unilaterally blocking murein synthesis results in autolysin-mediated **autolysis** and cell death. The molecular events that initiate autolysis are still poorly understood. One theory holds that bacterial exposure to antibiotics inhibiting cell wall synthesis leads to leakage and loss of an endogenous autolysin inhibitor, perhaps **lipoteichoic acid** in Gram-positive bacteria, and that this loss, in turn, results in the activation of autolysins and the eventual lysis of the cell. The **bactericidal effect** of many antibiotics discussed in this chapter is thought to result from drug-mediated disruption of the balance between cell wall synthesis and cell wall degradation.

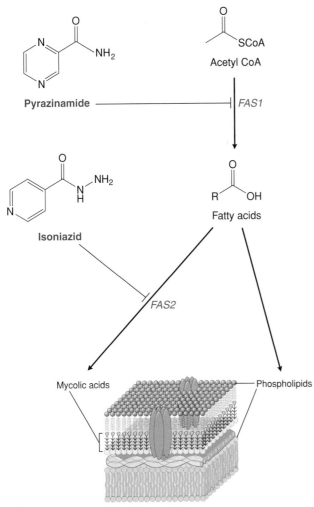

Figure 33-4. Mycolic acid synthesis and antimycobacterial drug action. Mycolic acids are produced by the crosslinking of fatty acid chains derived from acetyl coenzyme A (Acetyl CoA). Each of the arrows in this simplified representation denotes multiple synthetic steps; the focus is on the fatty acid synthetases (FAS1 and FAS2) because of their importance as drug targets. Specifically, FAS1 is inhibited by pyrazinamide, and FAS2 is inhibited by isoniazid.

PHARMACOLOGIC CLASSES AND AGENTS

The pharmacology of the drug classes that inhibit bacterial cell wall synthesis is discussed in the same order as the physiology of cell wall synthesis (Fig. 33-2). Although drugs have been identified that inhibit a number of steps in the biochemistry of cell wall synthesis, the polymer crosslinking (transpeptidation) step is, by far, the most clinically important biochemical target. For this reason, most of the discussion focuses on the panoply of agents that inhibit the crosslinking of peptidoglycan polymers.

INHIBITORS OF MUREIN MONOMER SYNTHESIS

Fosfomycin and Fosmidomycin

Two agents inhibit the production of murein monomers by inhibiting the synthesis of UDP-NAM from UDP-NAG. **Fosfomycin** (also written **phosphomycin**) is a phosphoenol-pyruvate (PEP) analogue that inhibits bacterial enol pyruvate transferase (also known as MurA) by covalent modification of the enzyme's active site. Given that PEP is a key intermediate in (mammalian) glycolysis, it may come as a surprise that this agent does not interfere with carbohydrate metabolism in human cells; this selectivity of antibacterial action is likely caused by structural differences between the mammalian and bacterial enzymes that act on PEP. Thus, fosfomycin has no appreciable effect on human enolase, pyruvate kinase, or carboxykinase, and the drug is relatively nontoxic. Fosfomycin has been shown to have antibacterial synergy in vitro with β-lactams, aminoglycosides, and fluoroquinolones.

Fosfomycin enters the cell via transporters for glycerophosphate or glucose-6-phosphate that are normally used by bacteria to take up these nutrients from the environment. Fosfomycin is especially effective against Gram-negative bacteria that infect the urinary tract, including *E. coli* and *Klebsiella* and *Serratia* species, because it is excreted unchanged in the urine. A single 3-g oral dose has been shown to be as effective as multiple doses of other agents in the treatment of urinary tract infections. As a rule, fosfomycin is less effective against Gram-positive bacteria because these bacteria generally lack selective glycerophosphate and glucose-6-phosphate transporters. Although resistance is typically caused by mutations in these transporters, a temperature-sensitive *E. coli* strain has been found in which a mutation in enol pyruvate transferase results in reduced affinity of the enzyme for PEP and therefore for fosfomycin. Adverse effects of fosfomycin are uncommon; between 1% and 10% of patients develop headache, diarrhea, or nausea. Significant drug interactions are also rare; the drug can precipitate when coingested with antacids or calcium salts, and its absorption can be decreased by coadministration with promotility agents such as metoclopramide.

Fosmidomycin, another PEP analogue, acts by the same mechanism as fosfomycin, and resistance typically arises via mutations in glycerophosphate or glucose-6-phosphate transporters. Again, however, there are exceptions: at least one strain of resistant *E. coli* appears to contain a protein that actively pumps fosmidomycin out of the cell. Fosmidomycin also has activity against malaria, but the drug has a different mechanism of action against the parasite and is not currently in clinical use for that organism.

Cycloserine

Cycloserine, a structural analogue of D-Ala, is a second-line agent used to treat multidrug resistant *M. tuberculosis* infection (Fig. 33-5). Cycloserine inhibits both the alanine racemase that converts L-Ala to D-Ala and the D-Ala-D-Ala synthetase that joins together two D-Ala molecules (Fig. 33-2). Cycloserine is an irreversible inhibitor of these enzymes and, in fact, binds these enzymes more tightly than does their

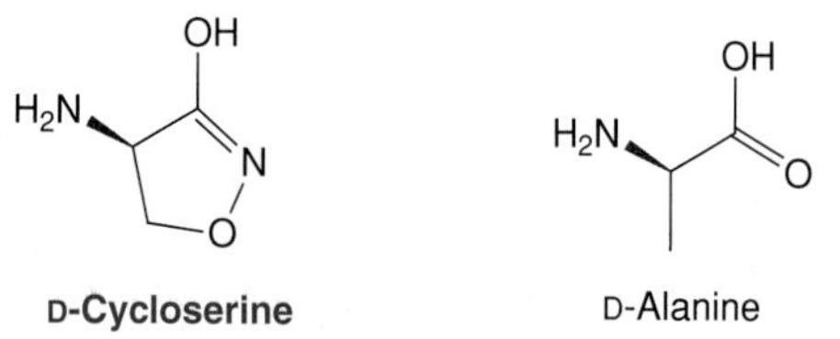

Figure 33-5. Structure of cycloserine. Cycloserine is a structural analogue of D-alanine that inhibits the racemic interconversion of L-alanine to D-alanine by alanine racemase. Cycloserine also inhibits the activity of D-Ala-D-Ala synthetase, the enzyme that catalyzes the formation of the D-Ala-D-Ala dipeptide that is subsequently utilized in the synthesis of murein monomers (see Fig. 33-2).

natural substrate, D-Ala. Resistance to cycloserine occurs by multiple mechanisms, some of which are still unknown; known mechanisms include the overexpression of alanine racemase and mutations in the alanine uptake system. As with many small molecules, including fosfomycin, cycloserine is excreted in the urine. Adverse effects include seizures, neurological syndromes including peripheral neuropathy, and psychosis. Patients with underlying neuropsychiatric disease, alcoholism, and chronic kidney disease should avoid the drug. Alcohol, isoniazid, and ethionamide potentiate its toxicity; pyridoxine may mitigate cycloserine-induced peripheral neuropathy. Cycloserine inhibits the hepatic metabolism of phenytoin.

Bacitracin

So named because it was first identified in a species of *Bacillus,* **bacitracin** is a peptide antibiotic that interferes with the dephosphorylation of bactoprenol pyrophosphate, rendering this lipid carrier useless for further rounds of murein monomer translocation (Fig. 33-2). Bacitracin is therefore notable among the anti-cell wall agents for having a lipid, rather than a protein or peptide, as its target. Bacitracin inhibits dephosphorylation by forming a complex with bactoprenol pyrophosphate that involves bacitracin's imidazole and thiazoline rings. This interaction requires a divalent metal ion, usually Zn^{2+} or Mg^{2+}; hence, drugs that act as metal chelators could interfere with the activity of bacitracin. Due to its significant kidney, neurological, and bone marrow toxicity, bacitracin is not used systemically. It is most commonly used topically for superficial dermal or ophthalmologic infections. Because bacitracin is not absorbed orally, it remains within the gut lumen and is occasionally administered orally to treat *Clostridium difficile* colitis or to eradicate **vancomycin-resistant enterococci** (**VRE**) in the gastrointestinal tract. It should not be coadministered with other nephrotoxic medications or neuromuscular blocking agents, since the latter may result in synergistic neuromuscular blockade.

INHIBITORS OF MUREIN POLYMER SYNTHESIS

Vancomycin and Teicoplanin

Vancomycin and **teicoplanin** are glycopeptides with bactericidal activity against Gram-positive rods and cocci. Gram-

negative rods are resistant to the action of these drugs. These agents interrupt cell wall synthesis by binding tightly to the D-Ala-D-Ala terminus of the murein monomer unit, inhibiting **transglycosidase** and thereby blocking the addition of murein units to the growing polymer chain. Intravenous vancomycin is most commonly used to treat sepsis or endocarditis caused by methicillin-resistant *Staphylococcus aureus* (MRSA) (see discussion below). Oral vancomycin is used to treat gastrointestinal infections with *C. difficile*; like bacitracin (see above), the drug is poorly absorbed and therefore stays within the gastrointestinal tract. Teicoplanin is not used clinically in the United States.

As a rule, the toxicity of vancomycin causes this agent to be used only when an infection is found to be resistant to other agents. Its adverse effects include skin flushing or rash—the so-called **red-man syndrome**—which can be avoided by slowing the rate of intravenous infusion or preadministering antihistamines. Vancomycin has also been associated with nephrotoxicity and ototoxicity, particularly when other nephrotoxic or ototoxic medications such as gentamicin are coadministered. Patients with underlying renal dysfunction may need reduced dosing as well as measurement of drug levels in order to prevent further nephrotoxicity. Drug fever, hypersensitivity rash, and drug-induced neutropenia can also occur. Resistance to vancomycin most commonly arises through the acquisition of DNA encoding enzymes that catalyze the formation of D-Ala-D-lactate instead of D-Ala-D-Ala. As with D-Ala-D-Ala, D-Ala-D-lactate is incorporated into the murein monomer unit and participates readily in the transpeptidase reaction, but the D-Ala-D-lactate dipeptide is not bound by vancomycin. Two enzymes mediate the synthesis of D-Ala-D-lactate: VanH, a dehydrogenase that generates D-lactate from pyruvate, and VanA, a ligase that links D-Ala to D-lactate. VanH and VanA are encoded on a transposable element that can be found on either the bacterial chromosome or an extrachromosomal plasmid. This element also encodes enzymes that degrade D-Ala-D-Ala, thereby removing any residual targets of vancomycin. In clinical practice, bacteria resistant to vancomycin (such as VRE) are often resistant to most other antibacterials; plasmid-mediated spread of vancomycin resistance is therefore a serious medical problem. A few cases of vancomycin-resistant *S. aureus* (VRSA) due to acquisition of enterococcal resistance genes have been reported. Vancomycin-intermediate *S. aureus* (VISA) has also been described; these organisms have a thicker murein layer in which increased amounts of free D-Ala-D-Ala act as a decoy target for vancomycin.

INHIBITORS OF POLYMER CROSSLINKING

Beta-Lactam Antibiotics: General Considerations

With more than 30 different agents currently in use, including the original **penicillin** used in the attempt to treat Pvt. H, the β-lactams are the largest and most widely prescribed class of antibiotics that inhibit bacterial cell wall synthesis. The different agents in this class vary in chemical structure (Fig. 33-6), and consequently in spectrum of action, but all β-lactams share the same antibiotic mechanism of action: inhibition of murein polymer crosslinking.

Chemically, the key to this mechanism of action is the presence of a four-membered **β-lactam ring** (Fig. 33-6).

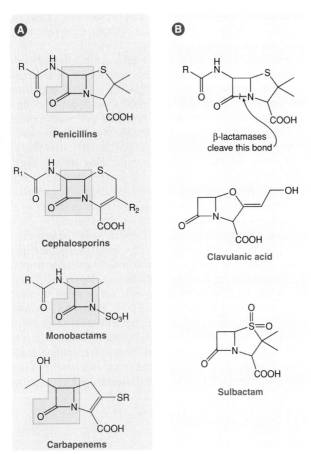

Figure 33-6. Structural features of β-lactam antibiotics and β-lactamase inhibitors. A. The β-lactam family members (penicillins, cephalosporins, monobactams, and carbapenems) differ from one another in their backbone structures; individual drugs within these subclasses also differ in their R groups. Note the four-membered β-lactam ring that is common to all four families *(blue boxes)*; it is this ring that gives the agents their ability to block the transpeptidation reaction (and also their name). **B.** Bacteria expressing β-lactamases are able to cleave the β-lactam bond *(blue line)* that is required for antibiotic action. The β-lactamase inhibitors clavulanic acid and sulbactam act as decoys by binding to (and thereby inhibiting) β-lactamase enzymes. Note the structural similarity between the β-lactamase inhibitors and the β-lactam antibiotics.

This ring makes every β-lactam a structural analogue of the terminal D-Ala-D-Ala dipeptide of the Park peptide, and hence a substrate for one or more bacterial transpeptidases. As with the Park peptide, the β-lactam is able to bind the transpeptidase covalently and thereby form an acyl enzyme intermediate. Unlike the Park peptide in the normal substrate reaction, however, the β-lactam ring renders the carboxy terminal end of the β-lactam unable to be cleaved from the rest of the molecule. As a result, the incoming amino terminal end of the adjacent peptide cannot attack the acyl enzyme intermediate, and the transpeptidase reaches a **"dead-end"** complex (Fig. 33-3). (This mode of irreversible enzyme inhibition is sometimes called **suicide substrate inhibition.**) Provided that the cells are growing, transpeptidase inhibition results in autolysin-mediated autolysis and cell death. Hence, as a rule, β-lactams are **bactericidal** for actively dividing bacteria.

The different subclasses of β-lactam agents fall into four families—the **penicillins,** the **cephalosporins** (which are further subdivided into four "generations"), the **monobactams,** and the **carbapenems.** Each of these subclasses differs structurally in the chemical substituents that are attached to the β-lactam ring (see Fig. 33-6). In general, these families resulted from pharmacologists' efforts in the laboratory to improve on penicillin's antibiotic **spectrum of action** and to stay ahead of the spread of **antibiotic resistance,** as was seen in the case of Pvt. H. (Recall that spectrum of action refers to the number and variety of bacterial species against which an antibiotic shows bactericidal or bacteriostatic activity. Hence, broad spectrum β-lactams are typically active against Gram-negative as well as Gram-positive bacteria, whereas narrow spectrum β-lactams are typically effective only against Gram-positive organisms.)

Because bacterial transpeptidases are located in the periplasmic space between the cytoplasmic membrane and the cell wall, β-lactams must traverse the cell wall, and, in the case of Gram-negative bacteria, the outer membrane, to exert their effect. Hence, a β-lactam's spectrum of action is determined by two factors: the degree to which it can penetrate the outer membrane and cell wall and, once in the periplasmic space, its ability to bind to specific transpeptidases. Both hydrophilic and (to a lesser extent) hydrophobic agents diffuse through the thick murein layer of Gram-positive bacteria, but hydrophilic agents pass through the outer membrane pores of Gram-negative bacteria much more readily than do hydrophobic agents. As a result, hydrophilic agents such as **ampicillin, amoxicillin,** and, especially, **piperacillin, ticarcillin, carbenicillin,** and **mezlocillin** tend to have broad spectra of action, whereas hydrophobic agents such as **oxacillin, cloxacillin, dicloxacillin, nafcillin, methicillin,** and **penicillin G**—a close relative of the agent that was available to soldiers during the Korean War—tend to have narrow spectra of action (see discussion below for details). This means that some Gram-negative bacteria are inherently resistant to narrow spectrum β-lactams simply by virtue of the permeability barrier presented by their outer membrane. (Similarly, **intracellular bacteria,** that is, bacteria that live within human cells, such as *Chlamydia* are, in general, also inherently resistant to β-lactams, both because mammalian cells tend to lack β-lactam uptake mechanisms and because these bacteria tend either to have unique cell wall architectures or to lack cell walls altogether.)

The second factor that determines a β-lactam's spectrum of action is the extent to which the drug, after accessing the periplasmic space, inhibits a particular transpeptidase. In large part, this is determined by the β-lactam's affinity for the transpeptidase. As noted above, bacteria typically have several transpeptidases that differ subtly in their substrate specificity and crosslinking activity; these differences are especially prominent between rods and cocci. Most β-lactams have selectivity for several different transpeptidases; others, such as the penicillin analogue methicillin that is used against *S. aureus,* are specific for just one.

Antibiotic resistance can be encoded by either **chromosomal (intrinsic)** or **acquired (extrinsic)** genes. For β-lactams, chromosomal resistance in Gram-positive bacteria is most commonly conferred by a chromosomally encoded mutation in a transpeptidase-encoding gene that abolishes the transpeptidase's ability to bind a particular β-lactam, or by acquisition of a gene encoding a transpeptidase with low affinity for the β-lactam. This mechanism is the cause of resistance to methicillin in *S. aureus* and the mechanism by which pneumococci acquire resistance to penicillin. Resistance to β-lactams by altered transpeptidases is the exception, not the rule, because most β-lactams are active against multiple transpeptidases that would all need to be altered in order to abolish the drugs' effectiveness.

Most resistance to β-lactams is conferred by proteins called **β-lactamases** that are encoded on the chromosome or on extrachromosomal DNA **plasmids.** Acquisition of such a plasmid is probably the mechanism by which resistance emerged in the *C. perfringens* that infected Pvt. H. As their name implies, β-lactamases are enzymes that inactivate β-lactams via (hydrolytic) cleavage of the β-lactam ring. More than 100 different β-lactamases have been identified, each with activity against a particular β-lactam or set of β-lactams. Beta-lactamases are secreted in Gram-positive bacteria, whereas, in Gram-negative bacteria, these enzymes are retained in the periplasmic space between the cell wall and outer membrane. Gram-negative bacteria produce much less β-lactamase than Gram-positive bacteria, but, because the Gram-negatives concentrate the β-lactamase where it is needed, the β-lactamase is more effective at conferring resistance. This concentration effect, coupled with the strong permeability barrier to penicillins afforded by the bacterial outer membrane, makes Gram-negative bacteria largely refractory to penicillin therapy.

That many β-lactamases are encoded on plasmids is of special clinical importance. Because plasmids are easily transferred by conjugation from one bacterium to another, the resistance conferred by the plasmid can sweep rapidly through a bacterial population. Moreover, plasmids can "jump strains," spreading resistance from one strain to another. Organisms such as *Klebsiella pneumoniae* and *E. coli* may also produce **extended-spectrum β-lactamases (ESBLs),** which render them resistant to most β-lactam antibiotics, including the penicillins and cephalosporins and the monobactam **aztreonam.** Other bacteria, such as *Enterobacter* species, may overexpress a chromosomally encoded β-lactamase that produces similarly broad resistance to β-lactams. Pharmacologists' response to β-lactamases has been twofold. First, as noted above, has been the development of new families of β-lactams whose structures make them less susceptible to cleavage by existing β-lactamases. Second has been the coadministration of β-lactams with **β-lactamase inhibitors,** which are β-lactam-like molecules that bind to β-lactamases and thereby prevent the β-lactamases from destroying the β-lactam antibiotics with which the lactamase inhibitors are coadministered. Three examples of β-lactamase inhibitors are **clavulanic acid (clavulanate), sulbactam,** and **tazobactam** (Fig. 33-6).

Beta-lactams act synergistically with **aminoglycosides,** the bactericidal inhibitors of protein synthesis discussed in Chapter 32. (For more on synergy, see Chapter 39, Principles of Combination Chemotherapy.) Aminoglycosides inhibit protein synthesis by binding to the 30S ribosomal subunit in the cytoplasm of the cell. To access the cytoplasm, aminoglycosides must diffuse passively across the cell wall before being transported actively across the cytoplasmic membrane. It is thought that the cell walls of some bacteria, such as enterococci, are poorly permeable to aminoglycosides when these drugs are administered as single agents. Because the

β-lactams act to increase cell wall permeability, coadministration of a β-lactam facilitates the uptake of an aminoglycoside and thus enhances its effect.

An interesting question is whether the aminoglycosides reciprocate by potentiating the activity of β-lactams, or whether, instead, the aminoglycosides antagonize β-lactams by inhibiting the synthesis of autolysins. From work on *Bacillus subtilis,* it appears that bacterial cell walls contain a lethal amount of autolysins throughout cell growth, and that cells actively restrain autolytic activity by controlling the state of activation of these proteins. This finding suggests that autolysis does not require de novo autolysin synthesis and, therefore, that aminoglycosides should not antagonize β-lactams. Regardless, the important point is that *clinically, β-lactams and aminoglycosides are synergistic.*

The most common adverse effects of β-lactam therapy are hypersensitivity reactions. As small molecules, β-lactams would not be expected to stimulate immune responses by themselves, and indeed they do not. However, β-lactam rings can react with amino groups on proteins to create a hapten-carrier complex (Fig. 33-7). The β-lactam-protein conjugate can then provoke a hypersensitivity response. The most dreaded of these reactions is **anaphylaxis,** which typically occurs within an hour of administration and leads to bronchospasm, angioedema, and/or cardiovascular collapse. Urticaria, morbilliform drug rash, serum sickness, and drug

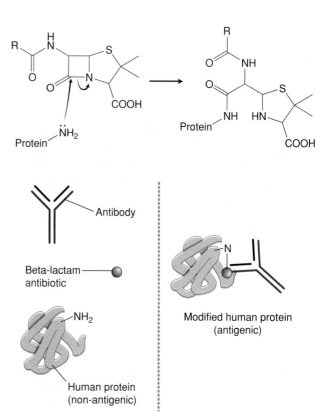

Figure 33-7. Beta-lactam toxicity. Upper panel: Beta-lactams can modify amino groups on human proteins, creating an immunogenic β-lactam hapten. **Lower panel:** In the absence of modification, human proteins are generally nonantigenic. Modification of endogenous proteins by the addition of a β-lactam antibiotic results in the formation of a new antigenic determinant that can be recognized as "nonself" by antibodies of the host immune system.

fever also may occur. Proteins on the surface of red blood cells can also be modified by penicillin, leading to drug-induced autoimmune hemolytic anemia. Rarely, β-lactam antibiotics cause drug-induced lupus. For most individuals, this process is strongly dose-dependent: the likelihood of a hypersensitivity reaction increases with each administration of a β-lactam. Beta-lactams of a given class often cross-react with each other, but β-lactams of one class are less often cross-reactive with β-lactams of another class. Patients with a penicillin allergy should not receive ampicillin or a carbapenem due to the high risk of cross-reactivity. Patients with a penicillin allergy other than anaphylaxis may receive a cephalosporin. **Aztreonam** (a monobactam) is unique in that it has no cross-reactivity with either the penicillins or carbapenems; however, cross-reactivity between aztreonam and ceftazidime (a cephalosporin) due to a shared side-chain is well described.

Beta-Lactam Antibiotics: Specific Agents

Penicillins

As noted above, there are four structurally distinct subclasses of β-lactam antibiotics (see Fig. 33-6A). The first of these subclasses, the penicillins, can be further divided into five groups according to their spectra of action.

The first group of penicillins includes **penicillin G**, which is intravenously administered, and **penicillin V,** its oral counterpart. Penicillin G is in more widespread use than penicillin V; the latter is used mostly to treat mixed aerobic-anaerobic infections of the head and neck, such as dental abscesses. Additionally, penicillin V is used to prevent recurrent rheumatic fever in patients with a prior episode and recurrent streptococcal cellulitis in patients with lymphedema. Penicillin G is used to treat serious infections with Gram-positive bacteria such as pneumococcus and *S. pyogenes* (some strains of each), Gram-negative diplococci such as *Neisseria* species (except penicillinase-producing *N. gonorrhoeae*), Gram-positive rods of the genus *Clostridium*, most anaerobes (except *Bacteroides*), and spirochetes such as syphilis and *Leptospira*. High-dose penicillin G may cause seizures, in addition to the already mentioned hypersensitivity reactions and rash. All penicillins can cause acute interstitial nephritis. Drug-drug interactions are rare, but the anticoagulant effects of warfarin may be potentiated by concomitant penicillin administration.

The second group consists of the **antistaphylococcal penicillins**, including **oxacillin, cloxacillin, dicloxacillin, nafcillin,** and **methicillin**. These drugs are structurally resistant to staphylococcal β-lactamase, which is encoded by plasmid genes in most clinical isolates. Because of their relative hydrophobicity, however, antistaphylococcal penicillins lack activity against Gram-negative bacteria. (Recall also that methicillin binds to only a single transpeptidase.) Thus, these agents are used mostly for skin and soft-tissue infections or documented methicillin-sensitive S. *aureus* infections. Use of the oral antistaphylococcal penicillins (cloxacillin and dicloxacillin) is limited by their gastrointestinal adverse effects (nausea, vomiting, and antibiotic-associated diarrhea) as well as secondary development of *C. difficile* colitis. Adverse effects of IV nafcillin include phlebitis at the injection site; agranulocytosis and acute interstitial nephritis

occur at a higher rate than with the other penicillins. Oxacillin use is limited by hepatotoxicity, which is reversible with discontinuation of the drug. The utility of antistaphylococcal penicillins in treating *S. aureus* has been compromised by the emergence of MRSA strains. When a case of MRSA is found in the hospital, special precautions are taken to prevent its spread to other patients. Patients with MRSA infection are typically treated with vancomycin.

Ampicillin and **amoxicillin** are members of the third group of penicillins, the amino penicillins, which have a positively charged amino group on the side chain. This positive charge enhances diffusion through porin channels but does not confer resistance to β-lactamases. These agents are effective against a variety of Gram-positive cocci, Gram-negative cocci such as *Neisseria gonorrhoeae* and *N. meningitidis,* and Gram-negative rods such as *E. coli* and *H. influenzae*, but their spectrum is limited by sensitivity to most β-lactamases. IV ampicillin is used most commonly to treat invasive enterococcal infections and *Listeria* meningitis; oral amoxicillin is used to treat uncomplicated ear, nose, and throat infections, to prevent endocarditis in high-risk patients undergoing dental work, and as a component of combination therapy for *Helicobacter pylori* infection. Nonurticarial rash is the most common adverse effect. The spectrum of both agents is broadened when they are coadministered with β-lactamase inhibitors such as clavulanic acid (with amoxicillin) or sulbactam (with ampicillin) to treat β-lactamase-producing organisms such as *S. aureus, Haemophilus influenzae, E. coli, Klebsiella, Acinetobacter, Enterobacter*, and anaerobes.

Agents in the fourth group of penicillins, the carboxy penicillins, are also broad in spectrum. The carboxyl group on the side chain provides a negative charge that confers resistance to some β-lactamases but is less effective than a positively charged amino group in facilitating diffusion across porin channels. To overcome this limitation in diffusion, high doses are used. Resistance to the chromosomally encoded β-lactamases of *Enterobacter* and *Pseudomonas* adds these organisms to the spectrum of the carboxy penicillins. This group has two members, **carbenicillin** and **ticarcillin**.

A fifth group, the ureido penicillins, is represented by **piperacillin** and **mezlocillin**. These drugs have both positive and negative charges on their side chains and are generally more potent than the carboxy penicillins. Their spectrum of action is similar to that of the carboxy penicillins; in addition, they have activity against *Klebsiella* and enterococci.

Cephalosporins

Cephalosporins differ structurally from penicillins by having a six-membered rather than a five-membered accessory ring attached to the β-lactam ring (Fig. 33-6).

The first-generation cephalosporins (**cefazolin** and **cephalexin**) are active against Gram-positive species as well as the Gram-negative rods *Proteus mirabilis* and *E. coli,* both of which cause urinary tract infections, and *Klebsiella pneumoniae,* which causes pneumonia in addition to urinary tract infections. These agents are sensitive to many β-lactamases but are resistant to the chromosomally encoded β-lactamase of *K. pneumoniae* and the common staphylococcal β-lactamase. Cephalexin and cefazolin are both used to treat skin and soft tissue infections; cefazolin is also used for surgical prophylaxis.

The second-generation cephalosporins can be divided into two groups. **Cefuroxime,** which represents the first group, has increased activity against *H. influenzae* compared to the first-generation cephalosporins; **cefotetan** and **cefoxitin,** which represent the second group, demonstrate increased activity against *Bacteroides*. Also, second-generation cephalosporins are generally resistant to more β-lactamases than are first-generation cephalosporins. Thus, cefuroxime is often used to treat community-acquired pneumonia, and cefotetan is used to treat intra-abdominal and pelvic infections, including pelvic inflammatory disease. The adverse effects of these agents include diarrhea, mild liver enzyme elevation, and hypersensitivity reactions; rarely, agranulocytosis or interstitial nephritis can occur.

Third-generation cephalosporins (**ceftriaxone** and **cefotaxime**) are resistant to many β-lactamases and are thus highly active against Enterobacteriaceae (*E. coli,* indole-positive *Proteus, Klebsiella, Enterobacter, Serratia,* and *Citrobacter*) as well as *Neisseria* and *H. influenzae.* The third-generation cephalosporins are less active against Gram-positive organisms than are the first-generation drugs; despite that, they have good activity against penicillin-intermediate *S. pneumoniae* (although cephalosporin resistance can occur). Common uses include treatment of lower respiratory tract infection, community-acquired meningitis due to *S. pneumoniae,* uncomplicated gonococcal infection, culture-negative endocarditis, and complicated Lyme disease. In addition to the adverse effects already mentioned, ceftriaxone can cause cholestatic hepatitis. **Ceftazidime** is the last commonly used third-generation cephalosporin; its spectrum differs from the other two agents in that it has significant antipseudomonal activity and minimal activity against Gram-positive organisms. It is used predominantly to treat hospital-acquired Gram-negative bacterial infections and documented infections with *P. aeruginosa* and as empiric therapy for neutropenic patients with fever. Gram-negative bacteria that have acquired extended-spectrum β-lactamase activity, however, are resistant to third-generation cephalosporins.

Cefepime is the only fourth-generation cephalosporin currently available. Like ceftriaxone, it is highly active against Enterobacteriaceae, *Neisseria, H. influenzae,* and Gram-positive organisms; additionally, it is as active as ceftazidime against *P. aeruginosa.* Cefepime is also more resistant to the chromosomally encoded β-lactamases of *Enterobacter* than are third-generation cephalosporins. Unlike ceftazidime, however, cefepime is not approved for treatment of meningitis. An uncommon adverse effect is the development of autoantibodies against red blood cell antigens, typically without significant hemolysis.

As noted above, cephalosporins can generally be used in patients with non–life-threatening allergy to penicillins. Nevertheless, cephalosporins can cause hypersensitivity reactions themselves and should be avoided in patients with known cephalosporin hypersensitivity. Interestingly, **cefotetan** and **cefoperazone** contain an N-methylthiotetrazole (NMTT) side chain that causes two unique adverse effects. The first is an alcohol intolerance syndrome known as the **disulfiram-like reaction** (disulfiram is a drug that inhibits alcohol metabolism; see Chapter 17, Pharmacology of Drug

Dependence and Addiction). The second involves an effect on vitamin K metabolism and results in decreased synthesis of vitamin K-dependent coagulation factors; thus, cefotetan and cefoperazone should be used with caution in patients taking warfarin and in patients with underlying coagulation abnormalities (see Chapter 22, Pharmacology of Hemostasis and Thrombosis). Cefotetan, like most of the cephalosporins, can also cause antibody-mediated hemolysis.

Monobactams and Carbapenems

The only available monobactam, **aztreonam,** is active against most Gram-negative bacteria, including *P. aeruginosa,* but it has no activity against Gram-positive organisms. Gram-negative bacteria with extended-spectrum β-lactamases are, however, resistant. Aztreonam is particularly useful in patients with serious penicillin allergy who have infections due to resistant Gram-negative organisms; its use is limited by IV-site phlebitis, and its short half-life necessitates frequent dosing.

There are three carbapenems used in clinical practice: **imipenem, meropenem,** and **ertapenem.** All three are broad spectrum and cover most Gram-positive, Gram-negative, and anaerobic organisms. None is active against MRSA, VRE, or *Legionella.* Importantly, ertapenem is much less active against *P. aeruginosa* and *Acinetobacter* than the other two agents; the benefit of ertapenem is its once-daily dosing. Because imipenem is inactivated by the human renal enzyme dehydropeptidase I, this drug is always coadministered with the dehydropeptidase inhibitor **cilastatin.** Neither meropenem nor ertapenem is inactivated by the renal enzyme. All three agents can cause hypersensitivity reactions and IV-site phlebitis; at high plasma drug levels, imipenem and meropenem can cause seizures. Probenecid can increase meropenem levels, and all three agents can decrease valproate levels.

ANTIMYCOBACTERIAL AGENTS

Ethambutol, Pyrazinamide, and Isoniazid

Ethambutol, pyrazinamide, and **isoniazid (INH)** are three of the five first-line agents used to treat tuberculosis (rifampin and streptomycin, discussed in Chapter 32, are the other two). Patients with active tuberculosis and without a history of prior therapy are started on a four-drug regimen if the local prevalence of isoniazid resistance is greater than 4%. If isoniazid resistance is rare, a three-drug regimen without ethambutol can be used (see Chapter 39).

Ethambutol, a bacteriostatic agent, decreases arabinogalactan synthesis by inhibiting the arabinosyl transferase that adds arabinose units to the growing arabinogalactan chain. Pyrazinamide and INH inhibit mycolic acid synthesis. Pyrazinamide is a prodrug; it must be converted to its active form, pyrazinoic acid, by the enzyme pyrazinamidase. Pyrazinoic acid inhibits FAS1, the enzyme that synthesizes the fatty acid precursors of mycolic acid. Isoniazid and the related second-line agent **ethionamide** target the FAS2 complex and are bactericidal, although the exact mechanism of action of bacterial killing is unknown. The targets of two antimycobacterials are summarized in Figure 33-4.

Treatment of active tuberculosis requires multidrug therapy. Since resistance to antimycobacterial agents usually occurs by mutation, a powerful argument in favor of this strategy is based on the frequency of resistance mutations and the number of bacteria present in a clinical infection. Each tuberculous lesion in an infected lung can contain 10^8 bacteria. The frequency of mutants resistant to any single antimycobacterial drug is about 1 in 10^6 bacteria. This frequency means that, in each tuberculous lesion, an average of about 100 bacteria will already be resistant to an antimycobacterial drug, even before that drug is administered. Combination therapy with just two drugs reduces the likelihood of encountering pre-existing resistance to just one bacterium in 10^{12}; treatment with four drugs lowers this probability to 1 in 10^{24} (see Chapter 39). Although these numbers were not yet available when Dr. Pierce put in his request for isoniazid, he knew from qualitative analysis that he could maximize his patients' chances for survival and recovery from tuberculosis by combining streptomycin with isoniazid, a selective antimycobacterial agent that had been introduced in 1952.

Antimycobacterial agents can cause a number of adverse effects. Ethambutol is associated with optic neuritis; patients report impaired visual acuity, loss of color discrimination, constricted visual fields, and/or central and peripheral scotomata. Symptoms usually occur after more than a month of therapy and are reversible; however, sudden-onset irreversible blindness has been reported. Therefore, patients taking ethambutol must be seen monthly for eye examination to assess both visual acuity and color discrimination. Pyrazinamide is associated with arthralgias and (usually asymptomatic) hyperuricemia; more importantly, it commonly causes hepatotoxicity that can be severe and irreversible. Whereas patients who experience mild hepatotoxicity due to INH may be rechallenged with the drug, patients who experience pyrazinamide-induced hepatotoxicity should not be rechallenged. Isoniazid is associated with hepatitis as well as peripheral neuropathy. INH-induced hepatotoxicity can be mild, manifesting only as minor liver enzyme elevation not requiring cessation of the drug (occurs in 10% to 20% of patients), or it can be severe, leading to symptomatic hepatitis (occurs in 0.1% of patients overall, with increased risk in older patients with underlying liver disease who are also taking rifampin). Neurological manifestations of INH toxicity include paresthesias, peripheral neuropathy, and ataxia; this toxicity is due to competitive inhibition by INH of pyridoxine in neurotransmitter synthesis and can be prevented by pyridoxine supplementation. Isoniazid can also inhibit or induce cytochrome P450 enzymes and thereby interact with a number of other drugs, including rifampin, the antiseizure medications carbamazepine and phenytoin, azole-type antifungals, and alcohol.

Resistance to these drugs, and to antimycobacterial agents in general, results from chromosomal mutations. Ethambutol resistance most often results from mutations in the arabinosyl transferase gene, some of which cause overexpression of the target enzyme. Resistance to isoniazid usually results from an inactivating mutation in the mycobacterial enzyme **catalase-peroxidase,** which converts isoniazid into its antimycobacterial form. Mutations in the INHA gene, which is required for mycolic acid synthesis, also confer resistance to INH. Resistance to pyrazinamide is generally due to mutations in the pyrazinamidase gene, which result in the inability to convert the prodrug into its active form.

Conclusion and Future Directions

The bacterial cell wall presents a number of unique antibacterial targets to clinicians and pharmacologists. This structure consists of a three-dimensional mat of crosslinked peptide-sugar polymers called *murein* and is synthesized in three phases: (1) synthesis of murein monomers; (2) polymerization of monomers into murein polymers; and (3) crosslinking of polymers to complete the wall.

Antibacterial agents act in all three phases of cell wall synthesis: fosfomycin and cycloserine act in the first phase; vancomycin, teicoplanin, and bacitracin act in the second phase; and the β-lactams, the largest and most important group, act in the third phase. Beta-lactams—which include the penicillins, cephalosporins, monobactams, and carbapenems—are bactericidal; autolytic cell death most likely results from the unopposed action of wall remodeling proteins, called *autolysins*. Structural and chemical differences among the β-lactams determine their spectra of activity against bacteria with different cell wall architectures.

Resistance to β-lactam antibiotics is generally conferred by plasmid-encoded β-lactamases. Pharmacologists have addressed this mechanism of resistance: (1) by developing new β-lactam agents, for example, the second- and third-generation cephalosporins that are resistant to degradation by many β-lactamases; and (2) by coadministering β-lactam "decoys," such as clavulanic acid and sulbactam, that serve as β-lactamase inhibitors. Because β-lactamases can be encoded on plasmids, they can spread through bacterial (and human) populations with great speed, making antibiotic development an ongoing "arms race."

Antimycobacterial agents act by blocking various steps in the synthesis of molecules, such as mycolic acid and arabinogalactan, that are unique to the mycobacterial cell wall. Resistance to these agents is typically due to chromosomal mutation, but combination therapy is critically important for avoiding the development of mutational resistance. Future innovations will likely include the development of new agents directed against the additional unique molecular targets that are presented by the biochemistry of the bacterial cell wall.

Suggested Reading

Brennan PJ. The envelope of mycobacteria. *Annu Rev Biochem* 1995;64:29–63. (*Reviews the structure, composition, and synthesis of the mycobacterial cell wall.*)

Cosgrove SE, Carroll KC, Perl TM. Staphylococcus aureus with reduced susceptibility to vancomycin. *Clin Infect Dis* 2005;39:539–545. (*Recent report on VISA and VRSA, including definitions, risk factors, and mechanisms of resistance.*)

El Zoeiby A, Sanschagrin F, Levesque RC. Structure and function of the Mur enzymes: development of novel inhibitors. *Mol Microbiol* 2003;47:1–12. (*Reviews the structure, catalytic action, and inhibition of MurA-MurF.*)

Gale EF, Cundliffe E, Reynolds PE, et al. *The Molecular Basis of Antibiotic Action.* 2nd ed. London: John Wiley; 1981. (*Classic on antibiotics that describes the experiments that led to the deter-*

mination of many of the mechanisms of action discussed in this chapter.)

Jacoby GA, Munoz-Price LS. The new beta-lactamases. *N Engl J Med* 2005;352:380–391. (*Reviews the pharmacology of recently developed beta-lactamases.*)

Kelkar PS, Li JT. Cephalosporin allergy. *N Engl J Med* 2001;345: 804–809. (*Comprehensive literature review of cephalosporin reactions in patients with a history of penicillin allergy.*)

Paterson DL, Bonomo DA. Extended-spectrum beta-lactamases: a clinical update. *Clin Microbiol Rev* 2005;18:657–686. (*Reviews the microbiology, transmission, and treatment of extended-spectrum beta-lactamase producing organisms.*)

Rattan A, Kalia A, Ahmad N. Multidrug-resistant *Mycobacterium tuberculosis:* molecular perspectives. *Emerg Infect Dis* 1998; 4:195–209. (*Discusses the problem of resistance in tuberculosis.*)

Drug Summary Table   Chapter 33 Pharmacology of Bacterial Infections: Cell Wall Synthesis

Drug	Clinical Applications	*Serious* and Common Adverse Effects	Contraindications	Therapeutic Considerations
INHIBITORS OF MUREIN MONOMER SYNTHESIS				
Mechanism—See specific drug				
Fosfomycin Fosmidomycin	Gram-negative urinary tract infections: *E. coli, Klebsiella, Serratia, Clostridia*	Headache, diarrhea, nausea	Hypersensitivity to fosfomycin or fosmidomycin	Phosphoenolpyruvate (PEP) analogues that inhibit bacterial enol pyruvate transferase by covalent modification of the enzyme's active site, thereby inhibiting the synthesis of UDP-NAG from UDP–NAG Synergistic with beta-lactams, aminoglycosides, and fluoroquinolones Decreased absorption when coadministered with antacids or motility agents
Cycloserine	*M. tuberculosis* *M. avium* complex	*Seizures* Somnolence, peripheral neuropathy, psychosis	Epilepsy Depression, anxiety, psychosis Severe renal insufficiency Alcohol abuse	Inhibits both alanine racemase and D-Ala-D-Ala synthetase Alcohol, isoniazid and ethionamide potentiate cycloserine toxicity Pyridoxine may prevent cycloserine-induced peripheral neuropathy Cycloserine inhibits hepatic metabolism of phenytoin
Bacitracin	Cutaneous and eye infections (topical) GI decontamination of *C. difficile* or vancomycin-resistant enterococci (oral)	*If systemic absorption occurs: nephrotoxicity, neurotoxicity, bone marrow suppression* With topical application: contact dermatitis, blurred vision, red eye	Coadministration with nephrotoxic agents or neuromuscular blocking agents (contraindication for orally administered bacitracin)	Inhibits dephosphorylation of bactoprenol pyrophosphate
INHIBITORS OF MUREIN POLYMER SYNTHESIS				
Mechanism—Bind to the D-Ala-D-Ala terminus of the murein monomer unit and inhibit transglycosidase, thereby preventing addition of murein units to the growing polymer chain				
Vancomycin Teicoplanin	Methicillin-resistant *S. aureus* infections (IV) *C. difficile* enterocolitis (oral)	*Neutropenia, ototoxicity, nephrotoxicity, anaphylaxis* "Red-man syndrome" (flushing and erythroderma), drug fever, hypersensitivity rash	Solutions containing dextrose in patients with known corn allergy	Increased nephrotoxicity with aminoglycosides "Red man syndrome" can be avoided by slowing infusion rate or pre-administering antihistamines Resistance to vancomycin most commonly arises through acquisition of DNA encoding enzymes that catalyze formation of D-Ala-D-lactate Teicoplanin is not used clinically in the US

(Continued)

Drug Summary Table **Chapter 33 Pharmacology of Bacterial Infections: Cell Wall Synthesis** *(Continued)*

INHIBITORS OF POLYMER CROSSLINKING: PENICILLINS

Mechanism—β-lactams inhibit transpeptidase by forming a covalent ("dead-end") acyl enzyme intermediate. Penicillins have a five-membered accessory ring attached to the beta-lactam ring.

Drug	Clinical Applications	Serious and Common Adverse Effects	Contraindications	Therapeutic Considerations
Penicillin G Penicillin V	Penicillin-sensitive *S. aureus* and *S. pyogenes*, oral anaerobes, *N. meningitidis*, *Clostridia* species Syphilis Yaws Leptospirosis Prophylaxis of rheumatic fever (penicillin V)	Seizures, pseudomembranous enterocolitis, drug-induced eosinophilia, hemolytic anemia, neuropathy, acute interstitial nephritis, anaphylaxis Rash, fever, injection site reaction, Jarisch Herxheimer reaction when used to treat syphilis	Hypersensitivity to penicillins	Penicillin G is the intravenous preparation; penicillin V is the oral preparation Anticoagulant effects of warfarin may be potentiated by concomitant penicillin administration Intravenous penicillin G is preferred to oral penicillin V in hospital settings Beta-lactamase sensitive
Oxacillin Cloxacillin Dicloxacillin Nafcillin Methicillin	Skin and soft-tissue infections or systemic infection with beta-lactamase-producing, methicillin-sensitive *S. aureus*	Diarrhea, nausea, vomiting, pseudomembranous enterocolitis (cloxacillin, dicloxacillin) Hepatitis (oxacillin) Interstitial nephritis, phlebitis (nafcillin)	Hypersensitivity to penicillins	Beta-lactamase resistant Narrow spectrum anti-bacterial activity; used mainly to treat skin and soft-tissue infections or documented methicillin-sensitive *S. aureus* infections
Ampicillin Amoxicillin Amoxicillin/ clavulanic acid Ampicillin/ sulbactam	Invasive enterococcal infections and *Listeria* meningitis (ampicillin) Uncomplicated ear, nose, and throat infections, endocarditis prevention, dental-surgery prophylaxis, component of combination therapy for *Helicobacter pylori* infection (amoxicillin) Beta-lactamase-producing organisms such as *S. aureus*, *H. influenzae*, *E. coli*, *Klebsiella*, *Acinetobacter*, *Enterobacter*, anaerobes (amoxicillin/clavulanic acid, ampicillin/sulbactam)	Rash, nausea, vomiting, diarrhea	Hypersensitivity to penicillins	Broad-spectrum anti-bacterial activity Ampicillin and amoxicillin are beta-lactamase sensitive as single agents; clavulanic acid and sulbactam are beta-lactamase inhibitors Positively charged amino group on side chain enhances diffusion through porin channels of Gram-negative bacteria
Carbenicillin Ticarcillin Piperacillin Mezlocillin	Primarily used as treatment or prophylaxis against *P. aeruginosa* infection Hospital-acquired pneumonia due to resistant Gram-negative organisms	Same as ampicillin and amoxicillin	Hypersensitivity to penicillins	Broad-spectrum anti-bacterial activity, but primarily used against *P. aeruginosa* Generally beta-lactamase sensitive Carbenicillin and ticarcillin have a carboxyl group on side chain, which confers resistance to some beta-lactamases Piperacillin and mezlocillin are generally more potent than carbenicillin and ticarcillin against a similar spectrum of organisms; unlike carbenicillin and ticarcillin, piperacillin and mezlocillin are also active against *Klebsiella* and enterococci

INHIBITORS OF POLYMER CROSSLINKING: CEPHALOSPORINS				
Mechanism—β-lactams inhibit transpeptidase by forming a covalent ("dead-end") acyl enzyme intermediate. Cephalosporins have a six-membered accessory ring attached to the beta-lactam ring.				
Cefazolin Cephalexin	*Proteus mirabilis, E. coli, Klebsiella pneumoniae* Skin and soft tissue infections Surgical prophylaxis	*Pseudomembranous enterocolitis, leukopenia, thrombocytopenia, hepatotoxicity* Nausea, vomiting, diarrhea, rash	Hypersensitivity to cephalosporins (rarely cross-react with penicillins)	First-generation cephalosporins Relatively good Gram-positive coverage Sensitive to many beta-lactamases
Cefuroxime Cefotetan Cefoxitin	*H. influenzae* (cefuroxime) *H. influenzae, Enterobacter* spp., *Neisseria* spp., *P. mirabilis, E. coli, K. pneumoniae* (cefotetan and cefoxitin)	Same as cefazolin, except cefotetan may produce disulfiram-like reaction with alcohol ingestion and block synthesis of vitamin K-dependent coagulation factors	Hypersensitivity to cephalosporins (rarely cross-react with penicillins)	Second-generation cephalosporins Relatively broader Gram-negative coverage than first-generation cephalosporins More beta-lactamase resistant than first-generation cephalosporins Cefuroxime is primarily used in community-acquired pneumonia Cefotetan and cefoxitin are primarily used in intra-abdominal and pelvic infections
Cefotaxime Ceftizoxime Ceftriaxone Cefoperazone Ceftazidime	*N. gonorrhoeae, Borrelia burgdorferi, H. influenzae,* most *Enterobacteriaceae* (ceftriaxone) *H. influenzae* (cefotaxime) *P. aeruginosa* (ceftazidime)	Same as cefazolin, except ceftriaxone may cause cholestatic hepatitis, and cefoperazone may produce disulfiram-like reaction with alcohol ingestion and block synthesis of vitamin K-dependent coagulation factors	Hypersensitivity to cephalosporins (rarely cross-react with penicillins)	Third-generation cephalosporins Highest CNS penetration of the cephalosporins Resistant to many beta-lactamases Highly active against *Enterobacteriaceae*, but less active against Gram-positive organisms than are first-generation cephalosporins
Cefepime	*Enterobacteriaceae, Neisseria, H. influenzae, P. aeruginosa,* Gram-positive organisms	Same as cefazolin, except cefepime may produce erythrocyte autoantibodies without significant hemolysis	Hypersensitivity to cephalosporins (rarely cross-react with penicillins)	Fourth-generation cephalosporin Resistant to many beta-lactamases
INHIBITORS OF POLYMER CROSSLINKING: MONOBACTAMS / CARBAPENEMS				
Mechanism—β-lactams inhibit transpeptidase by forming a covalent ("dead-end") acyl enzyme intermediate				
Aztreonam	Gram-negative bacteria Used in penicillin-allergic patients	Same as penicillins	Hypersensitivity to aztreonam	A monobactam No Gram-positive coverage
Imipenem/cilastatin Meropenem Ertapenem	Gram-positive and Gram-negative bacteria except MRSA, VRE, and *Legionella* (ertapenem is not active against *Pseudomonas* or *Acinetobacter*)	Same as penicillins. Additionally, high plasma levels of imipenem and meropenem may cause seizures	Hypersensitivity to imipenem, meropenem, or ertapenem	Cilastatin inhibits renal dehydropeptidase I, which would otherwise inactivate imipenem Probenecid may increase meropenem levels All three agents decrease valproate levels
ANTIMYCOBACTERIAL AGENTS				
Mechanism—See specific drug				
Ethambutol	*Mycobacterium* species	*Optic neuritis, blindness, peripheral neuropathy, neutropenia, thrombocytopenia* Hyperuricemia, mania, nausea, vomiting	Known optic neuritis Patients unable to report visual changes, such as young children Coadministration with antacids	Decreases arabinogalactan synthesis by inhibiting the arabinosyl transferase that adds arabinose units to the growing arabinogalactan chain Mycobacteriostatic, and used in combination with other antimycobacterials, including rifampin and streptomycin

(Continued)

Drug Summary Table **Chapter 33 Pharmacology of Bacterial Infections: Cell Wall Synthesis** *(Continued)*

Drug	Clinical Applications	Serious and Common Adverse Effects	Contraindications	Therapeutic Considerations
Pyrazinamide	*Mycobacterium* species	Anemia, hepatotoxicity Arthralgias, hyperuricemia (usually asymptomatic)	Acute gout Severe hepatic dysfunction	Pyrazinamide is a prodrug that must be converted to its active form pyrazinoic acid, which inhibits fatty acid synthetase 1 (FAS1) Used in combination with other antimycobacterials, including rifampin and streptomycin
Isoniazid **Ethionamide**	*Mycobacterium* species	*Hepatitis, neurotoxicity (paresthesias, peripheral neuropathy, ataxia), systemic lupus erythematosus, seizure, hematologic abnormalities*	Active liver disease	Inhibit mycolic acid synthesis by targeting fatty acid synthetase 2 (FAS2) Can inhibit or induce cytochrome P450 enzymes and thus interact with other drugs, such as rifampin, antiseizure medications (carbamazepine and phenytoin), azole antifungals, alcohol Mycobactericidal, and used in combination with other antimycobacterials, including rifampin and streptomycin Isoniazid neurotoxicity can be prevented by pyridoxine supplementation

34

Pharmacology of Fungal Infections

April W. Armstrong and Charles R. Taylor

INTRODUCTION

Fungi are free-living micro-organisms that exist as **yeasts** (single-cell, round fungi), **molds** (multicellular filamentous fungi), or a combination of the two (so-called *dimorphic fungi*). All fungi are **eukaryotic** organisms. Because of their phylogenetic similarity, fungi and humans have homologous metabolic pathways for energy production, protein synthesis, and cell division. Consequently, *there is greater difficulty in developing selective antifungal agents than in developing selective antibacterial agents.* The success of many antibacterial agents has resulted from the identification of unique molecular targets in bacteria, emphasizing the necessity for identifying unique fungal targets that can be exploited.

Certain patient populations are particularly susceptible to fungal infections (mycoses). These populations include surgical and intensive care unit (ICU) patients, patients with prostheses, and patients with compromised immune defenses. In the past 3 decades, the extensive use of broad-spectrum antibiotics, the wider use of long-term intravenous catheters, and infection with human immunodeficiency virus (HIV) have correlated with an increasing incidence of opportunistic and systemic mycoses. Additionally, the successes of organ transplantation, immunosuppressive therapy, and

cancer chemotherapy have contributed to an increasing number of chronically immunosuppressed patients, who are particularly susceptible to fungal infections.

Traditionally, the diagnosis of fungal infections has relied on culture-based methods and direct examination of specimens under light microscopy. However, the indolent growth of fungi makes culturing inefficient, while direct microscopic examination may not be reliable or provide definitive speciation. These disadvantages have important clinical implications, because prognosis often correlates inversely with the duration of time from clinical presentation to accurate diagnosis. Consequently, one major focus of modern mycology is the development of rapid, nonculture-based methods of early diagnosis. New diagnostic techniques rely on the polymerase chain reaction (PCR), western blot, antigen detection, and identification of fungal metabolites. Because these techniques are still investigational, they must be performed in parallel with traditional culture-based methods.

The treatment options for opportunistic and systemic fungal infections were once thought to be limited. These options are now expanding, however. Fungal processes that have been exploited in the development of antifungal agents include nucleic acid synthesis, mitosis, and membrane synthesis and stability. Traditional antifungal agents, such as azoles and polyenes, are directed against molecular targets involved in the synthesis and stability of the fungal membrane. The echinocandins, a new class of antifungal agents, target an enzyme complex involved in the synthesis of the fungal cell wall. As the emergence of resistant fungi increases, it will become increasingly important to identify and exploit new molecular targets for antifungal therapy.

■ Case

James F, a 31-year-old HIV-positive man, presents to his physician with a 3-week history of fever, cough, and chest pain after touring Southern California. His history is notable for past intravenous drug use. Clinical evaluation and chest x-ray reveal a left lower lobe infiltrate and left paratracheal adenopathy. Sputum cultures are positive for *Coccidioides immitis,* and blood tests are notable for an elevated titer of antibodies directed against this fungal pathogen. The physician makes a preliminary diagnosis of pulmonary coccidioidomycosis and prescribes a course of amphotericin B.

Over the next several days, however, Mr. F does not improve. He goes to the emergency department with fever, chills, sweats, cough, fatigue, and headaches. His temperature is 100°F, but he shows no evidence of meningitis or peripheral adenopathy. Lung examination reveals diffuse wheezing over the left lung fields, noted on both inspiration and expiration. Bronchoscopy shows narrowing of the tracheal lumen by numerous mucosal granulomas from the left main-stem bronchus to the level of the midtrachea. Fungal culture grows *Coccidiodes immitis,* a definitive diagnosis of chronic pulmonary coccidioidomycosis is made, the granulomas are bronchoscopically removed, and amphotericin B is continued. A week later, Mr. F's symptoms begin to subside, amphotericin B is discontinued, and a course of fluconazole is initiated.

QUESTIONS

■ **1.** What factors predisposed Mr. F to fungal infection?
■ **2.** What are the mechanisms of action of amphotericin B and fluconazole?
■ **3.** What adverse effects could Mr. F experience as a consequence of treatment with amphotericin B and fluconazole?

BIOCHEMISTRY OF THE FUNGAL MEMBRANE AND CELL WALL

Although fungi have a cellular ultrastructure similar to that of animal cells, there are a number of unique biochemical differences that have been exploited in the development of antifungal drugs. To date, the most important biochemical difference lies in the principal sterol used to maintain plasma membrane structure and function. Mammalian cells use cholesterol for this purpose, whereas fungal cells use the structurally distinct sterol **ergosterol**. The biosynthesis of ergosterol involves a series of steps, two of which are targeted

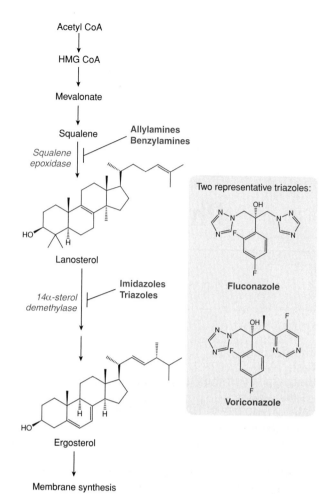

Figure 34-1. Ergosterol synthesis pathway. Ergosterol is synthesized in fungal cells from acetyl CoA building blocks. One of the intermediates, squalene, is converted to lanosterol by the action of squalene epoxidase. Allylamines and benzylamines inhibit the action of squalene epoxidase. 14α-Sterol demethylase, a cytochrome P450 enzyme not expressed in mammalian cells, catalyzes the first step in the conversion of lanosterol to the unique fungal sterol ergosterol. Imidazoles and triazoles inhibit 14α-sterol demethylase and thereby prevent the synthesis of ergosterol, which is the principal sterol in fungal membranes. Fluconazole and voriconazole are two representative triazoles.

by currently available antifungal drugs (Fig. 34-1). The enzymes that catalyze ergosterol synthesis are localized in fungal microsomes, which contain an electron transport system nearly identical to that found in mammalian liver microsomes. The first targeted step, the conversion of **squalene** to **lanosterol**, is catalyzed by the enzyme **squalene epoxidase**. This enzyme is the molecular target of the **allylamine** and **benzylamine** antifungal agents. The fungus-specific cytochrome P450 enzyme **14α-sterol demethylase** mediates the key reaction in the second targeted step, the conversion of lanosterol to ergosterol. **Imidazole** and **triazole** antifungal agents inhibit 14α-sterol demethylase. Therefore, allylamine, benzylamine, imidazole, and triazole antifungal agents all inhibit the biosynthesis of ergosterol. Because ergosterol is necessary for the maintenance of plasma membrane structure and function, these agents compromise fungal membrane integrity. Ergosterol synthesis inhibitors suppress fungal cell growth under most circumstances (**fungistatic** effect), although they can sometimes cause fungal cell death (**fungicidal** effect).

Fungal cells are surrounded by a cell wall, a rigid structure that has been studied intensively as a new and important target for antifungal therapy. The major components of the fungal cell wall are **chitin, β-(1,3)-D-glucan, β-(1,6)-D-glucan,** and cell wall glycoproteins (especially proteins containing complex mannose chains, or **mannoproteins**). Chitin is a linear polysaccharide consisting of more than 2,000 N-acetylglucosamine units joined by β-(1,4) linkages; these chains are bundled into microfibrils that form the fundamental scaffold of the cell wall. β-(1,3)-D-glucan and β-(1,6)-D-glucan, which are polymers of glucose units joined by β-(1,3) and β-(1,6) glycosidic linkages, respectively, are the most abundant components of the cell wall. These glucan polymers are covalently linked to the chitin scaffold. The cell wall glycoproteins comprise a diverse group of proteins that are noncovalently associated with other cell wall components or are covalently linked to chitin, glucan, or other cell wall proteins. Because mammalian cells do not have cell walls, drugs directed against the fungal cell wall would be expected to have a high therapeutic index. **Echinocandin** antifungal agents target **β-(1,3)-D-glucan synthase**, the enzyme that adds glucose residues from the donor molecule UDP-glucose to the growing polysaccharide chain. By inhibiting cell wall biosynthesis, echinocandins disrupt fungal cell wall integrity. Echinocandins often have fungicidal activity, although these agents are fungistatic under some circumstances (see Suggested Reading).

Fungal adhesion represents a third potential target for antifungal drugs. Adhesion to host cells is mediated by the binding of fungal **adhesins** to host cell receptors. In yeasts, for example, aspartyl proteases and phospholipases mediate adhesion. Compounds that block adhesive interactions between fungal cells and mammalian cells are currently under development.

PATHOPHYSIOLOGY OF FUNGAL INFECTIONS

Mycoses (fungal infections) can be divided into superficial, cutaneous, subcutaneous, systemic or primary, and opportunistic infections. Few fungi possess sufficient virulence to be considered primary pathogens capable of initiating serious infections in immunocompetent hosts. However, immunocompromised hosts can develop serious systemic infections with fungi that are not pathogenic in normal individuals. Thus, the pathogenesis of fungal infections is based on the interplay between a host's immune system and the pathogenicity of the particular fungal organism. Polymorphonuclear leukocytes, cell-mediated immunity, and humoral immunity are all important components of the host immune defense against fungal pathogens.

The pathogenesis of fungal infections is only partly understood, and different fungi possess distinct virulence factors that are unique to the pathogen. Adhesion is an initial step in the early stages of infection. Adhesion and localization can occur on skin, mucosal, and prosthetic device surfaces. For example, *Candida* species adhere to a variety of surfaces via a combination of specific ligand-receptor interactions as well as nonspecific forces such as van der Waals and electrostatic interactions. Virulent pathogens are subsequently able to invade the colonized surface and proliferate in deep tissue, sometimes reaching the systemic circulation. Systemic dissemination can be accelerated by local tissue injury, such as that caused by cancer chemotherapy, ischemia, or the presence of a prosthetic device. In addition, some pathogens secrete lytic enzymes to enable invasive growth and systemic dissemination. *C. immitis* breaches the respiratory mucosa by producing an alkaline proteinase capable of digesting structural proteins in lung tissue. *C. immitis* also produces a 36-kDa extracellular proteinase capable of degrading human elastin, collagen, immunoglobulins, and hemoglobin.

Fungal cell wall composition plays an important role in the pathogenesis of fungal infections. Pathogens such as *Blastomyces dermatitidis, Histoplasma capsulatum, and Paracoccidioides brasiliensis* modulate the complement of glycoproteins in their cell walls in response to host immune system interactions. For example, the cell wall of *B. dermatitidis* contains a 120-kDa glycoprotein, WI-1, which elicits a potent humoral and cellular immune response. Avirulent strains of *B. dermatitidis* have increased expression of WI-1, which is recognized by the host immune system and leads to elimination of the pathogen through phagocytosis. In contrast, the cell wall of virulent strains of *B. dermatitidis* contains high levels of α-(1,3)-glucan, which is inversely correlated with the amount of WI-1 detectable on the cell surface. It is speculated that the increased amount of α-(1,3)-glucan in the cell wall effectively masks the WI-1 surface glycoprotein, thereby allowing the virulent strains to evade host immune detection and destruction.

The ability of a fungal pathogen to change from one morphotype to another is termed **phenotype switching**. By responding to changes in the microenvironment, *Candida* species are capable of undergoing yeast-to-hyphae transformation. The hyphal forms of *Candida* species possess a ''sense of touch'' that allows them to grow in crevices and pores, thereby increasing their infiltrative potential. Similarly, *B. dermatitidis* undergoes transformation from conidia (small, asexual reproductive structures) to the larger yeast forms. The larger forms offer an important survival advantage, since these are capable of resisting the phagocytic action of neutrophils and macrophages.

PHARMACOLOGIC CLASSES AND AGENTS

The ideal antifungal agent would possess four characteristics: broad spectrum of action against a variety of fungal pathogens, low drug toxicity, multiple routes of administration, and excellent penetration into the cerebrospinal fluid (CSF), urine, and bone. With the recent expansion in identifying novel targets of antifungal therapy, treatment options for superficial and deep fungal infections are improving.

Some antifungal agents can be used to treat both superficial and deep mycoses using different formulations, while others are restricted to narrower indications. In this section, the currently available antifungal drugs are categorized according to their molecular targets and mechanisms of action. The primary molecular targets for antifungal therapy are enzymes and other molecules involved in fungal DNA synthesis, mitosis, plasma membrane synthesis, and cell wall synthesis (Fig. 34-2). Because the clinical trials used to support regulatory approval of new drugs often exclude children and women of childbearing potential (see Chapter 49, Clinical Drug Evaluation and Regulatory Approval), the safety of some of the newer antifungal agents is not precisely determined in these patient populations. The treating physician must therefore weigh the risks of treatment against the expected benefits.

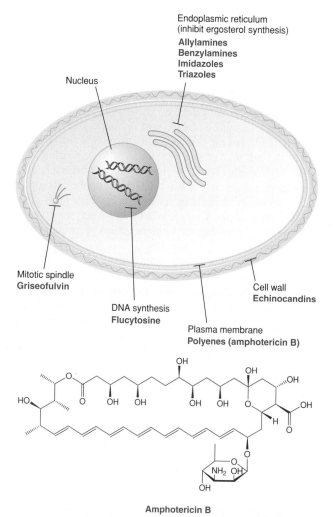

Figure 34-2. Cellular targets of antifungal drugs. The currently available antifungal agents act on distinct molecular targets. Flucytosine inhibits fungal DNA synthesis. Griseofulvin inhibits fungal mitosis by disrupting mitotic spindles. Allylamines, benzylamines, imidazoles, and triazoles inhibit the ergosterol synthesis pathway in the endoplasmic reticulum. Polyenes bind to ergosterol in the fungal membrane and thereby disrupt plasma membrane integrity. Amphotericin B is a representative polyene. Echinocandins inhibit fungal cell wall synthesis.

INHIBITOR OF FUNGAL NUCLEIC ACID SYNTHESIS: Flucytosine

Flucytosine is the name of the fluorinated pyrimidine 5-fluorocytosine. Flucytosine is selectively taken up by fungal cells via cytosine-specific permeases that are expressed only in fungal membranes. Lacking these transporters, mammalian cells are protected. Inside the fungal cell, the enzyme cytosine deaminase converts flucytosine to 5-fluorouracil (5-FU). (5-FU is itself an antimetabolite that is used in cancer chemotherapy; see Chapter 37, Pharmacology of Cancer: Genome Synthesis, Stability, and Maintenance.) Subsequent reactions convert 5-FU to 5-fluorodeoxyuridylic acid (5-FdUMP), which is a potent inhibitor of **thymidylate synthase**. Inhibition of thymidylate synthase results in inhibition of DNA synthesis and cell division (Fig. 34-3). Flucytosine appears to be fungistatic under most circumstances. Although mammalian cells lack cytosine-specific permeases and cytosine deaminase, fungi and bacteria in the intestine can convert flucytosine into 5-fluorouracil, which can cause adverse effects in host cells.

Flucytosine is typically used in combination with amphotericin B to treat systemic mycoses; when the drug is used as a single agent, resistance emerges rapidly due to mutations in fungal cytosine permease or cytosine deaminase. Although flucytosine has no intrinsic activity against *Aspergillus,* synergistic killing of *Aspergillus* by the combination of flucytosine and amphotericin B can be demonstrated experimentally. The mechanism of this synergistic interaction appears to involve enhancement of flucytosine uptake by fungal cells due to amphotericin-induced damage to the fungal plasma membrane. The spectrum of activity of flucytosine as a single agent is limited to candidiasis, cryptococcosis, and chromomycosis. The pharmacokinetic advantage of this drug is its large volume of distribution, with excellent penetration into the central nervous system (CNS), eyes, and urinary tract. Dose-dependent adverse effects include bone marrow suppression leading to leukopenia and thrombocytopenia, nausea, vomiting, diarrhea, and hepatic dysfunction. Flucytosine is contraindicated during pregnancy.

INHIBITOR OF FUNGAL MITOSIS: Griseofulvin

Derived from *Penicillium griseofulvum* in the 1950s, **griseofulvin** inhibits fungal mitosis by binding to tubulin and a microtubule-associated protein and thereby disrupting assembly of the mitotic spindle. The drug is also reported to inhibit fungal RNA and DNA synthesis. Griseofulvin accumulates in keratin precursor cells and binds tightly to keratin in differentiated cells. The prolonged and tight association of griseofulvin with keratin allows new growth of skin, hair, or nail to be free of dermatophyte infection. Griseofulvin appears to be fungistatic under most circumstances.

The therapeutic use of oral griseofulvin is currently limited, due to the availability of topical antifungal medications as well as other oral antifungal agents with fewer adverse effects. Griseofulvin can be used to treat fungal infection of the skin, hair, and nail due to *Trichophyton, Microsporum,* and *Epidermophyton.* The drug is not effective against yeast (such as *Pityrosporum*) and dimorphic fungi. Doses should

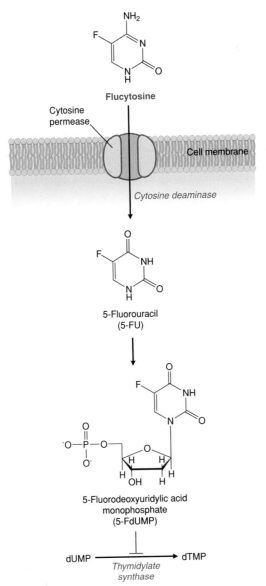

Figure 34-3. Mechanism of action of flucytosine. Flucytosine enters the fungal cell via a transmembrane cytosine permease. Inside the cell, cytosine deaminase converts flucytosine to 5-fluorouracil (5-FU), which is subsequently converted to 5-fluorodeoxyuridylic acid monophosphate (5-FdUMP). 5-FdUMP inhibits thymidylate synthase and thereby blocks the conversion of deoxyuridylate (dUMP) to deoxythymidylate (dTMP). In the absence of dTMP, DNA synthesis is inhibited.

be taken at 6-hour intervals because blood levels of griseofulvin can be variable; absorption is enhanced if the drug is taken with a fatty meal. It is important to continue treatment until the infected skin, hair, or nail is completely replaced by normal tissue.

Griseofulvin use is not associated with a high incidence of serious adverse effects. A relatively common (up to 15%) adverse effect of griseofulvin is headache, which tends to disappear as the therapy continues. Other nervous system effects include lethargy, vertigo, and blurred vision; these adverse effects can be exacerbated by the consumption of alcohol. Occasionally, hepatotoxicity or albuminuria without renal insufficiency can be observed. Hematologic ad-

verse effects—including leukopenia, neutropenia, and monocytosis—can occur during the first month of therapy. Serum sickness, angioedema, exfoliative dermatitis, and toxic epidermal necrolysis are extremely rare but potentially life-threatening adverse effects. Chronic use can sometimes result in increased fecal protoporphyrin levels. Concurrent administration with barbiturates decreases the gastrointestinal absorption of griseofulvin. Because griseofulvin induces hepatic cytochrome P450 enzymes, it can increase the metabolism of warfarin and potentially reduce the efficacy of low-estrogen oral contraceptive medications. Griseofulvin should be avoided during pregnancy, since fetal abnormalities have been reported.

INHIBITORS OF THE ERGOSTEROL SYNTHESIS PATHWAY

Inhibitors of Squalene Epoxidase

Allylamines and Benzylamines

In the ergosterol synthesis pathway (Fig. 34-1), squalene is converted to lanosterol by the action of **squalene epoxidase**. Inhibitors of squalene epoxidase prevent the formation of lanosterol, which is a precursor for ergosterol. These drugs also promote accumulation of the toxic metabolite squalene in the fungal cell, making them fungicidal under most circumstances. The antifungal agents that inhibit squalene epoxidase can be divided into **allylamines** and **benzylamines** based on their chemical structures: **terbinafine** and **naftifine** are allylamines, whereas **butenafine** is a benzylamine.

Terbinafine is available in both oral and topical formulations. When taken orally, the drug is 99% protein-bound in the plasma and it undergoes first-pass metabolism in the liver. Because of this first-pass metabolism, the oral bioavailability of terbinafine is 40%. The drug's elimination half-life is extremely long, approximately 300 hours, because terbinafine accumulates extensively in the skin, nails, and fat. The oral form of terbinafine is used in the treatment of onychomycosis, tinea corporis, tinea cruris, tinea pedis, and tinea capitis. Terbinafine is not recommended in patients with renal or hepatic failure and in pregnant women. Very rarely, the oral form of terbinafine can lead to hepatotoxicity, Stevens-Johnson syndrome, neutropenia, and exacerbation of psoriasis or subacute cutaneous lupus erythematosus. Liver function enzymes should be monitored during the treatment course. Plasma levels of terbinafine are increased by coadministration with cimetidine (a cytochrome P450 inhibitor) and decreased by coadministration with rifampin (a cytochrome P450 inducer). Topical terbinafine is available in cream or spray form and is indicated for tinea pedis, tinea cruris, and tinea corporis.

Similar to terbinafine, **naftifine** is a squalene epoxidase inhibitor that has broad-spectrum antifungal activity. Naftifine is only available topically as a cream or gel; it is effective in tinea corporis, tinea cruris, and tinea pedis.

Butenafine, a benzylamine, is a topical antifungal agent with a mechanism of action and spectrum of antifungal activity similar to that of the allylamines. Topical allylamines and benzylamines are more effective than topical azole agents against common dermatophytes, especially those causing tinea pedis. However, topical terbinafine and butenafine are less effective than topical azoles against *Candida* skin infections.

Inhibitors of 14α-Sterol Demethylase

Imidazoles and Triazoles

Another important molecular target in the ergosterol synthesis pathway is **14α-sterol demethylase**, a microsomal cytochrome P450 enzyme that converts lanosterol to ergosterol. The **azoles** are antifungal agents that inhibit fungal 14α-sterol demethylase. The resulting decrease in ergosterol synthesis and accumulation of 14α-methyl sterols disrupt the tightly packed acyl chains of the phospholipids in fungal membranes. Destabilization of the fungal membrane leads to dysfunction of membrane-associated enzymes, including those in the electron transport chain, and may ultimately lead to cell death. Azoles are not completely selective for the fungal P450 enzyme, however, and they can also inhibit hepatic P450 enzymes. While the extent of hepatic P450 enzyme inhibition varies among the azoles, *drug-drug interactions are an important consideration whenever an azole antifungal agent is prescribed.* For example, cyclosporine is an immunosuppressant drug used to prevent graft rejection in recipients of allogeneic kidney, liver, and heart transplants. It is metabolized by hepatic P450 enzymes and excreted in the bile. To minimize the risk of cyclosporine-associated nephrotoxicity and hepatotoxicity, patients concomitantly receiving an azole antifungal agent should be treated with lower doses of cyclosporine.

As a group, the azoles have a wide range of antifungal activity and are clinically useful against *B. dermatitidis*, *Cryptococcus neoformans*, *H. capsulatum*, *Coccidioides* species, *P. brasiliensis*, dermatophytes, and most *Candida* species. Azoles have intermediate clinical activity against *Fusarium*, *Sporothrix schenckii*, *Scedosporium apiospermum*, and *Aspergillus* species. Pathogens mediating zygomycosis (invasive fungal infections caused by *Zygomycetes* species) and *Candida krusei* are resistant to azoles. The azoles are generally fungistatic rather than fungicidal against susceptible organisms.

The azole antifungal agents can be categorized into two broad classes, **imidazoles** and **triazoles**, which share the same mechanism of action and similar antifungal spectrum. Because systemically administered triazoles tend to have less effect than systemically administered imidazoles on human sterol synthesis, recent drug developments have focused primarily on the triazoles.

The imidazole antifungal class includes **ketoconazole, clotrimazole, miconazole, econazole, butoconazole, oxiconazole, sertaconazole,** and **sulconazole. Ketoconazole** was introduced in 1977 as the prototypic drug in this class. Ketoconazole is available in both oral and topical formulations. Its broad spectrum of action includes *C. immitis, C. neoformans, Candida* species, *H. capsulatum, B. dermatitidis,* and a variety of dermatophytes. The pharmacokinetic and adverse-effect profiles of ketoconazole limit its clinical utility. (In fact, oral ketoconazole has been replaced by itraconazole for the treatment of many mycoses; see discussion below.) Gastrointestinal absorption of oral ketoconazole depends on conversion of the drug to a salt in the acidic environment of the stomach. Thus, ketoconazole cannot be used if the patient has achlorhydria or is receiving bicarbon-

ate, antacids, H2-blockers, or proton pump inhibitors. Ketoconazole has little penetration into the CSF and urine, which limits its efficacy in CNS and urinary tract infections. In approximately 20% of patients, the drug causes nausea, vomiting, or anorexia; hepatic dysfunction occurs in 1% to 2% of patients.

Ketoconazole potently inhibits hepatic P450 enzymes and therefore affects the metabolism of many other drugs. At therapeutic doses, it also inhibits the P450 enzymes 17,20-lyase and side-chain cleavage enzyme in the adrenal gland and gonads and thereby decreases steroid hormone synthesis. Persistent adrenal insufficiency has been reported in association with ketoconazole therapy; at high doses of the drug, significant inhibition of androgen synthesis can result in gynecomastia and impotence. This dose-dependent adverse effect has been exploited therapeutically by some clinicians, who prescribe ketoconazole to inhibit androgen production in patients with advanced prostate cancer and to inhibit corticosteroid synthesis in patients with advanced adrenal cancer.

Topical ketoconazole is widely used to treat common dermatophyte infections and seborrheic dermatitis. Topical ketoconazole has been shown to have anti-inflammatory activity comparable to that of hydrocortisone. The cream formulation contains sulfites and therefore should be avoided in patients with sulfite hypersensitivity because cases of asthma and even anaphylaxis have been reported.

Clotrimazole, miconazole, econazole, butoconazole, oxiconazole, sertaconazole, and **sulconazole** are topical imidazole antifungal agents used to treat superficial fungal infections of the stratum corneum, squamous mucosa, and cornea. All of these agents are comparable to one another in efficacy. In addition to inhibiting 14α-sterol demethylase, miconazole affects fatty acid synthesis and inhibits fungal oxidative and peroxidase enzymes. The currently available topical azoles are generally not effective against hair or nail fungal infections, and topical azoles should not be used to treat subcutaneous or systemic mycoses. Topical azole agents are available for cutaneous and vaginal application, and selection of a particular agent should be based on cost and availability. Rare adverse effects of these agents include itching, burning, and sensitization.

The triazole class of antifungal agents includes **itraconazole, fluconazole, voriconazole, terconazole,** and **posaconazole**; one additional member of this class, **ravuconazole**, is currently in clinical trials. **Itraconazole** is available in both oral and intravenous formulations. Given its broad spectrum of activity, itraconazole has largely replaced oral ketoconazole for the treatment of many mycoses. The absorption of oral itraconazole is maximized in an acidic gastric environment. However, because the oral bioavailability of itraconazole is unpredictable, intravenous administration is sometimes preferred. Itraconazole is oxidized in the liver to the active metabolite hydroxy-itraconazole, which is more than 90% bound to plasma protein. Hydroxy-itraconazole inhibits fungal 14α-sterol demethylase. Compared to ketoconazole and fluconazole, itraconazole shows increased activity in aspergillosis, blastomycosis, and histoplasmosis. Itraconazole is not efficiently transported into the CSF, urine, or saliva; however, itraconazole can be used in certain meningeal fungal infections due to the high drug levels achieved in the meninges. Hepatotoxicity is the major adverse effect associated with itraconazole therapy. Other adverse effects include nausea, vomiting, abdominal pain, diarrhea, hypokalemia, pedal edema, and hair loss. Of note, **posaconazole** is a triazole developed from itraconazole. Posaconazole demonstrates potent in vitro fungicidal activity against *Aspergillus*, and it has in vitro and in vivo activity against *Zygomycetes*.

Although expensive, **fluconazole** is currently the most widely used antifungal drug. Fluconazole is a hydrophilic triazole that is available in both oral and intravenous formulations. The bioavailability of oral fluconazole is nearly 100%, and, unlike ketoconazole and itraconazole, its absorption is not influenced by gastric pH. Once absorbed, fluconazole diffuses freely into CSF, sputum, urine, and saliva. Fluconazole is excreted primarily by the kidneys.

Its relatively low adverse-effect profile (see below) and excellent CSF penetration make fluconazole the drug of choice for systemic candidiasis and cryptococcal meningitis. Due to the morbidity associated with intrathecal amphotericin B administration, fluconazole is also the drug of choice for coccidioidal meningitis. While fluconazole is active against blastomycosis, histoplasmosis, and sporotrichosis, it is less effective than itraconazole against these infections. Fluconazole is not effective against aspergillosis.

Fungal resistance to fluconazole develops readily, and *Candida* species are the most notable pathogens to develop resistance. Mechanisms of drug resistance include mutation of fungal P450 enzymes and overexpression of multidrug efflux transporter proteins.

Numerous drug interactions have been noted with fluconazole. As examples, fluconazole can increase the levels of amitriptyline, cyclosporine, phenytoin, and warfarin, while the levels and effects of fluconazole can be decreased by carbamazepine, isoniazid, and phenobarbital. Adverse effects of fluconazole include nausea, vomiting, abdominal pain, and diarrhea in about 10% of patients, as well as reversible alopecia with prolonged oral therapy. Rare cases of Stevens-Johnson syndrome and hepatic failure have been reported.

Ravuconazole, a fluconazole derivative that is currently in clinical trials, demonstrates an expanded spectrum of antifungal activity in vitro against multiple fungal species, including *Aspergillus* and the relatively resistant Candida species *Candida krusei* and *Candida glabrata*.

Voriconazole is a triazole antifungal agent that is available in both oral and parenteral forms. It is the drug of choice in the treatment of invasive aspergillosis and other molds such as *Fusarium* and *Scedosporium*. Voriconazole is fungicidal against essentially all species of *Aspergillus*, and its spectrum of activity also includes *Candida* species and a number of newly emerging fungi. It is ineffective in the treatment of zygomycosis. Compared to amphotericin, voriconazole is associated with significantly better outcomes, particularly in difficult-to-treat cases such as allogeneic bone marrow transplant recipients, patients with CNS infections, and patients with disseminated infections. Voriconazole inhibits hepatic P450 enzymes to a significant extent, and lower doses of cyclosporine or tacrolimus are used when these drugs are combined with voriconazole. Due to accelerated voriconazole metabolism, coadministration with ritonavir, rifampin, and rifabutin is contraindicated. The intravenous formulation of voriconazole should not be used in patients with renal failure because the cyclodextrin excipient accumulates and causes CNS toxicity. Hepatic toxicity is common but can usually be managed by decreasing the dose. Unusual visual symptoms (photophobia and colored lights) can occur at peak plasma concentrations of voriconazole; typically, these symptoms last for 30 to 60 minutes.

Terconazole is a topical triazole used to treat vaginal candidiasis. Its mechanism of action and spectrum of antifungal activity are similar to those of the other topical azoles. Terconazole is available as a vaginal suppository that is inserted at bedtime.

INHIBITORS OF FUNGAL MEMBRANE STABILITY: Polyenes

Amphotericin B and **nystatin** are **polyene** macrolide antifungal agents that were developed in the 1950s. These drugs act by binding to ergosterol and disrupting fungal membrane stability. Both agents are natural products derived from *Streptomyces* species. For decades, amphotericin B provided the only effective treatment for systemic mycoses. Both its therapeutic effect and its toxicity are related to its affinity for plasma membrane sterols. Fortunately, *the affinity of amphotericin B for ergosterol is 500 times greater than its affinity for cholesterol*. The binding of amphotericin B to ergosterol produces channels or pores that alter fungal membrane permeability and allow for leakage of essential cellular contents, leading ultimately to cell death. The concentration of membrane-associated ergosterol in a given fungal species determines whether amphotericin B is fungicidal or fungistatic for that species. Resistance to amphotericin B, although less frequent than with other antifungal agents, is attributable to a decrease in the ergosterol content of the fungal membrane. In addition to its pore-forming activity, amphotericin B appears to destabilize fungal membranes by generating toxic free radicals upon oxidation of the drug.

Because amphotericin B is highly insoluble, it is supplied as a buffered deoxycholate colloidal suspension. This suspension is poorly absorbed from the gastrointestinal tract and must be administered intravenously. Once in the bloodstream, more than 90% of the drug binds rapidly to tissue sites, while the remainder binds to plasma proteins. Penetration of amphotericin B into the CSF is extremely low. Hence, intrathecal therapy may be necessary for treatment of serious meningeal disease. The drug also diffuses poorly into vitreous humor and amniotic fluid.

The toxicity of amphotericin B limits its clinical use. Adverse effects associated with amphotericin B are divided into three groups: immediate systemic reactions, renal effects, and hematologic effects. Systemic reactions can include cytokine storm, in which amphotericin B elicits release of tumor necrosis factor-alpha (TNF-α) and interleukin-1 (IL-1) from cells of the host immune system. In turn, TNF-α and IL-1 cause fever, chills, and hypotension within the first several hours after drug administration. These responses can usually be minimized by decreasing the rate of drug administration or by pretreatment with antipyretic agents (e.g., acetaminophen, nonsteroidal anti-inflammatory drugs [NSAIDs], or hydrocortisone).

Renal toxicity of amphotericin B is a serious adverse event. The mechanism of renal toxicity is unknown but may be related to amphotericin-mediated vasoconstriction of afferent arterioles leading to renal ischemia. Renal toxicity is often the limiting factor in determining the extent of the therapeutic response to amphotericin B. It may be necessary to discontinue therapy temporarily if the blood urea nitrogen (BUN) exceeds 50 mg/dL or the serum creatinine exceeds 3 mg/dL. (BUN and creatinine are surrogate measures of renal function.) Renal tubular acidosis, cylindruria (the presence of renal cell casts in the urine), and hypokalemia can occur to the extent that electrolyte replacement is required. In the introductory case, treatment with amphotericin B was discontinued as soon as Mr. F's acute symptoms had resolved, in order to prevent renal toxicity.

Hematologic toxicity of amphotericin B is also common; anemia is probably secondary to decreased production of erythropoietin. The renal and hematologic toxicities of amphotericin B are cumulative and dose-related. Therapeutic measures that can minimize these toxicities include avoidance of other nephrotoxic drugs, such as aminoglycosides and cyclosporine, and maintenance of euvolemia to provide adequate renal perfusion.

Attempts to reduce nephrotoxicity have also led to the development of lipid formulations of amphotericin B. The strategy is to package amphotericin B in liposomes or other lipid carriers, with the goal of preventing high drug exposure to the proximal tubule of the nephron. **Amphotec®**, **Abelcet®**, and **AmBisome®** are all FDA-approved lipid-containing preparations of amphotericin B. They are equal in efficacy to each other and to native amphotericin deoxycholate. These formulations are less toxic than the native compound, but more expensive.

Nystatin, a structural relative of amphotericin B, is a polyene antifungal agent that also acts by binding ergosterol and causing pore formation in fungal cell membranes. The drug is used topically to treat candidiasis involving the skin, vaginal mucosa, and oral mucosa. Nystatin is not absorbed systemically from the skin, vagina, or gastrointestinal tract.

INHIBITORS OF FUNGAL WALL SYNTHESIS: Echinocandins

The key components of the fungal cell wall are chitin, β-(1,3)-D-glucan, β-(1,6)-D-glucan, and cell wall glycoproteins. Because human cells do not have a cell wall, fungal cell wall components represent unique targets for antifungal therapy, and antifungal agents directed at these targets are likely to be relatively nontoxic. **Echinocandins** are a new class of antifungal agents that target fungal cell wall synthesis by noncompetitively inhibiting the synthesis of β-(1,3)-D-glucans. Disruption of cell wall integrity results in osmotic stress, lysis of the fungal cell, and ultimately fungal cell death. The three antifungal agents in the echinocandin class are **caspofungin, micafungin,** and **anidulafungin**; all are semisynthetic lipopeptides derived from natural products. The echinocandins have in vitro and in vivo antifungal activity against *Candida* and *Aspergillus* species. All three echinocandins are fungicidal against *Candida* species, including *Candida glabrata* and *Candida krusei*, and fungistatic against *Aspergillus* species. All three agents are cur-

rently available only in parenteral form because they are insufficiently bioavailable for oral use.

Caspofungin was the first echinocandin to be approved. The drug is used as primary therapy for esophageal candidiasis and candidemia, as salvage therapy for *Aspergillus* infections and as empiric therapy for febrile neutropenia. Like the other echinocandins, caspofungin is highly protein-bound (97%) in the plasma; it is metabolized in the liver via peptide hydrolysis and N-acetylation; and it penetrates poorly into the CSF (although animal data indicate that the echinocandins do have some activity in the CNS). Caspofungin does not require dose adjustment for renal insufficiency, but dose adjustment is required for patients with moderate hepatic dysfunction. Because coadministration with cyclosporine significantly increases the plasma concentration of caspofungin and elevates liver function enzymes, this drug combination is generally not recommended unless the expected benefits outweigh the risks. To achieve therapeutic plasma concentrations, caspofungin dosing may need to be increased in patients receiving nelfinavir, efavirenz, phenytoin, rifampin, carbamazepine, or dexamethasone.

Micafungin is approved for the treatment of esophageal candidiasis and as antifungal prophylaxis for recipients of hematopoietic stem cell transplants. **Anidulafungin** is approved for the treatment of esophageal candidiasis and candidemia. Several small case series have reported the use of echinocandins in combination with amphotericin B, flucytosine, itraconazole, or voriconazole in patients with refractory fungal infections.

Echinocandins are generally well tolerated; their adverse-effect profile is comparable to that of fluconazole. Because echinocandins contain a peptide backbone, symptoms related to histamine release can be observed (see Suggested Reading). Other adverse effects include headache, fever (more common with caspofungin), abnormal liver function tests, and, rarely, hemolysis.

Conclusion and Future Directions

The development of antifungal agents has progressed significantly since the introduction of amphotericin B. As the population of immunocompromised patients increases, opportunistic fungal infections that are resistant to conventional antifungal therapy pose new challenges to researchers and clinicians. For example, new antifungal therapy is greatly needed in the treatment of zygomycosis. Effective *topical* antifungal agents are eagerly sought for the treatment of nail and hair dermatophytosis, because oral therapies for these superficial fungal infections carry risks of adverse effects. As novel and unique molecular targets are identified in fungal pathogens, newer antifungal agents will be developed with the goal of minimizing mechanism-based ("on-target") toxicity while expanding antifungal spectrum of action.

Suggested Reading

Boucher HW, Groll AH, Chiou CC, et al. Newer systemic antifungal agents. *Drugs* 2004;64:1997–2020. (*Discusses pharmacokinetics, safety, and efficacy of echinocandins and new azole antifungals.*)

Morrison VA. Echinocandin antifungals: review and update. *Expert Rev Anti Infect Ther* 2006;4:325–342. *(Summarizes clinical trials and pharmacology of echinocandins.)*

Patterson TF. Advances and challenges in management of invasive mycosis. *Lancet* 2005;366:1013–1025. *(Focused discussion of fungal pathogens that occur in immunocompromised hosts and management strategies for these opportunistic pathogens.)*

Ruiz-Herrera J, Victoria Elorza M, Valentin E, et al. Molecular organization of the cell wall of *Candida albicans* and its relation to pathogenicity. *FEMS Yeast Res* 2006;6:14–29. *(Comprehensive review of the fungal cell wall.)*

Sarosi GA, Davies SF. *Fungal Diseases of the Lung.* 3rd ed. Philadelphia: Lippincott Williams & Wilkins; 2000. *(Extensive discussion of general mycology and pathophysiology of fungal pathogens in the lung.)*

Drug Summary Table | Chapter 34 Pharmacology of Fungal Infections

Drug	Clinical Applications	Serious and Common Adverse Effects	Contraindications	Therapeutic Considerations
INHIBITOR OF FUNGAL NUCLEIC ACID SYNTHESIS: FLUCYTOSINE				
Mechanism—Flucytosine is converted in several steps to 5-FdUMP, which inhibits thymidylate synthase and thereby interferes with DNA synthesis				
Flucytosine	Candidiasis Cryptococcosis Chromomycosis	Bone marrow suppression (leukopenia, thrombocytopenia), cardiotoxicity Gastrointestinal disturbance, hepatic dysfunction	Pregnancy	Mutations in cytosine permease or cytosine deaminase account for the development of resistance The combination of flucytosine and amphotericin B exhibits synergistic killing of *Aspergillus* Use with caution in patients with renal impairment
INHIBITOR OF FUNGAL MITOSIS: GRISEOFULVIN				
Mechanism—Binds to tubulin and a microtubule-associated protein, thereby disrupting assembly of the mitotic spindle				
Griseofulvin	Fungal infection of the skin, hair, or nail due to *Trichophyton, Microsporum,* or *Epidermophyton*	*Hepatotoxicity, albuminuria, leukopenia, neutropenia, monocytosis, serum sickness, angioedema, toxic epidermal necrolysis* Headache, lethargy, vertigo, blurred vision, increased fecal protoporphyrin levels	Pregnancy Porphyria and hepatic failure	Continue treatment until the infected skin, hair, or nail is completely replaced by normal tissue For adults, the recommended daily dose is 500 mg microsize (250–330 mg ultramicrosize) for skin and 1,000 mg microsize (500–600 mg ultramicrosize) for hair and nail dermatophytes For children, the recommended dose is 5–10 mg/kg/day for cutaneous infections and 15–20 mg/kg/day for hair and nail infections Concurrent administration with barbiturates decreases gastrointestinal absorption of griseofulvin Griseofulvin induces hepatic P450 enzymes, which may result in increased metabolism of warfarin and reduced efficacy of low-estrogen oral contraceptives
INHIBITORS OF SQUALENE EPOXIDASE: ALLYLAMINES AND BENZYLAMINES				
Mechanism—Inhibit conversion of squalene to lanosterol by inhibiting squalene epoxidase				
Terbinafine Naftifine Butenafine	Onychomycosis (terbinafine) Tinea corporis Tinea cruris Tinea pedis Tinea capitis	*Hepatotoxicity, Stevens-Johnson syndrome, neutropenia, exacerbation of psoriasis or subacute cutaneous lupus erythematosus (oral terbinafine)* Gastrointestinal disturbance (oral terbinafine) Burning sensation and local irritation of the skin (topical applications)	Hypersensitivity to terbinafine, naftifine, or butenafine	Terbinafine and naftifine are allylamines, whereas butenafine is a benzylamine Terbinafine dosage for onychomycosis is 250 mg by mouth daily for 12 weeks for fingernails or for 16 weeks for toenails Plasma levels of terbinafine are increased by coadministration with cimetidine and decreased by coadministration with rifampin Naftifine is only available topically as a cream or gel Topical allylamine and benzylamine agents are more effective than topical azole agents against common dermatophytes, especially those causing tinea pedis

INHIBITORS OF 14α-STEROL DEMETHYLASE: IMIDAZOLES AND TRIAZOLES

Mechanism—Inhibit ultimate conversion of lanosterol to ergosterol by inhibiting 14α-sterol demethylase; the resulting decrease in ergosterol synthesis and accumulation of 14α-methyl sterols disrupt the tightly packed acyl chains of the phospholipids in the fungal membrane

Drug	Uses	Serious and Common Adverse Effects	Contraindications	Therapeutic Considerations
Imidazole antifungals: Ketoconazole Butoconazole Clotrimazole Econazole Miconazole Oxiconazole Sertaconazole Sulconazole	*Coccidioides immitis, Cryptococcus neoformans, Candida* species, *Histoplasma capsulatum, Blastomyces dermatitidis,* and a variety of dermatophytes (ketoconazole) Superficial fungal infections of the stratum corneum, squamous mucosa, and cornea (butoconazole, clotrimazole, econazole, miconazole, oxiconazole, sertaconazole, sulconazole)	Gastrointestinal disturbance, hepatic dysfunction, gynecomastia, decreased libido, menstrual irregularities (ketoconazole) Pruritus and burning (butoconazole, clotrimazole, econazole, miconazole, oxiconazole, sertaconazole, sulconazole)	Concurrent administration of amphotericin B or oral triazolam (ketoconazole) Hypersensitivity to ketoconazole, butoconazole, clotrimazole, econazole, miconazole, oxiconazole, sertaconazole, or sulconazole	Ketoconazole is available both orally and topically and increases P450 3A4 and increases levels of many drugs, including warfarin, tolbutamide, phenytoin, cyclosporine, H1-antihistamines, and others Agents that decrease gastric acidity interfere with ketoconazole absorption Butoconazole, clotrimazole, econazole, miconazole, oxiconazole, sertaconazole, and sulconazole are topical imidazole antifungal agents Topical azoles should be applied to the skin twice a day for 3 to 6 weeks, whereas vaginal preparations should be used once a day for 1 to 7 days at bedtime
Triazole antifungals: Fluconazole Itraconazole Posaconazole Terconazole Voriconazole	Aspergillosis, blastomycosis, candidiasis, histoplasmosis, onychomycosis (itraconazole) Candidiasis, cryptococcal meningitis (fluconazole) Aspergillosis, candidiasis, *Fusarium, Monosporium apiospermum* (voriconazole) Vulvovaginal candidiasis (terconazole)	*Hepatic toxicity, Stevens-Johnson syndrome* Gastrointestinal disturbance, rash Hypokalemia, hypertension, edema, headache (itraconazole)	Coadministration with dofetilide, oral midazolam, pimozide, levacetylmethadol, quinidine, lovastatin, simvastatin, or triazolam (itraconazole and fluconazole) Coadministration with ergot alkaloids metabolized by P450 3A4, such as dihydroergotamine, ergotamine, ergonovine, and methylergonovine (itraconazole and fluconazole) Pregnancy Hypersensitivity to fluconazole, itraconazole, posaconazole, terconazole, or voriconazole	Itraconazole dosage for onychomycosis is 400 mg twice daily for one week per month, repeated to complete a 3-month course for fingernail infections or a 4-month course for toenail infections Fluconazole and itraconazole inhibit P450 3A4 The 0.4% terconazole cream is used for 7 days, whereas the 0.8% cream is used for 3 days for vulvovaginal candidiasis Ravuconazole is in clinical trials

INHIBITORS OF FUNGAL MEMBRANE STABILITY: POLYENES

Mechanism—Bind to ergosterol and form pores that alter fungal membrane permeability and stability

Drug	Uses	Serious and Common Adverse Effects	Contraindications	Therapeutic Considerations
Amphotericin B	Potentially life-threatening aspergillosis, cryptococcosis, North American blastomycosis, systemic candidiasis, coccidioidomycosis, histoplasmosis, systemic candidiasis, zygomycosis	*Renal toxicity (renal tubular acidosis, cylindruria, hypokalemia), cytokine storm (fever, chills, hypotension), anemia* Weight loss, gastrointestinal disturbance	Hypersensitivity to amphotericin B	Amphotericin B is supplied as a buffered deoxycholate colloidal suspension, which must be administered intravenously; intrathecal therapy may be necessary for serious meningeal disease Lipid formulations of amphotericin B are designed to reduce drug exposure to the proximal tubule of the nephron and thereby minimize nephrotoxicity Amphotec®, Abelcet®, and Ambisome® are all FDA-approved lipid-containing preparations of amphotericin B

(Continued)

Drug Summary Table | **Chapter 34 Pharmacology of Fungal Infections** (*Continued*)

Drug	Clinical Applications	*Serious* and Common Adverse Effects	Contraindications	Therapeutic Considerations
Nystatin	Mucocutaneous candidiasis	Rare contact dermatitis	Hypersensitivity to nystatin	Nystatin is not absorbed systemically from the skin, vagina, or gastrointestinal tract Nystatin is used clinically for topical treatment of candidiasis involving the skin, vaginal mucosa, or oral mucosa

INHIBITORS OF FUNGAL WALL SYNTHESIS: ECHINOCANDINS
Mechanism—Noncompetitively inhibit synthesis of β-(1,3)-D-glucans, which leads to disruption of cell wall integrity

Drug	Clinical Applications	*Serious* and Common Adverse Effects	Contraindications	Therapeutic Considerations
Caspofungin Micafungin Anidulafungin	Esophageal candidiasis, candidemia, salvage therapy of *Aspergillus* infections, empiric therapy of febrile neutropenia (caspofungin) Esophageal candidiasis, antifungal prophylaxis for recipients of hematopoietic stem cell transplants (micafungin) Esophageal candidiasis, candidemia (anidulafungin)	*Pruritus, rash, gastrointestinal disturbance, increased liver enzymes, thrombophlebitis, headache, fever*	Hypersensitivity to caspofungin, micafungin, or anidulafungin	All three echinocandins are fungicidal against *Candida* species, including *Candida glabrata* and *Candida krusei*, and fungistatic against *Aspergillus* species Coadministration of cyclosporine with caspofungin significantly increases plasma concentration of caspofungin and elevates liver function enzymes Caspofungin dose should be adjusted for patients with moderate liver dysfunction

35

Pharmacology of Parasitic Infections

Louise C. Ivers and Edward T. Ryan

INTRODUCTION

More than one billion people worldwide are infected with parasites. Parasites of medical importance include protozoa (such as the organisms that cause malaria, toxoplasmosis, giardiasis, amebiasis, leishmaniasis, and trypanosomiasis) and helminths (''worms''). Worms that infect humans include cestodes (''flat worms'' or ''tape worms,'' such as the worm that causes taeniasis), nematodes (''round worms,'' which cause filariasis, strongyloidiasis, and ascariasis), and trematodes (''flukes,'' such as the worm that causes schistosomiasis).

Ideally, antiparasitic drugs should be targeted to structures or biochemical pathways present or accessible only in parasites. Many antiparasitic drugs act by unknown or poorly defined mechanisms of action, however. This chapter focuses on a number of the better-defined agents, including

those active against *Plasmodia* species (which cause malaria), *Entamoeba histolytica* (which causes amebiasis), and *Onchocerca volvulus* (which causes onchocerciasis, a filarial infection referred to as ''river blindness''). In each of these cases, antiparasitic agents interfere with metabolic requirements of the parasite: the dependence of malarial plasmodia on heme metabolism, the dependence of luminal parasites on specific fermentation pathways, and the dependence of helminths on neuromuscular activity. These three examples are not all-inclusive, but rather emphasize opportunities to use or design pharmacologic agents to interrupt metabolic requirements specific to parasites.

MALARIAL PLASMODIA

Each year, 300 to 500 million individuals in more than 90 countries develop malaria, and 1.3 to 2.7 million individuals die of malaria. Malaria is the most important parasitic disease of humans and one of the most important infections of humans. Human malaria is caused by one of four species of plasmodial parasites: ***Plasmodium falciparum, P. vivax, P. malariae,*** and ***P. ovale.*** The most serious type of malaria is that caused by *P. falciparum.*

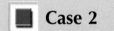

Case 1

Binata, a 3-year-old girl living in Senegal, is in good health when, one day, she begins to feel hot, has sweats and shaking chills, stops eating, and becomes intermittently listless and lethargic. Several days later, these symptoms climax in a seizure and coma, prompting Binata's parents to rush her to the local health care clinic. In the clinic, the unconscious child's neck is supple, but she is febrile to 103°F. Her lungs are clear to auscultation, and there is no rash. A smear of Binata's peripheral blood discloses *P. falciparum* ring trophozoites in approximately 10% of her erythrocytes. Binata is given the only antimalarial medicines available at the clinic, chloroquine and pyrimethamine-sulfadoxine; however, the child does not improve, and she dies within 24 hours.

QUESTIONS

■ **1.** Why did Binata die?
■ **2.** Why did Binata not improve after receiving antimalarial drugs?
■ **3.** How often does a child die of malaria?

Case 2

Mr. G is a 36-year-old married software engineer who was born and raised in India. He comes to the United States and is completely well for 6 months. He then begins to experience episodes of fever, headache, and body aches. One week later, he goes to his physician, who examines a smear of Mr. G's blood, diagnoses malaria, and prescribes chloroquine for treatment. Therapy with chloroquine resolves his symptoms completely. However, Mr. G notes recurrence of fevers and the other symptoms 3 months later and returns to his doctor's office.

QUESTIONS

■ **1.** What is a likely explanation for the return of Mr. G's fever?
■ **2.** How can Mr. G's treatment be modified so that his illness will not return?

PHYSIOLOGY OF MALARIAL PLASMODIA

Life Cycle

The life cycle of malaria involves a parasite, a mosquito vector, and a human host (Fig. 35-1). An ***Anopheles*** spp.

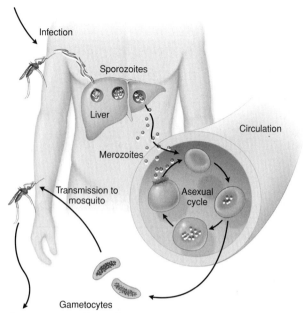

Figure 35-1. Life cycle of malaria. Malarial plasmodia have a complex life cycle that relies on both humans and *Anopheles* spp. mosquitoes. Gametocytes from an infected human are transferred to a mosquito during a blood meal. In the mosquito stomach, a zygote forms and matures to become an oocyst on the outside wall of the stomach (*not shown*). Sporozoites released from the oocyst migrate to the salivary glands. During its next blood meal, the mosquito transfers *Plasmodium* spp. sporozoites from its saliva to another human. Sporozoites enter the host's bloodstream and travel to the liver. Sporozoites replicate in the liver and then lyse infected hepatocytes, releasing merozoites into the circulation. Merozoites infect erythrocytes, undergoing asexual cycles of erythrocytic infection and lysis. Some merozoites differentiate into gametocytes, which can be ingested by another mosquito and thereby continue the cycle of infection. *P. vivax* and *P. ovale* can also form dormant hypnozoites, which can remain in infected hepatocytes for months to years before release into the circulation (*not shown*).

mosquito can ingest sexual forms of malarial parasites (gametocytes) when taking a blood meal from an infected human. After fusion of the male and female gametocytes and maturation of the zygote within the mosquito, **sporozoites** are released from an oocyst. The sporozoites, which migrate to the mosquito's salivary glands, can be inoculated into the blood of another human host during a subsequent blood meal. In the human, sporozoites leave the blood and multiply in the liver, forming **tissue schizonts.** This *exo-erythrocytic hepatic stage* is asymptomatic. In a typical *P. falciparum* infection, 1 to 12 weeks after the infective bite, the liver cells release parasites into the bloodstream as **merozoites.** A single sporozoite can produce more than 30,000 merozoites. Merozoites invade erythrocytes, multiply asexually, and form **blood schizonts.** This is the *erythrocytic stage.* Infected erythrocytes eventually rupture, releasing another generation of merozoites that continue the erythrocytic cycle. Rare merozoites also mature into gametocytes. Ingestion of these circulating gametocytes by an appropriate mosquito completes the life cycle. The clinical symptoms of malaria, most distinctively fever, are caused by the intravascular lysis of erythrocytes and subsequent release of merozoites into the blood. The fevers that Binata and Mr. G experienced were associated with these hemolytic episodes. Binata, unfortunately, developed cerebral malaria due to *P. falciparum.*

P. falciparum-infected erythrocytes express "knobs" on their surface that are composed of both host and parasite proteins. Parasite proteins include PfEMP-1, a protein family comprised of approximately 100 to 150 gene products that mediate attachment of infected erythrocytes to cellular receptors—including CD36, ICAM-1, ELAM-1, and chondroitin sulfate—on endothelial surfaces in the human host. This intravascular binding during a malarial episode occurs only during *P. falciparum* infection and contributes to intravascular "sludging" of erythrocytes. Endothelial attachment lessens the amount of time over which infected erythrocytes circulate systemically, thereby decreasing the likelihood that infected erythrocytes will be cleared via splenic sequestration. Sludging also accounts, in large part, for the pathophysiology of malaria caused by *P. falciparum.* Sludging can affect any organ, including the brain, lungs, and kidneys; damage to these organs leads to tissue hypoxia, focal necrosis, and hemorrhage. In Binata's case, the brain was involved (so-called *"cerebral malaria"*).

Untreated, cerebral malaria is almost uniformly fatal, and, even with optimal treatment, cerebral malaria has a case fatality rate exceeding 20%. Binata was treated with two drugs that have historically been quite important in treating individuals with malaria, but which, unfortunately, are now ineffective in many places in the world because of widespread drug-resistant *P. falciparum.* Largely because of their low cost and availability, these drugs (chloroquine and a fixed combination of pyrimethamine and sulfadoxine) have been widely used in many developing areas of the world to treat older children and adults with partial immunity to malaria, but these agents have little clinical use in treating nonimmune individuals such as Binata. Due to the increasing ineffectiveness of these older agents, it is now recommended that individuals in Sub-Saharan Africa with malaria be treated with an artemisinin derivative in combination with a second agent (see below).

Unfortunately, Binata's story is all too common. On average, worldwide, a child dies of malaria every 20 seconds; of these deaths, more than 90% occur in Sub-Saharan Africa, more than 90% occur in children under 5 years of age, and more than 95% are caused by *P. falciparum* infection. No pharmacologic agent has yet been developed that interferes with the recently elucidated role of PfEMP-1 in the endothelial attachment of malarially infected erythrocytes.

In Mr. G's case, a peripheral blood smear showed *P. vivax* parasites inside his erythrocytes. Because *P. falciparum* and *P. malariae* infections involve only one cycle of hepatic cell invasion, drugs that eliminate these species from erythrocytes are usually sufficient to clear the infection. Unfortunately, *P. vivax* and *P. ovale* also have dormant hepatic forms (**hypnozoites**) that release merozoites over months to 1 or 2 years. Therefore, individuals infected with *P. vivax* or *P. ovale* should be treated with agents that are effective against not only blood-stage plasmodia, but also liver-stage parasites (see below). Because chloroquine does not eliminate hepatic forms of *P. vivax* and *P. ovale*, Mr. G's *P. vivax* infection recurred.

Heme Metabolism

Plasmodia have a limited capacity for de novo amino acid synthesis; instead, they rely on amino acids released from ingested host **hemoglobin** molecules. Within red blood cells, plasmodia degrade hemoglobin in a digestive vacuole, which is an elaborate lysosome with an acidic pH (Fig. 35-2). Hemoglobin is sequentially degraded to its constituent amino acids by plasmodial aspartic proteases (plasmepsins), a cys-

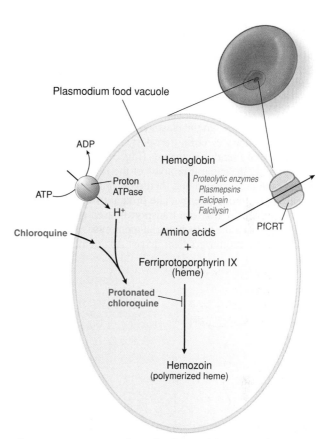

Figure 35-2. Proposed mechanisms of heme metabolism in the plasmodial food vacuole. Malarial plasmodia possess a specialized food vacuole that maintains an acidic intravacuolar environment by the action of a proton ATPase in the vacuolar membrane. Within the vacuole, human hemoglobin is used as a food source. Hemoglobin is proteolyzed to amino acids by several plasmodial-derived proteolytic enzymes, including plasmepsins, falcipain, and falcilysin. Protonated amino acids are then removed from the food vacuole through the PfCRT transporter. Degradation of hemoglobin also releases heme (ferriprotoporphyrin IX). Free ferriprotoporphyrin IX can react with oxygen to produce superoxide (O_2^-); oxidant defense enzymes, which may include plasmodial-derived superoxide dismutase and catalase, convert the potentially cytotoxic superoxide to H_2O *(not shown)*. Plasmodia polymerize ferriprotoporphyrin IX into the nontoxic derivative hemozoin; evidence suggests that polymerization requires the activity of positively charged histidine-rich proteins *(not shown)*. The iron moiety in ferriprotoporphyrin IX can also be oxidized from the ferrous (Fe^{2+}) to the ferric (Fe^{3+}) state, with concomitant production of hydrogen peroxide (H_2O_2). Many antimalarial agents are thought to disrupt the process of malarial heme metabolism; proposed mechanisms of drug action include inhibition of heme polymerization, enhancement of oxidant production, and reaction with heme to form cytotoxic metabolites. The inhibition of ferriprotoporphyrin IX polymerization by protonated chloroquine is shown.

teine protease (falcipain), and a metalloprotease (falcilysin). Degradation of hemoglobin releases protonated basic amino acids and a toxic heme metabolite, ferriprotoporphyrin IX. Ferriprotoporphyrin IX is detoxified by polymerization to crystalline hemozoin. If ferriprotoporphyrin IX does not polymerize, it causes lysosomal membrane damage and toxicity to the malarial parasite. Quinoline antimalarials (see below) are believed to act by inhibiting heme polymerization, thereby creating an environment that is toxic to intraerythrocytic plasmodia.

Electron Transport Chain

Malarial plasmodia also possess mitochondria with a tiny genome (approximately 6 kb) that encodes only three **cytochromes** (large protein complexes involved in electron transport and oxidative phosphorylation). These cytochromes, together with a number of mitochondrial-targeted proteins derived from the plasmodial nuclear genome, make up a rudimentary electron transport chain similar in organization to that found in mammals (Fig. 35-3). In this electron transport chain, integral proteins of the mitochondrial inner membrane are reduced and then oxidized as they transport electrons from one intermediate protein to another. The energy liberated by electron transport is used to drive proton pumping across the mitochondrial membrane, and the energy stored in the proton gradient drives ATP synthesis. In this electron transport chain, oxygen is the final electron acceptor, resulting in the reduction of oxygen to water.

Plasmodia derive most of their ATP directly from glycolysis and probably do not use mitochondrial electron transport as a significant source of energy. However, plasmodia do rely on electron transport for the oxidation of key enzymes involved in nucleotide synthesis. For example, **dihydro-orotate dehydrogenase** (DHOD), the enzyme that mediates an early step in pyrimidine synthesis (see Chapter 37, Pharmacology of Cancer: Genome Synthesis, Stability, and Maintenance), catalyzes the oxidation of dihydro-orotate to orotate. As part of this reaction, DHOD is reduced, and the enzyme must be reoxidized before it can continue with another cycle of catalysis. **Ubiquinone,** an integral membrane protein located near the beginning of the electron transport chain, accepts electrons from reduced DHOD, thus regenerating the oxidized form of DHOD necessary for pyrimidine synthesis. Because plasmodia depend on de novo pyrimidine synthesis for DNA replication, interrupting the ability of ubiquinone to oxidize DHOD can disrupt plasmodial DNA replication (see below).

PHARMACOLOGY OF ANTIMALARIAL AGENTS

The currently available antimalarial agents target four physiologic pathways in plasmodia: heme metabolism (**chloroquine, quinine, mefloquine,** and **artemisinin**), electron transport (**primaquine** and **atovaquone**), protein translation (**doxycycline, tetracycline,** and **clindamycin**), and folate metabolism (**sulfadoxine-pyrimethamine** and **proguanil**). The following section discusses the pharmacologic agents that target these pathways.

Clinically, antimalarials can be classified into agents used for prophylaxis (to prevent malaria in individuals residing in or traveling through a malaria zone), agents used for treating individuals with acute blood-stage malaria, and agents used to eliminate hypnozoite liver-stage malarial infections. Generally, agents used for prophylaxis must be well tolerated and easy to administer.

Inhibitors of Heme Metabolism

For many centuries, agents that disrupt intraerythrocytic malarial parasites have been the foundation of antimalarial treatment regimens. Most of these compounds are congeners of quinoline and, as a result, are all believed to possess similar mechanisms of action. Artemisinin, discussed at the end of this section, is also thought to act by inhibiting heme metabolism, although its structure is different from that of the quinolines.

Chloroquine

For the past 2,000 years, humans have used the roots of *Dichroa febrifuga* or the leaves of hydrangea in the treatment of individuals with malaria. More recently, the bark of the **cinchona** tree was found to be a more effective remedy. In all these plants, a **quinoline** compound is the pharmacologically active antiplasmodial agent. **Chloroquine,** a 4-aminoquinoline, was introduced in 1935 for use in the treatment of malaria. Chloroquine is a weak base that, in its

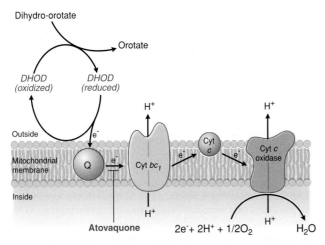

Figure 35-3. The mitochondrial electron transport chain in plasmodia. The electron transport chain consists of a series of oxidation/reduction steps that culminate in the donation of electrons to oxygen, forming water. In plasmodia, the electron transport chain acts as an electron acceptor for reduced dihydro-orotate dehydrogenase (DHOD), an enzyme that is essential for plasmodial pyrimidine synthesis. In this cascade, reduced ubiquinone *(Q)* transfers electrons to the cytochrome bc_1 complex *(Cyt bc_1)*, which then passes electrons to cytochrome c *(Cyt c)* and, finally, to cytochrome c oxidase *(Cyt c oxidase)*. In a 4-electron reduction of molecular oxygen *(shown here as the half-reaction)*, cytochrome c oxidase donates electrons to oxygen to form water. This chain of electron transfers also involves the pumping of protons across the mitochondrial membrane by Cyt bc_1 and Cyt c oxidase; the resulting electrochemical gradient of protons is used to generate ATP *(not shown)*. Atovaquone antagonizes the interaction between ubiquinone and the plasmodial cytochrome bc_1 complex, thereby disrupting pyrimidine synthesis by preventing the regeneration of oxidized DHOD.

neutral form, freely diffuses across the membrane of the parasite's food vacuole. Once inside the acidic environment of the vacuole, chloroquine is rapidly protonated, making it unable to diffuse out of the vacuole. As a result, protonated chloroquine accumulates to high concentrations inside the parasite's food vacuole, where it binds to ferriprotoporphyrin IX and inhibits the polymerization of this heme metabolite. Accumulation of unpolymerized ferriprotoporphyrin IX leads to oxidative membrane damage and is toxic to the parasite. *Chloroquine thus poisons the parasite by preventing the detoxification of a toxic product of hemoglobin catabolism* (Fig. 35-2).

Chloroquine is concentrated by as much as 100-fold in parasitized erythrocytes compared to uninfected erythrocytes. In addition, the concentration of chloroquine required to alkalinize lysosomes of mammalian cells is much higher than that needed to raise the pH in malarial food vacuoles. Therefore, chloroquine is relatively nontoxic to humans, although the drug commonly causes pruritus in darkly pigmented individuals and it can exacerbate psoriasis and porphyria. Taken in supratherapeutic doses, however, chloroquine can cause vomiting, retinopathy, hypotension, confusion, and death. In fact, chloroquine is used globally in suicides each year (largely because it is inexpensive, available, and toxic at high doses), and accidental ingestion by children can be fatal.

When initially introduced, chloroquine was a first-line drug used against all types of malaria; however, it is now ineffective against most strains of *P. falciparum* in Africa, Asia, and South America (Fig. 35-4). Hypotheses regarding the mechanisms responsible for chloroquine resistance are based on the finding that chloroquine-resistant plasmodia accumulate less chloroquine inside food vacuoles than chloroquine-sensitive plasmodia do. In the food vacuole, protonated amino acids are generated by the parasite as it degrades hemoglobin. These protonated amino acids exit the lysosome by means of a transmembrane protein called PfCRT,

encoded by *pfcrt* on *P. falciparum* chromosome 7. A number of mutations in PfCRT have been associated with chloroquine resistance; for example, a substitution of threonine for lysine at position 76 (K76T) is highly correlated with chloroquine resistance. This mutated PfCRT probably pumps protonated chloroquine out of the food vacuole. This altered pump action could also be detrimental to the parasite, perhaps because of altered amino acid export and/or changes in vacuole pH. Many *P. falciparum* strains with mutations in *pfcrt* carry a second mutation in the gene *pfmdr1* encoding Pgh1, a food vacuole membrane protein involved in pH regulation. It is speculated that this second mutation provides a "corrective" action that allows chloroquine-resistant *P. falciparum* to continue growth in the presence of a *pfcrt* mutation.

Strains of *P. vivax* with decreased susceptibility to chloroquine are now reported with increasing frequency in areas of Papua New Guinea, Indonesia, and other focal areas of Oceania and Latin America, although the exact mechanism of decreased susceptibility to chloroquine in these strains has not yet been established. Despite concerns regarding increasing resistance, chloroquine remains the drug of choice for treating most individuals with malaria caused by *P. vivax, P. ovale, P. malariae,* and chloroquine-sensitive strains of *P. falciparum.* It can also be used prophylactically to prevent malaria caused by sensitive strains of plasmodia.

Quinine and Quinidine

Quinine is an alkaloid that consists of a quinoline ring linked by a secondary carbinol to a quinuclidine ring. Its optical isomer, **quinidine,** has identical pharmacologic actions. Because of quinine's structural similarity to other antimalarial quinolines, quinine is thought to attack plasmodia by the mechanism described above. Quinine has also been shown

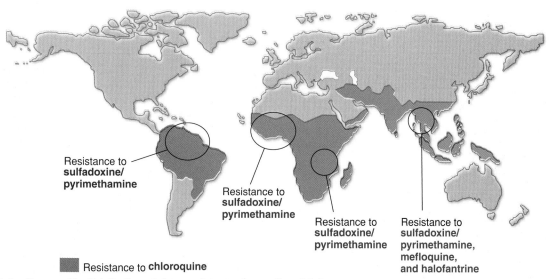

Figure 35-4. Geographic distribution of drug-resistant *Plasmodium falciparum.* Historically, chloroquine has been the drug of choice for prophylaxis and treatment of individuals with *P. falciparum* malaria. Unfortunately, *P. falciparum* is now resistant to chloroquine in most areas of the world *(blue shading)*. In many areas, *P. falciparum* is also resistant to other antimalarial agents, including sulfadoxine-pyrimethamine, mefloquine, and halofantrine. (Halofantrine is associated with potentially lethal cardiac toxicity and is therefore seldom used.)

to intercalate into DNA through hydrogen bonding, thus inhibiting DNA strand separation, transcription, and translation. The overall effect is a decrease in the growth and replication of the erythrocytic form of plasmodia. Quinine and quinidine are used to treat individuals with acute blood-stage malaria but are not used prophylactically. Use of quinine can cause **cinchonism,** a syndrome that includes tinnitus, deafness, headaches, nausea, vomiting, and visual disturbances. Quinine and quinidine can also prolong the cardiac QT interval (see Chapter 18, Pharmacology of Cardiac Rhythm).

Mefloquine

Mefloquine is a quinoline compound that is structurally related to other antimalarial agents. Unlike quinine, mefloquine does not bind to DNA. Its exact mechanism of action is unknown, although mefloquine appears to disrupt polymerization of hemozoin in intraerythrocytic malarial parasites. Mefloquine has a number of adverse effects, which are not sufficiently common to preclude its beneficial use. These include nausea, cardiac conduction abnormalities (including bradycardia, prolongation of the QT interval, and arrhythmia), and neuropsychiatric effects, including vivid dreams/nightmares, insomnia, anxiety, depression, hallucinations, seizures, and, rarely, psychosis. The mechanism(s) responsible for these adverse effects is unknown. Mefloquine can be used both therapeutically and prophylactically. Strains of *P. falciparum* resistant to both chloroquine and mefloquine have been reported in areas of Southeast Asia.

Artemisinin

Artemisinin has been used in China (where it is known as *qinghao*) for centuries in the treatment of individuals with fever. The compound is a cyclic endoperoxide that, when activated by free or heme-bound iron, forms a carbon-centered free-radical compound (Fig. 35-5). This free radical has the ability to alkylate many proteins as well as heme. The mechanism of specificity of the drug for plasmodia-infected erythrocytes is unknown—two potential sources of specificity include artemisinin's requirement for heme for free radical formation and artemisinin's preferential accumulation in plasmodia. Administration of artemisinin and its derivatives (**artesunate, artemether, artemotil, dihydroartemisinin**) is associated with a rapid decrease in the level of malaria parasites in the blood of an infected individual and rapid resolution of symptoms in patients with blood-stage malaria. Artemisinin is not effective as a prophylactic agent against malaria.

Because of widespread resistance to other antimalarial agents, first-line therapy for uncomplicated and complicated malaria in Sub-Saharan Africa involves a combination of artemisinin and a second antimalarial agent. Although there has been evidence of in vitro resistance to artemisinin in field isolates of *P. falciparum*, clinical cases of resistant infection have not yet been reported. Because of concerns over the development of resistance and over the short half-life of artemisinin derivatives (from 1 to 11 hours), it is recommended that artemisinin compounds be coadministered with a second agent with a different mechanism of action and a longer half-life. Addition of the second agent will hopefully delay the development of artemisinin resistance and prolong the therapeutic effect of the combination (see section on antimalarial drug resistance below).

Artemisinin and its derivatives are generally well tolerated but can have neurotoxic and cardiotoxic adverse effects. In laboratory animals, artemisinin has been shown to cause

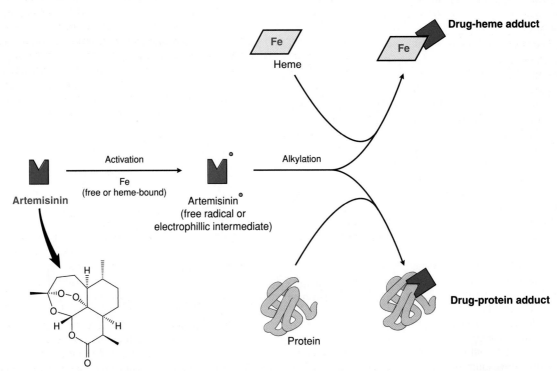

Figure 35-5. Proposed mechanism of action of artemisinin. Artemisinin is a cyclic endoperoxide compound that forms a free radical after activation by iron (Fe). This free radical is able to alkylate macromolecules such as heme and proteins, resulting in the formation of artemisinin-heme adducts and artemisinin-protein adducts that are toxic to plasmodia.

brainstem neuropathy; although this potentially lethal effect has not been observed in humans, accumulating evidence suggests that artemisinins may indeed be associated with auditory impairment and other neurotoxic effects. Hypoglycemia occurs less often than with quinine-based therapy. Safety data in pregnancy are lacking.

Inhibitors of Electron Transport

Although the electron transport chain is a ubiquitous feature of eukaryotic cells, two agents have been developed that appear to interrupt the plasmodial electron transport chain selectively. This selectivity is due to different molecular structures of the same biochemical target, rather than the presence of a unique enzymatic pathway in plasmodia (see Chapter 31, Principles of Antimicrobial and Antineoplastic Pharmacology).

Primaquine

Primaquine was approved in 1952 for the treatment of individuals with malaria. Because primaquine attacks the hepatic forms of malaria caused by *P. vivax* and *P. ovale,* it is used to prevent recrudescence of these infections and is the only standard drug currently available for this use. Primaquine severely disrupts the metabolic processes of plasmodial mitochondria. The antimalarial activity is probably attributable to **quinone,** a primaquine metabolite that interferes with the function of **ubiquinone** as an electron carrier in the respiratory chain. Another potential mechanism of action involves the ability of certain primaquine metabolites to cause nonspecific oxidative damage to plasmodial mitochondria.

Primaquine is predominantly used to clear hepatic hypnozoites from individuals with malaria caused by *P. vivax* or *P. ovale.* Strains of *P. vivax* have intrinsic variability in their susceptibility to primaquine. For example, the Chesson strain, first isolated from an American soldier in Papua New Guinea in the 1940s, is less susceptible than other strains to primaquine. Because of this variability, an increased dose of primaquine (compared to the most common dose administered historically) is now recommended as standard treatment. Primaquine may also be used as a prophylactic agent.

Individuals with **glucose-6-phosphate dehydrogenase (G6PD) deficiency** have a limited ability to protect their erythrocytes against oxidative damage. G6PD is needed to reduce $NADP^+$ to NADPH, which converts oxidized **glutathione** to reduced glutathione. Reduced glutathione protects erythrocytes by catalyzing the breakdown of toxic oxidant compounds. The administration of primaquine causes significant oxidative stress because of the formation of numerous oxidized compounds. As a result, primaquine can induce massive and potentially fatal **hemolysis** in individuals with G6PD deficiency. Therefore, primaquine should never be administered to an individual without first confirming adequate G6PD activity in that individual's erythrocytes. *Primaquine should never be administered to pregnant women,* because primaquine crosses the placenta and can induce fatal hemolysis in fetal erythrocytes independent of the maternal G6PD status. Primaquine can also cause gastrointestinal disturbances, methemoglobinemia and, very rarely, neutropenia, hypertension, arrhythmias, and neurological symptoms.

Atovaquone

Atovaquone is a structural analogue of ubiquinone, the shuttling protein in the electron transport chain. Under physiologic conditions, the transfer of two electrons from reduced ubiquinone to the cytochrome bc_1 complex oxidizes the ubiquinone (Fig. 35-3). Atovaquone inhibits the interaction between reduced ubiquinone and the cytochrome bc_1 complex and thereby disrupts electron transport. Because plasmodia depend on the electron transport chain to regenerate oxidized dihydro-orotate reductase, treatment with atovaquone disrupts pyrimidine synthesis and thereby prevents plasmodia from replicating their DNA. It is likely that inhibition of the electron transport chain also disrupts other steps in intermediary metabolism that depend on oxidation/reduction cycling of proteins.

The cytochrome bc_1 complex is a ubiquitous feature of eukaryotic organisms. The selectivity of atovaquone for plasmodia likely relies on differences in the sequences of amino acids between human and plasmodial ubiquinone-cytochrome bc_1 binding regions. Atovaquone inhibits the activity of plasmodial cytochrome bc_1 with approximately 100-fold selectivity compared to the human form of the protein. However, this selectivity is easily disrupted; a single point mutation in the cytochrome bc_1 complex can render plasmodia resistant to atovaquone. For this reason, atovaquone is not used as a single agent. Atovaquone can be coadministered with **doxycycline,** a protein synthesis inhibitor, or as a fixed combination with **proguanil,** a dihydrofolate reductase inhibitor (see discussion below). Proguanil and atovaquone are synergistic in their antimalarial activity. Interestingly, this synergy may not be related to proguanil's action as an antifolate, because other inhibitors of dihydrofolate reductase do not have synergistic effects with atovaquone. Instead, when administered with atovaquone, proguanil may act as an uncoupling agent in mitochondrial membranes, thereby enhancing atovaquone-mediated mitochondrial depolarization. Atovaquone is generally well tolerated; its use is associated with a low incidence of adverse gastrointestinal effects and an occasional rash. In combination with a second antimalarial drug, atovaquone can be used both therapeutically and prophylactically.

Inhibitors of Translation
Doxycycline, Tetracycline, and Clindamycin

Agents that disrupt parasite protein synthesis include **doxycycline, tetracycline,** and **clindamycin.** Doxycycline is a structural isomer of tetracycline and is produced semisynthetically from oxytetracycline or methacycline. Doxycycline inhibits parasite protein synthesis by binding to the 30S ribosomal subunit, thereby blocking the binding of aminoacyl tRNA to mRNA (see Chapter 32). By virtue of its high lipophilicity, doxycycline penetrates well into body tissues, has a large volume of distribution, and is reabsorbed in renal tubules and the gastrointestinal tract, resulting in a long half-life. Doxycycline's oral bioavailability and long half-life make it a useful drug (in combination with quinine) for the treatment of individuals infected with chloroquine-resistant *P. falciparum.* Doxycycline should not be used as a single antimalarial agent. Adverse effects include cutaneous photosensitivity, tooth discoloration in children, and vaginal candidiasis; gastrointestinal effects (including nausea, diarrhea, and dyspepsia) are typically mild, although esophageal ulceration can occur rarely.

Tetracycline and doxycycline have similar pharmacologic profiles, but tetracycline must be taken four times a day. Tetracycline may be used in combination with quinine for the treatment of individuals with chloroquine-resistant malaria; however, it is not recommended as a malaria chemoprophylactic.

Clindamycin inhibits protein synthesis by binding to the 50S ribosomal subunit. Clindamycin is used in combination with quinine for the treatment of individuals with malaria when the use of tetracycline or doxycycline is contraindicated (for example, in pregnant women or children less than 8 years of age). Clindamycin is usually well tolerated, especially in children; its major adverse effect is an increased risk of antibiotic-associated diarrhea and colitis caused by *Clostridium difficile*. Clindamycin is not used as a malaria chemoprophylactic.

Inhibitors of Folate Metabolism

Folic acid is a vitamin involved in the transfer of one-carbon units in a variety of biosynthetic pathways, including those of DNA and RNA precursors and certain amino acids (see Chapter 31). In humans, folate is an essential vitamin and must be ingested in the diet. In parasites and bacteria, folate is synthesized de novo, providing a useful target for selective drug action. Inhibition of folate metabolism can result in successful treatment of parasitic infections. In the context of malaria, antifolate drugs act against parasite-specific isoforms of dihydropteroate synthetase and dihydrofolate reductase. Combination therapies that include a sulfonamide and pyrimethamine are used. Two antimalarial formulations are available, **sulfadoxine-pyrimethamine** and the less frequently used **sulfalene-pyrimethamine**.

Sulfadoxine-Pyrimethamine

Sulfadoxine is a para-aminobenzoic acid (PABA) analogue that competitively inhibits parasite dihydropteroate synthetase, an essential enzyme in the folic acid synthesis pathway. **Pyrimethamine** is a folate analogue that competitively inhibits parasite dihydrofolate reductase, the enzyme that converts dihydrofolate to tetrahydrofolate (Figs. 31-6 and 31-7). In combination, sulfadoxine and pyrimethamine act synergistically to inhibit growth of the malarial parasite.

Sulfonamide-pyrimethamine combinations are highly effective against blood schizont stages of *P. falciparum* malaria, but not against gametocytes, and are less effective against other species of malaria. Both drugs are highly protein-bound, resulting in long elimination half-lives. The long half-life of the combination provides selective pressure for the development of drug resistance in areas with high-level malaria transmission, and increasing resistance to this combination has made it less effective for treatment and prophylaxis in many parts of the world (Fig. 35-4).

Sulfadoxine-pyrimethamine may be administered as a convenient single dose. Unfortunately, widespread resistance of malarial parasites to this combination has markedly limited its utility. The most serious drug reactions involve hypersensitivity to the sulfonamide component of the combi-nation. Severe skin reactions such as Stevens-Johnson syndrome or erythema multiforme have been reported, but the incidence of these adverse effects is rare after single dose therapy for malaria. Adverse hematologic effects include megaloblastic anemia, leukopenia, and thrombocytopenia. Sulfonamide-pyrimethamine is not used as a chemoprophylactic agent against malaria.

Proguanil

Proguanil is a derivative of pyrimidine and, like pyrimethamine, is an inhibitor of dihydrofolate reductase. Proguanil acts against the hepatic, pre-erythrocytic forms of *P. falciparum* and *P. vivax*. Proguanil has been used for prophylaxis in combination with chloroquine in areas of the world where chloroquine resistance is not widespread. However, other prophylactic agents are significantly more effective, and this combination should rarely be used, if ever. Proguanil may also be used in a synergistic combination with atovaquone for both treatment and prevention of malaria (discussed above). Proguanil is usually well tolerated, but it has been associated with oral ulcerations, pancytopenia, thrombocytopenia, and granulocytopenia.

ANTIMALARIAL DRUG RESISTANCE

Antimalarial drug resistance is a major public health problem and a significant barrier to the effective treatment of individuals with malaria. In association with the collapse of effective prevention efforts, lack of political will, and socioeconomic factors, the waning efficacy of antimalarial drugs has contributed significantly to the increasing burden of malaria morbidity and mortality worldwide.

Chloroquine was the standard therapy for treating individuals with malaria for many years after its introduction in 1946. Resistance was first reported in the 1950s and has steadily increased since then; at present, resistance has been reported everywhere in the world except on the island of Hispaniola and in focal parts of Central America, South America, and Asia. The risk of therapeutic failure with chloroquine is as high as 64% in some areas of Sub-Saharan Africa and up to 85% in Southeast Asia. Childhood mortality doubled in Eastern and Southern Africa in the 1980s and 1990s as chloroquine and sulfadoxine-pyrimethamine resistance increased; chloroquine resistance has been associated with an overall doubling of childhood mortality from malaria, with increases as high as 11-fold in certain areas. *P. vivax* resistance to chloroquine was unknown until 1989 but is now endemic in Indonesia and Papua New Guinea. Reports of chloroquine-resistant *P. vivax* have also emerged in South America, Brazil, Myanmar, and India.

Resistance to sulfadoxine-pyrimethamine was reported after the combination was introduced in 1971 as a second-line therapy for treating individuals with chloroquine-resistant *P. falciparum*. Resistance to sulfadoxine-pyrimethamine was initially reported in Southeast Asia but is now relatively widespread in South America and increasingly prevalent in Africa as well.

Strains of *P. falciparum* resistant to mefloquine were noted in Southeast Asia following the widespread introduction of this agent in the 1980s. Mefloquine resistance has not spread more widely as yet, in large measure due to the fact that the drug is not now routinely used to treat individuals with malaria.

Many factors contribute to the development of drug resistance by malaria parasites, including inappropriate and/or unsupervised drug use, inconsistent drug availability, poor adherence to treatment regimens due to adverse effects and other factors, inconsistent quality of drug manufacturing, presence of counterfeit drugs, and prohibitive drug costs. Combining therapies to reduce the development of resistance is a strategy that has long been employed in the treatment of individuals with tuberculosis, leprosy, and HIV infection, and this approach is strongly recommended in the treatment of individuals with malaria. For example, the World Health Organization (WHO) has demanded cessation of production of all stand-alone artemisinin products and has requested that only two-drug, fixed combination, artemisinin-containing products be produced. Although rapidly acting artemisinins reduce parasite burden by a factor of 10^4 with every treatment cycle, resulting in rapid clearance of parasites from the bloodstream, the short half-life of artemisinins favors the possibility of recrudescence of infection and the risk of selective pressure for drug resistance. To counter these risks, the WHO recommends combining an artemisinin with a slowly eliminated blood schizonticidal agent.

OTHER PROTOZOA

In addition to plasmodium, other medically important protozoa include *Entamoeba histolytica,* the organism that causes amebiasis; *Giardia lamblia,* the organism that causes giardiasis; *Cryptosporidium parvum,* the organism that causes cryptosporidiosis; *Trypanosoma brucei rhodesiense* and *T. b. gambiense,* the causative agents of African sleeping sickness; *Trypanosoma cruzi,* the causative agent of Chagas' disease; and *Leishmania* spp., the causative agents of leishmaniasis. Because more is known about *E. histolytica,* the following physiology section focuses on this parasite; however, the pharmacology section includes not only agents effective against amebiasis, but also agents effective against African sleeping sickness, Chagas' disease, and leishmaniasis.

■ Case 3

Mr. S, a 29-year-old American journalist, returns from a trip to Southeast Asia. He feels fine for 5 weeks but then begins to experience mild diarrhea, abdominal pain, and malaise. He does not attribute his symptoms to the trip, because they developed well after he returned home. Furthermore, Mr. S's wife shared the same food and water during the trip, and she remains well. As a result, Mr. S ignores the symptoms for a week, but he eventually goes to his physician when the symptoms do not abate spontaneously. Physical examination reveals tenderness in the right upper quadrant of the abdomen. Blood tests are notable for ele-

vated liver enzymes, and a computed tomography (CT) scan reveals a liver abscess. Stool examination is positive for heme and for *E. histolytica* cysts.

QUESTIONS

■ **1.** Why is Mr. S's wife asymptomatic?
■ **2.** What are the potential complications if Mr. S's condition is left untreated?

PHYSIOLOGY OF LUMINAL PROTOZOA

The enteric protozoa *Entamoeba dispar* and *E. histolytica* are morphologically indistinguishable, although these two species can be differentiated using specific monoclonal antibodies. *E. dispar* does not cause invasive disease (i.e., it does not compromise the gut epithelium), but *E. histolytica* can cause an asymptomatic carrier state, invasive colitis, or so-called *metastatic infections* (usually hepatic abscesses).

Five percent to 10% of individuals who live in poverty in the developing world have serologic evidence of previous *E. histolytica* infection. It is estimated that 50 million cases of dysentery are caused by *E. histolytica* each year, resulting in 40,000 to 100,000 deaths. Because Mr. S's wife shared the same food and water with her husband, she was also likely infected with *E. histolytica*. For unclear reasons, she excreted *E. histolytica* asymptomatically, while her husband developed invasive disease.

Life Cycle of *Entamoeba histolytica*

Colonic infection with *E. histolytica* occurs as a result of ingestion of cysts through the fecal-oral route, for example, drinking contaminated water. Whether intestinal invasion occurs may be a function of the number of cysts ingested, the strain of the parasite, the motility of the host gastrointestinal tract, and the presence of appropriate enteric bacteria to serve as nourishment for the ameba. Disease results when active trophozoites invade the intestinal epithelium, and secondary spread to the liver can occur via the portal circulation (Fig. 35-6). As its name implies, *E. histolytica* lyses and destroys human tissue. Trophozoites typically multiply superficial to the muscularis mucosae of the intestines and spread laterally. They may also penetrate more deeply, occasionally perforating the intestinal wall and spreading locally. Seeding of the liver is also common. In Mr. S's case, a CT scan revealed involvement of the liver with formation of an abscess.

E. histolytica exists in two forms: the inactive but infective **cyst** and the active **trophozoite**. Cysts are ingested in contaminated food or water. Excystation occurs in the small intestine, where the trophozoites mature. The trophozoite form is capable of invading host tissue. Inside the human body, the trophozoites move using pseudopods and ingest bacteria, other protozoa, and host red blood cells. A trophozoite can convert to a binucleated cyst form, which matures into a tetranucleated cyst that travels through the colon but is not capable of mucosal invasion (Fig. 35-6).

Symptoms due to amebiasis vary from diarrhea and abdominal cramps to fulminant dysentery and hepatic abscess formation. Fewer than 40% of individuals with amebic dysentery develop fever, and microscopic evaluation of the stool

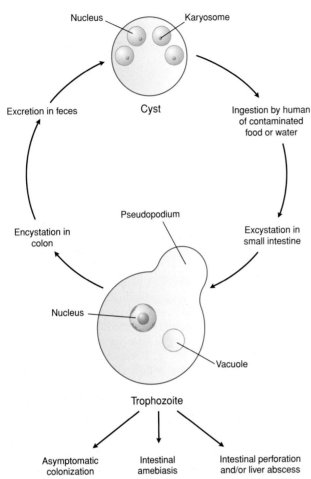

Figure 35-6. Manifestations of amebiasis. Ingestion of *Entamoeba histolytica* cysts can result in several different clinical outcomes, ranging from asymptomatic excretion of the cysts to invasive disease. Asymptomatic infection occurs when the ingested cysts excyst (mature) in the small intestine but do not invade the intestinal mucosa. These trophozoites then encyst in the colon, and excretion occurs in the feces. Invasive disease results when active trophozoites invade the intestinal epithelium. This invasion can result in asymptomatic colonization, intestinal amebiasis (amebic dysentery)—which is characterized by diarrhea and abdominal cramps—or intestinal perforation. Spread of infection via the portal vein can cause liver abscesses.

typically discloses few neutrophils. The onset of symptoms can range from a few days to a year after exposure, or symptoms may never occur. Mr. S's symptoms did not develop until at least a month after exposure, giving him reason not to attribute his symptoms to his travels.

Fermentation Pathways

E. histolytica and other luminal parasites are a diverse group of eukaryotes with novel adaptations to their anaerobic niche. For example, *E. histolytica* lacks **fermentation enzymes** (lactate dehydrogenase and pyruvate decarboxylase) that are present in yeast and other eukaryotes. Ameba also lack enzymes of oxidative phosphorylation, the Krebs cycle, and pyruvate dehydrogenase. Instead, ameba (and many anaerobic organisms) utilize novel enzymes to provide a source for the electron transfers that drive metabolism.

Ameba are obligate fermenters of glucose to ethanol (Fig. 35-7). Many of these fermentation enzymes, which are missing in humans, yeast, and most eubacteria, contain a set of iron-sulfur centers called **ferredoxins** that transfer electrons under strongly reducing (anaerobic) conditions. This is in contrast to heme and cytochromes that use iron centers to transfer electrons under oxidizing (aerobic) conditions. Pyruvate-ferredoxin oxidoreductase (**PFOR**), which contains a single ferredoxin domain, catalyzes the decarboxylation of pyruvate to acetyl CoA, with the production of CO_2. PFOR activity also produces reduced ferredoxin, which can reduce protons to form hydrogen gas or reduce $NADP^+$ to NADPH. Acetyl CoA is reduced to ethanol via alcohol dehydrogenase E (ADHE), with the recovery of two NAD^+ cofactors. Anaerobic bacteria (e.g., *Helicobacter* spp. and *Clostridia* spp.) express PFORs, ferredoxins, and ADHEs similar to those of luminal protozoa. Indeed, phylogenetic analyses suggest that most of the genes encoding parasite fermentation enzymes, and many of the genes encoding parasite enzymes involved in core energy metabolism, have been laterally transferred from anaerobic bacteria. Although lateral gene transfer is extraordinarily frequent between bacteria, it is extremely rare between bacteria and higher eukaryotes, which maintain their gametes in a sterile environment.

PHARMACOLOGY OF ANTIPROTOZOAL AGENTS

Metronidazole

Metronidazole is inactive until it is reduced within host or microbial cells possessing a large negative redox potential; such redox potentials are present in many anaerobic or microaerophilic luminal parasites. Activation can occur by interaction with reduced ferredoxin or with specific nitroreductases (Fig. 35-7). Activated metronidazole forms reduced cytotoxic compounds that bind to proteins, membranes, and DNA in target cells, causing severe damage.

Metronidazole sensitivity is directly related to the presence of PFOR activity. Most eukaryotes and eubacteria lack PFOR and therefore fail to activate metronidazole. However, in poorly oxygenated tissues such as abscesses, metronidazole can be activated. Because PFOR is expressed in protozoa but has no counterpart in mammalian systems, the drug is selectively toxic for ameba and anaerobic organisms.

The widespread use of metronidazole has led to drug resistance in *Helicobacter pylori,* a common bacterial cause of gastritis and peptic ulcers (see Chapter 45, Integrative Inflammation Pharmacology: Peptic Ulcer Disease). This resistance is due to a null mutation in the *rdxA* gene, which encodes an oxygen-insensitive NADPH nitroreductase. Low-level resistance to metronidazole has also been observed in a number of anaerobic protozoa, including trichomonads (caused by decreased expression of ferredoxin), giardia (caused by decreased PFOR activity and decreased drug permeability), and ameba (caused by increased expression of **superoxide dismutase**). Metronidazole resistance among luminal parasites has not yet become clinically important, however.

There are three explanations for the slow development of resistance to metronidazole among luminal parasites. First, luminal parasites are generally diploid, so a single mutation

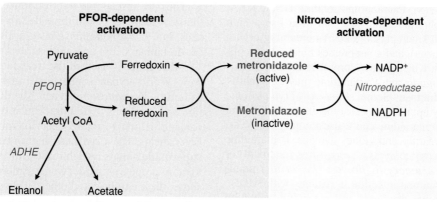

Figure 35-7. Fermentation enzymes of anaerobic organisms and mechanisms of metronidazole activation. Anaerobic organisms metabolize pyruvate to acetyl CoA; this conversion is catalyzed by the enzyme pyruvate-ferredoxin oxidoreductase (PFOR). Acetyl CoA is then either hydrolyzed to acetate or oxidized to ethanol by alcohol dehydrogenase E (ADHE). Metronidazole is a prodrug; it contains a nitro group that must be reduced for the drug to become active. Reduced metronidazole is highly effective against anaerobic organisms, probably because of the formation of cytotoxic intermediates that cause DNA, protein, and membrane damage. Two aspects of anaerobic metabolism provide opportunities for selective reduction of the nitro group. First, the reaction catalyzed by PFOR results in the reduction of ferredoxin; reduced ferredoxin can then transfer its electrons to metronidazole, resulting in reduced (active) metronidazole and reoxidized ferredoxin. Second, many anaerobic organisms express nitroreductase enzymes that selectively reduce metronidazole and, in the process, oxidize NADPH to NADP⁺.

will not typically confer resistance. This contrasts with the case of haploid bacteria and certain haploid stages of *P. falciparum,* in which resistance develops more quickly. Second, luminal parasites have few metabolic alternatives to PFOR activity. Third, metronidazole is hydrophilic, so overexpression or modification of P-glycoprotein, which confers resistance to hydrophobic drugs, does not increase metronidazole efflux.

Adverse effects of metronidazole include gastrointestinal discomfort, headaches, occasional neuropathy, a metallic taste, and nausea. Metronidazole also causes nausea and flushing when taken concomitantly with alcohol (a so-called *disulfiram-like effect,* caused by inhibition of ethanol metabolism). Metronidazole is active against *E. histolytica* trophozoites in tissues, but it has much less activity against intraluminal ameba (probably, in large part, because of the drug's extensive absorption in the upper gastrointestinal tract, leading to its low drug concentration in the lumen of the colon, where the ameba live). Therefore, individuals with invasive amebiasis are typically treated first with metronidazole (to eradicate trophozoites that are actively invading human tissue) and then with a second agent that has more intraluminal activity, such as **iodoquinol** or **paromomycin.** The latter two agents kill ameba by unknown mechanisms but are poorly absorbed from the gastrointestinal tract and therefore reach high concentrations in the lumen of the colon.

Tinidazole

Tinidazole, a second-generation nitroimidazole related to metronidazole, has recently been approved for use in the United States, although it has been available for many years in other countries. It is effective against a number of protozoa and is licensed for the treatment of giardiasis, amebiasis, and vaginal trichomoniasis. Its mechanism of action is unclear but is believed to be similar to that of metronida-

zole and related to the generation of cytotoxic free radicals. A particular benefit of tinidazole is that the duration of a therapeutic course of the drug is shorter than that of metronidazole. Tinidazole is also better tolerated than metronidazole, but it is similarly ineffective as a luminicidal agent for the treatment of ameba infections. Adverse effects are rare and mild, including gastrointestinal discomfort and the occasional development of a metallic taste. Tinidazole is not recommended for use during the first trimester of pregnancy, during breast-feeding, and in children less than 3 years of age.

Nitazoxanide

Nitazoxanide is a nitrothiazolyl-salicylamide derivative structurally related to metronidazole. Nitazoxanide has a broad spectrum of action, including activity against protozoa, anaerobic bacteria, and helminths. It is approved in the United States for use in children with giardiasis and in adults and children with cryptosporidiosis. As a structural analogue of thiamine pyrophosphate, nitazoxanide inhibits the PFOR that converts pyruvate to acetyl CoA in protozoa and anaerobic bacteria. Its mechanism of action against helminths is unclear. After oral administration, nitazoxanide is rapidly hydrolyzed to the active metabolite tizoxanide. The active metabolite is excreted in urine, bile, and feces. Nitazoxanide is usually well tolerated with few reported adverse effects.

Other Antiprotozoal Agents

Pentamidine can be used to treat individuals with early-stage African trypanosomiasis (African sleeping sickness), which is caused by ***Trypanosoma brucei gambiense*** and certain strains of ***T. b. rhodesiense.*** Early-stage trypanosomiasis is defined as disease that does not involve the central nervous system (CNS). Pentamidine inhibits DNA, RNA, protein, and phospholipid synthesis. The drug has a high affinity for DNA in kinetoplasts (a DNA-containing organelle in certain protozoa), and it suppresses kinetoplast replication and function. Kinetoplastida protozoa include *Trypanosoma* and *Leishmania* spp. Pentamidine may also inhibit **dihydrofolate reductase**. Some strains of *Trypanosoma* have a high-affinity uptake system for the drug, contributing to its selectivity. Pentamidine can cause fatigue, dizziness, hypotension, pancreatitis, and kidney damage. Pentamidine is now used most commonly as a second-line treatment for individuals with **Pneumocystis jiroveci (P. carinii) pneumonia** (PCP), a common infection in patients with AIDS.

Suramin is another drug used to treat individuals with early-stage African trypanosomiasis. Suramin interacts with many macromolecules and inhibits numerous enzymes, including those involved in energy metabolism (e.g., glycerol phosphate dehydrogenase). It also inhibits RNA polymerase and thus interferes with parasite replication. Suramin can cause pruritus, paresthesias, vomiting, and nausea. The biochemical basis for suramin's relative selectivity for African trypanosomiasis is not well understood.

Melarsoprol is used as a first-line drug in the treatment of individuals with late-stage African trypanosomiasis (i.e., disease that involves the CNS). Melarsoprol was developed by conjugating the heavy-metal chelator dimercaptopropanol to the trivalent arsenic of melarsen oxide. The drug is insoluble in water and is instead dissolved in propylene glycol. Blood trypanosomes lack a functional tricarboxylic acid cycle and are entirely dependent on glycolysis for ATP production. Melarsoprol inhibits trypanosomal pyruvate kinase, thereby inhibiting glycolysis and decreasing ATP production. Affected trypanosomes quickly lose motility and lyse. Melarsoprol also inhibits the uptake of adenine and adenosine by trypanosomal transporters. Mammalian cells are less permeable to the drug than are trypanosomes, and the drug has some selectivity on this basis. Unfortunately, melarsoprol is still quite toxic to humans (4% to 6% death rate). Melarsoprol is administered intravenously and can cause severe phlebitis. It is also corrosive to plastics, limiting storage and administration options. In addition, 5% to 10% of individuals with late-stage African trypanosomiasis develop intense inflammation of the brain after administration of melarsoprol (''*reactive encephalopathy*''); this complication is associated with a mortality of greater than 50%. Concomitant administration of corticosteroids lessens the likelihood of reactive encephalopathy. Polyneuropathy after melarsoprol administration is also common (10%) and can be lessened by concomitant administration of thiamine.

Eflornithine (α-difluoromethylornithine) is a much less toxic alternative to melarsoprol in the treatment of individuals with African trypanosomiasis caused by *T. b. gambiense* (West Africa sleeping sickness). Eflornithine is highly effective against both early- and late-stage West African sleeping sickness but not against East African trypanosomiasis (caused by *T. b. rhodesiense*). Eflornithine is a selective and irreversible inhibitor of **ornithine decarboxylase** and thus of polyamine synthesis. Ornithine decarboxylase converts ornithine to putrescine; this is a rate-limiting step in the synthesis of putrescine and the polyamines spermine and spermidine. Polyamines are involved in nucleic acid synthesis and the regulation of protein synthesis. *T. b. gambiense* or-

ganisms are susceptible to eflornithine, possibly because of the slow turnover of ornithine decarboxylase in these parasites, but *T. b. rhodesiense* have a higher rate of turnover (as do human cells) and are less sensitive.

Nifurtimox is used in the treatment of individuals with New World trypanosomiasis (Chagas' disease), which is caused by **Trypanosoma cruzi.** The drug undergoes reduction and generates toxic intracellular oxygen radicals in the parasite. It first forms reduced intermediates such as nitro aryl radicals. These radicals can then be oxidized to generate **superoxide** anions, which react with water to produce cytotoxic hydrogen peroxide. Some parasites, such as trypanosomes, lack **catalase** and other enzymes capable of degrading hydrogen peroxide. Such parasites are thus sensitive to the toxicity of nitro aromatic drugs. Mammalian cells are protected because of their complement of antioxidant enzymes such as catalase, glutathione peroxidase, and superoxide dismutase. Nifurtimox can cause anorexia, vomiting, memory loss, sleep disorders, and convulsions.

Sodium stibogluconate and **meglumine antimonate** are used to treat individuals with leishmaniasis, which is caused by parasites of the genus *Leishmania*. These agents contain pentavalent antimony and act by an unknown mechanism. It is postulated that these drugs inhibit the glycolytic pathway and fatty acid oxidation, processes that are crucial for intermediary metabolism. Pentavalent antimony can also have many nonspecific effects, such as modification of sulfhydryl groups. These drugs can cause bone marrow suppression, a prolonged QT interval, pancreatitis, and rash.

Resistance of leishmania to antimonial agents is being recognized with increasing frequency, especially in South Asia. Alternative agents include **amphotericin** and **miltefosine.** The mechanism of action of miltefosine is unknown. It is a synthetic ether phospholipid analogue that is chemically similar to natural phospholipids present in cell membranes. Miltefosine has been shown to have antineoplastic, immunomodulatory, and antiprotozoal activity. It is presumed that the cytostatic and cytotoxic effects of miltefosine are caused by inhibition of enzyme systems associated with plasma membranes (such as protein kinase C) and inhibition of phosphatidylcholine biosynthesis. Miltefosine may also inhibit platelet activating factor-induced responses and inositol phosphate formation. The immunomodulatory effects of miltefosine include T cell activation, interferon-gamma production in peripheral mononuclear cells, and increased interleukin-2 receptor and HLA-DR expression. The drug can be administered orally and can be used in the treatment of individuals with visceral leishmaniasis.

HELMINTHS

Helminths are multicellular worms with digestive, excretory, nervous, and reproductive systems. Parasitic helminths can infect the liver, blood, intestines, and other tissues in human hosts. Clinically significant worms can be divided phylogenetically into three classes: **nematodes** (roundworms), **trematodes** (flukes), and **cestodes** (tapeworms). The presence of a rudimentary nervous system provides a number of possible targets for antihelminthic agents. The physiology of **Onchocerca volvulus,** which causes onchocerciasis (''river blindness''), provides an example of potential targets for antihelminthic drugs. Although the majority of the following discussion focuses on the physiology and pharmacology of onchocerciasis, several other antihelminthic agents are also presented.

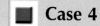 **Case 4**

Thumbi is a boy who enjoys fishing in a river near his village in the Democratic Republic of Congo. At the age of 13, he emigrates with his family to the United States. Shortly thereafter, he begins to scratch his arms and legs vigorously. Six months later, his mother brings him to a dermatologist. Physical examination reveals a macular and papular rash with excoriations on the arms and legs, as well as a few subcutaneous nodules. Examination of peripheral blood discloses high-level eosinophilia. A nodule is excised and examined by a pathologist, leading to a diagnosis. Thumbi begins treatment with ivermectin but returns the next day feverish and feeling more itchy than before.

QUESTIONS

1. What did the pathologist see in the subcutaneous nodule?

2. Why did Thumbi feel worse immediately after treatment with ivermectin?

PHYSIOLOGY OF HELMINTHS

Humans can become infected with helminths when they ingest food or water contaminated with eggs or larvae. In addition, larvae in soil can penetrate human skin, and insects can transmit still other larvae through bites. If humans are the definitive host, the eggs or larvae develop into adult worms that can migrate through tissues and enter the sexual stage. During the sexual stage, adult worms release additional eggs or larvae, which can then pass out of the host through the gastrointestinal or urinary tracts. Larvae in humans can also be ingested by insects during a blood meal. In the environment or within vector hosts, eggs or larvae then become infective for humans, and the cycles start over.

Life Cycle of *Onchocerca volvulus*

Onchocerciasis is one of eight human filarial infections (a specific type of nematodal worm infection). In Thumbi's case, an infected *Simulium* spp. blackfly bit and inoculated *O. volvulus* larvae into his skin in Africa. Adult worms then developed in Thumbi's subcutaneous tissues. These adult male and female filarial worms came to rest in subcutaneous nodules, in which they mated (Fig. 35-8). Adult worms are large (3 to 80 cm in length), look like spaghetti pasta, and can live for 10 to 15 years. The nodules have a characteristic appearance that was recognized by the pathologist. From these nodules (''onchocercomata''), gravid females release

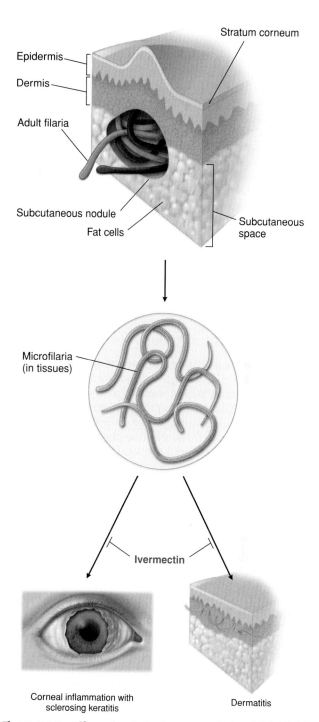

Figure 35-8. Life cycle of *Onchocerca volvulus.* Adult filarial worms mate in subcutaneous nodules in humans, releasing microfilariae that cause dermatitis and pruritus as they migrate through the skin and subcutaneous tissues. Microfilariae migrating through the eye induce ocular inflammation, which can lead to corneal scarring and blindness (''river blindness''). Ivermectin, the agent of choice for treating individuals with onchocerciasis, is effective only against microfilariae; the drug does not kill adult filarial worms.

millions of microfilariae, which migrate freely through the skin and cornea. If ingested by a *Simulium* fly, additional maturation can occur, and the cycle can continue. The diagnosis of onchocerciasis is usually based on microscopic detection of microfilariae in skin snips, not on pathological examination of excised onchocercomata. Microfilariae are small (200 to 400 μm); as they degenerate and die, they cause local inflammatory reactions, provoking itching, dermatitis, and, eventually, scarring. When microfilariae die in the cornea, they induce a punctate keratitis that, over years, leads to scarring and blindness. Such ocular involvement has made onchocerciasis the second leading cause of infectious blindness in the world (after trachoma) and is the reason onchocerciasis is also referred to as "river blindness" (also reflecting the fact that the blackflies carrying the larvae inhabit areas with flowing streams, such as the one in which Thumbi enjoyed fishing). Without treatment, Thumbi could well become one of the more than 500,000 individuals in the world who are currently blind or visually impaired from onchocerciasis.

Neuromuscular Activity

The subcuticular layer of longitudinal muscle in nematodes is inhibited by **GABAergic** transmitters and excited by **cholinergic** transmitters. The motor neurons of invertebrates are unmyelinated, making them more vulnerable to neurotoxins than the myelinated somatic motor neurons of humans. (See Chapter 7, Principles of Nervous System Physiology and Pharmacology, for more information on the human nervous system.) Many antihelminthic agents modulate parasite neuromuscular activity by enhancing inhibitory signaling, antagonizing excitatory signaling (nondepolarizing block), or tonically stimulating excitatory signaling (depolarizing block).

PHARMACOLOGY OF ANTIHELMINTHIC AGENTS

Agents That Interrupt Neuromuscular Activity

Ivermectin

Ivermectin is a semisynthetic macrocyclic lactone that acts against a broad range of helminths and arthropods and that has been used most extensively to treat and control onchocerciasis. Ivermectin's exact mechanism of action is unclear, but studies in *Caenorhabditis elegans* (a soil helminth that is studied extensively in eukaryotic biology as a simple model organism) suggest that the mechanism of action involves potentiation and/or direct activation of **glutamate-gated chloride channels** in nematode plasma membranes. This results in hyperpolarization of neuromuscular cells and pharyngeal paralysis. Ivermectin is also thought to affect **gamma-aminobutyric acid (GABA)** inhibitory transmission by potentiating the release of GABA from presynaptic terminals, directly activating GABA receptors and potentiating the binding of GABA to its receptor. All of these effects increase GABA-mediated transmission of signals in peripheral nerves, resulting in hyperpolarization. The net effect is variable, depending on the nematode model system under

study, but *the ultimate result is blockade of neuromuscular transmission and paralysis of the worm.*

Pharyngeal paralysis of *O. volvulus* inhibits nutrient uptake and kills developing larvae (microfilariae). Unfortunately, ivermectin does not kill adult filarial worms. It does, however, destroy microfilariae in utero, thereby preventing production and release of new microfilariae from adult female worms for at least 6 months. Thus, ivermectin is used to prevent microfilaria-mediated ocular damage and to decrease human-to-vector transmission (because microfilariae are infectious to *Simulium* flies), but it cannot cure human hosts of *O. volvulus* infection. Because the drug is noncurative, it is typically administered to infected humans every 6 to 12 months for the life expectancy of the adult worms (5 to 10 years).

Ivermectin does interact with GABA receptors in vertebrates, but its affinity for invertebrate GABA receptors is about 100-fold greater. Cestodes and trematodes lack high-affinity ivermectin receptors, which may explain the resistance of these organisms to the drug. GABA receptors in humans are present mainly in the CNS, but because ivermectin does not cross the blood-brain barrier, the drug is generally well tolerated. When the blood-brain barrier is hyperpermeable, as in patients with meningitis, ivermectin can be more toxic and can result in headaches, ataxia, and coma. Adverse effects of ivermectin are usually attributable to inflammatory or allergic responses to dying microfilariae ("*Mazzotti-type reaction*") and include headaches, dizziness, weakness, rash, pruritus, edema, abdominal pain, hypotension, and fever. This is why Thumbi felt worse the day after initiation of his treatment.

Ivermectin is widely used to treat animals with nematode infections, and resistance to ivermectin is already recognized in livestock parasites. Although the exact mechanism of resistance is unknown, the P-glycoprotein may be involved. In studies of mice, hypersensitivity to ivermectin results from disruption of the *mdr1a* gene, which encodes a P-glycoprotein membrane transporter. Furthermore, analysis of P-glycoprotein cDNA from *Haemonchus contortus* (a nematode of veterinary importance) shows 65% homology to P-glycoprotein/multidrug resistance (MDR) protein sequences in mice and humans. P-glycoprotein mRNA expression is higher in ivermectin-selected strains of *H. contortus* than in unselected strains, and verapamil, which reverses multidrug resistance by blocking P-glycoprotein channels, increases the efficacy of ivermectin. Fortunately, clinically important resistance in humans has not yet been documented.

In addition to its use in the treatment of individuals with onchocerciasis, ivermectin is used to treat individuals with strongyloidiasis and cutaneous larva migrans (both are nematodal infections) and individuals with scabies (an ectoparasitic infestation).

Piperazine and Pyrantel Pamoate

Piperazine and **pyrantel pamoate** are antihelminthic agents of primarily historical interest. They are discussed further in the Drug Summary Table.

Other Antihelminthic Agents

Albendazole, mebendazole, and **thiabendazole** inhibit tubulin polymerization by binding to β-tubulin. Evidence suggests that these agents are selective for the nematodal isoform of β-tubulin, thus decreasing host toxicity. Inhibition of tubulin polymerization disrupts nematodal motility and DNA replication (see Chapter 37), leading to degenerative changes in integumental and intestinal cells of helminths, and, eventually, causing immobilization and death of the worms. The effects of the drugs against immotile tissue forms of cestodal larval parasites (e.g., cysticercosis and echinococcosis) are less well understood but may also involve β-tubulin binding. In this case, the drugs disrupt the integumental integrity of the protoscolex, a larval structure that eventually becomes the "head" of the adult cestode. Thiabendazole causes significant nausea, vomiting, and anorexia at therapeutic doses, and is rarely used. Mebendazole and albendazole are better tolerated, and albendazole has the highest bioavailability of the three drugs after oral administration.

Praziquantel is the drug of choice for treating individuals infected with adult cestode (tapeworm) and trematode (fluke) infections. Most importantly, praziquantel is the drug of choice for treating individuals with schistosomiasis, a trematodal infection that causes considerable morbidity and mortality worldwide. Although the exact mechanism of praziquantel's action is unknown, it appears to increase parasite membrane permeability to calcium, resulting in contraction and paralysis of the worms. The main adverse effects of praziquantel include nausea, headache, and abdominal discomfort.

Diethylcarbamazine (DEC), a piperazine derivative, is the drug of choice for treating individuals with certain filarial infections, including lymphatic filariasis. Its use in the treatment of individuals with filarial onchocerciasis has been largely supplanted by the use of ivermectin (predominantly because of ivermectin's improved tolerability and ease of administration). Unlike ivermectin, however, DEC kills adult filarial worms and is thus a curative agent. DEC's mechanism of action is unknown; current hypotheses include stimulation of innate immune mechanisms, inhibition of microtubule polymerization, and inhibition of arachidonic acid metabolism. DEC is reasonably well tolerated at low doses; its major adverse effects include anorexia, headache, and nausea. Administration of DEC can, however, precipitate Mazzotti reactions in individuals with heavy microfilarial burdens, and such reactions can be fatal. Administration of gradually increasing doses of DEC minimizes this possibility. DEC is excreted by the kidneys, and dosing may need to be adjusted in individuals with decreased renal function.

Antibacterial agents may also have a role in treating individuals with certain helminthic infections. For example, *O. volvulus* has been found to contain an obligate symbiont (*Wolbachia* endobacteria) important in helminth fertility, and the use of doxycycline to treat individuals with onchocerciasis leads to decreased fertility, embryogenesis, and viability of *O. volvulus*.

Conclusion and Future Directions

The development of new antiparasitic agents will rely on continued exploitation of molecular and metabolic differences between parasites and hosts. Recent advances in the application of molecular biological and genetic techniques to study parasitic eukaryotes, and detailed knowledge of parasite, vector, and host genomes, transcriptomes, and proteomes, should facilitate the development of more selective agents effective against many parasitic infections. The development of resistance to antiparasitic agents is of increasing concern, most notably among malarial and leishmanial parasites, and will necessitate both the judicious use of currently available agents and the development of new agents, including antiparasitic vaccines.

Despite long-standing efforts to develop effective treatments for individuals infected with malaria, the disease remains a major global cause of morbidity and mortality. Development of an effective malaria vaccine could have a major impact on this global burden. However, the development of an effective vaccine has been hampered by a number of difficult scientific challenges, including the diversity of parasite species and strains, the diversity of parasite life forms, the intracellular location of the parasites, and the ability of *P. falciparum* to undergo antigenic variation. The situation has been worsened by the lack of meaningful economic incentives for vaccine development. Unfortunately, the complexity of the parasites and of their intimate relationship with infected hosts suggests that the development of effective antiparasite vaccines (especially against malaria) will be difficult.

Suggested Reading

Baird JK. Effectiveness of antimalarial drugs. *N Engl J Med* 2005; 352:1565–1577. (*Reviews current antimalarial agents.*)

Fox LM, Saravolatz LD. Nitazoxanide: a new thiazolide antiparasitic agent. *Clin Infect Dis* 2005;40:1173–1180. (*Reviews a recently approved antiparasitic agent.*)

Hoerauf A, Mand S, Volkmann L, et al. Doxycycline in the treatment of human onchocerciasis: kinetics of *Wolbachia* endobacteria reduction and of inhibition of embryogenesis in female *Onchocerca* worms. *Microbes Infect* 2003;5:261–273. (*Reports antibacterial treatment for onchocerciasis.*)

Jambou R, Legrand E, Niang M, et al. Resistance of *Plasmodium falciparum* field isolates to in vitro artemether and point mutations of the SERCA-type PfATPase6. *Lancet* 2005;366: 1960–1963. (*Reports disturbing harbinger of resistance to artemisinin derivatives used as single agents.*)

Moorthy VS, Good MF, Hill AV. Malaria vaccine developments. *Lancet* 2004;363:150–156. (*Discusses difficulties involved in development of an effective malaria vaccine.*)

Sidhu AB, Verdier-Pinard D, Fidock DA. Chloroquine resistance in *Plasmodium falciparum* malaria parasites conferred by *pfcrt* mutations. *Science* 2002;298:210–213. (*Provides a possible molecular explanation for malarial drug resistance.*)

Upcroft P, Upcroft J. Drug targets and mechanisms of resistance in the anaerobic protozoa. *Clin Microbiol Rev* 2001;14:150–164. (*Discusses mechanisms of resistance to metronidazole; predicts new targets for antiprotozoal agents.*)

Drug Summary Table   Chapter 35 Pharmacology of Parasitic Infections

Drug	Clinical Applications	Serious and Common Adverse Effects	Contraindications	Therapeutic Considerations
ANTIMALARIAL AGENTS: INHIBITORS OF HEME METABOLISM _Mechanism—Decrease the metabolism and/or removal of toxic heme products, resulting in increased toxicity to the plasmodia_				
Chloroquine	Malaria, all species	Retinopathy, prolonged QT interval, methemoglobinemia, amnesia, death (in supratherapeutic doses) Pruritus, muscle weakness, worsening of psoriasis and porphyria	Visual field changes	Protonated chloroquine accumulates inside the parasite's food vacuole, where it binds to ferriprotoporphyrin IX (heme) and inhibits its polymerization; accumulation of unpolymerized ferriprotoporphyrin IX leads to oxidative membrane damage Most strains of _P. falciparum_ in Africa, Asia, and South America have developed resistance to chloroquine Kills only erythrocytic stage of plasmodial infections Used therapeutically and prophylactically
Quinine Quinidine (See Chapter 18)	Malaria, especially _P. falciparum_	Cinchonism (tinnitus, deafness, headaches, nausea, vomiting, visual disturbances), prolonged QT interval, disseminated intravascular coagulation, thrombocytopenia, hepatotoxicity, hemolytic uremic syndrome, interstitial nephritis Rash, hypoglycemia, gastrointestinal disturbance, headache	Glucose-6-phosphate dehydrogenase (G6PD) deficiency Myasthenia gravis	Mechanism similar to chloroquine; additionally, quinine intercalates into DNA Used to treat acute blood-stage malaria, but not used prophylactically
Mefloquine	Chloroquine-resistant malaria	Seizure, neuropsychiatric symptoms (vivid dreams, insomnia, depression, hallucinations, psychosis), cardiac conduction abnormalities (bradycardia, prolonged QT interval, arrhythmia) Gastrointestinal disturbance, dizziness	Depression Generalized anxiety disorder Psychosis Schizophrenia Convulsions	Appears to disrupt polymerization of heme to hemozoin inside intra-erythrocytic malarial parasites Used therapeutically and prophylactically
Artemisinin Artesunate Artemether Artemotil Dihydroartemisinin	Malaria, all species	Hemolytic anemia, bradycardia, potential neurotoxic effects	Hypersensitivity to artemisinin and its derivatives	Form carbon-centered free radicals that alkylate heme First-line therapy for uncomplicated and complicated malaria in combination with a second antimalarial agent in Africa and frequently in Asia Not used prophylactically Not currently available in the United States
ANTIMALARIAL AGENTS: INHIBITORS OF ELECTRON TRANSPORT _Mechanism—Inhibit structurally distinct molecular targets of the plasmodial electron transport chain_				
Primaquine	_P. vivax_ _P. ovale_	Hemolytic anemia, leukopenia, methemoglobinemia Gastrointestinal distress	Glucose-6-phosphate dehydrogenase (G6PD) deficiency Pregnancy Concomitant medications that cause bone marrow suppression Rheumatoid arthritis Lupus erythematosus	Disrupts metabolism in plasmodial mitochondria, likely by inhibiting ubiquinone and by nonspecific oxidative damage Used to eradicate hypnozoites of _P. vivax_ and _P. ovale_; sometimes used as primary prophylaxis against all malarial plasmodia Kills both liver and erythrocyte-stage malarial parasites

Drug	Clinical Applications	Adverse Effects	Contraindications	Notes
Atovaquone	P. falciparum Toxoplasmosis Babesiosis	Gastrointestinal distress, headache, elevated liver function enzymes	Hypersensitivity to atovaquone	Inhibits the interaction between reduced ubiquinone and the cytochrome bc_1 complex Used in combination with proguanil or doxycycline

ANTIMALARIAL AGENTS: INHIBITORS OF TRANSLATION
Mechanism—Inhibit protein synthesis by binding to 30S ribosomal subunit (doxycycline and tetracycline) or 50S ribosomal subunit (clindamycin)

Drug	Clinical Applications	Adverse Effects	Contraindications	Notes
Doxycycline Tetracycline Clindamycin	Malaria, all species (See Chapter 32 for other indications)	Photosensitivity, gastrointestinal disturbance, esophageal ulceration, tooth discoloration in children, bulging fontanelle in neonates, vaginal candidiasis (doxycycline and tetracycline) Gastrointestinal disturbance and increased risk of C. difficile colitis (clindamycin)	Hypersensitivity to doxycycline, tetracycline, or clindamycin Last half of pregnancy, and childhood up to 8 years of age (doxycycline and tetracycline)	In combination with quinine, doxycycline or tetracycline is used for the treatment of chloroquine-resistant P. falciparum Clindamycin is used in combination with quinine when the use of doxycycline or tetracycline is contraindicated (for example, in pregnant women and children less than 8 years old)

ANTIMALARIAL AGENTS: INHIBITORS OF FOLATE METABOLISM
Mechanism—See specific drug

Drug	Clinical Applications	Adverse Effects	Contraindications	Notes
Sulfadoxine-pyrimethamine Sulfalene-pyrimethamine	P. falciparum	*Stevens-Johnson syndrome, toxic epidermal necrolysis, megaloblastic anemia, leukopenia, thrombocytopenia, nephrotoxicity* Gastrointestinal distress, urticaria	Blood dyscrasias Infants less than 2 months old Pregnancy or breastfeeding Severe liver or renal disease	Sulfadoxine and sulfalene are PABA analogues that competitively inhibit plasmodial dihydropteroate synthetase. Pyrimethamine is a folate analogue that competitively inhibits plasmodial dihydrofolate reductase Effective against blood schizont stages of *P. falciparum*, but not against gametocytes Sulfadoxine-pyrimethamine can be administered as a single dose, but worldwide resistance to this combination has markedly restricted its utility
Proguanil	Malaria, all species	*Pancytopenia, thrombocytopenia, granulocytopenia* Oral ulcerations, gastrointestinal distress, pruritus, headache	Prophylaxis of P. falciparum malaria in patients with severe renal impairment	Pyrimidine derivative that inhibits plasmodial dihydrofolate reductase Primarily active against the hepatic, pre-erythrocytic forms of P. falciparum and P. vivax In combination with chloroquine, used for prophylaxis in areas where chloroquine resistance is not widespread Also used in combination with atovaquone for treatment and prevention of malaria

ANTIPROTOZOAL AGENTS
Mechanism—See specific drug

Drug	Clinical Applications	Adverse Effects	Contraindications	Notes
Metronidazole Tinidazole	Anaerobic bacteria Amebiasis Giardiasis Trichomoniasis	*Leukopenia, thrombocytopenia, ototoxicity, Disulfiram-like effect with alcohol,* gastrointestinal disturbance, headache, neuropathy, metallic taste, vaginitis	Hypersensitivity to metronidazole or other nitroimidazole agents Hypersensitivity to parabens (gel formulation) First trimester of pregnancy Concomitant alcohol administration leads to disulfiram-like reaction	Metronidazole is activated by enzymes in parasites and anaerobic bacteria to form reduced cytotoxic compounds that damage microbial proteins, membranes, and DNA Active against E. histolytica trophozoites in tissues, but has less activity against intraluminal ameba Individuals with invasive amebiasis are typically treated first with metronidazole and then with a second agent such as iodoquinol or paromomycin

(Continued)

Drug Summary Table | **Chapter 35 Pharmacology of Parasitic Infections** (*Continued*)

Drug	Clinical Applications	Serious and Common Adverse Effects	Contraindications	Therapeutic Considerations
Nitazoxanide	Giardiasis Cryptosporidiosis	Gastrointestinal upset, headache	Hypersensitivity to nitazoxanide	Structurally related to metronidazole Inhibits the pyruvate-ferredoxin oxidoreductase (PFOR) enzyme that converts pyruvate to acetyl CoA in protozoa and anaerobic bacteria Mechanism of action against helminths unclear
Pentamidine	African trypanosomiasis *Pneumocystis carinii (jiroveci)* pneumonia	*Pancreatitis, nephrotoxicity, cardiac arrhythmia, hypotension, hypoglycemia, leukopenia, thrombocytopenia* Rash, liver function enzyme abnormalities, bronchospasm, dizziness	Hypersensitivity to pentamidine	Inhibits DNA, RNA, protein, and phospholipid synthesis, and dihydrofolate reductase activity Has a high affinity for DNA in kinetoplasts and suppresses kinetoplast replication and function Commonly used as a second-line treatment for individuals with *Pneumocystis carinii (jiroveci)* pneumonia
Suramin	Early-stage African trypanosomiasis	Pruritus, paresthesias, vomiting, nausea	Hypersensitivity to suramin	Inhibits RNA polymerase and glycerol phosphate dehydrogenase
Melarsoprol	Late-stage African trypanosomiasis	*Reactive encephalopathy, death* Fever, phlebitis, neuropathy	Hypersensitivity to melarsoprol	First-line drug for late-stage African trypanosomiasis, in which the disease involves the central nervous system Melarsoprol inhibits trypanosomal pyruvate kinase, thereby inhibiting glycolysis and decreasing ATP production; melarsoprol also inhibits adenine and adenosine uptake by trypanosomal transporters Treatment can be associated with 4%–6% death rate Concomitant administration of corticosteroids lessens the likelihood of reactive encephalopathy Concomitant administration of thiamine lessens the likelihood of polyneuropathy
Eflornithine	West African trypanosomiasis (intravenous) Hair removal (topical)	*Myelosuppression, thrombocytopenia, seizure, ototoxicity*	Hypersensitivity to eflornithine	Active against early- and late-stage West African trypanosomiasis (caused by *T. b. gambiense*), but not effective against East African trypanosomiasis (caused by *T. b. rhodesiense*) Eflornithine is a selective and irreversible inhibitor of ornithine decarboxylase; *T. b. gambiense* organisms are susceptible to eflornithine possibly because of their slow turnover of ornithine decarboxylase In the United States, topical formulation of eflornithine is used for hair removal
Nifurtimox	New World trypanosomiasis (Chagas' disease)	*Pancytopenia, neuropathy, convulsions* Vomiting, anorexia, memory loss, sleep disorders	Hypersensitivity to nifurtimox	Generates toxic intracellular oxygen radicals in the parasite; mammalian cells are protected by the activity of antioxidant enzymes such as catalase, glutathione peroxidase, and superoxide dismutase

Drug	Clinical uses	Contraindications	Adverse effects	Mechanism
Sodium stibogluconate Meglumine antimonate	Leishmaniasis	Hypersensitivity to sodium stibogluconate or meglumine antimonate	*Myelosuppression, chemical pancreatitis, prolonged QT interval, renal dysfunction* Rash	Contain pentavalent antimony and act by an unknown mechanism; postulated to inhibit the glycolytic pathway and fatty acid oxidation
Miltefosine	Visceral leishmaniasis (oral) Cutaneous lymphomas and skin metastases from breast cancer (topical)	Breastfeeding Concurrent radiation therapy of affected skin Large, deep metastases Not recommended for areas so small and well-defined that surgery or radiation would be successful Pregnancy	*Leukocytosis, thrombocytosis* Gastrointestinal upset, pruritus, rash	A synthetic ether phospholipid analogue similar to natural phospholipids in cell membranes Has antineoplastic, immunomodulatory, and antiprotozoal activity May inhibit enzyme systems associated with plasma membranes (such as protein kinase C) and phosphatidylcholine biosynthesis May also inhibit platelet activating factor-induced responses and inositol phosphate formation Immunomodulatory effects include T cell activation, interferon-gamma production, and increased interleukin-2 receptor and HLA-DR expression

ANTIHELMINTHIC AGENTS
Mechanism—All mechanisms lead to paralysis and death of worms; see specific drug for individual mechanisms

Drug	Clinical uses	Contraindications	Adverse effects	Mechanism
Ivermectin	Onchocerciasis Lymphatic filariasis Strongyloidiasis Scabies Cutaneous larva migrans	Hypersensitivity to ivermectin	*Seizure* Inflammatory or allergic responses to dying microfilariae (''Mazzotti-type reaction''), including itching, fever, dizziness, headache	Potentiates both glutamate-gated chloride channels in nematode cell membranes and release of GABA from presynaptic terminals → hyperpolarization of neuromuscular cells and pharyngeal paralysis Does not kill adult filarial worms and therefore cannot cure human hosts of *O. volvulus* infection Ivermectin does not cross the blood–brain barrier; however, the drug has increased CNS toxicity (headaches, ataxia, coma) when the blood–brain barrier is hyperpermeable (as in meningitis) Ivermectin resistance has been found in livestock parasites but not (to date) in humans; in livestock parasites, the P-glycoprotein may be involved in ivermectin resistance
Albendazole Mebendazole Thiabendazole	Nematode infections Cysticercosis Echinococcosis	Hypersensitivity to albendazole, mebendazole, thiabendazole	*Agranulocytosis, leukopenia, pancytopenia, thrombocytopenia, hepatotoxicity, acute renal failure* Gastrointestinal disturbance, headache	Inhibit tubulin polymerization by binding to β-tubulin → degenerative changes in integumental and intestinal cells of helminths Thiabendazole causes significant nausea, vomiting, and anorexia at therapeutic doses, and is rarely used Mebendazole and albendazole are better tolerated; albendazole has the highest bioavailability of the three drugs after oral administration Dose reduction is required for patients with renal insufficiency
Praziquantel	Schistosomiasis Tapeworm infections Liver fluke infections	Hypersensitivity to praziquantel	Headache, gastrointestinal disturbance	Increases parasite membrane permeability to calcium → contraction and paralysis of worms

(Continued)

Drug Summary Table   Chapter 35 Pharmacology of Parasitic Infections (Continued)

Drug	Clinical Applications	Serious and Common Adverse Effects	Contraindications	Therapeutic Considerations
Diethylcarbamazine	Filariasis	"Mazzotti-type reactions" in individuals with heavy microfilarial burdens Anorexia, headache, nausea	Hypersensitivity to diethylcarbamazine	Mechanism of action unknown; postulated to stimulate innate immune system, inhibit microtubule polymerization, and inhibit arachidonic acid metabolism Kills adult filarial worms and is considered a curative agent Excreted by the kidneys; consider dose adjustment in individuals with decreased renal function
Pyrantel pamoate	Pinworm, roundworm, and hookworm infections	Gastrointestinal disturbance, dizziness	Hypersensitivity to pyrantel pamoate	Causes constant release of acetylcholine → persistent activation of parasite nicotinic acetylcholine receptors → tonic paralysis Largely replaced by more effective and better tolerated agents
Piperazine	Roundworm infection	Gastrointestinal disturbance, pruritus	Hypersensitivity to piperazine	GABA agonist → flaccid paralysis Rarely used

36

Pharmacology of Viral Infections

Robert W. Yeh and Donald M. Coen

INTRODUCTION

Viral infections are among the leading causes of morbidity and mortality worldwide. Although progress has been made on antiviral drug development, public health measures and prophylactic vaccines remain the primary means by which society controls the spread of viral infections. The acquired immunodeficiency syndrome (AIDS) epidemic makes this painfully clear. Despite advances in anti-HIV drug therapies, AIDS is an increasingly common cause of death, particularly in some African nations, where as many as one person in five is infected with human immunodeficiency virus (HIV). This enormous prevalence is largely attributable to failures in public health measures and the lack of an effective vaccine against HIV, in a setting where anti-HIV drugs are too expensive.

Despite this bleak statistic, the array of drugs available to combat viruses has been instrumental in saving millions of lives each year and in improving the quality of life for countless others afflicted by viral illnesses. This chapter describes the physiology of viral replication and the steps in the viral life cycle that are targeted by current antiviral medications. Key concepts for the chapter include: (1) viruses replicate intracellularly by utilizing host cell machinery; (2) the intracellular mode of replication reduces the number of potential targets for antiviral drug therapy; and (3) current antiviral drugs exploit differences between the structures and functions of viral and human proteins to achieve selectivity of antiviral action.

Case

The year is 1993. Mr. M, a 26-year-old man, complains to Dr. Rose, his primary care physician, of a sore throat, fever, and tiredness for the past several weeks. On physical examination, Dr. Rose notes bilateral cervical lymphadenopathy, consistent with the patient's "flu-like symptoms." Dr. Rose thinks it likely that Mr. M has an infection, possibly a simple "cold," the "flu," or strep throat. Because of Mr. M's mononucleosis-like symptoms, Dr. Rose also includes cytomegalovirus (CMV), Epstein-Barr virus (EBV), toxoplasmosis, and HIV in her differential diagnosis. Laboratory tests for *Streptococcus,* CMV, EBV, toxoplasmosis, and HIV are negative. Mr. M is concerned about the possibility of HIV infection, although he denies any unprotected sexual activity, IV drug use, and other potential exposure risks. Dr. Rose tells Mr. M that his symptoms will soon resolve with rest, but that he should return for follow-up within 6 months. She explains to Mr. M that, if he has recently contracted HIV, his body would not yet have produced sufficient antibodies to become evident on an anti-HIV antibody test.

Five years later, Mr. M returns to Dr. Rose's office. He has not seen any physician in the interim and now presents with a number of new symptoms. There are multiple open lesions on his lips and in his mouth, and he confides that he has similar lesions in his genital area. An ELISA test is positive for anti-HIV antibodies, and a viral load measurement shows high levels of HIV RNA in his blood. Mr. M's CD4 count is 100 per mm^3 (normal range, 800 to 1,200 per mm^3). Dr. Rose immediately prescribes a drug regimen of zidovudine (AZT), lamivudine (3TC), and ritonavir, explaining to Mr. M that a combination of anti-HIV drugs is his best option for reducing the viral load and forestalling more serious disease. In addition, Dr. Rose prescribes oral acyclovir to treat Mr. M's oral and genital herpes.

Over the next 3 years, Mr. M's HIV viral load falls to undetectable levels and his condition improves. The herpes infections are also kept in check. Today, Mr. M appears in good health, and, although it takes considerable effort, he takes his medications diligently.

QUESTIONS

■ **1.** What are the mechanisms of action of the three anti-HIV drugs prescribed by Dr. Rose?
■ **2.** What is acyclovir, and how does it work?
■ **3.** Why does acyclovir not cause significant toxicity in humans, while AZT does?
■ **4.** What are the risks and benefits of prescribing three anti-HIV drugs and just one antiherpesvirus drug?

PHYSIOLOGY OF VIRAL REPLICATION

Viruses replicate by co-opting the host cell's metabolic machinery. As a result, there are fewer differences between viruses and their human hosts to exploit for drug development than between bacteria and humans. It is also more difficult to develop agents that are active against a broad spectrum of viruses than it is against bacteria. This difficulty arises because viruses are a heterogeneous group of infectious agents, whereas most bacteria share a common cell wall structure and distinct transcriptional and translational machinery.

Despite these obstacles, all viruses encode proteins that are substantially different from their human counterparts. In principle, antiviral drugs could target many of these proteins. In practice, however, only a few viral proteins have thus far served as useful targets for therapy.

Viruses exist as small particles called **virions.** Virions, in turn, consist of a nucleic acid genome packaged into a virus-encoded protein shell called a **capsid.** In some viruses, the capsid is surrounded by an **envelope,** a lipid bilayer membrane that contains virus-encoded envelope proteins. Viral genomes can consist of DNA or RNA and can be single- or double-stranded.

VIRAL LIFE CYCLE

Almost all viruses have the same general life cycle for replication. Figure 36-1 presents this cycle for the example of a typical DNA-containing virus. Figure 36-2 illustrates the cycle for HIV, which, as a retrovirus, contains RNA that is copied into DNA. (A somewhat different illustration would be drawn for an RNA-containing virus, such as influenza, in which the viral RNA itself is replicated and transcribed.) At the start of infection, the virus attaches to the host cell. This **attachment** is mediated by proteins on the viral surface that bind specifically to a particular host membrane component. For example, the HIV viral envelope contains the glycoprotein gp120, a transmembrane protein that mediates binding and attachment of the virus to host cells expressing CD4 and chemokine receptors such as CCR5 or CXCR4 (Fig. 36-2). Next, the virion undergoes **entry** by crossing the host cell membrane. In the case of HIV, the process of entry depends on gp41, a viral envelope protein that fuses together the membranes of HIV and the target cell.

The virion then loses enough of its capsid proteins—the stage of **uncoating**— that its nucleic acid becomes available for **transcription** into mRNAs, which then undergo **translation** on cellular ribosomes. For retroviruses, uncoating allows reverse transcription to occur. For certain RNA viruses, uncoating is followed directly by translation of the viral RNA.

Genome replication is the next step of the cycle. This step requires a supply of ribonucleoside triphosphates for RNA viruses and deoxyribonucleoside triphosphates for DNA viruses. For DNA viruses, the generation of these deoxyribonucleoside triphosphates occurs via two pathways: the salvage pathway, which employs the pharmacologically relevant enzyme thymidine kinase, and the de novo pathway, which includes the enzyme thymidylate kinase. Nucleoside triphosphates are incorporated into new viral genomes by a viral or cellular polymerase (see Chapter 37, Pharmacology of Cancer: Genome Synthesis, Stability, and Maintenance, for more detail on nucleotide metabolism). In the case of herpes simplex virus (HSV), the generation of deoxyribonucleoside triphosphates involves phosphorylation of nucleosides via the salvage pathway by a viral thymidine kinase; a viral DNA polymerase then adds deoxyribonucleoside triphosphates to the growing DNA genome. Exploitation of this two-step process has led to the development of some of the most effective and safe antivirals currently available, because *differences between human and viral kinases and*

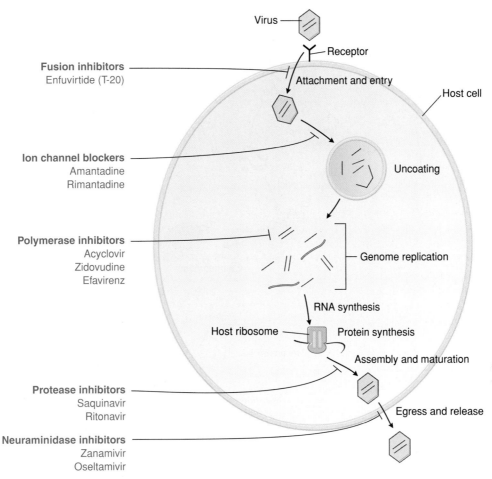

Figure 36-1. Viral life cycle and pharmacologic intervention. The viral life cycle can be divided into a sequence of individual steps, each of which is a potential site for pharmacologic intervention. Shown is a generic replication cycle of viruses in cells, alongside which are listed the names of drug classes and examples of individual agents that block each step. The majority of the currently approved antiviral agents are nucleoside analogues that target genome replication, typically by inhibiting viral DNA polymerase or reverse transcriptase. Several other drug classes target other steps in the viral life cycle, including attachment and entry, uncoating, assembly and maturation, and egress and release. It should be noted that the details of viral replication differ for each type of virus, often presenting unique targets for pharmacologic intervention and drug development. For example, the life cycle of HIV (and other retroviruses) includes additional steps such as integration (see Fig. 36-2).

polymerases allow drugs to take advantage of two different steps in a single pathway.

Viral proteins that are synthesized intracellularly assemble with viral genomes within the host cell in a process known as **assembly.** For a number of viruses, assembly is followed by a process known as viral **maturation,** which is essential for newly formed virions to become infectious. This process typically involves cleavage of viral polyproteins by proteases. For some viruses, maturation occurs within the host cell; for others, such as HIV, it occurs outside the host cell. Viruses **egress** from the cell either by cell lysis or by budding through the cell membrane. For influenza viruses, the newly formed virions require an additional step of **release** from the extracellular surface of the host cell membrane.

In summary, nearly all viruses replicate via the following steps: attachment, entry, uncoating, transcription, translation, genome replication, assembly, and egress. Some vi-

ruses have additional steps such as maturation and release. The steps of retrovirus infection occur in a different order from those of most other viruses, and retroviruses have additional steps in their life cycle. For example, replication of HIV includes the additional step of **integration,** in which the viral genome is incorporated into the host genome (Fig. 36-2). Specific host and/or viral proteins are involved in each of these steps. Differences between viral and host proteins at any of these steps can be targeted for antiviral therapy.

Different viruses have vastly different arrays of genes. Some, such as hepatitis B virus (HBV), have compact genomes that encode only coat proteins and a few proteins used in gene expression and genome replication. Others, such as herpes viruses, encode scores of proteins that perform many different functions. The viral proteins that have thus far served as the best targets for antiviral drugs are enzymes involved in genome replication or maturation, although other steps in the viral life cycle can also serve as targets for antiviral agents.

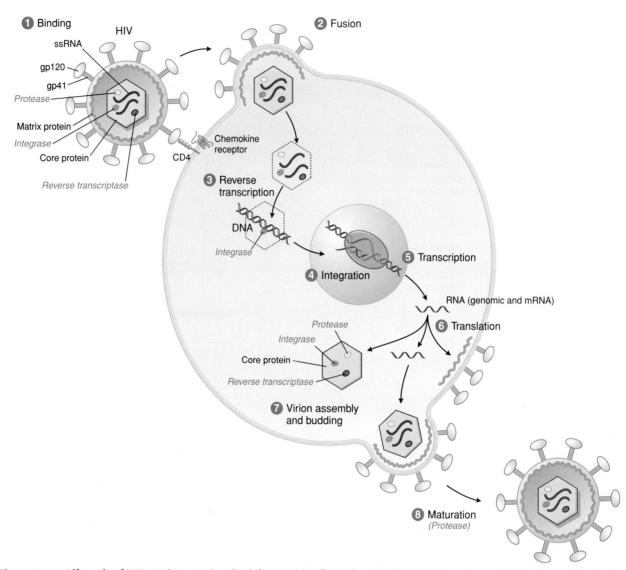

Figure 36-2.   Life cycle of HIV. HIV is a retrovirus that infects CD4⁺ cells. **1.** Virus attachment is dependent on binding interactions between viral gp160 (composed of gp41 and gp120 proteins) and host cell CD4 and certain chemokine receptors. **2.** Fusion of the viral membrane (envelope) with the host cell plasma membrane allows the HIV genome complexed with certain virion proteins to enter the host cell. **3.** Uncoating permits the single-stranded RNA (ssRNA) HIV genome to be copied by reverse transcriptase into double-stranded DNA. **4.** The HIV DNA is integrated into the host cell genome, in a reaction that depends on HIV-encoded integrase. **5.** Gene transcription and posttranscriptional processing by host cell enzymes produce genomic HIV RNA and viral mRNA. **6.** The viral mRNA is translated into proteins on host cell ribosomes. **7.** The proteins assemble into immature virions that bud from the host cell membrane. **8.** The virions undergo proteolytic cleavage, maturing into fully infective virions. Currently approved anti-HIV drugs target viral fusion, reverse transcription, and maturation. The development of drug resistance can be significantly retarded by using combinations of drugs that target a single step (e.g., two or more inhibitors of reverse transcription) or more than one step in the HIV life cycle (e.g., reverse transcriptase inhibitors and protease inhibitors). The diagram shows additional potential targets for future anti-HIV therapy, including proteins involved in HIV binding to CD4⁺ cells (e.g., gp120, gp41, chemokine receptors) and proteins required for integration of HIV DNA into the host cell genome (e.g., integrase).

PHARMACOLOGIC CLASSES AND AGENTS

INHIBITION OF VIRAL ATTACHMENT AND ENTRY

All viruses must infect cells to replicate. Therefore, inhibiting the initial step of viral attachment and entry provides a conceptual ''preventive'' measure against infection and

could limit the spread of virus throughout the body. **Enfuvirtide (T-20),** an anti-HIV peptide, is the first drug that acts by inhibiting viral entry to be approved by the FDA. This agent is structurally similar to a segment of gp41, the HIV protein that mediates membrane fusion. The proposed mechanism for gp41-mediated membrane fusion and T-20 action is illustrated in Figure 36-3. The native gp41 protein is trapped in the virion in a conformation that prevents its ability to fuse membranes or to bind T-20. Binding of HIV to its cellular receptors triggers a conformational change in gp41 that exposes the fusion-active segment (fusion peptide), a

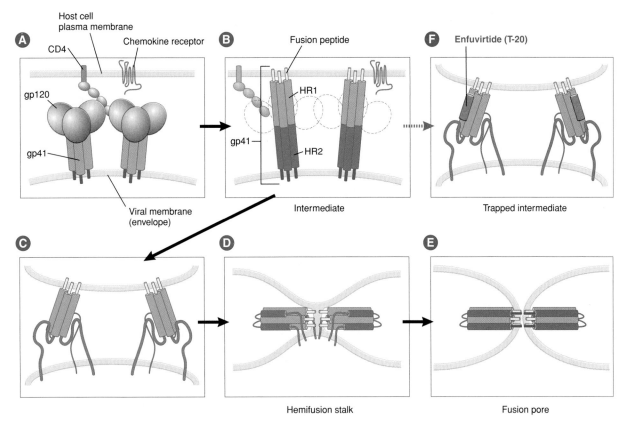

Figure 36-3. Model for HIV gp41-mediated fusion and enfuvirtide (T-20) action. A. HIV glycoproteins exist in trimeric form in the viral membrane (envelope). Each gp120 molecule is depicted as a ball attached noncovalently to gp41. **B.** The binding of gp120 to CD4 and certain chemokine receptors in the host cell plasma membrane causes a conformational change in gp41 that exposes the fusion peptide, heptad-repeat region 1 (HR1) and heptad-repeat region 2 (HR2). The fusion peptide inserts into the host cell plasma membrane. **C.** gp41 undergoes further conformational changes, characterized mainly by unfolding and refolding of the HR2 repeats. **D.** Completed refolding of the HR regions creates a hemifusion stalk, in which the outer leaflets of the viral and host cell membranes are fused. **E.** Formation of a complete fusion pore allows viral entry into the host cell. **F.** Enfuvirtide (T-20) is a synthetic peptide drug that mimics HR2, binds to HR1, and prevents the HR2-HR1 interaction *(dashed arrow)*. Therefore, the drug traps the virus host cell interaction at the attachment stage, preventing membrane fusion and viral entry.

heptad repeat region, and a second heptad repeat region mimicked by T-20. The gp41 then refolds, so that the segments mimicked by T-20 bind to the first set of heptad repeats. If the fusion peptide has properly inserted into the host cell membrane, this refolding brings the virion envelope and the cell membrane into close proximity, allowing membrane fusion to occur (by mechanisms that remain poorly understood). When T-20 is present, however, the drug binds to the first set of heptad repeats and prevents the refolding process, thereby preventing fusion of the HIV envelope with the host cell membrane.

Because T-20 is a peptide, it must be administered parenterally, typically by twice daily subcutaneous injections. A number of other inhibitors of HIV attachment and entry are under development, including both gp41 inhibitors and chemokine receptor antagonists. Continued clinical trials will be necessary to determine the efficacy and safety of these agents.

INHIBITION OF VIRAL UNCOATING

Amantadine and **rimantadine** (structures in Fig. 36-4) are inhibitors of viral uncoating that are active exclusively

against influenza A virus (and not against influenza B or C viruses).

A well-supported model for the mechanism of action of these drugs is diagrammed in Figure 36-4. Influenza virions enter cells via receptor-mediated endocytosis and are internalized into endosomes (see Chapter 1, Drug-Receptor Interactions). As endosomes acidify because of the action of an endosomal proton pump, two events occur. First, the conformation of the viral envelope protein **hemagglutinin** changes drastically. This conformational change permits fusion of the influenza virus envelope with the endosome membrane (see the above discussion of HIV-mediated membrane fusion). By itself, this action could liberate viral ribonucleoprotein (including the virion's RNA genome), but that would not be sufficient to permit its transcription. Rather, a second pH-dependent event within the virion is also required. This entails the influx of protons through a proton channel called **M2** in the viral envelope, which causes dissociation of the virion **matrix protein** from the rest of the ribonucleoprotein. Amantadine and rimantadine inhibit the influx of protons through M2. Exactly how this inhibition occurs is not clear. As hydrophobic molecules with a positive charge at one end, these drugs resemble blockers of cellular ion channels (see

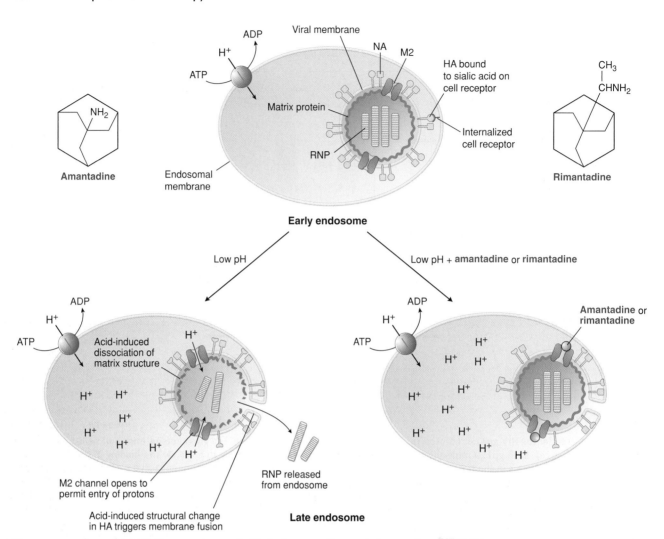

Figure 36-4. Uncoating of influenza virus and effect of amantadine and rimantadine. The structures of amantadine and rimantadine are shown. Influenza virus enters host cells by receptor-mediated endocytosis (not shown) and is contained within an early endosome. The early endosome contains an H⁺-ATPase that acidifies the endosome by pumping protons from the cytosol into the endosome. A low pH-dependent conformational change in the viral envelope hemagglutinin (HA) protein triggers fusion of the viral membrane with the endosomal membrane. HA binding alone is not sufficient to cause viral uncoating, however. In addition, protons from the low-pH endosome must enter the virus through M2, a pH-gated proton channel in the viral envelope that opens in response to acidification. The entry of protons through the viral envelope causes dissociation of matrix protein from the influenza virus ribonucleoprotein (RNP), releasing RNP and thus the genetic material of the virus into the host cell cytosol. Amantadine and rimantadine block M2 ion channel function and thereby inhibit acidification of the interior of the virion, dissociation of matrix protein, and uncoating. NA, neuraminidase; ADP, adenosine diphosphate.

Chapters 10 and 18). They may simply "plug" (physically occlude) the channel, but exactly where on the channel they bind and exactly how they inhibit proton flux are not yet known.

Amantadine can cause lightheadedness and difficulty concentrating; these adverse effects are likely due to its effects on host ion channels. Indeed, the unintended effects of amantadine on host channels likely account for this drug's other therapeutic use—the treatment of Parkinson's disease (see Chapter 12, Pharmacology of Dopaminergic Neurotransmission). Rimantadine is an analogue of amantadine that has a similar antiviral mechanism and has gained much wider use than amantadine in clinical practice because of its relative lack of adverse effects, especially the neurological effects that can be problematic in the elderly. Rimantadine is commonly used as a prophylactic agent in settings where

there is a large population at risk from influenza morbidity (e.g., nursing homes).

INHIBITION OF VIRAL GENOME REPLICATION

The vast majority of drugs that inhibit viral genome replication inhibit a polymerase. Every virus uses a polymerase to replicate its genome. A few viruses (e.g., papillomaviruses) use cellular DNA polymerases; for these viruses, drugs targeting the polymerases would also inhibit cellular DNA replication and would be unacceptably toxic. Most viruses, however, encode their own polymerases, making this step an excellent target for antiviral drugs. Viruses whose polymerases have been successfully targeted to yield FDA-approved drugs include certain human herpesviruses, the retrovirus HIV, and the hepadnavirus HBV. Most of these drugs are so-called **nucleoside analogues** (Fig. 36-5). A few, as discussed below, are **nonnucleoside inhibitors** of DNA polymerase or reverse transcriptase. The latter below do not structurally resemble physiologic nucleosides, but instead inhibit the activity of DNA polymerase or reverse transcriptase by binding at a site other than the deoxyribonucleoside triphosphate-binding site.

All nucleoside analogues must be activated by phosphorylation, usually to the triphosphate form, in order to exert their effect. Phosphorylation allows these agents to mimic deoxyribonucleoside triphosphates, which are the natural substrates of DNA polymerases. *Nucleoside analogues inhibit polymerases by competing with the natural triphosphate substrate; these analogues are also typically incorporated into the growing DNA chain, where they often terminate elongation.* Either or both of these features—enzyme inhibition and incorporation into DNA—can be important for antiviral activity.

The more efficiently cellular enzymes phosphorylate the nucleoside analogue, and the more potent the phosphorylated forms are against cellular enzymes, the more toxic the nucleoside analogue will be. Therefore, selectivity depends on how much more efficiently viral enzymes phosphorylate the drug than do cellular enzymes, as well as how much more potently and effectively viral DNA synthesis is inhibited than are cellular functions. The challenge in designing nucleoside analogues is to make the drug appear enough like a natural nucleoside that it is activated by cellular enzymes, but not so much like a natural nucleoside that it inhibits cellular processes. All nucleoside analogues employ variations on this theme to achieve their respective degrees of selectivity. The two main categories of nucleoside analogues are the antiherpesvirus agents and the anti-HIV agents. Two anti-HIV agents (**adefovir** and **lamivudine**) and a third drug, **entecavir** (Fig. 36-5), are also approved for use against hepatitis B virus.

Antiherpesvirus Nucleoside and Nucleotide Analogues

Although the diseases caused by herpesviruses are not life threatening for most people, some—such as genital herpes, caused by HSV, and shingles, caused by varicella zoster virus (VZV)—can be painful and emotionally debilitating. For immunocompromised patients such as Mr. M, however, herpesvirus diseases such as HSV esophagitis and CMV pneumonia or retinitis can cause devastating or even fatal illnesses. Herpesviruses also have the property of **latency**, in which viral genomes reside inside a cell and express, at most, a few genes, thus avoiding immune surveillance. The viruses can then reactivate long after the primary infection and cause disease. No currently available antiviral drug attacks viruses during latency; rather, all available drugs act only on actively replicating virus.

HSV is the best understood herpesvirus in terms of its replication, which corresponds to the schematic in Figure 36-1. Like all herpesviruses, HSV is a large virus that contains double-stranded DNA encoding a variety of proteins involved in DNA replication. These proteins are categorized in two groups. The first group, which includes the viral **DNA polymerase,** participates directly in DNA replication and is absolutely essential for virus replication; the second group, which includes viral **thymidine kinase,** helps catalyze formation of the deoxyribonucleoside triphosphates necessary for DNA replication. Proteins in the second group are not essential for virus replication in cell culture or in certain cells in mammalian hosts, because cellular enzymes can substitute for their activities. Viral DNA polymerase and thymidine kinase are sufficiently different from their cellular counterparts to permit development of selective antiviral nucleoside analogues.

Acyclovir

Acyclovir (ACV) is a drug used against HSV and VZV. Acyclovir illustrates the fundamental mechanisms of nucleoside analogues and it is the drug that convinced the medical community that antivirals could be safe and effective. Acyclovir was discovered in a screen of compounds for activity against HSV replication. It exhibits a high therapeutic index (toxic dose/effective dose) because of its high selectivity.

The structure of acyclovir consists of a guanine base attached to a broken and incomplete sugar ring (Fig. 36-5). This acyclic sugar-like molecule accounts for the name of the compound and for aspects of its action.

HSV and VZV each encode a thymidine kinase (TK) that is able to phosphorylate not only thymidine (dT), but also other pyrimidines such as dU and dC, thymidylate (dTMP), and a variety of nucleoside analogues—including some, like acyclovir, that do not contain a pyrimidine base. No mammalian enzyme phosphorylates acyclovir nearly as efficiently as the HSV and VZV thymidine kinases do. Therefore, HSV- and VZV-infected cells contain much more phosphorylated acyclovir than do uninfected cells; this finding accounts for much of acyclovir's antiviral selectivity. Some phosphorylation also occurs in uninfected cells, perhaps accounting for some of acyclovir's toxicity (which is relatively uncommon).

Phosphorylation of ACV produces the compound ACV monophosphate. This compound is then converted to ACV diphosphate and ACV triphosphate, probably exclusively by cellular enzymes (Fig. 36-6A). ACV triphosphate then inhibits the herpesvirus DNA polymerase; moreover, it inhibits viral DNA polymerase more potently than cellular DNA polymerase. In vitro, inhibition of HSV DNA polymerase is a three-step process. In the first step, ACV triphosphate competitively inhibits dGTP incorporation (high concentrations of dGTP can reverse inhibition at this early step). Next, ACV triphosphate acts as a substrate and is incorporated into the growing DNA chain opposite a C residue. The polymerase translocates to the next position on the template but cannot add a new deoxyribonucleoside triphosphate because there is no 3′-hydroxyl on ACV triphosphate; hence, ACV triphosphate is also a chain terminator. Finally, provided that the next deoxyribonucleoside triphosphate is present, the viral polymerase freezes in a "dead-end complex," leading to apparent inactivation of the enzyme (Fig. 36-6B). (The mechanism of polymerase "freezing" remains unknown.) Interestingly, cellular DNA polymerase α does not undergo inactivation to the dead-end complex. It is not yet known whether the inactivating step is important in vivo, or whether ACV incorporation and chain termination are sufficient to

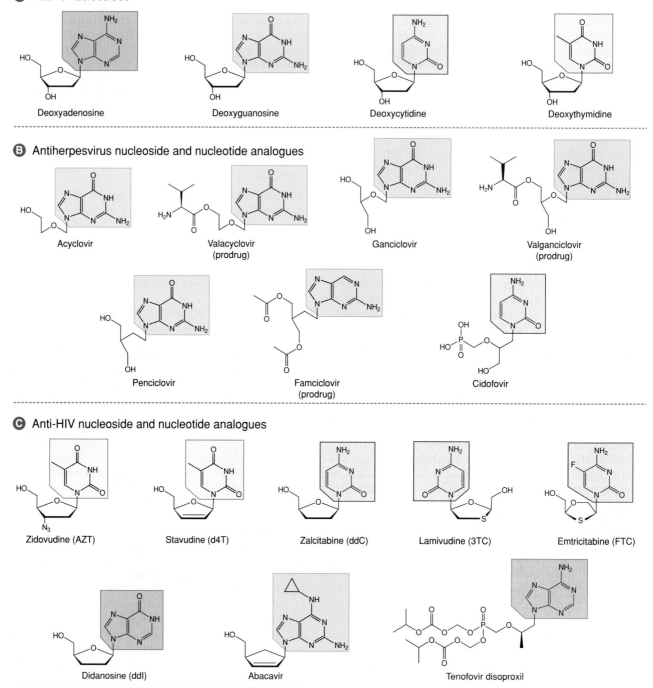

A Native nucleosides

Deoxyadenosine   Deoxyguanosine   Deoxycytidine   Deoxythymidine

B Antiherpesvirus nucleoside and nucleotide analogues

Acyclovir   Valacyclovir (prodrug)   Ganciclovir   Valganciclovir (prodrug)

Penciclovir   Famciclovir (prodrug)   Cidofovir

C Anti-HIV nucleoside and nucleotide analogues

Zidovudine (AZT)   Stavudine (d4T)   Zalcitabine (ddC)   Lamivudine (3TC)   Emtricitabine (FTC)

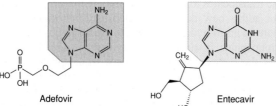

Didanosine (ddI)   Abacavir   Tenofovir disoproxil

D Anti-hepatitis B nucleoside and nucleotide analogues

Adefovir   Entecavir

E Anti-RNA virus nucleoside analogue

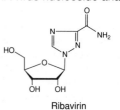

Ribavirin

Figure 36-5. Antiviral nucleoside and nucleotide analogues. A. The nucleosides used as precursors for DNA synthesis are depicted here in their *anti* conformations. Each nucleoside consists of a purine (adenine and guanine) or pyrimidine (cytosine and thymidine) base attached to a deoxyribose sugar. These deoxynucleosides are phosphorylated in stepwise fashion to the triphosphate forms *(not shown)* for use in nucleic acid synthesis. **B.** Except for cidofovir, the antiherpesvirus nucleoside and nucleotide analogues shown here are structural

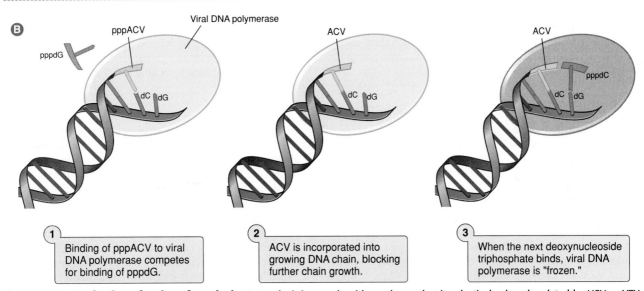

Figure 36-6. Mechanism of action of acyclovir. A. Acyclovir is a nucleoside analogue that is selectively phosphorylated by HSV or VZV thymidine kinase to generate acyclovir monophosphate. Host cellular enzymes then sequentially phosphorylate acyclovir monophosphate to its diphosphate and triphosphate (pppACV) forms. **B.** Acyclovir triphosphate has a three-step mechanism of inhibition of herpesvirus DNA polymerase in vitro: (1) it acts as a competitive inhibitor of dGTP (pppdG) binding; (2) it acts as a substrate and is base-paired with dC in the template strand to become incorporated into the growing DNA chain, causing chain termination; and (3) it traps the polymerase on the ACV-terminated DNA chain when the next deoxyribonucleoside triphosphate *(shown here as dCTP, or pppdC)* binds.

mimics of deoxyguanosine. For example, acyclovir consists of a guanine base attached to an acyclic sugar. Cidofovir, which mimics the deoxynucleotide deoxycytidine monophosphate, uses a phosphonate (C-P) bond to mimic the physiologic P-O bond of the native nucleotide. Valacyclovir, famciclovir, and valganciclovir are orally bioavailable prodrugs of acyclovir, penciclovir, and ganciclovir, respectively. **C.** Anti-HIV nucleoside and nucleotide analogues mimic a variety of endogenous nucleosides and nucleotides and contain variations not only in the sugar but also in base moieties. For example, AZT is a deoxythymidine mimic that has a 3′-azido group in place of the native 3′-OH. Stavudine, zalcitabine, and lamivudine also contain modified sugar moieties linked to normal base moieties. Tenofovir, which is shown as its prodrug tenofovir disoproxil, is a phosphonate analogue of deoxyadenosine monophosphate. Of the analogues that contain modified base moieties, didanosine mimics deoxyinosine and is converted to dideoxyadenosine, while emtricitabine contains a fluoro-modified cytosine and abacavir contains a cyclopropyl-modified guanine. **D.** Adefovir is a phosphonate analogue of the endogenous nucleotide deoxyadenosine monophosphate, while entecavir is a deoxyguanosine analogue with an unusual moiety substituting for deoxyribose. These two compounds and lamivudine (see **panel C**) are approved for use in the treatment of HBV infection. **E.** Ribavirin, which contains a purine mimic attached to ribose, is approved for use against the RNA viruses HCV and RSV.

inhibit viral replication. Regardless, studies of ACV-resistance mutations in the viral DNA polymerase gene show that the effects of ACV triphosphate on viral polymerase constitute a major component of acyclovir selectivity.

All acyclovir-resistant mutants studied to date contain mutations in the thymidine kinase (TK) gene, the DNA polymerase gene, or both. Because TK is not essential for virus replication in cell culture, mutations that completely or partially inactivate the enzyme do not prohibit virus replication. Also, some TK mutations render the enzyme incapable of phosphorylating acyclovir while permitting the phosphorylation of thymidine. Because DNA polymerase is essential for virus replication, resistance mutations do not inactivate but instead only alter this enzyme, so that higher concentrations of ACV triphosphate are required to inhibit the enzyme.

Clinically, acyclovir-resistant HSV is mainly a problem in immunocompromised hosts. In animal models of HSV infection, acyclovir-resistant mutants are frequently attenuated to reduce pathogenicity, but the degree of attenuation depends greatly on the type of mutation. These studies suggest that there are multiple mechanisms by which the virus can mutate to retain both drug resistance and pathogenicity.

Valacyclovir is a prodrug form of acyclovir that has approximately fivefold greater oral bioavailability than acyclovir (Fig. 36-5). This compound, which contains an acyclovir structure covalently attached to a valine moiety, is rapidly converted to acyclovir after oral administration.

Famciclovir and Penciclovir

Famciclovir (Fig. 36-5) is the diacetyl 6-deoxy analogue of **penciclovir,** the active form of the drug. Famciclovir is well absorbed orally, and subsequently modified by an esterase and an oxidase to yield penciclovir. In humans, this results in approximately 70% oral bioavailability. Like acyclovir, the structure of penciclovir consists of a guanine linked to an acyclic sugar-like molecule that lacks a 2' CH_2 moiety.

Penciclovir's mechanism of action is similar to that of acyclovir (Fig. 36-6), with only quantitative differences detected by both biochemical assays and analyses of resistant mutants. Penciclovir is more efficiently activated by HSV and VZV TK than is acyclovir, but penciclovir triphosphate is a less selective inhibitor of the viral DNA polymerases than is ACV triphosphate. Famciclovir is used in the treatment of HSV infections and shingles (which are caused by reactivation of VZV), and penciclovir ointment is used to treat cold sores caused by HSV.

Ganciclovir

Human CMV infections are unapparent in most adults, but CMV can cause life-threatening diseases such as pneumonia or sight-threatening retinitis in immunocompromised individuals. CMV is much less sensitive to acyclovir than are HSV and VZV, primarily because much less phosphorylated acyclovir accumulates in CMV-infected cells than in HSV- or VZV-infected cells. **Ganciclovir** is a nucleoside analogue that was originally synthesized as a derivative of acyclovir, with the intention of developing another anti-HSV drug. It turned out, however, that ganciclovir is much more potent than acyclovir against CMV, and ganciclovir was the first antiviral drug approved for use against CMV.

Like acyclovir, ganciclovir contains a guanine linked to an acyclic sugar-like molecule that lacks a 2' moiety. However, ganciclovir contains the 3' CHOH group that is missing in acyclovir (Fig. 36-5). Thus, ganciclovir more closely resembles the natural compound, dG, and this resemblance may account for its greater toxicity. (In fact, ganciclovir is so toxic that it should be used only for serious infections.)

CMV does not encode a homolog of the HSV TK (which phosphorylates ganciclovir very efficiently). However, genetic studies have revealed the existence of a viral protein kinase called UL97 that phosphorylates ganciclovir, leading to a 30-fold increase in the amount of phosphorylated ganciclovir in infected versus uninfected cells. Ganciclovir triphosphate inhibits CMV DNA polymerase more potently than it does cellular DNA polymerases. Thus, as with acyclovir and HSV, *ganciclovir is selective against CMV at two steps: phosphorylation and DNA polymerization.* However, the selectivity against CMV at each step is not as great as the selectivity of acyclovir against HSV; accordingly, the drug is more toxic than acyclovir. Toxicity is most commonly manifested as bone marrow suppression, especially neutropenia. As with acyclovir, ganciclovir resistance is a clinical problem in a minority of patients.

Valganciclovir is a prodrug form of ganciclovir that has greater oral bioavailability than ganciclovir. Valganciclovir is a valine ester of ganciclovir, making the relationship between valganciclovir and ganciclovir similar to that between valacyclovir and acyclovir (Fig. 36-5).

Cidofovir

Also known as hydroxyphosphonylmethoxypropylcytosine (HPMPC), this phosphonate-containing acyclic cytosine analogue represents a twist on the mechanism of action of antiherpes nucleoside analogues. Indeed, HPMPC can be considered a nucleotide rather than a nucleoside analogue. With its phosphonate group, **cidofovir** mimics deoxycytidine monophosphate; thus, in effect, it is already phosphorylated (Fig. 36-5). Therefore, cidofovir does not require viral kinases for its phosphorylation, and, accordingly, it is active against kinase-deficient viral mutants that are resistant to ganciclovir. Although cidofovir structurally resembles a phosphorylated compound, this drug enters cells with reasonable efficiency. It is further phosphorylated (twice) by cellular enzymes to yield an analogue of dCTP, which inhibits herpesvirus DNA polymerases more potently than cellular DNA polymerases. Selectivity has been confirmed by mapping HPMPC-resistance mutations to the DNA polymerase gene in CMV.

Cidofovir has been approved for use in the treatment of CMV retinitis in patients with HIV/AIDS. Cidofovir diphosphate has a long intracellular half-life. Therefore, its use requires relatively infrequent dosing (only once each week or less). Because of its mechanism of renal clearance, cidofovir must be administered with probenecid. (Probenecid inhibits a proximal tubule anion transporter and thereby decreases cidofovir excretion.) Nephrotoxicity is a major problem, and great care must be taken in administering this drug.

Two related phosphonate-containing drugs are the acyclic deoxyadenosine monophosphate analogues, **tenofovir** and **adefovir** (Fig. 36-5). Tenofovir, which was approved as an anti-HIV drug in 2001, can be administered just once each day, an important advantage for HIV-infected individuals who must comply with complex combination chemotherapy regimens. Adefovir was approved as an anti-HBV drug in 2002. The mechanisms of action of these drugs against their respective viruses are similar to that of cidofovir against CMV. (See discussions below of HIV and HBV replication, and of other drugs active against these viruses.)

Other Antiherpesvirus Nucleoside Analogues

Several other nucleoside analogues with antiherpesvirus activity were developed and approved before the development of acyclovir. These agents have greater toxicity than acyclovir, and so are not widely used, but are listed in the Drug Summary Table.

Anti-HIV and HBV Nucleoside and Nucleotide Analogues

HIV is a retrovirus. All retroviruses contain an RNA genome within a capsid surrounded by a lipid envelope studded with glycoproteins. The capsid also contains a small number of enzymes; two that are especially important from a pharmacologic perspective are reverse transcriptase and protease. Both enzymes are essential for HIV replication (Fig. 36-2). **Reverse transcriptase (RT)** is a DNA polymerase that can copy both DNA and RNA. RT copies the RNA retrovirus genome into double-stranded DNA after the virus enters a new cell. Once the viral DNA is integrated, through the action of the viral enzyme **integrase**, cellular RNA polymerase copies it back into RNA to make both full-length genomic viral RNA and the mRNAs that encode the various viral proteins. The structural proteins assemble onto the full-length genomic RNA and, soon thereafter, the virus buds through the cell membrane and matures into a form capable of infecting new cells. The **protease** cleaves viral proteins during assembly and maturation (see discussion below). Without these cleavages, the viral particles that are formed remain functionally immature and noninfectious.

Similar to herpesviruses, HIV forms latent infections in humans, and it appears that no available antiviral drug attacks HIV during latency. Rather, the available drugs act only on replicating virus.

Zidovudine

As with the antiherpesvirus drugs described above, **zidovudine (azidothymidine, AZT)** is a nucleoside analogue with an altered sugar moiety. Specifically, AZT contains a thymine base attached to a sugar in which the normal 3′ hydroxyl has been converted to an azido group (Fig. 36-5). Thus, as with acyclovir, AZT is an obligatory chain-terminator.

AZT is an excellent substrate for cellular thymidine kinase (K_m = 3 µM), which phosphorylates AZT to AZT monophosphate. (Unlike herpesviruses, HIV does *not* encode its own kinase.) AZT monophosphate is then converted to the diphosphate form by cellular thymidylate kinase and to the triphosphate form by cellular nucleoside diphosphate kinase. Thus, unlike acyclovir and ganciclovir, there is no selectivity at the activation step, and *phosphorylated AZT accumulates in almost all dividing cells in the body, not just infected cells.*

AZT triphosphate targets HIV RT and is a substantially more potent inhibitor of HIV RT than of the human DNA polymerases that have been tested. The detailed mechanism by which AZT inhibits RT is not entirely resolved, but, as with acyclovir, incorporation of AZT triphosphate into the growing DNA chain is important.

Thus, AZT can be compared with acyclovir and ganciclovir (Table 36-1). Acyclovir is the most selective of these drugs because it is highly selective at both the activation and inhibition steps. AZT is probably the least selective because it is nonselective at the activation step. Although AZT is relatively selective at the inhibition step, phosphorylated forms of AZT inhibit important cellular enzymes. For example, AZT monophosphate is both a substrate and an inhibitor of cellular thymidylate kinase, which is essential for cellular replication. Ganciclovir is intermediate in selectivity, with modest selectivity at both the activation and inhibition steps.

Especially because phosphorylated AZT accumulates in almost all dividing cells in the body, its toxicity is a serious clinical issue. In particular, AZT causes bone marrow suppression, which is manifested most commonly as neutropenia and anemia. AZT toxicity appears to be caused not only by the effects of AZT triphosphate on cellular polymerases, but also by the effects of AZT monophosphate on cellular thymidylate kinase (see above). The limited clinical effectiveness of AZT, and problems with its toxicity and resistance, have led to the development of other anti-HIV drugs and to the use of combination chemotherapy for HIV (Box 36-1).

Lamivudine

Several other anti-HIV nucleoside analogues are available, all of which use cellular rather than viral enzymes for activation

---

TABLE 36-1	Selectivity of Action of Antiviral Nucleoside Analogues Is Determined by Specificity of Viral and Cellular Kinases and Polymerases

DRUG	KINASE SPECIFICITY	POLYMERASE SPECIFICITY
Acyclovir	Viral TK >> Cellular kinases	Viral DNA polymerase >> Cellular DNA polymerase
Ganciclovir	Viral UL97 > Cellular kinases	Viral DNA polymerase > Cellular DNA polymerase
Zidovudine (AZT)	Cellular TK	Viral RT >> Cellular DNA polymerase

Drugs are presented in order of selectivity of action: >>, large difference in specificity; >, modest difference in specificity. TK, thymidine kinase; RT, reverse transcriptase.

BOX 36-1. Combination Chemotherapy in the Treatment of HIV

When AZT was first introduced, monotherapy with this drug delayed disease progression in HIV-infected individuals and prolonged the survival of patients with advanced AIDS. In the late 1980s and early 1990s, this was a major advance in treatment. Since then, however, the drawbacks of AZT as monotherapy have become well recognized. AZT causes considerable toxicity—including anemia, nausea, headache, insomnia, arthralgia, and, rarely, lactic acidosis—and it effects only a modest (3- to 10-fold) and transient decrease in the viral load of HIV in plasma. Most patients treated with AZT as monotherapy inexorably progress to AIDS. AZT-resistant virus can be detected in most of these patients, and it is generally accepted that these AZT-resistant variants contribute to the low long-term efficacy of AZT monotherapy.

Similar problems have been encountered with the use of most other anti-HIV drugs as monotherapy. When 3TC, the NNRTIs, or protease inhibitors are used as single agents, although the initial antiviral efficacy is greater than that of AZT (>30-fold reduction in the amount of HIV in plasma), it is still incomplete, and resistance develops even more quickly than it does with AZT. Toxicity, unfavorable pharmacokinetic properties, and drug-drug interactions are also significant problems with many of the available agents.

Because of these drawbacks, combination chemotherapy (i.e., the use of ''drug cocktails''; see Chapter 39, Principles of Combination Chemotherapy) has become the standard of care for HIV-infected individuals. The cocktails are more efficacious than single agents, inducing larger decreases in the viral load of HIV. Combination chemotherapy also decreases the emergence of resistance, both because virus replication is more efficaciously inhibited and, therefore, the chances for mutations to arise during replication are reduced, and because multiple mutations are required to confer resistance to all the drugs in the cocktail. In theory, combination chemotherapy can permit each drug to be used at lower doses, thereby reducing toxicity. It is now widely accepted that patients infected with HIV should start therapy with combination chemotherapy rather than with a single drug. Indeed, all new anti-HIV drugs are now approved by the FDA for combination use only, and certain drugs are combined into single pills. Still under debate is whether patients should be treated with combination chemotherapy as early as possible (''hit early, hit hard'')—which also subjects patients to unpleasant adverse effects and increases the risks of poor compliance (e.g., resistance)—or whether viral loads

should be allowed to exceed certain thresholds (or CD4$^+$ T cell counts to drop below certain thresholds) before combination chemotherapy is started. To resolve this question, long-term studies that include a significant period of follow-up may be required. In 2006, a single pill containing three anti-HIV drugs—tenofovir, emtricitabine, and efavirenz—was approved for use on a once-a-day basis, which is expected to improve compliance.

In antibacterial and antineoplastic combination chemotherapy, it is typical that only agents affecting different targets are combined (see Chapter 39, Principles of Combination Chemotherapy). However, in anti-HIV combination chemotherapy, two or even three RT inhibitors (e.g., tenofovir, emtricitabine, and efavirenz) have been combined with evident benefit. One factor accounting for this success could be the low efficacy of each drug alone; combining these drugs could allow for greater efficacy. (Because some of these drugs have toxicity profiles that differ from one another, it is possible to combine these agents without a significant increase in overall toxicity.) A second factor is that mutations conferring resistance to one drug do not necessarily confer resistance to the other drugs. For example, AZT-resistant mutants remain sensitive to NNRTIs and even to some other nucleoside analogues. A third possible factor is that mutations conferring resistance to one drug can suppress the effects of mutations conferring resistance to another drug, although the clinical significance of this finding is controversial. A fourth possible factor is that certain resistance mutations decrease the ''fitness'' of the virus; that is, its ability to replicate in the patient. Thus, it may be beneficial to include in a combination therapy regimen a drug to which the virus is resistant, in order to maintain selective pressure in favor of that drug-resistant virus.

In many patients undergoing combination anti-HIV therapy (often called highly active antiretroviral therapy or **HAART**), the amount of virus in the blood drops below the limit of detection (fewer than 50 copies of HIV RNA/mL in a standard test). Some scientists have speculated that the virus could be eradicated with drug cocktails if treatment were maintained for a sufficiently long period of time. However, anti-HIV drugs, like antiherpesvirus drugs, attack only replicating virus and not latent virus, and the best evidence is that latent virus can remain in the body for many years. Despite this limitation, and the sometimes prohibitive cost of anti-HIV drugs, combination therapy has been perhaps the best news in AIDS care since the beginning of the epidemic.

---

to their triphosphate forms. These analogues are shown in Figure 36-5 and listed in the Drug Summary Table. Like AZT, all of these analogues are obligatory chain terminators. Most exhibit toxicities that are thought to be due to inhibition of mitochondrial DNA polymerase by drug triphosphates. Of these analogues, **lamivudine,** or **3TC,** appears to exhibit the least toxicity. This may be related to its highly unusual structure: 3TC is an L-stereoisomer, not the standard D-stereoisomer of biologic nucleosides, and it contains a sulfur atom in

its five-membered ring (Fig. 36-5). 3TC's lack of certain toxicities may also be attributable to its relatively weak inhibition of mitochondrial DNA polymerase. Indeed, 3TC triphosphate is a substantially more potent inhibitor of HIV RT than of cellular polymerases. However, resistance to 3TC develops quickly in patients treated with this drug alone, so it is used in combination with other anti-HIV drugs (Box 36-1).

Emtricitabine (FTC) is a structural relative of 3TC (Fig. 36-5). This compound can be administered just once each day, which is an important advantage in patients with HIV.

In addition to its use in treating HIV infections, 3TC is used in patients with chronic HBV infections and evidence of active virus replication. HBV is an unusual DNA virus. Within the HBV virion is a partially double-stranded DNA genome and a viral DNA polymerase that also functions as a RT. Upon entry into the cell nucleus, this polymerase completes the synthesis of the viral DNA. The resulting DNA does not ordinarily integrate; rather, it serves as an episomal template for transcription by cellular RNA polymerase, which copies it into RNA to make both full-length genomic RNA and the mRNAs that encode the various viral proteins. Structural proteins, including the viral polymerase, then assemble onto the full-length genomic RNA. Within the resulting particles, which are still inside the infected cell, the polymerase copies the RNA into partially double-stranded DNA. Finally, the virus particle buds out of the cell, acquiring a lipid envelope. 3TC triphosphate is a very potent inhibitor of the HBV polymerase.

Nonnucleoside DNA Polymerase Inhibitors

Nucleoside analogues can inhibit cellular as well as viral enzymes. As a result, efforts have been made to discover compounds with different structures that can selectively target viral enzymes. The first such compound to be used clinically was **foscarnet (phosphonoformic acid, PFA**; Fig. 36-7). Foscarnet inhibits both DNA and RNA polymerases encoded by a wide variety of viruses. It has a relatively broad spectrum of activity in vitro (including against HIV), but clinically it is used for certain serious HSV and CMV infections where therapy with acyclovir or ganciclovir has not succeeded (e.g., because of resistance). It should also be noted that certain acyclovir-resistant and ganciclovir-resistant polymerase mutants exhibit at least moderate resistance to foscarnet.

Mechanistically, foscarnet differs from nucleoside analogues in that it does not require activation by cellular or viral enzymes: rather, foscarnet inhibits viral DNA polymerase directly by mimicking the pyrophosphate product of DNA polymerization. Selectivity results from the increased sensitivity of viral DNA polymerase relative to cellular enzymes; this biochemical result was confirmed by the existence of foscarnet-resistant DNA polymerase mutants. As might be expected of a compound that so closely mimics a natural compound (pyrophosphate), foscarnet's selectivity is not as high as acyclovir's; it inhibits cell division at concentrations not much higher than its effective antiherpesvirus concentration. Major drawbacks to foscarnet use include its lack of oral bioavailability and its poor solubility; renal impairment is its major dose-limiting toxicity.

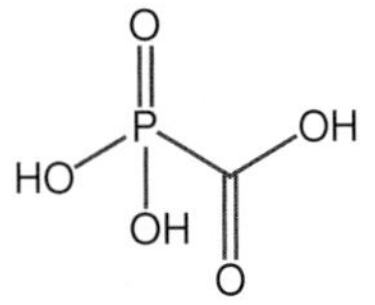

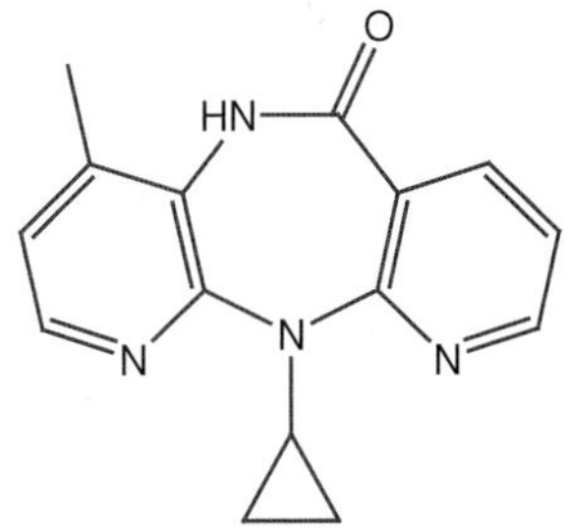

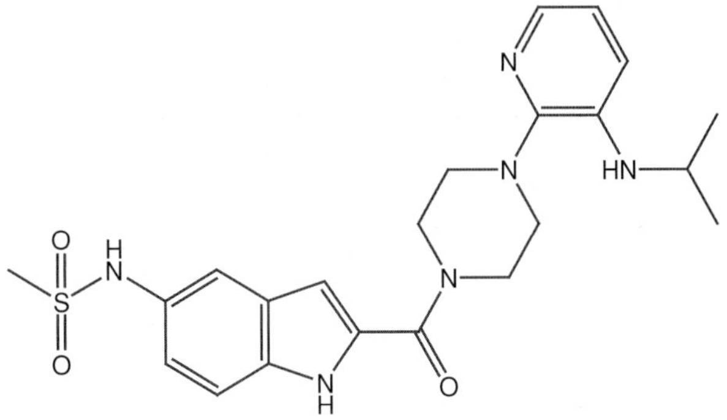

Nonnucleoside Reverse Transcriptase Inhibitors (NNRTIs)

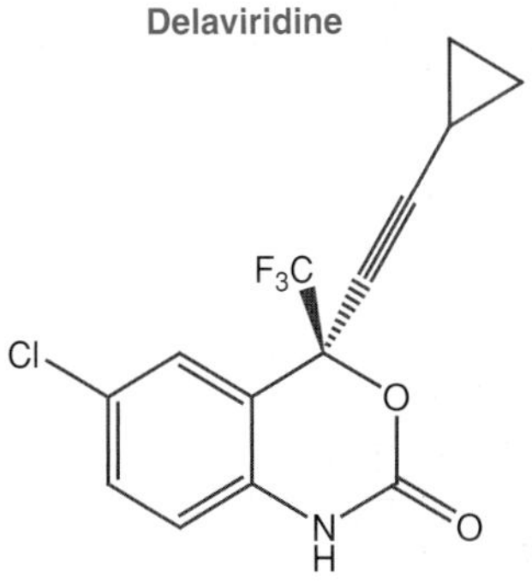

The nonnucleoside reverse transcriptase inhibitors (NNRTIs) **efavirenz, nevirapine,** and **delavirdine** have been developed by using a rational approach of target-based, high-throughput screening (Box 36-2 and Fig. 36-7). These

Figure 36-7. Nonnucleoside DNA polymerase and reverse transcriptase inhibitors. Foscarnet is a pyrophosphate analogue that inhibits viral DNA and RNA polymerases. Foscarnet is approved for the treatment of HSV and CMV infections that are resistant to antiherpesvirus nucleoside analogues. The nonnucleoside reverse transcriptase inhibitors (NNRTIs) efavirenz, nevirapine, and delavirdine inhibit HIV-1 reverse transcriptase. The NNRTIs are approved in combination with other antiretroviral drugs for the treatment of HIV-1 infection. Note that the structures of the NNRTIs are significantly different from those of the anti-HIV nucleoside and nucleotide analogues (compare with Fig. 36-5).

drugs inhibit their target directly, without the need for chemical modification. X-ray crystallographic studies have revealed that NNRTIs bind near the catalytic site of RT. NNRTIs permit RT to bind a nucleoside triphosphate and primer-template but inhibit the joining of the two. The NNRTIs are orally bioavailable, and their adverse effects (most commonly, rash) are typically less serious than those of foscarnet and most nucleoside analogues. The main limitation of NNRTI use is that resistance develops rapidly, requiring the use of these drugs in combination with other anti-HIV drugs (Box 36-1). One NNRTI, **efavirenz,** was the

first anti-HIV drug to be taken once a day. In 2006, a single
pill combining efavirenz, tenofovir, and FTC was approved
by the FDA for once-a-day administration.

INHIBITION OF VIRAL MATURATION

For many viruses, including HIV, the assembly of proteins
and nucleic acid into particles is not sufficient to produce
an infectious virion; rather, an additional step called **maturation** is required. In most cases, the viruses encode proteases that are essential for maturation. Consequently, there
has been a great effort to discover drugs active against the
viral proteases. Much of the impetus for this effort has resulted from the successes and lessons learned from the development of the **HIV protease inhibitors**. The approved antiviral drugs that target HIV protease—**saquinavir, ritonavir,
amprenavir, indinavir, nelfinavir, lopinavir, atazanavir,
tipranavir,** and **darunavir** (all but darunavir are shown in
Fig. 36-8)—are successful examples of rational drug design
(Box 36-3 and Fig. 36-9).

HIV protease was (and remains) an attractive target for
pharmacologic intervention for several reasons. First, it is
essential for HIV replication. Second, a point mutation is
sufficient to inactivate the enzyme, suggesting that a small
molecule could successfully inhibit activity. Third, the substrates of HIV protease are conserved and somewhat unusual, suggesting both specificity and a starting point for drug
design. Fourth, HIV protease—unlike the human proteases
most closely related to it—is a symmetric dimer of two identical subunits, each of which contributes to the active site,
again suggesting both specificity and a starting point for
drug design. Fifth, the enzyme can be easily overexpressed
and assayed, and its crystal structure has been solved. All
of these factors increased the likelihood that a drug discovery
effort would be successful.

The HIV protease inhibitor ritonavir provides an example
of rational drug design. Ritonavir is a peptidomimetic (i.e.,
it mimics the structure of a peptide; see Box 36-3 and Fig.
36-9). Its design began with the identification of one of the
natural substrates of HIV protease, a site for cleaving a
longer protein into RT. This site is unusual in that it contains
a phenylalanine-proline (Phe-Pro) bond (Fig. 36-9, top);
mammalian enzymes rarely, if ever, cleave at such a site.
To take advantage of the symmetrical dimer feature of the
HIV protease structure, correspondingly symmetrical inhibitors were designed in which the Pro was replaced with a
Phe. Moreover, CHOH was used in place of the native C=O
of the peptide bond in order to mimic the transition state of
protease catalysis, which is the catalytic intermediate that
binds the enzyme most tightly (Fig. 36-9). The designed
inhibitors, unlike the original peptide and the native transition state, cannot be cleaved by the enzyme. How these symmetric inhibitors evolved into ritonavir is discussed in Box
36-3 (also see Fig. 36-9).

Although clever design is no guarantee that a drug will
be active against a virus by the expected mechanism, the
protease inhibitors do act as expected. The compounds are
potent in cell culture, albeit often less potent against virus
replication than against the enzyme in vitro. As expected,
HIV-infected cells exposed to protease inhibitors continue
to make viral proteins, but these proteins are not processed
efficiently. Viral particles bud from the infected cells, but
these particles are immature and noninfectious. Compelling
evidence that protease inhibitors function as expected comes
from the observation that mutations conferring drug resistance map to HIV sequences encoding the protease.

Used in combination with other anti-HIV drugs, protease
inhibitors have had a major impact on AIDS therapy (Box
36-1). However, they have also had unexpected adverse effects involving fat distribution and metabolic abnormalities,
and the mechanisms of these adverse effects remain poorly
understood.

INHIBITION OF VIRAL RELEASE

Rational design has also led to the development of inhibitors
of influenza virus neuraminidases. The rationale for these
inhibitors, which block viral release from the host cell, follows from the mechanism of viral attachment and release.
Influenza virus attaches to cells via interactions between
hemagglutinin, a protein on the viral envelope, and sialic
acid moieties, which are present on many cell surface glycoproteins. Upon egress of influenza virus from cells at the
end of a round of replication, the hemagglutinin on nascent
virions again binds to the sialic acid moieties, thereby teth-
ering the virions to the cell surface and preventing viral release. To overcome this problem, influenza virus encodes
an envelope-bound enzyme, called **neuraminidase,** which
cleaves sialic acid from the membrane glycoproteins and
thereby permits release of the virus. Without neuraminidase,
the virus remains tethered and cannot spread to other cells.
In 1992, the structure of the neuraminidase-sialic acid complex was solved. The structure showed that sialic acid occupies two of three well-formed pockets on the enzyme. Based
largely on this structure, a new sialic acid analogue was

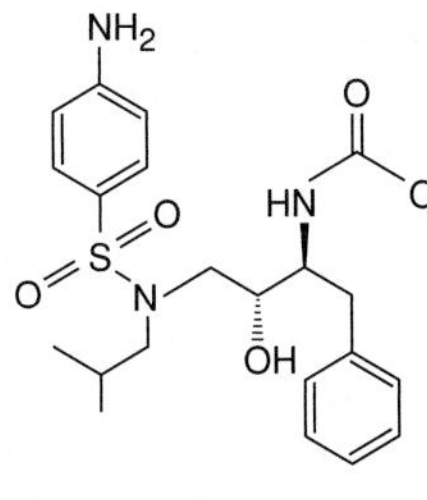

Amprenavir

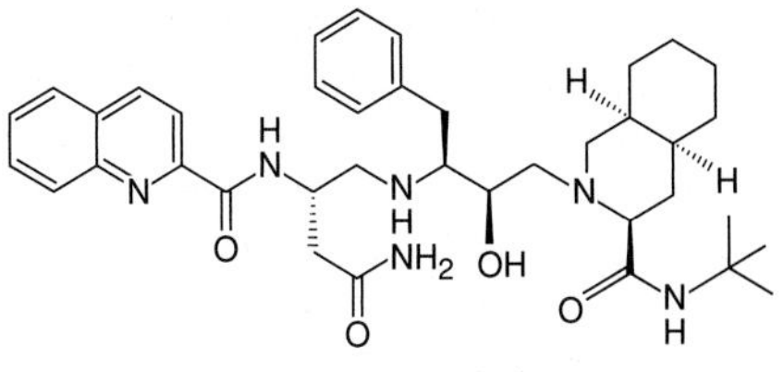

Saquinavir

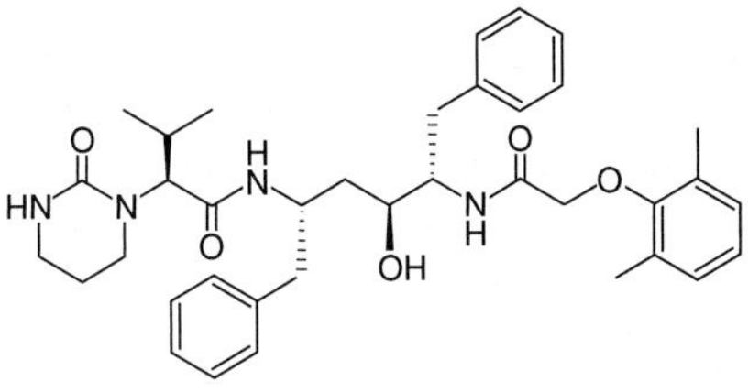

Lopinavir

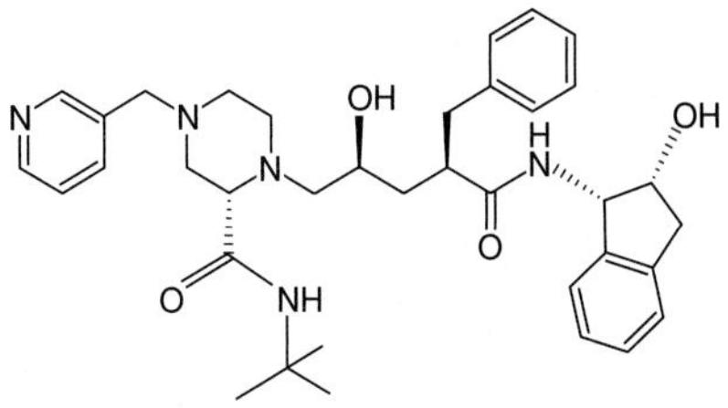

Indinavir

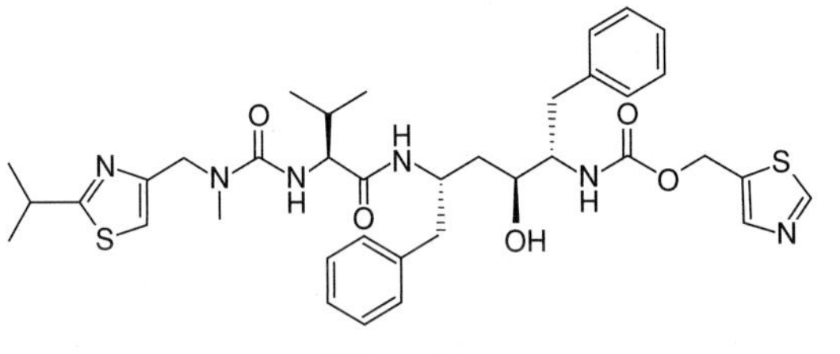

Ritonavir

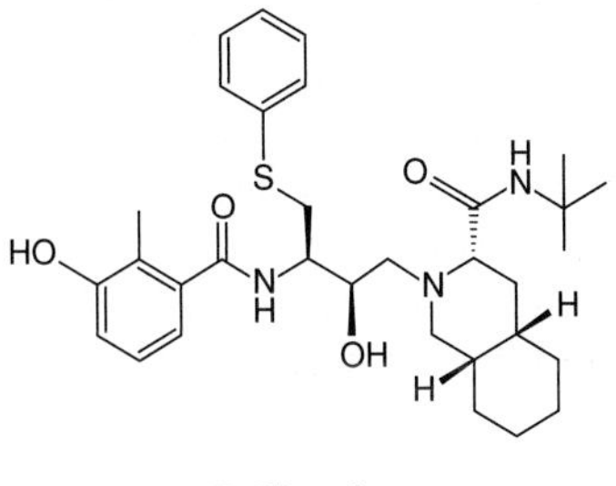

Nelfinavir

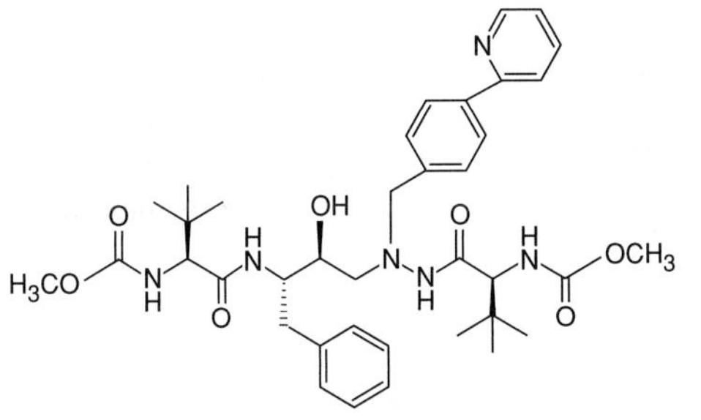

Atazanavir

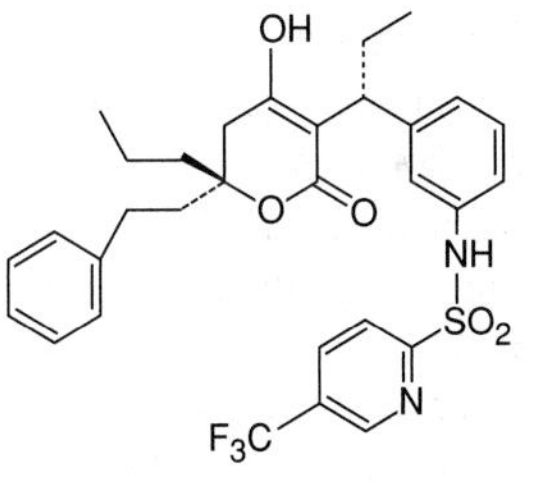

Tipranavir

Figure 36-8. Anti-HIV protease inhibitors. Shown are the structures of the approved anti-HIV protease inhibitors amprenavir, saquinavir, lopinavir, indinavir, ritonavir, nelfinavir, atazanavir, and tipranavir. These compounds mimic peptides (peptidomimetics), and all but tipranavir contain peptide bonds. A ninth anti-HIV protease inhibitor, darunavir, was approved in 2006 *(not shown).*

designed to maximize energetically favorable interactions in all three of the potential binding pockets (Fig. 36-10). This compound, now known as **zanamivir,** inhibits neuraminidase with a K_i of about 0.1 nM. Zanamivir is active against both influenza A and influenza B, with potencies of about 30 nM. Studies of resistant mutants confirm the mechanism of action described above. (Thus far, resistance to neuraminidase inhibitors has not emerged as a major clinical problem.) However, zanamivir has poor oral bioavailability and must be administered by inhaler.

Efforts to improve on zanamivir's pharmacokinetics resulted in a new drug, **oseltamivir** (Fig. 36-10), whose oral availability is approximately 75%. Oseltamivir binds well to two of the three binding pockets of the neuraminidase. When taken prophylactically, oseltamivir reduces the number of flu cases in susceptible populations (e.g., nursing home residents). Both oseltamivir and zanamivir reduce the duration of flu symptoms in patients who are already infected with the virus. However, this reduction is only 1 day on average, and even this modest effect requires that the drugs be taken within 2 days of the onset of symptoms. Although it is universally acknowledged that even 1 day less of ''the flu'' is a benefit, there is considerable disagreement about whether that benefit is worth the cost of these drugs and their potential adverse effects. Perhaps better known is oseltamivir's apparent effectiveness in preventing human mortality due to H5N1 avian influenza (''bird flu''), which has led to its stockpiling in advance of a potential influenza pan-

---

BOX 36-3. Development of Ritonavir

The development of ritonavir is an example of structure-based (''rational'') drug design. Scientists began with a model of the transition state that forms during the cleavage of a substrate by HIV protease (Fig. 36-9). An analogue of the transition state was designed, using just one residue on each side of the cleavage site. Knowing that HIV protease is a symmetric dimer, the scientists chose to use the same residue—phenylalanine—on both sides of the cleavage site, with a CHOH group that mimics the transition state as the center of symmetry. This molecule, A-74702, was a very weak inhibitor of HIV protease, but adding symmetric groups at both ends to form A-74704 (Fig. 36-9, where Val is valine and Cbz is carbobenzyloxy) resulted in a >40,000-fold increase in potency (IC$_{50}$ = 5 nM). All attempts to modify A-74704 to improve aqueous solubility also reduced potency, however, so a related potent inhibitor, A-75925, in which the center of symmetry was a C-C bond between two CHOH groups, became the scaffold for further modifications. Symmetric changes to both ends of the molecule resulted in a soluble, highly potent inhibitor, A-77003. This compound was not orally bioavailable, however. Further modifications, which removed a central OH group and altered other moieties at each end of the molecule, resulted in a compound—ritonavir—that was less soluble but had improved antiviral activity and good oral bioavailability. Therapeutically achievable plasma concentrations of ritonavir greatly exceed the concentration required for antiviral activity. In the process of structure-based drug design, successive modifications to these molecules took advantage of x-ray structures of HIV protease complexed to each inhibitor. By examining these structures, scientists were able to make informed guesses about specific chemical groups to add or subtract. The result was the therapeutically useful HIV protease inhibitor, ritonavir.

---

demic. Regardless, the neuraminidase inhibitors represent a triumph of rational drug design.

ANTIVIRAL DRUGS WITH UNKNOWN MECHANISMS OF ACTION

Despite the increasing success of rational drug design, a number of antiviral agents act by unknown or only partially understood mechanisms. Some of these agents, such as fomivirsen, were originally designed to act by a specific mechanism but later found to have other pharmacologic effects. Others, such as ribavirin, were discovered empirically.

Fomivirsen

A new anti-CMV drug, **fomivirsen,** was designed to be an antisense oligonucleotide. Antisense oligonucleotides target specific RNAs. Statistically, an oligonucleotide that is complementary to a viral RNA and more than 15 bases long will

have a binding site that is unique to the virus relative to the entire human genome. Such an oligonucleotide should be able to base-pair to the virus-specific segment of RNA and disrupt its function by inhibiting RNA processing or translation or by promoting RNA degradation. If the viral RNA is an mRNA, binding of the oligonucleotide should prevent the synthesis of the protein encoded by the mRNA.

Fomivirsen is the first FDA-approved oligonucleotide drug. It is a phosphorothioate oligonucleotide (i.e., sulfur replaces one of the oxygens in the phosphodiester backbone) designed to bind to an mRNA that encodes **IE2,** a gene-regulatory protein of CMV. Despite their large negative charge, oligonucleotides enter cells efficiently. In cell culture, under the right conditions, fomivirsen is more potent than ganciclovir against CMV, with activity at submicromolar concentrations.

Despite its design, it is not at all certain that fomivirsen acts by binding to IE2 mRNA. Alterations in the sequence of fomivirsen that substantially reduce base pairing do not significantly reduce antiviral activity, whereas alterations that do not substantially reduce base pairing can greatly reduce antiviral activity. A resistant CMV mutant has been isolated, but its mutation is not in the region complementary to fomivirsen. Regardless, the drug is approved for treatment of ophthalmic CMV disease and it is used mainly in CMV retinitis. The patient must be highly motivated to receive therapy, however, because the drug is administered intravitreally.

Despite its limitations, fomivirsen may pave the way for development of other oligonucleotide drugs. Eventually, antisense RNA, other inhibitory RNAs, antiviral ribozymes, or even inhibitory proteins may be deliverable through gene therapy approaches. Antisense and gene therapy approaches may also foster understanding of viral and host cell gene function.

Ribavirin

Ribavirin has been touted as a ''broad-spectrum antiviral'' and, indeed, it exhibits activity against many viruses in vitro and efficacy against several in vivo. In patients, however, ribavirin has been approved only in aerosol form (in effect, topical application to the lungs) for severe respiratory syncytial virus (RSV) infection, and only in combination with an interferon for chronic hepatitis C virus (HCV) infection.

Structurally, ribavirin differs from the other nucleoside analogues in that it has a natural sugar moiety (ribose) attached to a nonnatural base-like moiety that most resembles purines (adenine or guanine) (Fig. 36-5). Its mechanism of action is still not well understood. Ribavirin is converted to a monophosphate by cellular adenosine kinase and is known to inhibit cellular inosine monophosphate dehydrogenase, thereby lowering cellular GTP pools (see Chapter 37). That this mechanism should confer selective antiviral activity might seem unlikely at first, although there is some support for this notion from studies of viral mutants. It is possible that certain viral enzymes, such as the enzyme that adds 7-methylguanosine caps to mRNA, have higher K$_m$ values (and thus lower affinities) for GTP than do most cellular

A

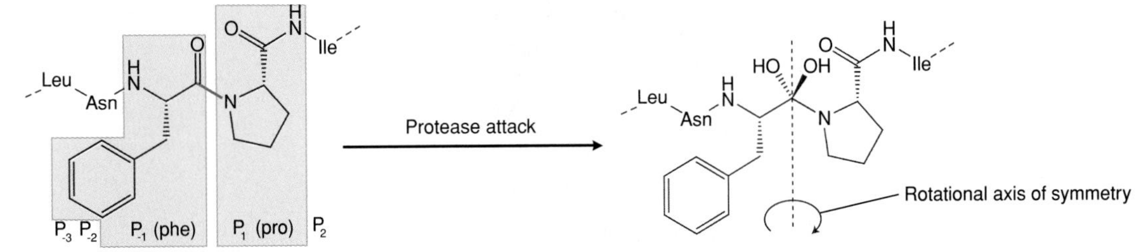

Protease attack

pol Substrate sequence

Rotational axis of symmetry

Model of transition state
on substrate sequence

B

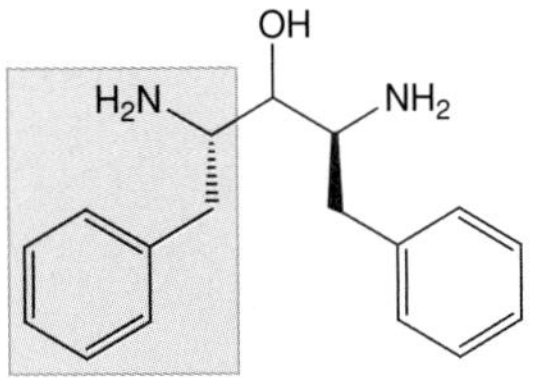

A-74702
Protease IC$_{50}$ > 200 μM

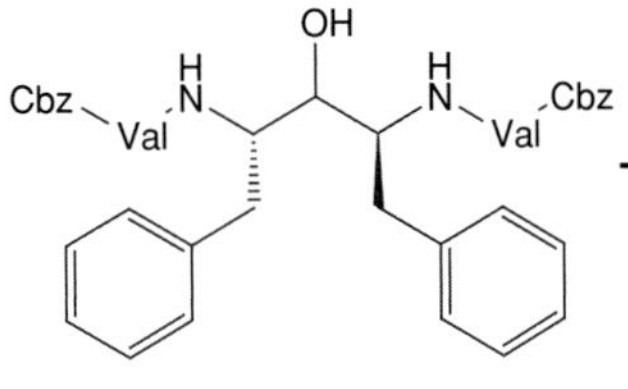

A-74704
Protease IC$_{50}$ = 5 nM
Antiviral activity < 1 μM

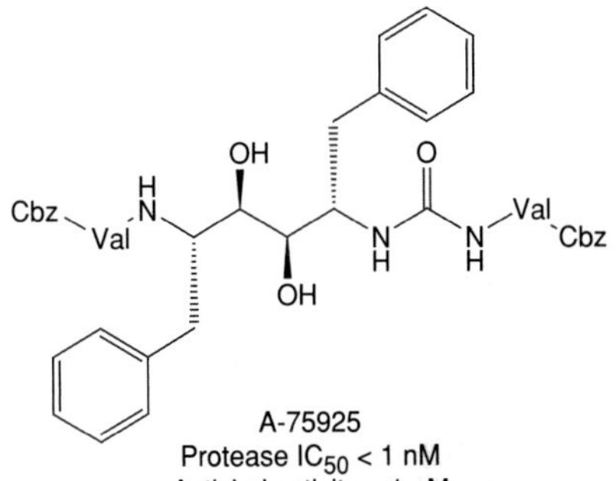

A-75925
Protease IC$_{50}$ < 1 nM
Antiviral activity < 1 μM
Poor aqueous solubility

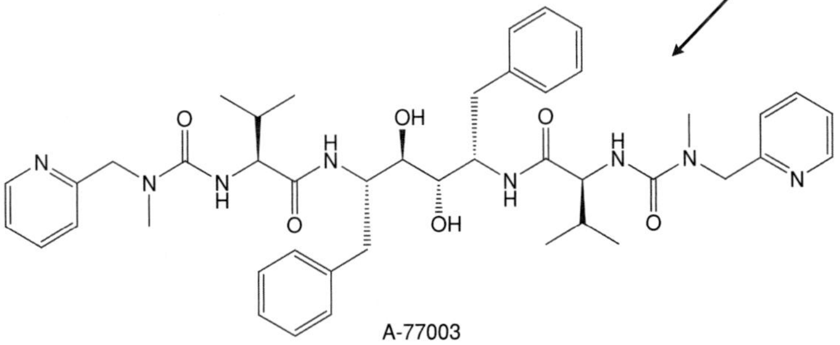

A-77003
Protease IC$_{50}$ < 1 nM
Antiviral activity = 0.1 μM
Good solubility
Poor oral bioavailability

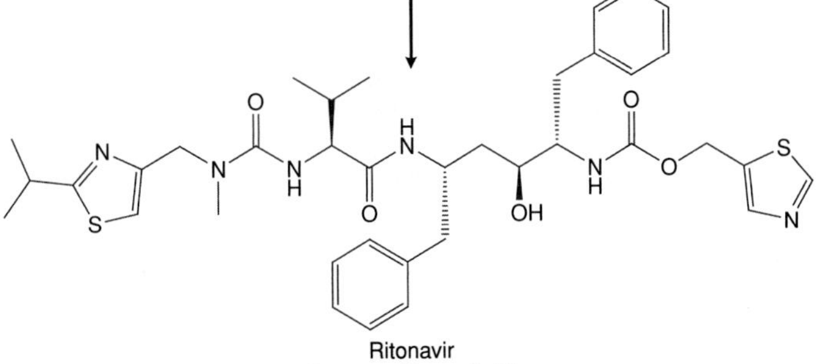

Ritonavir
Protease IC$_{50}$ < 1 nM
Antiviral activity = 25 nM
Fair solubility
Good oral bioavailability

Figure 36-9. Steps in the evolution of ritonavir. A. The HIV *pol* gene product has a phenylalanine (Phe)-proline (Pro) sequence that is unusual as a cleavage site for human proteases. HIV protease cleaves this Phe-Pro bond. The transition state of the protease reaction includes a rotational axis of symmetry. **B.** Structure-based development of a selective HIV protease inhibitor began with a compound (A-74702) that contained two phenylalanine analogues and a CHOH moiety between them. This compound, which had weak inhibitory activity, was then modified to maximize antiprotease activity while also maximizing antiviral activity, aqueous solubility, and oral bioavailability. The maximization of antiprotease activity was measured as a progressive reduction in IC$_{50}$, the drug concentration required to cause 50% inhibition of the enzyme. See Box 36-3 for details.

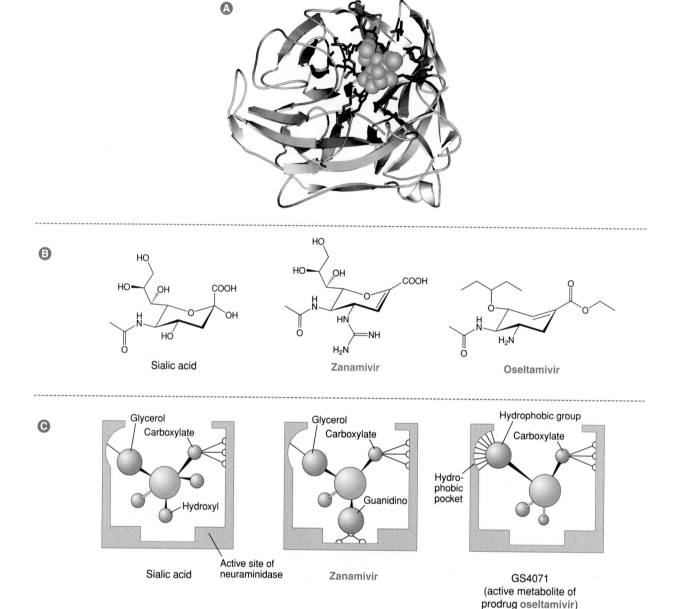

Figure 36-10. Structure-based design of neuraminidase inhibitors. A. Shown is a model of sialic acid (space-filling structure) bound to the influenza A virus neuraminidase, with the amino acids that bind sialic acid depicted in stick form. This structure was used to design transition state analogues that bind more tightly to neuraminidase than sialic acid does, resulting in potent inhibitors of the enzyme. **B.** Structures of sialic acid and the neuraminidase inhibitors zanamivir and oseltamivir. **C.** Schematic diagram of the active site of influenza virus neuraminidase, depicting the binding of sialic acid, zanamivir, and GS4071 to several different features of the active site. (Oseltamivir is the ethyl ester prodrug of GS4071.)

enzymes. Hence, lowering intracellular GTP concentrations below the K_m values of these viral enzymes could have a selective antiviral effect.

Inhibition of viral RNA polymerase could represent a second possible selective mechanism for ribavirin action. Interestingly, both ribavirin diphosphate and ribavirin triphosphate have inhibitory activity against the RNA polymerase from certain viruses.

A third possible mechanism also involves viral RNA polymerase. The error-prone nature of this enzyme leads to high mutation rates, and ribavirin has been shown to increase the mutation rates of several viruses (including HCV) when studied in an in vitro replication system. The increased mutation rates are thought to be caused by incorporation of ribavirin into RNA (without chain termination), although ribavirin's effects on GTP pools could also contribute. The proposed mechanism, called "error catastrophe," postulates that the increased mutation rate pushes the already high error rate of the polymerase "over the edge" of an "error threshold," so that few or no functional viral genomes are produced. This concept is interesting but controversial. For example, mutations that cause replication of HCV RNA to become resistant to ribavirin have not been found in the viral RNA polymerase gene.

Whether any of the proposed mechanisms of ribavirin action are relevant for the therapeutic effect of the drug on human RSV or HCV infections is not known. Indeed, for HCV, it is possible that some of the therapeutic effects of ribavirin are mediated by the immune system. Learning more about the mechanisms of ribavirin action may lead to improved antiviral therapies.

DRUGS THAT MODULATE THE IMMUNE SYSTEM

Three classes of drugs that make explicit use of host immune processes are used to treat viral infections. These classes include immunization, interferons, and imiquimod. For background on the immune system, see Chapter 40, Principles of Inflammation and the Immune System.

Active and **passive immunization** inhibit viral infection by providing antibodies against viral envelope proteins; these antibodies then block the attachment and penetration of virions into cells and increase virion clearance. Some antibodies are directly virucidal, causing virions to be destroyed or inactivated before the virus can interact with its receptor(s) on target cells. There are, of course, many vaccines that are examples of active immunization against viruses (e.g., measles, mumps, rubella, hepatitis B), and most of these vaccines are used prophylactically. One example of a vaccine used therapeutically is **rabies vaccine**, which can save the lives of individuals who are already infected with rabies virus. Examples of passive immunization are the prophylactic use of either pooled human immune globulins with anti-RSV activity or a humanized monoclonal antibody, **palivizumab**, to prevent RSV infection in high-risk children.

The interferons and imiquimod make use of the innate immune response (see Chapter 40) and do not directly target viral gene products. Interferons were first recognized as proteins that were produced in response to virus infection and that could inhibit replication of the same or other viruses. There are two major types of interferons. **Type I interferons** include **interferon α** and **interferon β**, which are produced by many cell types and interact with the same cell-surface receptor. **Type II interferons** include **interferon γ**, which is typically produced by cells of the immune system, especially T cells, and interacts with a separate receptor. Interaction of interferons with their receptors induces a series of signaling events that activate and/or induce the expression of proteins that combat virus infections. One relatively well-understood example of such a protein is a protein kinase, called **PKR**, which is activated by double-stranded RNA. (Double-stranded RNA is often produced during virus infections.) PKR phosphorylates a component of the host translational machinery, thereby turning off protein synthesis and thus the production of virus in infected cells.

Interferon α is used as a therapeutic agent in the treatment of HCV, HBV, condyloma acuminata (which is caused by certain HPVs), and Kaposi's sarcoma (which is caused by Kaposi's sarcoma-associated herpesvirus [KSHV], also known as human herpesvirus 8). Interferon α is usually modified with polyethylene glycol (pegylated) to improve its pharmacokinetic profile following injection. Although the mechanism by which interferons inhibit the replication of certain viruses is reasonably well understood (e.g., by inducing PKR), the mechanisms by which interferons act against HCV, HBV, HPVs, and KSHV remain poorly understood. Interestingly, all of these viruses encode proteins that inhibit interferon action. Understanding the mechanism of this inhibition may aid understanding of the action of interferons in inhibiting virus replication. This is an active area of investigation.

Interferon α is also used to treat certain relatively rare tumors, and **interferon β** is used to treat multiple sclerosis. Again, the mechanisms by which interferons exert their therapeutic effects in these clinical settings are poorly understood.

Imiquimod is approved for the treatment of certain diseases caused by HPVs. Imiquimod interacts with the Toll-like receptors TLR7 and TLR8 to boost innate immunity, including the secretion of interferons. Toll-like receptors are cell surface proteins that recognize pathogen-associated molecular patterns. Activation of Toll-like receptors induces intracellular signaling events that are important for defense against pathogens. In the case of imiquimod, it is not clear exactly how this stimulation results in effective treatment of disease caused by HPV.

Conclusion and Future Directions

The various steps of the viral life cycle provide the basis for understanding the mechanisms of action of currently available antiviral drugs and for developing new antiviral therapies. The vast majority of antiviral drugs available today inhibit viruses at the genome replication stage, by taking advantage of structural and functional differences between viral and host polymerases. In addition, enfuvirtide (T-20) inhibits viral attachment and entry, amantadine and rimantadine inhibit viral uncoating, protease inhibitors inhibit viral maturation, and neuraminidase inhibitors inhibit viral release. It is important to bear in mind, however, that many of these drugs inhibit only one virus (e.g., HIV), and, in some cases, only one type of that virus (e.g., HIV-1 but not HIV-2). Only a tiny fraction of viruses known to cause human disease can be treated effectively with the antiviral therapies that are currently available. Nevertheless, great strides have been made. As in the case of Mr. M, the treatment of HIV with a combination of drugs can reduce viral loads to undetectable levels and delay the progression of AIDS for many years. Although antiviral therapies do not yet represent either prevention or cure for this disease, such therapies have already decreased the morbidity and mortality of HIV/AIDS in millions of individuals.

Suggested Reading

Coen DM, Richman DD. Antiviral agents. In: Knipe DM, Howley PN, Griffin DE, et al., eds. *Fields Virology*. 5th ed. Philadelphia: Lippincott Williams & Wilkins; 2006. (*Detailed review of the general and specific aspects of the mechanisms and uses of antiviral drugs.*)

Flexner CF. HIV-protease inhibitors. *N Engl J Med* 1998;338: 1281–1292. (*Detailed discussion of protease mechanisms and clinical aspects of protease inhibitors.*)

Hay AJ, Wolstenholme AJ, Skehel JJ, et al. The molecular basis of the specific anti-influenza inhibition of amantadine. *EMBO J* 1985;4:3021–3024. (*This classic paper illustrates how viral genetics can be used to identify a drug target.*)

LaBranche C, Galasso G, Moore JP, et al. HIV fusion and its inhibition. *Antiviral Res* 2001;50:95–115. (*Summarizes the understanding of HIV fusion and includes a discussion of fusion inhibitors under investigation.*)

von Itzstein M, Wu WY, Kok GB, et al. Rational design of potent sialidase-based inhibitors of influenza virus replication. *Nature* 1993;363:418–423. (*Describes the structure-based design of zanamivir.*)

Drug Summary Table	**Chapter 36 Pharmacology of Viral Infections**			
Drug	**Clinical Applications**	***Serious* and Common Adverse Effects**	**Contraindications**	**Therapeutic Considerations**

INHIBITORS OF VIRAL ATTACHMENT AND ENTRY

Mechanism—Block HIV attachment and entry by inhibiting gp41-mediated fusion of the HIV envelope with the host plasma membrane.

Drug	Clinical Applications	Serious and Common Adverse Effects	Contraindications	Therapeutic Considerations
Enfuvirtide (T20)	Human immunodeficiency virus (HIV)	*Guillain-Barre syndrome, renal insufficiency, thrombocytopenia, neutropenia, eosinophilia* Peripheral neuropathy, sixth nerve palsy, conjunctivitis	Hypersensitivity to enfuvirtide	Enfuvirtide is a peptide that must be administered parenterally, with twice-daily injections

INHIBITORS OF VIRAL UNCOATING

Mechanism—Inhibit influenza A uncoating by blocking M2, a proton channel that acidifies the interior of the virus; acidification is necessary for dissociation of viral matrix protein from the viral ribonucleoprotein

Drug	Clinical Applications	Serious and Common Adverse Effects	Contraindications	Therapeutic Considerations
Amantadine Rimantadine	Influenza A Parkinsonism (amantadine)	*Neuroleptic malignant syndrome, exacerbation of mental disorder* Orthostatic hypotension, peripheral edema, gastrointestinal disturbance, confusion, dizziness, insomnia, irritability, hallucination	Hypersensitivity to amantadine or rimantadine	Rimantadine causes fewer neurologic effects than amantadine

ANTIHERPESVIRUS NUCLEOSIDE AND NUCLEOTIDE ANALOGUES

Mechanism—Phosphorylation of drug by viral kinases leads to inhibition of DNA synthesis in virus-infected cells. Acyclovir, valacyclovir, famciclovir, penciclovir, ganciclovir, and valganciclovir are phosphorylated by viral kinases, and then inhibit viral DNA polymerase. Cidofovir is phosphorylated by cellular enzymes, but then inhibits CMV DNA polymerase.

Drug	Clinical Applications	Serious and Common Adverse Effects	Contraindications	Therapeutic Considerations
Acyclovir Valacyclovir	Herpes simplex virus (HSV) Varicella-zoster virus (VZV)	*Renal failure (intravenous administration), thrombotic thrombocytopenic purpura in immunocompromised patients, encephalopathic changes, hemolytic uremic syndrome* Gastrointestinal disturbance, agitation, dizziness	Hypersensitivity to acyclovir or valacyclovir	Valacyclovir is a prodrug of acyclovir with better oral bioavailability
Famciclovir Penciclovir	HSV VZV	*Erythema multiforme* Gastrointestinal disturbance, headache	Hypersensitivity to famciclovir or penciclovir	Famciclovir is a diacetyl 6-deoxy prodrug analogue of penciclovir, the active form of the drug
Ganciclovir Valganciclovir	Cytomegalovirus (CMV)	Neutropenia, thrombocytopenia, anemia, fever, phlebitis	Severe neutropenia Severe thrombocytopenia	Valganciclovir is a prodrug of ganciclovir with better oral bioavailability
Cidofovir	CMV retinitis	*Nephrotoxicity, neutropenia, metabolic acidosis, decreased intraocular pressure* Gastrointestinal disturbance, headache, rash	Renal insufficiency Concomitant nephrotoxic agents Direct intraocular injection	Must be coadministered with probenecid Long half-life, requiring only once weekly dosing
Vidarabine Idoxuridine Trifluridine	HSV keratitis Rarely vidarabine for severe HSV or VZV	Eye irritation, lacrimation, light intolerance	Hypersensitivity to vidarabine, idoxuridine, or trifluridine	Early anti-HSV drugs with increased toxicity relative to other agents Trifluridine used as ophthalmic preparation

(Continued)

Drug Summary Table   **Chapter 36 Pharmacology of Viral Infections** (*Continued*)

Drug	Clinical Applications	Serious and Common Adverse Effects	Contraindications	Therapeutic Considerations
ANTI-HIV AND HBV NUCLEOSIDE AND NUCLEOTIDE ANALOGUES				
Mechanism—The anti-HIV nucleoside analogues are phosphorylated by cellular kinases, and then inhibit viral reverse transcriptase. Anti-HBV nucleoside analogues are also phosphorylated by cellular enzymes, but then inhibit HBV polymerase.				
Zidovudine (AZT) Stavudine (d4T) Zalcitabine (ddC) Lamivudine (3TC) Emtricitabine (FTC) Didanosine (ddI) Abacavir	HIV Hepatitis B virus (HBV) (lamivudine)	Neutropenia, anemia, pancreatitis, lactic acidosis, hepatomegaly with steatosis, optic neuritis, peripheral neuropathy, fatal hypersensitivity (abacavir)	Hypersensitivity to zidovudine, stavudine, zalcitabine, lamivudine, emtricitabine, didanosine, or abacavir	Most toxicity is due to inhibition of mitochondrial DNA polymerase by drug triphosphates Lamivudine is least toxic, possibly due to L-stereoisomer structure Emtricitabine is administered once daily
Tenofovir Adefovir Entecavir	HIV (tenofovir) HBV (adefovir, entecavir)	Lactic acidosis, hepatotoxicity (tenofovir), renal toxicity (adefovir)	Hypersensitivity to tenofovir, adefovir, or entecavir	Entecavir dose should be adjusted for patients with moderate renal insufficiency
NONNUCLEOSIDE DNA POLYMERASE INHIBITORS				
Mechanism—Inhibit viral DNA polymerase directly by mimicking the pyrophosphate product of the DNA polymerization reaction				
Foscarnet	HSV CMV	Renal impairment, electrolyte imbalance, seizures Anemia, fever, gastrointestinal disturbance	Concurrent administration of arsenic trioxide, bepridil, levomethadyl, mesoridazine, pimozide, probucol, thioridazine, ziprasidone, intravenous pentamidine	Renal impairment is the major dose-limiting toxicity
NONNUCLEOSIDE REVERSE TRANSCRIPTASE INHIBITORS (NNRTIs)				
Mechanism—Bind near the catalytic site of reverse transcriptase, and thereby prevent the enzyme from joining deoxyribonucleotides with the primer-template strand				
Efavirenz Nevirapine Delavirdine	HIV	Rash, psychiatric effects (depression, suicidal ideation), dizziness, insomnia	Concurrent administration of drugs metabolized by P450 3A4 is contraindicated for all of the NNRTIs—must verify metabolism of concurrent medications before prescribing NNRTIs	Resistance develops rapidly, requiring the use of these drugs in combination with other anti-HIV drugs
INHIBITORS OF VIRAL MATURATION				
Mechanism—Inhibit HIV protease required for viral maturation; HIV virions replicate and bud from the cell, but these particles are noninfectious				
Saquinavir Ritonavir Amprenavir Indinavir Nelfinavir Lopinavir Atazanavir Tipranavir Darunavir	HIV	Dyslipidemia (↑ cholesterol, ↑ triglycerides), lipodystrophy, hyperglycemia	Severe hepatic impairment Concurrent administration of P450 3A4 substrates with narrow therapeutic indices, including ergot derivatives, pimozide, midazolam, triazolam	Lopinavir is administered in combination with ritonavir; ritonavir inhibits P450 3A4, thus increasing plasma levels of lopinavir Many protease inhibitors are inducers and/or inhibitors of P450 enzymes, especially P450 3A4, with numerous pharmacokinetic drug interactions

INHIBITORS OF VIRAL RELEASE

Mechanism—Inhibit influenza virus neuraminidase, causing newly-synthesized virions to remain attached to host cell

Drug	Clinical Applications	Adverse Effects	Contraindications	Therapeutic Considerations
Zanamivir Oseltamivir	Influenza A and B	Bronchospasm, respiratory depression Gastrointestinal disturbance, headache, nasal symptoms	Hypersensitivity to zanamivir or oseltamivir	Inhibit both influenza A and influenza B Zanamivir is administered by inhaler Oseltamivir is approved for both prophylaxis and treatment; zanamivir is indicated only for treatment

ANTIVIRAL DRUGS WITH UNKNOWN MECHANISMS OF ACTION

Mechanism—See specific drug

Drug	Clinical Applications	Adverse Effects	Contraindications	Therapeutic Considerations
Fomivirsen	CMV retinitis (second-line)	Inflammatory disorders of the eye, transiently elevated intraocular pressure	IV or intravitreal cidofovir therapy within 2–4 weeks, due to risk for exaggerated ocular inflammation	Fomivirsen was designed as an antisense nucleotide, but the actual mechanism of action is uncertain Administered intravitreally
Ribavirin	Respiratory syncytial virus (RSV) Hepatitis C virus (in combination with interferons)	*Bradyarrhythmia, hypotension, pancreatitis, hemolytic anemia, thrombotic thrombocytopenic purpura, hepatotoxicity, bacterial infection, suicide* Rash, gastrointestinal disturbance, headache, conjunctivitis, fatigue	Pregnancy or women of child-bearing potential (inhalation) Creatinine clearance less than 50 mL/min (oral) Significant cardiac disease (oral) Hemoglobinopathies (oral) Autoimmune hepatitis (oral, in combination with peginterferon alfa-2a) Severe hepatic decompensation	Ribavirin may inhibit inosine monophosphate dehydrogenase, leading to lower cellular GTP levels; ribavirin may also inhibit viral RNA polymerases or make the polymerases more error-prone Administered in aerosol form for treatment of RSV

ANTIVIRAL DRUGS THAT MODULATE THE IMMUNE SYSTEM

Mechanism—Interferons activate signaling cascades that lead to production of anti-viral proteins, including protein kinase R, which turn off host translational machinery in virus-infected cells. Imiquimod interacts with Toll-like receptors to boost innate immunity, including the secretion of interferons.

Drug	Clinical Applications	Adverse Effects	Contraindications	Therapeutic Considerations
Interferon-α	HCV HBV Kaposi's sarcoma Chronic myeloid leukemia Hairy cell leukemia Malignant melanoma Renal cell carcinoma	*Gastric hemorrhage, aplastic anemia, neutropenia, thrombocytopenia, increased liver enzymes, autoimmune diseases, psychotic disorder* Depression, altered mental status, influenza-like symptoms	Hypersensitivity to interferon-α	Modified with polyethylene glycol to improve pharmacokinetic profile
Interferon-β	Multiple sclerosis	Same as interferon-α	Hypersensitivity to interferon-β or human albumin products	
Imiquimod	Human papilloma virus (HPV) Basal cell carcinoma Actinic keratosis	Skin irritation including erythema, superficial erosion and crusting, and burning sensation	Hypersensitivity to imiquimod	Wash hands before and after application

37

Pharmacology of Cancer: Genome Synthesis, Stability, and Maintenance

David A. Barbie and David A. Frank

INTRODUCTION

Cancer therapy has traditionally been based on the principle that tumor cells are traversing the cell cycle frequently and are thus more sensitive than normal cells to interference with DNA synthesis and mitosis. Indeed, the **antimetabolites**, a class of agents that are analogues of endogenous folates, purines, and pyrimidines, and that inhibit the enzymes of nucleotide synthesis, were some of the first drugs to be tested as chemotherapeutic agents. In the late 1940s, Sidney Farber and colleagues administered the antifolate compound **aminopterin** to patients with acute leukemia and observed temporary remissions in more than half of the patients. Because of their rapid growth and division, cancer cells are also

thought to be more sensitive than normal cells to the effect of DNA-damaging agents. Also in the late 1940s, **nitrogen mustards**—which had been found to cause bone marrow suppression through accidental wartime exposures—were tested in patients with lymphoma and leukemia and shown to induce remissions. These and other findings have since led to the development of multiple classes of antineoplastic drugs designed to interfere with the building blocks of DNA synthesis and mitosis, or to produce DNA damage and chromosomal instability, and thereby to promote cytotoxicity and programmed cell death **(apoptosis).** Unfortunately, the therapeutic window of these drugs is narrow because normal cells in tissues such as the gastrointestinal tract and bone marrow are undergoing cell division and are also susceptible to the effects of these agents. Use of combination chemotherapy with agents from different classes has helped to enhance efficacy while minimizing overlapping dose-limiting toxicities, but the ability to cure patients with most forms of advanced cancer remains limited. In part, this limited efficacy is due to the development of multiple **resistance** mechanisms, including the failure of tumor cells to undergo apoptosis in response to DNA damage or stress. In addition, it is increasingly apparent that populations of **cancer stem cells** may have low proliferation rates and other properties that render them resistant to cytotoxic chemotherapy.

■ Case

One day, J. L., a 23-year-old graduate student who had previously been in good health, noticed a hard lump in his left testis while showering. Concerned by the finding, J. L.'s physician ordered an ultrasound examination, which showed a solid mass suggestive of cancer. The testis was removed surgically; pathologic review confirmed the diagnosis of testicular cancer. A chest x-ray revealed several lung nodules, which were thought to represent metastatic spread of the cancer. J. L. was treated with several cycles of combination chemotherapy, including bleomycin, etoposide, and cisplatin. The lung nodules disappeared completely. One year later, J. L. was able to resume his studies, and there were no signs of recurrence of the cancer. Nonetheless, at every subsequent follow-up visit, J. L.'s physician asks him whether he is developing shortness of breath.

QUESTIONS

■ **1.** What is the molecular target of each of the drugs in J. L.'s combination chemotherapy regimen?
■ **2.** By what mechanisms could etoposide, bleomycin, and cisplatin act synergistically against J. L.'s testicular cancer?
■ **3.** Why does J. L.'s physician inquire about shortness of breath at each follow-up visit?
■ **4.** How did serendipity lead to the discovery of cisplatin, the most efficacious drug against testicular cancer?

BIOCHEMISTRY OF GENOME SYNTHESIS, STABILITY, AND MAINTENANCE

The central dogma of molecular biology states that DNA contains all the information necessary to encode cellular macromolecules—specifically, that DNA is transcribed into RNA, and RNA is then translated into proteins. Antimetabolites inhibit the synthesis of nucleotides, which are the building blocks of both DNA and RNA. Figure 37-1A provides an overview of nucleotide synthesis, and Figure 37-1B shows the steps at which some of the drugs discussed in this chapter inhibit nucleotide metabolism.

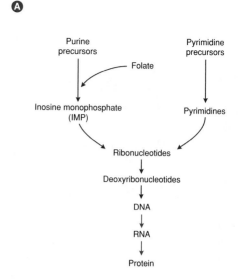

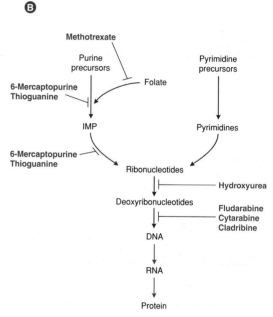

Figure 37-1. Overview of de novo nucleotide biosynthesis. A. Folate is an essential cofactor in the synthesis of inosine monophosphate (IMP), from which all purine nucleotides are derived. Pyrimidine synthesis does not require folate, although folate is required for the methylation of deoxyuridylate (dUMP) to deoxythymidylate (dTMP) (see Fig. 37-2). Ribonucleotides contain one of the purine or pyrimidine bases linked to ribose phosphate. Subsequent reduction of the ribose at the 2′ position produces deoxyribonucleotides. Deoxyribonucleotides are polymerized into DNA, while ribonucleotides are used to form RNA *(not shown)*. The central dogma of molecular biology states that the DNA code determines the sequence of RNA (transcription), and that RNA is then translated into protein *(blue arrows)*. **B.** Methotrexate inhibits dihydrofolate reductase (DHFR) and thereby prevents the utilization of folate in purine nucleotide and dTMP synthesis. 6-Mercaptopurine and thioguanine inhibit the formation of purine nucleotides. Hydroxyurea inhibits the enzyme that converts ribonucleotides to deoxyribonucleotides. Fludarabine, cytarabine, and cladribine are purine and pyrimidine analogues that inhibit DNA synthesis. 5-Fluorouracil inhibits the enzyme that converts dUMP to dTMP *(not shown)*.

NUCLEOTIDE SYNTHESIS

Nucleotides, the precursors of DNA and RNA, include the **purine** nucleotides and the **pyrimidine** nucleotides. Purines and pyrimidines are the bases that are used to determine the chemical code within DNA and RNA. Adenine and guanine are purines; cytosine, thymine, and uracil are pyrimidines. **Nucleosides** are derivatives of purines and pyrimidines that are conjugated to ribose or deoxyribose. **Nucleotides** are monophosphate, diphosphate, and triphosphate esters of the corresponding nucleosides. For example, an adenine base covalently linked to a ribose sugar and a diphosphate ester is called **adenosine diphosphate (ADP).** The various purine and pyrimidine bases, nucleosides, and nucleotides are shown in Table 37-1.

Nucleotide synthesis involves three general sets of sequential reactions: (1) synthesis of ribonucleotides; (2) reduction of ribonucleotides to deoxyribonucleotides; and (3) conversion of deoxyuridylate (dUMP) to deoxythymidylate (dTMP) (Fig. 37-2). Ribonucleotide synthesis differs for purines and pyrimidines; therefore, the synthesis of each class of molecules is discussed individually. All ribonucleotides are reduced to deoxyribonucleotides by a single enzyme, **ribonucleotide reductase.** Deoxyribonucleotides generated from ribonucleotides and from dUMP are used for DNA synthesis. Because folate is an essential cofactor for the synthesis of purine ribonucleotides and dTMP, folate metabolism is discussed separately (see Chapter 31, Principles of Antimicrobial and Antineoplastic Pharmacology).

Purine Ribonucleotide Synthesis

Adenine and **guanine,** the purine bases shown in Table 37-1, are synthesized as components of ribonucleotides (for RNA synthesis) and deoxyribonucleotides (for DNA synthesis). Derivatives of adenine and guanine, which include ATP,

---

TABLE 37-1 Purine and Pyrimidine Derivatives: Bases, Nucleosides, and Nucleotides

	BASE	RIBONUCLEOSIDE	RIBONUCLEOTIDE	DEOXYRIBONUCLEOSIDE	DEOXYRIBONUCLEOTIDE
Purines	Adenine (A)	Adenosine	Adenylate (AMP)	Deoxyadenosine	Deoxyadenylate (dAMP)
	Guanine (G)	Guanosine	Guanylate (GMP)	Deoxyguanosine	Deoxyguanylate (dGMP)
Pyrimidines	Cytosine (C)	Cytidine	Cytidylate (CMP)	Deoxcytidine	Deoxycytidylate (dCMP)
	Uracil (U)	Uridine	Uridylate (UMP)	Deoxyuridine	Deoxyuridylate (dUMP)
	Thymine (T)	NONE	NONE	Deoxythymidine	Deoxythymidylate (dTMP)

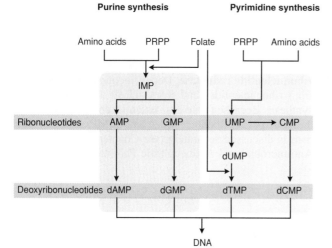

Figure 37-2. Nucleotide synthesis. Purine synthesis **(left)** begins with the formation of inosine monophosphate (IMP) from amino acids, phosphoribosylpyrophosphate (PRPP), and folate. IMP is aminated to adenylate (AMP) or oxidized to guanylate (GMP). The ribonucleotides AMP and GMP are reduced to form the deoxyribonucleotides deoxyadenosine monophosphate (dAMP) and deoxyguanosine monophosphate (dGMP), respectively. (The conversion of ribonucleotides to deoxyribonucleotides actually takes place at the level of the corresponding diphosphates and triphosphates, e.g., ADP → dADP and ATP → dATP.) Pyrimidine synthesis **(right)** begins with the formation of orotate from aspartate and carbamoyl phosphate (see Fig. 37-4). Orotate is ribosylated and decarboxylated to uridylate (UMP); amination of UMP yields cytidylate (CMP). (The conversion of UMP to CMP actually takes place at the level of the corresponding triphosphates, i.e., UTP → CTP.) The ribonucleotides UMP and CMP are reduced to form the deoxyribonucleotides deoxyuridine monophosphate (dUMP) and deoxycytidine monophosphate (dCMP). dUMP is converted to deoxythymidine monophosphate (dTMP) in a reaction that depends on folate. At the level of the corresponding triphosphates *(not shown)*, deoxyribonucleotides are incorporated into DNA, and ribonucleotides are incorporated into RNA *(not shown)*. Note the central role of folate as an essential cofactor in the synthesis of purine nucleotides and dTMP.

GTP, cAMP, and cGMP, are also used for energy storage and cell signaling. Purine synthesis begins with the assembly of **inosinate** (IMP) from a ribose phosphate, moieties derived from the amino acids glycine, aspartate, and glutamine, and 1-carbon transfers catalyzed by **tetrahydrofolate** (THF), as shown in Figure 37-2. Because of the central role of THF in purine synthesis, one important chemotherapeutic strategy is to reduce the amount of THF available to the cell and thereby to inhibit purine synthesis.

Figure 37-3 shows the central role of IMP in purine synthesis. IMP can be aminated to AMP or oxidized to GMP. In turn, AMP and GMP can be converted to ATP and GTP, respectively, and then incorporated into RNA, or reduced to dAMP and dGMP, respectively, as described below.

Purine bases, nucleosides, and nucleotides are readily interconverted by multiple enzymes within the cell. In one such reaction, the enzyme **adenosine deaminase** (ADA) catalyzes the irreversible conversion of adenosine or 2′-deoxyadenosine to inosine or 2′-deoxyinosine, respectively. Inhibition of ADA causes the intracellular stores of adenosine and 2′-deoxyadenosine to exceed those of the other purines,

ultimately resulting in metabolic effects that are toxic to the cell (see discussion of pentostatin below).

Pyrimidine Ribonucleotide Synthesis

Pyrimidine ribonucleotides are synthesized according to the metabolic pathway shown in Figure 37-4. The basic pyrimidine ring, orotate, is assembled from carbamoyl phosphate and aspartate. Orotate then reacts with a ribose phosphate; the decarboxylation product of this reaction yields **uridylate** (UMP). As with IMP in purine synthesis, UMP has a central role in pyrimidine synthesis. UMP is itself a nucleotide component of RNA, as well as the common precursor of the RNA and DNA components cytidylate (CMP), deoxycytidylate (dCMP), and deoxythymidylate (dTMP). CTP is formed by the amination of UTP.

Ribonucleotide Reduction and Thymidylate Synthesis

The ribonucleotides ATP, GTP, UTP, and CTP, which are required for RNA synthesis, are assembled on a DNA template and linked to form RNA. Alternatively, ribonucleotides can be reduced at the 2′ position on ribose to form the deoxyribonucleotides dATP, dGTP, dUTP, and dCTP. The conversion of ribonucleotides to deoxyribonucleotides is catalyzed by the enzyme **ribonucleotide reductase**. (In actuality, ribonucleotide reductase uses as substrates the diphosphate forms of the four ribonucleotides to produce dADP, dGDP, dUDP, and dCDP; nucleotides can, however, be readily interconverted among their monophosphate, diphosphate, and triphosphate forms.)

Note, in Figures 37-2 through 37-4, that ribonucleotide reductase catalyzes the formation of the DNA precursors dATP, dGTP, and dCTP. The DNA precursor dTTP is not synthesized directly by ribonucleotide reductase, however. Rather, dUMP must be modified to form dTMP. As can be seen in Table 37-1, dTMP is the product of dUMP methylation. The methylation of dUMP to dTMP is catalyzed by **thymidylate synthase,** with methylenetetrahydrofolate (MTHF) serving as the donor of the methyl group (Fig. 37-4). As MTHF donates its methyl group, it is oxidized to dihydrofolate (DHF). DHF must be reduced to THF by **dihydrofolate reductase** (DHFR) and then converted to MTHF in order to serve as the cofactor for another cycle of dTMP synthesis. Inhibition of DHFR prevents the regeneration of tetrahydrofolate and thereby inhibits the conversion of dUMP to dTMP, eventually resulting in an insufficient cellular level of dTMP for DNA replication.

NUCLEIC ACID SYNTHESIS

Provided that sufficient levels of nucleotides are available, DNA and RNA can be synthesized, and protein synthesis, cell growth, and cell division can occur. Many drugs, including the antimetabolites discussed in this chapter, can inhibit both DNA and RNA synthesis. To avoid repetition, a detailed discussion of DNA and RNA synthesis is provided in Chapter 32, Pharmacology of Bacterial Infections: DNA Replication, Transcription, and Translation. For the purposes of this chapter, the reader should be aware that *RNA and*

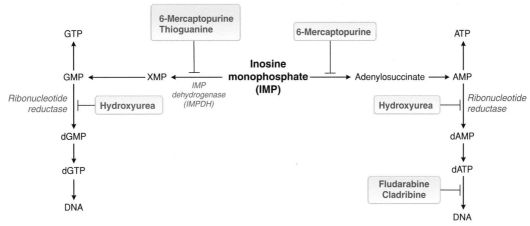

Figure 37-3.   Details of purine synthesis. Inosinate, or IMP, occupies a central position in the synthesis of purine nucleotides. IMP is oxidized by IMP dehydrogenase (IMPDH) to xanthylate (XMP), which is converted to guanosine monophosphate (GMP). GMP can be incorporated into DNA or RNA as deoxyguanosine triphosphate (dGTP) or guanosine triphosphate (GTP), respectively. Alternatively, IMP can be aminated to adenosine monophosphate (AMP) through an adenylosuccinate intermediate. AMP can be incorporated into DNA or RNA as deoxyadenosine triphosphate (dATP) or adenosine triphosphate (ATP), respectively. 6-Mercaptopurine and thioguanine inhibit IMPDH and thus interrupt GMP synthesis. 6-Mercaptopurine also inhibits the conversion of IMP to adenylosuccinate and thus interrupts AMP synthesis. Hydroxyurea inhibits ribonucleotide reductase and thus inhibits formation of the deoxyribonucleotides required for DNA synthesis. Fludarabine and cladribine are halogenated adenosine analogues that inhibit DNA synthesis.

DNA are formed by polymerization of ribonucleotides and deoxyribonucleotides, respectively. RNA polymers are elongated by the enzyme **RNA polymerase**, and DNA is elongated by **DNA polymerase**. Although antimetabolites primarily inhibit the enzymes that mediate nucleotide synthesis, some antimetabolites also inhibit DNA and RNA polymerases (see below).

DNA REPAIR AND CHROMOSOME MAINTENANCE

Mutations and other DNA lesions can arise spontaneously or as a result of exposure to DNA-damaging chemical agents

or radiation. Several general pathways exist for repair of these lesions, including **mismatch repair** (MMR) for DNA replication errors, **base excision repair** (BER) for small base modifications and single-strand breaks, **nucleotide excision repair** (NER) for removal of bulky adducts, and **homologous recombination** or **nonhomologous end-joining** for double-strand breaks (Fig. 37-5). DNA repair pathways are important not only because they can alter the efficacy of chemotherapy, but also because loss of these pathways frequently contributes to tumor development via impairment of genomic integrity and facilitation of mutations in oncogenes and tumor suppressor genes. On the chromosomal level, it has become apparent that **telomeres**, the repeat sequences that cap the ends of chromosomes, play an important

Figure 37-4.   Details of pyrimidine synthesis. Aspartate (an amino acid) and carbamoyl phosphate combine to form orotate, which then combines with phosphoribosylpyrophosphate (PRPP) to form uridylate (UMP). UMP occupies a central position in the synthesis of pyrimidine nucleotides. UMP can be sequentially phosphorylated to uridine triphosphate (UTP). UTP is incorporated into RNA *(not shown)* or aminated to form cytidine triphosphate (CTP). CTP is incorporated into RNA *(not shown)* or reduced by ribonucleotide reductase to deoxycytidine triphosphate (dCTP), which is incorporated into DNA. Alternatively, UMP can be reduced to deoxyuridylate (dUMP). Thymidylate synthase converts dUMP to deoxythymidylate (dTMP), in a reaction that depends on folate. dTMP is phosphorylated to deoxythymidine triphosphate (dTTP), which is incorporated into DNA. Hydroxyurea inhibits the formation of deoxyribonucleotides and thereby inhibits DNA synthesis. Cytarabine, a cytidine analogue, inhibits the incorporation of dCTP into DNA. 5-Fluorouracil inhibits dTMP synthesis by inhibiting thymidylate synthase. Methotrexate inhibits dihydrofolate reductase (DHFR), the enzyme responsible for regenerating tetrahydrofolate (THF) from DHF. By inhibiting DHF reductase, this drug inhibits the formation of methylenetetrahydrofolate (MTHF), which is the folate compound that is required for dTMP synthesis.

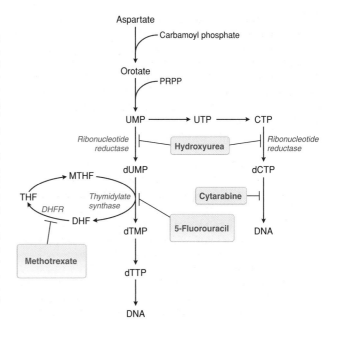

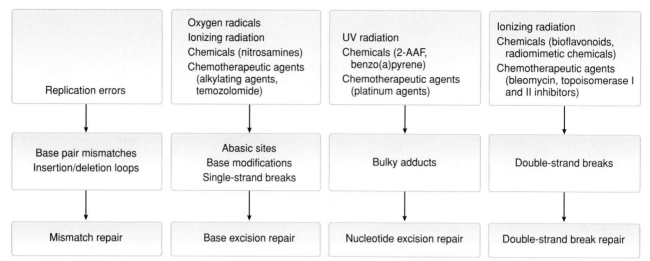

Figure 37-5. Mechanisms of DNA damage and repair. In response to DNA damage, there are several general pathways that mediate repair of DNA lesions. Replication errors typically result in base pair mismatches or insertion/deletion loops in regions of microsatellite DNA repeats; these lesions are repaired by the mismatch repair (MMR) pathway. Ionizing radiation, oxygen radicals, and various chemicals and chemotherapeutic agents can cause abasic site formation, base modifications, and single-strand breaks, which are repaired by the base excision repair (BER) pathway. UV irradiation and certain DNA-modifying chemicals and chemotherapeutic agents can cause the formation of bulky adducts that are excised and repaired by the nucleotide excision repair (NER) pathway. Ionizing radiation, radiomimetic chemicals, bleomycin, and natural (bioflavonoids) and chemotherapeutic (camptothecins, anthracyclines, epipodophyllotoxins) topoisomerase inhibitors can induce double-strand DNA breaks that trigger repair by the double-strand break repair (DSBR) pathway.

role in genome maintenance and prevention of chromosome fusion. The enzyme **telomerase**, which regulates telomere length, is emerging as a key component in the process of immortalization and oncogenic transformation.

Mismatch Repair

During DNA replication, errors such as single-base mismatches and insertions or deletions of microsatellite repeat sequences (microsatellite instability) are recognized and repaired by proteins of the mismatch repair (MMR) system. For single-base mismatches, recognition involves a heterodimer between the MSH2 protein and MSH6, while for insertion/deletion loops, MSH2 can partner with either MSH6 or MSH3 (Fig. 37-6). These complexes recruit the proteins MLH1 and PMS2 (as well as MLH3 for insertion/deletion loops), which, in turn, recruit exonucleases and components of the DNA replication machinery for excision and repair of the lesion. Germ-line mutations in MLH1, PMS2, MSH2, or MSH6 are associated with 70% to 80% of cases of **hereditary nonpolyposis colon cancer**. In addition, **microsatellite instability**, a hallmark of defective MMR, is observed in 15% to 25% of sporadic colorectal cancers.

Base Excision Repair

DNA single-strand breaks (SSB), which may be formed directly by ionizing radiation or indirectly due to enzymatic excision of a modified base by a DNA glycosylase, activate the enzyme **poly(ADP-ribose) polymerase 1 (PARP1)** (Fig. 37-7). At the site of the breakage, PARP1 transfers ADP-ribose moieties from NAD to a number of proteins involved in DNA and chromatin metabolism, including itself. The covalent addition of negatively charged ADP-ribose oligomers alters the interactions of these proteins with

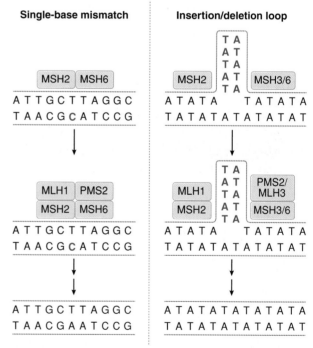

Figure 37-6. Mismatch repair pathway. Replication errors can result in single base pair mismatches or insertion/deletion loops in microsatellite repeat regions as a result of intrastrand complementary base-pairing. Single-base mismatches are recognized by an MSH2/MSH6 heterodimer, and insertion/deletion loops are recognized by an MSH2/MSH3 or MSH2/MSH6 heterodimer. Additional components of the mismatch repair machinery are then recruited, including MLH1/PMS2 for single-base mismatches or MLH1/PMS2 or MLH1/MLH3 for insertion/deletion loops. Exonucleases and components of the DNA replication machinery are subsequently recruited for excision and repair of the lesions.

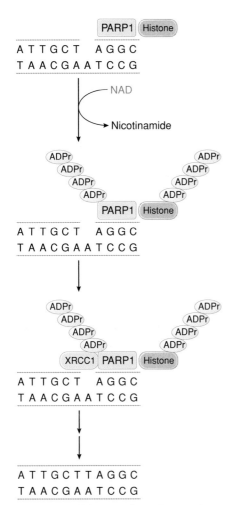

Figure 37-7. Base excision repair pathway. The enzyme poly (ADP-ribose) polymerase 1 (PARP1) is recruited to single-strand break sites resulting from ionizing radiation or base lesion excision. PARP1 poly-ADP ribosylates (ADPr) a variety of targets at the site of injury, including itself and histones. The ADPr-modified proteins then recruit additional proteins, such as XRCC1, which, in turn, recruit DNA polymerase β and DNA ligase III to repair the lesion.

DNA and with other proteins. PARP1 recruits the BER protein XRCC1; together with **DNA polymerase β** and **DNA ligase III**, XRCC1 facilitates repair of the lesion. PARP1 has also been implicated in the recognition of DNA double-strand breaks (DSB) and in the recruitment of **DNA-dependent protein kinase** in DSB repair (see below), as well as in cell death pathways, modification of chromatin structure, transcriptional regulation, and mitotic apparatus function.

Nucleotide Excision Repair

In response to the formation of bulky adducts that distort the DNA double helix, such as those induced by ultraviolet irradiation and DNA-damaging chemotherapeutic agents, a complex set of proteins recognizes and initiates repair of the lesion via a process termed **nucleotide excision repair** (NER). Repair involves local opening of the double helix around the site of the damage, incision of the damaged strand on both sides of the lesion, excision of the oligonucleotide containing the lesion, and, finally, DNA repair synthesis and

ligation. The proteins involved in this process were identified and derive their names from the clinical syndromes **xeroderma pigmentosa** and **Cockayne syndrome**, which are rare photosensitivity disorders that exhibit defects in NER.

Double-Strand Break Repair

In response to a double-strand break, activation of the ataxia telangiectasia mutated (ATM) kinase results in generation of the phosphorylated histone gamma-H2AX at the site of the break. Together with the protein MDC1, gamma-H2AX recruits to the locus of DNA damage a complex (MRN) containing the proteins Mre11, Rad50, and Nijmegen breakage syndrome gene 1 (NBS1) (Fig. 37-8). The breast and ovarian cancer susceptibility gene product **BRCA1** is also phosphorylated by the kinases ATM, ATR, and CHK2 in response to the double strand break, and phosphorylated BRCA1, RAD51, and **BRCA2** are also recruited to the break site. Subsequent repair is mediated either by **homologous recombination**, with formation and resolution of a Holliday junction (Fig. 37-8), or by **nonhomologous end joining** (NHEJ), in which DNA-dependent protein kinase and a complex of proteins, including XRCC4, catalyze nucleolytic processes that allow end joining by DNA ligase IV. The DNA repair effected by homologous recombination is more accurate than that mediated by NHEJ.

Telomere Biology

Human telomeres consist of the simple repeat sequence TTAGGG. These repeats are shaped, folded, and bound by a complex of proteins to form a unique structure termed a ''t-loop'' (Fig. 37-9). In the t-loop structure, a long single stranded overhang at the 3′ end of the DNA invades the proximal double-stranded DNA component; this process is facilitated by TRF1, TRF2, and other protein factors. The t-loop and its associated complex of proteins are thought to play important roles in capping and protecting the chromosome end, as well as protecting telomeres from recognition by the DNA damage checkpoint machinery.

Because DNA polymerase is unable to replicate the ends of linear chromosomes completely, telomeres shorten with each division in normal cells. Telomere shortening ultimately results in disruption of the telomeric caps, activation of a DNA damage checkpoint, and a state of cycle arrest termed **cellular senescence** (Fig. 37-10). When cells are able to bypass this checkpoint via inactivation of the **tumor suppressor protein p53**, which normally regulates cell cycle arrest or apoptosis in response to DNA damage, chromosome fusions are observed. It is thought that the progressive shortening of telomeres with age promotes genomic instability and contributes to oncogenesis. However, cells also continue to die under these conditions. Activation of the enzyme **telomerase**, which is a reverse transcriptase that uses an RNA template to synthesize TTAGGG repeats, allows cells to restore telomere length and divide indefinitely. Telomerase activation is observed in normal germ line cells and some stem cell populations, and has been shown to maintain the presence of the 3′ overhang in normal cells. The immortalization process associated with telomerase activation is also essential for tumor formation and maintenance. In a minority of tumors, an alternative lengthening of telomeres (ALT) pathway is activated.

MICROTUBULES AND MITOSIS

Once a cell has replicated its DNA, it is prepared to undergo mitosis. In this process, a single cell divides into two identical daughter cells. The cell-cycle transitions from DNA replication (S phase) to G2 phase and then to mitosis (M phase) are complex and depend on the coordinated action of a number of so-called **cyclin-dependent kinases** (CDKs; see Chapter 31). Many cancer cells exhibit dysregulation of cell-cycle timing. The biochemical control of the cell-cycle transitions between DNA replication and the initiation of mitosis is an active area of cancer research; it is hoped that, in the near future, cyclins will become pharmacologic targets for antineoplastic chemotherapy. Currently, however, microtubules are the only pharmacologically relevant structures that are targeted in mitosis.

Microtubules are cylindrical, hollow fibers composed of polymers of tubulin, which is a heterodimeric protein consisting of **α-tubulin** and **β-tubulin** subunits (Fig. 37-11). α-tubulin and β-tubulin are encoded by separate genes, but they have similar three-dimensional structures. Both α- and β-tubulin bind GTP; in addition, β-tubulin (but not α-tubulin) can hydrolyze GTP to GDP. Microtubules originate from a central microtubule organizing center (the centrosome, which includes two centrioles and associated proteins), where **γ-tubulin** (a protein with homology to α-tubulin and β-tubulin) nucleates tubulin polymerization. Nascent microtubules assemble into protofilaments, which are longitudinal polymers of tubulin subunits. Each protofilament interacts laterally with two other protofilaments to form a hollow-core tube, 24 nm in diameter, which consists of 13 protofilaments arranged concentrically. *Because tubulin is a heterodimer, this tube has inherent asymmetry;* the end of a microtubule nearest the centrosome is bordered by α-tubulin and is called the (−) ("minus") end, while the end of a microtubule extending from the centrosome is bordered by β-tubulin and is called the (+) ("plus") end (Fig. 37-11). Tubulin units are added at different rates to the (−) and (+) ends; the (+) end grows (adds tubulin) twice as fast as the (−) end.

Microtubules are not static structures. Rather, they possess an inherent property known as **dynamic instability** (Fig. 37-12). Tubulin heterodimers add to the end of the

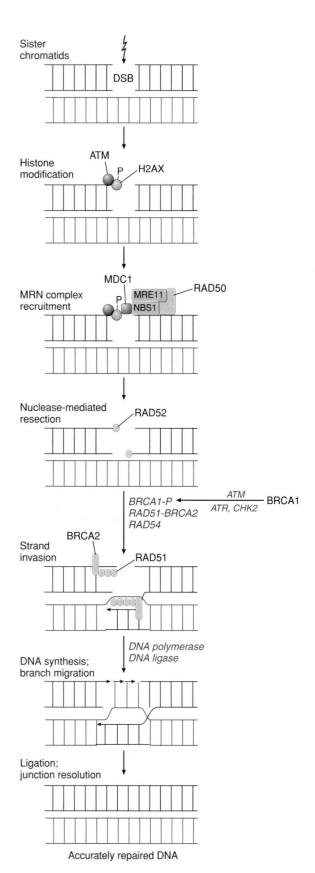

Figure 37-8. Double-strand break repair pathway. The ataxia telangectasia mutated (ATM) kinase recognizes and binds to double-strand DNA break sites. Upon activation, the ATM kinase marks the site by generating the phosphorylated histone gamma-H2AX. Gamma-H2AX and the protein MDC1 recruit the Mre11/Rad50/Nijmegen breakage syndrome gene 1 (NBS1) complex (MRN) to the site of injury. After RAD52 is recruited and nucleases mediate DNA resection, BRCA1 is recruited to the site and phosphorylated by ATM, ATR, and CHK2 kinases. Together with RAD51 and BRCA2, phosphorylated BRCA1 facilitates repair of the double-strand break by homologous recombination *(depicted in the figure)* or nonhomologous end joining *(NHEJ; not shown).*

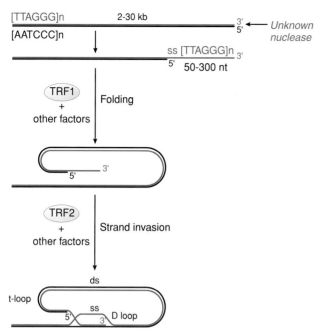

microtubule with GTP bound to both α-tubulin and β-tubulin subunits. As the microtubule grows, the β-tubulin of each tubulin heterodimer hydrolyzes its GTP to GDP. The hydrolysis of GTP to GDP introduces a conformational change in tubulin that destabilizes the microtubule. The exact mechanism of this destabilization is unknown, but it may be related to a decrease in the strength of lateral protofilament interactions or an increase in the tendency for protofilaments to "curve" away from the straight microtubule.

Therefore, microtubule stability is determined by the rate of microtubule polymerization relative to the rate of GTP hydrolysis by β-tubulin. If a microtubule polymerizes tubulin faster than β-tubulin hydrolyzes GTP to GDP, then, in the steady state, there is a cap of GTP-bound β-tubulin at the (+) end of the microtubule. This GTP cap provides stability to the microtubule structure, allowing further polymerization of the microtubule. Conversely, if tubulin polymerization proceeds more slowly than the hydrolysis of GTP to GDP by β-tubulin, then, in the steady state, the (+) end of the microtubule is enriched with GDP-bound β-tubulin. This GDP-bound tubulin conformation is unstable and causes rapid depolymerization of the microtubule. The ability of microtubules to assemble and disassemble rapidly is important for their many physiologic roles. Pharmacologic agents can disrupt microtubule function either by preventing the assembly of tubulin into microtubules or by stabilizing existing microtubules (and thereby preventing microtubule disassembly).

Microtubules have important physiologic roles in mitosis, intracellular protein trafficking, vesicular movement, and cell structure and shape. Mitosis is the physiologic role that is targeted pharmacologically; the other physiologic roles,

Figure 37-9. Telomere structure. Human telomeres are 2 to 30 kilobases (kb) in length and consist of the simple sequence repeats TTAGGG. A 3'-terminal 50- to 300-nucleotide (nt) single-stranded overhang is generated by an as yet unidentified nuclease. The telomere binding proteins TRF1, TRF2, and other factors facilitate folding and proximal invasion of double-stranded telomeric DNA by the single-stranded overhang to generate a stable "t-loop" structure. This structure plays an important role in capping and protecting the ends of chromosomes.

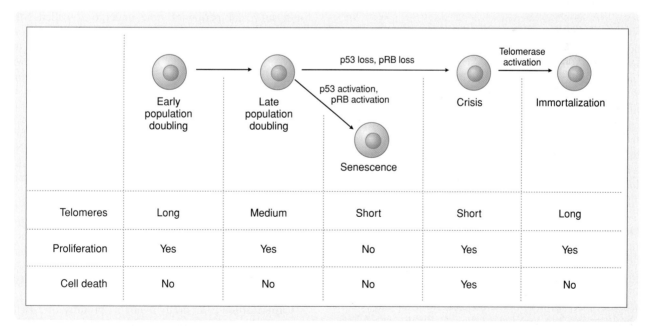

Figure 37-10. Chromosome maintenance and its relationship to immortalization. As primary cells undergo successive population doublings, telomeres progressively shorten due to the inability of DNA polymerase to replicate the ends of linear chromosomes. Ultimately, a checkpoint is triggered, mediated by the proteins p53 and pRB, which results in a state of growth arrest termed *cellular senescence.* Senescence can be bypassed by inactivation of p53 and pRB; ultimately, however, the critically short telomeres cause the cells to enter a state termed *crisis* and to die. Activation of telomerase allows cells to maintain adequate telomere length and divide indefinitely, resulting in immortalization. Notably, exogenous expression of telomerase alone in primary cells is sufficient for these cells to bypass senescence and become immortalized.

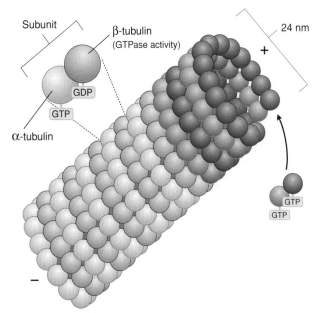

Figure 37-11. Microtubule structure. Microtubules are hollow cylindrical tubes that polymerize from tubulin subunits. Each tubulin subunit is a heterodimer composed of α-tubulin *(shades of gray)* and β-tubulin *(shades of blue)*. Both α-tubulin and β-tubulin bind GTP *(dark shades of gray and blue)*; β-tubulin hydrolyzes GTP to GDP after the tubulin subunit is added to the end of a microtubule *(lighter shades of gray and blue)*. Microtubules are dynamic structures that grow and shrink lengthwise; the cylindrical tubes are composed of 13 subunits arranged concentrically, resulting in a diameter of 24 nm. Note that microtubules have an inherent structural asymmetry. One end of a microtubule is limited by α-tubulin and is referred to as the (−) ("minus") end; the opposite end is limited by β-tubulin and is referred to as the (+) ("plus") end.

however, predict many of the adverse effects of drugs that interrupt microtubule function.

Recall that microtubules nucleate from centrosomes, which consist of centrioles and other associated proteins. In mitosis, the two centrosomes align at opposite ends of the cell. Microtubules are extremely dynamic during M phase; they grow and shrink during M phase at rates much greater than during other phases of the cell cycle. This increased dynamic instability during M phase allows microtubules to locate and attach to the chromosomes. The microtubules emanating from each centrosome bind to kinetochores, which are proteins that attach to the centromere of a chromosome. Once the kinetochore of each chromosome is attached to a microtubule, microtubule-associated proteins act as motors to align the kinetochore-bound chromosomes at the equator of the cell (defined by the midpoint between the two centrosomes). When every chromosome has aligned at the equator, the microtubules shorten, separating a diploid pair of chromosomes into each half of the cell. Finally, cytokinesis (division of the cytoplasm) occurs, and two daughter cells are formed. Although numerous other proteins are involved in the regulation of mitosis, microtubules have a critical role in the process. Disruption of microtubule function freezes cells in M phase, leading eventually to the activation of programmed cell death (apoptosis).

PHARMACOLOGIC CLASSES AND AGENTS

Traditional antineoplastic chemotherapy can be subdivided into several classes of agents. The antimetabolite drugs are compounds that either inhibit the enzymes involved in nucleotide synthesis and metabolism, or are incorporated as analogues into DNA and result in chain termination or strand breaks. These drugs act primarily during the S phase of the cell cycle, when cells are undergoing DNA replication. Another broad class of agents, which induce cytotoxicity by modification of DNA structure and generation of DNA damage, includes alkylating agents, platinum compounds, bleomycin, and topoisomerase inhibitors. These drugs exert their effects during multiple phases of the cell cycle. The final category of agents inhibits microtubule assembly or depolymerization, disrupting the mitotic spindle and interfering with mitosis.

INHIBITORS OF THYMIDYLATE SYNTHASE

Thymidylate (dTMP) is synthesized by the methylation of 2′-deoxyuridylate (dUMP). This reaction, which is catalyzed by thymidylate synthase, requires MTHF as a cofactor (Fig. 37-4). **5-Fluorouracil** (5-FU; Fig. 37-13) inhibits DNA synthesis, primarily by interfering with the biosynthesis of thymidylate. 5-FU is first converted to 5-fluoro-2′-deoxyuridylate (FdUMP) by the same pathways that convert uracil to dUMP. FdUMP then inhibits **thymidylate synthase** by forming, together with MTHF, a stable, covalent ternary enzyme-substrate-cofactor complex. Cells deprived of dTMP for a sufficient period of time undergo so-called "thymineless death." 5-FU can also be metabolized to floxuridine triphosphate (FUTP), which can be incorporated into mRNA in place of uridylate and can thereby interfere with RNA processing. Either inhibition of thymidylate synthase by FdUMP, or interference with RNA processing by FUTP, or a combination of the two mechanisms, could explain the toxic effect of 5-FU on cells. Recent evidence, however, demonstrates that certain 5-FU congeners, which inhibit thymidylate synthase but are not incorporated into RNA, show antitumor efficacy similar to that of 5-FU. This finding points to thymidylate synthase inhibition as the dominant mechanism of 5-FU action.

5-FU is used as an antineoplastic agent, especially in the treatment of carcinomas of the breast and gastrointestinal tract. 5-FU has also been used in the topical treatment of premalignant keratoses of the skin and of multiple superficial basal-cell carcinomas. Because 5-FU depletes thymidylate from normal cells as well as cancer cells, this agent is highly toxic and must be used with care.

Capecitabine is an orally available prodrug of 5-FU. It is absorbed across the gastrointestinal mucosa and converted by a series of three enzymatic reactions to 5-FU. Capecitabine is approved for the treatment of metastatic colorectal cancer and as second-line therapy in metastatic breast cancer. Clinical trials have demonstrated that the efficacy of oral capecitabine is similar to that of intravenous 5-FU.

Elucidation of the mechanism of action of 5-FU has led

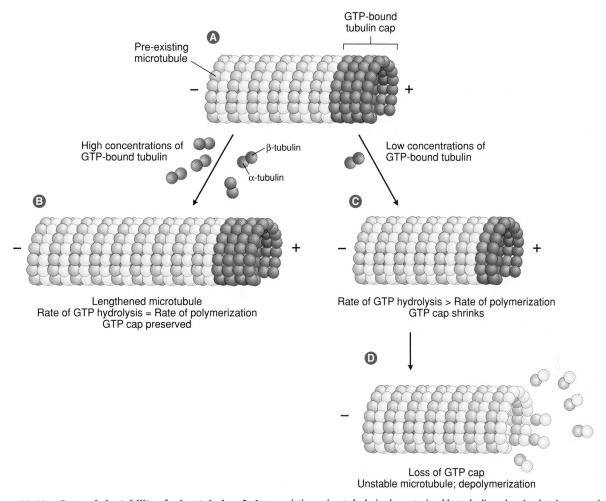

Figure 37-12. Dynamic instability of microtubules. A. A pre-existing microtubule is characterized by tubulin subunits that have predominantly hydrolyzed the GTP on β-tubulin to GDP *(light gray and light blue)*. However, β-tubulin subunits that have recently been added to the microtubule have not yet hydrolyzed GTP *(dark gray and dark blue)*. The GTP-bound tubulin subunits form a GTP-bound tubulin cap at the (+) end of the microtubule. **B.** In the presence of a high concentration of GTP-bound free tubulin subunits, new GTP-bound tubulin is added to the (+) end of the microtubule at a rate that equals or exceeds the rate of GTP hydrolysis by β-tubulin. Maintenance of a GTP-bound tubulin cap results in a stable microtubule. **C.** In the presence of a low concentration of GTP-bound free tubulin subunits, new GTP-bound tubulin is added to the (+) end of the microtubule at a rate less than the rate of GTP hydrolysis by β-tubulin. This results in shrinkage of the GTP-bound tubulin cap. **D.** A microtubule that lacks a GTP-bound tubulin cap is unstable and undergoes depolymerization.

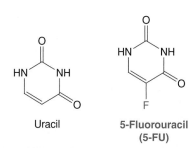

Figure 37-13. Structures of uracil and 5-fluorouracil. Note the structural similarity between uracil and 5-fluorouracil (5-FU). Uracil is the base in dUMP, the endogenous substrate for thymidylate synthase (see Fig. 37-4), and 5-FU is metabolized to FdUMP, an irreversible inhibitor of thymidylate synthase.

to the use of a **5-FU/folinic acid** (leucovorin) combination as first-line chemotherapy for colorectal cancer. Because 5-FU inhibits thymidylate synthase by forming a ternary complex involving the enzyme (thymidylate synthase), substrate (5-FdUMP), and cofactor MTHF, it was hypothesized that increasing the levels of MTHF would potentiate the activity of 5-FU. Clinical trials proved this hypothesis to be correct, by showing that the efficacy of the combined regimen is greater than that of 5-FU alone. This is an important example of the use of mechanistic knowledge to improve the clinical effectiveness of a drug.

Pemetrexed is a folate analogue that, similar to endogenous folate and the dihydrofolate reductase (DHFR) inhibitor methotrexate (see Chapter 31), is transported into cells by the reduced folate carrier and polyglutamated by the intracellular enzyme folylpolyglutamate synthase. Polyglutamated pemetrexed is a potent inhibitor of thymidylate synthase and a much weaker inhibitor of DHFR; similar to 5-FU, its cytotoxic effect is likely due to the induction of "thymineless" cell death. (Note that the 5-FU derivative 5-FdUMP inhibits thymidylate synthase by binding to the dUMP [substrate] site on the enzyme, whereas pemetrexed inhibits thymidylate synthase by binding to the MTHF [cofactor] site on the enzyme.) Pemetrexed is approved as a single agent in the second-line treatment of nonsmall cell lung cancer and in combination with cisplatin (see below) in the treatment of malignant pleural mesothelioma. To reduce toxicity to normal cells, patients treated with pemetrexed are also given folic acid and vitamin B_{12} supplementation.

INHIBITORS OF PURINE METABOLISM

6-Mercaptopurine (6-MP) and **azathioprine** (AZA), a prodrug that is nonenzymatically converted to 6-MP in tissues, are inosine analogues that inhibit interconversions among purine nucleotides (Fig. 37-14). 6-Mercaptopurine contains a sulfur atom in place of the keto group at C-6 of the purine ring. After its entry into cells, mercaptopurine is converted by the enzyme **hypoxanthine-guanine phosphoribosyl transferase** (HGPRT, see Chapter 47) to the nucleotide form, 6-thioinosine-5′-monophosphate (T-IMP). T-IMP is thought to inhibit purine nucleotide synthesis by several mechanisms. First, T-IMP inhibits the enzymes that convert IMP to AMP and GMP, including inosine monophosphate dehydrogenase (IMPDH) (Fig. 37-3). Second, T-IMP (as

with AMP and GMP) is a "feedback" inhibitor of the enzyme that synthesizes phosphoribosylamine, which is the first step in purine nucleotide synthesis. Both of these mechanisms lead to marked decreases in the cellular levels of AMP and GMP, which are essential metabolites for DNA synthesis, RNA synthesis, energy storage, cell signaling, and other functions. 6-MP may also inhibit DNA and RNA synthesis by less well-characterized mechanisms.

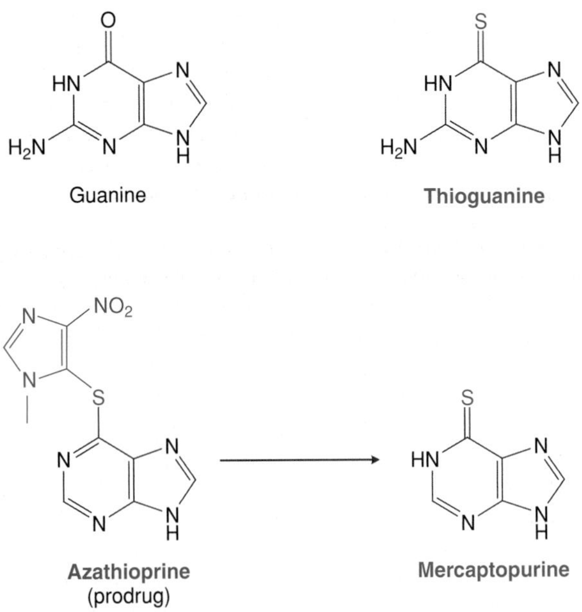

The major clinical application of 6-MP is in acute lymphoblastic leukemia (ALL), especially in the maintenance phase of a prolonged combination chemotherapy regimen. 6-MP is also active against normal lymphocytes and can be used as an immunosuppressive agent. For unknown reasons, the prodrug AZA is a superior immunosuppressant compared to 6-MP and is typically the drug of choice for this application. AZA is discussed in detail in Chapter 44, Pharmacology of Immunosuppression.

Both the effectiveness and the toxicity of 6-MP are potentiated by **allopurinol.** Allopurinol inhibits xanthine oxidase, thereby preventing the oxidation of 6-MP to its inactive metabolite 6-thiouric acid. (In fact, allopurinol was discovered in an effort to inhibit the metabolism of 6-MP by xanthine oxidase.) Coadministration of allopurinol with 6-MP allows the dose of 6-MP to be reduced by two-thirds (although toxicity is proportionally increased as well). Allopurinol is often used as a single agent to prevent the hyperuricemia that could result from the destruction of cancer cells by chemotherapeutic agents (**tumor lysis syndrome**). The use of allopurinol in the treatment of gout is presented in Chapter 47, Integrative Inflammation Pharmacology: Gout.

Pentostatin (Fig. 37-15) is a selective inhibitor of ADA. The drug is a structural analogue of the intermediate in the reaction catalyzed by ADA and binds to the enzyme with high affinity. The resulting inhibition of ADA causes an increase in intracellular adenosine and 2′-deoxyadenosine levels. The increased adenosine and 2′-deoxyadenosine have multiple effects on purine nucleotide metabolism. In particular, 2′-deoxyadenosine irreversibly inhibits S-adenosylhomocysteine hydrolase, and the resulting increase in intracellular S-adenosylhomocysteine is toxic to lymphocytes. This action may account for the effectiveness of pentostatin against some leukemias and lymphomas. Pentostatin is especially effective against hairy cell leukemia.

INHIBITORS OF RIBONUCLEOTIDE REDUCTASE

Hydroxyurea inhibits ribonucleotide reductase by scavenging a tyrosyl radical at the active site of the enzyme. In the absence of this free radical, ribonucleotide reductase is unable to convert nucleotides to deoxynucleotides, and DNA synthesis is thereby inhibited.

Hydroxyurea is approved for use in the treatment of adult sickle cell disease and certain neoplastic diseases. The mechanism of action of hydroxyurea in the treatment of sickle cell disease may or may not be related to inhibition of ribonucleotide reductase. As an alternative to this mechanism, hydroxyurea has been shown to increase the expression of the fetal isoform of hemoglobin (HbF), which inhibits the polymerization of sickle hemoglobin (HbS) and thereby decreases red blood cell sickling under conditions of hypoxia.

Figure 37-14. Structures of guanine, thioguanine, azathioprine, and mercaptopurine. Thioguanine, azathioprine, and mercaptopurine are structural analogues of purines. Thioguanine resembles guanine and can be ribosylated and phosphorylated in parallel with endogenous nucleotides. The nucleotide forms of thioguanine irreversibly inhibit IMPDH (see Fig. 37-3) and, upon incorporation into DNA, inhibit DNA replication. Azathioprine is a prodrug form of mercaptopurine; azathioprine reacts with sulfhydryl compounds in the liver (e.g., glutathione) to release mercaptopurine. The nucleotide form of mercaptopurine, thioinosine monophosphate (T-IMP), inhibits the enzymes that convert IMP to AMP and GMP (see Fig. 37-3). T-IMP also inhibits the first committed step in purine nucleotide synthesis.

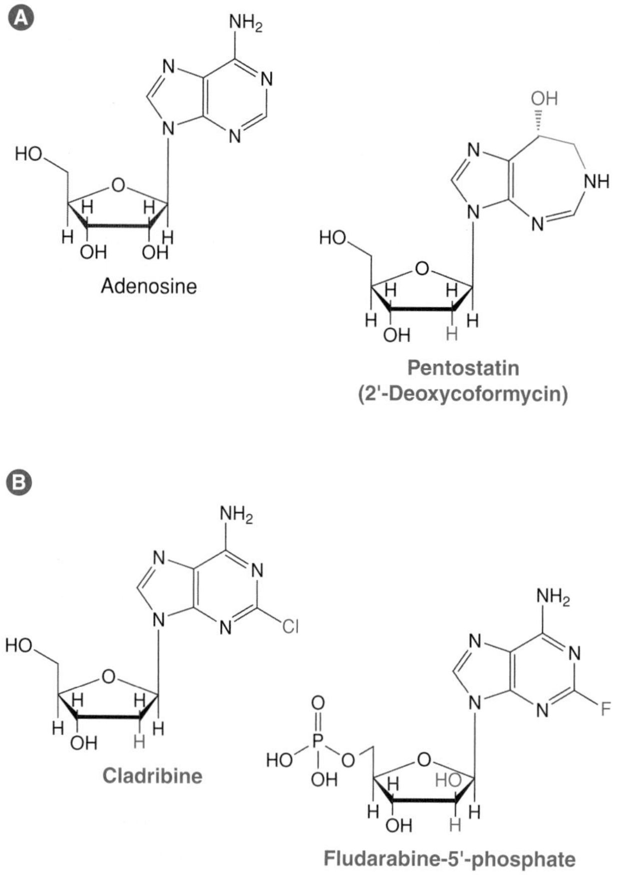

Figure 37-15. Structures of adenosine, pentostatin, cladribine, and flurabine. A. Pentostatin inhibits adenosine deaminase (ADA), the enzyme that converts adenosine and 2′-deoxyadenosine to inosine and 2′-deoxyinosine, respectively. Pentostatin binds to ADA with very high affinity ($K_d = 2.5 \times 10^{-12}$ M) because it structurally resembles the intermediate (transition state) in this enzymatic reaction. **B.** Cladribine and fludarabine-5′-phosphate are also adenosine analogues. Cladribine is a chlorinated purine analogue that is incorporated into DNA and causes DNA strand breaks. Fludarabine phosphate is a fluorinated purine analogue that is incorporated into DNA and RNA; this drug also inhibits DNA polymerase and ribonucleotide reductase.

Hydroxyurea significantly decreases the incidence of painful (vaso-occlusive) crisis in patients with sickle cell disease. The mechanism by which hydroxyurea increases HbF production is unknown. The role of hydroxyurea in the treatment of sickle cell anemia is discussed further in Chapter 43, Pharmacology of Hematopoiesis and Immunomodulation.

The neoplastic applications of hydroxyurea include head and neck cancer and myeloproliferative disorders such as polycythemia vera and essential thrombocytosis. In head and neck cancer, hydroxyurea is used as a radiosensitizing agent (i.e., an agent that increases the effectiveness of radiation therapy). The mechanism of radiosensitization is unknown; current theories suggest that hydroxyurea could increase tumor cell sensitivity to radiation by decreasing DNA repair or by synchronizing the cell-cycle timing of tumor cells. In myeloproliferative disorders, hydroxyurea can be used as a single agent or in combination with other agents to inhibit the excessive growth of myeloid cells in the bone marrow. The applications of hydroxyurea for these indications have been limited somewhat by concerns that long-term hydroxyurea use may be leukemogenic; this is an example of the phenomenon that certain antitumor agents can also cause cancer.

PURINE AND PYRIMIDINE ANALOGUES THAT ARE INCORPORATED INTO DNA

A number of antimetabolites exert their major therapeutic effect by acting as "rogue" nucleotides. These drugs are substrates for the various pathways of nucleotide metabolism, including ribosylation, ribonucleotide reduction, and nucleoside and nucleotide phosphorylation. The sugar triphosphate forms of these drugs can then be incorporated into DNA. Once incorporated into DNA, these compounds disrupt the structure of DNA, resulting in DNA chain termination, DNA strand breakage, and inhibition of cell growth. **Thioguanine** is a guanine analogue in which a sulfur atom replaces the oxygen atom at C-6 of the purine ring (Fig. 37-14). As with mercaptopurine, thioguanine is converted by HGPRT to its nucleotide form, 6-thioguanosine-5′-monophosphate (6-thioGMP). Unlike T-IMP, the nucleotide form of mercaptopurine, 6-thioGMP is a good substrate for guanylyl kinase, the enzyme that catalyzes the conversion of GMP to GTP. By this mechanism, 6-thioGMP is converted to 6-thioGTP, which is incorporated into DNA. Within the structure of DNA, 6-thioGTP interferes with RNA transcription and DNA replication, resulting in cell death. 6-ThioGMP also irreversibly inhibits IMPDH and thereby depletes cellular pools of GMP (Fig. 37-3). Thioguanine is used in the treatment of acute myelocytic leukemia. Major adverse effects of thioguanine include bone marrow suppression and gastrointestinal injury.

Fludarabine phosphate (Fig. 37-15) is a fluorinated purine nucleotide analogue that is structurally related to the antiviral agent vidarabine (see Chapter 36, Pharmacology of Viral Infections). The triphosphate form of fludarabine is incorporated into DNA and RNA, causing DNA chain termination. Fludarabine triphosphate also inhibits DNA polymerase and ribonucleotide reductase and thereby decreases nucleotide and nucleic acid synthesis in cells. The relative importance of these actions in mediating the cellular toxicity of the drug remains to be elucidated. Fludarabine phosphate is used in the treatment of lymphoproliferative disorders, especially chronic lymphocytic leukemia (CLL) and low-grade B-cell lymphomas.

Cladribine is a chlorinated purine analogue that is structurally related to fludarabine phosphate (Fig. 37-15). Cladribine triphosphate is incorporated into DNA, causing strand breaks. Cladribine also depletes intracellular pools of the essential purine metabolites NAD and ATP. Cladribine is approved for use in the treatment of hairy cell leukemia and has been used experimentally in the treatment of other types of leukemia and lymphoma.

Cytarabine (araC) is a cytidine analogue that is metabolized to araCTP (Fig. 37-16). AraCTP competes with CTP for DNA polymerase, and incorporation of araCTP into DNA results in chain termination and cell death (Fig. 37-

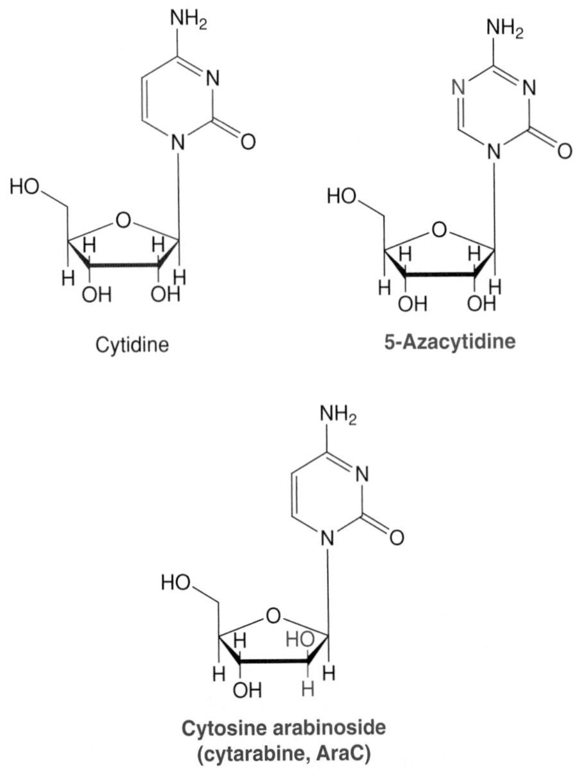

Figure 37-16. Structures of cytidine, cytarabine, and azacytidine. Cytarabine and azacytidine are both analogues of the nucleoside cytidine. Cytarabine has an arabinose sugar in place of ribose (note the chirality of the hydroxyl group *highlighted in blue*). The incorporation of cytarabine triphosphate (araCTP) into DNA inhibits further nucleic acid synthesis, because the replacement of 2′-deoxyribose by arabinose interrupts strand elongation. Azacytidine has an azide group *(highlighted in blue)* within the pyrimidine ring; this drug is incorporated into nucleic acids and interferes with the methylation of cytosine bases.

4). Synergism between cytarabine and cyclophosphamide has been noted, presumably because of the reduced DNA repair caused by cytarabine's inhibition of DNA polymerase. Cytarabine is used to induce and maintain remission in acute myelocytic leukemia; it is especially effective for this indication when combined with an anthracycline.

5-Azacytidine is a cytidine analogue whose triphosphate metabolite is incorporated into DNA and RNA (Fig. 37-16). Once incorporated into DNA, azacytidine interferes with cytosine methylation, altering gene expression and promoting cell differentiation. Azacytidine is currently used in the treatment of myelodysplasia and is under investigation for use in the treatment of acute leukemias.

Gemcitabine is a fluorinated cytidine analogue in which the hydrogen atoms on the 2′ carbon of deoxycytidine are replaced by fluorine atoms. The diphosphate form of gemcitabine inhibits ribonucleotide reductase; the triphosphate form of gemcitabine is incorporated into DNA, interfering with DNA replication and resulting in cell death. Gemcitabine is active in several solid tumors, including pancreatic cancer and nonsmall cell lung cancer, and is being evaluated in regimens for hematologic malignancies such as Hodgkin's disease.

AGENTS THAT DIRECTLY MODIFY DNA STRUCTURE

Alkylating Agents

The advent of modern chemotherapy dates to the 1940s, when highly reactive alkylating agents were first noted to induce remissions in otherwise untreatable malignancies. The clinical use of these agents was sparked by observations in sailors who had inadvertently been exposed to nitrogen mustards during World War II. These men were found to have dramatic suppression of their hematopoietic cells, suggesting that alkylating agents could have therapeutic utility in blood-derived malignancies such as leukemias and lymphomas. Soon thereafter, it was suggested that alkylating agents could also be useful in treating epithelial tumors, mesenchymal tumors, carcinomas, and sarcomas; in fact, alkylating agents are commonly used against all of these diseases today.

Alkylating agents—such as **cyclophosphamide, mechlorethamine, melphalan, chlorambucil,** and **thiotepa**—are electrophilic molecules that are attacked by nucleophilic sites on DNA, resulting in the covalent attachment of an alkyl group to the nucleophilic site. Depending on the particular agent, alkylation can take place on nitrogen or oxygen atoms of the base, the phosphate backbone, or a DNA-associated protein. The N-7 and O-6 atoms of guanine bases are particularly susceptible to alkylation. Alkylating agents typically have two strong leaving groups (Fig. 37-17). This structure confers the ability to *bis*-alkylate (perform two alkylating reactions), enabling the agent to crosslink the DNA molecule either to itself—by linking two guanine residues, for example—or to proteins. *Bis*-alkylation (crosslinking) seems to be the major mechanism of cytotoxicity (Fig. 37-18A). Alkylation of guanine residues can also result in cleavage of the guanine imidazole ring, in abnormal base-pairing between the alkylated guanine and thymine, or in depurination (i.e., excision of the guanine residue) (Fig. 32-18B–D). Ring cleavage disrupts the molecular structure of DNA; anomalous DNA base-pairing causes miscoding and mutation; and depurination leads to scission of the sugar-phosphate DNA backbone. Importantly, the mutations caused by these processes can increase the risk of developing new cancers.

Although all nitrogen mustards are relatively reactive, the

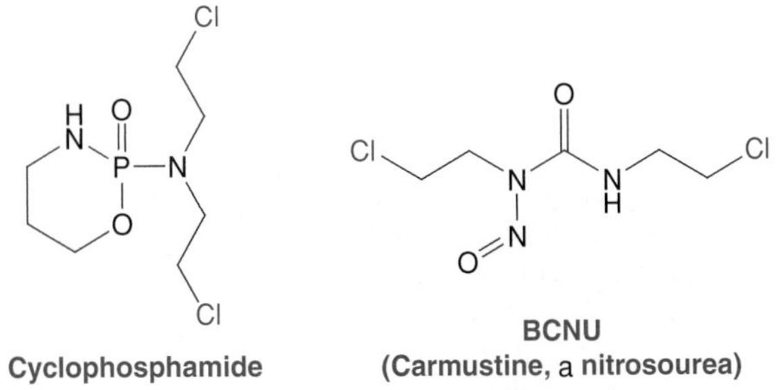

Figure 37-17. Structures of cyclophosphamide and BCNU. Cyclophosphamide and BCNU (carmustine) each have two chloride leaving groups. The presence of two leaving groups allows these alkylating agents to *bis*-alkylate and thereby crosslink macromolecules such as DNA. The ability to crosslink DNA is crucial to the DNA damage caused by these agents.

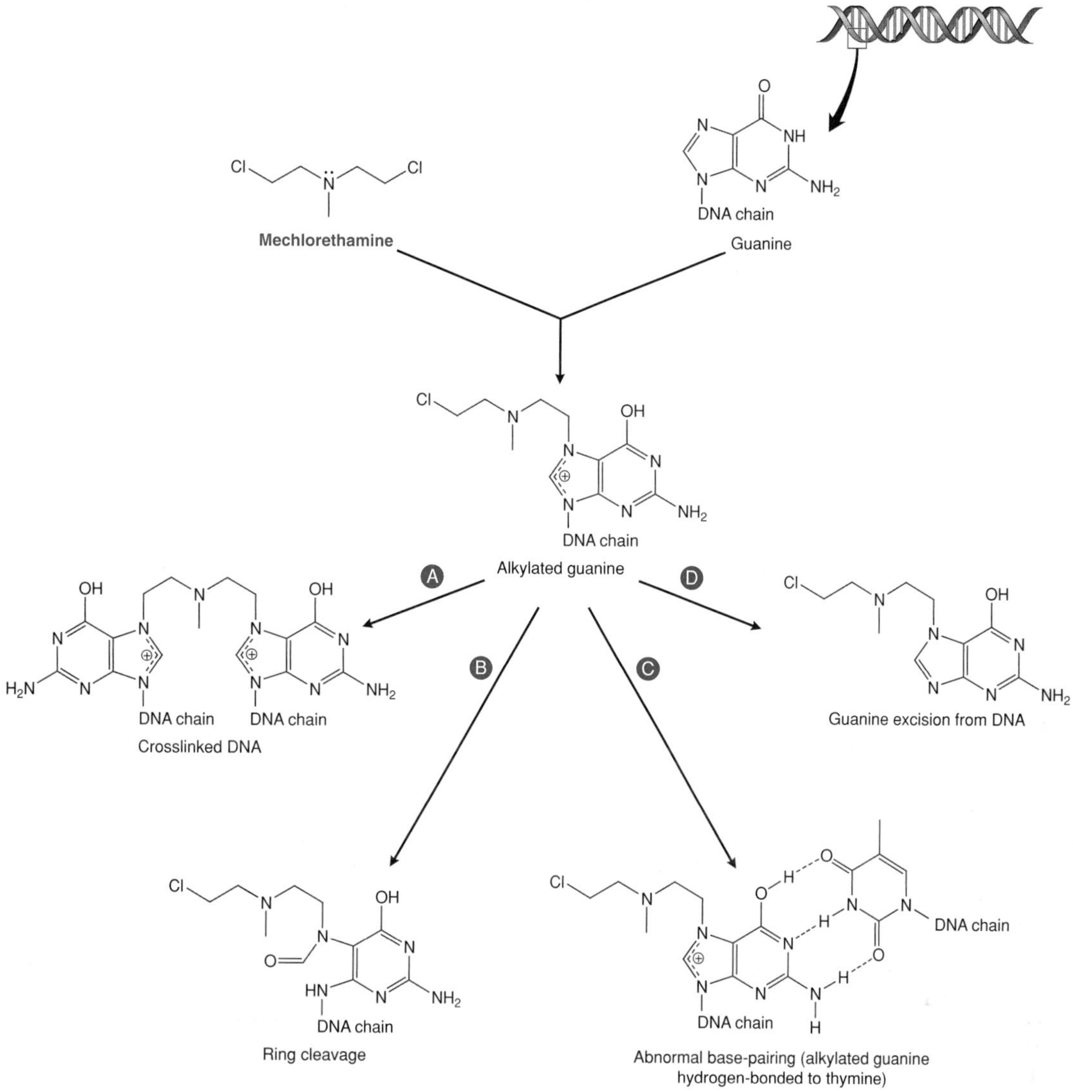

Figure 37-18. Biochemical outcomes of guanine alkylation. In reactions such as those exemplified here with mechlorethamine, guanine alkylation can cause several types of DNA damage. The nitrogen of mechlorethamine performs a nucleophilic attack on one of its own β-carbons, resulting in an unstable intermediate that is highly electrophilic *(not shown)*. The nucleophilic N-7 of guanine reacts with this unstable intermediate, resulting in an alkylated guanine. There are four potential outcomes that can result from this initial alkylation, all of which cause structural damage to DNA. **A.** The process of alkylation can be repeated, with a second guanine acting as a nucleophile. The resulting crosslinking of DNA appears to be a major mechanism by which alkylating agents damage DNA. **B.** Cleavage of the imidazole ring disrupts the structure of the guanine base. **C.** The alkylated guanine can hydrogen-bond to thymine rather than cytosine, leading to a mutation in the DNA. **D.** Excision of the alkylated guanine residue results in a depurinated DNA strand.

individual agents vary in the speed with which they react with nucleophiles; this fact has significant impact on their clinical use. Highly unstable compounds, such as mechlorethamine, cannot be administered orally because such agents alkylate target molecules within seconds to minutes. Because of this high reactivity, these molecules are powerful vesicants (causing blisters) and can severely damage skin and soft tissue if they leak outside of blood vessels. The rapid reactivity of alkylating agents can be exploited by infusing the drug directly into the site of a tumor. For example, thiotepa can be instilled into the bladder to treat superficial bladder cancers. In contrast to mechlorethamine and thiotepa, chlorambucil and melphalan are much less reactive and can be administered orally. Cyclophosphamide is particularly useful because it is a nonreactive prodrug that requires acti-

vation by the hepatic cytochrome P450 system; this agent can be administered either orally or intravenously (Fig. 37-19).

Nitrosoureas, such as BCNU (**carmustine**), target DNA in much the same way as do cyclophosphamide and other alkylating agents. Like cyclophosphamide, these compounds require bioactivation. Unlike most alkylating agents, however, nitrosoureas also attach carbamoyl groups to their DNA-associated targets. It is not clear whether carbamoylation contributes significantly to the activity of nitrosoureas.

Some alkylating agents are better than others at targeting specific tumors. For example, nitrosoureas are useful in the treatment of brain tumors, because their high lipid solubility enables them to cross the blood-brain barrier. Similarly, the alkylating antibiotic **mitomycin** targets hypoxic tumor cells,

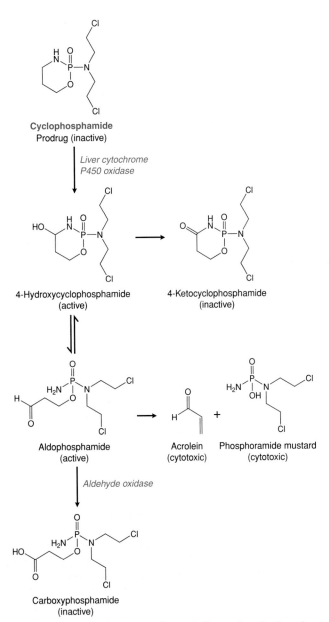

Cyclophosphamide
Prodrug (inactive)

*Liver cytochrome
P450 oxidase*

4-Hydroxycyclophosphamide
(active)

4-Ketocyclophosphamide
(inactive)

Aldophosphamide
(active)

Acrolein
(cytotoxic)

Phosphoramide mustard
(cytotoxic)

Aldehyde oxidase

Carboxyphosphamide
(inactive)

Figure 37-19. Activation and metabolism of cyclophospha-mide. Cyclophosphamide is a prodrug that must be oxidized by P450 enzymes in the liver to become pharmacologically active. Hydroxylation converts cyclophosphamide to 4-hydroxycyclophosphamide; this active metabolite can be further oxidized to the inactive metabolite 4-ketocyclophosphamide, or undergo ring cleavage to the active metabolite aldophosphamide. Aldophosphamide can be oxidized by aldehyde oxidase to the inactive metabolite carboxyphosphamide or be converted to the highly toxic metabolites acrolein and phosphoramide mustard. Accumulation of acrolein in the bladder can cause hemorrhagic cystitis; this adverse effect of cyclophosphamide can be ameliorated by coadministration of mesna, a sulfhydryl compound that inactivates the acrolein *(not shown).*

combination chemotherapy regimen for Hodgkin's disease. Dacarbazine also has some activity in treating melanoma and sarcomas. **Procarbazine** is an orally active drug that is used against Hodgkin's disease. A metabolite of procarbazine functions as a monoamine oxidase inhibitor, and toxicity related to this activity—such as tyramine sensitivity, hypotension, and dry mouth—can occur. Finally, **altretamine** is useful for treating refractory ovarian cancer. Although it is structurally related to alkylating agents of the triethylenemelamine class (such as thiotepa), whether the mechanism of action of this drug involves DNA alkylation remains controversial.

Through natural selection, tumor cells can develop resistance to a single alkylating agent as well as cross-resistance to other drugs in the same class. Several mechanisms for resistance have been reported. Highly reactive drugs can be deactivated by intracellular nucleophiles such as **glutathione.** Alternatively, cells can become resistant by reducing uptake of the drug or accelerating DNA repair. One enzyme, **O^6-alkylguanine-DNA alkyltransferase**, prevents permanent DNA damage by removing alkyl adducts to the O^6 position of guanine before DNA crosslinks are formed. Increased expression of this enzyme in neoplastic cells is associated with resistance to alkylating agents.

Alkylating agent toxicity is dose-dependent and can be severe. As a rule, adverse effects result from damage to DNA of normal cells. Three cell types are preferentially affected by alkylating agents. First, toxicity typically manifests in rapidly proliferating tissues, such as bone marrow, gastrointestinal and genitourinary tract epithelium, and hair follicles. This results in myelosuppression, gastrointestinal distress, and alopecia (hair loss). Second, organ-specific toxicity can result from low activity of a DNA damage repair pathway in that tissue. Third, a tissue can be preferentially affected because the toxic compound accumulates in that tissue; for example, **acrolein** (a by-product of the activation of cyclophosphamide or its analogue **ifosfamide**) can produce hemorrhagic cystitis because of accumulation and concentration in the bladder. This toxicity can be treated by using the sulfhydryl-containing molecule **mesna,** which is also concentrated in the urine and rapidly inactivates the acrolein.

The immune response requires rapid proliferation of lymphocytes; this makes lymphocytes especially vulnerable to damage by alkylating agents. Thus, in addition to their anticancer activity, alkylating agents such as cyclophosphamide are also effective at immunosuppression. This ''toxicity'' has been put to clinical use: when administered at doses lower than those needed for antineoplastic therapy, alkylating agents are used to treat autoimmune diseases and organ rejection (see Chapter 44, Pharmacology of Immunosuppression).

One approach to limiting toxicity has been to develop agents that accumulate preferentially inside tumor cells. An example of one such agent is melphalan, or phenylalanine mustard; this agent was designed to target melanoma cells, which accumulate phenylalanine for the biosynthesis of melanin. Another example is **estramustine,** in which the mustard component is conjugated to estrogen; this agent was designed to target breast cancer cells that express the estrogen receptor. Interestingly, neither melphalan nor estramustine works as intended, although they both have clinical utility; through mechanisms that are still poorly understood,

such as those at the center of a solid tumor, because it requires bioreductive activation, which occurs more readily in low-oxygen environments.

Three nonclassical alkylating agents also deserve mention as clinically useful drugs. The first is **dacarbazine,** a synthetic molecule that is a component of a potentially curative

melphalan is active against multiple myeloma, and estramustine is used to treat prostate cancer.

Platinum Compounds

The introduction of **cisplatin** (*cis*-diaminedichloroplatinum [II]) into clinical use in the 1970s transformed previously intractable tumors, such as testicular cancer, into curable ones. As with the alkylating agents, the anticancer properties of cisplatin were discovered by a chance observation. While studying the effects of electricity on bacteria, it was found that a product of the platinum electrode was inhibiting DNA synthesis in the microbes. The compound was purified and found to be cisplatin, which consists of a platinum atom bound to two amines and two chlorines in the *cis* conformation. This serendipitous finding led to the clinical use of cisplatin, which is now the most active drug used to treat testicular cancer (see the case of J. L.). As an antitumor agent, cisplatin is thought to act similarly to *bis*-alkylating agents (i.e., alkylating agents with two leaving groups) by targeting nucleophilic centers in guanine (N-7 and O-6), adenine (N-1 and N-3), and cytosine (N-3).

The *cis* conformation of cisplatin (Fig. 37-20) allows the drug to form intrastrand crosslinks between adjacent guanine residues, resulting in DNA damage (Fig. 37-21B). This structural feature is critical to the action of cisplatin; the *trans* isomer, although capable of binding covalently to DNA, has little antitumor activity. Tumor cells can develop resistance to cisplatin by enhancing the repair of DNA lesions, decreasing drug uptake, or enhancing drug inactivation through up-regulated synthesis of nucleophiles such as glutathione.

As J. L.'s case demonstrates, cisplatin is efficacious in the treatment of genitourinary cancers, including cancers of the testis, bladder, and ovary. Cisplatin and the related compound **carboplatin** (Fig. 37-20) are also among the most efficacious drugs used against lung cancer. As with many chemotherapeutic agents, the rationale for the efficacy of cisplatin and carboplatin in the treatment of certain tumor types over others is not clear.

Cisplatin can be administered intravenously, but it can also be effective when exposed directly to tumor cells. One example is in treating ovarian cancer, which spreads along the inner lining of the peritoneal cavity. For this application, cisplatin can be infused directly into the peritoneal cavity to achieve high local concentrations of the drug while decreasing systemic toxicity.

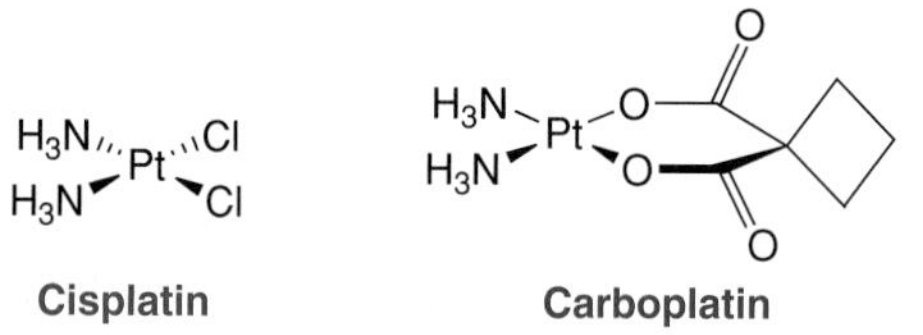

Figure 37-20. Structures of cisplatin and carboplatin. Cisplatin and carboplatin are coordinated complexes of platinum (Pt). The *cis* structure of these molecules (i.e., the presence of the two leaving groups on the same side of the molecule, rather than on opposite corners) provides them with the ability to crosslink adjacent guanines on the same DNA strand (intrastrand crosslink) or, much less frequently, on opposite DNA strands (interstrand crosslink). Similar compounds with *trans* conformations cannot effectively crosslink adjacent guanines.

J. L.'s oncologist considered cisplatin toxicities carefully in determining the dose of this drug to administer and the other agents that would be included in the combination chemotherapy regimen. Because the dose-limiting toxicities of cisplatin, bleomycin, and etoposide differ from one another, each of these drugs could be used at the maximum tolerated dose (see Chapter 39, Principles of Combination Chemotherapy). For cisplatin, the dose-limiting toxicity is **nephrotoxicity.** Gastrointestinal symptoms such as nausea and vomiting are also common; this is of concern because dehydration due to protracted vomiting can exacerbate cisplatin-induced kidney damage and lead to irreversible renal failure. Neurotoxicity, primarily manifested as paresthesias of the hands and feet and hearing loss, also occur frequently. Thiol-containing compounds, such as **amifostine,** can ameliorate cisplatin nephrotoxicity without diminishing its antitumor effects. **Carboplatin,** a cisplatin analogue associated with less nephrotoxicity, has replaced cisplatin in many chemotherapy regimens. **Oxaliplatin,** a third platinum compound, has activity in the treatment of colorectal cancer. Like cisplatin, oxaliplatin causes cumulative neurotoxicity; oxaliplatin also induces a unique acute neurotoxicity that is exacerbated by exposure to cold temperatures.

Bleomycin

The **bleomycins,** a family of natural glycopeptides synthesized by a species of *Streptomyces,* have prominent cytotoxic activity. A mixture of several of these glycopeptides, differing only in side chains, is used clinically (Fig. 37-21A). Bleomycin binds DNA and chelates iron (II), leading to the formation of free radicals that cause single- and double-strand DNA breaks. As with many chemotherapeutic agents, multidrug resistance mechanisms, such as increased drug efflux from tumor cells, can reduce tumor susceptibility to bleomycin.

In chelating iron, bleomycin forms a heme-like ring. It is believed that the chelated complex abstracts a hydrogen radical from the 4′ position of a nearby pyrimidine residue (thymine or cytosine). The unstable intermediate decomposes in the presence of oxygen to produce an abstracted pyrimidine and a free phosphodiester at one or both DNA strands (Fig. 37-21A).

Relative to other DNA-damaging agents, bleomycin causes less myelosuppressive toxicity. Because of its reactivity with oxygen, however, bleomycin can cause **pulmonary fibrosis,** the drug's most problematic and dose-limiting toxicity. The effects of bleomycin on pulmonary function are cumulative and irreversible. Therefore, this agent's use is largely restricted to potentially curative combination chemotherapy regimens for testicular carcinoma and Hodgkin's disease. In J. L.'s case, it was concern regarding pulmonary toxicity that led his physician to monitor his lung function closely throughout therapy and to inquire about shortness of breath on each visit. Worsening lung function would have required adjustments in J. L.'s therapy.

TOPOISOMERASE INHIBITORS

Several chemotherapeutic agents damage DNA by exploiting the natural nuclease/ligase function of topoisomerases;

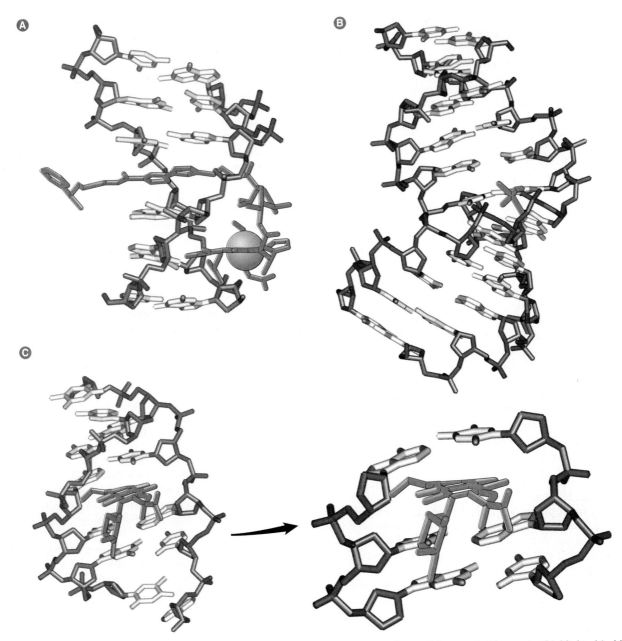

Figure 37-21. Interactions of bleomycin, platinum compounds, and anthracyclines with DNA. A. Bleomycin *(highlighted in blue)* binds to the DNA double helix and thereby exposes nucleotides in the DNA to the iron (II) atom *(large blue ball)* that is complexed to bleomycin. In the presence of molecular oxygen, the iron–bleomycin complex generates activated oxygen species that cause single-stranded and double-stranded breaks in the DNA by a free radical mechanism. **B.** Platinum complexes *(highlighted in blue)* crosslink N-7 atoms on adjacent guanine residues, forming intrastrand DNA crosslinks. **C.** Daunorubicin, an anthracycline *(highlighted in blue)*, intercalates into DNA structure *(see expanded view on right)* and thereby prevents the strand passage and religation steps that are part of the catalytic cycle of type II topoisomerase (see Fig. 32-4). Anthracyclines may also damage DNA by a free radical mechanism.

the basic physiology of this process is discussed in Chapter 32. The antineoplastic **camptothecins, anthracyclines, epipodophyllotoxins,** and **amsacrine** act in this manner. These compounds interfere with the proper function of topoisomerases and cause cellular topoisomerases to participate in DNA destruction.

Camptothecins

The camptothecins are semisynthetic molecules derived from alkaloid extracts of *Camptotheca* plants. Camptothe-

cins target **topoisomerase I**, causing DNA strand damage.

Topoisomerase I modulates supercoiling by complexing with DNA and nicking one of its two strands (see Fig. 32-3). The camptothecins act by stabilizing this nicked DNA complex and preventing topoisomerase I from religating the strand break. Other replication enzymes then bind to the camptothecin-DNA-topoisomerase complex, converting the single-strand DNA lesion to a double-strand break. Neoplastic cells are often unable to repair the resulting damage.

Two camptothecin derivatives, **irinotecan** and **topotecan,** have clinical utility. Irinotecan was initially introduced for the treatment of advanced colon cancer, although it may also be effective in treating other tumor types. It is a water-soluble prodrug that is cleaved by the enzyme carboxylesterase to release the lipophilic metabolite **SN-38**. Although SN-38 is approximately 1,000-fold more active than irinotecan in inhibiting topoisomerase I, it is more highly protein-bound than irinotecan and has a much shorter half-life in vivo. Thus, the relative contribution of SN-38 to the anticancer effects of irinotecan is unclear. Irinotecan use is limited by severe gastrointestinal toxicity, leading to potentially life-threatening diarrhea. As with many other chemotherapeutic agents, irinotecan also causes dose-dependent bone marrow suppression.

Topotecan has been used in the treatment of metastatic ovarian cancer, small cell lung cancer, and other neoplasms. Specifically, this agent has shown effectiveness in treating ovarian neoplasms that are resistant to cisplatin, which are otherwise difficult to treat effectively.

Anthracyclines

Anthracyclines, natural antitumor antibiotics isolated from a species of the fungus *Streptomyces,* are among the most clinically useful cytotoxic cancer chemotherapeutic agents. Although several mechanisms appear to be involved in their activity, the ability of the anthracyclines to damage DNA most likely results from their intercalation into DNA (Fig. 37-21C). This intercalation interferes with the action of **topoisomerase II**, resulting in DNA lesions such as strand scission and, ultimately, in cell death (see Fig. 32-4).

As with many other antineoplastic agents, anthracyclines cause myelosuppression and alopecia. Anthracyclines are excreted in bile, and their dose must be reduced in patients with hepatic dysfunction. These agents are major components of chemotherapy regimens for a variety of malignancies, particularly hematologic cancers (such as leukemias and lymphomas) and breast cancer.

The best known drug in this group, **doxorubicin (Adriamycin®),** is associated with **heart failure**. It is thought that doxorubicin facilitates the excessive production of free radicals in the myocardium and thereby damages cardiac cell membranes. Cardiotoxicity is related to both the peak plasma concentration and the cumulative dose of doxorubicin. Cardiotoxicity can be reduced by coadministration of **dexrazoxane,** which is thought to inhibit free radical formation by chelating intracellular iron and preventing iron-mediated free radical generation.

Epipodophyllotoxins

Like anthracyclines, **epipodophyllotoxins** appear to act primarily by inhibiting topoisomerase II-mediated religation of double-strand DNA breaks (see Fig. 32-4). The antineoplastic agents **etoposide (VP-16)** and **teniposide (VM-26)** are semisynthetic derivatives of a compound isolated from the plant *Podophyllum.* These drugs bind topoisomerase II and DNA, trapping the complex in its cleavable state. Tumor cells often develop resistance to etoposide by increasing their expression of **P-glycoprotein.** This protein normally serves as an efflux pump to rid the cell of toxic molecules such as natural metabolic side-products, but it can also remove chemotherapeutic agents derived from natural products be-

fore those agents have exerted their cytotoxic effect. Etoposide is useful for treating testicular cancer, lung cancer, and leukemia, while both etoposide and teniposide are used to treat various lymphomas. Bone marrow suppression is the chief toxicity of the two epipodophyllotoxins in clinical use.

Combining drugs that damage DNA directly, such as cisplatin and bleomycin, with drugs that inhibit topoisomerase II, such as etoposide, can have powerful synergistic anticancer effects. This synergy may relate to the role of topoisomerases in repairing DNA damage, or to the combined ability of these drug classes to induce sufficient DNA damage to trigger apoptosis. In practice, drugs of these classes are coadministered in many successful antineoplastic regimens. As J. L.'s case demonstrates, the combination of etoposide, bleomycin, and cisplatin can cure most cases of metastatic testicular cancer.

Amsacrine

Amsacrine is another example of a chemotherapeutic agent that acts primarily by inhibiting topoisomerase II-mediated religation of double-strand DNA breaks. This compound targets DNA by intercalating between base pairs, distorting the double helix, producing DNA-protein crosslinks, and creating both single- and double-strand DNA lesions. Its clinical use is generally restricted to the treatment of recurrent leukemia and ovarian cancer.

MICROTUBULE INHIBITORS

Microtubules depend on dynamic instability for physiologic functioning. Without the ability to change length quickly, microtubules can do little other than lend structural support to a quiescent cell. Although microtubules play important roles in numerous aspects of cellular physiology, drugs that inhibit microtubule function are preferentially toxic to M-phase cells. Vinca alkaloids inhibit microtubule polymerization, while taxanes inhibit microtubule depolymerization. Other inhibitors of microtubule polymerization, including griseofulvin and colchicine, are discussed in Chapters 34 and 47, respectively.

Inhibitors of Microtubule Polymerization: Vinca Alkaloids

The vinca alkaloids **vinblastine** and **vincristine** are natural products originally isolated from the periwinkle plant, *Vinca rosea.* Vinca alkaloids bind to β-tubulin on a portion of the molecule that overlaps with the GTP-binding domain (Fig. 37-22). The binding of vinca alkaloids to β-tubulin at the (+) end of microtubules inhibits tubulin polymerization and thereby prevents microtubule extension. Because microtubules must constantly add tubulin to maintain stability (i.e., they must retain a GTP-bound tubulin cap), inhibition of tubulin addition eventually leads to the depolymerization of existing microtubules (Fig. 37-12).

Vinblastine is used to treat certain lymphomas and, as part of a multidrug regimen (with cisplatin and bleomycin), to treat metastatic testicular cancer. Pharmacologic doses of the drug cause nausea and vomiting. **Myelosuppression** is the dose-limiting adverse effect of vinblastine.

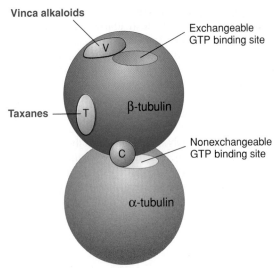

Figure 37-22. Tubulin binding sites of microtubule-inhibiting drugs. The tubulin heterodimer is composed of α-tubulin *(gray)* and β-tubulin *(blue).* α-Tubulin and β-tubulin both bind GTP. The GTP on α-tubulin is not hydrolyzed; for this reason, the GTP binding site on α-tubulin is referred to as the nonexchangeable GTP binding site. β-Tubulin hydrolyzes GTP to GDP; for this reason, the GTP binding site on β-tubulin is referred to as the exchangeable GTP binding site. The two classes of antineoplastic microtubule inhibitors bind to distinct sites on the tubulin heterodimer. Vinca alkaloids, which inhibit microtubule polymerization, bind to a site on β-tubulin located near the exchangeable GTP binding site *(V).* Vinca alkaloids associate preferentially at the (+) end of microtubules and thereby inhibit the addition of new tubulin subunits to the microtubule. Taxanes, which stabilize polymerized microtubules, bind to a different site on β-tubulin *(T).* Taxanes may stabilize either the interactions between tubulin subunits or the shape of microtubule protofilaments. Colchicine binds to a site located at the interface between α-tubulin and β-tubulin *(C).* Colchicine is not used in cancer chemotherapy but is used in the treatment of gout (see Chapter 47).

Vincristine plays an important role in the chemotherapy of pediatric leukemias. It is also a component of chemotherapy regimens used to treat Hodgkin's disease and some non-Hodgkin's lymphomas. Pharmacologic doses of vincristine cause nausea and vomiting. Vincristine causes some myelosuppression but not to the same degree as vinblastine. **Peripheral neuropathy** is usually the dose-limiting adverse effect of vincristine; this toxicity may result from inhibition of the microtubule trafficking function in long peripheral nerves that extend from the spinal cord to the extremities.

Inhibitors of Microtubule Depolymerization: Taxanes

The taxanes, which include **paclitaxel** and **docetaxel,** are natural products originally derived from the bark of the western yew tree. Taxanes bind to the β-tubulin subunit of microtubules at a site distinct from the vinca alkaloid binding site (Fig. 37-22). Paclitaxel has been shown to bind to the *inside* of microtubules. Unlike the vinca alkaloids, taxanes promote microtubule polymerization and inhibit depolymerization. Stabilization of the microtubules in a polymerized state arrests cells in mitosis and eventually leads to the activation of apoptosis.

There are two leading hypotheses for the apparent microtubule-stabilizing properties of taxanes. First, taxanes could strengthen the lateral interactions between microtubule protofilaments. Increased lateral interactions would decrease the tendency for protofilaments to "peel away" from the microtubule cylinder. Second, taxanes could straighten individual protofilaments. Once β-tubulin hydrolyzes GTP to GDP, protofilaments have a tendency to "curl," which produces a strain on the integrity of the microtubule cylinder. By straightening protofilaments, taxanes could reduce the tendency for the protofilaments to separate from the intact microtubule. In vivo, both of these mechanisms may be important for taxane-mediated stabilization of microtubules; alternative mechanisms are also possible.

Paclitaxel is used as an antineoplastic agent in the treatment of many solid tumors, especially breast, ovarian, and nonsmall cell lung cancer. Paclitaxel has a number of important adverse effects. An acute hypersensitivity reaction occurs commonly in response to paclitaxel, or more likely to the vehicle in which paclitaxel is solubilized; this effect can be obviated by administration of dexamethasone (a glucocorticoid receptor agonist) and a histamine H1 receptor antagonist before treatment with paclitaxel. Many patients experience myalgias and myelosuppression from paclitaxel, and high doses of the drug can cause pulmonary toxicity. **Peripheral neuropathy,** typically manifesting as a "stocking and glove" sensory deficit in the extremities, can limit the cumulative amount of drug that can be administered safely.

Abraxane® is an albumin-bound form of paclitaxel with a mean particle size of 130 nanometers. The albumin-bound paclitaxel nanoparticles do not cause a hypersensitivity reaction, do not require premedication, and cause less myelosuppresion than traditional, solvent-based paclitaxel. Preliminary studies in metastatic breast cancer also sugggest that this formulation of paclitaxel may have greater antineoplastic activity than solvent-based paclitaxel.

Docetaxel has found recent application in breast cancer and nonsmall cell lung cancer. As with paclitaxel, docetaxel causes an acute hypersensitivity reaction that can be obviated by preadministration of glucocorticoids. Docetaxel occasionally exhibits the drug-specific adverse effect of fluid retention, which likely arises from increased capillary permeability. Docetaxel does not cause neuropathy as frequently as paclitaxel. The myelosuppression associated with docetaxel is profound, however, and is usually dose-limiting.

◼ *Conclusion and Future Directions*

The antineoplastic agents described in this chapter exert their effects on the genome by preventing efficient DNA replication, inducing DNA damage, and interfering with mitosis. Because many normal cells as well as cancer cells are transiting through the cell cycle, these agents are associated with multiple dose-limiting toxicities. In addition, although cancer cells are susceptible to DNA damage, in some instances, mutations in key checkpoint proteins such as p53 can prevent the apoptosis that would otherwise be induced by these agents.

Novel approaches are being developed to target DNA damage more specifically. For example, it has been shown that mice deficient in PARP1 are able to overcome the defect in single-strand break repair by converting single-strand breaks to double-strand breaks and then repairing the DNA by the DSBR pathway. Furthermore, normal human cells treated in culture with PARP1 inhibitors are capable of undergoing normal cell division, although these cells do manifest increased susceptibility to DNA damage as a consequence of defective single-strand break repair. In contrast, cells deficient in BRCA1 or BRCA2, which are involved in DSB repair, are killed in response to treatment with PARP1 inhibitors; compared to normal cells, BRCA1$^-$ or BRCA2$^-$ cells are up to 1,000-fold more sensitive to the action of PARP1 inhibitors. Presumably, the BRCA1$^-$ and BRCA2$^-$ cells are more sensitive due to impairment of both single-strand break and DSB repair pathways, resulting in lethal accumulation of DNA damage. Based on these findings, **PARP1 inhibitors** are thought to represent promising new agents in the treatment of BRCA1- or BRCA2-deficient breast or ovarian cancer, and may be effective in other tumors in which the DNA damage response is compromised.

The observation that telomerase is expressed in most cancer cells and is a key component of the process of immortalization highlights this enzyme as an important target in future cancer therapy. Although telomerase is expressed to some degree in stem cells and in normally cycling cells, most normal cells lack telomerase expression. Therefore, the dependency of tumor cells on the immortalized state could provide **telomerase inhibitors** with a favorable therapeutic index. One concern is that multiple cell divisions may be required for telomere length to shorten to a level that is critical for cell survival. Small-molecule telomerase inhibitors are being developed, as are viral vectors utilizing the telomerase promoter to drive the expression of genes that promote apoptosis or increase sensitivity to agents that induce cell killing. In addition, combinations of telomerase inhibitors with traditional cytotoxic agents or newer molecularly targeted therapies could yield synergistic effects. Such strategies, as well as those described in Chapter 38, Pharmacology of Cancer: Signal Transduction, will help to advance cancer therapy by moving beyond general cytotoxic approaches and focusing treatment instead on the molecular abnormalities responsible for driving oncogenesis.

Suggested Reading

Brody LC. Treating cancer by targeting a weakness. *N Engl J Med* 2005;353:949–950. (*Advances in targeted cancer therapy.*)

DeBoer J, Hoeijmakers JH. Nucleotide excision repair and human syndromes. *Carcinogenesis* 2000;21:453–460. (*Molecular mechanisms of excision repair.*)

Hahn WC. Role of telomeres and telomerase in the pathogenesis of human cancer. *J Clin Oncol* 2003;21:2034–2043. (*Possible therapeutic applications of telomerase inhibitors.*)

Peltomaki P. Role of DNA mismatch repair defects in the pathogenesis of human cancer. *J Clin Oncol* 2003;21:1174–1179. (*Insights into pathophysiology of DNA repair mechanisms.*)

Venkitaraman AR. Cancer susceptibility and the functions of BRCA1 and BRCA2. *Cell* 2002;108:171–182. (*Pathophysiology of BRCA1 and BRCA2.*)

| Drug Summary Table | Chapter 37 Pharmacology of Cancer: Genome Synthesis, Stability, and Maintenance |

Drug	Clinical Applications	Serious and Common Adverse Effects	Contraindications	Therapeutic Considerations
INHIBITORS OF THYMIDYLATE SYNTHASE				
Mechanism—Inhibit thymidylate synthase, thereby decreasing cellular availability of dTMP and causing ''thymineless'' cell death				
Fluorouracil (5-FU)	Breast cancer Gastrointestinal cancers Skin cancer (topical application)	*Coronary atherosclerosis, thrombophlebitis, gastrointestinal ulcer, myelosuppression, cerebellar syndrome, visual changes, stenosis of lacrimal system* Alopecia, rash, pruritus, photosensitivity, gastrointestinal disturbance, stomatitis, headache	Severe bone marrow depression Poor nutritional state Serious infection Dihydropyrimidine dehydrogenase deficiency Pregnancy	5-FU is a uracil analogue that, after intracellular modification, inhibits thymidylate synthase by binding to the deoxyuridylate (substrate) site on the enzyme In addition to inhibiting thymidylate synthase, 5-FU interferes with protein synthesis after the drug metabolite FUTP is incorporated into mRNA Folinic acid can be used to potentiate the action of 5-FU
Capecitabine	Metastatic colorectal cancer Breast cancer	Same as fluorouracil	Dihydropyrimidine dehydrogenase deficiency Severe renal impairment	Orally available prodrug form of 5-FU
Pemetrexed	Nonsmall cell lung cancer Malignant pleural mesothelioma (in combination with cisplatin)	*Myelosuppression, angina, myocardial infarction, stroke, thrombophlebitis, liver damage, bullous skin rash* Fatigue, nausea, vomiting, diarrhea, stomatitis	Hypersensitivity to pemetrexed Severe renal impairment	Pemetrexed is a folate analogue that, after intracellular modification, inhibits thymidylate synthase by binding to the methylenetetrahydrofolate (cofactor) site on the enzyme Coadministered with folic acid and vitamin B12 to reduce hematologic and gastrointestinal toxicity
INHIBITORS OF PURINE METABOLISM				
Mechanism—Drug metabolites inhibit IMPDH and other synthetic enzymes, thereby interfering with AMP and GMP synthesis				
6-Mercaptopurine (6-MP) Azathioprine	Acute lymphoid leukemia, acute myeloid leukemia, Crohn's disease (6-MP) Immunosuppression in renal transplantation, rheumatoid arthritis, inflammatory bowel disease (azathioprine)	*Pancreatitis, myelosuppression, hepatotoxicity, infection* Gastritis	Pregnancy	Effectiveness and toxicity increased by allopurinol Azathioprine is a less toxic prodrug of 6-MP Azathioprine is used for immunosuppression of autoimmune diseases
Pentostatin	Hairy cell leukemia T-cell lymphoma	*Cardiac arrhythmia, heart failure, myelosuppression, hepatotoxicity, neurotoxicity, nephrotoxicity, pulmonary toxicity* Rash, shaking chills, vomiting, myalgia, upper respiratory infection, fever	Hypersensitivity to pentostatin	Selective inhibitor of adenosine deaminase (ADA)
INHIBITORS OF RIBONUCLEOTIDE REDUCTASE				
Mechanism—Inhibit ribonucleotide reductase, the enzyme that converts ribonucleotides to deoxyribonucleotides				
Hydroxyurea	Hematologic malignancies Head and neck cancers Melanoma Ovarian carcinoma Sickle cell anemia (adults only)	*Myelosuppression, secondary leukemia with long-term use* Gastrointestinal toxicity, skin ulcer	Severe bone marrow depression	Reduces tyrosine free radical critical to mechanism of action of ribonucleotide reductase In sickle cell anemia, hydroxyurea is thought to act by increasing hemoglobin F

PURINE AND PYRIMIDINE ANALOGUES THAT ARE INCORPORATED INTO DNA
Mechanism—Incorporation into DNA and RNA results in inhibition of DNA polymerase, thereby causing cell death

Drug	Clinical Applications	Serious and Common Adverse Effects	Contraindications	Therapeutic Considerations
Thioguanine	Acute myelocytic leukemia	*Myelosuppression, hyperuricemia, intestinal perforation, hepatotoxicity, infection* Gastrointestinal disturbance	Prior resistance to thioguanine or mercaptopurine	Guanine analogue
Fludarabine phosphate	B-cell chronic lymphocytic leukemia Non-Hodgkin's lymphoma	*Aplasia of skin, autoimmune hemolytic anemia, myelosuppression, neurotoxicity; pneumonia, infection* Edema, gastrointestinal disturbance, asthenia, fatigue	Hypersensitivity to fludarabine	Purine nucleotide analogue
Cladribine	Hairy cell leukemia Multiple sclerosis	*Febrile neutropenia, myelosuppression, neurotoxicity; infection* Rash, injection site reaction, nausea, headache	Hypersensitivity to cladribine	Purine analogue
Cytarabine (araC)	Acute lymphoid leukemia Acute myeloid leukemia Chronic myeloid leukemia Meningeal leukemia Hodgkin's disease Non-Hodgkin's lymphoma	*Myelosuppression, neuropathy; nephrotoxicity; liver dysfunction; infection* Thrombophlebitis, rash, hyperuricemia, gastrointestinal disturbance, ulcers of mouth or anus	Hypersensitivity to cytarabine	Cytidine analogue
Azacytidine	Myelodysplastic syndrome	*Myelosuppression, renal failure* Peripheral edema, gastrointestinal disturbance, hepatic coma, lethargy, cough, fever	Advanced malignant hepatic tumors	Cytidine analogue
Gemcitabine	Pancreatic cancer Nonsmall cell lung cancer Breast cancer Ovarian cancer Bladder cancer Sarcoma Hodgkin's disease	*Myelosuppression, febrile neutropenia, pulmonary toxicity; hepatotoxicity; hemolytic uremic syndrome* Fever, gastrointesinal disturbance, liver enzyme elevation, edema, rash, paresthesias	Hypersensitivity to gemcitabine Pregnancy	Cytidine analogue

AGENTS THAT DIRECTLY MODIFY DNA STRUCTURE: ALKYLATING AGENTS
Mechanism—Covalently bind DNA, often crosslink to DNA or associated proteins

Drug	Clinical Applications	Serious and Common Adverse Effects	Contraindications	Therapeutic Considerations
Cyclophosphamide	Autoimmune diseases Leukemias and lymphomas Advanced mycosis fungoides Neuroblastoma Ovarian cancer Retinoblastoma Breast cancer Malignant histiocytosis	*Myelosuppression, cardiomyopathy; Stevens-Johnson syndrome; hemorrhagic cystitis, azoospermia; interstitial pneumonia, infection* Alopecia, gastrointestinal disturbance, leukopenia, amenorrhea	Severely depressed bone marrow function	Acrolein, a metabolite of cyclophosphamide, causes hemorrhagic cystitis; this adverse effect can be prevented by coadministration with mesna

(Continued)

Drug Summary Table | **Chapter 37 Pharmacology of Cancer: Genome Synthesis, Stability, and Maintenance** (*Continued*)

Drug	Clinical Applications	Serious and Common Adverse Effects	Contraindications	Therapeutic Considerations
Mechlorethamine Melphalan Estramustine Chlorambucil Mitomycin Thiotepa Carmustine Dacarbazine Procarbazine Altretamine	Leukemia and Hodgkin's disease (mechlorethamine) Lymphoma (melphalan) Prostate cancer (estramustine) Leukemia (chlorambucil) Gastric and pancreatic cancer (mitomycin) Bladder cancer (thiotepa) Brain cancer (carmustine) Hodgkin's disease (dacarbazine) Hodgkin's disease (procarbazine) Ovarian cancer (altretamine)	*Same as cyclophosphamide*	Presence of known infectious disease (mechlorethamine) Active thrombophlebitis or thromboembolic disorder (estramustine) Coagulation disorder or renal impairment (mitomycin) Hepatic, renal or bone marrow dysfunction (thiotepa) Severe bone marrow depression (procarbazine, altretamine) Severe neurologic toxicity (altretamine)	Thiotepa is instilled directly in the bladder Carmustine is a nitrosurea that attaches a carbamoyl group to target proteins

AGENTS THAT DIRECTLY MODIFY DNA STRUCTURE: PLATINUM COMPOUNDS

Mechanism—Crosslink intrastrand guanine bases

Drug	Clinical Applications	Serious and Common Adverse Effects	Contraindications	Therapeutic Considerations
Cisplatin Carboplatin	Genitourinary cancers Lung cancers	*Nephrotoxicity (cisplatin), myelosuppression, peripheral neuropathy, ototoxicity* Electrolyte imbalance	Severe bone marrow depression Renal or hearing impairment	Cisplatin can be injected intraperitoneally for treatment of ovarian cancer Coadministration of amifostine with cisplatin can limit nephrotoxicity
Oxaliplatin	Colorectal cancer	*Acute and persistent neurotoxicity, myelosuppression, colitis, hepatic dysfunction* Gastrointestinal disturbance, back pain, cough, fever	Hypersensitivity to oxaliplatin	Acute neurotoxicity is exacerbated by exposure to cold temperatures

AGENTS THAT DIRECTLY MODIFY DNA STRUCTURE: BLEOMYCIN

Mechanism—Binds oxygen and chelates Fe(II); binds DNA and leads to strand breaks via generation of oxidative intermediates

Drug	Clinical Applications	Serious and Common Adverse Effects	Contraindications	Therapeutic Considerations
Bleomycin	Testicular cancer Hodgkin's disease Non-Hodgkin's lymphoma Squamous cell carcinoma	*Pulmonary fibrosis, vascular disease, myocardial infarction, stroke, Raynaud's, hepatotoxicity, nephrotoxicity, rare myelosuppression* Alopecia, rash, hyperpigmentation, skin tenderness, gastrointestinal disturbance, stomatitis	Hypersensitivity to bleomycin	Effects on pulmonary function are dose-limiting and irreversible

TOPOISOMERASE INHIBITORS

Mechanism—Inhibit topoisomerase I or topoisomerase II, leading to DNA strand breakage

Drug	Clinical Applications	Serious and Common Adverse Effects	Contraindications	Therapeutic Considerations
Irinotecan Topotecan	Colorectal cancer (irinotecan) Small cell lung cancer, cervical carcinoma, ovarian cancer (topotecan)	*Life-threatening diarrhea, myelosuppression, febrile neutropenia, liver dysfunction, interstitial lung disease* Alopecia, eosinophilia	Severe bone marrow depression	Irinotecan and topotecan are camptothecins that inhibit topoisomerase I Action is specific to S phase

Drug	Clinical Applications	Serious and Common Adverse Effects	Contraindications	Therapeutic Considerations
Doxorubicin Daunorubicin Epirubicin	Leukemias, lymphomas, breast cancer, bladder cancer, thyroid cancer, GI cancer, nephroblastoma, osteosarcoma, ovarian cancer, small cell carcinoma of lung, soft tissue sarcoma (doxorubicin) Acute lymphoid leukemia and acute myeloid leukemia (daunorubicin) Breast cancer (epirubicin)	*Heart failure (especially doxorubicin), myelosuppression* Alopecia, rash, gastrointestinal disturbance	Pre-existing heart failure Severe bone marrow depression Severe hepatic dysfunction (epirubicin)	Doxorubicin, daunorubicin, and epirubicin are anthracyclines that inhibit topoisomerase II Excreted in bile (reduce dose in patients with hepatic dysfunction) Action is specific to G2 phase
Etoposide Teniposide	Testicular and lung cancer, leukemia (etoposide) Acute lymphoid leukemia, non-Hodgkin's lymphoma (teniposide)	Same as doxorubicin	Hypersensitivity to etoposide or teniposide	Etoposide and teniposide are epipodophyllotoxins that inhibit topoisomerase II Action is specific to late S and G2 phases
Amsacrine	Recurrent leukemia Ovarian cancer	*ECG changes including QT prolongation, paralytic ileus, myelosuppression, convulsion, azoospermia, hepatotoxicity* Alopecia, gastrointestinal disturbance	Hypersensitivity to amsacrine	Inhibits topoisomerase II

AGENTS THAT INHIBIT MICROTUBULE POLYMERIZATION
Mechanism—Bind tubulin subunits and prevent microtubule polymerization

Drug	Clinical Applications	Serious and Common Adverse Effects	Contraindications	Therapeutic Considerations
Vinblastine	Metastatic testicular cancer Lymphoma AIDS-related Kaposi's sarcoma Breast cancer Choriocarcinoma Malignant histiocytosis Mycosis fungoides	*Myelosuppression, hypertension, neurotoxicity, azoospermia* Alopecia, bone pain, gastrointestinal disturbance	Bacterial infection Significant granulocytopenia	Bone marrow suppression is dose-limiting
Vincristine	Leukemias Hodgkin's disease Non-Hodgkin's lymphoma Rhabdomyosarcoma Nephroblastoma	*Peripheral neuropathy, myopathy, myelosuppression* Alopecia, gastrointestinal disturbance, diplopia	Charcot-Marie-Tooth syndrome Intrathecal use	Peripheral neuropathy is dose-limiting

AGENTS THAT INHIBIT MICROTUBULE DEPOLYMERIZATION
Mechanism—Bind polymerized tubulin and inhibit microtubule depolymerization

Drug	Clinical Applications	Serious and Common Adverse Effects	Contraindications	Therapeutic Considerations
Paclitaxel Albumin-bound paclitaxel	Ovarian cancer Breast cancer Nonsmall cell lung cancer AIDS-related Kaposi's sarcoma	*Myelosuppression, pulmonary toxicity, severe hypersensitivity reaction, myopathy, peripheral neuropathy* Alopecia, gastrointestinal disturbance, arthralgia	Severe neutropenia	Peripheral neuropathy is dose-limiting
Docetaxel	Breast cancer Gastric cancer Prostate cancer Nonsmall cell lung cancer	*Myelosuppression, Stevens-Johnson syndrome, fluid retention syndrome leading to severe edema, neuropathy, hepatotoxicity, colitis* Alopecia, gastrointestinal disturbance, asthenia, fever	Severe neutropenia	Myelosuppression is dose-limiting

38

Pharmacology of Cancer: Signal Transduction

David A. Barbie and David A. Frank

INTRODUCTION

Traditional antineoplastic therapy has consisted of agents directed against DNA replication and cell division. These drugs exhibit some degree of selectivity against cancer cells, which tend to have a higher growth fraction and in some cases an increased susceptibility to DNA damage compared to normal cells. However, the therapeutic window of these drugs is narrow, resulting in toxicity to normal stem cells and in hematologic and gastrointestinal adverse effects. With the impressive advances in basic tumor cell biology over the last several decades and the identification of numerous oncogenes and tumor suppressor genes, the potential exists for development of agents that are targeted more specifically at the molecular circuitry responsible for the dysregulated proliferation of cancer cells. An early example of such a drug is the selective estrogen receptor modulator **tamoxifen** (see Chapter 28, Pharmacology of Reproduction), which has been one of the most active agents in the treatment of hormone receptor positive breast cancer, with a relatively modest adverse effect profile. More recently, the remarkable suc-

cess of **imatinib mesylate** in the treatment of chronic myelogenous leukemia has suggested that, in some cases, tumor cells are dependent on oncogenes such as BCR-ABL for their survival. This chapter highlights basic principles of targeted cancer therapy, detailing recent advances and directions for the future.

Case

M. W. is a 65-year-old woman with metastatic nonsmall cell lung cancer. She has never smoked, and her primary tumor is an adenocarcinoma with bronchioalveolar features. She is initially treated with cisplatin and paclitaxel, but her tumor progresses. After discussions with her oncologist, M. W. is treated with the oral epidermal growth factor receptor (EGFR) inhibitor erlotinib. She develops a skin rash and diarrhea, but otherwise tolerates this medication well. Restaging computed tomography scans are performed 2 months after starting treatment with erlotinib. These scans reveal a dramatic reduction in M. W.'s tumor burden, and after 6 months there is no residual evidence of cancer.

Sequencing of the EGFR gene from her primary tumor reveals a mutation in the kinase domain at codon 858, resulting in a substitution of arginine for leucine (L858R). Unfortunately, M. W. subsequently develops resistance to erlotinib and recurrence of her disease. A repeat biopsy reveals a new mutation in the EGFR kinase domain in codon 790 (T790M). She decides to participate in a clinical trial of HKI-272, an irreversible EGFR inhibitor that has shown activity in vitro against lung cancer cells with this mutation.

QUESTIONS

1. How does signaling through the EGFR promote cell growth and survival?

2. By what mechanism does erlotinib inhibit the EGFR and inhibit cancer cell growth?

3. How might subsets of patients be selected for effective targeted therapy?

4. What mechanisms are responsible for resistance to targeted therapy, and how might such resistance be overcome?

BIOCHEMISTRY OF INTERCELLULAR AND INTRACELLULAR SIGNAL TRANSDUCTION

GROWTH FACTORS AND GROWTH FACTOR RECEPTORS

Stimulation of cell growth and proliferation by external signals is mediated by the interaction of growth factors with specific cell surface receptors. Growth factor receptors typically contain an extracellular ligand-binding domain, a hydrophobic transmembrane domain, and a cytoplasmic tail that has either intrinsic tyrosine kinase activity or an associated protein tyrosine kinase (Fig. 38-1A,B). In general, binding of the growth factor ligand results in receptor oligomerization, a conformational change in the cytoplasmic domain of the receptor, and tyrosine kinase activation. Intracellular targets are subsequently phosphorylated, propagating a signal that culminates in progression through the cell cycle and cellular proliferation.

One example of a receptor tyrosine kinase is the **epidermal growth factor receptor (EGFR),** which possesses intrinsic tyrosine kinase activity and is a member of the broader ErbB family of proteins, including EGFR (ErbB1), HER-2/*neu* (ErbB2), ErbB3, and ErbB4. Binding of epidermal growth factor (EGF) or transforming growth factor-α (TGF-α) to EGFR results in receptor homodimerization and propagation of a growth signal. In addition, heterodimerization between family members can occur, yielding further diversity in the signal that is transduced. ErbB receptors are expressed on epithelial cells and are often activated or overexpressed in a variety of carcinomas (e.g., EGFR in nonsmall cell lung cancer and HER-2/*neu* in breast cancer).

Other examples of receptor tyrosine kinases include the platelet-derived growth factor receptor (PDGFR), fibroblast

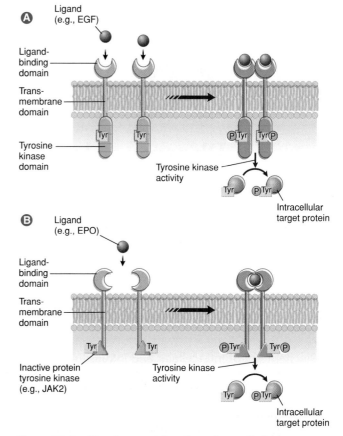

Figure 38-1. Structure and function of growth factor receptors. A. Growth factor receptors exemplified by the epidermal growth factor (EGF) receptor contain an extracellular ligand binding domain, a hydrophobic transmembrane domain, and a cytoplasmic domain with intrinsic tyrosine kinase activity. Binding of ligand results in receptor homodimerization (or heterodimerization with other family members), triggering activation of the tyrosine kinase, autophosphorylation of the receptor, and phosphorylation of intracellular target proteins. **B.** Growth factor receptors exemplified by the type I cytokine receptors (such as the erythropoietin [EPO] receptor) lack intrinsic tyrosine kinase activity. Instead, the receptors are associated with intracellular protein tyrosine kinases such as JAK2. Upon ligand-induced receptor dimerization, the associated kinase is activated and autophosphorylated, resulting in recruitment and phosphorylation of intracellular target proteins.

growth factor receptor (FGFR), c-KIT, and FMS-like tyrosine kinase (FLT-3). Signaling through these receptors activates the growth of certain hematopoietic and mesenchymal tissues, and dysregulation of these receptors is frequently observed in specific myeloproliferative disorders, leukemias, and sarcomas (Table 38-1).

Other hematopoietic receptors rely on interaction with an associated cytoplasmic tyrosine kinase for transduction of a growth signal. For example, type I cytokine receptors such as the erythropoietin receptor (EpoR), thrombopoietin receptor (TpoR), and G-CSF receptor (GCSFR) form specifically oriented homodimers upon binding of ligand, resulting in activation of the associated tyrosine kinase JAK2, which leads to further signaling and ultimately to cell growth. Activating mutations of the receptors themselves (e.g., EpoR) have been implicated in conditions such as congenital polycythemia.

TABLE 38-1 **Receptor Tyrosine Kinases Associated with Cancer**

RECEPTOR TYROSINE KINASE	MALIGNANCY OR MYELOPROLIFERATIVE DISORDER
EGFR (ErbB1)	Nonsmall cell lung cancer
	Head and neck cancer
	Colon cancer
	Pancreatic cancer
	Glioblastoma
HER-2/neu (ErbB2)	Breast cancer
	Ovarian cancer
	Head and neck cancer
PDGFR	Hypereosinophilic syndrome
	Mast cell disease
	Dermatofibrosarcoma protuberans
	Gastrointestinal stromal tumor (GIST)
FGFR3	Multiple myeloma
	Bladder cancer
c-KIT	Gastrointestinal stromal tumor (GIST), systemic mastocytosis
FLT-3	Acute myelogenous leukemia
RET	Multiple endocrine neoplasia type 2
	Familial medullary thyroid carcinoma
c-MET	Hepatocellular carcinoma
	Melanoma
	Glioblastoma
	Epithelial malignancies

Recently, an activating mutation in JAK2 resulting in the conversion of valine to phenylalanine at position 617 (V617F) has been found in a majority of patients with the myeloproliferative disorder polycythemia vera and in a significant proportion of patients with essential thrombocythemia and myeloid metaplasia with myelofibrosis.

INTRACELLULAR SIGNAL TRANSDUCTION PATHWAYS

Activation of a growth factor receptor initiates the transduction of a series of intracellular signals, culminating in events such as cell cycle entry, promotion of protein translation and cell growth, and enhanced cell survival. Two broad categories of pathways activated by receptor tyrosine kinases include the **RAS-MAP kinase** pathway and the **phosphatidylinositol-3-kinase** (PI3K)-AKT pathway (Fig. 38-2).

The Kirsten *ras* gene was initially identified as a retroviral oncogene in rats and subsequently found to have several human homologues, including K-*ras*, H-*ras*, and N-*ras*. The protein (RAS) encoded by *ras* is targeted to the plasma membrane by the farnesyltransferase-mediated addition of a hydrophobic farnesyl group to its COOH-terminus; this targeting brings RAS into close proximity to activated receptor tyrosine kinases. Other intracellular nonreceptor tyrosine kinases such as ABL and SRC, also originally identified as oncogene products, can activate signaling through RAS as well (Fig. 38-2A).

Upon activation by binding to GTP, RAS triggers a series of phosphorylation events through the kinases RAF, MEK, and ERK (MAP kinase), the targets of which include transcription factors that promote activation of genes involved in proliferation. For example, activation of cyclin D transcription results in cyclin D expression and binding to its catalytic partners, cyclin-dependent kinases 4 and 6 (CDK4 and CDK6) (Fig. 38-3). These complexes initiate phosphorylation of the **retinoblastoma protein** (pRB), thereby lifting pRB's repression of the transcription factor E2F. E2F mediates the expression of components of the DNA replication machinery and enzymes involved in nucleotide synthesis. Thus, phosphorylation of pRB by cyclin D/CDK4/6 and subsequent cyclin-CDK complexes results in the transition from G1 to S phase and progression through the cell cycle. While it might seem unnecessarily complicated, such signaling cascades allow for the integration of diverse extracellular and intracellular signals, the opportunity for multiple points of feedback control, and tight regulation of critical events such as cellular proliferation.

A second key intracellular signaling pathway is controlled by the lipid kinase **PI3K**. Stimulation of receptors for growth factors such as insulin or insulin-like growth factor (IGFs) commonly leads to activation of PI3K via an associated insulin receptor substrate protein (IRS). ErbB family members can also activate this pathway via phospholipase C-γ (PLC-γ), and RAS can also promote signaling through this pathway (Fig. 38-2B). Activation of PI3K results in generation of phosphatidylinositol-3,4,5-trisphosphate (PIP3) from plasma membrane phospholipids, activation of phosphoinositide dependent kinase-1 (PDK-1) via translocation to the cell membrane, and phosphorylation of AKT by PDK-1. This pathway is negatively regulated by the lipid phosphatase PTEN, which degrades PIP3. Downstream effects of AKT activation include promotion of translation and cell growth by the mammalian target of rapamycin (mTOR). In addition, phosphorylation of the forkhead family of transcription factors (FOXO) by AKT results in their exclusion from the nucleus, preventing expression of genes involved in cell cycle arrest, stress resistance, and apoptosis. Thus, a net effect of activating the PI3K-AKT pathway is the promotion of cell survival.

Signaling via type I cytokine receptors is associated with activation of the **JAK-STAT** pathway (Fig. 38-2C). Growth factor receptors such as EGFR, as well as intracellular tyrosine kinases such as SRC, can also signal through activation of **STATs**, a family of proteins that shuttle from the cytoplasm to the nucleus to regulate transcription directly. Activation of JAKs, or Janus kinases, via transphosphorylation induced by receptor dimerization, allows the recruitment of STAT proteins through their SH2 domains. STAT proteins are then phosphorylated, leading to the formation of SH2 domain-mediated homo- or heterodimers that translocate to the nucleus and regulate transcription.

PROTEASOME STRUCTURE AND FUNCTION

Key cellular processes such as cell cycle progression and apoptosis are also regulated at the posttranslational level by

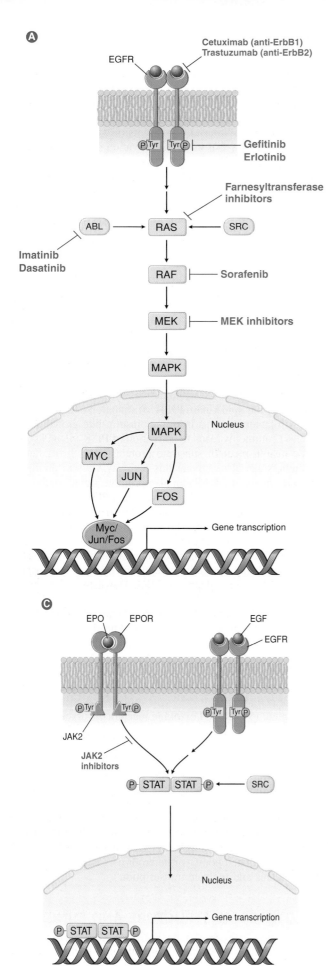

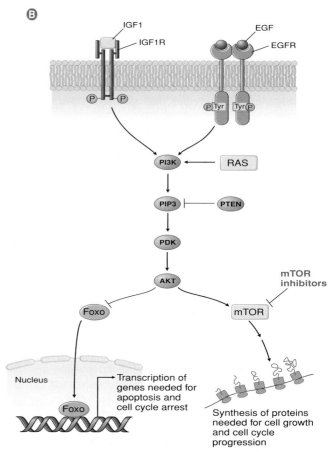

Figure 38-2. Intracellular signaling pathways. A. The RAS-MAP kinase pathway is activated by multiple growth factor receptors (here exemplified by the EGF receptor, EGFR) as well as several intracellular tyrosine kinases such as SRC and ABL. RAS is recruited to the plasma membrane by farnesylation and activated by binding to GTP. Activated RAS stimulates a sequence of phosphorylation events mediated by RAF, MEK, and ERK (MAP) kinases. Activated MAP kinase (MAPK) translocates to the nucleus and activates proteins such as MYC, JUN, and FOS that promote the transcription of genes involved in cell-cycle progression. Cetuximab and trastuzumab act as antagonists at the EGF receptor (ErbB1) and HER-2 receptor (ErbB2), respectively. Gefitinib and erlotinib inhibit the receptor tyrosine kinase. Farnesyltransferase inhibitors prevent RAS activation. Imatinib and dasatinib inhibit ABL kinase; sorafenib inhibits RAF kinase; and several agents under development (see text) inhibit MEK kinase. **B.** The PI3 kinase (PI3K) pathway is activated by RAS and by a number of growth factor receptors (here exemplified by the insulin-like growth factor receptor 1 [IGF1R] and the epidermal growth factor receptor [EGFR]). Activated PI3K generates phosphatidylinositol-3,4,5-triphosphate (PIP3), which activates phosphoinositide dependent kinase-1 (PDK). In turn, PDK phosphorylates AKT. PTEN is an endogenous inhibitor of AKT activation. Phosphorylated AKT transduces multiple downstream signals, including activation of the mammalian target of rapamycin (mTOR) and inhibition of the FOXO family of transcription factors. mTOR activation promotes the synthesis of proteins required for cell growth and cell-cycle progression. Because the FOXO family of transcription factors activates the expression of genes involved in cell-cycle arrest, stress resistance, and apoptosis, inhibition of FOXO promotes cell proliferation and resistance to apoptosis. Rapamycin (sirolimus) and its derivatives are mTOR inhibitors that inhibit cell-cycle progression and promote apoptosis. **C.** The STAT pathway is activated by SRC and by a number of growth factor receptors (here exemplified by the erythropoietin receptor [EPOR], which signals to STAT proteins through JAK2 kinase, and by the EGF receptor [EGFR], which signals to STAT proteins indirectly). Phosphorylation of STAT induces SH2 domain-mediated homodimerization, and phosphorylated STAT homodimers translocate to the nucleus and activate transcription. JAK2 inhibitors are under development for the treatment of polycythemia vera and other myeloproliferative disorders, many of which share a common activating mutation in JAK2 (V617F).

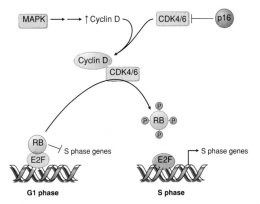

Figure 38-3. Regulation of the G1/S cell cycle transition. Activation of MAP kinase results in increased expression of the D-type cyclins. Cyclin D binds to its catalytic partners cyclin-dependent kinase 4 and 6 (CDK4 and CDK6), which phosphorylate the retinoblastoma protein (RB). Phosphorylation of RB releases its transcriptional repression of S-phase genes, allowing the transcription factor E2F to activate the transcription of genes needed for entry into S phase. These genes include cyclin E as well as DNA polymerase and the enzymes involved in nucleotide synthesis. Cyclin E binds to its catalytic partner CDK2, which further phosphorylates RB, creating a positive feedback loop that drives cells into S phase (not shown). The CDK2/CDK4/CDK6 system is counterbalanced by cyclin-dependent kinase inhibitors (CDKIs) such as p16, which inhibits CDK4/6, and p21 and p27, which inhibit CDK2 (not shown).

protein degradation. One of the major systems involved in this control is the **ubiquitin-proteasome pathway**, which comprises three enzymes that targets specific proteins for ubiquitin conjugation and destruction by the proteasome (Fig. 38-4A). **Ubiquitin** is a 9-kDa protein that derives its name from its widespread distribution in tissues and its conservation across eukaryotes. The first enzyme involved in the process, E1, uses ATP to activate ubiquitin. The second enzyme in the cascade, E2, is a ubiquitin-conjugating enzyme that transiently carries ubiquitin and acts in conjunction with the third enzyme, the ubiquitin ligase E3, to form a polyubiquitin chain that is transferred to the target protein on an internal lysine residue.

E1 is nonspecific, and there are a number of different E2 ubiquitin-conjugating enzymes with a limited degree of specificity. The E3 ubiquitin ligase component is largely responsible for target protein specificity. The RING family of E3 ligases contains a characteristic RING finger domain with conserved histidine and cysteine residues complexed with two central Zn^{2+} ions. RING E3 ligases can be subdivided into single-subunit E3 ligases and multisubunit complexes such as the Skp1-Cullin-F-box protein family (SCF) E3 ligases. In the latter complexes, the RING finger component, Rbx, is distinct from the specificity component, the F-box protein, which is so named because of a characteristic motif first identified in cyclin F.

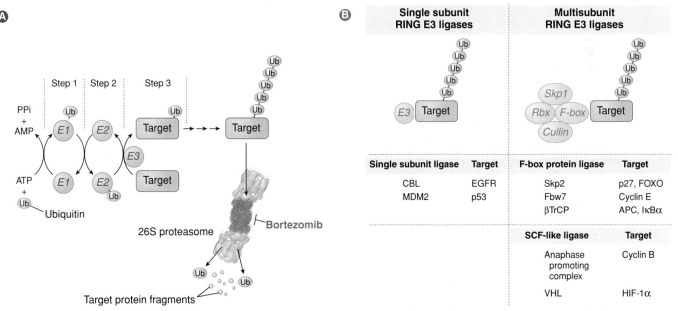

Figure 38-4. The ubiquitin-proteasome pathway. A. Ubiquitin (Ub) is activated by ATP-dependent conjugation to E1, the first enzyme in the pathway. Activated ubiquitin is then passed from the active-site cysteine of E1 to the active-site cysteine of the ubiquitin-conjugating enzyme E2, which functions coordinately with the ubiquitin ligase E3 to attach ubiquitin to protein targets. Polyubiquitination of target proteins results in their recognition by the 26S proteasome, which consists of a 19S outer regulatory subunit and a 20S internal core chamber. The proteasome mediates proteolytic degradation of the target protein into short peptide fragments. Bortezomib is a proteasome inhibitor that has been approved for use in multiple myeloma and is under investigation for use in other malignancies. **B.** The RING family of E3 ubiquitin ligases consists of single subunit enzymes **(left)** and multisubunit protein complexes **(right)**. Single subunit ligases include CBL, which targets EGFR for degradation, and MDM2, which targets p53 for degradation. Multisubunit RING E3 ligase complexes include SCF and SCF-like family members, which are named for their Skp1, Cullin, and F-box protein subunits. The F-box protein component mediates target protein specificity; for example, SKP2 targets p27 and FOXO for degradation, Fbw7 targets cyclin E for degradation, and βTrCP targets APC and IκBα for degradation. SCF-like ligase complexes include the anaphase promoting complex, which targets cyclin B for degradation, and VHL, which targets the α subunit of hypoxia inducible factor-1 (HIF-1α) for degradation.

Once proteins are selectively ubiquitinated, they are targeted for degradation by the 26S proteasome, which is a cylindrical particle present in both the cytoplasm and nucleus. The core 20S subunit is the catalytic component with multiple proteolytic sites, while the 19S regulatory component mediates binding to ubiquitin-conjugated proteins and has multiple ATPases involved in substrate unfolding and delivery to the central 20S chamber. Substrates are cleaved progressively, with one protein being completely degraded before the next protein enters. Short peptide segments, on average 6 to 10 amino acids in length, are extruded and subsequently hydrolyzed to individual amino acids in the cytosol.

Regulation of protein degradation occurs largely at the level of the E3 ubiquitin ligase and governs key aspects of cell cycle control, apoptosis, and other important cellular processes (Fig. 38-4B). For example, CBL is a single-subunit RING E3 ubiquitin ligase that targets phosphorylated EGFR family members for degradation. In addition, both cyclins and cyclin-dependent kinase inhibitors are major targets for ubiquitin-mediated proteasomal degradation. The anaphase-promoting complex is a complex multiprotein RING-containing E3 ligase that is activated by phosphorylation late in mitosis, triggering degradation of cyclin B and progression through mitosis. Regulation of the G1-S phase transition is in part mediated by the cyclin-dependent kinase inhibitor p27, which inhibits cyclin E/CDK2 and cyclin A/CDK2 complexes. Degradation of p27 is regulated by another SCF E3 ligase, which binds p27 via its F-box specificity component Skp2. Thus, overexpression of Skp2, which is found in a number of tumor types, can promote cell cycle progression by degrading p27. Degradation of FOXO by Skp2 is a second mechanism by which overexpression of Skp2 may promote tumorigenesis. Yet another SCF E3 ligase complex regulates cyclin E activity by targeting it for degradation via the F-box protein Fbw7. Loss of Fbw7 has been implicated in tumor progression due to high levels of cyclin E.

Another example of an E3 ligase with a critical role in the regulation of apoptosis and cell cycle regulation is MDM2, a single-subunit RING finger E3 ligase that targets p53 for degradation. Activation of MDM2 is linked to impairment of apoptosis and promotion of tumorigenesis via loss of p53. MDM2 is also inhibited by the p14^{ARF} protein, which shares the same genomic locus as the CDK4/6 inhibitor p16. Disruption of this locus, which is one of the most common events in cancer, leads ultimately to both p53 and pRB inactivation.

Other key cellular pathways regulated by ubiquitin-mediated proteasomal degradation include the WNT signaling and nuclear factor-kappa B (NFκB) pathways. Both pathways are targeted by the common F-box protein βTrCP, which recognizes phosphorylated substrates (Fig. 38-5). Activation of WNT signaling prevents phosphorylation of β-catenin, which allows it to escape recognition by βTrCP and SCF E3 mediated ubiquitin ligation, leading to translocation of β-catenin to the nucleus with its partners TCF/LEF and activation of transcription of genes such as myc and cyclin D1. This pathway is also regulated by the *adenomatous polyposis coli* (APC) gene, which forms part of the

complex that promotes phosphorylation and subsequent destruction of β-catenin. Loss of APC in colorectal cells prevents phosphorylation of β-catenin, leading to its accumulation and promotion of cancer. The F-box protein βTrCP also regulates signaling through NFκB, which is inhibited by its association with the inhibitor of NFκB (IκB). Phosphorylation of IκB by IκB kinase allows βTrCP to bind to and activate proteasome-mediated destruction of IκB. This release of IκB activity allows NFκB to translocate to the nucleus and activate transcription of genes involved in proliferation and inflammation.

ANGIOGENESIS

Solid tumors require development of a neovasculature in order to sustain growth and survive conditions of hypoxia. Tumor angiogenesis is a complex process involving a number of different pro- and anti-angiogenic factors. The **vascular endothelial growth factor** (VEGF) family of proteins and receptors has emerged as a key regulator of this process. The VEGF family consists of seven ligands, including VEGF-A, -B, -C, -D, -E, and placenta growth factor (PlGF)-1 and -2 (Table 38-2). These ligands have varying affinities for the major VEGF receptors, VEGFR1 (also known as Flt-1), VEGFR2 (Flk-1/KDR), and VEGFR3 (Flt-4). The VEGF receptors are receptor tyrosine kinases. Neuropilins (NRP-1 and -2) are coreceptors that lack an intracellular signaling domain and enhance the binding of ligand to VEGFR1 and VEGFR2. VEGFR1 and VEGFR2 are expressed on the vascular endothelium and play key roles in angiogenic signaling, while signaling through VEGFR3 appears to play a major role in lymphangiogenesis (i.e., development of new lymphatic vessels). VEGFR2, which appears to be the major proangiogenic receptor that is targeted by VEGF-A, has been shown to signal via both a RAF/MAP kinase pathway to promote proliferation of endothelial cells, and a PI3K/AKT pathway to promote endothelial cell survival. VEGF also potently induces vascular permeability, utilizing similar signaling pathways both to promote the formation of transendothelial cell vesicular organelles and to open interendothelial junctions. Invasion and migration of endothelial cells is promoted by activation of matrix metalloproteinases and serine proteases and by reorganization of intracellular actin.

Activation of VEGF is mediated by stimuli such as hypoxia, cytokines and growth factors, and by a variety of oncogenes and tumor suppressor genes. Regulation of the response to hypoxia is mediated by **von Hippel Lindau** protein (VHL), a component of an SCF-like RING E3 ubiquitin ligase complex that targets **hypoxia inducible factor-1α (HIF-1α)** for destruction (Fig. 38-6). Loss of VHL is the defining event in the inherited VHL syndrome and is a frequent finding in sporadic clear cell renal carcinoma.

Under normoxic conditions, HIF-1α undergoes oxygen-dependent hydroxylation, which allows VHL binding and subsequent ubiquitin-mediated degradation. During hypoxia, VHL is unable to bind HIF-1α, allowing it to translocate to the nucleus and pair with its binding partner HIF-1β to activate transcription of hypoxia-inducible genes such as

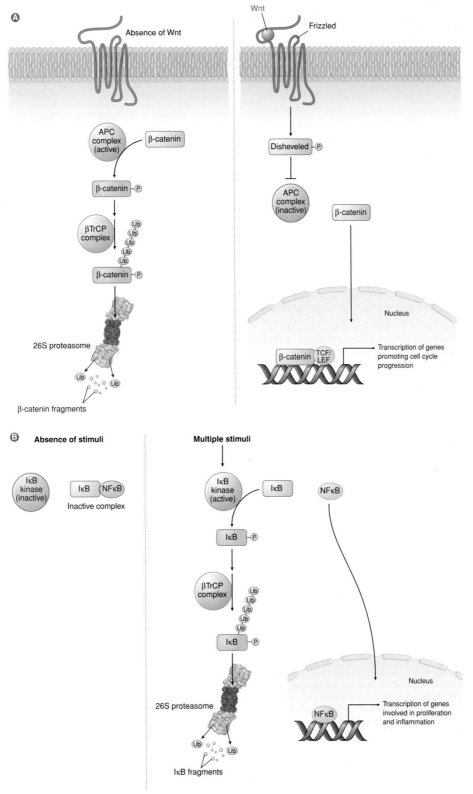

Figure 38-5. WNT signaling and NFκB pathways. A. In the absence of WNT signaling, β-catenin is phosphorylated by the adenomatous polyposis coli (APC) protein complex. Phosphorylated β-catenin is recognized by βTrCP and thereby targeted for ubiquitin-mediated proteasomal degradation. Activation of WNT signaling inhibits APC function, allowing β-catenin to accumulate and translocate to the nucleus. In the nucleus, β-catenin complexes with its partners TCF/LEF and activates the transcription of genes promoting cell-cycle progression. Hereditary or acquired loss of APC allows accumulation of β-catenin, contributing to oncogenesis in colon cancer. **B.** Similarly, the IκB protein is targeted for ubiquitin-mediated proteasomal degradation as a result of phosphorylation by IκB kinase and recognition by βTrCP. In the absence of stimuli, IκB binds to and inhibits NFκB. In the presence of stimuli, proteasomal degradation of IκB allows NFκB to translocate to the nucleus and activate the transcription of genes involved in proliferation and inflammation.

TABLE 38-2	Vascular Endothelial Growth Factor Receptors		
RECEPTOR	**TISSUE EXPRESSION**	**CORECEPTORS**	**LIGANDS**
VEGFR1	Vascular endothelium	Neuropilin-1	VEGF-A
	Hematopoietic cells	Neuropilin-2	VEGF-B
	Smooth muscle cells		PlGF-1
	Osteoclasts		PlGF-3
VEGFR2	Vascular endothelium	Neuropilin-1	VEGF-A
	Neuronal cells	Neuropilin-2	VEGF-E
VEGFR3	Vascular endothelium	None	VEGF-C
	Lymphatic endothelium		VEGF-D
	Monocytes and macrophages		

VEGFR, vascular endothelial growth factor receptor.

VEGF, PDGF-β, and TGF-α. In this manner, angiogenesis is stimulated by hypoxic conditions or by inappropriate activation of HIF-1 due to loss of VHL expression in tumors.

Cytokines such as IL-1 and IL-6, as well as prostaglandins and COX-2 activation, can also stimulate VEGF production. Signaling via EGFR family members, PDGFR, and the insulin like growth factor-1 receptor (IGF-1R) have also been shown to induce VEGF expression. Finally, activation of oncogenes such as RAS, SRC, and BCR-ABL, and inactivation of tumor suppressor genes such as p53 and PTEN, can result in VEGF production and thus promote angiogenesis and tumor maintenance.

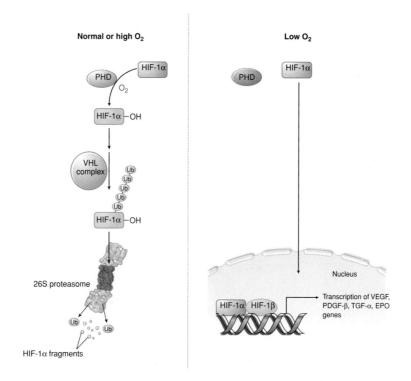

Figure 38-6. Regulation of the response to hypoxia. Under normal or high oxygen conditions, hypoxia inducible factor-1α (HIF-1α) is hydroxylated (in an oxygen-dependent reaction) by the prolyl hydroxylase PHD. Hydroxylated HIF-1α is recognized by VHL and thereby targeted for ubiquitin-mediated proteasomal degradation. PHD is inactive under low oxygen conditions, allowing HIF-1α to accumulate and translocate to the nucleus. In the nucleus, HIF-1α complexes with HIF-1β and activates the transcription of hypoxia-inducible genes such as VEGF, PDGF-β, TGF-α, and erythropoietin (EPO).

PHARMACOLOGIC CLASSES AND AGENTS

GROWTH FACTOR RECEPTOR AND SIGNAL TRANSDUCTION ANTAGONISTS

The identification of specific pathways that are dysregulated in certain tumors affords the potential to target key components of these pathways in a more selective manner. While the growth factor and signal transduction pathways described above are active during normal cell physiology, some tumors may become dependent on one pathway in particular for their growth and survival. Conversely, in normal cells the redundancy of signaling pathways allows for compensation, exemplified by the observation that inactivation of the EGFR gene in the mouse causes minimal defects. Thus, the therapeutic window of these newer targeted agents tends to be wider than that of traditional cytotoxic chemotherapy, with a different spectrum of adverse effects.

EGF Receptor Antagonists

Gefitinib and Erlotinib

The expression of EGFR on epithelial cells and its amplification and/or activation in a significant proportion of nonsmall cell lung cancers (NSCLCs) led to the development and testing of small-molecule EGFR inhibitors in patients with advanced NSCLC. The first of these agents to be tested was **gefitinib**, an orally bioavailable drug that competes with ATP binding to the cytoplasmic tyrosine kinase domain of the EGFR and is a reversible inhibitor of tyrosine kinase activity. In patients with metastatic NSCLC who had received multiple prior chemotherapy regimens, response rates to gefitinib were on the order of 10% in studies conducted in the United States and 20% in trials conducted in Japan and Europe. During the course of these studies, it was noted that patients who tended to respond were female, non-smokers, Asian, and with bronchoalveolar histology.

Given the dramatic responses in some cases, sequencing of the EGFR gene was carried out in tumors from these patients. Common activating mutations were found in the kinase domain of the EGFR, including L858R and in-frame deletions spanning positions 746 and 753. These mutations enhance tyrosine kinase activity in response to EGF and increase sensitivity to gefitinib. Signals generated by these mutant EGFRs selectively activate AKT and STAT pathways, leading to promotion of cell survival. Thus, screening tumors for these mutations could allow the selection of patients most likely to have an enhanced response to gefitinib.

Erlotinib is a clinically active oral small-molecule EGFR inhibitor similar to gefitinib. Both drugs yielded similar results in phase II studies, with similar adverse effects, including skin rash and diarrhea. Pivotal randomized phase III studies, however, demonstrated a statistically significant survival benefit for erlotinib but not for gefitinib. Thus, erlotinib is FDA-approved for second- or third-line treatment of metastatic NSCLC. In the randomized studies, response was not limited to patients with EGFR mutations but also occurred in patients with EGFR gene amplification. Furthermore, randomized comparisons of standard chemotherapy with or without EGFR inhibitors have not shown a benefit to the

population as a whole but have revealed increased response rates in patients carrying EGFR mutations. Trials are currently underway to determine the effectiveness of treatment with gefitinib or erlotinib earlier in the course of therapy in patients whose tumors express activating EGFR mutations.

Patients who initially respond to erlotinib or gefitinib but subsequently develop resistance have been found to carry a single secondary mutation, T790M, within the EGFR kinase domain. EGF receptors carrying both activating mutations and T790M exhibit reduced sensitivity to inhibition by erlotinib and gefitinib. Newer, irreversible EGFR inhibitors that act by covalently crosslinking to the receptor have been found to overcome resistance generated by the T790M mutation. In addition, the development of resistance in vitro is impaired by initial treatment with these irreversible EGFR inhibitors. One of these inhibitors, HKI-272, is currently in clinical testing in patients who have developed resistance to erlotinib or gefitinib. Other approaches to enhance the efficacy of small-molecule EGFR inhibition include the development of inhibitors such as **lapatinib**, which inhibits both EFGR and ErbB2 (HER-2).

Erlotinib has shown activity in a wide variety of other epithelial malignancies in which EGFR is overexpressed, including colon cancer, pancreatic cancer, and head and neck cancer. EGFR is frequently amplified, mutated, or overexpressed in patients with glioblastoma, but response rates of only 10% to 20% are seen with EGFR inhibitors, similar to patients with advanced NSCLC. A constitutively active EGFR genomic deletion variant, EGFRvIII, has been identified in a significant proportion of patients with glioblastoma. Because this mutant receptor also relies on PI3K/AKT signaling, it was hypothesized that loss of PTEN might impair response to EGFR inhibitors in this setting by activating AKT independently (Fig. 38-2B). Indeed, co-expression of EGFRvIII and PTEN in glioblastoma correlates with response to erlotinib.

Cetuximab and Trastuzumab

Strategies to target signaling by EGFR family members have also included the development of monoclonal antibodies that bind with high affinity to the extracellular ligand-binding domain of the receptor. One example is **cetuximab**, a chimeric mouse/human IgG1 monoclonal antibody that binds EGFR (ErbB1) with high specificity and an affinity greater than that of the physiologic ligands EGF or TGF-α. Cetuximab, when administered in combination with irinotecan, has been shown to improve response rates in EGFR-expressing colorectal cancers.

The principal adverse effects of cetuximab are similar to those of the small-molecule EGFR inhibitors, including skin rash and diarrhea. Interestingly, the development of skin rash due to cetuximab has been shown to be predictive of tumor response, perhaps reflecting the degree of EGFR blockade by cetuximab. As a single agent, cetuximab enhances the efficacy of radiation therapy in locally advanced head and neck cancer, improving locoregional control and overall survival compared to radiation therapy alone. Less dramatic effects have thus far been seen in NSCLC, where EGFR mutations do not predict responsiveness to cetuximab.

Trastuzumab, another chimeric mouse/human IgG monoclonal antibody, is directed against ErbB2 (HER-2). Approximately 25% to 30% of breast cancers are associated with amplification and overexpression of *Her2/neu*; these cancers also display more aggressive behavior. HER2 amplifies the signal generated by other ErbB family members via the formation of heterodimers. Trastuzumab down-regulates HER-2 and thereby disrupts this signaling. Trastuzumab has significant activity in breast tumors with high levels of HER-2 amplification. In vivo, trastuzumab also appears to induce antibody-dependent cellular cytotoxicity and inhibit angiogenesis. In addition to its intrinsic activity in the advanced and metastatic cancer settings, treatment of HER-2 amplified breast cancers with trastuzumab in the adjuvant setting following resection enhances the efficacy of chemotherapy and reduces rates of recurrence by 50%. The principal adverse effect of trastuzumab is cardiotoxicity, particularly when used in combination with anthracyclines.

Pertuzumab is another novel antibody under development. This agent binds to an epitope on HER-2 different from the epitope recognized by trastuzumab, and sterically hinders the association of HER-2 with other ErbB family members. Since HER-2 is one of the major dimerization partners used by this family of growth factor receptors, inhibition by pertuzumab is proposed to disrupt signaling by all EGFR family members and may be effective at lower levels of HER-2 expression.

BCR-ABL/C-KIT/PDGFR Inhibition

Imatinib mesylate

Imatinib mesylate is a small-molecule tyrosine kinase inhibitor that was initially developed as a 2-phenylaminopyrimidine derivative specific for PDGFR. Imatinib was subsequently found to be a potent inhibitor of ABL kinases, including the BCR-ABL fusion protein generated as a result of the t(9;22) chromosomal translocation (Philadelphia chromosome) found in **chronic myelogenous leukemia** (CML), and was also found to inhibit the receptor tyrosine kinase C-KIT. *Imatinib mesylate is the canonical example of a targeted therapeutic agent, because BCR-ABL is uniquely expressed by leukemic cells and is essential for their survival.*

Initial in vitro studies demonstrated that imatinib mesylate potently and specifically inhibits growth of BCR-ABL-expressing cells. Subsequent evaluation of an oral formulation in mice demonstrated suppression of growth of human BCR-ABL-positive tumors with minimal adverse effects. A phase I study of imatinib mesylate in patients with chronic-phase CML yielded impressive results, with normalization of blood counts (a hematologic response) in 95% of patients and significant reduction in Philadelphia chromosome-positive cells (a cytogenetic response) in 41% of patients. In a phase III study comparing imatinib mesylate with standard treatment with interferon and cytarabine in patients with chronic-phase CML, imatinib mesylate was superior, with a hematologic response rate of 95% and complete cytogenetic responses in 76% of patients. Treatment of accelerated or blast-phase CML with imatinib mesylate is less effective but associated with some responses. Imatinib mesylate is relatively well tolerated; its principal adverse effects are superficial edema, nausea, muscle cramps, skin rash, and diarrhea.

Despite impressive hematologic and cytogenetic response rates in chronic phase CML, evaluation of residual BCR-ABL transcript by reverse transcriptase PCR (RT-PCR) reveals that only 39% of patients have a complete molecular response, a much more sensitive measure of residual leuke-

mia cells. Preliminary results suggest that, compared with the standard dose of 400 mg, initial treatment with 800 mg of imatinib mesylate may increase the frequency of molecular responses but at the expense of a higher frequency of adverse effects, and this is currently being evaluated in a randomized study. Given the relatively recent development of imatinib mesylate, longer-term follow-up is needed to determine how sustained the responses will be over time.

Mutation of C-KIT, the receptor for stem cell factor (SCF), is found frequently in **gastrointestinal stromal tumors** (GIST) and in the myeloproliferative disorder **systemic mastocytosis**. In GIST, mutations and in-frame deletions of C-KIT are typically found in the juxtamembrane domain, resulting in constitutive activation of the tyrosine kinase in the absence of ligand. In contrast, in systemic mastocytosis, the characteristic D816V activating C-KIT mutation is within the kinase domain itself. Whereas imatinib mesylate has shown significant activity in advanced gastrointestinal stromal tumors, it has proven largely ineffective in the treatment of systemic mastocytosis due to ineffective targeting of C-KIT kinases with the D816V mutation.

The **idiopathic hypereosinophilic syndrome**, as well as a variant of systemic mastocytosis with eosinophilia, is characterized by the expression of the FIPL1-PDGFRA fusion protein, which is generated by an interstitial chromosomal deletion and results in constitutive signaling through PDGFRA. Inhibition of PDGFRA by treatment with imatinib mesylate has been a successful therapeutic approach in both conditions.

Dasatinib and Nilotinib

Crystallographic studies show that imatinib mesylate targets the ATP binding site of ABL only when the activation loop of the kinase is closed, thereby stabilizing the protein in an inactive conformation. Clinical resistance to imatinib mesylate has been recognized in some patients with CML, occasionally due to amplification of BCR-ABL, but more commonly due to the acquisition of resistance mutations. Only a fraction of these mutations directly interfere with drug binding, with most mutations instead affecting the ability of ABL to adopt the closed conformation to which imatinib mesylate binds.

A second class of tyrosine kinase inhibitors, the dual SRC-ABL inhibitors, can bind to the ATP-binding site in ABL irrespective of the conformational status of the activation loop. One of these drugs, **dasatinib** (BMS-354825), has significantly greater efficacy than imatinib mesylate against wild type BCR-ABL, and it inhibits the activity of most clinically relevant imatinib mesylate-resistant BCR-ABL isoforms, with the exception of the T315I mutation.

Another structure-based approach to improve the efficacy of imatinib mesylate has been to substitute alternative binding groups for the N-methylpiperazine group, resulting in the development of **nilotinib** (AMN107). Similar to dasatinib, the affinity of nilotinib for wild type BCR-ABL is significantly higher than that of imatinib mesylate, and nilotinib inhibits most imatinib-resistant mutants with the exception of T315I. Both dasatinib and nilotinib have shown activity in patients with CML who have developed resistance to imatinib mesylate, and both are undergoing further clinical testing. Both drugs also overcome resistance of the C-KIT D816V mutation in vitro and are being tested in patients with systemic mastocytosis.

FLT3 Inhibitors

One of the most common mutations in **acute myelogenous leukemia** (AML), occurring in approximately 25% to 30% of patients, involves internal tandem duplication within the juxtamembrane domain of the receptor tyrosine kinase FLT3. This mutation results in ligand-independent dimerization and activation of signaling via the RAS/MAPK and STAT pathways. A number of FLT3 inhibitors have been developed and demonstrate anti-leukemia cell activity in vitro. Several experimental agents, such as PKC412, have demonstrated single-agent activity in patients with relapsed/refractory AML carrying FLT3 mutations. Studies are underway to examine whether FLT3 inhibitors may improve outcomes in combination with standard chemotherapy. One of these agents, PKC412, is also a potent inhibitor of C-KIT and the D816V resistance mutation, and is also being examined in patients with systemic mastocytosis.

JAK2 Inhibitors

Despite the success of imatinib mesylate in the treatment of CML, the genetic basis of the other major **myeloproliferative disorders** (polycythemia vera, essential thrombocythemia, and myeloid metaplasia with myelofibrosis) has, until recently, remained obscure. It is now apparent that a common activating mutation in JAK2 (V617F) underlies the aberrant signaling and proliferation in most cases, although how one mutation leads to this spectrum of disorders remains unclear. The V617F mutation is found in the pseudokinase domain of JAK2, and disruption of this autoinhibitory region leads to unchecked activity of the kinase. Cells containing the JAK2 V617F mutation are growth inhibited and undergo apoptosis in response to specific JAK2 inhibitors in vitro. Thus, JAK2 inhibitors are under development for the treatment of polycythemia vera, essential thrombocythemia, and myeloid metaplasia with myelofibrosis.

RAS/MAP Kinase Pathway Inhibition

Oncogenic mutation of *ras* is one of the most common events in malignancy, occurring in approximately 30% of human cancers. K-*ras* mutations are frequently observed in non-small cell lung cancer, colorectal cancer, and pancreatic carcinoma, while H-*ras* mutations are found in kidney, bladder, and thyroid cancers, and N-*ras* mutations occur in melanoma, hepatocellular carcinoma, and hematologic malignancies. However, despite the frequency of these mutations, inhibition of RAS has thus far been difficult to achieve and has yielded minimal clinical success. Most efforts have been focused on targeting farnesylation of RAS and inhibiting downstream effectors.

Farnesylation of RAS is essential for its association with the plasma membrane and subsequent activation. A number of farnesyltransferase inhibitors (FTIs) have been developed that inhibit RAS farnesylation. While these inhibitors demonstrate activity against RAS in vitro, some RAS mutants exhibit resistance, and there are numerous other targets of farnesylation that could be inhibited by FTIs and are likely responsible for the cytotoxic effects of these drugs. FTIs that have been tested clinically include **tipifarnib** and **lonafarnib**. Tipifarnib has demonstrated activity in relapsed/refractory AML, although responses appear to be independent of *ras* mutations. Clinical testing of FTIs in solid tumors has not yet met with success.

Immediately downstream of RAS is the serine/threonine kinase RAF, which phosphorylates MEK, which in turn phosphorylates MAP kinase leading to transcription factor activation (Fig. 38-2A). There are three RAF family members—A-RAF, B-RAF, and C-RAF. Activating mutations in B-RAF have recently been found in a significant proportion of malignant melanomas and are also observed at a lower frequency in lung, colorectal, ovarian, and thyroid cancers. **Sorafenib** was initially designed as a C-RAF inhibitor but also demonstrates high inhibitory activity on both wild-type and mutant B-RAF. Sorafenib has shown significant activity against melanoma cell lines that contain activating B-RAF mutations, and the drug is currently in clinical testing for use in melanoma. Sorafenib also inhibits the tyrosine kinase activity of VEGFR-2 and PDGFR-β and has demonstrated clinical efficacy in the treatment of renal cell carcinoma.

There are two MEK homologues, MEK1 and MEK2, both of which have dual serine-threonine and tyrosine kinase activity, phosphorylating and activating ERK1 and ERK2. CI-1040 is a highly active inhibitor of both MEK1 and MEK2. Early clinical testing of CI-1040 in patients with solid tumors has shown some activity but unfavorable pharmacokinetic characteristics. More potent and bioavailable second-generation MEK inhibitors have been developed and are entering clinical trials.

An important emerging concept is the need to identify specific subsets of tumors that are susceptible to specific targeted agents, exemplified by the sensitivity of EFGR-mutant NSCLC to gefitinib and erlotinib. One current approach is to identify gene expression profiles that are markers of oncogene activation. For example, a specific gene expression profile has been characterized for RAS activation, and this profile correlates with RAS mutation and RAS pathway activation in cell lines and tumor specimens. Only cell lines displaying gene expression profiles concordant with RAS activation respond to FTIs in vitro. Thus, selection of patients for clinical trials based on such an approach may enrich for clinical activity of agents such as FTIs. Another approach has been to identify subsets of RAS pathway activation profiles that predict responsiveness to downstream inhibition of targets such as MEK. Comparison of cell lines with activating N-RAS mutations and those with activating B-RAF mutations has shown that only the latter cell lines exhibit high sensitivity to the MEK inhibitor CI-1040, possibly because MEK is more immediately downstream of RAF. Therefore, selection of patients with tumors containing B-RAF mutations for clinical trials of MEK inhibitors will potentially yield greater efficacy.

mTOR Inhibitors

Signaling via the PI3K/AKT pathway leads to downstream activation of the mammalian target of rapamycin (mTOR). mTOR is a serine-threonine kinase that regulates multiple cellular functions, including cell growth and proliferation, via activation of translation. mTOR regulation is accomplished in part by activation of the 40S ribosomal protein S6 kinase (p70^{S6k}) and inactivation of the 4E-binding protein (4E-BP1), which regulates translation of certain mRNAs. Dysregulated mTOR activity is seen in a wide variety of malignancies in which the PI3K pathway is activated or PTEN is lost. In addition, hamartoma syndromes such as tuberous sclerosis result in activation of mTOR. The tuberous sclerosis protein complex (TSC1/2) act as an intermediary between AKT and mTOR: native TSC1/2 inhibits mTOR, and activation of AKT results in phosphorylation of TSC1/2 and subsequent derepression of mTOR.

TOR was originally identified by a screen for mutations in yeast that conferred resistance to rapamycin, and mTOR was subsequently discovered as its mammalian homologue. **Rapamycin** (also known as **sirolimus**) binds to FKBP12, a member of the FK506-binding protein family, and the rapamycin-FKBP12 complex binds to mTOR and inhibits its activity. In addition to its immunosuppressive properties, rapamycin promotes cell cycle inhibition, apoptosis, and inhibition of angiogenesis by blocking translation of downstream targets of mTOR such as cyclin D1, c-MYC, the antiapoptotic protein BAD, and HIF-1α.

A number of rapamycin derivatives are currently undergoing clinical testing in a wide variety of malignancies, including **temsirolimus** (CCI-779) and **everolimus** (RAD001). Both are soluble ester analogues of rapamycin that demonstrate dose-dependent inhibition of tumor cell growth in vitro. Temsirolimus has shown evidence of activity in several phase II clinical studies in renal cell carcinoma, breast cancer, and mantle cell non-Hodgkin's lymphoma. Toxicities have included skin rash, mucositis, thrombocytopenia, and leukopenia.

It is likely that particular subsets of patients will benefit from mTOR inhibitors, and future clinical trials will be designed accordingly. For example, in renal cell carcinoma, activation of HIF-1α due to loss of VHL expression has been shown to sensitize cells to mTOR inhibition and may explain the clinical activity of temsirolimus in a subset of patients. Patients with glioblastoma and PTEN loss may be particularly responsive to mTOR inhibition, given the PI3K/AKT pathway activation in this malignancy. Furthermore, because EGFR signaling is dependent on this pathway as well, combination therapy using EGFR inhibitors and mTOR inhibitors is being explored.

PROTEASOME INHIBITORS

Given the role of ubiquitin-mediated proteasomal degradation in regulating the cell cycle, apoptosis, and a number of other processes involved in neoplastic transformation, proteasome inhibitors have been tested in vitro and in vivo for antitumor effects. The small molecule **bortezomib**, a dipeptide with a linked boronate moiety, targets with high affinity and specificity an active site N-terminal threonine residue within the 20S catalytic subunit of the proteasome (Fig. 38-4A). Bortezomib induces growth inhibition and apoptosis of tumor cells with relatively few toxic effects on normal cells. Clinically, the effects of bortezomib are reversible, requiring intravenous dosing on a twice-weekly schedule.

Bortezomib displays marked in vitro efficacy against cell lines derived from multiple myeloma, lymphoma, chronic lymphocytic leukemia, head and neck cancer, prostate cancer, and a variety of other solid-tumor malignancies. Bortezomib has also demonstrated considerable efficacy in clinical trials involving patients with relapsed or refractory multiple myeloma, with an overall response rate of 35% and a complete response rate of 10% in a phase II study, and superior response rates and survival compared with standard glucocorticoid therapy in a phase III study. Principal adverse effects include neuropathy, thrombocytopenia, and neutro-

penia. Based on these results, bortezomib has been approved for the treatment of refractory multiple myeloma. Given its relatively modest adverse effect profile, bortezomib has also been incorporated into combination regimens for primary therapy of multiple myeloma, with some of the highest response rates seen to date in this disease. In addition, bortezomib is being tested alone and in combination with standard chemotherapy in a wide variety of other malignancies.

Several mechanisms have been proposed to explain the efficacy of bortezomib in multiple myeloma. One mechanism involves inhibition of NFκB through stabilization of IκB (Fig. 38-5B). Given that NFκB activates the transcription of genes promoting cell proliferation and blocking apoptosis in response to inflammation and other stimuli, antagonism of these actions by bortezomib would be expected to lead to growth inhibition and apoptosis. A second proposed mechanism involves accumulation of misfolded proteins leading to cell death. Like the plasma cells from which they arise, multiple myeloma cells synthesize large amounts of immunoglobulin. The proteasome may play an important role in degrading misfolded proteins in these cells, and inhibition of proteasome function by bortezomib could be lethal in this setting. It has also been proposed that bortezomib can lead to stabilization of CDK inhibitors and of p53. Indeed, mutation of p53 is associated with resistance to bortezomib. A second mechanism of bortezomib resistance involves increased expression of heat shock protein-27 (HSP-27), and approaches designed at inhibiting heat shock proteins are underway both to overcome bortezomib resistance and to enhance its efficacy.

ANGIOGENESIS INHIBITORS

Recognition of the primary role of VEGF and its receptors in the regulation of angiogenesis has led to strategies to block VEGF function as a means of disrupting tumor vasculature. The most successful approaches to date have included the development of neutralizing antibodies against VEGF or VEGFR and small-molecule inhibitors of the VEGFR tyrosine kinase domain.

Anti-VEGF Antibodies

Bevacizumab is a recombinant humanized mouse monoclonal IgG1 antibody directed against VEGF-A, one of the major proangiogenic VEGF family members. In mouse models, blocking VEGF with a monoclonal antibody inhibits angiogenesis and growth of human tumor xenografts. Early clinical studies were designed to test the efficacy of bevacizumab in metastatic renal cell carcinoma, because most of these cancers overexpress VEGF as a consequence of VHL loss and HIF-1 activation. Treatment of patients with refractory renal cell carcinoma with single-agent bevacizumab resulted in a significant improvement in progression-free survival, although the response rate was only 10%.

Incorporation of bevacizumab into standard chemotherapy regimens has yielded further success in a number of tumor types. Addition of bevacizumab to chemotherapy for metastatic colon cancer has shown significant improvements in response rates and in median survival from approximately 15 to 20 months. Improvement in median survival has also resulted from the addition of bevacizumab to carboplatin and paclitaxel for the treatment of metastatic NSCLC, although patients with cerebral metastasis, squamous cell histology, and central tumors were excluded from these studies because intratumoral bleeding could lead to potentially fatal cerebral hemorrhage or severe hemoptysis. Benefits have also been seen in breast cancer, and clinical trials are ongoing to determine efficacy in other solid tumors such as ovarian cancer and pancreatic cancer.

The potentiation of cytotoxic chemotherapy by bevacizumab and its modest activity as a single agent suggest that its mechanism of action may not be as simple as induction of tumor hypoxia and starvation of nutrients. Activation of VEGFR signaling has been shown to increase vascular permeability, resulting in high interstitial fluid pressures in tumors. This high interstitial fluid pressure is postulated to prevent optimal delivery of chemotherapy to the tumor, and indeed, inhibition of VEGF with bevacizumab has been shown to decrease vascular permeability, reduce interstitial fluid pressure, and improve drug delivery to tumors.

Adverse effects of bevacizumab include proteinuria, hypertension, risk of thrombosis or bleeding, and impairment of wound healing.

VEGFR Inhibitors

Other strategies designed to inhibit VEGF signaling have included the development of monoclonal antibodies against VEGFR and small-molecule inhibitors of VEGFR tyrosine kinase activity. The small-molecule inhibitors of VEGFR are of special interest because a number of these agents inhibit multiple receptor tyrosine kinases (Table 38-3). For example, ZD6474 inhibits VEGFR-1, VEGFR-2, and VEGFR-3 as well as EGFR. Given the demonstrated efficacy of bevacizumab and erlotinib in the treatment of NSCLC, presumably via inhibition of VEGF and EGFR, respectively, ZD6474 is being evaluated in combination regimens for patients with NSCLC.

The treatment of clear cell renal cell carcinoma provides another example of how the broad activity of these agents could be utilized. Loss of VHL and activation of HIF-1 result in expression of VEGF, PDGF-β, and TGF-α in a significant proportion of these tumors, and inhibition of VEGF alone with bevacizumab has yielded only modest benefit in patients with metastatic renal carcinoma. More significant activity has recently been seen with the receptor tyrosine kinase inhibitors **sunitinib** (SU11248), which inhibits VEGFR-1, VEGFR-2, and PDGFR, and **sorafenib**, which inhibits not only B-RAF but also VEGFR-1, VEGFR-2, and PDGFR. Given the refractory nature of renal cell carcinoma to traditional chemotherapy, the development and use of these new agents, based on a deeper understanding of the tumor cell biology, represents a major advance in the treatment of this tumor. Further improvements in response rates may be seen by combining these agents with drugs that provide additional blockade of TGF-α signaling through EGFR, such as erlotinib.

Other small-molecule VEGF inhibitors have not shown equivalent responses to bevacizumab. In metastatic colorectal cancer, for example, combination regimens involving **vatalanib** (PTK-787), which inhibits VEGFR-1 and VEGFR-2, have yet to demonstrate an improvement in progression-free survival. Further studies with similar agents are underway, and it is likely that activity of these agents will be context-specific.

Thalidomide and Lenalidomide

Thalidomide is a synthetic glutamic acid derivative that was found to have sedative and antiemetic properties and was marketed outside the United States during the mid-1950s as a treatment for morning sickness in pregnant women. Tragically, thalidomide was discovered to be teratogenic, causing severe developmental deformities including stunted limb development (phocomelia). Thalidomide was subsequently shown to have immunomodulatory properties, inhibiting the synthesis of TNF-α and demonstrating efficacy in the treatment of erythema nodosum leprosum (ENL). In addition, it was hypothesized that the abnormal limb development caused by thalidomide was due to antiangiogenic properties, and indeed it has since been shown that thalidomide inhibits basic fibroblast growth factor (bFGF)-induced angiogenesis. Thalidomide has also been shown to costimulate T cells. Given its combination of properties, thalidomide is now termed an **immunomodulatory drug** (IMiD).

Because increased microvascular density in the bone marrow is associated with poor outcomes in multiple myeloma, thalidomide was initially tested in patients with advanced disease and found to have an overall response rate of 32%. Currently, the combination of thalidomide and dexamethasone is a standard first-line regimen for patients with multiple myeloma, with response rates of 60% to 70%. Principal adverse effects include risk of thrombosis, neuropathy, constipation, and somnolence. Evidence is accumulating that the efficacy of thalidomide in the treatment of multiple myeloma is related to both its immunomodulatory and antiangiogenic properties.

Lenalidomide is a synthetic second-generation IMiD analogue of thalidomide. While maintaining the antiangiogenic activity of thalidomide, lenalidomide exhibits enhanced inhibition of TNF-α and costimulation of T cells as well as direct antitumor activity with induction of apoptosis. Lenalidomide has demonstrated activity even in thalidomide-refractory multiple myeloma, and in primary treatment has resulted in overall response rates of 90% when used in combination with dexamethasone. The incidence of thrombosis with lenalidomide is markedly reduced compared to that with thalidomide, and lenalidomide causes less neuropathy, constipation, and somnolence as well. Lenalidomide has also shown significant activity in the treatment of myelodysplastic syndromes, principally in patients with a deletion of the long arm of chromosome 5 (del 5q) or with normal cytogenetics.

TABLE 38-3	**Vascular Endothelial Growth Factor Receptor Inhibitors**
VEGFR TYROSINE KINASE INHIBITORS	**TARGETS**
Sunitinib (SU11248)	VEGFR-1, VEGFR-2, PDGFR
Sorafenib (Bay 93-4006)	VEGFR-1, VEGFR-2, PDGFR, B-RAF
AG013736	VEGFR-1, VEGFR-2
Vatalanib (PTK-787)	VEGFR-1, VEGFR-2
ZD-6474	VEGFR-1, VEGFR-2, VEGFR-3, EGFR

VEGFR, vascular endothelial growth factor receptor.

The principal adverse effects of lenalidomide are myelosuppression and thrombocytopenia.

TUMOR-SPECIFIC MONOCLONAL ANTIBODIES

Most hematologic malignancies express specific cell-surface markers that have been used to subclassify the malignancies by immunohistochemistry and flow cytometry. The development of chimeric monoclonal antibodies against several of these antigens has provided the opportunity for targeted antibody therapy in a number of these disorders (Table 53-1).

Although the mechanism of action of monoclonal antibodies is incompletely understood, it is likely related to the induction of antibody-dependent cell-mediated cytotoxicity and apoptosis. For example, B-cell lymphomas characteristically express the CD20 cell-surface antigen, which is normally found almost exclusively on mature B cells. The anti-CD20 IgG1 monoclonal antibody **rituximab** has demonstrated significant single-agent activity and enhancement of the effects of chemotherapy in B-cell non-Hodgkin's lymphoma (NHL), and is now routinely incorporated in the therapy of this disorder. Principal adverse effects include immunosuppression due to the targeting of normal mature B cells, and hypersensitivity reactions related to the chimeric nature of the antibody.

Conjugation of radioactive isotopes to anti-CD20 antibodies, such as iodine-131 (I^{131}) **tositumomab** and yttrium-90 (Y^{90}) **ibritumomab tiuxetan**, has allowed targeted radioimmunotherapy of B-cell NHL. These agents are being incorporated into treatment regimens of patients with refractory disease and as induction therapy for stem cell transplantation.

Alemtuzumab is a humanized monoclonal antibody directed against the pan-leukocyte antigen CD52. This agent has been used in the treatment of chronic lymphocytic leukemia (CLL) and as part of conditioning regimens for stem cell transplantation. Because alemtuzumab induces lysis of both T-cell and B-cell populations, its principal adverse effect is significant immunosuppression, including risk for *Pneumocystis carinii* pneumonia, fungal, cytomegalovirus, and herpesvirus infections. Therefore, prophylaxis for opportunistic infections is required.

Two additional examples of antibody conjugates are denileukin diftitox and gemtuzumab ozogamicin. **Denileukin diftitox**, a recombinant fusion protein composed of fragments of diphtheria toxin and human IL-2, targets the CD25 component of the IL-2 receptor and has demonstrated activity in T-cell NHL. **Gemtuzumab ozogamicin** is a conjugate between the antitumor antibiotic calicheamicin and a monoclonal antibody directed against CD33, which is found on the surface of leukemic blasts in more than 80% of patients with AML.

Conclusion and Future Directions

Elucidation of the molecular and biochemical circuitry that regulates normal cell proliferation and identification of the key mutations that promote oncogenesis have provided the ability to target specific pathways that are dysregulated in tumors. The success of imatinib mesylate in the treatment of CML demonstrates that cancers can become dependent on oncogenes such as BCR-ABL, requiring oncoprotein signaling for continued proliferation and survival. Although inhibitors of receptor tyrosine kinases and intracellular kinases have a wider therapeutic index than traditional antineoplastic therapies and have had some success in certain tumors, in many cases responses are neither durable nor complete. The identification of subsets of tumors in which specific pathways are activated, such as the EFGR mutation in NSCLC, will guide therapy and improve response rates. Oncogenic microarray signatures and correlations between specific mutations and sensitivity to targeted agents will facilitate the design of clinical trials focusing on subsets of patients with the highest likelihood of response. Efficacy will also be improved with second- and third-generation drugs that have higher specificity for targets and the ability to overcome resistance mutations.

It is clear, however, that multiple factors contribute to tumor development, including downstream mutations in pathways regulating cell cycle progression, apoptosis, proteasomal degradation, and angiogenesis. The biology of these processes and of tumor cell invasion and acquisition of metastatic potential will likely provide novel targets for directed therapy. As with combination chemotherapy, the successful targeted therapies of the future will likely involve inhibition of multiple pathways using a combination of agents directed at the defects found in individual tumors. The higher degree of specificity inherent in such strategies will likely give them a superior therapeutic index compared to traditional combination antineoplastic chemotherapy and will hopefully be met with a greater degree of clinical success.

Suggested Reading

Adjei AA, Hidalgo M. Intracellular signal transduction pathway proteins as targets for cancer therapy. *J Clin Oncol* 2005;23: 5386–5403. (*Future directions in targeting of intracellular signaling.*)

Bartlett JB, Dredge K, Dagleish AG. The evolution of thalidomide and its IMiD derivatives as anticancer agents. *Nat Rev Cancer* 2004;4:314–322. (*Historic and scientific overview of thalidomide and its derivatives.*)

Hanahan D, Weinberg RA. The hallmarks of cancer. *Cell* 2000;100: 57–70. (*Seminal overview of the characteristic genetic changes leading to oncogenesis.*)

Hicklin DJ, Ellis LM. Role of the vascular endothelial growth factor pathway in tumor growth and angiogenesis. *J Clin Oncol* 2005; 23:1011–1027. (*Overview of VEGF pathways.*)

Krause DS, van Etten RA. Tyrosine kinases as targets for cancer therapy. *N Engl J Med* 2005;353:172–187. (*Advances in tyrosine kinase inhibition.*)

Mani A, Gelmann EP. The ubiquitin-proteasome pathway and its role in cancer. *J Clin Oncol* 2005;23:4776–4789. (*Biochemical details of ubiquitin pathways.*)

Wullchleger S, Loewith R, Hall M. TOR signaling in growth and metabolism. *Cell* 2006;124:471–484. (*Possible applications of mTOR inhibitors.*)

Drug Summary Table   Chapter 38 Pharmacology of Cancer: Signal Transduction

Drug	Clinical Applications	Serious and Common Adverse Effects	Contraindications	Therapeutic Considerations
INHIBITORS OF EGFR (ErbB1) AND HER2/neu (ErbB2) *Mechanism—Small-molecule and monoclonal antibody inhibitors of EGFR and HER2/neu; see specific drug*				
Gefitinib	Nonsmall cell lung cancer	*Interstitial lung disease, corneal erosion* Rash, diarrhea	Hypersensitivity to gefitinib	Reversible inhibitor of the EGFR (ErbB1) cytoplasmic tyrosine kinase domain; competes with ATP binding to the kinase domain More favorable response in patients with bronchoalveolar cell carcinoma
Erlotinib Lapatinib (investigational)	Nonsmall cell lung cancer Carcinoma of pancreas	*Myocardial infarction, gastrointestinal hemorrhage, deep vein thrombosis, microangiopathic hemolytic anemia, elevated liver enzymes, stroke, conjunctivitis, keratitis* Rash, diarrhea	Hypersensitivity to erlotinib or lapatinib	Erlotinib is a reversible inhibitor of the EGFR (ErbB1) cytoplasmic tyrosine kinase domain; competes with ATP binding to the kinase domain Erlotinib has a statistically greater survival benefit compared to gefitinib Lapatinib, an inhibitor of EGFR and ErbB2, is under development
Cetuximab	Colorectal cancer Head and neck cancer	*Cardiac arrest, leukopenia, renal failure, interstitial lung disease, pulmonary embolism, infection* Rash, diarrhea, hypomagnesemia, gastrointestinal disturbance, asthenia, headache	Hypersensitivity to cetuximab	Monoclonal antibody that binds to extracellular domain of EGFR (ErbB1) Improved response rates in EGFR-expressing colorectal cancer when combined with irinotecan Development of rash is predictive of tumor response
Trastuzumab Pertuzumab (investigational)	Breast cancer with HER2 overexpression	*Cardiotoxicity, nephrotic syndrome, interstitial pneumonia* Diarrhea, anemia, leukopenia	Hypersensitivity to trastuzumab or pertuzumab	Monoclonal antibodies against ErbB2 (HER2) Treatment with trastuzumab in the adjuvant setting enhances the efficacy of chemotherapy and reduces rates of recurrence Pertuzumab, which binds to a different epitope of HER2 than trastuzumab, is under development
INHIBITORS OF BCR-ABL, C-KIT, AND PDGFR *Mechanism—Small-molecule tyrosine kinase inhibitors active against ABL kinases (including BCR-ABL fusion protein), C-KIT, and PDGFR*				
Imatinib mesylate	Chronic myeloid leukemia (CML) with Philadelphia chromosome positivity Gastrointestinal stromal tumor (GIST) with Kit (CD117) positivity Idiopathic hypereosinophilic syndrome	*Edema, myelosuppression, hepatotoxicity* Nausea, muscle cramps, diarrhea, rash	Hypersensitivity to imatinib mesylate	Hematologic and cytogenetic response (disappearance of Philadelphia chromosome) is observed in a large fraction of patients with chronic-phase CML; molecular response (disappearance of BCR-ABL) is observed in a smaller fraction
Dasatinib (investigational) Nilotinib (investigational)	Dasatinib is a dual SRC-ABL kinase inhibitor that binds to the ATP-binding site in ABL irrespective of the conformational status of the activation loop Nilotinib substitutes alternative binding groups for the N-methylpiperazine group Dasatinib and nilotinib have greater efficacy than imatinib mesylate against wild-type BCR-ABL in vitro, and they inhibit imatinib mesylate-resistant BCR-ABL isoforms with the exception of the T315I mutation			

(Continued)

Drug Summary Table | **Chapter 38 Pharmacology of Cancer: Signal Transduction** *(Continued)*

Drug	Clinical Applications	*Serious and Common* Adverse Effects	Contraindications	Therapeutic Considerations
INHIBITORS OF RAS/MAP KINASE PATHWAYS				
Mechanism—See specific drug				
Tipifarnib (investigational) Lonafarnib (investigational)	Inhibit farnesyltransferase, which is important for farnesylation of RAS and recruitment of RAS to the plasma membrane Tipifarnib has demonstrated activity in relapsed/refractory acute myeloid leukemia (AML)			
Sorafenib	Renal cell carcinoma	*Cardiovascular disease, erythema multiforme, hemorrhage, thromboembolic disorder, acute renal failure* Hypertension, alopecia, hand-foot rash and pain due to cytotoxic therapy, rash, gastrointestinal disturbance, elevated amylase and lipase levels, depressed blood cell counts, neuropathy	Hypersensitivity to sorafenib	Initially developed as a C-RAF inhibitor, sorafenib demonstrates high inhibitory activity on both wild-type and mutant B-RAF Significant activity against melanoma cell lines that have activating B-RAF mutations Also inhibits VEGFR-2 and PDGFR-beta
mTOR INHIBITORS				
Mechanism—mTOR is a serine-threonine kinase that regulates cell growth and proliferation via activation of translation; rapamycin binds to FKBP12, and the rapamycin-FKBP12 complex binds to mTOR and inhibits its activity				
Rapamycin (sirolimus)	Prophylaxis for renal transplant rejection	*Deep vein thrombosis, pulmonary embolism, pancytopenia, hepatotoxicity, interstitial lung disease* Hypertension, peripheral edema, asthenia, arthralgia	Hypersensitivity to rapamycin	In addition to inhibiting mTOR, rapamycin also blocks downstream targets of mTOR such as cyclin D1, c-MYC, the antiapoptotic protein BAD, and HIF-1
Temsirolimus (investigational) Everolimus (investigational)	Temsirolimus and everolimus are ester analogues of rapamycin In phase II clinical studies, temsirolimus has shown activity against renal cell carcinoma, breast cancer, and mantle cell non-Hodgkin's lymphoma			
PROTEASOME INHIBITOR				
Mechanism—Inhibits an active site N-terminal threonine residue within the 20S catalytic subunit of the proteasome				
Bortezomib	Multiple myeloma Mantle cell lymphoma	*Heart failure, neutropenia, thrombocytopenia* Neuropathy, hypotension, rash, gastrointestinal disturbance, arthralgia	Hypersensitivity to bortezomib, boron, or mannitol	Because of its relatively modest adverse effects, bortezomib is incorporated into combination regimens for primary therapy of multiple myeloma, with good response rates
ANGIOGENESIS INHIBITORS				
Mechanism—Neutralizing antibodies against VEGF or VEGFR and small-molecule inhibitors of the VEGFR tyrosine kinase domain; see specific drug				
Bevacizumab	Metastatic colorectal cancer Metastatic breast cancer Nonsmall cell lung cancer	*Arterial thromboembolism, hypertensive crisis, impaired wound healing, gastrointestinal perforation, nephrotic syndrome* Neuropathy, dizziness, headache, gastrointestinal disturbance	Hypersensitivity to bevacizumab	Monoclonal IgG1 antibody against VEGF-A Clinical trials are ongoing to determine efficacy in other solid tumors such as ovarian and pancreatic cancer

Drug	Clinical Applications	Serious and Common Adverse Effects	Contraindications	Therapeutic Considerations
Sunitinib	Renal cell carcinoma Gastrointestinal stromal tumor	*Left ventricular dysfunction, anemia, hemorrhage, neutropenia, thrombocytopenia, lymphopenia* Yellow skin, inflammation of mucous membrane, neuropathy, gastrointestinal disturbance	Hypersensitivity to sunitinib	Sunitinib inhibits VEGFR-1, VEGFR-2, and PDGFR
Vatalanib (investigational)	Inhibits VEGFR-1 and VEGFR-2 Under investigation in metastatic colorectal cancer			
Thalidomide	Multiple myeloma Erythema nodosum leprosum	*Teratogenesis, thrombotic disorder; neutropenia, leukopenia, Stevens-Johnson syndrome* Peripheral neuropathy, edema, hypocalcemia, constipation, somnolence	Pregnancy Women capable of becoming pregnant Males not using latex condom	An immunomodulatory drug that inhibits basic fibroblast growth factor (bFGF)-induced angiogenesis; also, co-stimulates T cells Combination of thalidomide with dexamethasone is a standard first-line regimen for multiple myeloma, with response rates of 60%–70%
Lenalidomide	Multiple myeloma Myelodysplastic syndrome	*Same as thalidomide, except for lower incidence of thrombosis, neuropathy, constipation and somnolence*	Pregnancy Women capable of becoming pregnant Males not using latex condom	Analogue of thalidomide with enhanced inhibition of TNF-α and improved T-cell costimulatory properties, while maintaining anti-angiogenic activity Combination of lenalidomide with dexamethasone has response rates of 90% in multiple myeloma

TUMOR-SPECIFIC MONOCLONAL ANTIBODIES AND OTHER RECOMBINANT PROTEINS

Mechanism—See specific drug

Drug	Clinical Applications	Serious and Common Adverse Effects	Contraindications	Therapeutic Considerations
Rituximab Tositumomab Ibritumomab Alemtuzumab Denileukin diftitox Gemtuzumab	B cell non-Hodgkin's lymphoma (rituximab, tositumomab, ibritumomab) Chronic lymphocytic leukemia (alemtuzumab) T cell non-Hodgkin's lymphoma (denileukin diftitox) Acute myeloid leukemia (gemtuzumab)	*Significant immunosuppression (including the risk of developing opportunistic bacterial, fungal, and viral infections), hypersensitivity, anaphylactoid reaction related to chimeric antibody* Hematologic abnormalities, infusion reactions	Hypersensitivity reactions	Rituximab: anti-CD20 antibody Tositumomab: anti-CD20 antibody Ibritumomab: anti-CD20 antibody Alemtuzumab: anti-CD52 antibody Denileukin diftitox: fusion protein of diphtheria toxin and IL-2 Gemtuzumab: conjugate of an anti-CD33 antibody and calicheamicin (antitumor antibiotic)

39

Principles of Combination Chemotherapy

Ryan L. Albritton, Donald M. Coen, and David E. Golan

INTRODUCTION

Upon identifying the infectious agent or cell type responsible for an infectious or neoplastic illness, the physician may choose a single-drug therapy that specifically and potently targets that agent or cell type. Provided that the pathogen or tumor is susceptible, the emergence of resistance is rare, and the therapeutic index is high, such monotherapies, as compared to multidrug combinations, can minimize unwanted adverse effects. However, when pathogens or tumors are resistant to a chemotherapeutic agent or quickly develop resistance to others, when multiple pathogens with different drug susceptibilities are present simultaneously, or when the dose of the therapeutic agent is limited by toxicity, single-drug regimens often fail. Under these circumstances, combination chemotherapy may offer decisive advantages over monotherapy. The drugs in a multidrug regimen can interact synergistically to enhance the antimicrobial or antineoplastic effectiveness of the combination, and can decrease the likelihood that resistance will emerge. Combinations are fre-

quently used when treatment must be initiated before the definitive identification of the pathogen, and synergistic combinations can be used to reduce toxicity when the individual drugs in the combination have low therapeutic indices. Although combination chemotherapy opens new avenues for the expedient elimination of a pathogen or tumor from the body, it also introduces an extra level of complexity, with the potential for multiple adverse effects and drug interactions. The goal of any combination drug regimen should be to enable the efficient removal of the offending pathogen or tumor without incurring unacceptable toxicity in the host.

Case

Mr. M is a 27-year-old man from rural Haiti who presents to a clinic with a chronic cough. He could not afford treatment at a private clinic, so he went to a drugstore and asked the pharmacist for some appropriate medicines. The pharmacist thought that Mr. M could have tuberculosis, and he sold Mr. M a 2-week supply of isoniazid and rifampin. Mr. M took both drugs for a couple of days, but they made him nauseated, and he therefore decided to take just the isoniazid for 2 weeks. His symptoms resolved.

Three months later, Mr. M's cough returned. This time, he noticed blood in his sputum and he had night sweats. He took the remainder of the 2-week supply of rifampin and experienced a brief lull in his symptoms. Within a few days, however, his cough, bloody sputum, and night sweats returned. Because he did not have enough money to buy additional drugs, he traveled to the nearest government hospital to seek free care and medications. The government doctor took three sputum samples, all of which were positive for acid-fast bacilli. The doctor also sent sputum to the laboratory for culture, but since the causative agent of tuberculosis, *Mycobacterium tuberculosis*, is slow-growing, he also started Mr. M on a drug regimen consisting of isoniazid, rifampin, pyrazinamide, and ethambutol for 2 months, followed by isoniazid and rifampin for 4 months.

After several weeks, however, the culture revealed that Mr. M's tuberculosis was not susceptible to either isoniazid or rifampin. He is now seeking a new recommendation for treatment.

QUESTIONS

■ **1.** Why were Mr. M's initial efforts at treatment unsuccessful? What treatment strategy could have been employed to avoid Mr. M's treatment failure?

■ **2.** Why did the government doctor prescribe four different drugs for Mr. M?

■ **3.** How is resistance transferred from one generation of tubercle bacilli to the next? How does this resistance-transfer mechanism compare to the mechanism by which penicillin resistance is transferred from one generation of bacteria to the next?

■ **4.** Does Mr. M have multidrug-resistant tuberculosis (MDR-TB)? Should he stay on the four-drug regimen that includes isoniazid and rifampin? If not, how should his treatment be modified?

ANTIMICROBIAL COMBINATION THERAPY

Microbial infections are commonly treated with drug combinations for a variety of reasons, including the threat of drug resistance, the need to treat immunocompromised patients, and the polymicrobial nature of many infections. Because microbes are genetically distant from humans, antimicrobial drug combinations can also offer the advantage of targeting several different molecules that are specific to the microbe(s), without a concomitant increase in adverse effects. This rationale is in stark comparison to the use of many antineoplastic drugs (see below), where adverse effects often limit the dose of an agent. The following discussion provides conceptual background on the different types of antimicrobial drug interactions, and then discusses specific examples of antimicrobial combination therapy.

MINIMUM INHIBITORY CONCENTRATION AND MINIMUM BACTERICIDAL CONCENTRATION

Antimicrobial agents with activity against a particular pathogenic microorganism (bacterial, protozoal, or fungal) can be characterized by the **minimum inhibitory concentration** (MIC) and the **minimum bactericidal concentration** (MBC) for that drug-pathogen pair. The MIC is defined as the lowest concentration of drug that inhibits growth of the microorganism after 18 to 24 hours of incubation in vitro. The MBC is defined as the lowest concentration of drug at which 99.9% of a culture of bacteria or some other microorganism is killed after 18 to 24 hours of incubation in vitro. In general, the MBC is greater than the MIC. Comparisons between the MICs or MBCs and the clinically achievable concentrations of antimicrobial drugs allow these drugs to be grouped broadly into two categories: *cidal* and *static* (Table 39-1; see Chapter 31, Principles of Antimicrobial and Antineoplastic Pharmacology). An antimicrobial agent is *static* (e.g., bacterio*static*, fungi*static*) if its MIC is within the therapeutic range of the drug but its MBC is not, and the agent is *cidal* (e.g., bacteri*cidal*, fungi*cidal*) if its MBC is within the therapeutic range of the drug. It is important to note that the MIC and MBC refer to a specific drug-microbe pair under a specific set of conditions. Many drugs with activity against an organism are static in one growth medium but cidal in another growth medium, or are cidal at sufficiently high concentrations in vitro. In addition, for any particular drug, the MIC and MBC may differ from one microbe to the next. Indeed, a drug may be static against one organism and cidal against another. As an operating definition, we can state that, *at therapeutic concentrations, cidal drugs kill the microorganism, while static drugs merely arrest microbial growth*. In this definition, the therapeutic concentration refers to plasma drug levels that are sufficient for pharmacologic activity (here, killing or arresting the growth of the microorganism) without unacceptable toxicity to the patient. For example, most inhibitors of bacterial cell wall synthesis are bactericidal, whereas most inhibitors of bacterial protein synthesis are bacteriostatic (see Chapter 32, Pharmacology of Bacterial Infections: DNA Replication,

TABLE 39-1 Examples of Bactericidal and Bacteriostatic Antibiotics

BACTERICIDAL ANTIBIOTICS		BACTERIOSTATIC ANTIBIOTICS
CONCENTRATION-DEPENDENT	TIME-DEPENDENT	
Aminoglycosides	β-lactams	Chloramphenicol
Bacitracin	Isoniazid	Clindamycin
Quinolones	Metronidazole	Ethambutol
	Polymyxins	Macrolides
	Pyrazinamide	Novobiocin
	Rifampin	Sulfonamides
	Vancomycin	Tetracyclines
		Trimethoprim

Transcription, and Translation, and Chapter 33, Pharmacology of Bacterial Infections: Cell Wall Synthesis).

As noted in Chapter 31, an important distinction between static and cidal drugs lies in their clinical applications. In general, the successful use of static drugs to treat infections requires an intact host immune system. This is because static drugs do not themselves kill existing microorganisms but only prevent them from multiplying. Accordingly, such drugs rely on the host's immune and inflammatory mechanisms to effect clearance of existing organisms from the body. These drugs are more efficacious when initiated early in the course of an infection, at a time when the infectious burden is lower. Related to this observation is the possible reappearance of an infection if the static drug is removed before the immune system has completely cleared the infection. Under these circumstances, the microorganism can resume growth after removal of the drug (Fig. 39-1).

According to their mechanism of cell killing, bactericidal agents can be further characterized as either **time-dependent** or **concentration-dependent** (Fig. 39-2). Time-dependent bactericidal agents exhibit a constant rate of killing that is independent of drug concentration, provided that the drug concentration is greater than the minimum bactericidal concentration (MBC). Thus, the overriding consideration for the clinical use of such agents is not the absolute drug concentration that is achieved, but for how long the drug concentration remains in the therapeutic range (which is defined as [drug] > MBC). In contrast, concentration-dependent bactericidal agents have a rate of killing that increases with drug concentration for [drug] > MBC. For such agents, a single very large dose can have a profound therapeutic effect, and may be sufficient to eliminate the infection.

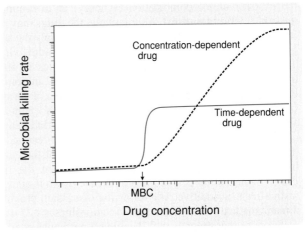

Figure 39-2. Relationship between rate of microbial killing and drug concentration for time-dependent and concentration-dependent bactericidal drugs. Time-dependent bactericidal agents exhibit a constant rate of microbial killing at concentrations of drug greater than the minimum bactericidal concentration (MBC) *(solid line)*. In contrast, concentration-dependent bactericidal agents show increased killing with increasing drug concentration *(dashed line)*. Note that the efficacy of concentration-dependent bactericidal agents eventually plateaus, because the effective concentration of the drug becomes limited by the rate of drug diffusion to its molecular target.

TYPES OF DRUG INTERACTIONS—SYNERGY, ADDITIVITY, AND ANTAGONISM

The discussion has thus far considered the general properties of drugs used as single agents to treat a microbial infection. When such drugs are used in combination with other agents, these effects can be modified (either enhanced or diminished). In fact, drugs that have little or no activity against an organism when used as single agents can show high activity when used in combination with another agent. One example of this concept involves the treatment of *Enterococcus faecalis,* a Gram-positive organism that exhibits little susceptibility to **aminoglycosides**. Recall that, according to the Davis model, aminoglycosides kill bacteria by inducing misreading of the genetic code and translation of defective proteins, which cause further cellular damage (see Chapter 32). In the case of *E. faecalis,* aminoglycosides are unable to penetrate the organism's thick cell wall to reach their target, the 30S ribosomal subunit. However, when used in combination with a cell wall synthesis inhibitor such as **vancomycin** or a **β-lactam** antibiotic, aminoglycosides are able to reach the bacterial ribosomes and effectively kill the bacteria (see Chapter 33). The potentiating effect of the cell wall synthesis inhibitor on the activity of the aminoglycoside is an example of the important pharmacologic concept of **synergy.**

From this example, one could ask whether combining two drugs with individual activity against a particular microbe always results in a more potent drug combination. Surprisingly, for many combinations, this turns out not to be the case. In fact, when two drugs with activity against the same pathogen are combined, the drugs can interact to enhance

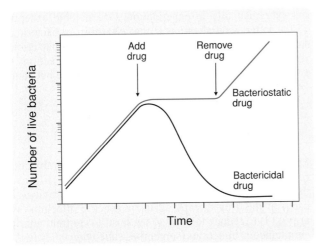

Figure 39-1. Comparison of the effects of bacteriostatic and bactericidal drugs on bacterial growth kinetics. In the absence of drug, bacteria grow with exponential (first-order) kinetics. A bactericidal drug kills the target organism, as demonstrated by the time-dependent decrease in the number of live bacteria. A bacteriostatic drug prevents microbial growth without killing the bacteria. Removal of a bacteriostatic drug is followed by an exponential increase in bacterial number as the previously inhibited bacteria resume growth. Bacteriostatic drugs eradicate infections by limiting the growth of the infecting organism for a long enough period of time to allow the host immune system to kill the bacteria.

the efficacy of the combination (synergy) or to diminish the efficacy (**antagonism**). Alternatively, the drugs may not interact, and the effect of the combination is simply the sum of the effects of each drug used individually (**additivity**). The interaction between two antimicrobial drugs is often quantified by selecting a particular endpoint (e.g., inhibition of bacterial growth) and then measuring the effect of various combinations of the two drugs that reach this endpoint. When such data are plotted, additional information can be obtained (Fig. 39-3). The x- and y-intercepts correspond to the MICs of the two drugs, and the concavity of the curve indicates the nature of the interaction between the two drugs—concave-up is synergistic; concave-down is antagonistic; linear is additive. The following discussion provides a mathematical rationale for these relationships.

Suppose that drugs A and B inhibit a particular enzyme required for bacterial growth and division. In this case, the ratio $[A]/MIC_A$ would represent the fraction of bacterial growth inhibition that can be attributed to the presence of drug A. This is known as the fractional inhibitory concentration of A (FIC_A). Similarly, $FIC_B = [B]/MIC_B$ is the fraction of growth inhibition that can be attributed to drug B. Now, suppose that the concentration of A is decreased by a small amount, $-d[A]$. To compensate for this loss of growth inhibition ($dFIC_A = -d[A]/MIC_A$), the concentration of B must be increased by an amount $+d[B]$.

For additive drugs, the ratio $-d[A]/d[B]$ (which is the same as the slope of the curve in Fig. 39-3) is a constant

because one unit of A has exactly the same activity as (MIC_A/MIC_B) units of B. For example, A and B could bind to independent sites on the enzyme (i.e., each drug has no effect on the binding of the other drug).

In contrast, if A and B are synergistic, then the amount of B ($d[B]$) required to compensate for a decrease in A ($-d[A]$) depends on the amount of A that is already present. Because of the potentiating effect of drug A on drug B, $d[B]$ is less for higher $[A]$ (i.e., $d^2[A]/d[B]^2 > 0$, which corresponds to the concave-up curve in Fig. 39-3). From a molecular perspective, this relationship could correspond to a situation in which the binding of A to the enzyme induces a conformational change in the binding site for B that enhances the binding of B.

By extension, A and B are antagonistic if the amount of B required to compensate for a small decrease in the concentration of A is larger for higher $[A]$ (i.e., $d^2[A]/d[B]^2 < 0$, which corresponds to the concave-down curve in Fig. 39-3). For example, the binding of A could result in a lower affinity for the binding of B to the enzyme.

Note that, because of its intuitiveness and simplicity, the mathematical model described above is often used to define synergy, additivity, and antagonism. It is not, however, the most general formulation of the quantitative analysis of the effects of multiple drugs, which is beyond the scope of this text. The interested reader is referred to the work of Chou and Talalay (1984) for more detailed coverage of this subject.

Several generalizations can be made concerning the nature of drug interactions between different classes of antimicrobial agents. First, many bacteriostatic drugs (e.g., **tetracycline**, **erythromycin**, **chloramphenicol**) antagonize the action of bactericidal drugs (e.g., **vancomycin**, **penicillin**) by inhibiting cell growth and/or preventing the cellular processes that are required for cidal drugs to act (described below in more detail). Second, two bactericidal drugs usually act synergistically in combination. One notable exception to the latter generalization is that **rifampin**, a bactericidal inhibitor of RNA polymerase, antagonizes other bactericidal drugs by inhibiting cell growth. Finally, the interactions between two bacteriostatic drugs are often additive but cannot be predicted in all cases.

EXAMPLES OF ANTIMICROBIAL COMBINATION THERAPY

There are several compelling reasons for using combinations of drugs to treat microbial infections, including (1) to prevent the emergence of resistance; (2) to enhance the activity (efficacy) of the drug therapy against a specific infection (synergy); (3) to reduce toxicity to the host; (4) to treat multiple simultaneous infections (sometimes called *polymicrobial infections*); and (5) to treat a life-threatening infection empirically before the microorganism causing the infection has been identified.

Tuberculosis

The treatment of tuberculosis illustrates one of the principal reasons combinations of drugs are used—to suppress the emergence of resistance. In the course of this illness, tuberculous bacilli (also called *mycobacteria*) are inhaled and phagocytosed by alveolar macrophages, where the bacilli

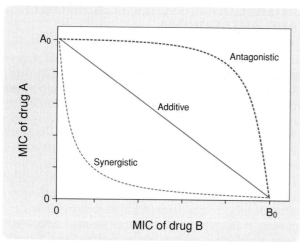

Figure 39-3. Quantification of additive, synergistic, and antagonistic drug interactions. Drug combinations can exhibit additive, synergistic, or antagonistic effects. The nature of this interaction can be depicted graphically by observing the effect that each drug has on the other's minimum inhibitory concentration (MIC). If two drugs have an additive interaction, then the addition of increasing amounts of Drug B to Drug A results in a linear decrease in the MIC of Drug A; in this case, each of the two drugs can be thought of as interchangeable. If two drugs have a synergistic interaction, then the addition of Drug B to Drug A results in a significantly lower MIC for Drug A (i.e., there is an increase in the potency of Drug A). If two drugs have an antagonistic interaction, then the addition of Drug B to Drug A does not significantly lower the MIC of Drug A; in some cases (*not shown*), much higher doses of each drug must be administered to achieve the same effect as that of each drug used alone. A_0 and B_0 are the MICs of Drugs A and B, respectively, when used as single agents.

multiply within intracellular vacuoles. A predominantly T-cell–mediated lymphocytic response is then elicited, and the macrophages and helper T cells form large granulomas that wall off the infected sites. Activated macrophages are usually able to keep the infection under control by killing the multiplying bacilli, but are unfortunately unable to eradicate the infection completely. Tissue damage is caused by the release of neutral proteases and reactive oxygen intermediates from activated macrophages, with the end result that central necrosis occurs in the tuberculous cavities in the lungs. Inside each of these cavities, as many as 10^8 to 10^9 living bacilli may be held in check by macrophages and helper T cells.

Successful cure of tuberculosis infections typically requires the use of combinations of drugs with antimycobacterial activity. Commonly used drugs include **isoniazid, rifampin, pyrazinamide**, and **ethambutol** (see Chapter 33). As illustrated in the case of Mr. M, a standard regimen could consist of 2 months of isoniazid, rifampin, pyrazinamide, and ethambutol, followed by 4 months of isoniazid and rifampin. **Streptomycin** and other second-line drugs are sometimes substituted for one or two drugs in this regimen if resistance develops. Isoniazid and rifampin are the preferred drugs because of their ability to kill intracellular as well as extracellular mycobacteria. The other drugs are either bacteriostatic (pyrazinamide and ethambutol), ineffective against intracellular bacilli (streptomycin), or hepatotoxic (pyrazinamide).

As noted in Chapter 33, resistance to antimycobacterial drugs develops primarily through chromosomal mutations, and the frequency of resistance to any one of the drugs is about 1 in 10^6 bacteria. These mutations are passed on to daughter cells when the bacteria replicate, leading to establishment of a drug-resistant population. Chapter 33 discusses the implications of the fact that a tuberculous cavity contains 10^8 to 10^9 bacteria, while the frequency of mutants resistant to a single drug is about 1 in 10^6. On average, 100 bacteria will already be resistant to each drug in any single lesion, even before that drug is administered. Moreover, treatment with only one drug would result in selection for bacilli that are resistant to that drug. In the case of Mr. M, his initial 2 weeks of isoniazid treatment likely killed all of the isoniazid-susceptible bacilli in his cavity. This accounts for the cessation in his symptoms after 2 weeks of treatment. However, the 100 or so isoniazid-resistant bacilli that were selected for by Mr. M's use of monotherapy remained and multiplied. If he had taken the rifampin as well as the isoniazid, only 1 in 10^{12} bacilli would have been resistant to both drugs.

Over the 3 months during which Mr. M stopped taking isoniazid, the isoniazid-resistant bacilli remaining in his lungs multiplied, creating another lesion of bacilli and leading to a relapse in his symptoms. He then began taking rifampin. Of these 10^8 to 10^9 isoniazid-resistant bacilli, again there was a 1 in 10^6 probability that a bacillus had mutated to acquire rifampin resistance. By taking rifampin for 2 weeks, he killed all the rifampin-susceptible bacilli but selected for rifampin-resistant organisms. He was therefore left with bacilli that were both isoniazid-resistant and rifampin-resistant—the phenotype of **multidrug-resistant tuberculosis (MDR-TB)**.

Mr. M should not now continue with the combination regimen he was initially prescribed, because it could cause further resistance by augmenting or amplifying the original resistance pattern. In other words, it could further select for isoniazid- and rifampin-resistant bacilli, eliminating any susceptible bacilli that remain. Furthermore, continuing to take drugs known to be ineffective would increase the chances of adverse effects without conferring therapeutic benefit. Importantly, Mr. M could also transmit MDR-TB to others.

Mr. M will therefore require a new drug regimen for treatment of MDR-TB. Ideally, the regimen should be constructed using drugs that have been shown to be effective in susceptibility tests. Also, drugs that have been part of his previously unsuccessful treatment plan should be avoided (i.e., pyrazinamide and ethambutol), even if they have demonstrated "susceptibility" in culture tests. Treatment for MDR-TB should begin with six new drugs to which Mr. M's TB isolate has proven susceptibility. Such regimens usually include daily dosing of an aminoglycoside (**streptomycin, kanamycin**, or **amikacin**) for at least 4 to 6 months. Four to five oral drugs should be administered along with the aminoglycoside for 24 months after the sputum culture converts to negative. **Fluoroquinolones, rifabutin, ethionamide**, and **clofazimine** are second-line drugs that could be included in the regimen. Note that, as a whole, the second-line regimen will be significantly more toxic and less well tolerated than the first-line regimen.

Considering all of the issues discussed above, MDR-TB is to be avoided at all costs. Patients with drug-susceptible tuberculosis require access to combination therapy as well as help in complying with the combination therapy to avoid the emergence of drug-resistant bacilli. This rationale is the basis for **DOTS** (Directly Observed Therapy Short Course), the WHO-recommended strategy for tuberculosis treatment. DOTS is a public health program that has five components: (1) political commitment and resources for TB control; (2) the use of sputum-smear microscopy for accurate diagnosis of TB infection; (3) a standardized 6- to 8-month treatment that is directly observed by a community health worker for at least the first 2 months; (4) a regular and uninterrupted supply of medicines; and (5) standardized recording and reporting of each patient's treatment and progress to central authorities. When used in cases of drug-susceptible TB, DOTS has a remarkable cure rate and can prevent the development of resistance. As noted above, treatment of MDR-TB requires therapy that is more intensive, more invasive, more toxic, and of longer duration than the standardized DOTS regimen.

Synergistic Combinations

A second reason for using a combination drug regimen is to take advantage of the synergy between the actions of the two drugs. This consideration is especially important in the setting of infections that are not readily handled by the immune defenses of immunocompromised patients. In the immunocompetent patient, bacteriostatic and bactericidal drugs are often equally efficacious in eliminating an infection. Bactericidal drugs are strongly preferred, however, in the setting of immunocompromised patients (e.g., HIV/AIDS patients, immunosuppressed transplant patients, and neutropenic cancer patients), endovascular infection (e.g., bacterial endocarditis), or meningitis. The reason for using bactericidal combinations in the immunocompromised patient should be obvious—the host does not have sufficient numbers of functioning lymphocytes and/or neutrophils to eliminate even a nondividing bacterial population. In the case of endocarditis, the reason is not so straightforward. In this case, although there is not a deficiency in the absolute number of leukocytes, the phagocytes are unable to penetrate efficiently the thick "vegetation"—composed of a meshwork of fibrin, platelets, and bacterial products—that surrounds the bacteria. Bactericidal drug combinations are often indicated for meningitis to maximize the probability of overcoming the poor opsonization of bacteria by antibody and complement in the immunologically privileged site of the meninges (see Chapter 7, Principles of Nervous System Physiology and Pharmacology).

One example of antibacterial synergy involves the use of a **penicillin** and an **aminoglycoside** to treat the most common causes of acute and subacute bacterial endocarditis, *Staphylococcus aureus* and *Streptococcus viridans,* respectively. As described above, the mechanism of synergy relies on the penicillin inhibiting cell wall biosynthesis, which allows the aminoglycoside to penetrate the thick peptidoglycan layer of these Gram-positive organisms.

Two other commonly used synergistic combinations include (1) the antifungal combination of **amphotericin B** and **flucytosine**, and (2) the antibacterial and antiprotozoal combination of a **sulfonamide** and **trimethoprim** or **pyrimethamine**. These classic examples serve to illustrate two basic mechanisms whereby one drug can potentiate the activity of another. It is thought that, analogous to the action of penicillins, which enhance the uptake of aminoglycosides by Gram-positive bacteria, amphotericin B enhances flucytosine uptake by fungal cells by damaging ergosterol-rich fungal cell membranes (see Chapter 34, Pharmacology of Fungal Infections). Only after penetrating the fungal membrane can flucytosine be converted into its active form (5-fluorouracil, which is converted to 5-FdUMP, an irreversible inhibitor of thymidylate synthase) by a fungal-specific deaminase. Because of the particularly low therapeutic index of amphotericin B (which is primarily a consequence of its nephrotoxicity), this combination has the great advantage of reducing the dose of amphotericin B required to treat a systemic fungal infection such as cryptococcal meningitis.

Sulfamethoxazole and **trimethoprim** are commonly used in combination in the treatment of *Pneumocystis carinii* pneumonia, an opportunistic infection frequently encountered in patients with AIDS, as well as many urinary tract infections caused by Gram-negative enteric organisms. An analogous combination, **sulfadoxine** and **pyrimethamine**, is used in the treatment of malaria, toxoplasmosis, and other protozoal infections. These combinations illustrate a second mechanism whereby drugs can exert a synergistic effect. The mechanism of synergy is based on the inhibition of two steps in folic acid biosynthesis affecting the cellular concentration of the same critical metabolite, dihydrofolate (see Chapter 31). The reduced form of this metabolite, tetrahydrofolate, is a required substrate for purine biosynthesis and for many one-carbon transfer reactions, and is thus necessary for DNA replication and cell division (see Fig. 31-7).

The sulfonamides are competitive inhibitors of dihydropteroate synthase, the enzyme that catalyzes the first step in the synthesis of tetrahydrofolate from PABA and pteridine. Trimethoprim and pyrimethamine inhibit a subsequent step in this pathway, acting as competitive inhibitors of the bacterial and protozoal isoforms of dihydrofolate reductase (DHFR), respectively. The sulfonamide-induced reduction in the cellular concentration of dihydrofolate acts synergistically with trimethoprim or pyrimethamine, because the latter drugs compete with dihydrofolate for binding to DHFR. (In other words, the action of trimethoprim or pyrimethamine is enhanced because the sulfonamide acts to decrease the concentration of dihydrofolate, the substrate that competes with these drugs for binding to the enzyme.) Moreover, resistance to this combination cannot develop easily because strains that are resistant to trimethoprim usually possess an altered DHFR that has a lower affinity for dihydrofolate. Under these circumstances, the lower concentration of dihydrofolate that results from the action of the sulfonamide is insufficient to allow the altered DHFR to meet the cellular needs for tetrahydrofolate. For resistance to develop to the drug combination, the cell would simultaneously have to overproduce PABA (to overcome the competitive inhibition by the sulfonamide) and mutate its DHFR (to decrease the affinity of this enzyme for trimethoprim). This combination of events is unlikely to occur in a single bacterial or protozoal cell.

Coadministration of Penicillins with β-Lactamase Inhibitors

The combination of a β-lactam antibiotic and a β-lactamase inhibitor (e.g., **clavulanic acid**, **sulbactam**, **tazobactam**) illustrates a mechanism of drug interaction that is not technically synergistic (because the β-lactamase inhibitor has no antibacterial activity of its own) but that shares a functional similarity with the drug combinations discussed above. Clavulanic acid is an inhibitor of β-lactamase, an enzyme used by many β-lactam-resistant Gram-positive and Gram-negative bacteria to inactivate penicillins (see Chapter 33). By preventing the hydrolysis and inactivation of penicillins, clavulanic acid (and other β-lactamase inhibitors) greatly increases the potency of penicillins (and other β-lactams) against bacteria that express β-lactamase. This combination has been effective in the treatment of infections due to penicillin-resistant *Streptococcus pneumoniae,* which is a common cause of otitis media in infants. Such organisms have typically acquired resistance to penicillins through a plasmid-encoded β-lactamase.

Polymicrobial and Life-Threatening Infections

Combinations of antimicrobial drugs are used not only to prevent the emergence of resistance and to act synergistically against a specific, known pathogen, but also to treat polymicrobial infections and infections in which treatment must be initiated before the microbe causing the infection is identified. Consider, for example, the case of a ruptured appendix or colonic diverticulum that has leaked bacteria into the peritoneal cavity. Such an intra-abdominal abscess is likely to contain a wide spectrum of microorganisms—much too broad to be targeted effectively by a single antibiotic. After draining the abscess, treatment with a combination of antibacterial agents such as an **aminoglycoside**—to kill aerobic Gram-negative Enterobacteriaceae (e.g., *E. coli*)—and **clindamycin** or **metronidazole**—to kill anaerobes (e.g., *Bacte-*

roides fragilis; see Chapter 35)—often results in clearance of the infection. In cases where presumptive treatment is indicated before the causative microorganism is identified, body fluids such as blood, sputum, urine, and cerebrospinal fluid (CSF) should be cultured before initiating therapy. A combination of drugs with activity against the microbes that are most likely to be involved in the infection (or that could result in the most serious outcome) is then administered until a positive bacteriologic identification is made and drug susceptibility results are obtained. At that point, it may be possible to discontinue unnecessary drugs and to implement specific and potent monotherapy.

UNFAVORABLE DRUG COMBINATIONS

Antagonism can sometimes result from combination chemotherapy, although this situation is to be avoided if possible. Antagonism is most commonly observed when static drugs are used in combination with cidal drugs. For example, **tetracyclines** are bacteriostatic antimicrobials that antagonize the bactericidal activity of **penicillins** (see Chapter 32). Recall that the bactericidal activity of penicillins depends on cell growth. By inhibiting the transpeptidation reaction involved in bacterial cell wall crosslinking, the penicillins create an imbalance between cell wall synthesis and autolysin-mediated cell wall degradation. If the bacterial cell continues to grow, this leads to spheroplast formation and eventually to osmotic lysis. A protein synthesis inhibitor such as tetracycline, which arrests cell growth, would therefore antagonize the effect of a β-lactam. Similarly, **imidazoles** and **triazoles** are fungistatic agents that antagonize the fungicidal activity of **amphotericin B** (see Chapter 34). The mechanism of antagonism can be appreciated by noting that amphotericin B acts by binding ergosterol and forming pores in the fungal membrane, whereas imidazoles and triazoles inhibit a microsomal cytochrome P450-dependent enzyme, 14α-sterol demethylase, which is involved in ergosterol biosynthesis. Thus, the imidazoles and triazoles oppose the action of amphotericin B by decreasing the concentration of the target for the latter drug. (Despite these considerations, static and cidal antimicrobial drugs are sometimes used clinically in combination when no good alternatives exist. In such cases, it may be required to increase the dose of the static and/or cidal drug to overcome the antagonistic drug-drug interaction. The resulting elevation in the level of one or both drugs in the combination can lead to an increased probability of adverse effects.)

ANTIVIRAL COMBINATION THERAPY: HIV

As discussed in Chapter 36, Pharmacology of Viral Infections, no anti-HIV drug shows long-term suppressive benefit when used individually. This is due largely to the development of drug resistance.

The viral life cycle is central to understanding the reason that monotherapy for HIV fails to suppress long-term viral replication (see Chapter 36; Fig. 36-2). After virus binding and fusion, the viral enzyme reverse transcriptase (RT) syn-thesizes double-stranded DNA from the single-stranded viral RNA genome. The DNA is then integrated into the host chromosome and transcribed over and over using the host cell's transcription machinery. These complete genomic transcripts are eventually packaged into virions that infect new cells. However, HIV RT is relatively unfaithful, so replication error rates are quite high. In addition, transcription of the integrated DNA into RNA is also error-prone. As a result, on average, every new HIV particle contains one mutation relative to its parental virus. Although the resulting error rate is not so high as to be intolerable to the virus, it is sufficiently high that, after repeated cycles of infection, reverse transcription, and transcription, a significant number of viruses encode altered targets of anti-HIV therapy and thereby acquire resistance, even prior to treatment.

In the setting of high mutation rates, combination chemotherapy is beneficial. Combinations of RT inhibitors (e.g., AZT and 3TC) are more effective than one RT inhibitor alone, in part because resistance to one nucleoside analogue does not necessarily confer resistance to another. The current standard of care for treatment of HIV infection is "triple therapy." Triple therapy can use a nucleoside analogue RT inhibitor in combination with a nonnucleoside reverse transcriptase inhibitor (NNRTI) and a protease inhibitor, or two nucleoside analogues and a protease inhibitor, or two nucleoside analogues and an NNRTI. Clinical trials have shown that such combinations are able to reduce viral RNA plasma levels below the limit of detection (currently, 50 copies/mL). At such low levels of viral replication, the probability of resistance emerging to any one of the drugs is greatly reduced. Thus, for example, it has been shown that combinations remain effective for much longer periods of time than does any single agent. However, the complicated administration schedules (which are improving) and adverse effects of such combinations can reduce compliance. Thus, although some investigators are optimistic that early aggressive treatment with combinations of drugs can suppress viral replication indefinitely, others prefer to wait before initiating such aggressive treatment.

ANTINEOPLASTIC COMBINATION CHEMOTHERAPY

Antineoplastic chemotherapy faces a number of intrinsic difficulties. *Cancer cells can be thought of as "altered self" cells that maintain a number of similarities to normal, noncancerous cells, making it difficult to target the cancer cells specifically.* Also, many of the currently available cancer chemotherapeutic agents have numerous adverse effects that often limit their dose and frequency of administration. Despite these hurdles, combination chemotherapy has led to remarkable advances in the treatment of cancer, including the examples of Hodgkin's disease and testicular cancer discussed at the end of this section. Table 39-2 provides an overview of the major antineoplastic drug classes, including their mechanisms of action, cell-cycle specificities, major resistance mechanisms, and dose-limiting toxicities. Note that all of these drug classes have been discussed in previous chapters; the following discussion integrates relevant information about the individual drugs in a clinical context.

TABLE 39-2   Classes of Cancer Chemotherapeutic Agents

DRUG CLASS	MECHANISM OF ACTION	CELL CYCLE SPECIFICITY	MAJOR RESISTANCE MECHANISM	DOSE-LIMITING TOXICITY
Alkylating agents	Crosslink DNA, RNA, protein	Nonspecific	↑ DNA repair, ↓ drug uptake, ↑ drug inactivation	Bone marrow
Platinum complexes	DNA intrastrand crosslinks (G-G)	Nonspecific	↑ DNA repair, ↓ drug uptake, ↑ drug inactivation	Renal
Antimetabolites	Disrupt nucleotide synthesis, utilization, incorporation	S	↓ drug uptake, ↓ drug activation, ↑ drug inactivation, ↑ or altered target enzyme, salvage pathway	Bone marrow
Hydroxyurea	Inhibits ribonucleotide reductase	S	↑ DNA repair, ↓ drug uptake, ↑ drug inactivation	Bone marrow
Natural products				
Bleomycin	DNA strand scission	G2	↑ drug inactivation?	Pulmonary fibrosis
Camptothecins	Inhibit topoisomerase I	S	↑ drug efflux?	Bone marrow
Anthracyclines	DNA intercalation, inhibit topoisomerase II, lipid peroxidation	G2	↑ drug efflux	Bone marrow/heart
Epipodophyllotoxins	Inhibit topoisomerase II	S/G2	↑ drug efflux	Bone marrow/diarrhea
Vinca alkaloids	Disrupt microtubule assembly	M	↑ drug efflux	Bone marrow/neuropathy
Taxanes	Disrupt microtubule disassembly	M	↑ drug efflux	Bone marrow (mild)
Hormones/antagonists				
Prednisone	Glucocorticoid receptor agonist	G1	Loss of hormone sensitivity (↑ or altered target receptor)	Cushingoid syndrome
Tamoxifen	Estrogen receptor antagonist		Loss of estrogen-dependent growth	Endometrial cancer/thrombosis
Anastrozole	Aromatase inhibitor		Loss of estrogen-dependent growth	Osteoporosis
Flutamide	Androgen receptor antagonist		Loss of androgen-dependent growth	
Leuprolide	GnRH receptor "superagonist"		Loss of androgen-dependent growth	

Agent	Mechanism	Molecular marker	Toxicity
Monoclonal antibodies	Target tumor-specific antigen		Infusion reactions (fever/rash/dyspnea)
Toxin conjugates	Target tumor-specific antigen		
Biological response modifiers			
Interferon-alpha	Interferon receptor agonist		Bone marrow/neurotoxic/cardiotoxic
Interleukin-2	IL-2 receptor agonist (proliferation, differentiation of T cells)		Hypotension/pulmonary edema
Differentiating agents	Induce differentiation of cancer cells		
Tretinoin	Retinoic acid receptor α agonist	PML-RAR-α fusion gene mutation	Retinoic acid syndrome
Epidermal growth factor receptor (EGFR) antagonist	Inhibits EGFR tyrosine kinase domain or targets EGFR extracellular domain	EGFR kinase mutation	Skin/GI (diarrhea)
Trastuzumab	ErbB2 (Her-2)		Cardiotoxic
BCR-ABL/C-KIT/ PDGFR inhibitors	Inhibit protein tyrosine kinase domain	BCR-ABL mutation	Skin/GI (diarrhea)/fluid retention
Proteasome inhibitors	Inhibit protein degradation by proteasome	p53 mutation, ↑ HSP-27 expression	Neurotoxic/bone marrow
Angiogenesis inhibitors	Target vascular endothelial growth factor (VEGF) receptor extracellular domain		Renal (proteinuria)/hypertension
Immunomodulatory drugs	Inhibit TNF, inhibit fibroblast growth factor-mediated angiogenesis, costimulate T cells		Thrombosis (thalidomide)/bone marrow (lenalidomide)

GI, gastrointestinal.

GENERAL CONSIDERATIONS

It has been said that cancer is a disorder of the cell cycle. To appreciate the challenges that must be faced in treating cancer with drug therapies, it is useful to examine the current model for oncogenic transformation. Normal somatic cells undergo differentiation as they mature from a small regenerating stem cell population. Because cells lose the ability to divide as they progress further along their differentiation pathway, it is not surprising that malignancies tend to arise in populations of immature or undifferentiated cells (perhaps even stem cells). At the molecular level, the process of malignant transformation involves multiple steps, including the loss of tumor suppressor gene products (e.g., p53 and Rb) and the activation of proto-oncogenes (e.g., ras and c-myc) through such processes as somatic mutation, DNA translocation, and gene amplification. Acquired alterations in genes that regulate the progression of cells through the cell cycle confer a growth advantage on malignant cells, which proliferate in the absence of normal growth regulatory signals. Some of the most aggressive transformed cells multiply at a rate of about two divisions each day. At this rate, a single such cell could give rise to a clinically detectable mass of 1 g (10^9 cells) in just 15 days, and a tumor burden of 1 kg (10^{12} cells), which is often incompatible with life, could be achieved in 20 days.

Fortunately, oncogenesis usually occurs much more slowly than this—a fact that supports the concept of screening for many types of cancer (e.g., cervical, prostate, and colon). A malignant cell can give rise to a small colony of cells (10^6 cells) rather quickly, but further growth is held in check by the limited availability of oxygen and nutrients. Because oxygen can diffuse passively in tissues over a distance of only 2 to 3 mm, cells in the center of the growing tumor mass become hypoxic and enter the G_0 (resting) phase. Accordingly, the percentage of cells that are actively dividing (i.e., the growth fraction of the tumor) decreases as tumor size increases. Moreover, the continued proliferation of cells at the tumor margins causes a further decrease in the pO_2 in the center of the tumor, and hypoxic tumor cells begin to die (central necrosis). The tumor continues to grow, albeit at a slower rate, because the rate of cell division at the margins exceeds the rate of central necrosis. At some point, hypoxic tumor cells can express or induce the stromal expression of angiogenic factors (e.g., vascular endothelial growth factor, VEGF) that induce vascularization of the tumor. Vascularization can be accompanied by a sudden increase in the growth fraction, as cells are pulled out of G_0 phase and into the cell cycle.

Because a single malignant cell can expand clonally to give rise to a tumor, it is thought that every malignant cell must be destroyed to effect a cure of the cancer. This hypothesis, together with the "log-kill" hypothesis for tumor cell killing (see Chapter 31), suggests that *multiple cycles of chemotherapy must be administered at the highest tolerable doses and the most frequent tolerable intervals to achieve a cure*. Antineoplastic chemotherapy usually follows first-order kinetics (i.e., a constant *fraction* of tumor cells is killed with each cycle of chemotherapy). These kinetics of tumor cell killing are unlike the time-dependent killing characteristic of many antimicrobial drugs, which follows zero-order kinetics (i.e., a fixed *number* of microbes is killed per unit time).

Adding to the difficulty of successful cancer treatment is the phenomenon of tumor progression, in which a clonally derived population of malignant cells becomes heterogeneous through the accumulation of multiple genetic alterations (mutations). When subjected to selective pressure by immune surveillance or the administration of an antineoplastic agent, subclones of the tumor with relatively nonantigenic or drug-resistant phenotypes are selected for in Darwinian fashion. Mutations that confer drug resistance are of particular concern, because many transformed cells, having lost the ability to repair DNA damage, are characterized by genomic instability. Thus, deletions, gene amplifications, translocations, and point mutations are not infrequent events, and can result in antineoplastic drug resistance through any of the mechanisms shown in Table 39-3.

With the possible exception of recently developed classes of therapies that are based on molecular targets selectively expressed by a malignant clone of cells (e.g., a monoclonal antibody directed against a tumor cell antigen or an enzyme inhibitor directed against a mutated signal transduction molecule; see Chapter 1, Drug-Receptor Interactions; Chapter 38, Pharmacology of Cancer: Signal Transduction; and Chapter 53, Protein-Based Therapies), antineoplastic chemotherapy has focused on disrupting the cell cycle in rapidly dividing cells. Some of these agents act by inducing DNA damage and subsequent apoptosis in all phases of the cell cycle, whereas others act selectively in one phase of the cell cycle (see Chapter 31, especially Fig. 31-4). Unfortunately, such drugs are also associated with significant host toxicity, especially in tissues that normally have a high rate of cell turnover (e.g., bone marrow, hair follicles, intestinal epithelia). Accordingly, neutropenia, thrombocytopenia, anemia, alopecia, nausea, and oral and intestinal ulcerations are common adverse effects of many antineoplastic agents.

Although many rapidly growing lymphomas and leukemias seem to melt away with antineoplastic chemotherapy, more indolent solid tumors must be treated with adjuvant (i.e., chemotherapy-enhancing) radiation therapy and/or surgery. By the time these tumors come to clinical attention, they are often quite large and may have metastasized widely. In such cases, surgical removal of the primary tumor is often followed by radiation therapy and/or systemic chemotherapy, using agents that penetrate various tissues (e.g., brain, liver) that could be sites of metastatic disease.

In summary, cancer therapy must eliminate every malignant cell from the body, making high doses of chemotherapeutic agents desirable. (In practice, immune mechanisms may be able to clear small numbers of remaining cancer cells, if these cells are sufficiently immunogenic.) However, the toxicity of these relatively nonselective agents limits their achievable doses. Moreover, resistance to these drugs can develop through genetic alterations. Finally, because these agents target mainly rapidly dividing cells, antineoplastic drugs are much less effective against large solid tumors with low growth fractions. Each of these considerations points to the need for combination drug regimens to treat cancer. The basic pharmacologic principles for such regimens are discussed below.

TABLE 39-3	Mechanisms of Tumor Resistance to Chemotherapeutic Agents
MECHANISM OF TUMOR RESISTANCE	**EXAMPLES**
Pharmacokinetic Mechanisms	
Insufficient accumulation of drug	
Insufficient uptake of drug	Methotrexate, doxorubicin
Efflux of drug from tumor cell (MDR phenotype)	Vinca alkaloids, etoposides, doxorubicin
Insufficient distribution of drug	
Sanctuary sites (e.g., brain, testis)	Methotrexate, ara-C
Unfavorable metabolism of drug or prodrug	
Insufficient activation of prodrug	5-FU, 6-MP, ara-C, 6-TG
Increased inactivation of drug	
Cytidine deaminase overexpression	Ara-C
Alkaline phosphatase overexpression	6-TG, 6-MP
Pharmacodynamic Mechanisms	
Overexpression, alteration, or loss of target molecule*	
Dihydrofolate reductase	Methotrexate
Decreased concentration of cofactor	5-FU
Increased concentration of competing molecule	Ara-C metabolite (dCTP)
Repair of drug-induced lesions in DNA, proteins, or lipids (membranes)	Alkylating agents
Increased utilization of alternate pathways	Antimetabolites
Resistance to drug-induced apoptosis	Most antineoplastics

* Due to DNA mutation, amplification or deletion; altered transcription or posttranscriptional processing; altered translation or posttranslational modification; or altered target stability.

RATIONALE FOR COMBINATION CHEMOTHERAPY

In antineoplastic chemotherapy, combination drug regimens typically include agents that act on different molecular targets, at different phases of the cell cycle, and with different dose-limiting toxicities (Table 39-2). This strategy targets asynchronously dividing tumor cells, reduces the emergence of drug resistance, and allows each drug to be given at its highest tolerable dose, thereby maximizing efficacy without excessive toxicity. Recent advances in supportive therapy have also increased the maximum tolerated doses for many antineoplastic agents. For example, the routine use of antiemetics, autologous bone marrow transplantation, hematopoietic growth factors (e.g., **GM-CSF, G-CSF, erythropoietin**), and prophylactic broad-spectrum antibiotics has reduced the complications of myelosuppressive chemotherapy regimens. Similarly, **allopurinol** treatment to prevent the hyperuricemia that could result from widespread release and metabolism of purines from necrotic tumor cells (i.e., **tumor lysis syndrome**) has reduced morbidity associated with high doses of systemic chemotherapy (see Chapter 47, Integrative Inflammation Pharmacology: Gout). Finally, so-called "**leucovorin rescue**" after high-dose **methotrexate** administration selectively spares nonmalignant cells from death associated with tetrahydrofolate depletion (see Chapter 31).

Unlike the treatment of bacterial and viral infections, chemotherapy for cancer often employs an intermittent dosing strategy. The main rationale for this strategy is to avoid unacceptable toxicity to normal cells and tissues, for example, by allowing time for bone marrow recovery. Intermittent dosing may also have the advantage of "pulling" some nondividing cells out of G_0 and making them more susceptible to subsequent cycles of chemotherapy. The latter rationale has prompted the use of adjuvant radiation therapy and the inclusion of cell-cycle nonspecific drugs in certain combination chemotherapy regimens; both of these strategies have been noted to increase significantly the growth fractions of tumors in some studies. Despite these considerations, continuous delivery of chemotherapeutic agents is occasionally beneficial in treating slowly cycling tumors (e.g., multiple myeloma) or in cases where bolus infusion of drug is associated with significantly higher toxicity (e.g., **anthracyclines**).

Finally, some antineoplastic drug combinations take advantage of known synergies. A clinically important example is the interaction between **5-FU** and **methotrexate**. These drugs are used in combination in the treatment of many adenocarcinomas, including breast, colon, and prostate cancers. Both drugs are S-phase specific and have common dose-limiting toxicities (bone marrow and intestinal mucosal damage), so their use in combination may seem surprising (see Chapter 31 and Chapter 37, Pharmacology of Cancer: Genome Synthesis, Stability, and Maintenance). The mechanism of synergy appears to be the enhanced activation of 5-FU in the presence of methotrexate. Recall that 5-FU is metabolized by cellular salvage pathways that ultimately convert the drug into the active form 5-FdUMP, which irreversibly inhibits the enzyme thymidylate synthase. The first step in the activation of 5-FU is catalyzed by the enzyme phosphoribosyl transferase: 5-FU + PRPP → 5-FUMP + PP_i. Methotrexate, an inhibitor of purine biosynthesis, enhances these salvage pathways. In particular, cells treated with methotrexate have elevated levels of 5-phosphoribosyl-

1-pyrophosphate (PRPP), which favors the conversion of 5-FU to 5-FUMP, which is ultimately converted to 5-FdUMP by the action of ribonucleotide reductase.

EXAMPLES OF ANTINEOPLASTIC COMBINATION CHEMOTHERAPY

Hodgkin's Disease

The treatment of Hodgkin's disease (HD) illustrates the rational use of antineoplastic drug combinations. In this disease, there is clonal proliferation of Reed-Sternberg (RS) cells within a dense, reactive inflammatory cell background. HD originates in a single lymph node, and progresses in a contiguous fashion involving adjacent lymphoid tissues. The RS cell is the neoplastic cell; this cell seems to be of B-cell origin, making the disease a true lymphoma. Pathologic subtypes, defined on the basis of RS cell morphology and the pattern of surrounding reactive inflammatory changes, include nodular sclerosing, mixed cellularity, and lymphocyte-depleted HD.

Patients typically present with lymphadenopathy (cervical, supraclavicular, axillary, or inguinal) and/or systemic symptoms including fever, malaise, pruritus, night sweats, and weight loss. The stage of the disease determines treatment; patients with early-stage disease (stages I and II) receive radiation therapy with or without chemotherapy, and patients with advanced-stage disease (stages III or IV) require combination chemotherapy (Table 39-4).

Before the introduction of alkylating agents in the mid-1960s, single-agent chemotherapy for advanced HD resulted in a median survival of 1 year. With the development of **MOPP** (**mechlorethamine**, **vincristine**, **procarbazine**, and **prednisone**), the first successful antineoplastic drug combination, half of these patients were cured of their disease. Treatment remained limited by significant toxicity, however, including early gastrointestinal and neurological complications as well as late sterility and secondary malignancies (myelodysplastic syndrome, acute nonlymphocytic leukemia, and non-Hodgkin's lymphoma). Further investigation led to the development of the **ABVD** (**doxorubicin**, **bleomycin**, **vinblastine**, and **dacarbazine**) combination, which is often less toxic and at least as effective as MOPP. ABVD or an ABVD/MOPP combination remains the current standard of care for advanced stage HD. The rationale for the ABVD drug combination comes from the knowledge that it combines both cell-cycle selective and nonselective agents as well as drugs with different dose-limiting toxicities. Compared to MOPP, ABVD is associated with significantly fewer hematological and gonadal complications and secondary malignancies.

Testicular Cancer

The principles of antineoplastic combination chemotherapy are also exemplified in the treatment of testicular cancer. This tumor arises from the spermatogenic epithelium of the testis and is usually detected as a testicular mass on physical examination. The tumor metastasizes through lymphatic channels to pelvic and periaortic lymph nodes before disseminating widely through hematogenous routes. Treatment of local disease (without evidence of metastasis) involves surgical removal of the affected testis with or without pelvic radiation. Advanced disease requires systemic treatment with combination chemotherapy. The standard of care is **PVB** (Fig. 39-4). Of the three drugs used in this regimen (**cisplatin**, **vinblastine**, and **bleomycin**), cisplatin is the cell-cycle nonspecific drug that may draw nondividing tumor cells into the actively cycling pool, where they are susceptible to the action of the cell-cycle specific agents bleomycin and vinblastine. The drugs in this combination have different molecular targets, act on different phases of the cell cycle, and have different dose-limiting toxicities. Intermittent dos-

---

TABLE 39-4 **The Ann Arbor Staging System for Hodgkin's Disease**

STAGE	DESCRIPTION	SUBCLASSIFICATION
I	Involvement of a single lymph node region	IA: No systemic symptoms IB: Systemic symptoms (e.g., fever, night sweats, weight loss) IE: Extranodal contiguous extension
II	Involvement of two or more lymph node regions on the same side of the diaphragm	IIA: No systemic symptoms IIB: Systemic symptoms IIE: Extranodal contiguous extension
III	Involvement of nodal regions on both sides of the diaphragm	IIIA: No systemic symptoms IIIB: Systemic symptoms IIIS: Splenic involvement IIIE: Extranodal contiguous extension
IV	Disseminated disease involving multiple extralymphatic organs (e.g., liver, spleen, bone marrow)	IVA: No systemic symptoms IVB: Systemic symptoms

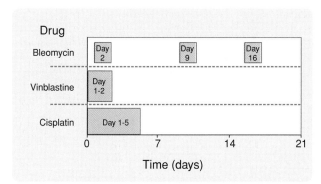

Figure 39-4. The platinum-vinblastine-bleomycin (PVB) combination chemotherapy regimen for testicular cancer. The PVB regimen used to treat testicular cancer consists of a combination of cisplatin, vinblastine, and bleomycin. Cisplatin is cell-cycle–nonspecific; this drug may draw nondividing cells into the cell cycle, where they can be killed by the G2-phase–specific agent bleomycin and the M-phase–specific agent vinblastine. The intermittent dosing schedule limits drug toxicity and allows time for the bone marrow to recover from drug-induced myelosuppression. The 3-week cycle shown here is typically administered four times in succession (12 weeks total).

ing allows each affected organ system (pulmonary, renal, and bone marrow) time to recover between cycles. After surgical removal of the primary tumor, such a regimen usually results in a cure.

TREATMENT OF REFRACTORY OR RECURRENT DISEASE

Although combination chemotherapy has resulted in vastly improved survival for some cancers, many cancers become refractory to standard combination chemotherapy. If a standard chemotherapy regimen fails, other options include experimental drug therapies, palliative care, or novel drugs approved for use after treatment failure. Many patients choose to enroll in experimental clinical trials. This decision may be based on the hope that an investigational agent could prove efficacious, but with the understanding that the true benefit may be realized only by future patients. Palliative and hospice care are alternatives to continued drug treatment in cases of advanced metastatic disease. An increasing number of agents with novel mechanisms of action are becoming available for disease that is otherwise treatment-refractory. Many of these agents selectively target tumor-specific antigens and signal transduction pathways, as discussed in Chapters 38 and 53. Optimizing combinations of these and other antineoplastic agents for efficacy and safety will be an important challenge for the future.

Conclusion and Future Directions

The principles of combination chemotherapy highlight the importance of combination drug treatment in a variety of clinical situations. The use of drug combinations has greatly enhanced the effectiveness of treatment of both infectious and neoplastic diseases. The advantages offered by multidrug regimens over individual drug therapy (monotherapy) include increased antimicrobial, antiviral, and antineoplastic efficacy, decreased overall drug resistance, decreased host

toxicity, and broader coverage of suspected pathogenic organisms. These advantages are illustrated in the rational use of drug combinations to treat infections with *Mycobacterium tuberculosis* and HIV, as well as neoplastic disorders such as Hodgkin's disease and testicular cancer. Treatment of multidrug-resistant microorganisms such as MDR-TB and MDR-HIV remains a special challenge, as does treatment of genetically heterogeneous cancers with low growth fractions such as lung, colon, breast, and prostate cancers. Continued refinement of combination chemotherapy regimens will rely on increased understanding of molecular targets and metabolic pathways used by microorganisms and cancer cells.

Suggested Reading

Canellos GP, Anderson JR, Propert KJ, et al. Chemotherapy of advanced Hodgkin's disease with MOPP, ABVD, or MOPP alternating with ABVD. *N Engl J Med* 1992;327:1478–1484. (*These antineoplastic drug combinations remain the standard of care for advanced Hodgkin's disease.*)

Centers for Disease Control and Prevention (CDC). Emergence of *Mycobacterium tuberculosis* with extensive resistance to second-line drugs—worldwide, 2000–2004. *MMWR Morb Mortal Wkly Rep* 2006;55:301–305. (*Surveys international network of tuberculosis [TB] laboratories for incidence and prevalence of multidrug-resistant [MDR] and extensively drug-resistant [XDR] TB isolates.*)

Chou R, Huffman LH, Fu R, et al. Screening for HIV: a review of the evidence for the U.S. Preventive Services Task Force. *Ann Intern Med* 2005;143:55–73. (*Compares benefits and risks of screening for HIV and reviews efficacy of highly active antiretroviral therapy [HAART] for patients with advanced HIV infection.*)

Chou TC, Talalay P. Quantitative analysis of dose-effect relationships: the combined effects of multiple drugs or enzyme inhibitors. *Adv Enzyme Regul* 1984;22:27–55. (*Detailed analysis of models for synergistic, antagonistic, and additive drug combinations.*)

Dancey JE, Chen HX. Strategies for optimizing combinations of molecular targeted anticancer agents. *Nat Rev Drug Discov* 2006; 5:649–659. (*Discusses principles for determining combinations of antineoplastic agents that could be most promising to test in preclinical and clinical trials.*)

Harvey RJ. Synergism in the folate pathway. *Rev Infect Dis* 1982; 4:255–260. (*Describes the kinetics of synergism between trimethoprim and the sulfonamides.*)

Koynov KD, Tzekova VI, Velikova MT, et al. Cisplatin, vinblastine and bleomycin in the treatment of disseminated testicular cancer. *Int Urol Nephrol* 1993;25:389–394. (*This antineoplastic drug combination remains the standard of care for metastatic testicular cancer.*)

Ormerod LP. Multidrug-resistant tuberculosis (MDR-TB): epidemiology, prevention and treatment. *Br Med Bull* 2005;73/74: 17–24. (*Reviews epidemiology, prevention, and treatment of multidrug-resistant tuberculosis.*)

Yazdanpanah Y, Sissoko D, Egger M, et al. Clinical efficacy of antiretroviral combination therapy based on protease inhibitors or non-nucleoside analogue reverse transcriptase inhibitors: indirect comparison of controlled trials. *Br Med J* 2004;328:249–256 (doi:10.1136/bmj37995.435787.A6). (*Reviews combination therapies used in the treatment of HIV.*)

Acknowledgment

The authors thank Shreya Kangovi and Gia Landry for initial drafts of the case of Mr. M and the discussion in the chapter related to his case.

VI

Principles of Inflammation and Immune Pharmacology

40

Principles of Inflammation and the Immune System

Ehrin J. Armstrong and Lloyd B. Klickstein

INTRODUCTION

Inflammation and the immune system are closely intertwined. Inflammation is a complex web of responses to tissue injury and infection, characterized by the classic signs of *rubor* (redness), *calor* (heat), *tumor* (swelling), *dolor* (pain), and *functio laesa* (loss of function). The immune system comprises the cells and soluble factors, such as antibodies and complement proteins, that mediate the inflammatory response; these cells and factors both eliminate the inciting inflammatory stimulus and initiate the process of immunologic memory.

A normal inflammatory response is an acute process that resolves after removal of the inciting stimulus. Diseases of inflammation and immunity can occur due to inappropriate inflammation or when the normal inflammatory response progresses to chronic inflammation, either because of a long-term inappropriate response to a stimulus (for example, allergies) or because the offending agent is not removed (for example, chronic infection, transplantation, and autoimmunity).

Two pharmacologic strategies are used to target the pathophysiology of immune diseases. The first involves modification of the signaling mediators of the inflammatory process or suppression of components of the immune system. This is the rationale for drugs that affect eicosanoid pathways (Chapter 41, Pharmacology of Eicosanoids), histamine (Chapter 42, Histamine Pharmacology), and cells of the immune system (Chapter 43, Pharmacology of Hematopoiesis and Immunomodulation, and Chapter 44, Pharmacology of Immunosuppression). This approach (because it is dependent on understanding the molecular events in the relevant pathways) is still in its infancy but promises to yield a number of new drugs in the foreseeable future.

The second pharmacologic approach, used in diseases such as peptic ulcer disease (Chapter 45, Integrative Inflammation Pharmacology: Peptic Ulcer Disease), asthma (Chapter 46, Integrative Inflammation Pharmacology: Asthma), and gout (Chapter 47, Integrative Inflammation Pharmacology: Gout), involves modification of the underlying pathophysiologic stimulus, thus removing the impetus for inflammation. The difference between these two approaches is, at times, indistinct, and will continue to blur as the pathophysiology of chronic inflammatory disease is better understood at a molecular level.

This chapter provides sufficient background in the physiology of inflammation and the immune system to understand the subsequent chapters in this section of the book. The treatment is necessarily brief, with an emphasis on pharmacologically relevant targets of the inflammatory response. The chapter is organized into four parts. First, a general overview of the immune system is presented. Second, the molecular signals mediating cellular communication and inflammation are introduced. Third, the immune and inflammatory cells and signaling molecules are discussed in the context of an integrated inflammatory response. Fourth, chronic inflammation, a pathologic state that is often associated with autoimmunity, is presented. For a more exhaustive presentation of this rapidly changing subject, see the Suggested Reading at the end of this chapter.

■ Case

Mark is stressed—he has to take the United States Medical Licensing Examination (USMLE) in 2 weeks, and he has barely begun to study. Throwing aside any pretense of a balanced lifestyle, Mark travels to the microbiology lab late one night to review techniques for performing a Gram stain. While applying the gentian violet component of the Gram stain, Mark cuts his thumb on the edge of the microscope slide. Fearing the worst, but thinking he lacks the time to clean his thumb properly, Mark continues to study furiously. Over the next 5 hours, Mark's thumb becomes progressively swollen, warm, red, and tender. Mark retains focus and continues to study through the evening. By that night, however, he develops a fever and increased swelling in the thumb. By the third day, pus builds up at the site. By the fourth day, however, Mark's body seems to have gotten the better of the offending agent. The swelling decreases, the site loses its distinctive angry red appearance, and his fever abruptly subsides. Relieved that he has not become a casualty of his own procrastination, Mark continues studying and performs well on his exam, not the least because his wound has provided him with fundamental insights into immunology.

QUESTIONS

■ **1.** What initial changes in the vasculature accounted for the immediate swelling of Mark's thumb?
■ **2.** What chemical signals mediated the inflammatory response in Mark's thumb?
■ **3.** What mediators accounted for Mark's fever?
■ **4.** Which pathways in the inflammatory cascade can be interrupted using currently available pharmacologic agents?

OVERVIEW OF THE IMMUNE SYSTEM

The fundamental role of the immune system is to distinguish self from nonself. "Nonself" can be an infectious organism,

a transplanted organ, or an endogenous tissue that is mistaken for something foreign. Because protection against infection is the classic role of the immune system, the phrases "infection" and "infectious agent" are generally used to denote the inciting stimulus for an immune response. It should be understood, however, that the immune system can be stimulated to react against any nonself entity.

Skin and barrier tissues form the first line of defense against any infection. (In the introductory case, Mark's infection occurred only after he cut his skin.) Once an offending agent penetrates these barriers, the immune system mounts a response. The immune response consists of innate and adaptive responses. **Innate** responses are stereotyped reactions to a stimulus (e.g., release of histamine, phagocytosis of a bacterium). In some cases, innate responses are sufficient to neutralize the offending agent. Cells of the innate immune system, especially antigen-presenting cells, can also process the offending agent into small fragments; this processing is necessary for activation of the adaptive immune system. **Adaptive** responses are neutralizing reactions that are specific to the offending agent (e.g., antibodies, cytotoxic T cells). In general, then, *the innate immune system initiates and activates the response to an offending agent, while the adaptive immune system creates a response that specifically neutralizes or kills that agent.*

There are many different cell types in the immune system, and these cell types interact in a complex web of signaling and communication to create the overall response. The cells of the immune system derive from two types of pluripotent cells in the bone marrow: **myeloid** stem cells and **lymphoid** stem cells. (The lymphoid stem cell is sometimes called the **common lymphoid stem cell** because it gives rise to both B cells and T cells.) Myeloid stem cells give rise to precursors of cells of the innate immune system, whereas lymphoid stem cells generate precursors of cells of the adaptive immune system. Figure 40-1 shows the myeloid and lymphoid stem cells and the mature cell types into which precursor cells differentiate. The derivation of these cell types is also discussed in Chapter 43.

INNATE IMMUNITY

Cells of the innate immune system are the first responders to an offending agent that has penetrated the skin or another barrier (Table 40-1). Innate immune cells perform three important tasks. First, these cells defend against bacterial and parasitic infections, either by neutralizing the infectious agent with secreted cytotoxic proteins, or by phagocytosis (engulfing) of the bacterium or parasite. Second, phagocytosis of the offending agent initiates proteolytic digestion of microbial macromolecules to fragments (antigens) that are then displayed, together with major histocompatibility complex (MHC) class II proteins, on the surface of antigen-presenting cells. In turn, these antigen-presenting cells, which include macrophages and dendritic cells, activate cells of the adaptive immune system. Third, the innate immune cells secrete numerous cytokines (see below) that further amplify the immune response. The major cell types of the innate immune system include **granulocytes** (neutrophils, eosinophils, and basophils), **mast cells**, and **antigen-presenting cells** (macrophages and dendritic cells).

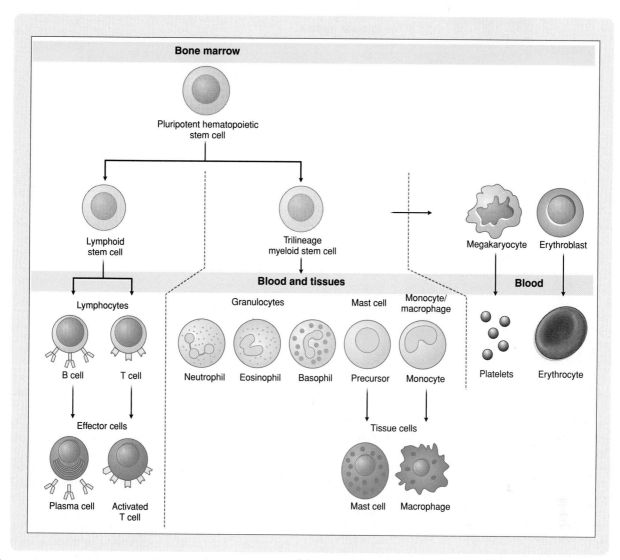

Figure 40-1. Development of cells of the immune system. All hematopoietic cells develop from the pluripotent hematopoietic stem cell. This cell gives rise to the lymphoid stem cell and the trilineage myeloid stem cell. The lymphoid stem cell and its progenitor cells *(not shown)* give rise to mature lymphocytes (B cells and T cells), the cells that mediate adaptive immune responses. When exposed to specific antigens, B cells differentiate into antibody-producing plasma cells, and T cells assume an activated phenotype. The myeloid stem cell and its progenitor cells, including megakaryocytes, erythroblasts, and myeloid precursors *(not shown)*, proliferate and differentiate into mature neutrophils, eosinophils, basophils, mast cells, monocytes, platelets, and erythrocytes. In the tissues, monocytes differentiate into macrophages, and mast cell precursors differentiate into mast cells. (See Fig. 43-1 for more details about the differentiation of cell lineages in the bone marrow.)

''Granulocyte'' is a descriptive term based on the appearance of the cytoplasmic granules within these cells. **Neutrophils,** the most abundant cell type of the innate immune system, are phagocytic cells primarily responsible for defense against bacterial infection. These cells envelop invading bacteria in phagocytic vesicles and destroy the bacteria within these vesicles using enzymes such as myeloperoxidase. **Eosinophils** are circulating granulocytes primarily involved in defense against parasitic infections. Because parasites are often too large to engulf, eosinophils attach to a parasite's exterior and secrete cytotoxic substances directly on the parasite. Both **basophils** (circulating) and **mast cells** (tissue-resident) bind IgE antibody, display this IgE on the cell surface, and maintain histamine-containing granules that are released when exogenous antigen binds to and crosslinks

the IgE. Basophils and mast cells are important in allergic responses. Eosinophils and basophils are so named because they exhibit eosinophilic and basophilic patterns, respectively, when stained with Wright-Giemsa stain.

Antigen-Presenting Cells

Antigen-presenting cells (APCs) process the macromolecules (especially proteins) of an invading agent to display the processed fragments on the surface of the APC. In this form, the fragments serve as molecular fingerprints used by cells of the adaptive immune system to recognize the invading agent. APCs are important initiators of immune responses because, in addition to displaying nonself antigens to T cells (see below), they provide the costimulatory signals

TABLE 40-1	Cells of the Immune System

CELL TYPE	FUNCTION
Innate Immunity	
Macrophage	Tissue-resident cell, derived from monocyte
	Phagocytoses cellular and foreign debris
	Involved in chronic inflammation
	Antigen-presenting cell
Dendritic cell	Transports and presents antigen to T cells in lymph nodes
	Antigen-presenting cell
Neutrophil	Phagocytoses and kills invading pathogens, especially bacteria
Eosinophil	Defends against parasites
Basophil/Mast cell	Release histamine, leukotrienes, and other mediators after exposure to antigen
Adaptive Immunity	
Cytotoxic T cell (T_C)	Effector of cellular adaptive immunity
Helper T cell (T_H)	Controls adaptive immune responses
B cell	Synthesizes and secretes antibody
	Antigen-presenting cell

that are necessary for T-cell activation. The concept of **costimulation,** in which two separate signals are required to initiate an immune response to a stimulus, is discussed below.

Monocytes that exit the bloodstream and take up residence in the tissues can differentiate into **macrophages.** As "professional APCs," macrophages process and present antigenic fragments of an invading pathogen for recognition by T cells. The ability of macrophages to envelop and destroy pathogens is enhanced by other components of the immune system, including antibodies that mediate opsonization and cytokines that enhance killing ability. In addition, macrophages produce cytokines such as TNF-α that modify immune responses. **Dendritic cells** are antigen-presenting cells that, in their mature form, are found primarily in the T-cell areas of lymphoid tissue. Dendritic cells are the most important APCs for the initiation of adaptive immune responses. Immature dendritic cells reside in nonlymphoid tissues, ready to engulf and process foreign antigens; the dendritic cells then transport these antigens to lymphoid tissues and present the antigens to T cells.

Activation of the Innate Immune Response

Innate immune cells respond to common determinants that are present on many invading agents (for example, lipopolysaccharide [LPS] in the outer membrane of Gram-negative bacteria). In this role, innate immune cells use **pattern recognition** to phagocytose a class of infectious agents rather than a specific infectious agent. In contrast, adaptive immune cells, as discussed below, mount a specific response to the three-dimensional conformation of a particular antigen, referred to as an **epitope.** From a teleological perspective, innate immunity provides a broad gating function, attempting to counteract harmful effects of foreign invaders in a rapid manner and to determine whether an infectious agent should be further attacked by adaptive immunity, while adaptive immunity provides a specialized response that is specific to the particular invading infectious agent. Innate immune cells lack memory; they respond in the same way and to the same extent to repeated infections with the same agent. In contrast, adaptive immune cells mount a faster and more intense response on re-exposure to the infectious agent.

The pattern recognition function of innate immune cells is mediated primarily by **Toll-like receptors (TLRs).** TLRs are transmembrane proteins that bind to common microbial components, such as LPS of Gram-negative bacteria, mannans expressed by fungi, and double-stranded RNA of viral pathogens. Ten TLRs are expressed in humans, and each has a characteristic immune cell distribution and set of ligands. For example, TLR4 expressed by antigen-presenting cells binds to LPS. Binding of TLRs to their ligands activates an intracellular signaling cascade that converges on the expression of proinflammatory cytokines, leading to further immune cell recruitment and activation of the inflammatory response. Several pharmaceutical agents are being investigated as modulators of TLR signaling. **Imiquimod,** discussed in Chapter 43, may function as a TLR agonist.

ADAPTIVE IMMUNITY

The main features of the adaptive immune system, specificity to foreign antigens and tolerance to self-antigens, rely on two factors. First, there must be a mechanism to generate a specific response to a foreign antigen. Second, adaptive immune cells must be able to distinguish native (self) cells and soluble factors from foreign (nonself) cells and soluble factors. The first property is provided by **major histocompatibility complex** (MHC) proteins along with somatic gene recombination in T cells and B cells, whereas the second property is provided by regulated immune cell development and costimulation.

Major Histocompatibility Complex

MHC proteins are transmembrane proteins that bind and display on their surface proteolytically degraded protein fragments and, in some cases, glycolipid antigens. There are two classes of MHC proteins, MHC class I and MHC class II. MHC class I proteins primarily display fragments of cytosolic proteins (Fig. 40-2). All nucleated cells express MHC class I proteins; the repertoire of protein fragments displayed by MHC class I proteins on a cell provides a fingerprint for all the proteins expressed within that cell. If a cell is expressing a recognizable pattern of proteins, then it will not be attacked by the immune system. However, if foreign (for example, viral) proteins are being generated within the cytosol of the cell, then proteolytic fragments of those viral proteins will be displayed on MHC class I proteins at the surface of the cell, and the immune system will recognize that cell as virally infected. Antigens presented by MHC class I proteins are recognized by T cells bearing the cell surface protein CD8. (The designation "CD" stands for "cluster of differentiation" or "cluster designation" and is a system for naming an ever-growing list of cell-associated antigens—now numbering in the hundreds—that are present on leukocytes and other cell types. Each antigen must be defined by at least two different monoclonal antibodies in order to earn the "CD" designation.)

MHC class II proteins display protein fragments derived from endocytic vesicles. In contrast to class I proteins, which are expressed on all nucleated cells, MHC class II proteins are expressed mostly on antigen-presenting cells (e.g., macrophages and dendritic cells), although some other cell types can be induced to express MHC class II proteins. Endocytic vesicles contain antigenic protein fragments derived from infectious agents after phagocytosis and proteolytic processing of those agents. Therefore, the protein fragments expressed on MHC class II proteins generally identify extracellular foreign agents (e.g., bacteria). As discussed below, T cells expressing the cell surface protein CD4 recognize antigens presented by MHC class II proteins. In the process, these T cells activate the antigen-presenting cells to produce soluble factors called *cytokines* and *chemokines* that, in turn, aid the T cells in responding to the antigen. In general, then, *the protein fragments bound to MHC class I identify infected cells, whereas the fragments bound to MHC class II identify infectious agents.* However, because of the phenomenon of cross-presentation, some proteins generated in the cytosol can be presented by MHC class II to CD4$^+$ T cells, and some phagocytosed antigens can be presented by MHC class I to CD8$^+$ T cells.

Immune Diversity

Whereas MHC proteins provide a means for distinguishing infected cells and infectious agents from uninfected cells, somatic gene recombination and other mechanisms for gen-

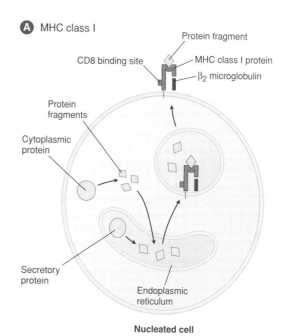

A MHC class I

Nucleated cell

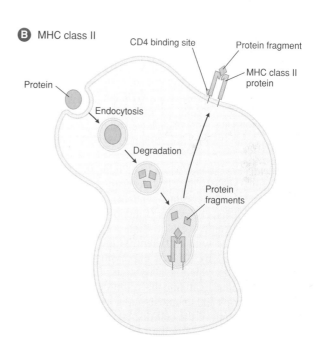

B MHC class II

Antigen-presenting cell

cytoplasmic or secretory protein in the ER. The MHC class I:protein fragment complex is transported to the cell surface, where it serves as a fingerprint for the diversity of proteins expressed by that cell. The CD8 binding site on MHC class I ensures that the class I protein: antigen complex interacts only with cytotoxic T cells, which express CD8. All nucleated human cells express MHC class I proteins. **B.** Antigen-presenting cells phagocytose and degrade bacteria and other foreign agents, generating protein fragments that bind to MHC class II protein in the ER. The MHC class II:protein fragment complex is transported to the cell surface, where it serves to display all the potentially nonself antigens that have been ingested by that cell. The CD4 binding site on MHC class II ensures that the class II protein:antigen complex interacts only with helper T cells, which express CD4. Professional antigen-presenting cells (B cells, macrophages, and dendritic cells) are usually the only cell types that express MHC class II proteins, but other cells can be induced to express class II proteins and present antigens under some circumstances.

Figure 40-2. Class I and class II major histocompatibility complex proteins. A. A representative fraction of cytoplasmic proteins are proteolytically degraded in the cytosol, and the protein fragments are transported to the endoplasmic reticulum (ER). A fraction of secretory proteins are degraded directly in the ER. MHC class I protein, in association with β_2 microglobulin, binds a fragment of the degraded

erating diversity provide a means for generating a specific response to an infection. By recombination, **immunoglobulin** and **T-cell receptor** genes semirandomly create millions of modular three-dimensional protein structures (referred to as *variable regions*) that, in the aggregate, can recognize almost any structure. This is one mechanism by which the immune system can generate an astounding diversity of immune responses.

Humoral and Cellular Immunity

Adaptive immunity is generally divided into **humoral immunity** and **cellular immunity.** The primary cells mediating these branches of the immune system are referred to as **B cells** and **T cells,** respectively (Table 40-1). The humoral response involves the production of **antibodies** specific for an antigen. These antibodies are secreted by plasma cells (differentiated B cells) and are therefore most effective against extracellular infectious agents such as bacteria. In contrast, the cellular response involves activation and clonal expansion of T cells that recognize a specific antigen. Some T cells recognize infected cells and then lyse those cells using cytotoxic proteins called **perforins** and **granzymes.** Cellular immune responses are effective against many intracellular infectious agents such as viruses.

In addition to their role in cellular immunity, T cells control the extent of immune responses. Each T cell evolves so that it is activated by only one specific MHC:antigen complex. All T cells express an MHC:antigen-specific T cell receptor (TCR). T cells are divided into cytotoxic T cells (T_C) and helper T cells (T_H), based on the type of coreceptor expressed and the function imparted by that coreceptor (Fig. 40-3).

T_C **cells** are the *mediators* of cellular adaptive immunity. These cells express the CD8 coreceptor, which recognizes a constant (i.e., antigen-independent) domain on MHC class I proteins. This coreceptor function allows the antigen-specific TCR on T_C cells to bind a specific class I MHC:antigen complex with sufficiently high affinity that the T_C cell is activated by the cell expressing the class I MHC:antigen complex. Specific activation of the T_C cell initiates a chain of events, including the secretion of membrane-penetrating perforins and apoptosis-inducing granzymes, that results in the death of the cell displaying the foreign antigen.

T_H **cells** are primarily the *regulators* of adaptive immunity. T_H cells are identified by their expression of the CD4 coreceptor, which recognizes an antigen-independent domain on MHC class II proteins. This coreceptor function allows the antigen-specific receptor on T_H cells to bind a specific class II MHC:antigen complex with sufficiently high affinity that the T_H cell is activated by the antigen-presenting cell. In addition to initiating and strengthening the immune response, T_H cells control the type of immune response by producing one or another set of cytokines. The T_H cells can be divided into T_H1 and T_H2 subtypes based on the cytokines produced by the cells. T_H1 cells characteristically produce IFN-γ and IL-2, and these cytokines influence the development of cell-mediated immune responses of both CD8$^+$ T_C cells and other CD4$^+$ T_H cells. In contrast, T_H2 cells characteristically produce IL-4, IL-5, and IL-10, and these cytokines enhance antibody production by B cells. The T_H2 cell subtype is more often associated with autoim-

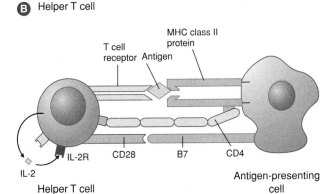

Ⓐ Cytotoxic T cell

Ⓑ Helper T cell

Figure 40-3. Activation of cytotoxic and helper T cells. T cells mediate and regulate the cellular immune response. **A.** Cytotoxic T cells (T_C) are the primary *mediators* of cellular immunity. These cells express T-cell receptors (TCR) and CD8. The TCR identifies nonself antigens bound to MHC proteins, whereas the CD8 ensures that T_C cells interact only with cells expressing MHC class I proteins. In the example shown, the interaction of a T_C cell with the MHC class I protein of a virus-infected cell leads to activation of the T_C cell and subsequent killing of the virus-infected cell. **B.** Helper T cells (T_H) are the primary *regulators* of cellular immunity. These cells express TCR and CD4. CD4 binds to MHC class II proteins on antigen-presenting cells (APC); this interaction ensures that T_H cells interact only with cells expressing MHC class II proteins. An additional degree of specificity is provided by the interaction of CD28 on T_H cells with proteins of the B7 family on APC; this "costimulatory signal" is required for T_H activation. In the example shown, the interaction of a T_H cell with the MHC class II and B7 proteins of an antigen-presenting cell leads to activation of the T_H cell. The activated T_H cell secretes IL-2 and expresses the IL-2 receptor (IL-2R); this autocrine pathway stimulates further T_H-cell proliferation and activation. IL-2 and other cytokines secreted by the T_H cell activate not only T_H cells, but also T_C cells and B cells.

munity (see Chapter 44). In addition to regulating adaptive immunity, T_H cells can mediate immunity by secreting cytokines that activate phagocytic cells to kill infecting microbes more efficiently.

Tolerance and Costimulation

The diversity in the variable regions of immunoglobulins and T-cell receptors creates the potential that some of these molecules could recognize and attack native proteins. In a process referred to as **tolerance,** cells of the immune system undergo a carefully regulated series of steps during development to ensure that mature immune cells do not recognize native proteins.

Costimulation—the requirement for multiple simultaneous signals to initiate an immune response—ensures that stimulation of a single immune receptor does not activate a damaging immune reaction. Signal 1 provides specificity, while signal 2 is permissive, ensuring that an inflammatory response is appropriate. Regulation of costimulatory molecules may be a mechanism whereby the immune system limits the extent of an immune response. If antigen is presented without a coincident costimulatory signal, anergy results, whereby a cell becomes unreactive and will not respond to further antigenic stimuli. *Induction of anergy could lead to long-term acceptance of an organ graft or limit the extent of an autoimmune disease.*

For T cells, signal 1 is mediated by the MHC:TCR interaction. Signal 2 is mediated predominantly by the interaction of CD28 on T cells with B7-1 (also called CD80) or B7-2 (CD86) on activated antigen-presenting cells (Fig. 40-4). Resting T cells present CD28, which can bind either B7-1 or B7-2. B7-1 and B7-2 are not normally present on antigen-presenting cells, but their expression is increased during an inflammatory response mediated by the innate immune system. The lack of expression of B7 molecules during noninflammatory states may help to limit inappropriate adaptive immune responses. Expression of IL-2, T-cell activation, and clonal expansion of T_H cells specific for that foreign epitope occur when a T cell receives both signal 1 and signal 2. Activated T cells eventually down-regulate CD28 expression and up-regulate CTLA-4 expression. **CTLA-4,** like CD28, binds B7-1 and B7-2 but with much higher affinity than CD28. In contrast to the activating CD28 signal, interac-

tion of CTLA-4 with B7-1 or B7-2 inhibits T-cell proliferation. This also may be a physiologic mechanism for self-limitation of the immune response.

CD40 ligand (CD40L) is another mediator of costimulation. Activated T cells express CD40L (CD154). CD40 is expressed on antigen-presenting cells, including macrophages and B cells (Fig. 40-5). The CD40–CD40L interaction on T cells promotes B-cell activation, isotype switching, and affinity maturation. Interaction of T_H cell CD40L with macrophage CD40 promotes macrophage expression of B7-1 and B7-2. These molecules, as mentioned above, are crucial for costimulation of T cells. This pathway thus provides a positive feedback mechanism whereby activated T cells can promote further expansion of activated T cells. In addition, the increased expression of B7-1 and B7-2 molecules on macrophages is important for promoting $CD8^+$ T_C cell activation.

Because the CD40–CD40L interaction promotes numerous costimulation pathways, it has been hypothesized that blockade of CD40L could also produce tolerance. Preliminary studies have recently demonstrated that blockade of CD40L with anti-CD40L antibody can produce tolerance and long-term graft survival in animal models of organ transplantation.

Increasing experimental evidence suggests that peripheral tolerance is maintained by a subset of T cells, referred to as regulatory T cells (T_{reg}). These cells, the best characterized of which are $CD4^+CD25^+$, elaborate inhibitory cytokines and thereby limit the immune response to self-antigens. Pharmacologic induction of T_{reg} cells may have application in transplantation and many autoimmune diseases, including Type I diabetes.

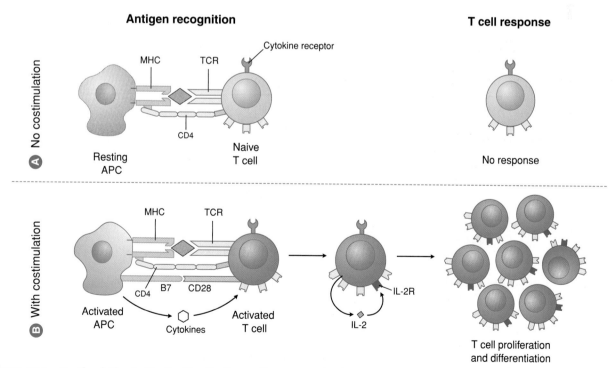

Figure 40-4. Costimulation in the T cell activation pathway. Two signals are required for activation of a T cell response to antigen. **A.** If an antigen-presenting cell (APC) presents an antigen to a T cell in the absence of an appropriate costimulatory signal, the T cell does not respond and may become anergic. **B.** If an APC presents both the antigen and a costimulatory molecule such as B7, the T cell proliferates and differentiates in response to the antigenic stimulus. Cytokines secreted by the activated APC augment T-cell activation.

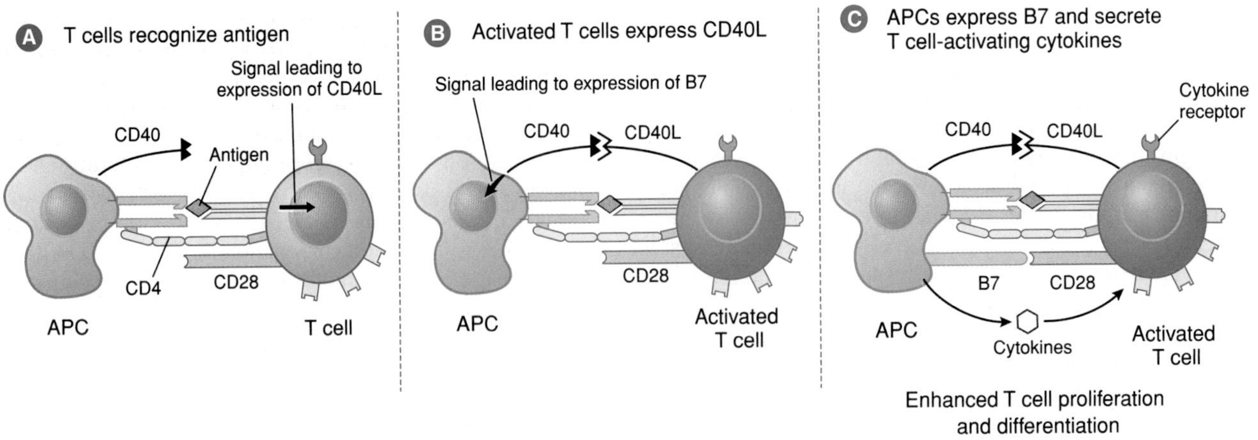

Figure 40-5. Costimulation and the CD40–CD40L interaction. A. An antigen-presenting cell (APC) presents MHC class II-bound antigen to a CD4$^+$ T cell. T-cell recognition of antigen initiates an intracellular signaling cascade that leads to expression of CD40 ligand (CD40L) at the T-cell surface. **B.** CD40L on the activated T cell binds to CD40 on the surface of the APC. Activation of CD40 generates an intracellular signaling cascade that leads to expression of B7 on the APC surface. **C.** Enhanced T-cell proliferation and differentiation are promoted by costimulation of the T cell by MHC class II-antigen (which binds to the T-cell receptor), CD40 (which binds to T-cell CD40L), and B7 (which binds to T-cell CD28). Cytokines secreted by the activated APC augment T-cell proliferation and differentiation.

CHEMICAL MEDIATORS OF INFLAMMATION

The discussion to this point has focused on the cells of the immune system and their roles in mounting an immune response. Equally important, and the main targets of pharmacologic intervention, are the molecular mediators of immune cell activity. The discussion below highlights endogenous molecules that regulate the inflammatory process. (Signaling pathways for immune cells are discussed mainly in Chapter 44, although there is some overlap among the endogenous mediators of inflammation and immunity, especially among the cytokines.) The list of mediators is long (Table 40-2), and essentially all of these signaling systems have been explored as potential pharmacologic targets. Only those most crucial to inflammation and those for which therapies already exist are discussed in detail here.

TABLE 40-2 **Chemical Mediators of the Inflammatory Response**

RESPONSE	MEDIATORS
Vasodilation	Prostaglandins (PG) PGI$_2$, PGE$_1$, PGE$_2$, PGD$_2$ Nitric oxide (NO)
Increased vascular permeability	Histamine C3a, C5a (complement components) Bradykinin Leukotrienes (LT), especially LTC$_4$, LTD$_4$, LTE$_4$ Platelet-activating factor Substance P Calcitonin gene-related peptide (CGRP)
Chemotaxis and leukocyte activation	C5a LTB$_4$, lipoxins (LX) LXA$_4$, LXB$_4$ Bacterial products
Tissue damage	Neutrophil and macrophage lysosomal products Oxygen radicals NO
Fever	Interleukin-1 (IL-1), IL-6, tumor necrosis factor (TNF) LTB$_4$, LXA$_4$, LXB$_4$
Pain	PGE$_2$, PGI$_2$ Bradykinin CGRP

HISTAMINE

Histamine, one of the initiators of the inflammatory response, is constitutively synthesized and stored in the granules of mast cells and basophils. These cells migrate through tissue on a continual basis. Any injury, from physical trauma to microbial invasion, stimulates mast cells to release histamine into the interstitium. Histamine is referred to as a ''vasoactive amine'' because its inflammatory effects occur mainly on the vasculature—histamine release stimulates dilation of arterioles and postcapillary venules, constriction of veins, and contraction of endothelial cells. These effects are responsible for the early changes in hemodynamics and vascular permeability discussed below. A number of pharmacologic agents modify histamine signaling; these agents are discussed in Chapter 42 and Chapter 45.

COMPLEMENT

Complement is a system of serine proteases that is one of the first innate mechanisms to be activated in response to injury. The complement system can be activated by antigen-antibody interactions (the classical pathway), by direct interactions with foreign surfaces (the alternative pathway), or by interactions with certain complex carbohydrates (the lectin pathway). In each pathway, a series of proteolytic reactions converts a complement precursor protein, referred to by the letter ''C'' followed by a number (for example, C3), into its active form(s), indicated by the letter ''a'' or ''b'' (for example, C3a and C3b; in this case, both forms are active). The general scheme of this pathway is analogous to that of the coagulation cascade (see Chapter 22, Pharmacology of Hemostasis and Thrombosis), in which precursor proteins are proteolytically cleaved to active products that contribute to the actions of the cascade.

After activation, complement triggers further inflammatory responses by two mechanisms. First, several cleavage products of the complement cascade are potent stimulators of inflammation. For example, C3b is an important opsonin, whereas C3a and C5a mediate leukocyte chemotaxis. Second, the final step in complement activation is the assembly of the **membrane attack complex.** This complex of complement proteins produces large pores in the outer membrane of Gram-negative bacteria, leading to lysis of the bacteria. A large number of complement regulatory proteins, both soluble and on the cell surface, carefully govern and localize complement activation to the site of inflammation. Inhibitors of complement activation are under development as potential inhibitors of the tissue injury associated with inappropriate inflammatory responses (for example, in paroxysmal nocturnal hemoglobinuria, age-related macular degeneration, and possibly myocardial infarction).

EICOSANOIDS

Eicosanoids are metabolites of arachidonic acid, a fatty acid component of phospholipids in the inner leaflet of the plasma membrane of many cell types. Inflammatory mediators such as cytokines and complement are able to stimulate the enzymatic release of arachidonic acid from the plasma mem-

brane. A number of biochemical reactions ensue, resulting in the formation of prostaglandins, leukotrienes, and other eicosanoids. Notably, certain arachidonic acid derivatives are proinflammatory, whereas others serve to limit the inflammatory process. This underscores the fact that acute inflammation is a self-limited process and that the process of pathogen destruction is intimately tied to the process of tissue repair. Chapter 41 is devoted to an in-depth discussion of eicosanoid physiology, pathophysiology, and pharmacology.

CYTOKINES

Cytokines are proteins that act in a paracrine manner to regulate leukocyte activity. **Interleukins** are cytokines secreted by cells of the hematopoietic lineage. Interleukin-1 (IL-1) and tumor necrosis factor-α (TNF-α) are two cytokines elaborated as part of an acute inflammatory response; these cytokines were two of the mediators responsible for Mark's fever. **Chemokines** are a subset of cytokines that promote immune cell trafficking and localization to sites of inflammation. For example, macrophage chemoattractant protein-1 (MCP-1) promotes monocyte transmigration and activation. Other notable cytokines include the hematopoietic growth factors granulocyte-monocyte colony stimulating factor (GM-CSF) and granulocyte colony stimulating factor (G-CSF) (see Chapter 43).

Because cytokines affect the proliferation and function of cells that mediate innate and adaptive immune responses, selective inhibition or stimulation of cytokine actions has the potential to modulate immune and inflammatory responses. Pharmacologic uses for cytokine and anticytokine therapies are discussed in Chapter 43 and Chapter 44, respectively.

OTHER AGENTS

As noted in Table 40-2, a number of other signaling molecules are also used to coordinate the inflammatory response. These include kinins, platelet-activating factor, nitric oxide, oxygen radicals, and other leukocyte and bacterial products released during phagocytosis. Although pharmacologic agents are being developed to modulate each of these pathways, there are, as yet, no approved anti-inflammatory drugs that specifically interrupt the action of these mediators.

THE INFLAMMATORY RESPONSE

The cells and soluble mediators of the immune system interact with one another to generate the **inflammatory response,** which typically occurs in four phases. First, the vasculature around a site of injury reacts to recruit cells of the immune system. Second, circulating immune cells migrate from these vessels into the injured tissues, and the mechanisms of innate and adaptive immunity (see above) serve to neutralize and remove the inciting stimulus. Next, the process of repair and tissue healing ensues and the acute inflammatory process is terminated. If the events of inflammation are not halted but continue to smoulder, chronic inflammation can occur.

DILATION OF VESSELS

Within hours of being cut, Mark's thumb begins to exhibit the five classic signs of inflammation presented in the Introduction. Initially, these signs and symptoms result from alterations in vascular hemodynamics at the site of injury. Injury to a tissue causes the release of inflammatory mediators (discussed above) that dilate arterioles and postcapillary venules; in turn, vasodilation leads to increased blood flow to the site of injury, causing the clinical signs of redness and warmth. Inflammatory mediators also cause contraction of vascular endothelial cells, leading to increased capillary permeability and to the development of an exudate (i.e., interstitial fluid with a high protein content); in turn, the exudate causes the clinical manifestations of swelling and pain from increased tissue pressure.

RECRUITMENT OF CELLS

Increased vascular permeability also allows cells from the blood to enter the interstitium. Cellular migration out of the blood is not random; rather, leukocyte recruitment is orchestrated to optimize clearing of the infection or local repair of the injured tissue (Fig. 40-6). At the onset of an inflammatory response, the endothelial cells at the site of injury are activated to express adhesion molecules that bind specific receptors expressed by leukocytes. For example, intercellular adhesion molecules (**ICAMs**) expressed by activated endothelial cells bind integrins expressed on the cell surface of leukocytes. This interaction causes the leukocytes, which normally roll along the surface of the endothelium by means

of loose, transient binding interactions, to adhere tightly to the activated endothelium at the site of injury. The adherent leukocytes then bind other endothelial cell receptors that promote **transmigration** (diapedesis) of the leukocytes from the vasculature into the interstitium. Specificity of the immune response is achieved according to the pattern of adhesion molecules expressed by the activated endothelium and the various types of leukocytes; for example, neutrophils dominate the early inflammatory response, while monocytes predominate after 24 hours.

CHEMOTAXIS

Once the cells of the immune system have crossed the endothelial barrier, they can migrate through the interstitium to the specific site of injury or infection. Immune cell targeting is accomplished by the process of **chemotaxis,** or chemical signaling. Inflammatory mediators released at the site of injury, such as C3a and leukotriene B4 (LTB_4), create a chemical gradient to which the leukocytes respond, allowing them to move preferentially toward the site of the inflammatory reaction.

PHAGOCYTOSIS

Upon their arrival at the site of injury or infection, the neutrophils, macrophages, and other cells of the immune system are ready to perform their duties. However, these cells require one further stimulus to activate their killing machinery. Foreign substances must be coated by an opsonin before they can be ingested (phagocytosed) by leukocytes. **Opsonins** are molecular adaptors that coat foreign surfaces and signal leukocytes that a particle should be attacked. The major opsonins consist of complement, immunoglobulins (antibod-

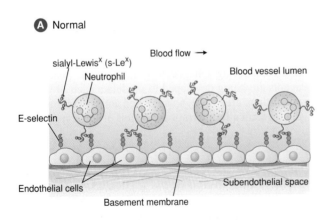

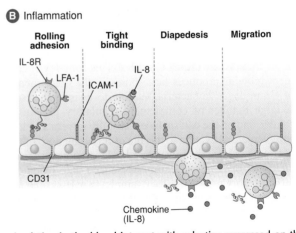

Figure 40-6. Overview of the inflammatory response. A. Leukocytes circulating in the blood interact with selectins expressed on the surface of vascular endothelial cells. In the absence of inflammation, the interaction between leukocytes and endothelial cells is weak, and leukocytes either flow past or roll along the endothelium. Neutrophil rolling is mediated by the interaction between endothelial cell E-selectin and neutrophil sialyl-Lewis^x (s-Le^x). **B.** During the inflammatory response, endothelial cells up-regulate their expression of intercellular adhesion molecules (ICAMs). ICAM expression increases the potential for strong binding interactions between leukocytes and the activated endothelial cells. For example, ICAM-1 on endothelial cells binds tightly to LFA-1 on neutrophils. The enhanced cell-cell interaction leads to margination of leukocytes onto endothelial cell surfaces and initiates the process of leukocyte diapedesis and transmigration from the vascular space into extravascular tissues. Leukocytes migrate through injured tissue in response to chemokines such as IL-8, which are inflammatory mediators released by injured cells and by other immune cells that have already reached the site of injury.

ies), and **collectins** (plasma proteins that bind to certain microbial carbohydrates). The interaction of a phagocytic cell with an opsonized particle initiates the engulfment and destruction of the offending agent. This step is also the crucial point of interaction between innate and adaptive immunity. Antigen-presenting cells process engulfed particles and present their antigens to B cells and T cells, which then react to the antigens. In the introductory case, Mark's cut presumably allowed bacteria to penetrate his skin barrier, leading to infection. The presence of these bacteria initiated an inflammatory response that included phagocytosis of bacteria by APCs, presentation of bacterial antigens to T_H cells, activation and expansion of T_H cells, T_H cell activation of further APC-mediated phagocytosis, and synthesis and secretion of antibodies specific for the bacteria.

RESOLUTION

Tissue repair and the re-establishment of homeostasis are the final events in the acute inflammatory response. The same mediators that activate inflammation also initiate a cascade of tissue repair; this process is mediated by the release of growth factors and cytokines, including epidermal growth factor (EGF), platelet-derived growth factor (PDGF), basic fibroblast growth factor-2 (bFGF-2), transforming growth factor-β1 (TGF-β1), IL-1, and TNF-α. These factors act as mitogens for endothelial cells and fibroblasts and ultimately stimulate healing and scar formation through angiogenesis (formation of new blood vessels) and the formation of granulation tissue. In the introductory case, the granulation tissue and eventual scar will be the only record of Mark's acute inflammatory event. Of note, angiogenesis can be a pathologic state when it is associated with tumor growth, and pharmacologic inhibitors of angiogenesis are currently being used as antineoplastic agents (see Chapter 38, Pharmacology of Cancer: Signal Transduction).

CHRONIC INFLAMMATION

Chronic inflammation is a pathologic state characterized by the continued and inappropriate response of the immune system to an inflammatory stimulus. Chronic inflammation accounts for the symptoms of many autoimmune diseases and may be an important cause of organ transplant rejection. In contrast to the acute inflammatory response, which is dominated by neutrophils, one of the hallmarks of chronic inflammation is the predominance of macrophages. Activated macrophages secrete inflammatory mediators such as proteases and eicosanoids, as well as collagenases and growth factors. These secreted products initiate and maintain a cycle of tissue injury and repair, leading to tissue remodeling. Over time, chronic inflammation can cause relentless tissue destruction. Promising areas of treatment for chronic inflammation include the use of cytokine inhibitors to neutralize mediators of the signaling cascades that perpetuate chronic inflammation. These agents are discussed in Chapter 44.

Conclusion and Future Directions

The immune system intricately regulates the response to tissue injury and infection. Innate immune mechanisms respond to patterned elements common to an infection, such as bacterial lipoproteins or viral particles. The innate immune system also processes these particles and presents them to lymphocytes, thereby activating the adaptive immune system. The adaptive immune system develops a response specific to an infectious agent or inflammatory stimulus. As part of the inflammatory response, the adaptive immune response also has mechanisms that mediate tolerance to distinguish self from nonself; dysregulation of these mechanisms may lead to chronic inflammation and autoimmune disease.

The chemical mediators of the inflammatory response—including histamine, complement, eicosanoids, and cytokines—are the major targets of current pharmacologic therapies. Macromolecules are playing an increasingly important role in modulation of these chemical mediators; for example, a number of anti-cytokine antibodies, including inhibitors of tumor necrosis factor-α, have been developed for the treatment of rheumatoid arthritis, psoriatic arthritis, and inflammatory bowel disease. A second approach to modulation of inflammatory responses has been to target the intracellular signaling cascades responsible for initiation of immune responses. Examples of such drugs include cyclosporine and mycophenolate mofetil, as discussed in Chapter 44. As the number of agents available for treatment of immune disorders grows, it will become increasingly important to determine whether macromolecular agents and small-molecule signaling inhibitors can be used in combination to target multiple steps in inflammatory pathways.

Suggested Reading

Akira S, Uematsu S, Takeuchi O. Pathogen recognition and innate immunity. *Cell* 2006;124:783–801. (*Recent advances in understanding of the innate immune system.*)

Delves PJ, Roitt IM. Advances in immunology: the immune system—first of two parts. *N Engl J Med* 2000;343:37–49. (*This article and subsequent articles in the series provide an excellent general introduction to immunology.*)

Ibelgaufts H. *COPE: Cytokines & Cells Online Pathfinder Encyclopaedia.* Available at: http://www.copewithcytokines.de/cope.cgi. (*Web site that describes all known actions of cytokines.*)

Janeway CA. *Immunobiology: The Immune System in Health and Disease.* 6th ed. New York: Garland Publishing; 2004. (*A general immunology textbook.*)

Pier GB, Lyczak JB, Wetzler L. *Immunology, Infection and Immunity.* Washington, DC: ASM Press; 2004. (*A detailed text covering current understanding of immunologic mechanisms.*)

Taams LS, Palmer DB, Akbar AN, et al. Regulatory T cells in human disease and their potential for therapeutic manipulation. *Immunology* 2006;118:1–9. (*Discusses possible therapeutic uses of regulatory T cells in transplantation and autoimmune disease.*)

Zola H, Swart B, Nicholson I, et al. CD molecules 2005: human cell differentiation molecules. *Blood* 2005;106:3123–3126. (*Recent report on molecules with the "CD" designation.*)

41

Pharmacology of Eicosanoids

David M. Dudzinski and Charles N. Serhan

INTRODUCTION

Autacoids are substances that are rapidly synthesized in response to specific stimuli, act quickly at the immediate locality, and remain active for only a short time before degradation. **Eicosanoids** represent a chemically diverse family of arachidonic acid-derived autacoids. Research on eicosanoids continues to reveal their critical roles in cardiovascular, inflammatory, and reproductive physiology. Numerous pharmacologic interventions in eicosanoid pathways—including the nonsteroidal anti-inflammatory drugs (NSAIDs), cyclooxygenase-2 (COX-2) inhibitors, and leukotriene inhibitors—are useful in the current clinical management of

inflammation, pain, and fever. Given the diverse bioactivities of eicosanoids, future research in eicosanoid physiology and pharmacology may lead to the development of new therapeutics for the treatment of inflammatory conditions, autoimmune diseases, asthma, glomerulonephritis, cancer, sleep disorders, and Alzheimer's disease.

 Case

Mrs. D, a 57-year-old Caucasian female, goes to her physician because of joint pain and chronic fatigue. Her history reveals general joint stiffness and pain, especially in the early morning, and pain in the left metatarsophalangeal joint of 3 weeks' duration. Mrs. D is advised to take ibuprofen as needed, and this medication provides relief of her pain for some time.

Two years later, Mrs. D notes indigestion and a few isolated instances of vomiting "coffee-grounds"–like material. Her physician recommends an upper gastrointestinal endoscopic examination, which reveals gastric mucosal erosion and hemorrhage. Based on this finding, Mrs. D is advised to discontinue ibuprofen therapy. Her physician is also concerned about the recent progression in Mrs. D's joint stiffness and pain, and refers her to a rheumatology clinic. Mrs. D reports to the rheumatologist that her pain has progressed to include both feet, both hands and wrists, both elbows, some cervical vertebrae, and the left hip. Over the past few months, she has noted difficulty with basic household tasks and has avoided physical activity. The metacarpophalangeal and proximal interphalangeal joints of both hands are found to be swollen, tender, and warm. Skin nodules are apparent on the extensor surface of both forearms. Laboratory tests show high erythrocyte sedimentation rate (ESR), low hematocrit, and positive rheumatoid factor (an immune complex formed from IgM and autoreactive IgG produced in joints). Synovial fluid aspirate is notable for leukocytosis.

Because the presentation is consistent with a diagnosis of rheumatoid arthritis, Mrs. D is started on a course of celecoxib (a COX-2 selective inhibitor), etanercept (a TNF-α antagonist), and prednisone (a glucocorticoid). Over the next several months, Mrs. D's joint pain, swelling, and tenderness decrease noticeably. Joint function in the hands is restored, and Mrs. D is able to resume some physical activity.

QUESTIONS

■ **1.** Why was ibuprofen sufficient to control Mrs. D's early symptoms? Explain the rationale for discontinuing ibuprofen.

■ **2.** What are the advantages and limitations of each of the classes of drugs to which celecoxib, etanercept, and prednisone belong?

PHYSIOLOGY OF ARACHIDONIC ACID METABOLISM

Eicosanoids are crucially involved in a number of metabolic pathways that have diverse roles in inflammation and cellular signaling. All of these pathways center on reactions involving the metabolism of arachidonic acid (Fig. 41-1). The following section considers the biochemical steps leading to arachidonic acid synthesis, and then discusses the cyclooxygenase, lipoxygenase, epoxygenase, and isoprostane pathways of arachidonic acid metabolism.

GENERATION OF ARACHIDONIC ACID

Arachidonic acid (cis-,cis-,cis-,cis-5,8,11,14-eicosatetraenoic acid), the common precursor to eicosanoids, must be

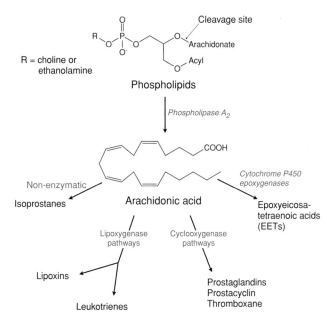

Figure 41-1. Overview of arachidonic acid pathways. Phospholipase A_2 acts on the phospholipids phosphatidylcholine *(PC)*, phosphatidylethanolamine *(PE)*, and phosphatidylinositol *(PI)* to release arachidonic acid. Unesterified arachidonic acid is then used as substrate for the cyclooxygenase, lipoxygenase, and epoxygenase pathways. The cyclooxygenase pathways produce prostaglandins, prostacyclin, and thromboxane. The lipoxygenase pathways produce leukotrienes and lipoxins. The epoxygenase pathway produces epoxyeicosatetraenoic acids (EETs). Nonenzymatic peroxidation of arachidonic acid can also produce isoprostanes. Phospholipase A_2 cleaves the ester bond marked by the *arrow* to release arachidonic acid.

biosynthesized from the essential fatty acid precursor **linoleic acid** (cis-,cis-9,12-octadecadienoic acid), which can be obtained only from dietary sources. In the cell, arachidonic acid does not exist as a free fatty acid, but rather is esterified to the sn_2 position of membrane phospholipids, predominantly phosphatidylcholine and phosphatidylethanolamine.

Arachidonic acid is released from cellular phospholipids by the enzyme **phospholipase A_2** (Fig. 41-1), which hydrolyzes the acyl ester bond. *This important reaction, which represents the first step in the arachidonic acid cascade, is the overall rate-determining step in the generation of eicosanoids.*

There are membrane-bound and soluble isoforms of phospholipase A_2, classified as secretory ($sPLA_2$) and cytoplasmic ($cPLA_2$), respectively. The phospholipase A_2 isoforms are differentiated based on molecular weight, pH sensitivity, regulation and inhibition characteristics, calcium requirements, and substrate specificity. The existence of multiple isoforms allows for tight regulation of the enzyme in different tissues to achieve selective biologic responses. Phospholipase A_2 isoforms, relevant in inflammation, are stimulated by cytokines such as TNF-α, GM-CSF, and IFN-γ; growth factors such as epidermal growth factor (EGF); and the MAP kinase-protein kinase C (MAPK-PKC) cascade. Although glucocorticoids were once thought to inhibit phospholipase A_2 activity directly, it has now been shown

TABLE 41-1A Comparison of COX-1 and COX-2

PROPERTY	COX-1	COX-2
Expression	Constitutive	Inducible; not normally present in most tissues
		Constitutive in parts of nervous system
Tissue location	Ubiquitous expression	Inflamed and activated tissues
Cellular localization	Endoplasmic reticulum	ER and nuclear membrane
Substrate selectivity	Arachidonic acid, eicosapentaenoic acids	Arachidonic acid, γ-linolenate, α-linolenate, linoleate, eicosapentaenoic acids
Role	Protection and maintenance functions	Proinflammatory and mitogenic functions
Induction	Generally no induction	Induced by LPS, TNF-α, IL-1, IL-2, EGF, IFN-γ
	hCG can up-regulate COX-1 in amnion	mRNA rises 20- to 80-fold upon induction
		Regulated within 1–3 hours
Inhibition	Pharmacologic: NSAIDs (low-dose aspirin)	In vivo: Anti-inflammatory glucocorticoids, IL-1β, IL-4, IL-10, IL-13
		Pharmacologic: NSAIDs, COX-2 selective inhibitors

TABLE 41-1B Major Adverse Effects of Nonselective COX Inhibitors and COX-2 Selective Inhibitors

ADVERSE EFFECT	NONSELECTIVE COX INHIBITORS (NSAIDS)	COX-2 SELECTIVE INHIBITORS
Gastric ulceration	Yes	Yes*
Inhibit platelet function	Yes	No
Inhibit labor induction	Yes	Yes
Impair renal function	Yes	Yes
Hypersensitivity reaction	Yes	?

* The gastrointestinal toxicity of COX-2 selective inhibitors may be less than that of nonselective COX inhibitors.

that glucocorticoids act by inducing the synthesis of **lipocortins,** a family of phospholipase A_2-regulatory proteins. One of the lipocortins, annexin 1, mediates some of the anti-inflammatory actions of glucocorticoids (see below).

CYCLOOXYGENASE PATHWAY

Unesterified intracellular arachidonic acid is rapidly converted by **cyclooxygenase, lipoxygenase,** or cytochrome-containing **epoxygenase** enzymes; the specific enzyme dictates the particular class of local eicosanoids that are generated. *The cyclooxygenase pathway leads to the formation of **prostaglandins, prostacyclin,** and **thromboxanes;** the li-poxygenase pathways lead to **leukotrienes** and **lipoxins;** and the epoxygenase pathways lead to epoxyeicosatetraenoic acids* (Fig. 41-1). Cyclooxygenases (also known as *prostaglandin H synthases*) are glycosylated, homodimeric, membrane-bound, heme-containing enzymes that are ubiquitous in animal cells from invertebrates to humans. *Two cyclooxygenase isoforms, denoted **COX-1** and **COX-2,** are found in humans.* Although COX-1 and COX-2 share 60% sequence homology and near-superimposable three-dimensional structures, the genes are located on different chromosomes, and the enzymes differ in cellular, genetic, physiologic, pathologic, and pharmacologic profiles (Table 41-1). Each cyclooxygenase catalyzes two sequential reactions. The first (cyclooxygenase) reaction is the oxygen-dependent cyclization of arachidonic acid to prostaglandin G_2 (PGG_2); the second (peroxidase) reaction is the reduction of PGG_2 to PGH_2.

As a result of differences in cellular localization, regulatory profile, tissue expression, and substrate requirement, COX-1 and COX-2 ultimately produce different sets of eicosanoid products that are involved in two different pathways. Constitutively expressed COX-1 is believed to function in physiologic, or "housekeeping," activities such as vascular homeostasis, maintenance of renal and gastrointestinal blood flow, renal function, intestinal mucosal proliferation, platelet function, and antithrombogenesis. A number of "as-needed," or specialized, functions are attributed to the inducible COX-2 enzyme, including roles in inflammation, fever, pain, transduction of painful stimuli in the spinal cord, mitogenesis (particularly in the gastrointestinal epithelium), renal adaptation to stresses, deposition of trabecular bone, ovulation, placentation, and uterine contractions of labor. The role of constitutive COX-2 expression in areas of the nervous system such as the hippocampus, hypothalamus, and amygdala remains to be elucidated.

Protein kinetic studies suggest that there may be a third functional cyclooxygenase isoform. The putative COX-3 isoform may be a product of the same gene as COX-1 but with different protein characteristics, possibly because of alternative mRNA splicing or posttranslational modification. Furthermore, COX-3 may be a potential site of action of **acetaminophen.** However, definitive proof of the existence of COX-3 remains elusive.

Prostaglandins

Prostaglandins are a large family of structurally similar compounds that each has potent and specific biological actions. The name of the family derives from their initial identification in the genitourinary system of male sheep. Prostaglandins all share a chemical structure, called a **prostanoid,** consisting of a 20-carbon carboxylic acid containing a cyclopentane ring and a 15-hydroxyl group (Fig. 41-2).

Prostaglandins are divided into three major subseries: PG_1, PG_2, and PG_3. The subscript numeral indicates the number of double bonds present in the molecule. The PG_2 series is the most prevalent because these are direct derivatives of arachidonic acid, an eicosa*tetra*enoic acid. The PG_1 series derive from the arachidonic acid precursor dihomo-γ-linolenic acid (DHGLA), an eicosa*trien*oic acid,

while the PG_3 series derive from an eicosa*penta*enoic acid (EPA).

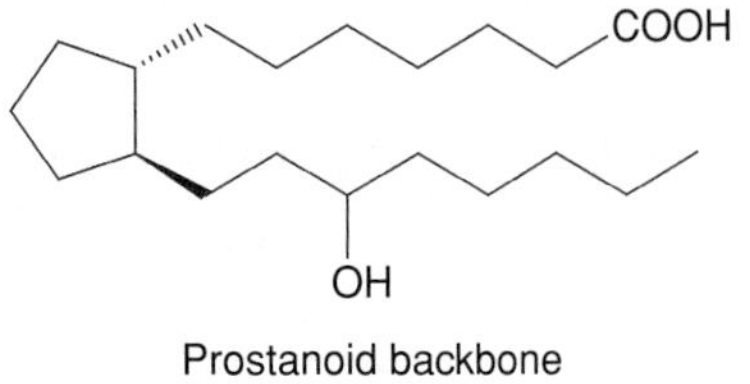

The prostaglandin PGH_2 represents the critical juncture of the cyclooxygenase pathway (Fig. 41-3) because it is the precursor to PGD_2, PGE_2, $PGF_{2\alpha}$, thromboxane A_2 (TxA_2), and prostacyclin (PGI_2). The distribution of these eicosanoids in various tissues is determined by the expression pattern of the different enzymes of prostaglandin synthesis (i.e., PG synthases).

The prostaglandins are important in many physiologic processes, most of which are not directly related to inflammation. All of these functions are highlighted in Table 41-2. Note especially the important housekeeping functions of PGE_2, broadly referred to as **cytoprotective** roles, in which organs such as gastric mucosa, myocardium, and renal parenchyma are shielded from the effects of ischemia by PGE_2-mediated vasodilation and regulation of blood flow. PGE_2 is also involved in inflammatory cell activation, and PGE_2 that is biosynthesized by COX-2 and PGE_2 synthase in cells near the hypothalamus appears to have a role in fever.

Thromboxane and Prostacyclin

Platelets express high levels of the enzyme thromboxane synthase but do not contain prostacyclin synthase. Therefore, *TxA_2 is the chief eicosanoid product of platelets.* TxA_2 has a half-life of only 10 to 20 seconds before it is nonenzymatically hydrolyzed to inactive TxB_2. TxA_2, which signals via a 7-transmembrane G protein-coupled G_q mechanism, is both a strong vasoconstrictor and a promoter of platelet adhesion and aggregation. In contrast, the vascular endothelium lacks thromboxane synthase but expresses prostacyclin synthase. Therefore, *PGI_2 is the primary eicosanoid product of the vascular endothelium.* PGI_2, which signals via G_s, functions as a vasodilator, venodilator, and inhibitor of platelet aggregation. In other words, PGI_2 is a physiologic antagonist of TxA_2. The vasodilatory actions of PGI_2, as with those of PGE_2, also confer cytoprotective properties.

TxA_2 is a relatively stronger vasoconstrictor and platelet activator than PGI_2 is a vasodilator and platelet inhibitor. Therefore, the local balance between TxA_2 and PGI_2 levels is critical in the regulation of systemic blood pressure and thrombogenesis. Imbalances can lead to hypertension, ischemia, thrombosis, coagulopathy, myocardial infarction, and stroke. In certain populations of the northern latitudes (including Inuit, Greenland, Irish, and Danish populations), the incidence of heart disease, stroke, and thromboembolic disorders is less than in populations further south. The diet of these northern peoples is richer in whale and fish oils and, as a result, contains relatively smaller amounts of arachidonic acid precursors but relatively larger amounts of EPAs. Analogous to the conversion of arachidonic acid into TxA_2 and PGI_2, EPA is converted into TxA_3 and PGI_3 (Fig. 41-4A). Importantly, the vasoconstricting and platelet aggregating effects of TxA_3 are relatively weak compared to the vasodilating and platelet inhibiting effects of PGI_3. As a result, the thromboxane-prostacyclin balance is tipped toward vasodilation, platelet inhibition, and antithrombogenesis, with a corresponding decline in the related diseases (Fig. 41-4B,C). This is one possible explanation for the observation that the northern populations have a lower inci-

Figure 41-2. Prostanoid structure. The generic prostanoid structure is a 20-carbon carboxylic acid with a cyclopentane ring and a 15-hydroxyl group. All prostaglandins, thromboxanes, and prostacyclins are derived from this common structure.

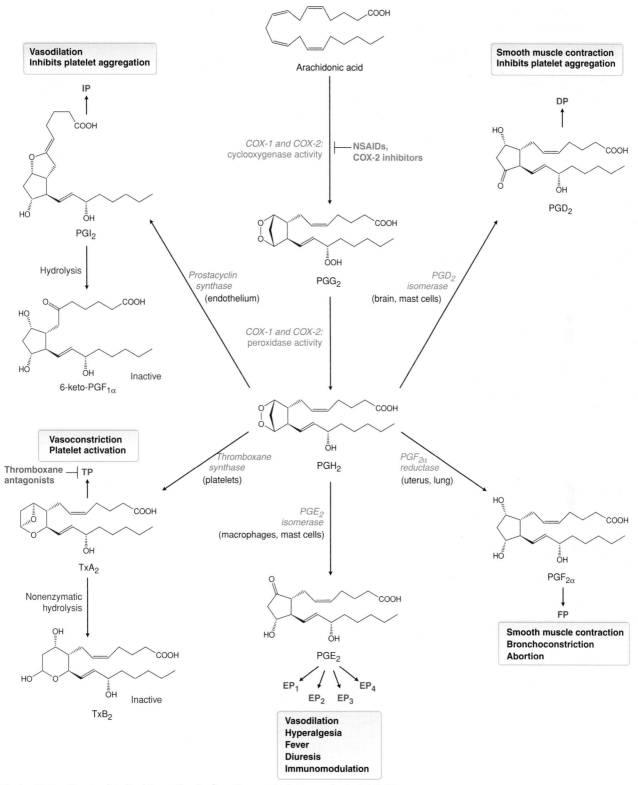

Figure 41-3. Prostaglandin biosynthesis, function, and pharmacologic inhibition. The biosynthetic pathways from arachidonic acid to prostaglandins, prostacyclin, and thromboxane are shown. Note that tissue-specific enzyme expression determines the tissues in which the various PGH$_2$ products are produced. NSAIDs and COX-2 inhibitors are the most important classes of drugs that modulate prostaglandin production. Thromboxane antagonists and PGE$_2$ synthase inhibitors are promising pharmacologic strategies that are currently in development. COX, cyclooxygenase; PG, prostaglandin; Tx, thromboxane; DP, PGD$_2$ receptor; EP, PGE$_2$ receptor; FP, PGF$_{2\alpha}$ receptor; IP, PGI$_2$ receptor; TP, TxA$_2$ receptor; NSAID, nonsteroidal anti-inflammatory drug.

TABLE 41-2	Prostaglandin Products, Synthesis, Receptors, and Functions			
PROSTAGLANDIN	**SYNTHETIC ENZYME**	**TISSUES EXPRESSING SYNTHETIC ENZYME**	**RECEPTOR TYPE AND SIGNALING MECHANISM**	**FUNCTIONS**
PGD_2	PGD_2 isomerase	Mast cells Neurons	DP G_s	Bronchoconstriction (asthma) Sleep control functions Alzheimer's disease
PGE_2	PGE_2 isomerase	Many tissues, including macrophages and mast cells	EP1 G_q EP2 G_s EP3 G_i EP4 G_s Other	Potentiation of responses to painful stimuli Vasodilation Bronchoconstriction Cytoprotective: modulates gastric mucosal acid secretion, mucus, and blood flow Vasodilation Bronchoconstriction Inflammatory cell activation Pyrexia Mucus production Possibly erectile function
$PGF_{2\alpha}$	$PGF_{2\alpha}$ reductase	Vascular smooth muscle Uterine smooth muscle	FP G_q	Vascular tone Reproductive physiology (abortifacient) Bronchoconstriction

The prostanoid receptors are all G protein-coupled receptors.

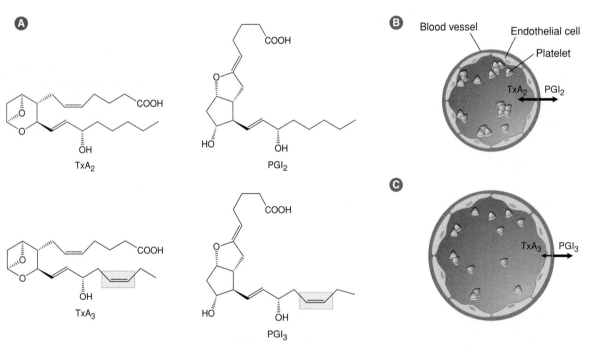

Figure 41-4. Control of vascular tone and platelet activation by thromboxanes and prostacyclins. A. In comparison to TxA₂, TxA₃ has a third double bond *(highlighted in blue box)* three carbons from the noncarboxylic acid end of the molecule (the "omega-3" position). By analogy, PGI₃ has an additional double bond *(highlighted)* compared to PGI₂. **B.** A cross section of a vessel is shown, with platelets in the vascular lumen. The *arrows* depict the relative balance between TxA₂-mediated vasoconstriction and PGI₂-mediated vasodilation. The figure also shows the relative balance between TxA₂-mediated platelet aggregation and PGI₂-mediated inhibition of platelet aggregation. TxA₂ is slightly more dominant than PGI₂, so there is net vasoconstriction and mild platelet aggregation. **C.** This panel shows the balance between thromboxane and prostacyclin action in an individual on a diet rich in fish oil (which contains high concentrations of omega-3 fatty acids). On this diet, there are relatively higher levels of TxA₃, which is considerably less potent than TxA₂, and PGI₃, which is approximately as potent as PGI₂. Therefore, the balance is shifted toward net vasodilation and net inhibition of platelet aggregation. This shift may lower the incidence of thrombogenic and ischemic diseases such as myocardial infarction and stroke.

dence of heart disease and is one rationale for increasing dietary fish consumption.

LIPOXYGENASE PATHWAY

The lipoxygenase pathways represent the second major fate of arachidonic acid. These pathways lead to the formation of leukotrienes and lipoxins. Lipoxygenases are enzymes that catalyze the insertion of molecular oxygen into arachidonic acid, using nonheme iron to generate specific hydroperoxides. Three lipoxygenases, 5-, 12-, and 15-lipoxygenases (5-LOX, etc.), are the major LOX isoforms found in humans (Table 41-3). The lipoxygenases are named for the position in arachidonic acid on which they catalyze the insertion of molecular O_2. The immediate products of lipoxygenase reactions are hydroperoxyeicosatetraenoic acids (**HPETEs**). HPETEs can be reduced to the corresponding hydroxyeicosatetraenoic acids (**HETEs**) by enzymes using glutathione peroxidase (GSP). 5-HPETE formed by 5-LOX is the direct precursor to LTA_4, which itself is the precursor to all potent bioactive leukotrienes (Fig. 41-5). Lipoxygenases are also involved in converting 15-HETE and LTA_4 to lipoxins (Fig. 41-6).

5-LOX requires translocation to the nuclear membrane for activity. The protein 5-lipoxygenase-activating protein (**FLAP**) helps 5-LOX translocate to the nuclear membrane, form an active enzyme complex, and accept the arachidonic acid substrate from phospholipase A_2.

Leukotrienes

Leukotriene biosynthesis begins with the 5-LOX-mediated conversion of 5-HPETE to leukotriene A_4 (LTA_4). Therefore, *5-LOX catalyzes the first two steps in leukotriene biosynthesis* (Fig. 41-5). It is not known whether the 5-HPETE diffuses out of the 5-LOX enzymatic active site between these steps or remains bound to the same 5-LOX enzyme for both reactions.

LTA_4 is next converted to either LTB_4 or LTC_4. The enzyme LTA_4 hydrolase converts LTA_4 to LTB_4 in neutrophils and erythrocytes. LTA_4 conversion to LTC_4 occurs in mast cells, eosinophils, basophils, and macrophages by the addition of a γ-glutamylcysteinylglycine tripeptide (glutathione). LTC_4, LTD_4, LTE_4, and LTF_4, which represent the **cysteinyl leukotrienes,** are interconverted by removal of amino acid portions of the γ-glutamylcysteinylglycine tripeptide (Fig. 41-5).

LTB_4 acts via two G protein-coupled receptors, BLT1 and BLT2. Binding of LTB_4 to BLT1, which is expressed mainly in tissues involved in host defense and inflammation (leukocytes, thymus, spleen), leads to proinflammatory sequelae, most importantly neutrophil chemotaxis, aggregation, and transmigration across epithelium and endothelium. LTB_4 up-regulates neutrophil lysosomal function and free-radical production, enhances cytokine production, and potentiates the actions of natural killer (NK) cells. The role of the ubiquitously expressed BLT2 remains unknown.

The cysteinyl leukotrienes (LTC_4 and LTD_4) bind to CysLT1 receptors to cause vasoconstriction, bronchospasm, and increased vascular permeability. Cysteinyl leukotrienes are responsible for the hyperreactivity to stimuli and airway and vascular smooth muscle contraction that occur in asthmatic, allergic, and hypersensitivity processes. Together, both arms of the leukotriene pathways (i.e., LTB_4 and LTC_4/LTD_4) play key roles in psoriasis, arthritis, and various inflammatory responses. They are also key mediators in vascular disease and atherosclerosis.

Lipoxins

Lipoxins (**lipox**ygenase **in**teraction products) are derivatives of arachidonic acid containing four conjugated double bonds and three hydroxyl groups. *The two main lipoxins, LXA_4 and LXB_4 (Fig. 41-6), modulate the actions of leukotrienes and cytokines and are important in resolution of inflammation.*

At sites of inflammation, there is typically an inverse relationship between the amounts of lipoxin and leukotriene

TABLE 41-3	Tissue Expression of Lipoxygenases and Products of Lipoxygenase Action			
LIPOXYGENASE	**TISSUE EXPRESSION**	**PRODUCTS**	**PATHWAYS**	**NOTES**
5-LOX	Neutrophils	5-HPETE/5-HETE	Leukotrienes/Lipoxins	Requires FLAP for activity
	Macrophages	LTA_4	Lipoxins	
	Mast cells	Epoxytetraene	Lipoxins/Aspirin-triggered lipoxins	
	Eosinophils			
12-LOX				
Platelet type	Platelets	12-HPETE/12-HETE	Lipoxins	
	Megakaryocytes (tumors)	Epoxytetraene		
Epidermal type	Skin			
Leukocyte type	Macrophages			
	GI system			
	Brain			
15-LOX	Macrophages	15-HPETE/15-HETE	Lipoxins	
	Monocytes	Epoxytetraene	Lipoxins	
	Airway epithelium			

FLAP, 5-lipoxygenase activating protein; GI, gastrointestinal; LOX, lipoxygenase.

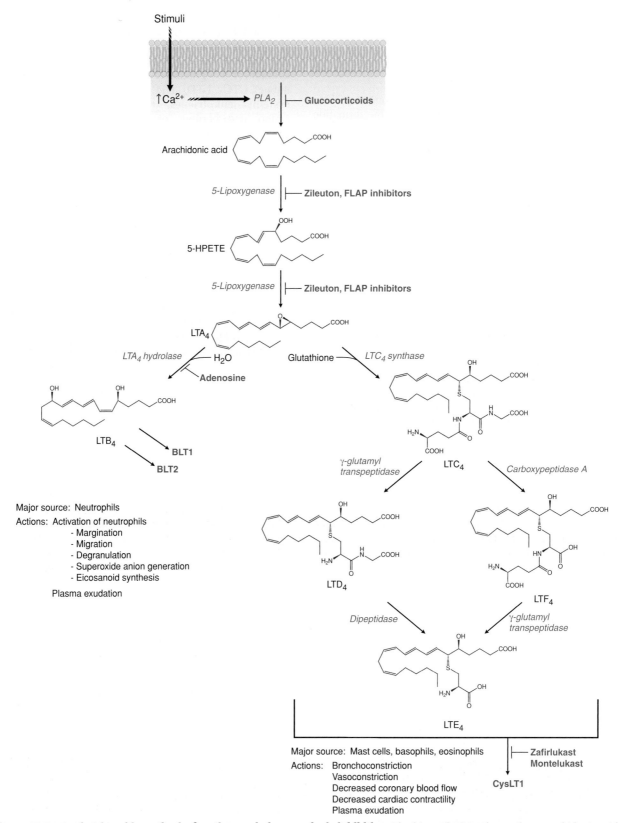

Figure 41-5. Leukotriene biosynthesis, function, and pharmacologic inhibition. The biosynthetic pathways from arachidonic acid to the leukotrienes are shown. Glucocorticoids decrease phospholipase A_2 (PLA$_2$) activity, thereby preventing the synthesis of all leukotrienes (LTs). Zileuton and 5-lipoxygenase activating protein (FLAP) inhibitors prevent the conversion of arachidonic acid to 5-HPETE and LTA$_4$; zileuton is used in the chronic management of asthma. Adenosine inhibits LTB$_4$ synthesis in neutrophils but is not used pharmacologically for this purpose. Zafirlukast and montelukast are antagonists at CysLT1, the receptor for all cysteinyl leukotrienes; these drugs are used in the chronic management of asthma. BLT1 and BLT2, LTB$_4$ receptors; CysLT1, receptor for LTC$_4$, LTD$_4$, LTE$_4$, and LTF$_4$.

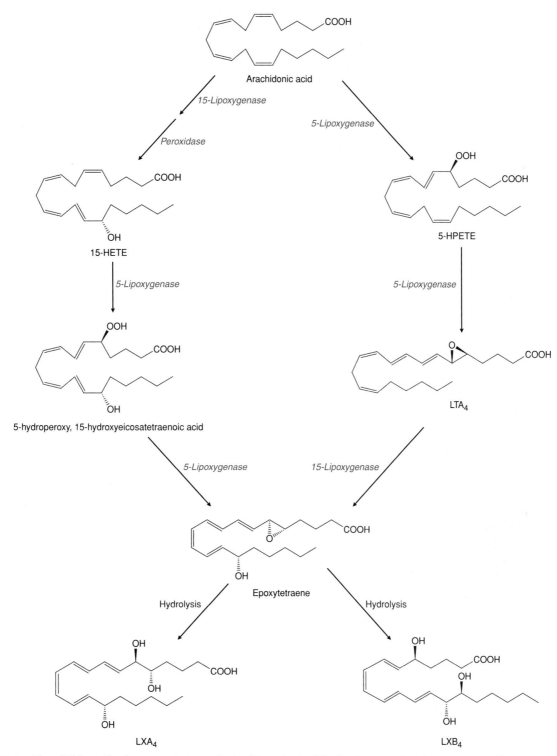

Figure 41-6. Lipoxin biosynthesis. Two main routes lead to biosynthesis of the lipoxins. In each pathway, sequential lipoxygenase reactions are required, followed by hydrolysis. The immediate precursor of the lipoxins is epoxytetraene; hydrolysis of epoxytetraene yields the lipoxins. **Left pathway:** Arachidonic acid is converted to 15-HETE by sequential activity of 15-lipoxygenase and peroxidase. 15-HETE is converted by 5-lipoxygenase to the chemical intermediate 5-hydroperoxy, 15-hydroxyeicosatetraenoic acid, and 5-lipoxygenase acts on this intermediate to form epoxytetraene. **Right pathway:** Arachidonic acid is converted to 5-HPETE by 5-lipoxygenase, and 5-HPETE is converted to LTA$_4$ by further action of 5-lipoxygenase. LTA$_4$ is converted to epoxytetraene by 15-lipoxygenase. **Common pathway:** Epoxytetraene is hydrolyzed to the active lipoxins LXA$_4$ and LXB$_4$. The lipoxins have an anti-inflammatory role, are counter-regulators of leukotriene action, and regulate many cytokines and growth factors.

present. This observation has led to the suggestion that lipoxins may act as counter-regulatory signals or negative regulators of leukotriene action. LXA_4 receptors are present on neutrophils and in the lung, spleen, and blood vessels. Lipoxins inhibit neutrophil chemotaxis, adhesion, and transmigration through endothelium (by decreasing P-selectin expression), inhibit eosinophil recruitment, stimulate vasodilation (by inducing synthesis of PGI_2 and PGE_2), inhibit LTC_4- and LTD_4-stimulated vasoconstriction, inhibit LTB_4 inflammatory effects, and inhibit the function of NK cells. Lipoxins stimulate the uptake and clearance of apoptotic neutrophils by macrophages and thereby mediate resolution of the inflammatory response. *Because lipoxin production appears to be important in the resolution of inflammation, an imbalance in lipoxin-leukotriene homeostasis may be a key factor in the pathogenesis of inflammatory disease.* For example, it is possible that Mrs. D's chronic joint inflammation involves an imbalance in the relative amounts of leukotrienes and lipoxins in her affected joints.

EPOXYGENASE PATHWAY

Microsomal cytochrome P450 epoxygenases oxygenate arachidonic acid, resulting in the formation of epoxyeicosatetraenoic acid (EET) and hydroxyacid derivatives (Fig. 41-1). The epoxygenase pathway is important in tissues that do not express COX or LOX, such as certain cells of the kidney. Epoxygenation of arachidonic acid produces four different EETs, depending on which double bond in arachidonic acid is modified. Dihydroxy derivatives of EETs, formed by hydrolysis, may regulate vascular tone by inhibiting the Na^+/K^+-ATPase in vascular smooth muscle cells and may affect renal function by regulating ion absorption and secretion. With respect to inflammation, dihydroxy EET derivatives inhibit platelet cyclooxygenase and inhibit the expression of **i**ntercellular **a**dhesion **m**olecules (**ICAMs**). Down-regulation of ICAMs inhibits platelet and inflammatory cell aggregation. Thus, *as with lipoxins, specific EETs (e.g., 11,12-EET) may play a role in regulating inflammation at certain sites and within select tissues.* Future research may reveal more definitive functions for EETs in human physiology.

ISOPROSTANES

Phospholipid-esterified arachidonic acid is susceptible to free-radical-mediated peroxidation; cleavage of these modified lipids from the phospholipid by phospholipase A_2 gives rise to the isoprostanes (Fig. 41-1). During oxidative stress, isoprostanes are found in the blood at levels much higher than those of cyclooxygenase products. Two isoprostanes in particular, 8-epi-$PGF_{2\alpha}$ and 8-epi-PGE_2, are potent vasoconstrictors. Isoprostanes can function in activating NF-κB, phospholipase Cγ, protein kinase C, and calcium flux. *Because the rate of formation of isoprostanes depends on cellular oxidation conditions, isoprostane levels may be indicative of oxidative stress and a wide range of pathology.* Urinary isoprostane levels are used as markers of oxidative stress in ischemic syndromes, reperfusion injury, atherosclerosis, and hepatic diseases. Isoprostanes are not, however, known to have any role in inflammation or host defense.

METABOLIC INACTIVATION OF LOCAL EICOSANOIDS

Prostaglandins, leukotrienes, thromboxanes, and lipoxins are inactivated by hydroxylation, β-oxidation (resulting in a loss of two carbons), or ω-oxidation (to dicarboxylic acid derivatives). These degradation processes render the molecules more hydrophilic and excretable in the urine.

INTEGRATED INFLAMMATION SCHEMA

As described above, eicosanoids are generated locally in numerous complex reactions. It is not necessary to remember every mediator, but rather to understand the general scheme of these synthetic pathways. This section, along with Table 41-4, provides a concise overview of the physiologic functions of eicosanoids relevant to inflammation and host defense.

Acute inflammation is the result of an intricate network of molecular and cellular interactions induced by responses to a variety of stimuli, such as trauma, ischemia, infectious agents, or antibody reactions. Acute superficial inflammation generates local pain, edema, erythema, and heat; inflammation in visceral organs can have similar symptoms and result in severe impairment of organ function.

Leukotrienes and lipoxins, as well as thromboxanes, prostaglandins, and prostacyclins, are critical for generating, maintaining, and mediating inflammatory responses. The inflammatory cascade is initiated when cells in a particular region are exposed to a foreign substance or are damaged. That insult stimulates a local cytokine cascade (including interleukins or TNF), which increases COX-2 mRNA and enzyme levels. COX-2 then facilitates production of the proinflammatory and vasoactive eicosanoids.

Locally high concentrations of PGE_2, LTB_4, and cysteinyl leukotrienes promote the accumulation and infiltration of inflammatory cells by increasing blood flow and vascular permeability. LTB_4 and 5-HETE are also important in attracting and activating neutrophils. LTB_4, formed by activated neutrophils at the site of inflammation, recruits and

TABLE 41-4	Roles of Eicosanoids in the Steps of Inflammation

ACTION	EICOSANOIDS INVOLVED
Vasoconstriction	$PGF_{2\alpha}$, TxA_2, LTC_4, LTD_4, LTE_4
Vasodilation (erythema)	PGI_2, PGE_1, PGE_2, PGD_2, LXA_4, LXB_4, LTB_4
Edema (swelling)	PGE_2, LTB_4, LTC_4, LTD_4, LTE_4
Chemotaxis, leukocyte adhesion	LTB_4, HETE, LXA_4, LXB_4
Increased vascular permeability	LTC_4, LTD_4, LTE_4
Pain and hyperalgesia	PGE_2, PGI_2, LTB_4
Local heat and systemic fever	PGE_2, PGI_2, LXA_4

activates additional neutrophils and lymphocytes so that these cells adhere to endothelial surfaces and transmigrate into the interstitial spaces. Increased vascular permeability also results in fluid leak and cellular infiltration, causing edema.

With the aggregation of a multitude of inflammatory cells, **transcellular biosynthetic routes** are exploited to generate eicosanoids (Fig. 41-7). *In transcellular synthesis, eicosanoid intermediates are donated from one cell type to another to generate a larger diversity of eicosanoids.* This demonstrates the importance of cellular adhesion and cell-cell interaction in inflammatory and immune responses.

The body tries to ensure that the inflammatory response cannot proceed unchecked. Lipoxins help resolve inflammation and promote the return of the tissue to homeostasis. COX-2–derived eicosanoids may also function in wound healing and resolution. Hence, the temporal sequence of events is important in an organized inflammatory response. PGE_2 inhibits the functions of B and T lymphocytes and NK cells, while LTB_4 and the cysteinyl leukotrienes regulate T-lymphocyte proliferation. PGE_2 and PGI_2 are potent pain sensitizers, and lipoxins reduce nociception. These factors coordinately mediate and regulate the transition from acute to chronic inflammation.

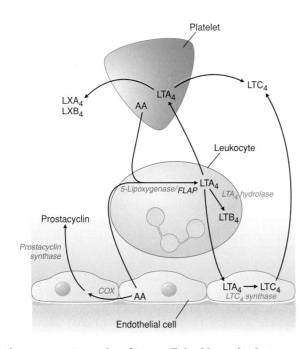

Figure 41-7. Examples of transcellular biosynthesis. Transcellular biosynthesis is used to generate lipoxins and cysteinyl leukotrienes locally. In the example shown here, the leukocyte (neutrophil) obtains arachidonic acid *(AA)* from platelets and uses this AA to synthesize leukotriene A_4 *(LTA_4)* and leukotriene B_4 *(LTB_4)*. Leukotriene A_4 is transferred from the leukocyte to platelets and endothelial cells, which synthesize and secrete leukotriene C_4 *(LTC_4)*. Platelets also synthesize lipoxins *(LXA_4, LXB_4)* from leukotriene A_4, and endothelial cells synthesize prostacyclin using AA from endogenous stores. Note that the eicosanoids synthesized within each cell type are determined by the enzymatic repertoire of that cell type: for example, neutrophils synthesize primarily LTA_4 and LTB_4 because they express 5-lipoxygenase and LTA_4 hydrolase, whereas endothelial cells biosynthesize prostacyclin and LTC_4 because they express COX-1, COX-2, prostacyclin synthase, and LTC_4 synthase.

PATHOPHYSIOLOGY

Inflammation and the immune response are the body's mechanisms for combating foreign invaders. This overall program is designed to remove the inciting stimulus and resolve tissue damage. In some cases, the response mechanism itself causes local tissue damage, such as when activated neutrophils inadvertently release proteases and reactive oxygen species into the local milieu. In other settings, if the inflammatory reactions persist for too long or if the immune system misidentifies a part of self as foreign, these misdirected immune responses can cause significant and chronic tissue injury.

Profiled below are selected inflammatory diseases in which eicosanoids are implicated, including asthma, inflammatory bowel disease, rheumatoid arthritis, glomerulonephritis, and cancer. Other diseases not discussed here, but having a possible eicosanoid-related inflammatory basis, include atherogenesis, myocardial infarction, certain skin disorders, reperfusion injuries, Alzheimer's disease, and adult respiratory distress syndrome.

ASTHMA

Asthma is a chronic inflammatory disorder typified by intermittent attacks of dyspnea, coughing, and wheezing. Symptoms result from chronic airway inflammation, hyperreactivity, constriction, and obstruction. In asthma, antigens in the lungs stimulate cytokine cascades leading to the generation of both prostaglandins (e.g., PGD_2) and leukotrienes. Elaboration of LTB_4 attracts inflammatory cells and promotes cellular aggregation. LTB_4 acts particularly on B lymphocytes to cause activation, proliferation, and differentiation. LTB_4 also promotes expression of $FC\epsilon RII$ receptors (i.e., receptors for the constant chain of IgE antibodies) on mast cells and basophils; these receptors bind IgE that is released by antigen-stimulated B lymphocytes. LTC_4 and LTD_4 are extremely potent bronchoconstrictive compounds (originally known as the slow-reacting substances of anaphylaxis, SRS-A), being over 1,000 times more potent than histamine. These cysteinyl leukotrienes also cause the airway epithelium to secrete mucus, while impairing the clearance of this mucus by inhibiting the beating of cilia on airway epithelium. Mucus secretion is exacerbated by neutrophils and eosinophils, which become part of the inflammatory exudate clogging the airways. LTD_4 and LTE_4 also recruit eosinophils to asthmatic airways; eosinophils integrate signals from T lymphocytes and, when activated, release factors that damage the airway epithelium and enhance local airway inflammation.

In a mouse model of asthma in which the 5-LOX gene was knocked out, no airway hyperresponsiveness or eosinophilia was observed. This result underscores the important role of the leukotriene products of 5-LOX activity in the pathogenesis of asthma. The role of leukotriene inhibitors in asthma treatment is discussed below; for additional information, refer to Chapter 46, Integrative Inflammation Pharmacology: Asthma.

INFLAMMATORY BOWEL DISEASE

Crohn's disease and ulcerative colitis are two idiopathic, chronic, relapsing, ulcerative, and inflammatory diseases of the gastrointestinal tract. Although the diseases are physiologically and pathologically distinct, elevated LTB_4 production in the affected mucosa results in abnormal leukocyte infiltration into the parenchyma in both conditions. Chronic inflammation and leukocyte infiltration lead to progressive mucosal damage, with overt histologic changes. Crohn's disease is characterized by focal damage, fissuring ulcers, and granulomas, while mucosal inflammation and colonic dilatation are found in ulcerative colitis. Both diseases increase the risk of adenocarcinoma of the colon in the affected areas. Stable analogues of lipoxin A_4 are effective treatments in mouse models of Crohn's disease and bowel inflammation and may represent a promising new pharmacologic approach to the treatment of inflammatory bowel disease.

RHEUMATOID ARTHRITIS

Rheumatoid arthritis is a chronic, systemic, autoimmune, and inflammatory disease that primarily attacks the joints but also affects the skin, cardiovascular system, lungs, and muscles. Rheumatoid arthritis affects up to 1.5% of North Americans and is three times more prevalent in females than in males. Autoimmune targeting of normal joint proteins results in inflammation, with local release of cytokines, TNF, growth factors, and interleukins, all of which induce COX-2 expression. *Levels of COX-2 enzyme and PGE_2 are markedly elevated in the synovial fluid of affected joints.* Other COX-2-derived eicosanoids activate the surrounding endothelium to help recruit inflammatory cells. Macrophages elaborate collagenase and proteases, while lymphocyte activity leads to immune complex formation; both processes further damage joint tissue and provide substrates that accelerate chronic inflammation. Common findings include synovitis, leukocytosis, rheumatoid nodules, and the presence of rheumatoid factor (a circulating antibody directed against IgG).

As an older Caucasian woman, Mrs. D is in a risk group for rheumatoid arthritis. Autoimmune destruction of her joints resulted in the findings of a high erythrocyte sedimentation rate and a low hematocrit, both of which indicate a state of chronic inflammation, synovial leukocytosis, and the progressive loss of joint mobility and function. For additional information on rheumatoid arthritis, refer to Chapter 44, Pharmacology of Immunosuppression.

GLOMERULONEPHRITIS

Glomerulonephritis represents a large group of inflammatory renal conditions that ultimately lead to renal failure through deterioration of renal hemodynamics and glomerular filtration. Local complement activation promotes neutrophil and macrophage infiltration. Infiltration of the glomerulus is a characteristic early pathologic finding that correlates with abnormal levels of LTB_4, which is biosynthesized by LTA_4 hydrolase located in the kidney mesangium, and which facilitates neutrophil adhesion to the glomerular mesangium and epithelium. LTA_4 is also a substrate for the biosynthesis of LTC_4 and LTD_4. All of the cysteinyl leukotrienes (LTC_4, LTD_4, LTE_4, and LTF_4) promote endothelial and mesangial proliferation. Cysteinyl leukotrienes also directly affect glomerular function; specifically, LTC_4 and LTD_4 decrease renal blood flow and glomerular filtration rate (GFR) by vasoconstricting arterioles and contracting mesangial spaces. Studies with inhibitors have confirmed the roles of leukotrienes in glomerulonephritis. LOX inhibitors administered at early stages of glomerulonephritis prevent glomerular inflammation and evidence of structural damage. Both LOX inhibitors and LTD_4 receptor antagonists improve GFR and decrease proteinuria.

Interestingly, the kidney mesangium expresses both LTA_4 hydrolase and 12-LOX, conferring the ability to synthesize either LTB_4 or LXA_4 from leukocyte-derived LTA_4. At low concentrations, LTA_4 is used primarily for LTB_4 formation; these conditions correspond to the initiation of inflammation or to a low level of chronic inflammation. Conversely, when LTA_4 concentrations are relatively high, as in long-standing inflammation, LTA_4 is converted mostly into LXA_4, which provides an autoinhibitory counter-regulatory impact on the inflammatory response. In the glomerulus, LXA_4 counteracts the deleterious proinflammatory consequences of leukotrienes as well as the effect of leukotrienes on GFR, in part by raising afferent arteriolar flow via vasodilation.

CANCER

Long-term epidemiologic studies have shown a correlation between chronic NSAID therapy and decreased incidence of colorectal cancer. Human colorectal adenomas and carcinomas express abundant COX-2; similar results have been obtained in gastric adenocarcinomas and breast tumors. In these tissues, COX-2 is believed to generate PGE_2 and other eicosanoids that promote tumor growth. The perinuclear localization of the COX-2 enzyme (Table 41-1) suggests the potential for an intracellular function of eicosanoid products in oncogenesis. Some eicosanoid derivatives can bind to homologues of the retinoic acid receptor (RXR) family of transcription factors, which are involved in many functions including the regulation of cell growth and differentiation. Overexpression of COX-2 would generate eicosanoids that could flood RXR signaling pathways and provide excessive growth stimuli. A COX-2 inhibitor is being sought as a prophylactic therapy for patients with familial adenomatous polyposis, who are at risk for colorectal cancer (see discussion of COX-2 inhibitors below).

CARDIOVASCULAR DISEASE

Platelet-derived thromboxane A_2 is an important mediator of thrombosis in myocardial infarction and other cardiovascular diseases, and the COX inhibitor aspirin is an effective antiplatelet agent in the prophylaxis and treatment of these diseases (see below and Chapter 22, Pharmacology of Hemostasis and Thrombosis). Intravascular leukotriene production during the rupture of atheromatous plaques is also thought to contribute to the pathophysiology of myocardial infarction. Recent studies have suggested that 5-lipoxygenase, FLAP, and LTA$_4$ hydrolase are genetically linked to myocardial infarction, and 5-lipoxygenase inhibitors, FLAP antagonists, and LTA$_4$ hydrolase inhibitors may represent new classes of therapeutics for the treatment of atherosclerosis and myocardial infarction.

PHARMACOLOGIC CLASSES AND AGENTS

Pharmacologic intervention in eicosanoid biosynthesis and action is particularly useful for controlling inflammation and aberrant immune responses. Pharmacologic interventions can be directed at any of a number of steps outlined above to achieve the desired effects with selectivity. Strategies considered here include altering the expression of key enzymes, competitively and noncompetitively inhibiting the activity of specific enzymes (e.g., PGE$_2$ synthase), activating receptors with exogenous receptor agonists, and preventing receptor activation with exogenous receptor antagonists. As always, the therapeutic benefits must be weighed against the possible adverse effects.

PHOSPHOLIPASE INHIBITORS

Inhibition of phospholipase A$_2$ prevents the generation of arachidonic acid, the rate-limiting step in eicosanoid biosynthesis. In the absence of proinflammatory mediators derived from arachidonic acid, inflammation is limited.

Glucocorticoids (also known as corticosteroids, of which **prednisone** is a member) are a mainstay of therapy in a multitude of autoimmune and inflammatory diseases. Glucocorticoids induce a family of secreted calcium- and phospholipid-dependent proteins called **lipocortins.** Lipocortins interfere with the action of phospholipase A$_2$ and thereby limit the release of arachidonic acid. Annexins, such as annexin 1 and annexin 1-derived peptides, are also induced by glucocorticoids. In turn, annexins act at G protein-coupled receptors on leukocytes to block proinflammatory responses and enhance endogenous anti-inflammatory mechanisms; one anti-inflammatory mechanism involves activation of the lipoxin A$_4$ receptor.

Small-molecule inhibitors of specific phospholipases are in development; these drugs may offer the potential for decreased adverse effects associated with glucocorticoid use. (See Chapter 27, Pharmacology of the Adrenal Cortex, for a more extensive discussion of the effects of glucocorticoids.)

CYCLOOXYGENASE INHIBITORS

Cyclooxygenase pathway inhibitors are some of the most frequently prescribed drugs in medicine. The nonsteroidal anti-inflammatory drugs (NSAIDs) and acetaminophen are the most commonly used agents in this class.

Traditional Nonselective Inhibitors: NSAIDs

NSAIDs are important because of their combined anti-inflammatory, antipyretic, and analgesic properties. The ulti-

mate goal of most NSAID therapies is to inhibit the COX-mediated generation of proinflammatory eicosanoids and to limit the extent of inflammation, fever, and pain. The drugs' antipyretic activity is likely related to their decreasing the levels of PGE$_2$, particularly in the region of the brain surrounding the hypothalamus. *Despite the benefits of current NSAIDs, these drugs only suppress the signs of the underlying inflammatory response.*

A multitude of NSAIDs have been developed over the last century; most are polycyclic carboxylic acid derivatives. Except for aspirin, all NSAIDs act as reversible, competitive inhibitors of cyclooxygenase. These drugs block the hydrophobic channel in cyclooxygenase in which the substrate arachidonic acid binds, thereby preventing access of arachidonic acid to the active site of the enzyme. Traditional NSAIDs inhibit both COX-1 and COX-2 to different degrees. Because of inhibition of COX-1, long-term NSAID therapy has many deleterious effects. The cytoprotective roles of the COX-1 eicosanoid products are eliminated, leading to a spectrum of **NSAID-induced gastropathy** including dyspepsia, gastrotoxicity, subepithelial damage and hemorrhage, gastric mucosal erosion, frank ulceration, and gastric mucosal necrosis. (As in Mrs. D's case, patients with gastric hemorrhage have bleeding into the stomach, where the digestion of hemoglobin produces a material that, when regurgitated, has the color and consistency of coffee grounds.) Regulation of blood flow to the kidney is likewise perturbed, decreasing GFR and potentially causing renal ischemia, papillary necrosis, interstitial nephritis, and renal failure. Epidemiologic studies suggest that 20% to 30% of hospitalizations of patients over the age of 60 are due to complications of NSAID use.

The organic acid functionality of NSAIDs confers important pharmacokinetic properties on these drugs, including near-complete absorption from the gut, binding to plasma albumin, accumulation in cells at the site of inflammation, and efficient renal excretion. NSAIDs can be divided into short (<6 hours) and long (>10 hours) half-life classes. NSAIDs with long elimination half-lives include **naproxen, salicylate, piroxicam,** and **phenylbutazone.**

Chemical classification of the NSAIDs is based on the structure of a key moiety in each subclass of drugs (Fig. 41-8). The following discussion groups the NSAIDs by chemical class; a discussion of the choice of a particular NSAID for a given clinical situation follows the descriptions of the individual agents.

Salicylates

Salicylates include **aspirin** (acetylsalicylic acid) and its derivatives. Aspirin is the oldest of the NSAIDs and is widely used to treat mild-to-moderate pain, headache, myalgia, and arthralgia. *In contrast to other NSAIDs, aspirin acts in an irreversible manner by acetylating the active-site serine residue in both COX-1 and COX-2.* Acetylation of COX-1 destroys the enzyme's cyclooxygenase activity, preventing the formation of COX-1-derived prostaglandins, thromboxanes, and prostacyclin. Salicylates (along with indomethacin, piroxicam, and ibuprofen) may also inhibit the neutrophil oxidative burst by reducing NADPH oxidase activity.

Daily low-dose aspirin is used as an anti-thrombogenic agent for prophylaxis and postevent management of myocar-

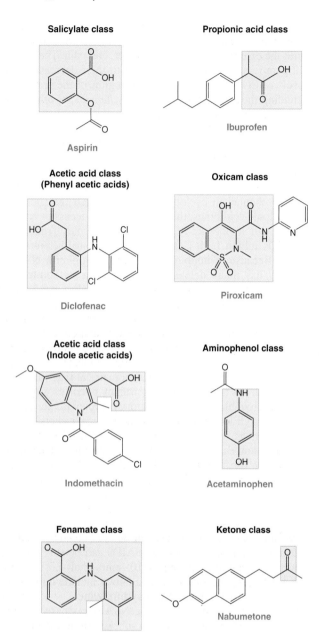

Figure 41-8. Structural classes of NSAIDs. NSAIDs are generally hydrophobic molecules, most of which have a carboxylic acid group. NSAIDs are categorized by classes depending on one or more of the key moieties in the structure. The moiety that is common to members of each class is highlighted by a box. The structure helps to determine the pharmacokinetic properties of each particular NSAID. Note that acetaminophen is not actually an NSAID, because it has only weak anti-inflammatory properties; this drug is included here because, as with NSAIDs, acetaminophen is commonly used for its analgesic and antipyretic effects.

ibly inhibited for their lifetime (about 10 days). Although aspirin also irreversibly inhibits vascular endothelial cell COX-1 and COX-2, the endothelial cells can synthesize new COX protein and thus can rapidly resume synthesis of PGI$_2$. *A single administration of aspirin decreases for several days the amount of thromboxane that can be generated, shifting the vascular TxA$_2$-PGI$_2$ balance toward PGI$_2$-mediated vasodilation, platelet inhibition, and antithrombogenesis.*

Aspirin-mediated inhibition of COX-2 prevents the generation of prostaglandins. Unlike COX-1, which is totally inactivated, aspirin-modified COX-2 retains a part of its catalytic activity and can form a new product, 15-(R)-HETE, from arachidonic acid. By analogy to normal lipoxin synthesis (Fig. 41-6), 5-LOX then converts 15-(R)-HETE to 15-epi-lipoxins, which are relatively stable stereoisomers (carbon 15-position epimers) of lipoxins that are collectively called **aspirin-triggered lipoxins** (**ATLs**). *15-Epi-lipoxins mimic the functions of lipoxins as anti-inflammatory agents.* 15-Epi-lipoxins may represent an endogenous mechanism of anti-inflammation, and their production is believed to mediate at least part of the anti-inflammatory effects of aspirin. Development of 15-epi-lipoxin analogues could lead to anti-inflammatory drugs that do not have the adverse effects associated with COX-1 inhibition.

Aspirin is generally well tolerated. Its major toxicities are the gastropathy and nephropathy common to all NSAIDs. Long-term aspirin therapy can lead to gastrointestinal ulceration and hemorrhage, nephrotoxicity, and hepatic injury. Two unique toxicities are **aspirin-induced airway hyperreactivity** in asthmatics (so-called *aspirin-sensitive asthma*) and **Reye's syndrome.** The prevalence of aspirin sensitivity among patients with asthma is estimated to be approximately 10%. Exposure to aspirin in these patients leads to ocular and nasal congestion along with severe airway obstruction. Aspirin-sensitive patients are also reactive to some other NSAIDs, including indomethacin, naproxen, ibuprofen, mefenamate, and phenylbutazone. One possible etiology of aspirin/NSAID sensitivity in asthmatics is that exposure to these drugs leads to increased levels of leukotrienes, which are implicated in the pathogenesis of asthma (see Fig. 41-1).

Reye's syndrome is a condition characterized by hepatic encephalopathy and liver steatosis in young children. Aspirin therapy during the course of a febrile viral infection has been implicated as a potential etiology of the liver damage. Although a causal link between aspirin and Reye's syndrome has not been definitively established, aspirin is generally not administered to children because of the fear of Reye's syndrome. Acetaminophen is widely used in children instead of aspirin.

Propionic Acid Derivatives

Propionic acid NSAIDs include **ibuprofen, naproxen, ketoprofen,** and **flurbiprofen.** Ibuprofen is a relatively potent analgesic used in rheumatoid arthritis (as in the case of Mrs. D, to relieve intermittent pain), osteoarthritis, ankylosing spondylitis, gout, and primary dysmenorrhea. Naproxen has a long plasma half-life, is 20 times more potent than aspirin, directly inhibits leukocyte function, and causes less severe gastrointestinal adverse effects than aspirin.

dial infarction and stroke. Recall that aspirin is antithrombogenic because of its irreversible inhibition of COX, which prevents platelets from biosynthesizing TxA$_2$. Within an hour of oral aspirin administration, the COX-1 activity in existing platelets is irreversibly destroyed. Platelets, lacking nuclei, cannot synthesize new protein. Therefore, the irreversibly acetylated COX-1 enzymes cannot be replaced by freshly synthesized proteins, and these platelets are irrevers-

Acetic Acid Derivatives

Acetic acid NSAIDs include the indole acetic acids—**indomethacin, sulindac,** and **etodolac**—and the phenylacetic acids **diclofenac** and **ketorolac** (a substituted phenylacetic acid derivative). Besides inhibiting cyclooxygenase, many of the acetic acid NSAIDs promote the incorporation of unesterified arachidonic acid into triglyceride, thus reducing the availability of the substrate for cyclooxygenase and lipoxygenase. Indomethacin is a direct inhibitor of neutrophil motility, but it is not tolerated by patients as well as ibuprofen. Diclofenac is a more potent anti-inflammatory than indomethacin and naproxen. Diclofenac also reduces intracellular arachidonic acid concentrations by altering cellular fatty acid transport and is used widely in the treatment of pain associated with renal stones. Ketorolac is primarily employed for its strong analgesic properties, particularly in postsurgical patients.

The acetic acid NSAIDs are mostly used to relieve symptoms in the long-term treatment of rheumatoid arthritis, osteoarthritis, ankylosing spondylitis, and other musculoskeletal disorders. Use of acetic acid NSAIDs causes gastrointestinal ulceration and, rarely, hepatitis and jaundice. Indomethacin also has a specific use in promoting the closure of a patent ductus arteriosus in newborns by inhibiting the vasodilatory eicosanoids PGE_2 and PGI_2.

Oxicam Derivatives

Piroxicam is as efficacious as aspirin, naproxen, and ibuprofen in the treatment of rheumatoid arthritis and osteoarthritis, but may be better tolerated. Piroxicam has additional effects in the modulation of neutrophil function by inhibiting collagenase, proteoglycanase, and the oxidative burst. Because of its extremely long half-life, piroxicam can be administered once daily. As with other NSAIDs, piroxicam displays gastrointestinal adverse effects such as ulceration, and it prolongs bleeding time because of its antiplatelet effect.

Fenamate Derivatives

The two fenamate NSAIDs are **mefenamate** and **meclofenamate.** Both inhibit cyclooxygenases but also antagonize prostanoid receptors to various degrees. Because fenamates have less anti-inflammatory activity and are more toxic than aspirin, there is little advantage to their use. Mefenamate is used only for primary dysmenorrhea, whereas meclofenamate is used in the treatment of rheumatoid arthritis and osteoarthritis.

Ketones

Nabumetone is a ketone prodrug that is oxidized in vivo to the active acid form. Compared to other nonselective NSAIDs, nabumetone has preferential activity against COX-2. The incidence of gastrointestinal adverse effects is relatively low, although headache and dizziness are frequently reported.

Acetaminophen

Acetaminophen, although sometimes classified with the NSAIDs, is technically not an NSAID: *although acetamino-* *phen has analgesic and antipyretic effects similar to aspirin, the anti-inflammatory effect of acetaminophen is insignificant because of its weak inhibition of cyclooxygenases.* Nonetheless, acetaminophen therapy can be valuable in patients, such as children, who are at risk for the adverse effects of aspirin. The most important adverse effect of acetaminophen is hepatotoxicity. Modification of acetaminophen by hepatic cytochrome P450 enzymes produces a reactive molecule, which is normally detoxified by conjugation with glutathione. An overdose of acetaminophen can overwhelm glutathione stores, leading to cellular and oxidative damage and, in severe cases, to acute hepatic necrosis (see Chapter 5, Drug Toxicity).

Selection of the Appropriate NSAID

The anti-inflammatory, analgesic, and antipyretic effects of the NSAIDs appear to vary among the many agents in this class. However, despite differences in chemistry, tissue selectivity, enzyme selectivity, pharmacokinetics, and pharmacodynamics, the differences in efficacy may not be clinically significant. Overall, the rationale and choice of NSAID do not generally make a substantial difference in treating rheumatoid arthritis or osteoarthritis. However, successful NSAID therapy is still considered more of an art than a science, and therapy for each patient should be directed at achieving the desired anti-inflammatory, analgesic, and antipyretic effects while minimizing adverse effects. The adverse gastric effects of long-term NSAID therapy can be reduced by coadministration of H2 receptor antagonists or proton pump inhibitors (refer to Chapter 45, Integrative Inflammation Pharmacology: Peptic Ulcer Disease).

COX-2 Inhibitors

Because of the sometimes severe gastrointestinal adverse effects associated with long-term NSAID therapy, thought to be caused by inhibition of gastrointestinal COX-1, recent strategies for inhibition of cyclooxygenase pathways have focused on selective inhibition of COX-2. This approach was thought to have the theoretical advantage of inhibiting the chemical mediators responsible for inflammation, while maintaining the cytoprotective effects of the products of COX-1 activity.

COX-2 Selective Inhibitors

Although COX-2 was identified only in the 1990s, intense research swiftly led to the development of COX-2 selective inhibitors for clinical use. *Compared with COX-1, COX-2 has a larger hydrophobic channel through which substrate (arachidonic acid) enters the active site.* Subtle structural differences between COX-2 and COX-1 allowed the development of drugs that act preferentially on COX-2.

The COX-2 selective inhibitors—**celecoxib, rofecoxib, valdecoxib,** and **meloxicam** (Fig. 41-9)—are sulfonic acid derivatives that display 100 times greater selectivity for COX-2 than for COX-1. The relative inhibition of the two cyclooxygenase isozymes in any given tissue is also a function of drug metabolism, pharmacokinetics, and possibly enzyme polymorphisms. The COX-2 selective inhibitors have anti-inflammatory, antipyretic, and analgesic properties similar to

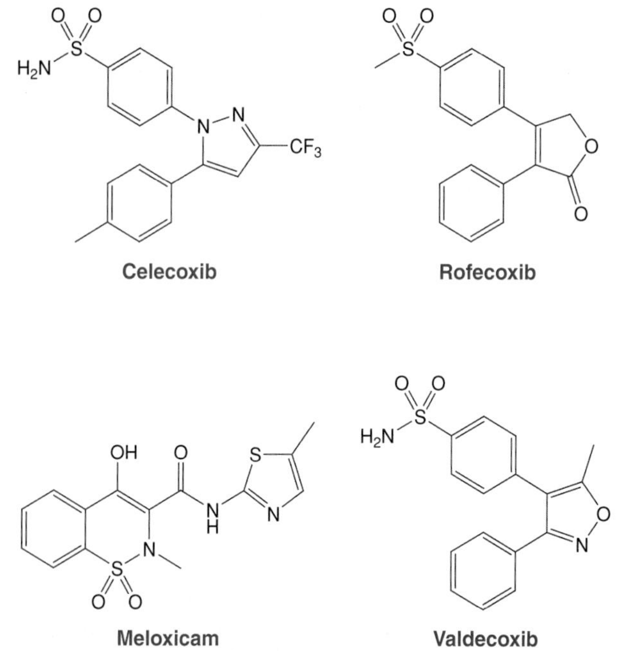

Figure 41-9. COX-2 selective inhibitors. COX-2 selective inhibitors are hydrophobic sulfonic acid derivatives. As with traditional NSAIDs, these molecules block the hydrophobic channel leading to the active site of cyclooxygenase and thus inhibit the enzyme. Note that the COX-2 selective inhibitors are generally larger molecules than NSAIDs. These drugs preferentially inhibit COX-2 compared to COX-1, because the hydrophobic channel of COX-2 is larger than that of COX-1. (That is, COX-2 selective inhibitors are too bulky to access the smaller hydrophobic channel of the COX-1 enzyme.) The COX-2 selective inhibitors display approximately 100-fold greater selectivity for COX-2 compared to COX-1.

the traditional NSAIDs, but they do not share the antiplatelet actions of the COX-1 inhibitors. Relative to other NSAIDs, the safety profile of the COX-2 selective inhibitors is uncertain. At the present time, only celecoxib is an approved drug. Rofecoxib was recently withdrawn because of an increase in thrombogenicity with prolonged use. Note that Mrs. D took advantage of the improved gastrointestinal safety of COX-2 selective inhibitors when she switched from ibuprofen to a COX-2 inhibitor, in part because of symptomatic and endoscopic evidence of NSAID-induced gastropathy. The long-term safety profiles of COX-2 inhibitors are in question, however; there are concerns that COX-2 inhibitors—in particular, rofecoxib—have deleterious effects on the cardiovascular and renal systems by inducing hypertension, renal failure, and cardiac failure. The increased thrombogenicity uncovered in clinical use may be due to prolonged inhibition of vascular COX-2 within endothelial cells, leading to reduced PGI_2 formation. In addition, inhibition of COX-2 may generate problems in wound healing, angiogenesis, and the resolution of inflammation. COX-2 selective inhibitors are much more expensive than equivalent doses of many NSAIDs, especially aspirin and indomethacin.

Celecoxib remains the COX-2 selective inhibitor currently approved for osteoarthritis, rheumatoid arthritis, acute pain in adults, and primary dysmenorrhea. This drug is also approved to reduce the number of adenomatous colorectal polyps in individuals with **familial adenomatous polyposis.** Celecoxib decreases the activity of peroxisome proliferator-

activated receptor δ (PPARδ), a transcription factor that heterodimerizes with the RXR transcription factors involved in growth regulation. It is not yet clear whether COX-2 inhibitors bind directly to PPARδ or whether they lead indirectly to the synthesis of other molecules that inhibit PPARδ. Nevertheless, inhibition of PPARδ prevents signaling through the PPARδ pathway and thus removes a potent mitogenic stimulus that could function in the development of colon cancer.

Valdecoxib was initially approved for osteoarthritis, rheumatoid arthritis, and primary dysmenorrhea. Rofecoxib was approved for osteoarthritis, acute pain in adults, and primary dysmenorrhea. Meloxicam was approved only for osteoarthritis.

It was hoped that the second-generation COX-2 inhibitors in development—such as parecoxib (a prodrug of valdecoxib), etoricoxib, and lumiracoxib—would demonstrate increased selectivity for COX-2 over COX-1 and would not have the adverse cardiovascular effects of the existing COX-2 inhibitors. However, further clinical development of this class of drugs is in question.

Glucocorticoids

Prednisone and other glucocorticoids inhibit the action of COX-2 and the formation of prostaglandins by several mechanisms: (1) repressing COX-2 gene and enzyme expression; (2) repressing the expression of cytokines that activate COX-2; and (3) limiting the available pool of COX-2 substrate (arachidonic acid) by indirectly blocking phospholipase A_2. Glucocorticoids also stimulate endogenous anti-inflammatory pathways. In combination, all of these mechanisms create a powerful anti-inflammatory effect. Because of this profound and global suppression of immune and inflammatory responses, glucocorticoids are indicated for the treatment of a number of autoimmune conditions (see Chapter 44, Pharmacology of Immunosuppression).

Cytokine Inhibitors

The proinflammatory cytokines TNF-α and IL-1 enhance prostaglandin production and up-regulate COX-2. Novel molecular technologies have provided the ability to inhibit the action of these cytokines and thus to inhibit the process whereby an injurious stimulus activates COX-2 and initiates the inflammatory response. Three TNF-α antagonists, **etanercept, infliximab,** and **adalimumab,** are currently used in the treatment of rheumatoid arthritis. Etanercept consists of the extracellular domain of the TNF-α receptor coupled to human IgG1; infliximab is a humanized mouse monoclonal antibody directed against TNF-α; and adalimumab is a fully humanized monoclonal IgG1 antibody directed against TNF-α. With few adverse effects, these drugs halt joint destruction and bone erosion, decrease pain, improve swollen and tender joints, and limit overall disease progression in rheumatoid arthritis. These drugs have also been approved for use in a variety of other autoimmune diseases (see Chapter 44). Lipoxins, ATLs, and lipoxin-stable analogues also block the actions of TNF-α, providing a potential new treatment approach (see below).

Anakinra is a recombinant form of the human IL-1 receptor produced in *E. coli;* this drug is approved for use in rheumatoid arthritis. Additional IL-1 antagonists are being developed for use in inflammatory and autoimmune diseases. For more information on these agents, refer to Chapter 44.

PROSTANOID RECEPTOR MIMETICS

Several interesting applications for prostanoid receptor agonists are listed in the Drug Summary Table at the end of this chapter.

THROMBOXANE ANTAGONISTS

Both TxA_2 receptor antagonists and thromboxane synthase inhibitors could represent extremely powerful and selective agents capable of inhibiting platelet activity and protecting against thrombosis and vascular disease. These thromboxane antagonists could theoretically serve as "super" platelet inhibitors in the management of patients with cardiovascular disease. TxA_2 receptor antagonists, unlike aspirin, would also be expected to block the vasoconstrictive action of the isoprostanes. Compounds such as **dazoxiben** and **pirmagrel** inhibit thromboxane synthase, whereas **ridogrel** is a TxA_2 receptor antagonist. These thromboxane antagonists have not yet found clinical utility, however, because the clinical benefit of these drugs is not significantly greater than that of aspirin, which is far less expensive.

LEUKOTRIENE INHIBITION

Lipoxygenase Inhibition

Inhibition of 5-lipoxygenase has the potential to represent a major therapeutic modality in diseases involving leukotriene-mediated pathophysiology, including asthma, inflammatory bowel disease, and rheumatoid arthritis. Lipoxygenase inhibition is an attractive therapeutic approach in these diseases because leukotrienes are potent, locally acting mediators.

Several strategies are possible for the design of lipoxygenase inhibitors, based on the structure, function, and mechanism of the lipoxygenase enzymes. Suicide inhibitors of lipoxygenase (e.g., derivatives of arachidonic acid with triple bonds instead of double bonds), which become covalently bound to the active site and render it inactive, have been developed but are not available for clinical use. Radical scavengers such as catechols, butylated hydroxytoluene (BHT), and α-tocopherol trap the radical intermediates in the lipoxygenase reaction and thereby prevent the functioning of the enzyme, but these nonspecific compounds cannot be used clinically for lipoxygenase inhibition.

Drugs that impair or alter the ability of lipoxygenase to utilize its nonheme iron properly would be expected to inhibit the activity of the enzyme. The only lipoxygenase inhibitor in clinical use is **zileuton** (Fig. 41-10A), a benzothiophene derivative of N-hydroxyurea that inhibits 5-LOX by chelating its nonheme iron. In asthma, zileuton induces bronchodilation, improves symptoms, and generates long-lasting improvement in pulmonary function tests. Zileuton is effective in the treatment of asthma induced by cold, drugs, and allergens. However, because of its low bioavailability, low potency, and significant adverse effects such as liver toxicity, zileuton is not as widely used as the other anti-leukotriene asthma drugs (see below).

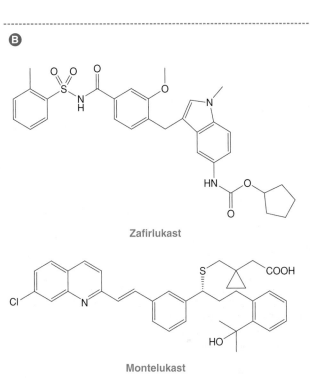

Figure 41-10. Leukotriene pathway inhibitors. A. Zileuton is a 5-lipoxygenase inhibitor that blocks the biosynthesis of leukotrienes from arachidonic acid. **B.** Zafirlukast and montelukast are leukotriene receptor antagonists. All three drugs were originally approved for the prevention and chronic treatment of asthma in both adults and children. None of these drugs, however, is effective in the treatment of acute asthma attacks.

5-Lipoxygenase Activating Protein (FLAP) Inhibition

Interfering with the role of FLAP could represent an approach to the selective inhibition of 5-LOX activity and leukotriene function. Recall that 5-LOX is activated after the enzyme translocates to the nuclear membrane and docks with FLAP; FLAP also binds arachidonic acid released by phospholipase A_2 and shuttles it to the 5-LOX active site. FLAP inhibitors have been developed that both prevent and reverse LOX binding to FLAP and block the arachidonic acid binding site, but no FLAP inhibitors are currently available for clinical use.

Leukotriene Synthesis Inhibitors

Other than zileuton, no specific inhibitors of the enzymes involved in leukotriene synthesis are available for clinical use. Specific LTA$_4$ hydrolase inhibitors, which block LTB$_4$ biosynthesis, are currently in development. **Adenosine**, acting via its receptors on neutrophils, inhibits LTB$_4$ biosynthesis by regulating arachidonic acid release and, possibly, by interfering with the influx of calcium. Furthermore, adenosine is thought to have a role in limiting cell and tissue injury during inflammation. High cell turnover at inflammatory sites generates high local concentrations of adenosine, which may decrease LTB$_4$ biosynthesis and reduce leukocyte recruitment and activation. Adenosine receptor agonists could be considered for development as pharmacologic agents in the control of inflammation.

Leukotriene Receptor Antagonists

Leukotriene receptor antagonism represents a receptor-based mechanism for inhibiting leukotriene-mediated bronchoconstriction and smooth muscle effects. Cysteinyl leukotriene receptor (CysLT1) antagonists are effective against asthma induced by antigen, exercise, cold, or aspirin. These agents significantly improve bronchial tone, pulmonary function tests, and asthma symptoms. **Montelukast** and **zafirlukast** (Fig. 41-10B) are the currently available cysteinyl leukotriene receptor antagonists; the main clinical application for these antagonists is in the treatment of asthma.

More potent CysLT1 antagonists are in development, including pobilukast, tomelukast, and verlukast. Further research will likely elucidate cysteinyl leukotriene receptor subtypes and their respective tissue distributions, which could offer the possibility of tissue-targeted antagonism and the application of these tissue-selective antagonists to other conditions such as rheumatoid arthritis, inflammatory bowel disease, and various allergic disorders.

LIPOXINS, ASPIRIN-TRIGGERED LIPOXINS, AND LIPOXIN-STABLE ANALOGUES

Lipoxins and ATLs offer the potential to antagonize the inflammatory actions of leukotrienes and other inflammatory mediators and to promote resolution of inflammation. Analogues of these compounds represent a new approach to treatment, since they are agonists of endogenous anti-inflammation and proresolution pathways rather than direct enzyme inhibitors or receptor antagonists. Because lipoxins are endogenous regulators, they are expected to have selective actions with few adverse effects. Stable analogues of lipoxins and ATLs are currently being developed, and second-generation lipoxin-stable analogues have shown efficacy in enhancing the resolution of recurring bouts of acute inflammation in skin inflammation and gastrointestinal inflammation models. This new approach to the treatment of inflammation remains to be established in human trials.

Conclusion and Future Directions

Eicosanoids are critical mediators of homeostasis and of many pathophysiologic processes, especially those involv-

ing host defense and inflammation. Arachidonic acid, the primary substrate, is converted into prostaglandins, thromboxanes, prostacyclin, leukotrienes, lipoxins, isoprostanes, and epoxyeicosatetraenoic acids. Prostaglandins have diverse roles in vascular tone regulation, gastrointestinal regulation, uterine physiology, analgesia, and inflammation. Prostacyclin and thromboxane coordinately control vascular tone, platelet activation, and thrombogenesis. Leukotrienes (LTC$_4$, LTD$_4$) are the chief mediators of bronchoconstriction and airway hyperactivity; LTB$_4$ is a major activator of leukocyte chemotaxis and infiltration. Lipoxins antagonize the effects of leukotrienes and reduce the extent of inflammation and activate resolution pathways.

Pharmacologic interventions at many critical points in these pathways are useful in limiting inflammatory sequelae. Glucocorticoids inhibit several steps in eicosanoid generation, including the rate-determining step involving phospholipase A$_2$. However, chronic glucocorticoid use is associated with many serious adverse effects, including osteoporosis, muscle wasting, and abnormal carbohydrate metabolism. Cyclooxygenase inhibitors block the first step of prostanoid synthesis and prevent the generation of prostanoid mediators of inflammation. Lipoxygenase inhibitors, FLAP inhibitors, leukotriene synthesis inhibitors, and leukotriene receptor antagonists prevent leukotriene signaling, thereby limiting inflammation and its deleterious effects. Future drug development efforts will allow selective targeting of eicosanoid pathways involved in many clinical conditions.

Suggested Reading

Brink C, Dahlen SE, Drazen J, et al. International Union of Pharmacology XXXVII. Nomenclature for leukotriene and lipoxin receptors. *Pharmacol Rev* 2003;55:195–227. (*International consensus report on eicosanoid receptors and their antagonists.*)

Gilroy DW, Perretti M. Aspirin and steroids: new mechanistic findings and avenues for drug discovery. *Curr Opin Pharmacol* 2005;5:1–7. (*Reviews the anti-inflammatory actions of aspirin-triggered lipoxins and the discovery of annexin and related compounds in the actions of glucocorticoids.*)

Helgadottir A, Manolescu A, Thorleifsson G, et al. The gene encoding 5-lipoxygenase activating protein confers risk of myocardial infarction and stroke. *Nat Genet* 2004;36:233–239. (*Association between leukotriene pathway enzyme and myocardial infarction.*)

Ostor AJ, Hazleman BL. The murky waters of the coxibs: a review of the current state of play. *Inflammopharmacology* 2005;13:371–380. (*Reviews coxib pharmacology and issues surrounding the ongoing use of COX-2 selective inhibitors.*)

Psaty BM, Furberg CD. COX-2 inhibitors—lessons in drug safety. *N Engl J Med* 2005;352:1133–1135. (*Reviews issues surrounding withdrawal of COX-2 selective inhibitors.*)

Serhan CN, Savill J. Resolution of inflammation: the beginning programs the end. *Nature Immunol* 2005;6:1191–1197. (*Advances in the role of eicosanoid pathways and novel lipid mediators in resolution programs of inflammation.*)

Vane JR, Bakhle YS, Botting RM. Cyclooxygenases 1 and 2. *Ann Rev Pharmacol Toxicol* 1998;38:97–120. (*Historic overview of prostaglandin research, including discussion of the pharmacologic manipulation of these pathways.*)

Drug Summary Table | Chapter 41 Pharmacology of Eicosanoids

NONSTEROIDAL ANTI-INFLAMMATORY DRUGS (NSAIDs)

Mechanism—Inhibit cyclooxygenase-1 (COX-1) and cyclooxygenase-2 (COX-2), decreasing the biosynthesis of downstream eicosanoids and thereby limiting the inflammatory response

Drug	Clinical Applications	Serious and Common Adverse Effects	Contraindications	Therapeutic Considerations
Aspirin	Mild to moderate pain Headache, myalgia, arthralgia Prophylaxis of stroke and myocardial infarction (antiplatelet effect)	*Gastrointestinal ulcer, bleeding, Reye's syndrome, asthma exacerbation, bronchospasm, angioedema* Gastrointestinal disturbance, tinnitus	Aspirin hypersensitivity Aspirin-triggered asthma Children and teenagers with chickenpox or flu symptoms, due to risk of Reye's syndrome	The oldest of the NSAIDs Widely used to treat mild to moderate pain, headache, myalgia, and arthralgia In contrast to other NSAIDs, aspirin acts in an irreversible manner by acetylating the active site serine residue in both COX-1 and COX-2 Aspirin increases plasma concentration of acetazolamide, which leads to CNS toxicity Ibuprofen may inhibit the antiplatelet effect of aspirin Limited reports suggest that salicylates may enhance methotrexate toxicity Aspirin increases the risk of bleeding in anticoagulated patients
Propionic acids: Ibuprofen Naproxen Ketoprofen Flurbiprofen *Acetic acids:* Indomethacin Sulindac Etodolac Diclofenac Ketorolac *Oxicams:* Piroxicam *Fenamates:* Mefenamate Meclofenamate *Ketones:* Nabumetone	Mild to moderate pain Fever Osteoarthritis, rheumatoid arthritis Dysmenorrhea Gout Patent ductus arteriosus closure (indomethacin)	*Gastrointestinal hemorrhage, ulceration, perforation; nephrotoxicity; Stevens-Johnson syndrome; pseudoporphyria (naproxen)* Gastrointestinal disturbance, tinnitus	Gastrointestinal or intracranial bleeding Coagulation defects Asthma, urticaria, or allergic-type reactions after taking NSAIDS, due to risk of severe, even fatal, anaphylactic reactions Significant renal insufficiency	Naproxen has a longer half-life, is 20 times more potent, and causes fewer gastrointestinal adverse effects than aspirin Ketorolac is used for analgesia in postsurgical patients Piroxicam has a long half-life; once daily dosing Nabumetone has the greatest selectivity of these agents for COX-2 Fenamates have limited use; compared to aspirin, fenamates have less anti-inflammatory activity and higher toxicity

ACETAMINOPHEN

Mechanism—Weak inhibitor of peripheral cyclooxygenases; predominant effect may be inhibition of cyclooxygenase-3 (COX-3) in the CNS

Drug	Clinical Applications	Serious and Common Adverse Effects	Contraindications	Therapeutic Considerations
Acetaminophen	Fever Mild to moderate pain	*Hepatotoxicity, nephrotoxicity (rare)* Rash, hypothermia	Hypersensitivity to acetaminophen	Although acetaminophen has analgesic and antipyretic effects similar to aspirin, the anti-inflammatory effect of acetaminophen is insignificant because of its weak inhibition of peripheral cyclooxygenases Generally safe for use in patients undergoing surgery and dental procedures May inhibit COX-3 isoform in CNS

(Continued)

Drug Summary Table **Chapter 41 Pharmacology of Eicosanoids** (*Continued*)

Drug	Clinical Applications	Serious and Common Adverse Effects	Contraindications	Therapeutic Considerations
				Acetaminophen overdose is a leading cause of hepatic failure Antidote for acetaminophen overdose is N-acetylcysteine
COX-2 SELECTIVE INHIBITORS *Mechanism—Selective inhibition of COX-2*				
Celecoxib	Osteoarthritis, rheumatoid arthritis Primary dysmenorrhea Acute pain in adults Familial adenomatous polyposis	Myocardial infarction; gastrointestinal bleeding, ulceration, perforation; renal papillary necrosis; exacerbation of asthma Gastrointestinal disturbance, peripheral edema	Hypersensitivity to sulfonamides Hypersensitivity to celecoxib Asthma, urticaria, or allergic-type reactions after taking NSAIDS, due to risk of severe, even fatal, anaphylactic reactions	Decreases efficacy of ACE inhibitors Incidence of gastropathy and nephropathy may be less than that associated with NSAIDs Valdecoxib and rofecoxib recently withdrawn from market due to possible increased cardiovascular mortality
GLUCOCORTICOIDS *Mechanism—Inhibit COX-2 action and prostaglandin biosynthesis by inducing lipocortins, activating endogenous anti-inflammatory pathways, and other mechanisms*				
Prednisone Prednisolone Methylprednisolone Dexamethasone	See Drug Summary Table: Chapter 27 Pharmacology of the Adrenal Cortex			
CYTOKINE ANTAGONISTS *Mechanism—Etanercept, infliximab, and adalimumab inhibit TNF-alpha; anakinra inhibits IL-1*				
Etanercept Infliximab Adalimumab	See Drug Summary Table: Chapter 44 Pharmacology of Immunosuppression			
Anakinra	See Drug Summary Table: Chapter 44 Pharmacology of Immunosuppression			
PROSTANOID MIMETICS *Mechanism—Prostanoid receptor agonists; see specific drug*				
Alprostadil	Maintenance of patent ductus arteriosus Erectile dysfunction	Heart failure, cardiac arrhythmia and conduction defects, disseminated intravascular coagulation (DIC), disorders of bone development, seizure, priapism, apnea in newborn Hypotension, penile fibrosis, penile discomfort	Sickle cell anemia or trait Leukemia, myeloma Neonatal respiratory distress syndrome Anatomical deformation of the penis, penile implant, Peyronie's disease	PGE1 analogue with vasodilator properties Used primarily for maintaining patent ductus arteriosus in tetralogy of Fallot, Eisenmenger pulmonary hypertension, and aortic valve atresia

Drug	Clinical Applications	Adverse Effects	Contraindications	Therapeutic Considerations
Misoprostol	Cytoprotective and antisecretory effects against gastric ulcers in long-term NSAID therapy; Abortifacient with mifepristone	*Rare anemia, rare cardiac arrhythmia*; Gastrointestinal disturbance	Pregnancy	PGE1 analogue with vasodilator properties. Also used in peptic ulcer disease (see Chapter 45); Cytoprotective effects likely mediated by increasing gastric mucus and bicarbonate production; antisecretory effects mediated via inhibition of basal and nocturnal gastric acid secretion by parietal cells
Carboprost	Abortion in second trimester; Postpartum hemorrhage	*Dystonia, pulmonary edema*; Gastrointestinal disturbance with prevalent diarrhea, headache, paresthesia, fever, breast tenderness	Acute pelvic inflammatory disease; Cardiac, pulmonary, renal, or hepatic disease	$PGF2\alpha$ analogue that stimulates uterine contraction for abortifacient activity; luteolytic activity controls fertility
Latanoprost Bimatoprost Travoprost	Ocular hypertension; Open-angle glaucoma	*Macular retinal edema*; Blurred vision, hyperpigmentation of eyelid, iris pigmentation	Hypersensitivity to latanoprost, bimatoprost, or travoprost	$PGF2\alpha$ analogues with vasodilator properties; ocular hypotensive agents
Epoprostenol	Pulmonary hypertension	*Supraventricular tachycardia, hemorrhage, thrombocytopenia*; Hypotension, rash, gastrointestinal disturbance, musculoskeletal pain, paresthesia, anxiety, influenza-like illness	Heart failure with severe left ventricular dysfunction; Chronic use in patients developing pulmonary edema	Prostacyclin analogue that stimulates vasodilation of pulmonary and systemic arterial vasculature; also inhibits platelet aggregation

THROMBOXANE ANTAGONISTS
Mechanism—Inhibit thromboxane synthase or antagonize thromboxane receptor; investigational agents

Drug	Clinical Applications	Adverse Effects	Contraindications	Therapeutic Considerations
Dazoxiben Pirmagrel Ridogrel				Dazoxiben and pirmagrel inhibit thromboxane synthase, whereas ridogrel is a thromboxane A2 receptor antagonist; Advantages of these agents over aspirin are unproven; Little effect on platelet aggregation

LIPOXYGENASE INHIBITOR
Mechanism—Inhibits 5-lipoxygenase, which catalyzes the formation of leukotrienes from arachidonic acid

Drug	Clinical Applications	Adverse Effects	Contraindications	Therapeutic Considerations
Zileuton	Asthma	*Increased liver function tests*; Urticaria, abdominal discomfort, dizziness, insomnia	Active liver disease; Elevated liver enzymes	

LEUKOTRIENE RECEPTOR ANTAGONISTS
Mechanism—Selective antagonists of the cysteinyl leukotriene (CysLT) type-I receptor

Drug	Clinical Applications	Adverse Effects	Contraindications	Therapeutic Considerations
Montelukast Zafirlukast	Chronic asthma; Perennial allergic rhinitis (montelukast); Seasonal allergic rhinitis (montelukast)	*Allergic granulomatosis angiitis, hepatitis*; Gastrointestinal distress, hallucinations, agitation	Hypersensitivity to montelukast or zafirlukast	Montelukast and zafirlukast are not indicated for acute asthma attacks and are generally not appropriate as monotherapy for asthma; Both drugs are excreted in breast milk

42

Histamine Pharmacology

April W. Armstrong and Joseph C. Kvedar

INTRODUCTION

Histamine is a biogenic amine found in many tissues. It is an autacoid—that is, a molecule secreted locally to increase or decrease the activity of nearby cells. *Histamine is a major mediator of inflammatory processes: it also has significant roles in regulating gastric acid secretion and in neurotransmission.* Knowledge of the diverse actions of histamine has led to the development of several important pharmacologic agents that regulate the effects of histamine in pathologic states. This chapter focuses on the pharmacologic actions of H1-antihistamines; H2-antihistamines are discussed in Chapter 45, Integrative Inflammation Pharmacology: Peptic Ulcer Disease.

■ Case

Ellen, a 16-year-old high school student, suffers from allergic rhinitis. Every spring, she develops a runny nose, itchy eyes, and sneezing. To relieve her symptoms, she takes an over-the-counter antihistamine, diphenhydramine. She is annoyed by the unpleasant effects that accompany her allergy medication. Every time she takes her antihistamine, Ellen feels drowsy and her mouth feels dry. She makes an appointment with her doctor who, after allergy testing, advises her to take loratadine. Upon taking her new allergy medication, Ellen's symptoms are relieved and she experiences no drowsiness or other adverse effects.

QUESTIONS

■ **1.** Why does Ellen develop seasonal rhinitis?
■ **2.** Why does diphenhydramine relieve Ellen's symptoms?
■ **3.** Why does diphenhydramine cause drowsiness?
■ **4.** Why doesn't loratadine cause drowsiness?

PHYSIOLOGY OF HISTAMINE

HISTAMINE SYNTHESIS, STORAGE, AND RELEASE

Histamine is synthesized from the amino acid L-histidine. The enzyme **histidine decarboxylase** catalyzes the decarboxylation of histidine to 2-(4-imidazolyl)ethylamine, commonly known as **histamine** (Fig. 42-1). The synthesis of

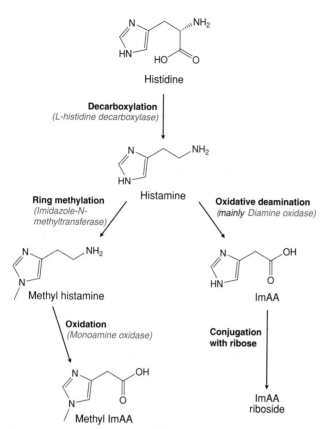

Figure 42-1. Histamine synthesis and degradation. Histamine is synthesized from histidine in a decarboxylation reaction catalyzed by L-histidine decarboxylase. The liver metabolizes histamine into inert byproducts. Histamine can be methylated on the imidazole ring or oxidatively deaminated. These degradation products can then undergo further oxidation or conjugation with ribose. Diamine oxidase is also known as histaminase. ImAA, imidazole acetic acid.

histamine occurs in mast cells and basophils of the immune system, enterochromaffin-like (ECL) cells in the gastric mucosa, and certain neurons in the central nervous system (CNS) that use histamine as a neurotransmitter. Oxidative pathways in the liver rapidly degrade circulating histamine to inert metabolites. One major metabolite of histamine, im-

idazole acetic acid, can be measured in the urine, and the level of this metabolite is used to determine the amount of histamine that has been released systemically.

Histamine synthesis and storage can be divided into two "pools": a slowly turning over pool and a rapidly turning over pool. The **slowly turning over pool** is located in mast cells and basophils. Histamine is stored in large granules in these inflammatory cells, and the release of histamine involves complete degranulation of the cells. This process is termed the *slowly turning over pool* because several weeks are required to replenish the stores of histamine after degranulation has occurred. The **rapidly turning over pool** is located in gastric ECL cells and in histaminergic CNS neurons. These cells synthesize and release histamine as required for gastric acid secretion and neurotransmission, respectively. Unlike mast cells and basophils, ECL cells and histaminergic neurons do not store histamine. Instead, the production and release of histamine in these cells depend on physiologic stimuli. In the gut, for example, histidine decarboxylase is activated after the ingestion of food.

ACTIONS OF HISTAMINE

Histamine has a wide spectrum of actions involving many organs and organ systems. To understand the roles of histamine, it is useful to consider the physiologic effects of histamine in each tissue (Table 42-1). These effects include actions on smooth muscle, vascular endothelium, afferent nerve terminals, heart, gastrointestinal tract, and CNS.

The cellular actions of histamine on smooth muscle cause some muscle fibers to contract and others to relax. Histamine causes contraction of **bronchial smooth muscle** in humans (although the effect varies in other species). The sensitivity of bronchial smooth muscle to histamine also varies among individuals; those with asthma may be up to 1,000 times more sensitive to histamine-mediated bronchoconstriction than nonasthmatic individuals. Additional actions of histamine on smooth muscle involve dilation or constriction of certain blood vessels. Histamine dilates all terminal arterioles and postcapillary venules. Veins, however, constrict on exposure to histamine. The dilatory effect on the postcapillary venule bed is the most prominent effect of his-

TABLE 42-1	Major Physiologic Actions of Histamine		
TISSUE	**EFFECT OF HISTAMINE**	**CLINICAL MANIFESTATIONS**	**RECEPTOR SUBTYPE**
Lungs	Bronchoconstriction	Asthma-like symptoms	H1
Vascular smooth muscle	Postcapillary venule dilation	Erythema	H1
	Terminal arteriole dilation		
	Venoconstriction		
Vascular endothelium	Contraction and separation of endothelial cells	Edema, wheal response	H1
Peripheral nerves	Sensitization of afferent nerve terminals	Itchiness, pain	H1
Heart	Minor increase in heart rate and contractility	Minor	H2
Stomach	Increased gastric acid secretion	Peptic ulcer disease, heartburn	H2
CNS	Neurotransmitter	Circadian rhythms, wakefulness	H3

CNS, central nervous system.

tamine on the vasculature. During infection or injury, hista-mine-induced venule dilation engorges the local microvascu-lature with blood, enhancing the access of immune cells that initiate repair processes in the damaged area. This engorge-ment explains the redness observed in inflamed tissues. Al-though other smooth muscles—such as those in the bowel, bladder, iris, and uterus—contract on exposure to histamine, these effects are not thought to play a large role physiologi-cally or clinically.

Histamine also causes contraction of vascular endothelial cells. *Histamine-induced contraction of vascular endothelial cells causes these cells to separate from one another, allow-ing the escape of plasma proteins and fluid from postcapil-lary venules and thereby causing edema.* Thus, histamine is a key mediator of local responses at sites of injury.

Peripheral sensory nerve terminals also respond to hista-mine. The sensations of itch and pain result from a direct depolarizing action of histamine on afferent nerve terminals. This effect is responsible for the pain and itch experienced after an insect bite, for example.

The combined actions of histamine on vascular smooth muscle, vascular endothelial cells, and nerve terminals are responsible for the **wheal and flare** response noted follow-ing histamine release in the skin. Endothelial cell contraction causes the edematous wheal response, while the red, painful flare results from vasodilatation and sensory nerve stimula-tion.

The cardiac effects of histamine consist of minor in-creases in the force and rate of cardiac contraction. Hista-mine enhances Ca^{2+} influx into cardiac myocytes, leading to increased inotropy. The increase in heart rate is caused by an increase in the rate of phase 4 depolarization in sino-atrial nodal cells.

The primary role of histamine in the gastric mucosa is to potentiate gastrin-induced acid secretion. *Histamine is one of three molecules that regulate acid secretion in the stom-ach, the others being gastrin and acetylcholine.* Activation of histamine receptors in the stomach leads to an increase in intracellular Ca^{2+} in parietal cells and results in increased secretion of hydrochloric acid by the gastric mucosa.

Histamine also functions as a neurotransmitter in the CNS. Both histidine decarboxylase and histamine receptors are expressed in the hypothalamus, and histaminergic CNS neurons have numerous diffuse projections throughout the brain and spinal cord. Although the functions of histamine in the CNS are not well understood, histamine is believed to be important in the maintenance of wakefulness and to act as an appetite suppressant.

HISTAMINE RECEPTORS

Histamine actions are mediated by the binding of histamine to one of four receptor subtypes: H1, H2, H3, and H4. All four subtypes are seven-transmembrane, G protein–coupled receptors. The receptor isoforms differ in their second mes-senger pathways and tissue distributions (Table 42-2).

The **H1 receptor** activates G protein–mediated hydroly-sis of phosphatidylinositol, leading to increased inositol tris-phosphate (IP_3) and diacylglycerol (DAG). IP_3 triggers the release of Ca^{2+} from intracellular stores, increasing cyto-solic Ca^{2+} concentration and activating downstream path-ways. DAG activates protein kinase C, leading to phosphory-lation of numerous cytosolic target proteins. In some tissues, such as bronchial smooth muscle, the increase in cytosolic Ca^{2+} causes smooth muscle contraction by Ca^{2+}/calmodu-lin-mediated phosphorylation of the myosin light chain. In other tissues, especially precapillary arteriolar sphincters and postcapillary venules, the increase in cytosolic Ca^{2+} causes smooth muscle relaxation by inducing the synthesis of nitric oxide (see Chapter 21, Pharmacology of Vascular Tone). H1 receptor stimulation also leads to the activation of NF-κB, an important and ubiquitous transcription factor that pro-motes the expression of adhesion molecules and proinflam-matory cytokines.

H1 receptors are expressed primarily on vascular endo-thelial cells and smooth muscle cells. These receptors me-diate inflammatory and allergic reactions. Tissue-specific re-sponses to H1 receptor stimulation include (1) edema, (2) bronchoconstriction, and (3) sensitization of primary affer-ent nerve terminals. H1 receptors are also expressed on pre-synaptic histaminergic neurons in the tuberomammillary nucleus of the hypothalamus, where they function as autore-ceptors to inhibit further release of histamine. These neurons may be involved in the control of circadian rhythms and wakefulness.

TABLE 42-2	Histamine Receptor Subtypes	
RECEPTOR SUBTYPE	**POSTRECEPTOR SIGNALING MECHANISM**	**TISSUE DISTRIBUTION**
H1	$G_{q/11}$→Increased IP_3, DAG, and intracellular Ca^{2+}, activated NF-κB	Smooth muscle, vascular endothelium, brain (autoreceptor)
H2	G_s→Increased cAMP	Gastric parietal cells, cardiac muscle, mast cells, brain
H3	$G_{i/o}$→Decreased cAMP	CNS and some peripheral nerves
H4	$G_{i/o}$→Decreased cAMP, increased intracellular Ca^{2+}	Hematopoietic cells, gastric mucosa

G, G protein; cAMP, cyclic adenosine monophosphate; IP_3, inositol trisphosphate; DAG, diacylglycerol; NF-κB, nuclear factor kappa B; CNS, central nervous system.

*The major function of the **H2 receptor** is to mediate gastric acid secretion in the stomach.* This receptor subtype is expressed on parietal cells in the gastric mucosa, where histamine acts synergistically with gastrin and acetylcholine to regulate acid secretion (see Chapter 45). H2 receptors are also expressed on cardiac muscle cells, on some immune cells, and on certain presynaptic neurons. H2 receptors on parietal cells activate a G protein–dependent cyclic AMP cascade, leading to enhanced proton pump-mediated delivery of protons into the gastric fluid.

Whereas H1 and H2 receptor subtypes have been well characterized, H3 and H4 receptor subtypes and their downstream actions are areas of active investigation. **H3 receptors** appear to provide *feedback inhibition* of certain effects of histamine. H3 receptors have been localized to several cell types, including presynaptic histaminergic neurons in the CNS and ECL cells in the stomach. On presynaptic nerve terminals, activated H3 receptors suppress neuronal firing and histamine release. H3 receptors also appear to limit histaminergic actions in gastric mucosa and bronchial smooth muscle. The downstream effects of H3 receptor activation are mediated via a decrease in Ca^{2+} influx.

H4 receptors are localized to cells of hematopoietic origin, primarily mast cells, eosinophils, and basophils. H4 receptors share 40% homology with H3 receptors and bind many H3 receptor agonists, although with lower affinity. Coupling of the H4 receptor to $G_{i/o}$ leads to decreased cAMP and activation of phospholipase Cβ, and downstream events result in increased intracellular Ca^{2+}. H4 receptors are of particular interest because they are thought to play an important role in inflammation; activation of H4 receptors has been shown to mediate histamine-induced mast cell chemotaxis as well as leukotriene B_4 production. H4 receptor antagonists are under development for the treatment of inflammatory diseases involving mast cells and eosinophils.

PATHOPHYSIOLOGY

Histamine is an essential mediator of immune and inflammatory responses. Histamine plays a prominent role in the **IgE-mediated hypersensitivity reaction,** also known as the **allergic reaction.** In a localized allergic reaction, an allergen (antigen) first penetrates an epithelial surface (e.g., skin, nasal mucosa). The allergen can also be delivered systemically, as in the case of an allergic response to penicillin. With the aid of T-helper (T_H) cells, the allergen stimulates B lymphocytes to produce IgE antibodies that are specific for that allergen. The IgE then binds to Fc receptors on mast cells and basophils, in a process known as *sensitization*. Once these immune cells are "sensitized" with IgE antibodies, they are able to detect and respond rapidly to a subsequent exposure to the allergen. Upon such an exposure, the allergen binds to and crosslinks the IgE/Fc receptor complexes, triggering cell degranulation (Fig. 42-2).

Histamine released by mast cells and basophils binds to H1 receptors on vascular smooth muscle cells and vascular endothelial cells. Activation of these receptors increases local blood flow and vascular permeability. This completes the initial stage of the inflammatory response. Prolonged inflammation requires the activity of other immune cells. The histamine-induced local vasodilatation allows such immune cells greater access to the injured area, while the increased vascular permeability facilitates movement of the immune cells into the tissue.

Mast cell degranulation can also occur as a response to local tissue damage, in the absence of a humoral immune response. For example, trauma or chemical damage can physically disrupt the mast cell membrane and thereby initiate the degranulation process. Histamine release allows for enhanced access of macrophages and other immune cells, which can begin to repair the damaged area.

CLINICAL MANIFESTATIONS OF HISTAMINE PATHOPHYSIOLOGY

The IgE-mediated hypersensitivity reaction is responsible for initiation of certain inflammatory disorders, including **allergic rhinitis** and **acute urticaria** (hives). In the introductory case, Ellen suffered from allergic rhinitis, with a runny nose, itchy eyes, and sneezing. In allergic rhinitis, an environmental allergen, such as pollen, crosses the nasal epithelium and enters the underlying tissue. There, the allergen encounters previously sensitized mast cells and crosslinks IgE/Fc receptor complexes on the mast cell surface. Consequently, the mast cell degranulates and releases histamine, which binds to H1 receptors in the nasal mucosa and local tissues. Stimulation of the H1 receptors causes blood vessel dilation and increases vascular permeability, leading to edema. This swelling in the nasal mucosa is responsible for the nasal congestion that is experienced in allergic rhinitis. The accompanying itching, sneezing, runny nose, and tearing result from the combined action of histamine and other inflammatory mediators, including kinins, prostaglandins, and leukotrienes. These molecules initiate the hypersecretion and irritation characteristic of allergic rhinitis.

Mast cell activation also occurs in acute urticaria. Here, an allergen, such as penicillin, enters the body, either through ingestion or parenterally, and reaches the skin through the circulation. Histamine release results in a disseminated wheal-and-flare response, creating pruritic, erythematous, and edematous plaques on the skin.

HISTAMINE AND ANAPHYLAXIS

Systemic mast cell degranulation can cause the life-threatening condition known as **anaphylaxis.** Typically, anaphylactic shock is initiated in a previously sensitized individual by a hypersensitivity reaction to an insect bite, an antibiotic such as penicillin, or ingestion of certain highly allergenic foods (e.g., nuts). An allergen that is distributed systemically, either by intravenous injection or by absorption into the circulation, can stimulate mast cells and basophils to release histamine throughout the body. The resulting sys-

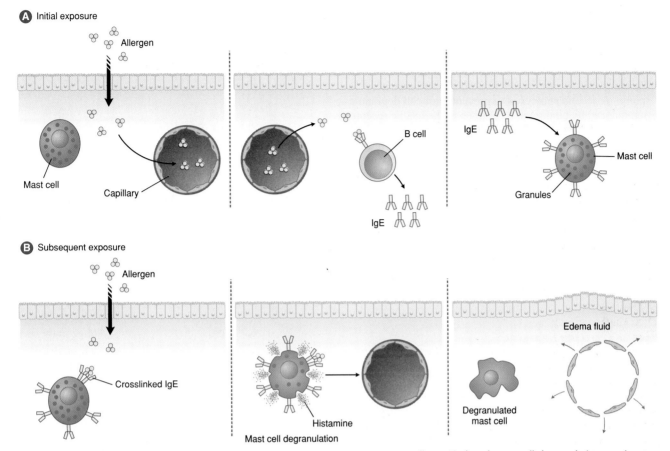

Figure 42-2. Pathophysiology of the IgE-mediated hypersensitivity reaction. Allergen-induced mast cell degranulation requires two separate exposures to the allergen. **A.** On initial exposure, the allergen must penetrate mucosal surfaces so that it can encounter cells of the immune system. Activation of the immune response causes B lymphocytes to secrete allergen-specific IgE antibodies. These IgE molecules bind to Fc receptors on mast cells, leading to sensitization of the mast cells. **B.** On subsequent exposure, the multivalent allergen crosslinks two IgE/Fc receptor complexes on the mast cell surface. Receptor crosslinking causes the mast cell to degranulate. Local histamine release results in an inflammatory response, shown here as edema.

temic vasodilatation causes a massive decrease in blood pressure; hypotension also results from the systemic pooling of fluid because of the extravasation of plasma into the interstitium. Severe bronchoconstriction and epiglottal swelling are also induced by massive histamine release. This state of anaphylactic shock can be lethal within minutes if not treated rapidly by the administration of epinephrine, as described below.

PHARMACOLOGIC CLASSES AND AGENTS

Histamine pharmacology employs three approaches, each of which leads to inhibition of histamine action (Table 42-3). The first, and the most frequently used, approach is to

TABLE 42-3	Strategies of Histamine Pharmacology	
STRATEGY	**EXAMPLE OF PHARMACOLOGIC AGENT**	**EXAMPLE OF DISEASE TREATED**
Administer inverse agonists of histamine receptor	Diphenhydramine	Allergies
Prevent mast cell degranulation	Cromolyn, nedocromil	Asthma
Administer physiologic antagonists to counter the pathologic effects of histamine	Epinephrine	Anaphylaxis

administer **antihistamines,** which typically are inverse agonists or competitive antagonists selective for the H1, H2, H3, or H4 receptor. H1-antihistamines are discussed below in detail: their mechanism of action involves stabilization of the inactive conformation of the H1 receptor to decrease signaling events that would lead to the inflammatory response. A second strategy is to prevent mast cell degranulation induced by binding of an antigen to the IgE/Fc receptor complex on mast cells. **Cromolyn** and **nedocromil** use this strategy to prevent asthma attacks (see Chapter 46, Integrative Inflammation Pharmacology: Asthma); these compounds disrupt the chloride current across mast cell membranes, which is a key step in the degranulation process. The third strategy is to administer a drug that functionally counteracts the effects of histamine. An example of this approach is the use of **epinephrine** to treat anaphylaxis. Epinephrine, an adrenergic agonist, induces bronchodilation and vasoconstriction (see Chapter 9, Adrenergic Pharmacology); these actions counter the bronchoconstriction, vasodilatation, and hypotension caused by histamine in anaphylactic shock.

H1-ANTIHISTAMINES

Mechanism of Action

Historically, H1-antihistamines were referred to as H1 receptor antagonists, based on experiments in tracheal smooth muscle that showed a parallel shift in the histamine concentration-response relationship. Recently, however, advances in histamine pharmacology have shown that *H1-antihistamines are inverse agonists rather than receptor antagonists.*

H1 receptors appear to coexist in two conformational states—the inactive and active conformations—which are in equilibrium with one another in the absence of histamine or antihistamine (Fig. 42-3). In the basal state, the receptor tends toward constitutive activation. Histamine acts as an agonist for the active conformation of the H1 receptor and shifts the equilibrium toward the active receptor state. In comparison, antihistamines are **inverse agonists**. Inverse agonists bind preferentially to the inactive conformation of the H1 receptor and shift the equilibrium toward the inactive state. Thus, even in the absence of endogenous histamine, inverse agonists reduce constitutive receptor activity.

Classification of First- and Second-Generation H1-Antihistamines

The finding that histamine is a major mediator of the allergic hypersensitivity reaction led to the discovery of the first **H1-antihistamines** by Bovet and Staub in 1937. Clinically useful drugs that inhibit the actions of histamine began to appear in the 1940s. *Currently, H1-antihistamines parse into two categories: first-generation and second-generation H1-antihistamines* (see the Drug Summary Table for details of H1-antihistamine classification).

The basic structure of the **first-generation H1-antihistamines** consists of two aromatic rings linked to a substituted ethylamine backbone. These drugs are divided into six main subgroups based on their substituted side chains—ethanolamines, ethylenediamines, alkylamines, piperazines, phenothiazines, and piperidines (Fig. 42-4). **Diphenhydramine,**

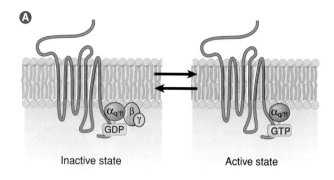

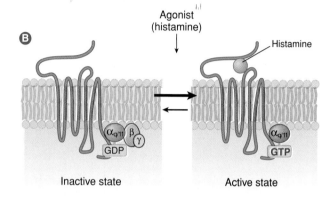

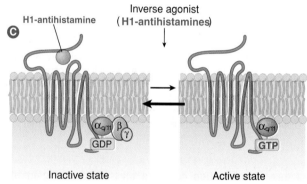

Figure 42-3. Simplified two-state model of H1 receptor. A. H1 receptors coexist in two conformational states—the inactive and active states—which are in conformational equilibrium with one another. **B.** Histamine acts as an agonist for the active conformation of the H1 receptor and shifts the equilibrium toward the active conformation. **C.** Antihistamines act as inverse agonists that bind and stabilize the inactive conformation of the H1 receptor, thereby shifting the equilibrium toward the inactive receptor state.

hydroxyzine, chlorpheniramine, and promethazine are among the most frequently used first-generation H1-antihistamines. First-generation H1-antihistamines are neutral compounds at physiologic pH and readily cross the blood-brain barrier.

The **second-generation H1-antihistamines** can be structurally categorized into four subclasses—alkylamines, piperazines, phthalazinones, and piperidines. Widely used second-generation H1-antihistamines include **loratadine, cetirizine,** and **fexofenadine**. Second-generation H1-antihistamines are ionized at physiologic pH and do not appreciably cross the blood-brain barrier. The differences in lipophilicity between the first- and second-generation H1-

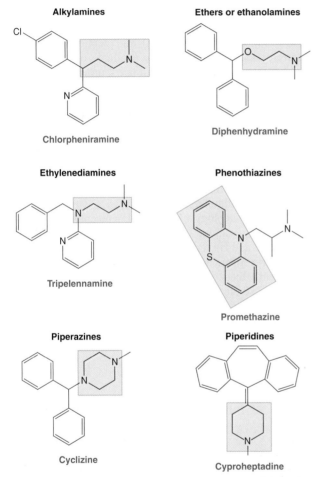

General structure
(X = C, O, or omitted)

Alkylamines

Chlorpheniramine

Ethers or ethanolamines

Diphenhydramine

Ethylenediamines

Tripelennamine

Phenothiazines

Promethazine

Piperazines

Cyclizine

Piperidines

Cyproheptadine

Figure 42-4. Structure of first-generation H1-antihistamines. The general structure of the first-generation H1-antihistamines consists of a substituted ethylamine backbone with two terminal aromatic rings. (Note the similarity between the ethylamine moiety in these drugs and the ethylamine side chain of histamine shown in Fig. 42-1.) Each of the six subclasses is a variation on this general structure. First-generation H1-antihistamines are neutral compounds at physiologic pH and readily cross the blood-brain barrier. In contrast, second-generation H1-antihistamines (e.g., loratadine, cetirizine, fexofenadine) are ionized at physiologic pH and do not appreciably cross the blood-brain barrier *(not shown)*. This difference in blood-brain barrier penetration underlies the differential extent of sedation associated with use of the first- and second-generation H1-antihistamines.

antihistamines account for their differential adverse-effect profiles, notably, the tendency to cause CNS depression (drowsiness).

Pharmacologic Effects and Clinical Uses

H1-antihistamines are most useful in the treatment of allergic disorders to relieve symptoms of rhinitis, conjunctivitis, urticaria, and pruritus. H1-antihistamines strongly block the increased capillary permeability necessary for the formation of edema and wheals. The anti-inflammatory properties of H1-antihistamines are attributable to suppression of the NF-κB pathway. The first- and second-generation H1-antihistamines are equally efficacious in the treatment of chronic urticaria; however, they are not effective against urticarial vasculitis or hereditary angioedema (C1 inhibitor deficiency).

Hydroxyzine and **doxepin** are potent antipruritic agents, and their clinical effectiveness is likely related to their pronounced CNS effects. Doxepin, a tricyclic antidepressant, is best used in patients with depression, since even small doses can cause confusion and disorientation in nondepressed patients. Compared to oral H1-antihistamines, topical H1-antihistamines (including nasal and ophthalmic preparations) have a more rapid onset of action, but they require multiple administrations each day. Cutaneous preparations of antihistamines, administered for pruritic dermatoses, may paradoxically cause allergic dermatitis. H1-antihistamines alone are frequently ineffective for systemic anaphylaxis or severe angioedema with laryngeal swelling. In these conditions, contributions from other local mediators are unaffected by H1-antihistamine treatment, and epinephrine remains the treatment of choice.

H1-antihistamines have limited efficacy in bronchial asthma and should not be used as the sole therapy for asthma. While H1-antihistamines appear to inhibit constriction of bronchial smooth muscles in guinea pigs, this therapeutic effect is much less pronounced in humans because of contributions from other mediators such as leukotrienes and serotonin.

H1-antihistamines can also be used to counter motion sickness, chemotherapy-related nausea and vomiting, and insomnia. By inhibiting histaminergic signals from the vestibular nucleus to the vomiting center in the medulla, H1-antihistamines such as **dimenhydrinate**, **diphenhydramine**, **meclizine**, and **promethazine** are useful as antiemetic agents. Due to their prominent CNS depressive effects, the first-generation H1-antihistamines such as **diphenhydramine**, **doxylamine**, and **pyrilamine** are also used to treat insomnia.

Pharmacokinetics

Oral H1-antihistamines are well absorbed from the gastrointestinal (GI) tract, and they reach peak plasma concentrations in 2 to 3 hours. The duration of effect varies depending on the particular H1-antihistamine agent. Whereas first-generation H1-antihistamines are distributed widely throughout the peripheral tissues as well as the CNS, second-generation H1-antihistamines have less penetration into the CNS. Most H1-antihistamines are metabolized by the liver, and dose adjustments should be considered in patients with severe liver disease. As inducers of hepatic cytochrome P450 enzymes, H1-antihistamines can facilitate their own metabolism. Loratadine, a second-generation H1-antihistamine, is metabolized by P450 enzymes into an active metabolite. Drugs that are substrates or inhibitors of P450 enzymes can affect the metabolism of loratadine, and antihistamines may affect the metabolism of other drugs that are substrates of the same P450s.

Adverse Effects

The major adverse effects of H1-antihistamines are CNS toxicity, cardiac toxicity, and anticholinergic effects. Whereas adverse-effect profiles of second-generation H1-antihistamines have been thoroughly investigated, long-term safety studies of first-generation H1-antihistamines are lacking despite their use for over 6 decades.

Because of their high lipophilicity, first-generation H1-antihistamines readily penetrate the blood-brain barrier. These drugs antagonize the neurotransmitter effects of histamine on H1 receptors in the CNS (especially the hypothalamus) and the periphery. As noted above, the high CNS penetration accounts for the sedating action of these drugs. In the introductory case, Ellen experienced sedation when she took diphenhydramine for her allergic rhinitis. Factors that increase the risk of developing CNS toxicity include low body mass, severe hepatic or renal dysfunction, and concomitant use of drugs such as alcohol that impair CNS function.

The low CNS penetration of second-generation H1-antihistamines is attributable to two features of the molecules. First, as noted above, these compounds are ionized at physiologic pH, and so do not diffuse readily across membranes. Second, they exhibit high binding to albumin, and thus are less free to diffuse into the CNS. Second-generation H1-antihistamines are often preferred for extended use because of their limited sedative effects. For example, the second-generation H1-antihistamines loratadine, desloratadine, and fexofenadine are the only oral H1-antihistamines permitted for use by airline pilots.

H1-antihistamines that prolong the QT interval can cause cardiac toxicity, especially in patients with pre-existing cardiac dysfunction. Some earlier second-generation H1-antihistamines had serious cardiotoxic effects at high plasma concentrations. Two of these drugs, terfenadine and astemizole, were withdrawn by the U. S. Food and Drug Administration (FDA) because they caused prolonged QT intervals that sometimes led to ventricular arrhythmias. The mechanism by which H1-antihistamines prolong the QT interval is thought to involve inhibition of the I_{Kr} current. The human ether-a-go-go-related gene (*HERG*) encodes the α subunit of the potassium channel mediating the I_{Kr} current, and in vitro testing using variants of HERG is now available for assessing whether a medication has the potential to inhibit the I_{Kr} current.

Anticholinergic adverse effects, which are more prominent with first-generation than with second-generation H1-antihistamines, include pupillary dilatation, dry eyes, dry mouth, and urinary retention and hesitancy. Fatal overdose of first-generation H1-antihistamines is more likely due to profound adverse CNS effects than to adverse cardiac effects.

OTHER ANTIHISTAMINES

Competitive antagonists and inverse agonists have also been developed against the H2, H3, and H4 receptors. Considerable interest was generated by the development of selective **H2 receptor antagonists** that inhibit histamine-induced gastric acid secretion. H2 receptor antagonists, which are discussed in detail in Chapter 45, differ in structure from the H1-antihistamines in that they contain an intact imidazole ring and an uncharged side chain (Fig. 42-5). These agents act as reversible, competitive antagonists of histamine binding to H2 receptors on gastric parietal cells, and thereby reduce gastric acid secretion. Clinical indications include acid-reflux disease (heartburn) and peptic ulcer disease. Many of these agents are also available over the counter for the symptomatic treatment of heartburn. **Cimetidine** and **ranitidine** are two of the most commonly used H2 receptor antagonists. A significant adverse effect of cimetidine involves inhibition of cytochrome P450-mediated drug metabolism, which can result in undesirable elevations in the plasma levels of certain concomitantly administered drugs. H2 receptors are also expressed in the CNS and in cardiac muscle, but the therapeutic doses of H2 receptor antagonists are sufficiently low that cardiovascular and CNS adverse effects are negligible.

The pharmacology of H3 and H4 receptors is an active area of investigation. To date, no drugs selectively directed against H3 and H4 receptors have been approved for clinical use. **H3 receptors** are thought to provide *feedback inhibition* of certain effects of histamine in the CNS and in ECL cells. In animal studies, H3 receptor antagonists induce wakefulness and improve attention, effects that are thought to be mediated by overstimulation of cortical H1 receptors. H3

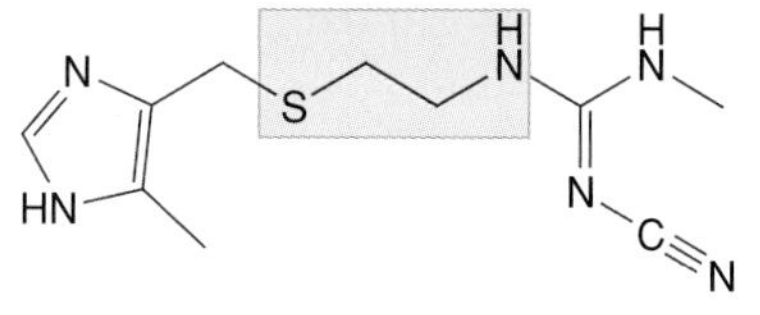

Cimetidine

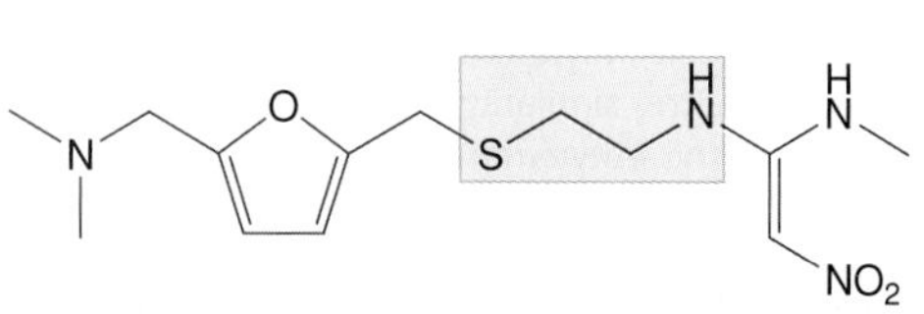

Ranitidine

Figure 42-5. Structure of H2 receptor antagonists. H2 receptor antagonists have a thioethanolamine backbone *(highlighted in blue box)* that is N-substituted with a bulky side chain and that terminates in a single five-membered ring. (Compare the bulky N-substituted side chain of the H2 antagonists with the simple tertiary amine of the H1-antihistamines in Fig. 42-4, and compare the small five-membered imidazole or furan ring of the H2 antagonists with the pair of bulky aromatic rings of the H1-antihistamines.) These structural differences enable cimetidine, ranitidine, and other H2 antagonists to bind selectively to H2 receptors in the gastric mucosa, thereby decreasing the production of gastric acid.

receptor antagonists that have been developed for experimental use include **thioperamide, clobenpropit, ciproxifan**, and **proxyfan**.

Similar to H3 receptors, **H4 receptors** couple with $G_{i/o}$ to decrease intracellular cAMP concentrations. Because H4 receptors are selectively expressed on cells of hematopoietic origin, especially mast cells, basophils, and eosinophils, there is considerable interest in elucidating the role of the H4 receptor in the inflammatory process. H4 receptor antagonists represent a promising area of drug development to treat inflammatory conditions that involve mast cells and eosinophils.

Conclusion and Future Directions

The discovery of histamine and its receptors has significantly increased the pharmacologic options for treatment of allergy and peptic ulcer disease. Selective receptor targeting allows specific treatment of each of these disease processes without affecting the other physiologic actions of histamine. Drug selectivity is achieved by the existence and targeting of histamine receptor subtypes (H1, H2, H3, and H4).

The identification and elucidation of H3 and H4 receptors will allow for the development of new antihistamines directed against these receptor subtypes. H3 antagonists have the potential to increase arousal as well as improve attention and learning. The H4 receptor is an especially exciting molecular target for drug development, as it is thought to play an important role in inflammatory conditions involving mast cells and eosinophils. Agents directed against H4 receptors might one day be employed to treat a wide variety of inflammatory conditions, such as asthma, allergic rhinitis, and rheumatoid arthritis.

Suggested Reading

Leurs R, Church MK, Taglialatea M. H1-antihistamines: inverse agonism, anti-inflammatory actions and cardiac effects. *Clin Exp Allergy* 2002;32:489–498. *(Mechanism-based discussion of H1-antihistamines as inverse agonists.)*

Nicolas JM. The metabolic profile of second-generation antihistamine. *Allergy* 2000;55:46–52. *(Discussion of differences among second-generation drugs.)*

Simons FE. Advances in H1-antihistamines. *N Engl J Med* 2004; 351:2203–2217. *(Comprehensively summarizes the mechanism of action and clinical uses of H1-antihistamines.)*

Simons FE. H1-antihistamines: more relevant than ever in the treatment of allergic disorders. *J Allergy Clin Immunol* 2003;112(4 Suppl):S42–S52. *(Evidence-based review of the use of H1-antihistamines in allergic disorders.)*

Timmerman H. Factors involved in the absence of sedative effects by the second generation antihistamines. *Allergy* 2000;55:5–10. *(Discussion of second-generation antihistamines.)*

Drug Summary Table　Chapter 42 Histamine Pharmacology

FIRST-GENERATION H1-ANTIHISTAMINES

Mechanism—*Inverse agonists that bind preferentially to the inactive conformation of the H1 receptor and shift the equilibrium toward the inactive receptor state*

Drug	Clinical Applications	*Serious* and Common Adverse Effects	Contraindications	Therapeutic Considerations
Ethanolamines: Diphenhydramine Carbinoxamine Clemastine Dimenhydrinate	Allergic rhinitis Anaphylaxis Insomnia Motion sickness Parkinsonism Urticaria	Sedation, dizziness, pupillary dilatation, dry eyes, dry mouth, urinary retention and hesitancy	Diphenhydramine: newborns or premature infants, nursing mothers Carbinoxamine: acute asthma attack, MAOI therapy, narrow-angle glaucoma, peptic ulcer, severe coronary artery disease, severe hypertension, urinary retention Clemastine: lactation, lower respiratory tract symptoms, MAOI therapy, newborn or premature infants Dimenhydrinate: hypersensitivity to dimenhydrinate	In general, first-generation H1-antihistamines have greater CNS and anticholinergic adverse effects than second-generation H1-antihistamines Diphenhydramine (trade name, Benadryl®) is available in oral solid, oral liquid, intramuscular, intravenous, and topical preparations Diphenhydramine may raise thioridazine plasma levels, thereby increasing the risk of arrhythmia
Ethylenediamines: Pyrilamine Tripelennamine	Same as diphenhydramine	Same as diphenhydramine	Pyrilamine: hypersensitivity to pyrilamine maleate Tripelennamine: narrow-angle glaucoma, stenosing peptic ulcer, symptomatic prostatic hypertrophy, bladder neck obstruction, pyloroduodenal obstruction, lower respiratory tract symptoms, premature infants, neonates, nursing mothers, concomitant therapy with MAO inhibitors	
Alkylamines: Chlorpheniramine Brompheniramine	Same as diphenhydramine	Same as diphenhydramine	Chlorpheniramine: hypersensitivity to chlorpheniramine Brompheniramine: concurrent MAOI therapy, focal CNS lesions, hypersensitivity to brompheniramine or related drugs	
Piperidines: Cyproheptadine Phenindamine	Same as diphenhydramine	Same as diphenhydramine	Cyproheptadine: angle-closure glaucoma, concurrent MAOI therapy, newborn or premature infants, nursing mothers, stenosing peptic ulcer, pyloroduodenal obstruction, symptomatic prostatic hypertrophy, bladder neck obstruction Phenindamine: children under 12	
Phenothiazines: Promethazine	Same as diphenhydramine	Same as diphenhydramine; in addition, photosensitivity and jaundice have been reported	Comatose states Lower respiratory tract symptoms, including asthma Pediatric patients less than 2 years of age Subcutaneous or intra-arterial injection	Promethazine is used primarily to relieve preoperative anxiety and reduce postoperative nausea and vomiting

Drug	Clinical Applications	Adverse Effects	Contraindications	Therapeutic Considerations
Piperazines: Hydroxyzine Cyclizine Meclizine	Pruritus, alcohol withdrawal, anxiety, vomiting (hydroxyzine) Motion sickness, vertigo (cyclizine, meclizine)	Same as diphenhydramine	Hydroxyzine: early pregnancy Cyclizine: hypersensitivity to cyclizine Meclizine: hypersensitivity to meclizine	Hydroxyzine is a potent anti-pruritic agent
Tricyclic dibenzoxepins: Doxepin	Anxiety Depression Pruritus	*Hypertension, hypotension, agranulocytosis, thrombocytopenia, worsening of depression, suicidal thoughts* Weight gain, constipation, dry mouth, somnolence, blurred vision, urinary retention	Glaucoma Urinary retention	Doxepin is a tricyclic antidepressant; it is best used in patients with depression, as even small doses can cause confusion and disorientation in nondepressed patients

SECOND-GENERATION H1-ANTIHISTAMINES

Mechanism—Inverse agonists that bind preferentially to the inactive conformation of the H1 receptor and shift the equilibrium toward the inactive receptor state

Drug	Clinical Applications	Adverse Effects	Contraindications	Therapeutic Considerations
Piperazines: Cetirizine	Allergic rhinitis Urticaria	Somnolence, dry mouth, headache, fatigue (have less anticholinergic effects and are less sedating than first-generation H1-antihistamines)	Hypersensitivity to cetirizine or hydroxyzine	In general, second-generation H1-antihistamines have less anticholinergic effects and are less sedating than first-generation H1-antihistamines because of reduced entry into the CNS
Alkylamines: Acrivastine	Allergic rhinitis	Same as cetirizine	Concurrent MAOI therapy Severe coronary artery disease Severe hypertension	Same as cetirizine
Phthalazinones: Azelastine	Allergic conjunctivitis and rhinitis	Same as cetirizine	Concurrent use of alcohol or other CNS depressants	Same as cetirizine
Piperidines: Loratadine Desloratadine Levocabastine Ebastine Mizolastine Fexofenadine	Allergic rhinitis Urticaria	Same as cetirizine	Loratadine: hypersensitivity to loratadine Desloratadine: hypersensitivity to desloratadine Levocabastine: soft contact lens Ebastine: hypersensitivity to ebastine Mizolastine: hypersensitivity to mizolastine Fexofenadine: hypersensitivity to fexofenadine	Same as cetirizine

H2 RECEPTOR ANTAGONISTS

Drug				
Cimetidine Famotidine Nizatidine Ranitidine	See Drug Summary Table: Chapter 45 Integrative Inflammation Pharmacology: Peptic Ulcer Disease			

43

Pharmacology of Hematopoiesis and Immunomodulation

Andrew J. Wagner, Ramy A. Arnaout, and George D. Demetri

INTRODUCTION

A number of clinical situations are characterized by deficiencies of red blood cells, white blood cells, or platelets—cells of the hematopoietic system. This chapter describes the pharmacologic agents that can be used to stimulate production of hematopoietic cells. (Nonpharmacologic alternatives include transfusion and bone marrow transplantation.) Blood cell production is controlled physiologically by hematopoietic growth factors, a diverse but functionally overlapping group of glycoproteins produced by the body in response to certain signals. For example, hypoxia stimulates production of the growth factor erythropoietin, which in turn stimulates the production of erythrocytes in an attempt to relieve the hypoxia.

The main pharmacologic strategy used to stimulate the production of blood cells is to administer exogenous growth factors or synthetic growth factor analogues. This chapter provides an introduction to the cells of the hematopoietic system and the growth factors that stimulate their production, and discusses the pharmacologic agents used to increase blood cell production. An outline of the immunomodulatory agents used in cancer chemotherapy is also presented.

 Case

Fifty-two-year-old Mrs. M presents with a lump in her left breast. Subsequent mammogram, core biopsy, and lumpectomy lead to the diagnosis of infiltrating ductal carcinoma that is localized but lymph-node–positive. She begins adjuvant chemotherapy with doxorubicin and cyclophosphamide. Ten days after the first cycle of chemotherapy, her white blood cell (WBC) count drops, as expected; over the next 9 days, her WBC recovers to its normal value. By the third cycle of chemotherapy, Mrs. M is moderately anemic, with a hematocrit of 28% (normal, 37% to 48%), and she feels quite fatigued. Seven days after the fourth cycle of chemotherapy, her WBC plummets to 800 cells per microliter (μL) of blood (normal, 4,300 to 10,800 cells/μL), and her absolute neutrophil count (ANC) is 300 cells/μL. In this setting, she develops shaking chills and a fever to 102 °F. She is admitted to the hospital, where she receives parenteral antibiotics, and she remains there for 5 days until her ANC rises to an acceptable level. Mrs. M completes her cycles of doxorubicin and cyclophosphamide chemotherapy, continues chemotherapy with paclitaxel, and receives local radiation therapy.

Mrs. M is well for 2 years but then presents with pain in the left leg. Workup reveals that the cancer has metastasized to her left femur and liver. She is again fatigued, and her hematocrit is 27%. She begins chemotherapy with doxorubicin and docetaxel but again develops severe neutropenia and fever. Thereafter, her chemotherapy is supplemented with recombinant human G-CSF (filgrastim) and recombinant human erythropoietin (epoetin alfa). Neutropenia and fever do not recur, and by 4 weeks after the initiation of erythropoietin therapy, her hematocrit rises to 34.5% and she feels less fatigued. The chemotherapy yields excellent palliative results. One year later, she is still in remission and leading an active life.

QUESTIONS

■ **1.** What types of molecules are G-CSF and erythropoietin, and what are their mechanisms of action?

■ **2.** How do recombinant hematopoietic growth factors differ from endogenous, "natural" hematopoietic growth factors?

■ **3.** What are some important adverse effects of recombinant hematopoietic growth factors?

PHYSIOLOGY OF HEMATOPOIESIS

The cells of the hematopoietic system are functionally diverse (Table 43-1). Red blood cells, or **erythrocytes,** carry oxygen; many types of white blood cells, from **granulocytes** and **macrophages** to **lymphocytes,** fight infection and help protect against cancer; and **platelets** help control bleeding. Nonetheless, these cells all have one feature in common: they all develop from a common cell in the bone marrow called the **pluripotent hematopoietic stem cell** (Fig. 43-1). Hematopoietic stem cells are induced to differentiate along committed lineages into red blood cells, white blood cells,

---

TABLE 43-1 Hematopoietic Cells, Growth Factors, and Growth Factor Analogues

CELL TYPE	MAJOR FUNCTION(S)	LINEAGE-SPECIFIC GROWTH FACTOR	DEFICIENCY STATE	THERAPEUTIC AGENTS
Red blood cell (erythrocyte)	Oxygen transport	Erythropoietin (EPO)	Anemia	rhEPO, darbepoetin
Platelet (thrombocyte)	Hemostasis	Thrombopoietin (TPO)	Thrombocytopenia	rhTPO, IL-11, PEG-rHuMGDF (TPO analogue)
Monocyte/ macrophage	Phagocytosis of bacteria and cellular and chemical debris, stimulation of T lymphocytes	M-CSF	—	—
Neutrophil	Phagocytosis of bacteria, immune stimulation	G-CSF	Neutropenia	Filgrastim, sargramostim
Eosinophil	Control of parasites	IL-5	—	—
Basophil	Phagocytosis of bacteria	—	—	Filgrastim, sargramostim
B lymphocyte	Production of antibody, stimulation of T lymphocytes	Specific interleukins	Various immunodeficiency syndromes	—
T lymphocyte	Killing of virus- and bacteria-infected cells, control of immune responses	Specific interleukins	Various immunodeficiency syndromes	rhIL-2
NK cell	Killing of cancer cells	—	—	—

NK, natural killer; M-CSF, monocyte colony-stimulating factor; G-CSF, granulocyte colony-stimulating factor; IL-5, interleukin-5; rhEPO, recombinant human erythropoietin; rhTPO, recombinant human thrombopoietin; IL-11, interleukin-11; rhIL-2, recombinant human interleukin-2.

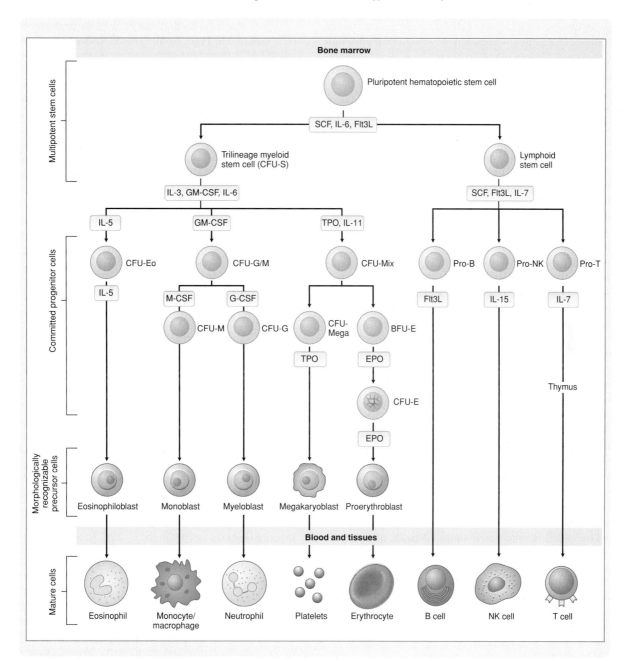

Figure 43-1. Development of cells of the hematopoietic system. Mature cells of the hematopoietic system all develop from pluripotent stem cells that reside in the bone marrow. The type of mature cell that develops is dependent on the extracellular milieu and the exposure of stem cells and progenitor cells to specific growth factors. The pluripotent stem cell differentiates into a trilineage myeloid stem cell (CFU-S) or a lymphoid stem cell. Depending on the growth factors that are present, CFU-S cells differentiate into granulocytes (eosinophils, monocyte/macrophages, neutrophils), platelets, or erythrocytes. Lymphoid stem cells differentiate into B cells, natural killer (NK) cells, or T cells. Except for the terminal differentiation of pro-T cells to mature T cells, which takes place in the thymus, the differentiation of all hematopoietic stem cells, progenitor cells, and precursor cells occurs in the bone marrow. Of the growth factors illustrated here, G-CSF, GM-CSF, erythropoietin *(EPO),* and IL-11 are currently used as therapeutic agents. BFU, burst forming unit; CFU, colony forming unit; CSF, colony stimulating factor; IL, interleukin; SCF, stem cell factor; TPO, thrombopoietin.

or platelets through interactions with glycoproteins called **hematopoietic growth factors.**

CENTRAL ROLE OF HEMATOPOIETIC GROWTH FACTORS

Hematopoietic growth factors and cytokines constitute a heterogeneous group of molecules. Nearly 36 growth factors have been identified, ranging in size from 9 to 90 kDa. The membrane-associated receptors for these growth factors belong to 6 receptor superfamilies, and genes encoding the growth factors are found on 11 chromosomes. Functionally, hematopoietic growth factors stimulate the proliferation, differentiation, and function of hematopoietic cells. Certain factors selectively stimulate the growth and differentiation of a single lineage, as **erythropoietin** does for the erythrocyte lineage. Others, such as **stem cell factor,** stimulate the proliferation of multiple lineages and are said to be **pleiotropic.** Many growth factors act synergistically with one another, often with overlapping effects. This overlapping functionality may serve a protective role to ensure that vitally important processes, such as hematopoiesis, would be maintained if a gene for a single growth factor were to be altered by mutation.

Conceptually, growth factors can be divided into two groups: **multilineage** (also called **general** or **early-acting**) growth factors, which stimulate multiple lineages, and **lineage-specific** (also called **lineage-dominant** or **late-acting**) growth factors, which stimulate differentiation and survival of a single lineage.

Multilineage Growth Factors

Multilineage growth factors include **stem cell factor** (also called **steel factor** or **c-kit ligand**), **interleukin-3 (IL-3), granulocyte-monocyte colony-stimulating factor (GM-CSF),** insulin-like growth factor 1, IL-9, IL-11, and others. Many of these growth factors are discussed below with respect to the development of individual hematopoietic cell types. The relevant pharmacologic principle is that multilineage growth factors are appropriate for treating conditions, such as **pancytopenia,** in which multiple hematopoietic lineages are affected.

The ability of multilineage growth factors to stimulate multiple lineages results from two features of their molecular and cellular physiology. First, the receptors for these growth factors are both structurally related and modular; this commonality makes them somewhat interchangeable. Second, the signal transduction cascades activated by binding of these growth factors to their receptors involve the same family of signaling proteins, the JAK-STAT proteins. It was recently shown that the JAK2 kinase is constitutively activated by a single amino acid mutation, V617F, in the myeloproliferative diseases polycythemia vera, essential thrombocytosis, and myeloid metaplasia with myelofibrosis. These diseases are characterized by clonal proliferation of all lineages, highlighting the general role of the JAK-STAT pathway in hematopoiesis. Pharmacologists have exploited the commonalities of multilineage growth factor signaling to design synthetic growth factors with novel properties (see below).

Lineage-Specific Growth Factors

For a growth factor to be lineage-specific, at least one of two conditions must be met: (1) the expression of the growth factor's receptor(s) must be limited to progenitor and/or precursor cells within a single lineage; and/or (2) the growth factor must induce inhibitory or apoptotic signals in cells of other lineages. **Erythropoietin** is one example of a lineage-specific growth factor; **thrombopoietin,** whose actions are essentially limited to the platelet lineage, is another. Other so-called lineage-specific growth factors are more properly considered lineage-selective, because they have secondary effects on lineage(s) different from the lineage of their primary action. Such factors include **G-CSF,** which primarily promotes the differentiation of neutrophils, and a number of **interleukins,** which have selective actions on certain myeloid and lymphoid lineages (see below). From a pharmacologic perspective, lineage-specific growth factors represent selective therapeutics that can be used to treat a deficiency of a single cell type. Some growth factors may also have unique effects against certain cancers, perhaps due to their prodifferentiation and promaturation properties.

ERYTHROCYTE PRODUCTION (ERYTHROPOIESIS)

Erythrocytes are uniquely suited to their role of transporting oxygen from the lungs to the tissues of the body. These cells contain high concentrations of **hemoglobin,** a protein that binds and releases oxygen molecules in response to the partial pressure of oxygen in the blood and tissues. Each hemoglobin molecule consists of four similar polypeptide chains, and each chain contains a binding site for molecular oxygen. (The protein gets its name from the iron-containing **heme group** at each oxygen binding site, although heme groups are also found in many other proteins.) The major form of adult hemoglobin, which has two alpha and two beta chains ($\alpha_2\beta_2$), is called **hemoglobin A (HbA).** Fetal hemoglobin, or **hemoglobin F (HbF),** contains gamma (γ) chains instead of β chains ($\alpha_2\gamma_2$); this form of hemoglobin predominates during the latter 6 months of fetal life. After birth, DNA methylation inactivates the γ globin gene, and expression of the β globin gene rises. It is important to note that expression of the α, β, and γ globin chains is regulated independently, making possible a multitude of **hemoglobinopathies** in which the α or β chains are abnormal or underexpressed because of an inherited mutation. In **sickle cell anemia,** a point mutation in the β globin gene results in the production of an abnormal hemoglobin—**hemoglobin S (HbS)**—that polymerizes upon deoxygenation, causing morphologic ''sickling'' of erythrocytes and leading to hemolytic anemia, painful vaso-occlusive crises, and profound end-organ damage. This autosomal recessive disease is the most common inherited blood disorder in the United States, affecting more than 70,000 individuals. Another common hemoglobinopathy is **β thalassemia,** in which the β chain is structurally and functionally normal but underexpressed.

Upon their release from the bone marrow, normal erythrocytes circulate in the blood with a lifespan of approximately 120 days. The number of erythrocytes in the blood is determined by the balance between new erythrocyte production in the bone marrow and erythrocyte loss because of cell destruction (hemolysis) or bleeding. This number is measured clinically as either the hemoglobin level (the concentration of hemoglobin per unit volume of blood) or the **hematocrit** (the percentage of blood volume that is composed of erythrocytes). The normal hematocrit ranges from 42% to 50% in men and 37% to 48% in women; the gender difference is often attributed to increased blood loss through physiologic—that is, menstrual—bleeding in women and enhanced erythropoiesis induced by androgens (through unclear mechanisms) in men. A hemoglobin level or hematocrit below the normal range is defined as **anemia.**

Erythropoietin

Erythrocyte production, or **erythropoiesis,** proceeds under the control of several growth factors. The major growth factor controlling erythropoiesis is erythropoietin, a heavily glycosylated protein that is produced mainly by the liver in the fetus and by the kidney after birth. A lineage-specific growth factor, erythropoietin has received great clinical attention because it stimulates all but the earliest intermediates in the erythroid lineage but does not significantly affect other lineages. Its physiologic importance is attested to by experiments in mice and pathologic conditions in humans, both of which show that the absence of erythropoietin results in severe anemia. Furthermore, rare activating mutations of the erythropoietin receptor have been described in patients with primary familial and congenital polycythemia, a disorder manifested by isolated erythrocytosis and increased responsiveness to erythropoietin. Such was the case for Eero Mantyranta, a Finnish cross-country skier who won several gold medals in the 1964 Olympics but was accused of blood "doping" (receiving erythrocyte transfusions to artificially increase oxygen-carrying capacity) because of an abnormally high hematocrit. He was exonerated 30 years later when researchers identified an activating mutation of the erythropoietin receptor in samples from him and his family.

Given the role of erythrocytes in transporting oxygen, it is not surprising that erythropoietin production is triggered by hypoxia. Erythropoietin expression is strongly induced by **hypoxia-inducible factor 1 alpha (HIF-1α)**, which binds to an enhancer element in the erythropoietin gene and activates gene transcription (Fig. 43-2). The amount of HIF-1α within a cell is heavily influenced by the local oxygen tension. Under normal or high oxygen conditions, HIF-1α is hydroxylated by prolyl hydroxylase (PHD) via its Fe (II)-dependent dioxygenase activity. Prolyl hydroxylation of HIF-1α facilitates its binding to the von Hippel-Lindau (pVHL) E3 ubiquitin ligase complex, thus targeting HIF-1α for proteasomal degradation. Under hypoxic conditions, prolyl hydroxylation of HIF-1α does not occur, HIF-1α does not associate with pVHL, and HIF-1α instead translocates to the nucleus, where it enhances transcription of the hypoxia-inducible genes, including erythropoietin. In the rare autosomal recessive disease familial erythrocytosis 2 (also called *Chuvash polycythemia*, after the ethnic population of the mid-Volga River region in which it was first described), both germ-line copies of pVHL are mutated so as to prevent association with HIF-1α, reducing the rate of degradation

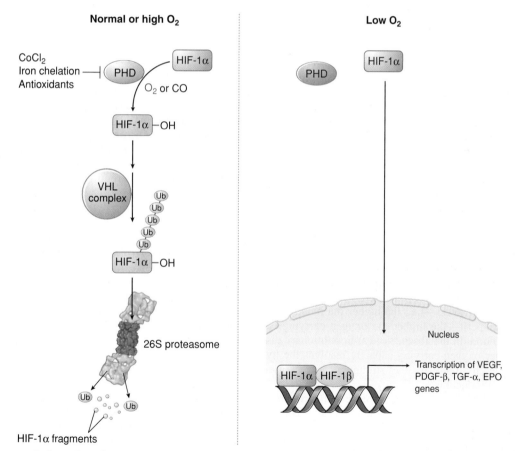

Figure 43-2. Regulation of erythropoietin synthesis. Synthesis of erythropoietin (EPO) by the kidney is increased when the oxygen content of the blood is low and decreased when the oxygen content of the blood is normal or high. The physiologic O_2 sensor is an iron-containing dioxygenase, prolyl hydroxylase (PHD). (In vitro experiments using $CoCl_2$, iron chelation, antioxidants, and CO demonstrated the identity of the O_2 sensor as an iron-containing protein.) Under conditions of normal or high O_2, activated PHD hydroxylates proline residues on hypoxia-inducible factor 1α (HIF-1α). This posttranslational modification enhances HIF-1α binding to the ubiquitin ligase pVHL (VHL complex), leading to ubiquitination (Ub) and proteolytic degradation of HIF-1α by the 26S proteasome. Under low oxygen conditions, the prolyl hydroxylase is inactivated, allowing HIF-1α to accumulate, translocate to the nucleus, and induce the expression of a number of genes, including the gene encoding erythropoietin (EPO). In pathologic conditions, such as chronic kidney disease, the cells of the kidney that normally synthesize EPO are injured. These injured cells cannot synthesize adequate amounts of EPO, even under conditions of hypoxia, and anemia ensues. Recombinant human EPO can be administered exogenously to supply the missing growth factor and thereby treat the anemia.

TABLE 43-2 Pathologic Conditions That Stimulate or Inhibit Erythropoiesis

CONDITION	MECHANISM
Stimulate Erythropoiesis:	
Bleeding	Induce tissue hypoxia
Hemolysis	
High altitude	
Pulmonary disease	
JAK2-activating mutations in myeloproliferative disorders	Increase intracellular JAK-STAT signaling cascade
Inhibit Erythropoiesis:	
Chronic kidney disease	Decreases erythropoietin synthesis in kidney
Iron, folate, or vitamin B_{12} deficiency	Decrease erythroblast differentiation and erythrocyte production
Chronic inflammatory conditions	
Sideroblastic anemia	
Thalassemia	
Malignant infiltration of bone marrow	
Aplastic anemia, pure red cell aplasia	
Drug-induced bone marrow toxicity	

of HIF-1α and leading to elevated levels of erythropoietin and other target genes.

Following transcription and translation, the 166-amino acid, 18-kDa erythropoietin protein is glycosylated to 34 to 39 kDa, its terminal arginine is cleaved, and the protein is secreted and transported in the circulation to the bone marrow. There, it binds to erythropoietin receptors expressed on the surface of BFU-E and all subsequent progenitor and precursor cells in the erythroid lineage, including the erythrocyte's immediate precursor cell, the **reticulocyte.** Then, through a complex intracellular signaling cascade mediated by JAK-STAT, erythropoietin receptor activation enhances the proliferation and differentiation of erythroid-lineage cells, including the terminal differentiation of reticulocytes to erythrocytes. Erythropoiesis completes a negative feedback loop on erythropoietin production, because the more erythrocytes in the blood—i.e., the higher the hemoglobin level and hematocrit—the higher the oxygen-carrying capacity of the blood. In the absence of cardiopulmonary disease, the higher oxygen-carrying capacity resolves the hypoxia and thereby removes the stimulus for increased erythropoietin production.

Table 43-2 lists the mechanisms of several prominent pathologic conditions that stimulate or inhibit erythropoiesis.

LEUKOCYTE PRODUCTION (MYELOPOIESIS AND LYMPHOPOIESIS)

White blood cells, or **leukocytes,** are essential cells of the immune system. There are two main categories of leukocytes, corresponding to the two main branches of the immune system. Cells of the **innate branch** of the immune system include granulocytes (**neutrophils, eosinophils,** and **basophils**), **monocyte/macrophages,** and variants of the macrophage lineage. Neutrophils target bacteria, while eo-

sinophils target parasites. Basophils participate in hypersensitivity responses. Macrophages also target bacteria, but these cells and their variants—**dendritic cells, Langerhans cells,** and **osteoclasts,** among others—have important additional functions. Macrophages have a key role in stimulating and regulating both branches of the immune system during infection and in clearing biological debris. Dendritic cells and Langerhans cells are important for initiating and targeting the immune response. These cells transport antigen from the site of inoculation to lymph nodes, where lymphocyte responses are coordinated. Osteoclasts are essential for bone resorption. Cells of the **adaptive branch** of the immune system are called **lymphocytes.** The two types of lymphocytes are B cells, which make antibodies, and T cells, which target virus-infected and neoplastic cells (among other functions). "Adaptive" refers to the ability of these cells to recognize and respond to specific infectious agents and other targets (see Chapter 40, Principles of Inflammation and the Immune System).

All white blood cells develop from pluripotent hematopoietic stem cells (Fig. 43-1). Under the influence of growth factors, these stem cells differentiate into either **myeloid stem cells** or **lymphoid stem cells.** Myeloid stem cells further differentiate into the various cells of the innate branch of the immune system (as well as erythrocytes and platelets), while lymphoid stem cells differentiate into cells of the adaptive branch of the immune system. The growth factors that regulate these differentiation pathways are discussed below.

Granulocyte-Stimulating Factors

The differentiation of pluripotent stem cells into myeloid stem cells is fostered by certain multilineage growth factors such as stem cell factor and IL-3. Further differentiation of myeloid stem cells into neutrophils and monocyte/macrophages is controlled by the multilineage growth factor **gran-**

ulocyte-monocyte colony-stimulating factor (GM-CSF) and the lineage-specific growth factors **granulocyte colony-stimulating factor (G-CSF)** and **monocyte colony-stimulating factor (M-CSF)**. The differentiation of myeloid stem cells into eosinophils is controlled by **interleukin-5 (IL-5)**.

GM-CSF has relatively broad effects on cells of the myeloid lineage. Produced mainly by macrophages and T cells, this 18- to 28-kDa glycoprotein stimulates the differentiation of myeloid stem cells and progenitor cells into morphologically recognizable precursors of eosinophils, monocyte/macrophages, and neutrophils. GM-CSF also enhances the activity of these mature leukocytes and promotes the differentiation of macrophages into Langerhans cells. Some of the effects of GM-CSF are indirect. For example, the effects of GM-CSF on neutrophil production and function may result not only from direct GM-CSF stimulation of neutrophil precursors, but also from GM-CSF-stimulated IL-1 secretion by other cells. Like other growth factors, GM-CSF signals through the JAK-STAT signaling pathway.

G-CSF has narrower effects than GM-CSF. G-CSF is an 18-kDa glycoprotein that, like GM-CSF, signals through the JAK-STAT signaling cascade. G-CSF is released into the circulation by monocytes, macrophages, epithelial cells, and fibroblasts at sites of infection. In the bone marrow, G-CSF stimulates the production of neutrophils, which in turn enhance the ability of the immune system to fight the infection. Locally released G-CSF stimulates neutrophil-mediated phagocytosis.

The effects of M-CSF are restricted to the differentiation and activation of monocyte/macrophages and their various related cells (including a subset of osteoclasts). In a positive feedback loop, these are also the cells that produce M-CSF. M-CSF exists in alternatively spliced 70- to 80-kDa and 40- to 50-kDa isoforms.

IL-5 is produced by a subset of helper T cells. This growth factor selectively promotes the differentiation, adhesion, degranulation, and survival of eosinophils. As such, IL-5 is believed to have an important role in the pathophysiology of allergic reactions and asthma.

Lymphocyte-Stimulating Factors

Regulatory proteins called **interleukins** control lymphocyte development and activation. To date, more than 30 members of this family have been defined. Family members are numbered IL-1, IL-2, and so forth. Interleukins regulate not only lymphocyte differentiation, but also multiple and overlapping aspects of the innate and adaptive immune responses, including stimulation of T cells and macrophages. Several interleukins are described above as granulocyte-stimulating factors; others are discussed below in the context of platelet production.

IL-2 and **IL-7** are two interleukins critical to white blood cell differentiation. IL-2 is a 45-kDa protein produced by T cells. Because it drives proliferation of T cells and B cells, IL-2 once received much attention as a potential immunostimulant. Investigations of this hypothesis showed, however, that mice lacking IL-2 exhibit lymphoproliferative rather than lymphopenic diseases. This unexpected finding underscores the principle that growth factors have diverse functions in vivo, including, as in this case, regulatory or suppressive (tolerogenic) effects as well as stimulatory effects. This

finding also points out that uncontrolled proliferation can ensue if differentiation is not regulated normally, a process that may underlie some types of cancer. IL-7, produced by cells in the spleen, thymus, and bone marrow stroma, is a multilineage lymphostimulatory growth factor that enhances the growth and differentiation of B cells and T cells.

The **interferons** constitute a second family of regulatory proteins that modulate lymphocyte growth and activity. Like the interleukins, these proteins can stimulate the activity of T cells and macrophages. Interferons have prominent antiviral actions and are used in the treatment of infections such as hepatitis B and C (see Chapter 36, Pharmacology of Viral Infections). Other effects of interferons include promoting the terminal differentiation of lymphocytes, suppressing cell division (in some situations), and exerting direct cytotoxic effects on cells under stress. The three types of interferons—called IFN-α, IFN-β, and IFN-γ—have different biological actions. The cellular effects of interferons, like those of the growth factors, are mediated by specific cell surface receptors and JAK-STAT signal transduction cascades.

PLATELET PRODUCTION (THROMBOPOIESIS)

Platelets—sometimes called **thrombocytes**—are essential for clot formation. These small cells, which lack a nucleus and do not synthesize new proteins, have a half-life of about 9 or 10 days in the circulation. The production of platelets, like that of all formed elements of the hematopoietic system, is controlled by both multilineage and lineage-specific growth factors (Fig. 43-3). The most important multilineage growth factors that stimulate platelet production are IL-11, IL-3, GM-CSF, stem cell factor, and IL-6. Not surprisingly, these factors also stimulate the production of erythrocytes because platelets and erythrocytes share a common progenitor, the CFU-Mix cell. Whether CFU-Mix cells become

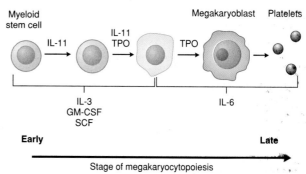

Figure 43-3. Growth factors involved in platelet production. A number of growth factors are involved in platelet production (megakaryocytopoiesis). IL-11 acts primarily in the early stages; this growth factor stimulates production of GM-CSF and acts synergistically with IL-3 and stem cell factor (SCF) to increase the proliferation and differentiation of megakaryocyte progenitors. IL-6 and thrombopoietin (TPO) act primarily in the late stages of megakaryocytopoiesis. Oprelvekin (recombinant human IL-11) can be used therapeutically to increase platelet production. Because IL-11 acts at an early stage of megakaryocytopoiesis, this drug requires a number of days to stimulate the production of new platelets. Recombinant TPO is in clinical development; this agent would be expected to increase platelet production within a shorter period of time.

erythrocytes or platelets depends on their subsequent exposure to lineage-specific growth factors. Differentiation into BFU-E and other cells of the erythroid lineage is promoted by erythropoietin. In contrast, differentiation into CFU-Mega cells and then into megakaryocytes (which then form platelets) is promoted by the lineage-specific growth factor thrombopoietin (Fig. 43-1).

Thrombopoietin

Thrombopoietin (TPO) is produced in the liver and, to a lesser extent, in the proximal convoluted tubule of the kidney. Like erythropoietin, thrombopoietin is a heavily glycosylated protein (35 kDa) that has its major effect on a single cell lineage; also like erythropoietin, thrombopoietin signals through a JAK-STAT transduction cascade. However, unlike erythropoietin, thrombopoietin is not regulated in its activity at the level of gene expression, because thrombopoietin is expressed constitutively. Instead, by an unusual mechanism, thrombopoietin levels are regulated by the thrombopoietin receptor (also known as *Mpl*), which is the protein product of the gene *c-mpl*.

Structurally and functionally, the thrombopoietin receptor resembles the receptors for IL-3, erythropoietin, and GM-CSF. It is found both on platelet progenitors—CFU-S, CFU-Mix, CFU-Mega, and megakaryocytes—and on platelets themselves. Thrombopoietin has different effects on these cell types, however. On platelet progenitors, the binding of thrombopoietin to its receptor promotes cell growth and differentiation. In contrast, thrombopoietin receptors on platelets act as molecular sponges to bind excess thrombopoietin and thereby prevent platelet overproduction if platelets are in adequate supply. Thrombopoietin also enhances platelet function by sensitizing these cells to the proaggregatory effects of thrombin and collagen (see Chapter 22, Pharmacology of Hemostasis and Thrombosis).

PHARMACOLOGIC CLASSES AND AGENTS

The hematopoietic growth factors used clinically can be divided into two groups. First, recombinant or synthetic growth factor analogues are used to treat deficiencies of the various hematopoietic cell populations. This group includes both the G-CSF and erythropoietin received by Mrs. M. Second, some growth factors have therapeutic use in the treatment of various malignancies.

AGENTS THAT STIMULATE ERYTHROCYTE PRODUCTION

The erythroid lineage-specific actions of erythropoietin make this growth factor an obvious candidate for use in the treatment of some forms of anemia. Anemia can result from any of a large number of underlying conditions that either interrupt the normal process of erythropoiesis or result in the premature loss or destruction of mature erythrocytes (Table 43-2). One common indication for erythropoietin

therapy is chronic kidney disease, in which the loss of functional kidney tissue results in loss of the cells responsible for erythropoietin production. Another potential indication for erythropoietin is cancer, which can induce a state of relative resistance to endogenous erythropoietin by mechanisms that may involve proinflammatory cytokines, oxidative stress, and antierythropoietin antibodies. (Cancer can also cause anemia through bleeding, poor nutrition, and infiltration of the bone marrow by tumor cells; these causes can often be diagnosed and treated directly.) Often, cancer-related anemia results from the bone marrow toxicity of the chemotherapeutic agents used to treat the cancer. The fatigue associated with cancer-related anemia, such as that experienced by Mrs. M, can therefore be treated with erythropoietin under some circumstances.

Recombinant Human Erythropoietin (rhEPO) and Darbepoetin (NESP)

There are currently two erythropoietic agents in clinical use in North America, **recombinant human erythropoietin (rhEPO)** (also known as **epoetin alfa**) and **darbepoetin** (formerly known as "novel erythropoiesis stimulating protein" or **NESP**). (Epoetin beta is a different bioengineered form of rhEPO that is available as a therapeutic agent in other parts of the world.) Like endogenous erythropoietin, epoetin alfa and darbepoetin act by stimulating the erythropoietin receptor and inducing erythropoiesis. rhEPO increases the hematocrit level by at least 6% in half to three-quarters of patients receiving the drug, depending on the etiology of the anemia and the dose of rhEPO administered.

rhEPO and darbepoetin are very similar in structure; in fact, the two agents differ only in the number of sialic acid (carbohydrate) groups that are attached to the protein. The development of darbepoetin began with the observation that more sialic acid groups confer higher potency on erythropoietin. Darbepoetin's two extra sialic acid groups also give this drug a threefold longer half-life than erythropoietin, enabling less frequent administration. Both agents are proteins and must therefore be administered parenterally.

In addition to its well-characterized role in stimulating erythropoiesis, erythropoietin may also play a role in glial and neuronal cell survival following noxious stimuli or ischemic injury. Clinical studies of the neuroprotective effects of erythropoietin are ongoing.

Administration of erythropoietin to non-anemic patients can lead to polycythemia, blood hyperviscosity, and stroke or myocardial infarction. Eighteen young cyclists died unexpectedly after the illegal introduction of erythropoietin into the world of professional cycling in the 1980s, possibly as a consequence of these adverse effects. Another serious adverse effect of certain preparations of recombinant erythropoietin became evident between 1998 and 2003. More than 200 patients who received one formulation of recombinant erythropoietin developed pure red cell aplasia and were found to have developed neutralizing antibodies against erythropoietin. The exact cause of the immune response is not well understood; one hypothesis involves the exposure of erythropoietin neoantigens as a result of partial denaturation of the therapeutic protein preparation. Erythropoietin and darbepoetin may also induce hypertension, and the use of these drugs is contraindicated in patients with uncontrolled hypertension. The mechanism responsible for erythropoietin-induced hypertension remains to be elucidated.

Recent limited studies have suggested that erythropoietin may decrease survival in patients with head and neck carcinoma or breast cancer, despite an improvement in the patients' chemotherapy-induced anemia. The mechanisms and implications of these findings remain controversial. Potential explanations could include expression of the erythropoietin receptor on some cancer cells, synergistic toxicity due to combining erythropoietin therapy with chemotherapy and radiation therapy, and increased thrombogenicity associated with the elevated hemoglobin levels induced by erythropoietin therapy. Nonetheless, it appears at the present time that use of rhEPO and darbepoetin within the labeled indications represents safe and effective supportive care for patients with chemotherapy-induced anemia.

AGENTS THAT INDUCE FETAL HEMOGLOBIN (HbF)

Sickle cell disease is marked by acute pain crises, increased susceptibility to infection, and profound hemolytic anemia. Sickle hemoglobin (HbS)-containing erythrocytes are the root cause of these clinical manifestations of disease, which begins in childhood when HbS is first produced. Newborns and infants with sickle cell disease are asymptomatic because fetal globin gene expression persists for many months after birth, keeping fetal hemoglobin (HbF) levels high. (In patients with sickle cell disease, typical HbF levels are 15% of total hemoglobin as late as age 2, and 1% to 5% of total hemoglobin in adults.) Consistent with this observation, adults in whom HbF expression persists at high levels have less frequent pain crises and milder anemia than those with low HbF expression. These observations have made increasing HbF levels a tantalizing therapeutic goal.

In principle, there are two approaches for increasing HbF: stimulating HbF expression in adults and preventing the switch from fetal (HbF) to adult (HbS) hemoglobin expression in children. Two drugs in current clinical practice, **5-azacytidine** and **hydroxyurea**, use the first approach; the **butyrates**, a class of drugs that are still in clinical trials, may utilize both approaches. Early studies suggest that 5-azacytidine and hydroxyurea could be synergistic with butyrates and with erythropoietin, although erythropoietin should be used with caution in patients with sickle cell disease because it stimulates erythropoiesis in HbS- as well as HbF-containing cells.

5-Azacytidine

5-Azacytidine is a DNA demethylating agent that, in the 1980s, was found to increase HbF production to over 20% of total globin expression in patients with sickle cell disease or beta-thalassemia. (Theoretical studies suggest that an HbF level of 30% to 40% would render a patient asymptomatic.) 5-Azacytidine is thought to act by reversing the methylation of the γ globin gene, but this mechanism remains unproven. Concern over the unknown mechanism of action and fear of long-term cancer risk (5-azacytidine also interferes with normal DNA synthesis; see Chapter 37, Pharmacology of Cancer: Genome Synthesis, Stability, and Maintenance)

have hindered the acceptance of this drug as a prophylactic therapy in sickle cell disease.

Hydroxyurea

The 1990s saw the first use of hydroxyurea to treat sickle cell disease. A cytostatic agent that blocks cell division by inhibiting ribonucleotide reductase, hydroxyurea had previously been used to treat clonal hematological disorders such as chronic myelogenous leukemia and polycythemia vera (see Chapter 37). From this experience, hydroxyurea was known to be relatively safe for long-term administration, even in children; myelosuppression of white blood cells and platelets was known to be its main adverse effect. The induction of HbF by hydroxyurea is slower than that by azacytidine; nevertheless, hydroxyurea has proved to be effective in about 60% of patients with sickle cell disease. In these patients, hydroxyurea increases HbF levels to 20% or more, decreases the frequency of painful crises by 50% (from 4.5 to 2.5 per year, on average), and decreases the number of transfusions required by patients who have three or more crises per year. However, hydroxyurea does not prevent endorgan damage or stroke. In 1998, hydroxyurea received approval from the U. S. Food and Drug Administration (FDA) for use in the treatment of sickle cell disease.

Despite its long history of use, hydroxyurea's mechanism of action in sickle cell disease remains uncertain. The current hypothesis is that hydroxyurea blocks the division of HbS-expressing erythroid precursors, and that this somehow triggers reversion to a fetal pattern of hemoglobin expression in an attempt to maintain erythrocyte production. Interestingly, it has been shown that the mechanism by which hydroxyurea increases HbF expression is independent of ribonucleotide reductase inhibition.

Butyrates

Butyrates (e.g., arginine butyrate, phenylbutyrate) are short-chain fatty acids that inhibit histone deacetylases, the enzymes that modify DNA to make it inaccessible to transcription factors. Butyrates have been shown to increase HbF levels from 2% to more than 20% in early clinical trials, although these agents are apparently not effective in patients whose baseline HbF level is less than 1%. Butyrates prevent the switch from HbF to HbS in experimental animals, and children born to diabetic mothers (whose blood contains elevated levels of butyrates) have higher than normal levels of HbF. Butyrates are thought to act by allowing certain transcription factors to maintain or resume activity. Although this mechanism could explain the increased HbF production in response to butyrates, it does not explain the selectivity of butyrates for HbF production over HbS expression in patients with sickle cell disease.

AGENTS THAT STIMULATE LEUKOCYTE PRODUCTION

A low neutrophil count, or **neutropenia,** is most often the result of interference with progenitor cell division (**myelosuppression**). Neutropenia frequently accompanies leukemia and other malignancies that invade the bone marrow, and it is a common adverse effect of cancer chemotherapy. Less common causes of neutropenia include bone marrow transplantation, congenital neutropenia, and HIV- or zidovudine-associated neutropenia. Three agents have been approved for use in the treatment of cancer- and chemotherapy-induced neutropenia: recombinant human G-CSF (**filgrastim**); its pegylated, long-acting form, PEG-G-CSF (**PEG-filgrastim**); and recombinant human GM-CSF (**sargramostim**).

Recombinant Human G-CSF (Filgrastim) and GM-CSF (Sargramostim)

Filgrastim and sargramostim are almost identical to the natural growth factors G-CSF and GM-CSF, and they act by the same mechanisms as the endogenous proteins. Although GM-CSF is a multilineage growth factor, the major clinical effect of GM-CSF or G-CSF administration is a dose-independent increase in the absolute neutrophil count. (GM-CSF also causes a mild and dose-dependent increase in eosinophils.) As noted above, G-CSF and GM-CSF enhance the microbicidal activity of neutrophils in addition to stimulating their production. For Mrs. M (see introductory case), filgrastim hastened the recovery of her neutrophils after chemotherapy and enhanced the ability of her neutrophils to combat infection. G-CSF and GM-CSF also mobilize hematopoietic stem cells from the bone marrow into the peripheral circulation; for this reason, they are often used before harvesting stem cells for transplantation. The immunostimulatory effects of GM-CSF have fostered research into its ability to increase anti-tumor immune activity.

A filgrastim analogue has been conjugated to polyethylene glycol (PEG). This analogue, PEG-filgrastim, is metabolized more slowly than the native molecule. PEG-filgrastim can therefore be administered as a single injection that is functionally equivalent to multiple daily doses of filgrastim.

The main adverse effect of recombinant human G-CSF is bone pain, which resolves upon discontinuation of the drug. The theoretical risk that G-CSF could induce acute myelogenous leukemia (AML) or myelodysplastic syndrome (MDS) remains controversial. In general, observational studies do not support an increased risk, but a study of breast cancer patients treated with chemotherapy did demonstrate a fivefold increased incidence of AML/MDS in patients who received G-CSF. Of note, however, these patients also received a higher dose of cyclophosphamide than patients who did not develop AML/MDS. GM-CSF is associated with fever, arthralgia, edema, and pleural and pericardial effusion. G-CSF and GM-CSF are proteins and must be administered parenterally, typically by daily injection over the course of several weeks.

AGENTS THAT STIMULATE PLATELET PRODUCTION

A low platelet count, or **thrombocytopenia,** is an important adverse effect of many cancer chemotherapeutic agents, occasionally limiting the doses that can be delivered with acceptable safety and tolerability. The complications of thrombocytopenia include increased bleeding risk and platelet transfusion requirement; in turn, platelet transfusion is associated with an increased risk of infection, febrile reaction, and, rarely, graft-versus-host disease.

Research into the pharmacologic management of chemotherapy-induced thrombocytopenia has focused on the thrombopoietin analogues **recombinant human thrombopoietin (rhTPO)** and **pegylated recombinant human megakaryocyte growth and development factor (PEG-rHuMGDF)**. A small-molecule oral drug that directly stimulates the TPO receptor is also in clinical trials. To date, however, only **recombinant human IL-11 (rhIL-11 or oprelvekin)** has been approved by the FDA for clinical use. These agents all have the potential to increase megakaryocytopoiesis (platelet production) in a dose-dependent fashion; although these drugs stimulate some multipotent as well as committed precursor cells, they do not significantly increase the hematocrit or white blood cell count. Importantly, these agents must all be administered prophylactically because their activity is delayed in onset, with a 1- to 3-week hiatus before the platelet count reaches its peak value. Current research has identified several small-molecule ligands for the TPO receptor, such as hydrazinonaphthalene and azonaphthalene, which could serve as lead compounds for the development of new drugs.

Thrombopoietin and Pharmacologic Analogues

Cloning of the thrombopoietin gene in 1994 led to the development of two thrombopoietin analogues. The first, rhTPO, is a full-length, glycosylated analogue; the second, PEG-rHuMGDF, consists of the N-terminal 163 amino acids of thrombopoietin conjugated to polyethylene glycol (PEG). Like natural thrombopoietin, both rhTPO and PEG-rHuMGDF bind to Mpl (the endogenous receptor for thrombopoietin, named for its role in murine myeloproliferative leukemia), and activation of Mpl is the basis for the effect of these drugs. Both rhTPO and PEG-rHuMGDF have been tested as prophylactic agents to minimize chemotherapy-induced thrombocytopenia, and both can cause a 2- to 10-fold increase in the platelet count.

One caution is that stimulation of platelet production could lead to thrombosis if the platelets that are produced are also activated. A small trial of PEG-rHuMGDF suggests that this drug is safe to use in treating the thrombocytopenia associated with AML, even though AML cells may also express the TPO receptor. The heavily bioengineered variants of natural TPO (e.g., PEG-rHuMGDF) have recently been dropped from clinical development because of an excess risk of developing anti-TPO autoantibodies, which could suppress natural platelet production. The testing of full-length rhTPO continues; there are no reports to date of neutralizing antibodies in patients who receive this lightly bioengineered agent, which differs from native human TPO only in its glycosylation pattern.

Interleukin-11 [rhIL-11 (Oprelvekin)]

Although IL-11's ability to stimulate the differentiation of myeloid stem cells could theoretically make this protein a multilineage growth factor, in clinical practice, recombinant human IL-11 (rhIL-11), also called **oprelvekin,** has been used to stimulate platelet production. The recombinant form of IL-11, which is produced in *Escherichia coli,* differs from natural IL-11 only in its lack of the N-terminal proline residue. rhIL-11 causes a dose-dependent increase in the platelet count and in the number of megakaryocytes in the bone marrow. The main clinical application of rhIL-11 is to prevent thrombocytopenia in patients who are about to receive chemotherapy. The practical goal of treatment is to maintain the platelet count above 20,000/μL (normal range, 150,000 to 450,000/μL) in order to minimize the risk of life-threatening bleeding.

The use of rhIL-11 is associated with significant adverse effects, especially fatigue and fluid retention. Atrial fibrillation has also been observed, and rhIL-11 should be used with caution in any patient with underlying heart disease. The undesirable actions of rhIL-11 likely result from pleiotropic effects of this factor on receptors distributed outside the hematopoietic system. It is unclear whether the therapeutic benefit of this agent outweighs the risk of adverse systemic effects.

IMMUNOMODULATORY AGENTS WITH ANTINEOPLASTIC APPLICATIONS

Interferons

Clinical investigation has led to the use of interferons as therapeutic agents against a number of different malignancies, with moderate success. However, the multiple and overlapping effects of these proteins have made it difficult to determine the drugs' mechanism of action in any given clinical situation. Induction of antitumor-directed immunity, terminal differentiation of cycling tumor cells, and direct cytotoxic effects have all been hypothesized to have important roles in the treatment of different malignancies. Interferons are also used to treat certain viral infections and are discussed in greater detail in Chapter 36.

Levamisole

Levamisole was known as an antihelminthic agent for decades before its anticancer effects were discovered. In combination with the antimetabolite 5-fluorouracil (see Chapter 37), this drug is now approved for use in the treatment of colon cancer. Although its mechanism of action remains uncertain, levamisole is thought to cause macrophages and T cells to secrete cytokines (such as IL-1) and other factors that suppress tumor growth.

Interleukin-2

Interleukin-2 (IL-2) is approved by the FDA for the treatment of melanoma. At therapeutic doses, however, this cytokine has relatively low efficacy and relatively high toxicity. See Chapter 44, Pharmacology of Immunosuppression, for more information about IL-2.

Tretinoin

Tretinoin, or all-trans retinoic acid (ATRA), is a ligand of the retinoic acid receptor (RAR). ATRA is used in the treatment of acute promyelocytic leukemia. This disease is characterized by a translocation t(15;17) in which part of the *RARα* gene is fused to the *PML* gene, creating a fusion protein that induces a block to differentiation and thereby allows development of the leukemia. Treatment with ATRA stimulates differentiation of these cells into more normal granulocytes. In some patients, the induction of differentiation can lead to a life-threatening overproduction of white blood cells. ATRA can also induce a rapidly progressive syndrome of fever, acute respiratory distress with pulmonary infiltrates, edema and weight gain, and multisystem organ failure. Often, therapy with high doses of glucocorticoids effectively treats this ATRA syndrome.

Conclusion and Future Directions

The production of cells of the hematopoietic system—red blood cells (erythrocytes), white blood cells (neutrophils, monocytes, lymphocytes, and other cell types), and platelets—is controlled by a variety of proteins called growth factors. Cancer chemotherapy, malignant infiltration of the bone marrow, and other conditions can cause deficiencies (anemia, neutropenia, and/or thrombocytopenia) in these cell populations. The agents currently used to treat these deficiencies are recombinant analogues of the natural growth factors. Thus, the erythropoietin analogues rhEPO and darbepoetin treat anemia; the G-CSF and GM-CSF analogues filgrastim and sargramostim treat neutropenia; and rhIL-11 and the thrombopoietin analogue rhTPO treat thrombocytopenia. Several agents affecting the hematopoietic system are also used to treat sickle cell disease, a common autosomal recessive disease caused by a point mutation in the β globin gene. These agents (hydroxyurea, 5-azacytidine) increase expression of fetal hemoglobin (HbF) and thereby restore normal erythrocyte structure and function. Several other drugs, including recombinant forms of the immunostimulatory interferon proteins, levamisole, and retinoic acid, are used to treat certain cancers, although their precise mechanisms of action remain unknown.

Other agents that activate hematopoiesis continue to be identified. Recent preclinical evidence suggests that daily injections of a parathyroid hormone analogue (PTH 1-34) promote blood cell development, perhaps by activating stimulatory receptors on osteoblasts that neighbor hematopoietic stem cells. These observations have led to ongoing clinical trials of PTH in enhancing stem cell production for transplantation and in protecting hematopoietic stem cells from the cytotoxic effects of chemotherapy. Studies designed to tease apart the complex overlapping functionalities of these hematopoietic regulatory proteins are likely to provide a source of more selective pharmacologic interventions in the future.

Suggested Reading

Demetri GD. Anaemia and its functional consequences in cancer patients: current challenges in management and prospects for improving therapy. *Br J Cancer* 2001;84:31–37. (*Reviews the use and effectiveness of recombinant human erythropoietin.*)

Demetri GD. Pharmacologic treatment options in patients with thrombocytopenia. *Semin Hematol* 2000;37:11–18. *(Reviews therapy for thrombocytopenia.)*

Egrie JC, Browne JJ. Development and characterization of novel erythropoiesis stimulating protein (NESP). *Br J Cancer* 2001; 84:3–10. *(Reviews the development of darbepoetin.)*

Henke M, Laszig R, Rube C, et al. Erythropoietin to treat head and neck cancer patients with anaemia undergoing radiotherapy: randomised, double-blind, placebo-controlled trial. *Lancet* 2003; 362(9392):1255–1260. *(Describes unfavorable outcome in head and neck cancer patients receiving epoetin beta.)*

Kaushansky K. Lineage-specific hematopoietic growth factors. *N Engl J Med* 2006;354:2034–2045. *(Reviews hematopoietic growth factors.)*

Leyland-Jones B. Breast cancer trial with erythropoietin terminated unexpectedly. *Lancet Oncol* 2003;4:459–460. *(Describes unfavorable outcome in breast cancer patients receiving epoetin alfa.)*

Smith TJ, Khatcheressian J, Lyman GH, et al. Update of recommendations for the use of white blood cell growth factors: an evidence-based clinical practice guideline. *J Clin Oncol* 2006;24: 3187–3205. *(American Society of Clinical Oncology guidelines for the use of myeloid growth factors.)*

Vansteenkiste J, Pirker R, Massuti B, et al. Double-blind, placebo-controlled, randomized phase III trial of darbepoetin alfa in lung cancer patients receiving chemotherapy. *J Natl Cancer Inst* 2002; 94:1211–1220. *(Evidence for clinical effectiveness of darbepoetin.)*

Drug Summary Table | Chapter 43 Pharmacology of Hematopoiesis and Immunomodulation

Drug	Clinical Applications	*Serious* and Common Adverse Effects	Contraindications	Therapeutic Considerations
AGENTS THAT STIMULATE ERYTHROCYTE PRODUCTION				
Mechanism—Activate the erythropoietin receptor and stimulate erythropoiesis				
Erythropoietin (epoetin alfa) Darbepoetin	Cancer-associated anemia Chemotherapy-induced anemia Anemia of chronic kidney disease	*Cardiac arrhythmia or heart failure in patients with renal failure, thrombotic disorder, dyspnea, dehydration, fever* Hypertension, edema, gastrointestinal disturbance, headache, fatigue	Uncontrolled hypertension and hypertensive encephalopathy	Darbepoetin has more sialic acid groups, giving it a longer half-life Epoetin beta available outside the US Administration of erythropoietin in non-anemic patients can lead to polycythemia, blood hyperviscosity, and stroke or myocardial infarction May be abused by athletes
AGENTS THAT INDUCE FETAL HEMOGLOBIN				
Mechanism—5-azacytidine may reverse methylation of the gamma globin gene, leading to increased HbF expression; hydroxyurea may block the division of HbS-expressing erythroid precursors, leading to increased HbF expression				
5-Azacytidine	See Chapter 37 Pharmacology of Cancer: Genome Synthesis, Stability, and Maintenance			
Hydroxyurea	Sickle cell anemia Refractory chronic myeloid leukemia Head and neck cancer Malignant melanoma Ovarian carcinoma	*Myelosuppression, skin ulcer, secondary leukemia with long-term use*	Severe bone marrow depression Live rotavirus vaccine	Mechanism of therapeutic effect in cancer treatment appears to involve inhibition of ribonucleotide reductase Mechanism of therapeutic effect in sickle cell anemia is uncertain
AGENTS THAT STIMULATE LEUKOCYTE PRODUCTION				
Mechanism—Multilineage (GM-CSF) or lineage-specific (G-CSF) growth factors that stimulate myelopoiesis. The major effect of GM-CSF and G-CSF is to raise neutrophil counts; GM-CSF also increases eosinophil counts.				
Filgrastim (rhG-CSF) PEG-Filgrastim	Neutropenia Peripheral blood stem cell harvest	*Hemoglobin S disease with crisis, vasculitis of the skin, acute respiratory distress syndrome, splenic rupture* Bone pain, influenza-like illness, nausea and vomiting	Hypersensitivity to *E. coli* derived proteins or filgrastim	PEG-filgrastim is a PEGylated formulation with a longer half-life G-CSF and GM-CSF enhance the microbicidal activity of neutrophils in addition to stimulating their production
Sargramostim (rhGM-CSF)	Neutropenia Peripheral blood stem cell harvest	*Allergic reaction, hypotension, tachycardia, dyspnea* Bone pain, fever, arthralgia, edema, pleural and pericardial effusion	Concomitant chemotherapy or radiation therapy (or within 24 hours before or after) Excess (>10%) leukemic myeloid blasts in the blood or bone marrow Hypersensitivity to GM-CSF or yeast-derived products	GM-CSF also causes a mild and dose-dependent increase in eosinophils

(Continued)

Drug Summary Table | **Chapter 43 Pharmacology of Hematopoiesis and Immunomodulation** (*Continued*)

Drug	Clinical Applications	Serious and Common Adverse Effects	Contraindications	Therapeutic Considerations
AGENTS THAT STIMULATE PLATELET PRODUCTION				
Mechanism—See specific drug				
Thrombopoietin analogues rhTPO PEG-rHuMGDF	Investigational agents for prevention of severe chemotherapy-induced thrombocytopenia	Investigational; theoretical risk of thrombosis	Investigational	Both rhTPO and PEG-rHuMGDF bind and activate Mpl, the endogenous receptor for thrombopoietin rhTPO is a full-length, glycosylated analogue of thrombopoietin PEG-rHuMGDF consists of the N-terminal 163 amino acids of thrombopoietin, conjugated to polyethylene glycol (PEG)
Oprelvekin (rhIL-11)	Prevention of severe chemotherapy-induced thrombocytopenia	*Fluid retention, atrial fibrillation* Oral candidiasis, conjunctival hyperemia, fatigue	Hypersensitivity to oprelvekin	Differs from natural IL-11 in that it lacks the N-terminal proline residue rhIL-11 causes a dose-dependent increase in the platelet count and in the number of megakaryocytes in the bone marrow
IMMUNOMODULATORY AGENTS WITH ANTINEOPLASTIC APPLICATIONS				
Mechanism—See specific drug				
Interferons	See Drug Summary Table: Chapter 36 Pharmacology of Viral Infections			
Levamisole	Colon cancer (in combination with 5-fluorouracil)	*Leukopenia, neutropenia, thrombocytopenia, convulsions, exfoliative dermatitis* Gastrointestinal disturbance, arthralgia, dizziness	Hypersensitivity to levamisole	Thought to cause macrophages and T cells to secrete cytokines (such as IL-1) and other factors that suppress tumor growth
IL-2	See Drug Summary Table: Chapter 44 Pharmacology of Immunosuppression			
Tretinoin	Acute promyelocytic leukemia Acne vulgaris Fine wrinkles of the face (topical)	*ATRA syndrome (fever, acute respiratory distress with pulmonary infiltrates, edema and weight gain, and multi-system organ failure), leukocytosis, pseudotumor cerebri, fever, bone pain, cardiac arrhythmias* Severe skin and mucosal dryness, hyperlipidemia, increased liver function tests, fatigue	Hypersensitivity to tretinoin or parabens	Tretinoin is an all-trans retinoic acid (ATRA) that allows differentiation of promyelocytic cells into more normal granulocytes Also used widely to treat moderate to severe acne vulgaris

44

Pharmacology of Immunosuppression

Ehrin J. Armstrong and Lloyd B. Klickstein

INTRODUCTION

Patients with autoimmune disease and patients who have received transplanted tissues or organs typically require therapy with immunosuppressive drugs. Immunosuppressive agents have been in use for more than 50 years, beginning with corticosteroids, antimetabolites, and alkylating agents. These early agents assisted in the treatment of previously incurable conditions, but their lack of specificity led to many serious adverse effects. Over the past 20 years, the field of immunosuppression has shifted to specific inhibitors of immunity that affect distinct immune pathways. This shift is important both because of the greater efficacy and reduced toxicity of these agents, and because, as the mechanisms of these agents are discovered, insights are gained into the operation of the immune system.

Case

Mrs. W is 59 years old when she undergoes heart transplantation in the spring of 1990 for heart failure resulting from chronic severe mitral valve regurgitation. Her initial immunosuppressant regimen consists of cyclosporine, glucocorticoids, and azathioprine. Progress during the first 3 months post-transplant is excellent, but then Mrs. W develops anorexia and an echocardiogram shows a significant drop in her cardiac ejection fraction. The glucocorticoid dose is increased, her ejection fraction improves, and she is discharged from the hospital.

Four months after surgery, Mrs. W is admitted to the hospital with dyspnea and fatigue. A right ventricular biopsy demonstrates evidence of moderate acute rejection, with localized areas of lymphocytic infiltration and necrosis. She is treated with a 10-day course of OKT3 (a monoclonal antibody against T cells), which produces adverse effects of fever, myalgias, nausea, and diarrhea. The patient also states, "This OKT3 makes me sleepy." Mrs. W is discharged following improvement of her cardiac status. A few months later, however, she returns to the hospital with dyspnea and fatigue. Although right ventricular biopsy shows no evidence of rejection, rejection is nonetheless suspected based on her history and symptoms. She is tested for the presence of anti-OKT3 antibodies; because no neutralizing antibodies are found, a second course of OKT3 is administered, and her symptoms abate.

In December 2000, Mrs. W arrives at the hospital for her regular annual examination. She is in good health on a baseline immunosuppressant regimen of cyclosporine, azathioprine, and glucocorticoids. There has been no evidence of rejection since 1990. Coronary angiography shows remarkably normal coronary arteries, perhaps as a result of the aggressive plasma lipid level maintenance by her physicians. However, Mrs. W's blood urea nitrogen (BUN) and creatinine levels are elevated, an indication of damage to her kidneys. Because of her kidney disease, Mrs. W's dose of cyclosporine is decreased and she is started on sirolimus. Over the next 2 years, her creatinine level remains stable, and she is able to enjoy time with her grandchildren.

QUESTIONS

■ **1.** How does each of the drugs prescribed for Mrs. W reduce the likelihood of rejection?

■ **2.** Why does Mrs. W develop fever, myalgias, nausea, and diarrhea after administration of OKT3?

■ **3.** Why is Mrs. W tested for neutralizing antibodies before receiving her second course of OKT3?

■ **4.** What is a likely cause of Mrs. W's renal disease? Why was her cyclosporine dose decreased and sirolimus added to her immunosuppressive regimen?

PATHOPHYSIOLOGY

TRANSPLANTATION

The first transplant performed successfully in humans was a kidney transplant between identical twins. No immunosuppression was used, and the individuals did well. Currently, most organ transplantation occurs between unrelated individuals. Donor and recipient tissues express different MHC class I molecules, and recipient immune cells therefore recognize the transplanted tissues as foreign. This is termed **alloimmunity,** and it occurs when the recipient's immune system attacks a transplanted organ. In the case of a bone marrow or stem cell transplant, **graft versus host disease (GVHD)** can result when donor lymphocytes mount an assault on recipient tissues.

Solid Organ Rejection

Transplant rejection of solid organs can be divided into three major phases according to the time to onset. These phases, **hyperacute, acute,** and **chronic rejection,** are caused by different mechanisms and are therefore treated differently. The following three sections examine each of these processes, and Table 44-1 summarizes their differences.

Hyperacute Rejection

Hyperacute rejection is mediated by pre-formed recipient antibodies against donor antigen. Because these antibodies are present at the time of organ implantation, hyperacute rejection occurs almost immediately after reperfusion of the transplanted organ. In fact, the surgeon can observe the changes in the organ minutes after restoration of blood flow. The normal, healthy, pink appearance of the transplanted

| TABLE 44-1 | Modes of Immune Rejection |

	HYPERACUTE REJECTION	ACUTE REJECTION	CHRONIC REJECTION
Mechanism	Preformed recipient antibodies react with donor antigen and activate complement	*Cellular*—Donor antigen activates recipient T cells *Humoral*—Recipient generates antibody response to donor antigen	Unknown but thought to be caused by chronic inflammation resulting from T-cell responses to donor antigen
Time course	Minutes to hours	Weeks to months	Months to years
How suppressed	Matching of donor and recipient blood types	Immunosuppression	Currently cannot be suppressed

organ rapidly becomes cyanotic, mottled, and flaccid. This rapid change is the result of complement activation by antibody binding to endothelial cells of the transplanted organ, resulting in thrombosis and ischemia. Most commonly, hyperacute rejection is mediated by recipient antibodies that react with blood group antigens in donor organs (e.g., type AB donor in a type O recipient). Matching of blood types between donor and recipient prevents hyperacute rejection; therefore, drug therapy for hyperacute rejection is typically not necessary. Hyperacute rejection also occurs in xenotransplantation (i.e., organ transplantation between species, such as a pig heart transplanted into a human recipient), due to the presence of pre-formed human antibodies that react against antigenic proteins and carbohydrates expressed by the donor species.

Acute Rejection

Acute rejection has cellular and humoral components. **Acute cellular rejection** is mediated by cytotoxic T cells and causes interstitial as well as vascular damage. This cellular response is most commonly seen in the initial months after transplantation. Immunosuppression of T cells is highly effective at preventing or limiting activation of the recipient immune system by the transplanted organ, thereby preventing acute cellular rejection. In **acute humoral rejection,** recipient B cells become sensitized to donor antigens in the transplanted organ and produce antibodies against these alloantigens after a period of 7 to 10 days. The antibody response is typically directed against endothelial cells and is thus also known as **acute vascular rejection.** Like acute cellular rejection, acute humoral rejection can usually be prevented by immunosuppression of the recipient after transplantation. Even with immunosuppression, however, episodes of acute rejection can occur months or even years after transplantation.

Chronic Rejection

Chronic rejection is believed to be both humoral and cellular in nature and does not occur until months or years after transplantation. Because hyperacute and acute rejection are generally well controlled by donor/recipient matching and immunosuppressive therapy, chronic rejection is now the most common life-threatening pathology associated with organ transplantation.

Chronic rejection is thought to result from chronic inflammation caused by the response of activated T cells to donor antigen. Activated T cells release cytokines that recruit macrophages into the graft. The macrophages induce chronic inflammation that leads to intimal proliferation of the vasculature and scarring of the graft tissue. The chronic changes eventually lead to irreversible organ failure. Other contributing nonimmune factors can include ischemia-reperfusion injury and infection.

No effective treatment regimens are currently available to eliminate chronic rejection. It is believed, however, that several experimental therapies have a reasonable chance of reducing chronic rejection. Especially promising is the possibility of developing tolerance through elimination of costimulation (see below).

Graft Versus Host Disease (GVHD)

Leukemia, primary immunodeficiency, and other conditions can be treated with bone marrow or peripheral stem cell transplantation. In this procedure, hematopoietic and immune function is restored after the patient's bone marrow has been eradicated by aggressive chemotherapy and/or radiation therapy. GVHD is a major complication of allogeneic bone marrow or stem cell transplantation. GVHD is an alloimmune inflammatory reaction that occurs when transplanted immune cells attack the cells of the recipient. The severity of GVHD ranges from mild to life-threatening and typically involves the skin (rash), gastrointestinal tract (diarrhea), lungs (pneumonitis), and liver (veno-occlusive disease). GVHD can often be ameliorated by removing T cells from the donor bone marrow before transplantation. Mild-to-moderate GVHD can also be beneficial when donor immune cells attack recipient tumor cells that have survived the aggressive chemotherapy and radiation therapy. (In the case of leukemia, this is called the **graft versus leukemia effect**, or **GVL**.) Therefore, although removing donor T cells from the ''graft'' reduces the risk of GVHD, this may not be the best approach for marrow transplants used in antineoplastic therapy.

AUTOIMMUNITY

Autoimmune diseases occur when the host immune system attacks its own tissues, mistaking self-antigen for foreign. The typical result is chronic inflammation in the tissue(s) expressing the antigen.

Autoimmune diseases are most commonly due to a breakdown of self-tolerance, both central and peripheral. **Central tolerance** refers to the specific clonal deletion of autoreactive T and B cells during their development from precursor cells in the thymus and bone marrow. Central tolerance ensures that the majority of immature autoreactive T and B cells do not develop into self-reactive clones. The thymus and bone marrow do not express every antigen in the body, however; a number of proteins are expressed only in specific tissues. For this reason, **peripheral tolerance** is also important. Peripheral tolerance results from deletion of autoreactive T cells by Fas-Fas ligand-mediated apoptosis, activation of T suppressor cells, or induction of T-cell anergy due to antigen presentation in the absence of costimulation.

Although breakdown in tolerance lies at the center of virtually all autoimmune diseases, the inciting stimulus leading to loss of tolerance is often unknown. Genetic factors may play a role, in that the presence of certain MHC subtypes may predispose T cells to the loss of self-tolerance. For example, human leukocyte antigen (HLA)-B27 is causally related to many forms of autoimmune spondylitis. Several other autoimmune diseases are linked to specific HLA loci, supporting an association, if not a causal role, for genetic predisposition to autoimmunity. **Molecular mimicry,** whereby epitopes from infectious agents are similar to self antigens, can also lead to a breakdown of tolerance and may be the mechanism underlying poststreptococcal glomerulonephritis. A number of other processes, including failure of T-cell apoptosis, polyclonal lymphocyte activation, and exposure of cryptic self-antigens, have also been hypothesized to lead to autoimmunity. The details of these mechanisms are beyond the scope of this book; however, the result of each is a *loss of tolerance.*

Once self-tolerance has been compromised, the specific expression of autoimmunity can take one of three general forms (Table 44-2). In some diseases, production of autoantibodies against a specific antigen causes antibody-dependent opsonization of cells in the target organ, with subsequent cytotoxicity. One example is Goodpasture's syndrome, which results from autoantibodies against collagen type IV in the renal glomerular basement membrane. In some autoimmune vasculitis syndromes, circulating antibody-antigen complexes deposit in blood vessels, causing inflammation and injury to the vessels. Two examples of immune-complex disease are mixed essential cryoglobulinemia and systemic lupus erythematosus. Finally, T-cell–mediated diseases are caused by cytotoxic T cells that react with a specific self-antigen, resulting in destruction of the tissue(s) expressing that antigen. One example is type I diabetes mellitus, in which the cytotoxic T cells react against self-antigens in pancreatic β cells.

The pharmacologic therapy for autoimmune diseases does not yet match the exquisite specificity of the offending biological process. Most currently available pharmacologic agents cause generalized immunosuppression and do not target the specific pathophysiology. Better understanding of the molecular pathways leading to autoimmune diseases should reveal new pharmacologic targets that can be used to suppress the specific autoimmune response before disease arises.

PHARMACOLOGIC CLASSES AND AGENTS

Pharmacologic suppression of the immune system utilizes eight mechanistic approaches (Fig. 44-1):
1. Inhibition of gene expression to modulate inflammatory responses
2. Depletion of expanding lymphocyte populations with cytotoxic agents
3. Inhibition of lymphocyte signaling to block activation and expansion of lymphocytes
4. Neutralization of cytokines essential for mediating the immune response
5. Depletion of specific immune cells, usually via cell-specific antibodies
6. Blockade of costimulation to induce anergy

TABLE 44-2	Representative Examples of Autoimmune Diseases, Categorized by Type of Tissue Damage

ANTIBODY TO SELF-ANTIGEN		
SYNDROME	**AUTOANTIGEN**	**CONSEQUENCE**
Acute rheumatic fever	Streptococcal cell wall antigens that cross-react with cardiac muscle	Arthritis, myocarditis
Autoimmune hemolytic anemia	Rh blood group antigens	Destruction of erythrocytes
Goodpasture's syndrome	Renal glomerular basement membrane collagen type IV	Glomerulonephritis, pulmonary hemorrhage
Immune thrombocytopenic purpura	Platelet GPIIb:IIIa	Excessive bleeding
Pemphigus vulgaris	Epidermal cadherin	Blistering of skin

IMMUNE-COMPLEX DISEASE		
SYNDROME	**AUTOANTIGEN**	**CONSEQUENCE**
Mixed essential cryoglobulinemia	Rheumatoid factor IgG complexes	Systemic vasculitis
Systemic lupus erythematosus	DNA, histones, ribosomes, snRNP, scRNP	Glomerulonephritis, vasculitis, arthritis

T-CELL MEDIATED DISEASE		
SYNDROME	**AUTOANTIGEN**	**CONSEQUENCE**
Experimental autoimmune encephalitis, multiple sclerosis	Myelin basic protein, proteolipid protein, myelin oligodendrocyte glycoprotein	Brain invasion by CD4 T cells, several CNS deficits
Rheumatoid arthritis	Unknown—possible synovial joint antigens	Joint inflammation and destruction
Type I diabetes mellitus	Pancreatic β-cell antigens	β-cell destruction, insulin-dependent diabetes mellitus

Rh, Rhesus factor; DNA, deoxyribonucleic acid; IgG, immunoglobulin G; CNS, central nervous system; snRNP, small nuclear ribonucleoprotein; scRNP, small cytoplasmic ribonucleoprotein.

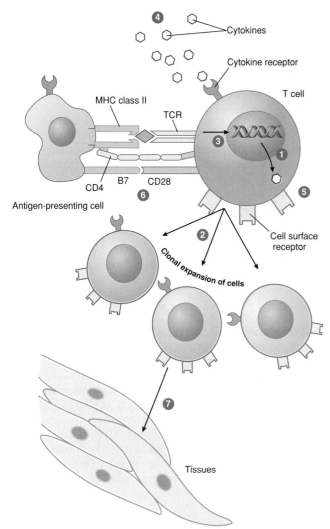

Figure 44-1. Overview of mechanisms of pharmacologic immunosuppression. The molecular mechanisms by which immune cells are activated and function provide eight major points for pharmacologic intervention by immunosuppressive agents. Blockade of T-cell activation can be accomplished by (1) inhibition of gene expression; (2) selective attack on clonally expanding lymphocyte populations; (3) inhibition of intracellular signaling; (4) neutralization of cytokines required for T-cell stimulation; (5) selective depletion of T cells (or other immune cells); (6) inhibition of costimulation by antigen-presenting cells; and (7) inhibition of lymphocyte–target-cell interactions. Suppression of innate immune cells and complement activation may also block the initiation of immune responses *(not shown).*

7. Blockade of cell adhesion to prevent migration and homing of inflammatory cells
8. Inhibition of innate immunity, including complement activation

INHIBITORS OF GENE EXPRESSION

Glucocorticoids

Glucocorticoids have broad anti-inflammatory effects. The intimate relationship between cortisol and the immune sys-

tem is discussed in Chapter 27, Pharmacology of the Adrenal Cortex. Briefly, glucocorticoids are steroid hormones that exert their physiologic actions by binding to the cytosolic glucocorticoid receptor. The glucocorticoid-glucocorticoid receptor complex translocates to the nucleus and binds to glucocorticoid response elements (GREs) in the promoter region of specific genes, either up-regulating or down-regulating gene expression.

Glucocorticoids have important metabolic effects on essentially all cells of the body, and in pharmacologic doses suppress the activation and function of innate and adaptive immune cells. Glucocorticoids down-regulate expression of many inflammatory mediators, including key cytokines such as TNF-α, interleukin-1 (IL-1), and IL-4. The role of glucocorticoids in suppressing eicosanoid biosynthesis and signaling is discussed in Chapter 41, Pharmacology of Eicosanoids. The overall effect of glucocorticoid administration is profoundly anti-inflammatory and immunosuppressive, explaining the use of glucocorticoids for the treatment of numerous inflammatory diseases such as rheumatoid arthritis and transplant rejection.

Long-term glucocorticoid administration has important adverse effects. *Diabetes, reduced resistance to infection, osteoporosis, cataracts, increased appetite leading to weight gain, hypertension and its sequelae, as well as the masking of inflammation* must be closely monitored in patients receiving glucocorticoids. *Abrupt cessation of glucocorticoid therapy can result in acute adrenal insufficiency* because the hypothalamus and pituitary gland require a number of weeks to months to re-establish adequate ACTH production. During this time, the underlying disease can worsen because of disinhibition of the immune system. To prevent the latter complications, glucocorticoid dosage should be tapered slowly as therapy is terminated.

CYTOTOXIC AGENTS

Cytotoxic agents are used for immunosuppression as well as for antineoplastic chemotherapy. Two classes of cytotoxic agents, **antimetabolites** and **alkylating agents,** are commonly used as immunosuppressants. Antimetabolites are structural analogues of natural metabolites that inhibit essential pathways involving these metabolites. Alkylating agents interfere with DNA replication and gene expression by conjugating alkyl groups to DNA. The therapeutic goal in both antineoplastic chemotherapy and immunosuppression is the elimination of undesirable cells.

Antimetabolites

For many years, antimetabolites have been a mainstay of immunosuppressive treatment. Their powerful effect on immunity is accompanied by many adverse effects related to their lack of specificity. The older antimetabolites, such as azathioprine and methotrexate, affect all rapidly dividing cells and can have damaging effects on the gastrointestinal mucosa and bone marrow as well as their intended immune targets. Newer antimetabolites, such as **mycophenolate mofetil** and **leflunomide**, cause fewer adverse effects and can be used therapeutically at lower doses. Mycophenolate mofetil may also be more specific for immune cells, further reducing its toxicity. Antimetabolites typically affect both cell-mediated and humoral immunity, rendering patients more susceptible to infection than would occur if only one of these systems were affected.

Antimetabolites are widely used in the treatment of cancer, and the underlying principles of their mechanisms are described in Chapter 37, Pharmacology of Cancer: Genome Synthesis, Stability, and Maintenance. Anti-inflammatory aspects of their mechanisms are briefly described below although Chapter 37 provides a more detailed description of their mechanisms of action.

Azathioprine

Azathioprine (AZA) was the first drug to be used for suppression of the immune system after transplantation, and it remains a mainstay for this indication. AZA is a prodrug of the purine analogue 6-mercaptopurine (6-MP), which is slowly released as AZA reacts nonenzymatically with sulfhydryl compounds such as glutathione (Fig. 44-2). *The slow release of 6-MP from AZA favors immunosuppression, while 6-MP itself is more useful as an antineoplastic drug.*

Although AZA does prolong organ graft survival, this drug is less efficacious than mycophenolate mofetil in improving the long-term survival of kidney allografts. AZA is also used as an immunosuppressant for patients with inflammatory bowel disease.

Methotrexate

Methotrexate (MTX) is a folate analogue used since the 1950s to treat malignancies. Since that time, methotrexate has also become an extremely versatile drug in treating a wide variety of immune-mediated diseases, including rheumatoid arthritis and psoriasis. In addition, MTX is used for the prevention of graft versus host disease.

MTX appears to have anti-inflammatory activity that is independent of its cytotoxic action. The mechanism by which MTX exerts its anti-inflammatory effect is uncertain, but does not appear to involve depletion of folate pools because the combination of MTX and folate is as effective as MTX alone in the treatment of rheumatoid arthritis. MTX may act as an anti-inflammatory agent by increasing adenosine levels. Adenosine is a potent endogenous anti-inflammatory mediator that inhibits neutrophil adhesion, phagocytosis, and superoxide generation.

MTX has also been shown to cause apoptosis of activated CD4 and CD8 T cells, but not of resting cells. Other immunosuppressive agents, including 5-fluorouracil, 6-mercaptopurine, and mycophenolic acid, also promote apoptosis. MTX may be such a versatile drug because of its combined antineutrophil, anti-T-cell, and antihumoral effects.

Mycophenolic Acid and Mycophenolate Mofetil

Mycophenolic acid (MPA) is an inhibitor of inosine monophosphate dehydrogenase (IMPDH), the rate-limiting enzyme in the formation of guanosine. Because MPA has low oral bioavailability, it is usually administered in its prodrug form, **mycophenolate mofetil (MMF),** which has much higher oral bioavailability (Fig. 44-3). MMF is increasingly used in the treatment of immune-mediated disease because of its high specificity and profound effect on lymphocytes.

MPA and MMF both act primarily on lymphocytes. Two main factors contribute to this specificity. First, as discussed in Chapter 37, lymphocytes are dependent on the de novo

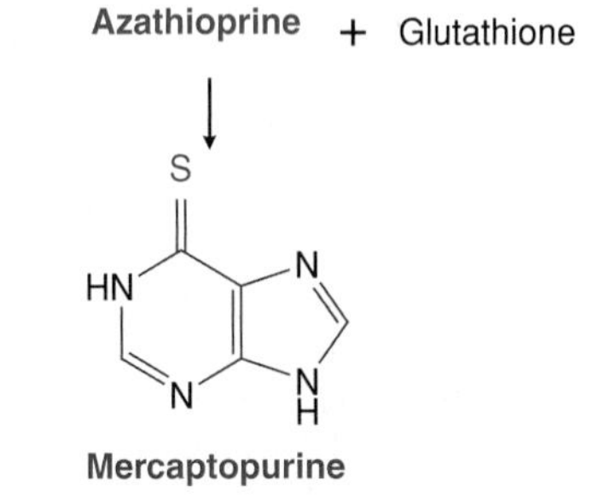

Figure 44-2. Formation of mercaptopurine from azathioprine. Azathioprine is a prodrug form of the antimetabolite 6-mercaptopurine. Mercaptopurine is formed by the cleavage of azathioprine in a nonenzymatic reaction with glutathione. Although mercaptopurine can also be used directly as a cytotoxic agent, azathioprine has a longer duration of action and is more immunosuppressive than mercaptopurine.

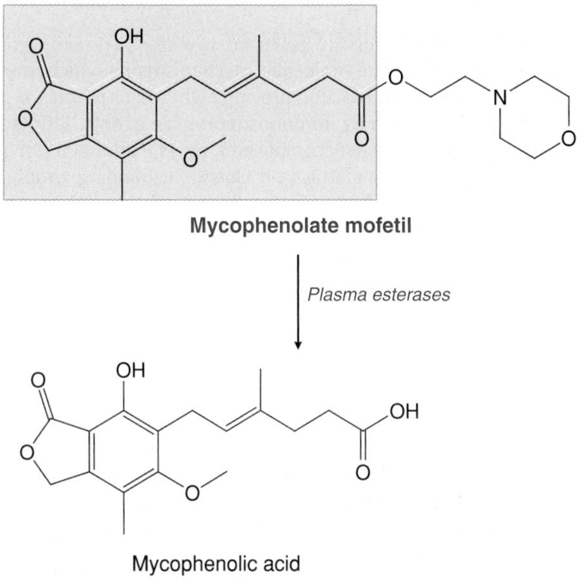

Figure 44-3. Mycophenolic acid and mycophenolate mofetil. Mycophenolate mofetil (MMF) has higher oral bioavailability than mycophenolic acid (MPA). Orally administered mycophenolate mofetil is absorbed into the circulation, where plasma esterases rapidly cleave the ester bond to yield mycophenolic acid. Both agents inhibit inosine monophosphate dehydrogenase type II (IMPDH II), an enzyme crucial for de novo synthesis of guanosine. Because of its higher oral bioavailability, MMF is typically used.

pathway of purine synthesis, whereas most other tissues rely heavily on the salvage pathway. Because IMPDH is required for de novo synthesis of guanosine nucleotides but not for the salvage pathway, MPA affects only cells such as lymphocytes that rely on de novo purine synthesis. Second, IMPDH is expressed in two isoforms, type I and type II. MPA preferentially inhibits type II IMPDH, the isoform expressed mainly in lymphocytes. Together, these factors confer on MPA and MMF selectivity against T and B cells, with low toxicity to other cells.

Inhibition of IMPDH by MPA reduces intracellular guanosine levels and elevates intracellular adenosine levels, with many downstream effects on lymphocyte activation and activity. MPA has a cytostatic effect on lymphocytes, but can also induce apoptosis of activated T cells leading to the elimination of reactive lines of proliferative cells. Because guanosine is required for some glycosylation reactions, the reduction in guanosine nucleotides leads to decreased expression of adhesion molecules that are required for recruitment of several immune cell types to sites of inflammation. Furthermore, because guanosine is a precursor of tetrahydrobiopterin (BH4), which regulates inducible nitric oxide synthase (iNOS), the reduction in guanosine levels leads to decreased NO production by neutrophils. Endothelial NOS (eNOS), which controls vascular tone and is regulated by Ca^{2+} and calmodulin, is not affected by changes in guanosine levels, again demonstrating the considerable specificity of MPA.

Clinical studies comparing MMF and AZA have shown MMF to be more efficacious in preventing acute rejection of kidney transplants. Animal models show that chronic rejection is also reduced more effectively in recipients treated with MMF than in those treated with AZA or cyclosporine. The efficacy of MMF in treating chronic rejection may be related to its inhibition of both the lymphocyte and smooth muscle cell proliferation characteristic of chronic rejection.

MMF is also efficacious in the treatment of autoimmune disease. In rheumatoid arthritis, levels of rheumatoid factor, immunoglobulin, and T cells are reduced by treatment with MMF. MMF is frequently used in the initial therapy of lupus nephritis. There have also been isolated reports of successful treatment of myasthenia gravis, psoriasis, autoimmune hemolytic anemia, and inflammatory bowel disease with MMF.

Leflunomide

Activated lymphocytes must both proliferate and synthesize large quantities of cytokines and other effector molecules, processes requiring increased DNA and RNA synthesis. Therefore, agents that reduce intracellular nucleotides have effects on these activated cells. **Leflunomide** is an inhibitor of pyrimidine synthesis, specifically blocking the synthesis of uridylate (UMP) by inhibiting dihydroorotate dehydrogenase (DHOD). DHOD is a key enzyme in the synthesis of UMP (Fig. 44-4), which is essential for the synthesis of all pyrimidines. (See Chapter 37 for a review of pyrimidine synthesis.) Experimentally, leflunomide has been shown to be most effective in reducing B-cell populations, but a significant effect on T cells has also been observed.

Leflunomide is currently approved for rheumatoid arthritis, but the drug has also shown significant efficacy in the

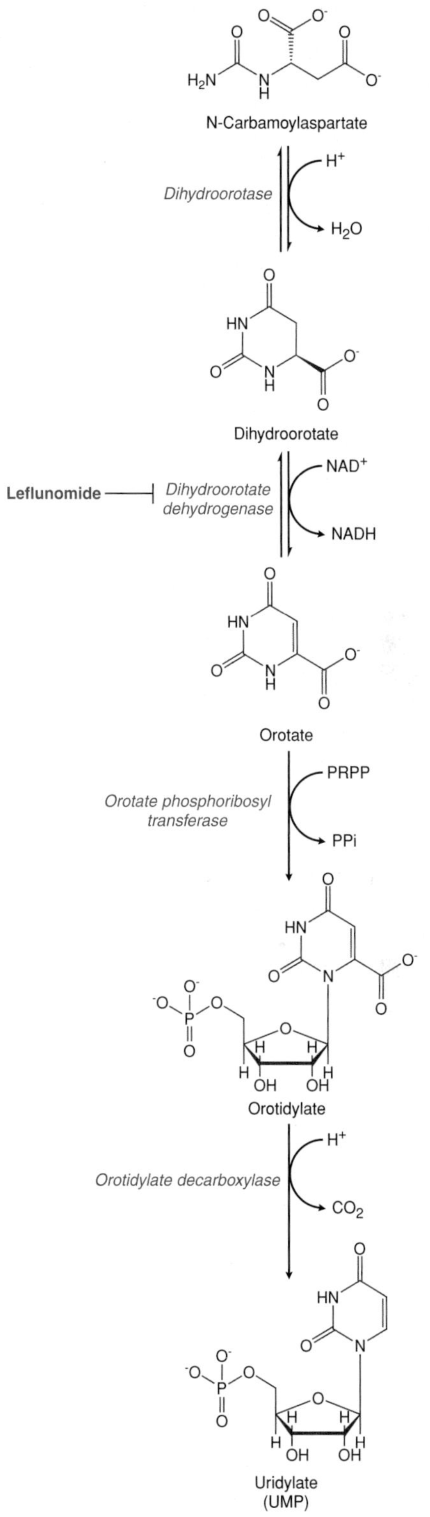

Figure 44-4. Inhibition of pyrimidine synthesis by leflunomide. De novo pyrimidine synthesis depends on the oxidation of dihydroorotate to orotate, a reaction that is catalyzed by dihydroorotate dehydrogenase. Leflunomide inhibits dihydroorotate dehydrogenase and thereby inhibits pyrimidine synthesis. Because lymphocytes are dependent on de novo pyrimidine synthesis for cell replication and clonal expansion after immune-cell activation, depletion of the pyrimidine pool inhibits lymphocyte expansion. Experimentally, leflunomide appears to inhibit preferentially the replication of B cells; the reason for this preferential action is unknown.

treatment of other immune diseases, including Wegener's granulomatosis, systemic lupus erythematosus, and myasthenia gravis. Leflunomide prolongs transplant graft survival and limits GVHD in animal models.

The most significant adverse effects of leflunomide are diarrhea and reversible alopecia. Leflunomide undergoes significant enterohepatic circulation, resulting in a prolonged pharmacologic effect. If leflunomide must be removed quickly from a patient's system, cholestyramine may be administered. By binding to bile acids, cholestyramine interrupts the enterohepatic circulation and causes a "washout" of leflunomide.

Alkylating Agents

Cyclophosphamide

Cyclophosphamide (Cy) is a highly toxic drug that alkylates DNA. The mechanism of action and uses of Cy are discussed extensively in Chapter 37; therefore, the discussion here is limited to Cy's utility in treating diseases of the immune system. Because Cy has a major effect on B-cell proliferation but can enhance T-cell responses, the use of Cy in immune diseases is limited to disorders of humoral immunity, particularly systemic lupus erythematosus. Another use under consideration for Cy is the suppression of antibody formation against xenotransplant grafts. Adverse effects of Cy are severe and widespread, including leukopenia, cardiotoxicity, alopecia, and an increased risk of cancer because of mutagenicity. The risk of bladder cancer is especially notable because Cy produces a carcinogenic metabolite, **acrolein**, which is concentrated in the urine. When high-dose Cy is administered by intravenous infusion, acrolein can be detoxified by coadministration of **mesna** (a sulfhydryl-containing compound that neutralizes the reactive moiety of acrolein).

SPECIFIC LYMPHOCYTE-SIGNALING INHIBITORS

Cyclosporine and Tacrolimus

The discovery in 1976 that **cyclosporine** (CsA; also referred to as *cyclosporin A*) is a specific inhibitor of T-cell–mediated immunity enabled widespread whole-organ transplantation. In fact, CsA made heart transplantation a legitimate alternative in the treatment of end-stage heart failure. CsA is a decapeptide isolated from a soil fungus, *Tolypocladium inflatum.*

CsA inhibits the production of IL-2 by activated T cells. IL-2 is an important cytokine that acts in an autocrine and paracrine manner to cause activation and proliferation of T cells (Fig. 44-5). Activated T cells increase their production of IL-2 via a pathway that begins with dephosphorylation of a cytoplasmic transcription factor, **NFAT** (nuclear factor of activated T cells). NFAT is dephosphorylated by the cytoplasmic phosphatase **calcineurin.** Upon dephosphorylation, NFAT translocates to the nucleus and enhances transcription of the IL-2 gene. CsA acts by binding to **cyclophilin**, and the CsA-cyclophilin complex binds to calcineurin and inhibits its phosphatase activity. By inhibiting calcineurin-mediated NFAT dephosphorylation, CsA prevents translocation of NFAT to the nucleus and thereby suppresses IL-2 production.

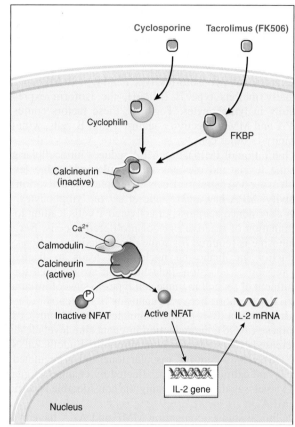

Figure 44-5. Mechanisms of action of cyclosporine and tacrolimus. The actions of cyclosporine and tacrolimus (also known as FK506) are mediated by blockade of intracellular T-cell signaling. In normal T-cell signaling **(bottom),** stimulation of T cells increases the level of intracellular calcium, and Ca^{2+}/calmodulin activates the calcineurin-mediated dephosphorylation of the cytoplasmic transcription factor NFAT. Activated NFAT translocates to the nucleus, where it induces IL-2 gene transcription. Cyclosporine and tacrolimus cross the plasma membrane and bind to the cytoplasmic immunophilins cyclophilin and FK-binding protein (FKBP), respectively **(top).** Both the cyclosporine-cyclophilin and tacrolimus-FKBP complexes bind to calcineurin, preventing the activation of calcineurin phosphatase activity by Ca^{2+}/calmodulin.

CsA is approved for use in organ transplantation, psoriasis, and rheumatoid arthritis. CsA is also used occasionally in the treatment of rare autoimmune diseases not responsive to other immunosuppressants. An ophthalmic preparation of CsA is approved for the treatment of chronic dry eyes.

The usefulness of CsA is limited by severe adverse effects, which include *nephrotoxicity, hypertension, hyperlipidemia, neurotoxicity, and hepatotoxicity.* Cyclosporine nephrotoxicity is the probable reason for Mrs. W's chronic kidney disease. The mechanism of CsA toxicity appears to relate to its stimulation of transforming growth factor-β (TGF-β) production. TGF-β causes cells to increase their production of extracellular matrix, resulting in interstitial fibrosis.

Tacrolimus (also known as FK506) is a more potent immunosuppressant drug than CsA; although its structure differs from that of CsA, it acts by a similar mechanism (Fig. 44-5). Tacrolimus is a macrocyclic triene isolated from the soil bacterium *Streptomyces tsukubaensis.* Tacrolimus acts by binding to FK-binding proteins (**FKBP**), and the tacrolimus–FKBP complex inhibits calcineurin. Tacrolimus inhibits IL-3, IL-4, IFN-γ, and TNF-α production in vitro, and it appears to inhibit cell-mediated immunity without suppressing B cell or natural killer (NK) cell function. Tacrolimus is generally 50 to 100 times more potent than CsA, but, like CsA, it is nephrotoxic.

Tacrolimus is approved as an immunosuppressant for transplantation. A topical formulation is used for the treatment of atopic dermatitis and other eczematous diseases.

Sirolimus

Sirolimus, also referred to as *rapamycin,* is a macrocyclic triene isolated from the soil bacterium *Streptomyces hygroscopicus.* Although they are structurally similar and are both used to prevent and treat organ rejection, tacrolimus and sirolimus have different mechanisms of action. Both bind to FKBP, but the sirolimus-FKBP complex does not inhibit calcineurin; instead, it blocks the IL-2 receptor signaling required for T-cell proliferation (Fig. 44-6). Sirolimus-

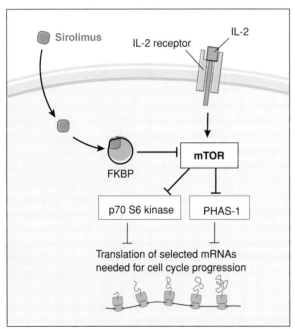

Figure 44-6. Mechanism of action of sirolimus. IL-2 receptor signal transduction involves a complex set of protein-protein interactions that lead to increased translation of selected mRNAs encoding proteins required for T-cell proliferation. Specifically, IL-2 receptor activation initiates an intracellular signaling cascade that leads to phosphorylation of the molecular target of rapamycin (mTOR). mTOR is a kinase that phosphorylates and thereby regulates the activity of PHAS-1 and p70 S6 kinase. PHAS-1 inhibits the activity of a factor (eiF4E) required for translation, and p70 S6 kinase phosphorylates proteins involved in protein synthesis *(not shown).* The net effect of mTOR activation is to increase protein synthesis, thereby promoting the transition from G1 to S phase of the cell cycle. Sirolimus (also known as rapamycin) crosses the plasma membrane and binds to intracellular FK-binding protein (FKBP). The sirolimus-FKBP complex inhibits mTOR, thereby inhibiting translation and causing T cells to arrest in G1.

FKBP binds to and inhibits molecular target of rapamycin (mTOR), a serine-threonine kinase that phosphorylates p70 S6 kinase and PHAS-1 (among other substrates). p70 S6 kinase and PHAS-1 regulate translation, the former by phosphorylating proteins (including the ribosomal S6 protein) involved in protein synthesis and the latter by inhibiting the activity of a factor (eiF4E) required for translation. By inhibiting mTOR, sirolimus-FKBP inhibits protein synthesis and arrests cell division in the G1 phase (Fig. 44-6). Major adverse effects of sirolimus include hyperlipidemia, leukopenia, and thrombocytopenia. Notably, however, the nephrotoxicity associated with CsA and tacrolimus is not observed with sirolimus. This was the rationale for adding sirolimus to Mrs. W's immunosuppressive regimen after she developed nephrotoxicity from cyclosporine.

Sirolimus-eluting stents have been approved for use in the treatment of coronary artery disease. In this unique drug delivery system, sirolimus elutes from stents during the first few weeks after stent placement, locally inhibiting proliferation of coronary artery smooth muscle cells and thereby reducing the rate of in-stent restenosis that results from neointimal proliferation of vascular smooth muscle cells.

CYTOKINE INHIBITION

Cytokines are critical signaling mediators in immune function. Cytokines are also pleiotropic; that is, they exert different effects depending on the target cell and overall cytokine milieu. For this reason, pharmacologic uses of cytokines or cytokine inhibitors may have unpredictable effects. Anticytokine therapy is still in its infancy, and a number of new drugs that inhibit proinflammatory cytokines are under development.

TNF-α Inhibitors

Tumor necrosis factor-α (TNF-α) is a cytokine central to many aspects of the inflammatory response. Macrophages, mast cells, and activated T$_H$ cells (especially T$_H$1 cells) secrete TNF-α. TNF-α stimulates macrophages to produce cytotoxic metabolites, thereby increasing phagocytic killing activity. TNF-α also stimulates production of acute-phase proteins, has pyrogenic effects, and fosters local containment of the inflammatory response. Some of these effects are indirect and are mediated by other cytokines induced by TNF-α.

TNF-α has been implicated in numerous autoimmune diseases. Rheumatoid arthritis, psoriasis, and Crohn's disease are three disorders in which inhibition of TNF-α has demonstrated therapeutic efficacy. Rheumatoid arthritis illustrates the central role of TNF-α in the pathophysiology of autoimmune diseases (Fig. 44-7). Although the initial stimulus for joint inflammation is still debated, it is thought that macrophages in a diseased joint secrete TNF-α, which activates endothelial cells, other monocytes, and synovial fibroblasts. Activated endothelial cells up-regulate adhesion molecule expression, resulting in recruitment of inflammatory cells to the joint. Monocyte activation has a positive feedback effect on T-cell and synovial fibroblast activation. Activated synovial fibroblasts secrete interleukins, which recruit additional inflammatory cells. With time, the synovium hypertrophies

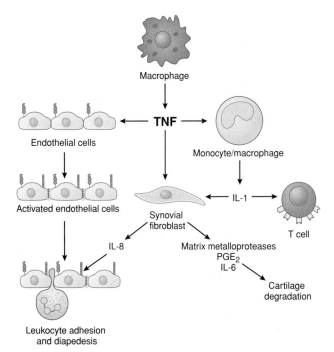

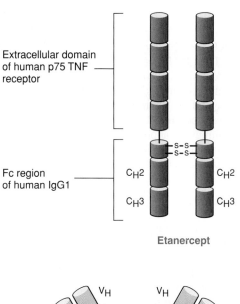

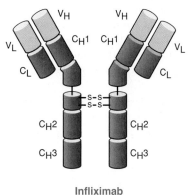

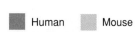

Figure 44-7. Proposed roles for tumor necrosis factor in rheumatoid arthritis. Tumor necrosis factor (TNF) is secreted by activated macrophages in an affected joint, where this cytokine has multiple proinflammatory effects. First, TNF activates endothelial cells to up-regulate their expression of cell surface adhesion molecules *(shown as projections on endothelial cells)* and undergo other phenotypic changes that promote leukocyte adhesion and diapedesis. Second, TNF has a positive feedback effect on nearby monocytes and macrophages, promoting their secretion of cytokines such as IL-1. In turn, IL-1 activates T cells (among other functions), and the combination of IL-1 and TNF stimulates synovial fibroblasts to increase their expression of matrix metalloproteases, prostaglandins (especially PGE$_2$), and cytokines (such as IL-6) that degrade the joint cartilage. Synovial fibroblasts also secrete IL-8, which promotes neutrophil diapedesis.

Figure 44-8. Anti-TNF agents. Shown is the molecular domain organization of etanercept and infliximab. Etanercept consists of the extracellular domain of the human TNF receptor fused to the F$_c$ region of human IgG1. This "decoy" receptor binds TNF-α and TNF-β in the circulation, preventing the access of these cytokines to target tissues. Infliximab is a partially humanized monoclonal antibody against TNF-α. The variable heavy chain *(V$_H$)* and variable light chain *(V$_L$)* regions are derived from mouse antihuman sequences, while the remainder of the antibody *(the constant regions, denoted by C$_H$ and C$_L$)* is composed of human antibody sequences. This modification of the original mouse monoclonal anti-TNF-α antibody reduces the development of neutralizing antibodies against infliximab. Adalimumab *(not shown)*, a fully humanized antibody against human TNF-α, has recently been developed.

and forms a pannus that leads to destruction of bone and cartilage in the joint, causing the characteristic deformity and pain of rheumatoid arthritis.

Three therapies interfering with TNF-α activity have been approved. **Etanercept** is a soluble TNF receptor dimer; **infliximab** is a partially humanized mouse antibody against human TNF-α; **adalimumab** is a fully humanized IgG1 antibody against TNF-α (Fig. 44-8). **Certolizumab** pegol, a pegylated anti-TNF-α antibody fragment lacking the F$_c$ portion of the antibody, is currently in late-stage clinical trials.

Although all of these agents target TNF-α, etanercept is somewhat less specific because it binds to both TNF-α and TNF-β. Infliximab and adalimumab are TNF-α–specific and do not bind TNF-β. The F$_c$ portions of infliximab and adalimumab may also have specific activity with respect to complement fixation and binding to F$_c$ receptors on effector cells.

Etanercept is approved for use in rheumatoid arthritis, juvenile rheumatoid arthritis, plaque psoriasis, psoriatic arthritis, and ankylosing spondylitis; infliximab is approved for use in rheumatoid arthritis, Crohn's disease, ulcerative colitis, and ankylosing spondylitis; and adalimumab is approved for use in rheumatoid arthritis and psoriatic arthritis.

It is important to recognize that high levels of TNF-α

are likely markers of underlying pathophysiologic processes. Treatment with etanercept, infliximab, or adalimumab improves disease symptoms but does not reverse the underlying pathophysiology. Therefore, the long-term efficacy of these therapies may be limited. In addition, etanercept, infliximab, and adalimumab are proteins and must be administered parenterally. Orally active inhibitors of TNF-α, such as **thalidomide**, and inhibitors of TNF-α converting enzyme (TACE) are under investigation.

A number of important adverse effects must be considered when administering TNF inhibitors. All patients should undergo screening for tuberculosis before initiating therapy because of a greatly increased risk of reactivating latent tuberculosis. Any patient developing an infection while taking a TNF-α inhibitor should undergo evaluation and aggressive antibiotic treatment. Epidemiologic surveillance has also suggested that there may be an increased risk of demyelinating disease with anti-TNF therapy, although it has not yet been determined whether the relationship is causal.

IL-1 Inhibitors

Interleukin-1 (IL-1) is an ancient cytokine, expressed in both vertebrates and invertebrates, that serves as a bridge between innate and adaptive immunity. Two forms of IL-1, IL-1α and IL-1β, are encoded on different genes. Most IL-1 is generated by activated mononuclear cells. IL-1 stimulates IL-6 production, enhances adhesion molecule expression, and stimulates cell proliferation. Modulation of IL-1 activity in vivo is accomplished in part by an endogenous IL-1 receptor antagonist (IL-1ra).

Anakinra, a recombinant form of IL-1ra, is approved for use in rheumatoid arthritis. Anakinra has modest effects on pain and swelling but significantly reduces bony erosions, possibly because it decreases osteoclast production and blocks IL-1–induced metalloproteinase release from synovial cells. A number of rare syndromes mediated in part by increased levels of IL-1, including Muckle-Wells syndrome and Hibernian fever, have also been treated effectively with anakinra. Anakinra may cause neutropenia and increase susceptibility to infection.

DEPLETION OF SPECIFIC IMMUNE CELLS

A number of antibodies deplete the immune system of reactive cells and thereby provide effective therapy for autoimmune diseases and transplant rejection. When the adaptive immune system reacts to an antigen, the resulting immunologic response includes the clonal expansion of cells specifically reactive against that antigen. Treatment with exogenous antibodies against cell-surface molecules that are expressed specifically on reactive immune cells can preferentially deplete the immune system of these reactive cells. Antibodies that target cell-surface receptors expressed specifically on malignant immune cells are discussed in Chapter 38, Pharmacology of Cancer: Signal Transduction.

Polyclonal Antibodies

Anti-thymocyte Globulin

Anti-thymocyte globulin (ATG) is a preparation of antibodies induced by injecting rabbits with human thymocytes. The rabbit antibodies are polyclonal and probably target many epitopes on human T cells. Because ATG targets essentially all T cells, ATG treatment results in broad immunosuppression that can predispose to infection. ATG is approved for use in acute renal transplant rejection and is administered intravenously over 1 to 2 weeks.

ATG therapy is often complicated by fever and headache as prominent components of the **cytokine release syndrome.** This syndrome, common to many antibody drugs that target lymphocytes, results from activation of T cells and release of T-cell cytokines before the antibody-coated T cells can be cleared by macrophages. The cytokine release syndrome typically occurs after the first few doses of ATG therapy, and the symptoms dissipate as T cells are eliminated. However, administration of successive ATG doses can be complicated by the development of antibodies against rabbit-specific epitopes on the administered immunoglobulins.

Monoclonal Antibodies

OKT3

OKT3 (muromonab-CD3, anti-CD3) is a mouse monoclonal antibody against human CD3, one of the cell-surface signaling molecules important for activation of the T-cell receptor. CD3 is specifically expressed on T cells (both CD4 and CD8 cells). Treatment with OKT3 depletes the available pool of T cells via antibody-mediated activation of complement and clearance of immune complexes. OKT3 is approved for use in acute renal transplant rejection and is considered a second-line agent for use when CsA or glucocorticoids fail.

Because OKT3 targets all T cells, OKT3 treatment can result in profound immunosuppression; however, the immunosuppression is transient and T-cell levels return to normal within a week after discontinuing therapy. Also, because OKT3 binds to CD3, and CD3 is important for T-cell activation, OKT3 therapy can sometimes broadly activate T cells resulting in the cytokine release syndrome. In the introductory case, the fever, myalgias, nausea, and diarrhea after administration of OKT3, as well as Mrs. W's complaint that "this OKT3 makes me sleepy," were likely manifestations of the cytokine release syndrome.

Another limitation is that OKT3 is a mouse–anti-human antibody. Because the mouse antibody is foreign, OKT3 treatment can induce the production of antibodies against the mouse-specific regions of OKT3. This is why Mrs. W was tested for anti-OKT3 antibodies when she returned to the hospital in December 1990. The presence of anti-OKT3 antibodies would reduce drug efficacy by sequestering OKT3 before it could exert its desired effect. To solve this clinical problem, a current approach is to **humanize** therapeutic antibodies. In this approach, the portions of the antibody not involved in binding to the antigen are changed to the corresponding human sequences. Antibodies can be partially or fully humanized, depending on the extent of these changes. Humanization limits the likelihood of production of human antibodies against the therapeutic antibody, increasing the clinical effectiveness of the antibody and allowing its long-term use (see Chapter 53, Protein-Based Therapies).

Anti-CD20 mAb

Rituximab is a partially humanized anti-CD20 antibody. CD20 is expressed on the surface of all mature B cells, and administration of rituximab causes profound depletion of circulating B cells. Originally approved for the treatment of CD20$^+$ non-Hodgkin's lymphoma (see Chapter 38), rituximab has also been approved for use in rheumatoid arthritis refractory to TNF-α inhibitors.

Anti-CD25 mAb

Daclizumab and **basiliximab** are antibodies against CD25, the high-affinity IL-2 receptor. IL-2 mediates early steps in T-cell activation. Because CD25 is expressed only on activated T cells, anti-CD25 antibody therapy specifically targets T cells that have been activated by an MHC-antigen stimulus.

Daclizumab is administered prophylactically in renal transplantation to inhibit acute organ rejection. It is also used as a component of general immunosuppressive regimens after organ transplantation. Daclizumab is typically administered in a five-dose regimen, with the first administration immediately after transplantation and then four additional doses at two-week intervals. This type of dosing regimen, in which drug is administered for only a short period after transplantation, is referred to as **induction therapy.**

Anti-CD52 mAb

Campath-1 (CD52) is an antigen expressed on most mature lymphocytes and on some lymphocyte precursors. An antibody against this antigen was originally tested in rheumatoid arthritis and found to cause prolonged and sustained depletion of all T cells, often lasting for years. Anti-CD52 mAb therapy did lead to some improvement in the symptoms of arthritis; however, the sustained depletion of lymphocytes and concern about infections precluded further study of this antibody in autoimmune conditions. Under the generic name **alemtuzumab**, anti-CD52 mAb has recently been approved as an adjunctive therapy in the treatment of B-cell chronic lymphocytic leukemia—a condition in which sustained suppression of the leukemic cells is desirable.

LFA-3

LFA-3 (also called **CD58**) is the counter-receptor for CD2, an antigen expressed at high levels on the surface of memory effector T cells. Interaction of CD2 on T cells with LFA-3 on antigen-presenting cells promotes increased T-cell proliferation and enhanced T-cell–dependent cytotoxicity. Because the memory effector T-cell population is elevated in patients with psoriasis, a pharmacologic agent that disrupts the CD2–LFA-3 interaction was tested for use in psoriasis.

Alefacept is an LFA-3/F$_c$ fusion protein that interrupts CD2–LFA-3 signaling by binding to T-cell CD2, and thereby inhibits T-cell activation. Additionally, the F$_c$ portion of alefacept may activate NK cells to deplete the immune system of memory effector T cells. Clinically, alefacept significantly decreases the severity of chronic plaque psoriasis. Because CD2 is expressed on other adaptive immune cells, administration of alefacept also causes a dose-dependent reduction in CD4 and CD8 T-cell populations. Its use is therefore contraindicated in patients with HIV, and patients taking alefacept may have an increased risk of serious infection. Alefacept therapy may also be associated with an increased risk of malignancy, primarily skin cancer.

INHIBITION OF COSTIMULATION

Costimulation refers to the paradigm that cells of the immune system typically require two signals for activation (see Chapter 40, Principles of Inflammation and the Immune System). If a first signal is provided in the absence of a second signal, the target immune cell may become anergic rather than activated. Because induction of anergy could lead to long-term acceptance of an organ graft or limit the extent of an autoimmune disease, inhibition of costimulation represents a viable strategy for immunosuppression. Several therapeutic agents inhibit costimulation by blocking the second signal required for cell activation, and more such agents are under development.

Abatacept

Abatacept consists of CTLA-4 fused to an IgG1 constant region. Abatacept complexes with costimulatory B7 molecules on the surface of antigen-presenting cells. When the antigen-presenting cell interacts with a T cell, MHC–TCR interaction (''signal 1'') occurs, but the complex of B7 with abatacept prevents delivery of a costimulatory signal (''signal 2'') and the T cell develops anergy or undergoes apoptosis. By this mechanism, abatacept therapy appears to be effective in down-regulating specific T-cell populations.

Abatacept is approved for the treatment of rheumatoid arthritis that is refractory to methotrexate or TNF-α inhibitors. Clinically, abatacept significantly improves symptoms of rheumatoid arthritis in patients who fail to respond to methotrexate or TNF-α inhibitors. The major adverse effects of abatacept are exacerbations of bronchitis in patients with pre-existing obstructive lung disease, and increased susceptibility to infection. Abatacept should not be administered concurrently with TNF-α inhibitors or anakinra because the combination carries an unacceptably high risk of infection.

Belatacept is a close structural congener of abatacept that has increased affinity for B7-1 and B7-2. In a large clinical trial, belatacept was as effective as cyclosporine at inhibiting acute rejection in renal transplant recipients. Belatacept is currently under further investigation as an immunosuppressant for organ transplantation.

BLOCKADE OF CELL ADHESION

The recruitment and accumulation of inflammatory cells at sites of inflammation is an essential element of most autoimmune diseases; the only exceptions to this rule are autoimmune diseases that are purely humoral, such as myasthenia gravis. Drugs that inhibit cell migration to sites of inflammation may also inhibit antigen presentation and cytotoxicity, thus providing multiple potential mechanisms of beneficial action.

Efalizumab

T-cell adhesion and migration are dependent on the interaction of cell-surface integrins with intercellular adhesion molecules (ICAMs). All T cells express LFA-1 (CD11a/CD18), an integrin that binds to ICAM-1. **Efalizumab** is a monoclonal antibody against LFA-1. By disrupting the LFA-1–ICAM-1 interaction, efalizumab limits T-cell adhesion, activation, and migration to sites of inflammation.

Efalizumab is approved for the treatment of chronic plaque psoriasis. Important adverse effects include immune-mediated thrombocytopenia, immune-mediated hemolytic anemia, an increased rate of infection, and a possible increased risk of malignancy. Unlike alefacept, which appears to deplete a pathogenic cell population, efalizumab blocks T-cell adhesion and migration without eradicating the cells. Thus, the symptoms of psoriasis return promptly after discontinuation of a course of efalizumab, whereas patients can maintain clinical improvement for many months following a 12-week course of alefacept.

Natalizumab

Alpha-4 integrins are critical to immune-cell adhesion and homing. The $\alpha_4\beta_1$ integrin mediates immune-cell interactions with cells expressing vascular cell adhesion molecule 1 (VCAM-1), while the $\alpha_4\beta_7$ integrin mediates immune-cell binding to cells expressing mucosal addressin cell adhesion molecule 1(MAdCAM-1). **Natalizumab** is a monoclonal antibody against α_4 integrin that inhibits immune-cell interactions with cells expressing VCAM-1 or MAdCAM-1.

Natalizumab was approved for the treatment of relapsing multiple sclerosis. During postmarketing surveillance of the drug, however, several patients treated with natalizumab developed progressive multifocal leukoencephalopathy (PML), a rare demyelinating disorder caused by infection with JC virus. This finding resulted in voluntary withdrawal of the drug. After further FDA investigation, it was decided to resume testing of natalizumab and to add a warning to the product label regarding the possible association. Natalizumab was subsequently reapproved for use in the treatment of multiple sclerosis.

INHIBITION OF COMPLEMENT ACTIVATION

The complement system mediates a number of innate immune responses (see Chapter 40). Recognition of foreign proteins or carbohydrates leads to sequential activation of complement proteins and eventual assembly of the **membrane attack complex**, a multiprotein structure that can cause cell lysis. Patients with paroxysmal nocturnal hemoglobinuria (PNH) have acquired defects in complement regulatory proteins, leading to inappropriate activation of complement and complement-mediated lysis of erythrocytes. **Eculizumab** is a humanized monoclonal antibody against C5, a complement protein that mediates late steps in complement activation and triggers assembly of the membrane attack complex. In clinical trials, eculizumab significantly decreased hemoglobinuria and the need for erythrocyte transfusions in patients with PNH. Phase III trials of eculizumab are currently ongoing. Genetic evidence indicates that complement activation may play an etiologic role in age-dependent macular degeneration, suggesting that inhibitors of the complement cascade could be useful local therapies for this disease.

 Conclusion and Future Directions

Several approaches are available for the pharmacologic suppression of adaptive immunity, ranging from the relatively low-specificity approaches represented by glucocorticoids and cytotoxic agents to the more specific approaches represented by cell-signaling inhibitors and antibody therapies. *Glucocorticoids* induce profound suppression of the inflammatory response and immune system, but cause many adverse effects. Glucocorticoid receptor modulators are being developed that retain the anti-inflammatory effects of glucocorticoids but have less severe adverse effects on metabolism and bone mineral homeostasis. *Cytotoxic agents* target DNA replication; although immune cells are highly susceptible to these drugs, so too are other normal cells such as those in the gastrointestinal epithelium. The cytotoxic agent mycophenolate mofetil is highly specific, both because lymphocytes depend on de novo purine synthesis and because mycophenolic acid preferentially targets the inosine monophosphate dehydrogenase isoenzyme expressed in lymphocytes. *Lymphocyte-signaling inhibitors*—such as cyclosporine, tacrolimus, and sirolimus, which target intracellular signal transduction pathways necessary for T-cell activation—are also reasonably specific. *Cytokine inhibitors* interrupt soluble signals mediating immune-cell activation. Etanercept, infliximab, and adalimumab, all of which block TNF-α activity, are examples of this rapidly expanding class of drugs. The concept of preventing immune-cell activation has also been extended to the *blockade of costimulation* represented by the antirheumatic agent abatacept. *Specific depletion of T cells* may be beneficial in organ transplantation: antithymocyte globulin, OKT3, and daclizumab are antibodies against T-cell–specific epitopes. Several antibody therapeutics are available that *block immune-cell adhesion* and homing, and more such agents are under development.

 Suggested Reading

Allison A. Immunosuppressive drugs: the first 50 years and a glance forward. *Immunopharmacology* 2000;47:63–83. (*General review of immunosuppressive drugs.*)

Allison A, Eugui E. Mycophenolate mofetil and its mechanisms of action. *Immunopharmacology* 2000;47:85–118. (*Review of mycophenolate mofetil.*)

Costa MA, Simon DI. Molecular basis of restenosis and drug-eluting stents. *Circulation* 2005;111:2257–2273. (*Overview of advances in drug-coated stents.*)

Janeway CA, Travers P, Walport M, et al. *Immunobiology: The Immune System in Health and Disease.* 6th ed. New York: Garland Publishing; 2005. (*Discussion of autoimmunity and transplantation immunity.*)

Nucleotide biosynthesis. In: Berg JM, Tymoczko JL, Stryer L, eds. *Biochemistry.* 6th ed. New York: W. H. Freeman and Company; 2007. (*Review of nucleotide biosynthesis.*)

Olsen NJ, Stein CM. New drugs for rheumatoid arthritis. *N Engl J Med* 2004;350:2167–2179. (*Review of cytokine therapy in rheumatoid arthritis.*)

Vincenti F, Larsen C, Durrbach A, et al. Costimulation with belatacept in renal transplantation. *N Engl J Med* 2005;353:770–781. (*Clinical trial demonstrating noninferiority of belatacept relative to cyclosporine.*)

Drug Summary Table   **Chapter 44 Pharmacology of Immunosuppression**

Drug	Clinical Applications	Serious and Common Adverse Effects	Contraindications	Therapeutic Considerations
INHIBITORS OF GENE EXPRESSION _Mechanism—Inhibit COX-2 expression; induce lipocortins and activate endogenous anti-inflammatory pathways_				
Prednisone Prednisolone Methylprednisolone Dexamethasone	See Drug Summary Table: Chapter 27 Pharmacology of the Adrenal Cortex			
CYTOTOXIC AGENTS _Mechanism—See specific drug_				
Mycophenolic acid Mycophenolate mofetil	Solid organ transplantation Lupus nephritis Rheumatoid arthritis Pemphigus	_Hypertension, peripheral edema, gastrointestinal hemorrhage, leukopenia, myelosuppression, neutropenia, increased risk of infection, lymphoma_ Gastrointestinal disturbance, headache	Hypersensitivity to mycophenolate mofetil or mycophenolic acid Hypersensitivity to polysorbate 80 (IV formulation)	Inhibitor of inosine monophosphate dehydrogenase (IMPDH), the rate-limiting enzyme in the formation of guanosine Avoid concurrent administration of oral iron because it markedly reduces the bioavailability of mycophenolate mofetil
Leflunomide	Rheumatoid arthritis	_Hypertension, hepatotoxicity, interstitial lung disease_ Alopecia, diarrhea, rash	Pregnancy	Inhibits dihydroorotate dehydrogenase (DHOD), leading to inhibition of pyrimidine synthesis Leflunomide undergoes significant enterohepatic circulation, resulting in a prolonged pharmacologic effect
Azathioprine Methotrexate Cyclophosphamide	See Drug Summary Table: Chapter 37 Pharmacology of Cancer: Genome Synthesis, Stability, and Maintenance			
SPECIFIC LYMPHOCYTE-SIGNALING INHIBITORS _Mechanism—See specific drug_				
Cyclosporine	Keratoconjunctivitis sicca (topical cyclosporine)	_Nephrotoxicity, hypertension, neurotoxicity, hepatotoxicity, infection_ Gingival hyperplasia, hyperlipidemia, hirsutism, gastrointestinal disturbance	Active ocular infection (topical cyclosporine)	Cyclosporine binds to cyclophilin, and the resulting complex inhibits the phosphatase activity of calcineurin, a cell-signaling protein that mediates T-cell activation Cyclosporine inhibits the production of IL-2 by activated T cells Danazol and other androgens can increase serum cyclosporine level Rifampin and St. John's wort reduce serum cyclosporine level
Tacrolimus	Organ transplantation Atopic dermatitis (topical tacrolimus)	_Nephrotoxicity, hypertension, prolonged QT interval, hyperglycemia, lymphoma, infection_ Alopecia, gastrointestinal disturbance, anemia, leukocytosis, thrombocytopenia, headache, insomnia, paresthesia, tremor, skin irritation (topical application)	Hypersensitivity to hydrogenated castor oil (IV formulation of tacrolimus)	Tacrolimus binds to FK-binding protein (FKBP), and the tacrolimus-FKBP complex inhibits calcineurin Topical tacrolimus is used widely to treat atopic dermatitis and other eczematous dermatitis St. John's wort markedly reduces serum tacrolimus level

Drug	Clinical Applications	Serious and Common Adverse Effects	Contraindications	Therapeutic Considerations
Sirolimus	Organ transplantation Coronary artery disease (cardiac stents)	*Hypertension, peripheral edema, thromboembolic disorder, hyperlipidemia, hepatotoxicity* Anemia, thrombocytopenia, arthralgia, asthenia, headache	Hypersensitivity to sirolimus	Sirolimus binds to FKBP, and the resulting sirolimus-FKBP complex inhibits mTOR, a regulator of protein translation Sirolimus-eluting stents are also used in the treatment of coronary artery disease Coadministration with voriconazole markedly increases serum sirolimus level

TUMOR NECROSIS FACTOR-ALPHA INHIBITORS
Mechanism—Etanercept is a soluble TNF receptor dimer, while infliximab and adalimumab are anti-TNF antibodies

Drug	Clinical Applications	Serious and Common Adverse Effects	Contraindications	Therapeutic Considerations
Etanercept	Rheumatoid arthritis Juvenile rheumatoid arthritis Psoriasis Psoriatic arthritis Ankylosing spondylitis	*Myelosuppression, heart failure, optic neuritis, reactivation of tuberculosis, increased risk of infection, demyelinating disease of central nervous system* Injection site reaction, upper respiratory infection, abdominal pain, vomiting	Sepsis Heart failure	All patients should undergo screening for tuberculosis before initiating therapy with a TNF inhibitor because of a greatly increased risk of reactivating latent tuberculosis Any patient developing an infection while taking a TNF inhibitor should undergo evaluation and aggressive antibiotic treatment Etanercept binds to both TNF-alpha and TNF-beta, whereas infliximab and adalimumab are TNF-alpha specific
Infliximab Adalimumab	Rheumatoid arthritis Crohn's disease (infliximab) Ulcerative colitis (infliximab) Ankylosing spondylitis (infliximab) Psoriatic arthritis (adalimumab)	Same as etanercept	Sepsis Heart failure	Infliximab is a partially humanized mouse antibody against human TNF-alpha; adalimumab is a fully humanized IgG1 antibody against TNF-alpha Certolizumab pegol, a pegylated TNF-alpha antibody, is currently in late-stage clinical trials

INTERLEUKIN-1 INHIBITORS
Mechanism—Recombinant IL-1 receptor antagonist

Drug	Clinical Applications	Serious and Common Adverse Effects	Contraindications	Therapeutic Considerations
Anakinra	Rheumatoid arthritis	*Neutropenia, increased risk of infection*	Hypersensitivity to anakinra or *E. coli* derived proteins	Reduces bony erosions, possibly by decreasing metalloproteinase release from synovial cells

DEPLETION OF SPECIFIC IMMUNE CELLS
Mechanism—See specific drug

Drug	Clinical Applications	Serious and Common Adverse Effects	Contraindications	Therapeutic Considerations
Antithymocyte globulin	Organ transplantation	*Cytokine release syndrome (fever, shivering, myalgia, headache, hypertension, anemia, leukopenia, thrombocytopenia, increased risk of infection*	Acute viral illness History of allergy or anaphylaxis to rabbit proteins	Polyclonal antibodies against human T-cell epitopes ATG treatment can result in a broad immunosuppression that can lead to infection
OKT3	Organ transplantation	Same as anti-thymocyte globulin	Anti-mouse antibody titers greater than 1:1000 Heart failure Seizures Pregnancy or breastfeeding Uncontrolled hypertension	Mouse monoclonal antibody against human CD3, a signaling molecule important for T cell receptor-mediated cell activation Treatment can result in antibodies against the mouse-specific regions of OKT3

(Continued)

Drug Summary Table | Chapter 44 Pharmacology of Immunosuppression (Continued)

Drug	Clinical Applications	Serious and Common Adverse Effects	Contraindications	Therapeutic Considerations
Daclizumab Basiliximab	Organ transplantation	Same as anti-thymocyte globulin	Hypersensitivity to daclizumab or basiliximab	Antibodies to CD25, the high-affinity IL-2 receptor
Alemtuzumab	B-cell chronic lymphocytic leukemia	Same as anti-thymocyte globulin	Active systemic infection Underlying immunodeficiency	Antibody to Campath-1 (CD52), an antigen expressed on most mature lymphocytes and some lymphocyte precursors
Alefacept	Psoriasis	Same as anti-thymocyte globulin	HIV infection Low CD4 T-cell count	LFA-3/Fc fusion protein that interrupts CD2/LFA-3 signaling by binding to T-cell CD2, leading to inhibition of T-cell activation

INHIBITION OF COSTIMULATION
Mechanism—CTLA-4 analogues fused to an IgG1 constant region; by forming a complex with cell-surface B7 molecules, the drug prevents delivery of a costimulatory signal and the T cell develops anergy or undergoes apoptosis

Abatacept	Rheumatoid arthritis refractory to methotrexate or TNF-alpha inhibitors	Exacerbation of chronic obstructive pulmonary disease (COPD), increased susceptibility to infection Nausea, headache, urinary tract infection (UTI)	Hypersensitivity to abatacept	Abatacept should not be administered concurrently with TNF-alpha inhibitors or anakinra due to increased risk of infection
Belatacept	Investigational Close structural congener of abatacept that has increased affinity for B7-1 and B7-2			

BLOCKADE OF CELL ADHESION
Mechanism—See specific drug

Efalizumab	Chronic plaque psoriasis	*Increased risk of serious infection, immune-mediated thrombocytopenia, immune-mediated hemolytic anemia, influenza-like symptoms* Acne, lymphocytosis, elevated alkaline phosphatase, antibody formation to efalizumab	Hypersensitivity to efalizumab	Monoclonal antibody against LFA-1 that inhibits the LFA-1/ICAM-1 interaction and thereby limits T-cell adhesion, activation, and migration to sites of inflammation
Natalizumab	Multiple sclerosis	*Cholelithiasis, progressive multifocal leukoencephalopathy, depression, pneumonia* Rash, arthralgia, headache, fatigue, UTI, lower respiratory tract infection	History of progressive multifocal leukoencephalopathy (PML) or existing PML	Monoclonal antibody against alpha-4 integrin that inhibits immune cell interaction with cells expressing VCAM-1 and MAdCAM-1

INHIBITOR OF COMPLEMENT ACTIVATION
Mechanism—Humanized antibody against C5, a complement protein that mediates late steps in complement activation and assembly of the membrane attack complex

Eculizumab	Investigational In late stage clinical trials for treatment of paroxysmal nocturnal hemoglobinuria			

45

Integrative Inflammation Pharmacology: Peptic Ulcer Disease

Dalia S. Nagel and Helen M. Shields

INTRODUCTION

A peptic ulcer is a break in the mucosa of the stomach (gastric ulcer) or duodenum (duodenal ulcer). Four-and-a-half million people in the United States suffer from active peptic ulcer disease, and 500,000 new cases of peptic ulcer disease are diagnosed each year. The lifetime prevalence of peptic ulcer disease is approximately 10%, and the estimated annual cost for treatment exceeds one billion dollars.

There are several different pathophysiologic mechanisms for peptic ulcer disease, and clinical management therefore requires multiple pharmacologic strategies. This chapter describes the physiology of gastric acid secretion and the pathophysiology underlying the formation of peptic ulcers. The corresponding pharmacologic agents used in the treatment of peptic ulcer disease are then discussed in relation to the pathophysiology that is interrupted by these drugs.

 Case

FIRST EPISODE

Tom is a 24-year-old graduate student. He is in good health, although he smokes approximately two packs of cigarettes and drinks five cups of coffee a day. He is currently under stress because of the impending deadline for his computer science thesis. He has also been taking two aspirin daily for the past 2 months because of a knee injury he sustained while skiing during winter vacation.

For the past 2 weeks, Tom has noted a burning pain in his upper abdomen that occurs 1 to 2 hours after eating. In addition, the pain frequently awakens him at approximately 3:00 A.M. His pain is usually relieved by eating and by taking over-the-counter antacids.

When the pain increases in intensity, Tom decides to visit his internist, Dr. Smith, at University Health Services. Dr. Smith notes that the abdominal examination is normal except for epigastric tenderness. Dr. Smith discusses diagnostic options with Tom, including an upper gastrointestinal

811

x-ray series and an endoscopic examination. Tom chooses to undergo the endoscopic examination. During the examination, an ulcer is identified in the proximal portion of the duodenum on the posterior wall. The ulcer is 0.5 cm in diameter. A mucosal biopsy of the gastric antrum is performed for detection of *Helicobacter pylori*.

Tom is diagnosed with a duodenal ulcer. Dr. Smith prescribes omeprazole, a proton pump inhibitor. The following day, when the pathology report indicates the presence of an *H. pylori* infection, Dr. Smith prescribes bismuth, clarithromycin, and amoxicillin in addition to the proton pump inhibitor. Dr. Smith also advises Tom to stop smoking and drinking coffee and, importantly, to avoid taking aspirin.

SECOND EPISODE

Tom has no medical problems for 10 years after the healing of his duodenal ulcer. At age 34, he develops carpal tunnel syndrome and begins to take several aspirin daily for the pain. One month later, Tom develops a burning pain in his upper abdomen. After vomiting "coffee grounds" material and noticing that his bowel movements are black, he decides to visit his internist. Dr. Smith discovers by endoscopy that Tom has a gastric ulcer and that the ulcer has recently bled. Dr. Smith explains to Tom that he has a recurrence of peptic ulcer disease. Tom's breath test is negative for *H. pylori,* and he is told that aspirin is the most likely cause of this recurrence. He is treated with antacids and ranitidine, an H2 receptor antagonist, and is told to stop taking aspirin. Dr. Smith goes over with Tom which pain-relieving medications are considered nonsteroidal anti-inflammatory drugs (NSAIDs).

Two weeks pass. Tom informs Dr. Smith that the pain in his wrist has become unbearable and that he must continue taking aspirin to be able to concentrate at work. Dr. Smith tells him that he can take aspirin as long as he switches his antiulcer medication from an H2 antagonist to a proton pump inhibitor.

QUESTIONS

■ **1.** What risk factors did Tom have for the development of peptic ulcer disease? What are the roles of *H. pylori* and NSAIDs in this disease?

■ **2.** Why was Tom given a proton pump inhibitor for his first episode of peptic ulcer disease? Why was an H2 antagonist prescribed for his second episode, and then a proton pump inhibitor when he insisted on using aspirin as an analgesic?

■ **3.** Why was Tom given clarithromycin rather than metronidazole for treatment of his *H. pylori* infection?

PHYSIOLOGY OF GASTRIC ACID SECRETION

NEUROHORMONAL CONTROL OF GASTRIC ACID SECRETION

Hydrochloric acid is secreted into the stomach by **parietal cells**, which are located in oxyntic glands of the fundus and body of the stomach. The parietal cell actively transports H^+ across its apical canalicular membranes via H^+/K^+-ATPases (proton pumps) that exchange intracellular H^+ for extracellular K^+. Three neurohormonal secretagogues regulate this process: **histamine, gastrin,** and **acetylcholine** (ACh). Each of these secretagogues binds to and activates specific receptors on the basolateral membrane of the parietal cell, thereby initiating the biochemical changes necessary for active transport of H^+ out of the cell.

Histamine, released by **enterochromaffin-like (ECL) cells** located in and adjacent to the oxyntic glands and by **mast cells** in the lamina propria, binds to histamine **H2 receptors** on the parietal cell. H2 receptor activation stimulates adenylyl cyclase and increases intracellular cyclic adenosine monophosphate (cAMP). In turn, cAMP activates cAMP-dependent protein kinase, which phosphorylates H^+/K^+-ATPase in the apical membrane of the cell. Phosphorylation of the exchanger activates extrusion of H^+ from the parietal cell into the gastric lumen (Fig. 45-1).

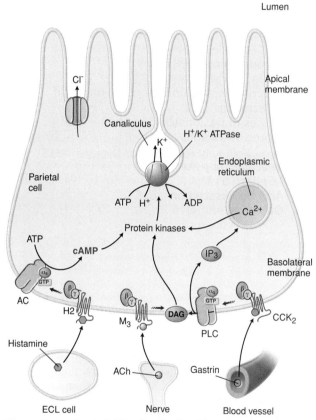

Figure 45-1. Control of parietal cell acid secretion. Stimulation of parietal cell acid secretion is modulated by paracrine (histamine), neuroendocrine (acetylcholine [ACh]), and endocrine (gastrin) pathways, which activate their respective receptors (H2, M_3, and CCK_2). H2 receptor activation increases cAMP, which activates protein kinases. M_3 and CCK_2 receptor activation stimulate release of Ca^{2+} by the G_q-mediated IP_3/DAG pathway; these signals also stimulate protein kinase activity. Protein kinase activation results in phosphorylation and activation of the canalicular membrane H^+/K^+-ATPase, which pumps H^+ ions into the stomach lumen. An apical membrane Cl^- channel couples Cl^- efflux to H^+ efflux, and an apical membrane K^+ channel *(not shown)* recycles K^+ out of the cell. The net result of this process is the rapid extrusion of HCl into the stomach lumen.

Gastrin is secreted into the bloodstream by **G cells** in the gastric antrum, whereas ACh is released from postganglionic nerves with cell bodies located in the submucosa (Meissner's plexus). These secretagogues bind to their respective receptors on the parietal cell and thereby increase intracellular calcium levels (Ca^{2+}). Ca^{2+} binds to calmodulin and stimulates adenylyl cyclase. Ca^{2+} also activates protein kinase C, which phosphorylates and activates H^+/K^+-ATPase to increase H^+ secretion (Fig. 45-1).

While histamine, gastrin, and ACh increase acid secretion by parietal cells, **somatostatin-secreting D cells** and **prostaglandins** limit the extent of gastric acid secretion. Somatostatin decreases acid secretion via three mechanisms: (1) inhibition of gastrin release from G cells by a paracrine mechanism; (2) inhibition of histamine release from ECL cells and mast cells; and (3) direct inhibition of parietal cell acid secretion. Prostaglandin E_2 (PGE_2) enhances mucosal resistance to tissue injury by: (1) reducing basal and stimulated gastric acid secretion; and (2) enhancing epithelial cell bicarbonate secretion, mucus production, cell turnover, and local blood flow.

PHASES OF GASTRIC ACID SECRETION

Gastric secretions increase considerably during a meal. There are three phases of gastric acid secretion.

The **cephalic phase** includes responses to sight, taste, smell, and thought of food. "Sham feedings," experiments in which food is chewed but not swallowed, trigger an increase in acid secretion mediated by vagal stimulation and increased gastrin secretion.

Mechanical distension of the stomach and ingestion of amino acids and peptides stimulate the **gastric phase.** Distension activates stretch receptors in the wall of the stomach that are linked to short intramural nerves and vagal fibers. Luminal nutrients, such as amino acids, are strong stimulants for gastrin release. Gastrin travels via the blood to the oxyntic mucosa and stimulates ECL cells to release histamine. An important negative feedback on acid secretion in this phase is acid (pH <3)-mediated inhibition of gastrin release from antral G cells. Acid secretion is also inhibited by release of somatostatin from antral D cells.

The **intestinal phase** involves stimulation of gastric acid secretion by digested protein in the intestine. Gastrin plays a major role in mediating this phase as well.

PROTECTIVE FACTORS

Factors that protect the gastric mucosa include gastric mucus, gastric and duodenal bicarbonate, prostaglandins (discussed above and in Chapter 41, Pharmacology of Eicosanoids), restitution (repair), and blood flow. The epithelial cells of the stomach secrete **mucus,** which acts as a lubricant that protects the mucosal cells from abrasions. Composed of hydrophilic glycoproteins that are viscous and have gel-forming properties, the mucus layer enables formation of an uninterrupted layer of water at the luminal surface of the epithelium. Together, the mucus and water layers attenuate potential damage due to the acidic environment of the gastric lumen. Prostaglandins stimulate mucus secretion, whereas

NSAIDs and anticholinergic medications inhibit mucus production. In addition, *H. pylori* disrupts the mucus layer (see below).

Bicarbonate, like mucus, protects the gastric epithelium by neutralizing gastric acid. Bicarbonate is secreted by epithelial cells at the luminal surface of the gastric mucosa, in gastric pits, and at the luminal surface of the duodenal mucosa. Bicarbonate secretion in the duodenum serves to neutralize acid entering the intestine from the stomach.

Restitution refers to the ability of the gastric mucosa to undergo repair. Damage is repaired through migration of undamaged epithelial cells along the basement membrane to fill defects created by the sloughing of injured cells.

The final protective factor is **blood flow.** Blood flow to the gastric mucosa removes acid that has diffused across a damaged mucus layer.

PATHOPHYSIOLOGY OF PEPTIC ULCER DISEASE

A peptic ulcer is a break in the lining of the stomach or duodenum. The break can involve the mucosa, muscularis mucosa, submucosa, and in some cases, the deeper layers of the muscle wall. This compromise of mucosal integrity can cause pain, bleeding, obstruction, perforation, and even death. Peptic ulcers are caused by an imbalance between protective factors and damaging factors in the gastrointestinal mucosa. This section describes the main pathophysiologic mechanisms involved in ulcer formation, the two most common of which are *H. pylori* infection and NSAID use.

HELICOBACTER PYLORI

H. pylori is a Gram-negative, spiral-shaped bacterium. *H. pylori* is the most common cause of non-NSAID–associated peptic ulcer disease. *H. pylori* has been found in the gastric antrum of a significant number of patients with duodenal ulcers and gastric ulcers, including Tom on his first presentation to Dr. Smith in the introductory case. Eradication of *H. pylori* leads to lower recurrence and relapse rates in patients with ulcers. The latter finding, together with the fact that many ulcer patients are infected with *H. pylori,* constitute the major evidence for *H. pylori*'s causal role in peptic ulcer disease.

H. pylori lives in the acidic environment of the stomach. The initial infection is transmitted by the oral route. Upon ingestion, the microaerophilic bacterium uses its four to six flagellae to move in corkscrew fashion through the gastric mucus layer. *H. pylori* attaches to adhesion molecules on the surface of gastric epithelial cells. In the duodenum, *H. pylori* attaches only to areas containing gastric epithelial cells that have arisen as a result of excess acid damage to the duodenal mucosa (gastric metaplasia). *H. pylori* is able to live in such a hostile environment partly because of its production of the enzyme **urease**, which converts urea to ammonia. The ammonia buffers the H^+ and forms ammonium hydroxide, creating an alkaline cloud around the bacterium and protecting it from the acidic environment of the stomach.

H. pylori's virulence factors cause damage to the host. Urease is one of these damaging factors because it is an antigen that causes a strong immune response. In addition, the ammonium hydroxide produced by urease causes gastric epithelial cell injury. Other virulence factors include lipopolysaccharides (endotoxins), which are components of the bacteria's outer membrane, as well as a lipase and a protease that are secreted by the bacteria and degrade the gastric mucosa. Cytotoxicity caused by *H. pylori* has also been linked to two proteins associated with vacuolating cytotoxins, cagA and vacA.

The persistence of *H. pylori* can be traced, in part, to the inappropriate immune response that it elicits. Instead of the normal T_H2 mucosal immunity response, which controls luminal infections by means of secretory (IgA) antibody, the *H. pylori* organism elicits a T_H1 response. Cytokines associated with the T_H1 response induce inflammation and epithelial cell damage.

Several additional mechanisms characterize *H. pylori*-induced peptic ulcer disease (Fig. 45-2). Acid secretion is increased in patients with *H. pylori*-associated duodenal ulcers. This is thought to result from increased levels of circulating gastrin, causing parietal cell proliferation and increased acid production. Gastrin secretion is elevated by two mechanisms: (1) the ammonia generated by *H. pylori* produces an alkaline environment near the G cells and thereby stimulates gastrin release; and (2) the number of antral D cells is lower than normal in *H. pylori*-infected patients, resulting in decreased somatostatin production and increased gastrin release. *H. pylori* also decreases duodenal bicarbonate secretion and thereby weakens the protective mechanisms of the duodenal mucosa.

The presence of *H. pylori* infection can be detected using the **^{13}C urea breath test,** which is based on the organism's production of urease. In this test, urease converts ingested ^{13}C-urea to ^{13}CO$_2$ if *H. pylori* is present in the stomach, and the ^{13}CO$_2$ is detected in the breath. The ^{13}C urea breath test is currently the best diagnostic test for *H. pylori*; other methods of detection include histologic examination of a gastric mucosal biopsy (as was performed initially in Tom's

case), serologic testing for *H. pylori* antibodies, and a stool antigen test.

NSAIDS

More than 100,000 patients are hospitalized each year for NSAID-associated gastrointestinal complications, and gastrointestinal bleeding has a 5% to 10% mortality rate in these patients. The gastrointestinal tract is the most common target for the adverse effects of NSAID use.

NSAID-associated gastrointestinal damage is attributable to both *topical injury* and *systemic effects* of the NSAID (Fig. 45-3). Most NSAIDs are weak organic acids. In the acidic environment of the stomach, these drugs are neutral compounds that can cross the plasma membrane and enter gastric epithelial cells. In the neutral intracellular environment, the drugs are re-ionized and trapped. The resulting intracellular damage is responsible for the local gastrointestinal injury associated with NSAID use.

NSAIDs also cause systemic injury to the gastrointestinal lining, largely because of decreased mucosal prostaglandin synthesis. As described in detail in Chapter 41, two cyclooxygenase enzymes catalyze the formation of prostaglandins from arachidonic acid. In general, cyclooxygenase-1 (COX-1) is constitutively expressed and produces the gastric prostaglandins responsible for mucosal integrity, whereas cyclooxygenase-2 (COX-2) is induced by inflammatory stimuli. Inhibition of COX-1 by NSAIDs can lead to mucosal ulceration because inhibition of PGE$_2$ synthesis removes one of the protective mechanisms maintaining the integrity of the gastric mucosa. Although **COX-2 selective NSAIDs** (coxibs) may carry a lower risk of ulcer formation than **nonselective NSAIDs**, the coxibs appear to be associated with an increase in myocardial infarction and stroke. Several of the COX-2 selective NSAIDs have been voluntarily withdrawn (rofecoxib and valdecoxib), and use of the third has been voluntarily limited (celecoxib). The adverse cardiovascular effects of the COX-2 selective inhibitors may result from their suppression of prostacyclin production by vascular endothelial cells (catalyzed by COX-1 and COX-2), allowing

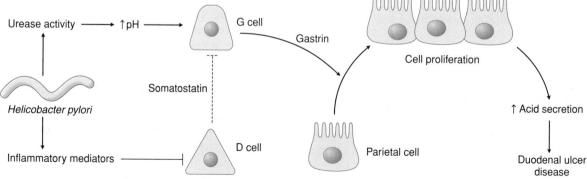

Figure 45-2. The role of *H. pylori* in duodenal peptic ulcer disease. Two of the mechanisms by which *H. pylori* infection predisposes to peptic ulcer disease are illustrated. First, the inflammatory mediators elicited by *H. pylori* inhibit somatostatin secretion by D cells in the antrum of the stomach. Decreased D cell somatostatin secretion causes disinhibition of gastrin release from G cells. Second, the ammonium hydroxide produced by *H. pylori*-derived urease increases gastric pH, which in turn stimulates gastrin secretion. Activation of gastrin release by both of these mechanisms leads to parietal cell proliferation, which increases the functional capacity of the gastric mucosa to secrete H$^+$ ions and thereby predisposes to the development of duodenal ulcer disease.

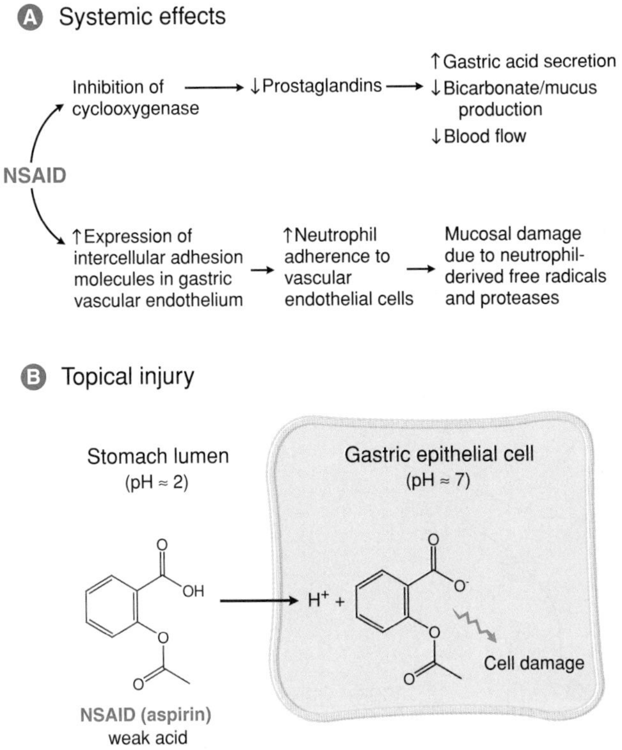

A Systemic effects

B Topical injury

Figure 45-3. Role of NSAIDs in peptic ulcer disease. NSAID-associated peptic ulcer disease is a result of both systemic effects and topical injury. **A.** Systemic effects: NSAIDs inhibit cyclooxygenase and thereby decrease the production of prostaglandins. Because prostaglandins activate G_i, and thereby decrease the generation of cAMP in gastric parietal cells, decreased prostaglandin production causes increased gastric acid secretion. Decreased prostaglandins also decrease bicarbonate production, mucus production, and blood flow in the stomach. An additional systemic effect involves the increased expression of intercellular adhesion molecules (ICAMs) in the vascular endothelium of the stomach, which increases neutrophil adherence to the vascular endothelial cells. Neutrophils release free radicals and proteases that cause mucosal damage. **B.** Topical effects: NSAIDs induce local injury via ion trapping. From the lumen of the stomach, the drug enters the gastric epithelial cell in its protonated (uncharged) form. In the neutral environment of the cytoplasm, the NSAID is ionized and trapped inside the cell, causing cell damage.

thromboxane produced by platelets (catalyzed by COX-1) to exert an unopposed prothrombotic effect (see Chapter 41).

Although there is much evidence for NSAID damage caused by inhibition of prostaglandin synthesis, there are other systemic mechanisms by which NSAIDs may cause ulcers. For example, NSAIDs increase expression of intercellular adhesion molecules in the vascular endothelium of the gastric mucosa. Increased adherence of neutrophils to the vascular endothelium causes release of free radicals and proteases that damage the gastric mucosa.

ACID HYPERSECRETION

Acid hypersecretion is an important causative factor in some patients with peptic ulcer disease. **Zollinger-Ellison syndrome** and **Cushing's ulcers** are two clinical examples in which hyperacidity leads to peptic ulcer disease. In

Zollinger-Ellison syndrome, a gastrin-secreting tumor of the non-beta cells of the endocrine pancreas leads to increased acid secretion. In Cushing's ulcers, seen in patients with severe head injuries, heightened vagal (cholinergic) tone causes gastric hyperacidity (see Fig. 45-1).

OTHER FACTORS

Pepsin is a digestive enzyme secreted by gastric chief cells as the inactive precursor pepsinogen. Studies have suggested a role for pepsin in ulcer formation. Cigarette smoking is associated with peptic ulcer disease because of its impairment of mucosal blood flow and healing and its inhibition of pancreatic bicarbonate production. Caffeine ingestion (increased acid secretion), alcoholic cirrhosis, glucocorticoid use, and genetic influences are also associated with peptic ulcer disease. Finally, chronic psychological stress may occasionally be an important cause of peptic ulcer disease. In the introductory case, Tom smoked cigarettes, drank a lot of coffee, and was under stress to finish his computer science thesis. These factors may have contributed to his development of an ulcer.

PHARMACOLOGIC CLASSES AND AGENTS

Because several pathophysiologic mechanisms can lead to peptic ulcer disease, clinical management requires consideration of multiple pharmacologic options. The available agents can be divided into drugs that: (1) decrease acid secretion; (2) neutralize acid; (3) promote mucosal defense; and (4) modify risk factors (Fig. 45-4).

AGENTS THAT DECREASE ACID SECRETION

H2 Receptor Antagonists

The discovery of **H2 receptor antagonists** by Black and colleagues in the 1970s significantly changed the treatment of peptic ulcer disease. These investigators identified a second histamine receptor and elucidated its role in gastric acid secretion. H2 receptor antagonists reversibly and competitively inhibit the binding of histamine to H2 receptors, resulting in suppression of gastric acid secretion. H2 receptor antagonists also indirectly decrease gastrin- and acetylcholine-induced gastric acid secretion.

Four H2 receptor antagonists are available: **cimetidine, ranitidine, famotidine,** and **nizatidine** (Fig. 45-5). H2 receptor antagonists are absorbed rapidly from the small intestine. Peak plasma concentrations are achieved within 1 to 3 hours. Elimination of H2 receptor antagonists involves both renal excretion and hepatic metabolism. It is therefore important to decrease the dose of these drugs for patients with liver or kidney failure. An exception is nizatidine, which is eliminated primarily by the kidney.

All four drugs are well tolerated in general. Occasional minor adverse effects include diarrhea, headache, muscle pain, constipation, and fatigue. H2 receptor antagonists may

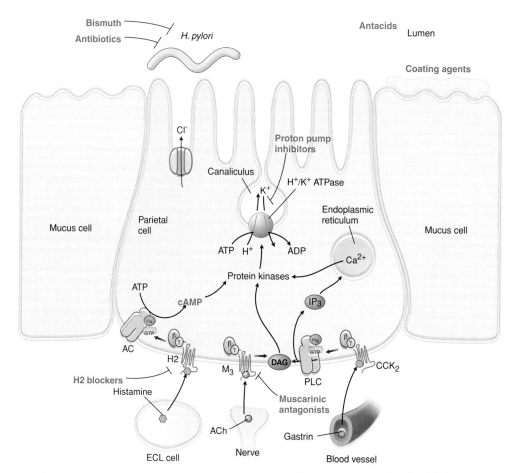

Figure 45-4. Sites of action of drugs used to treat peptic ulcer disease. H2 receptor antagonists (H2 blockers) inhibit activation of the histamine H2 receptor by endogenous histamine. Muscarinic antagonists inhibit signaling through the M_3 muscarinic acetylcholine (ACh) receptor. Proton pump inhibitors decrease the activity of the H^+/K^+-ATPase on the canalicular membrane of the parietal cell. Antacids neutralize acid in the stomach lumen. Coating agents provide a protective layer on the epithelial surface of the gastric mucosa. Bismuth and antibiotics act to eradicate *H. pylori* from the mucus layer coating the gastric mucosa. *H. pylori* infection is an important contributing factor in the pathogenesis of peptic ulcer disease.

induce confusion and hallucinations in some patients. These adverse effects in the central nervous system (CNS) are uncommon, however, and are typically associated with intravenous administration of the H2 receptor antagonist. Additional adverse effects specific to cimetidine, the first H2 receptor antagonist to be developed, are discussed below.

Several clinically significant drug-drug interactions can occur with H2 receptor antagonists. For example, ketoconazole, a drug that requires an acidic medium for gastric absorption, has reduced uptake in the alkaline environment created by H2 receptor antagonists. As a second example, H2 receptor antagonists compete for renal tubular secretion of procainamide and certain other drugs.

Cimetidine inhibits many cytochrome P450 enzymes and thus can interfere with hepatic metabolism of a number of drugs. For example, cimetidine can decrease the metabolism of lidocaine, phenytoin, quinidine, theophylline, and warfarin, allowing toxic levels of these drugs to accumulate. Cimetidine appears to inhibit P450 enzymes to a greater extent than the other H2 receptor antagonists, and an H2 receptor antagonist other than cimetidine may be preferred when the patient is receiving other medications.

Cimetidine crosses the placenta and is secreted into breast milk, and is therefore not recommended for use during pregnancy or when nursing. Cimetidine can have antiandrogenic effects because of its action as an antagonist at the androgen receptor, resulting in gynecomastia (enlarged breasts) in men and galactorrhea (discharge of milk) in women.

Proton Pump Inhibitors

Proton pump inhibitors block the parietal cell H^+/K^+-ATPase (proton pump). Compared to H2 receptor antagonists, proton pump inhibitors are superior at suppressing acid secretion and promoting peptic ulcer healing. **Omeprazole** is the prototype proton pump inhibitor. Several other proton pump inhibitors have also been developed, including **esomeprazole** (the [*S*]-enantiomer of omeprazole), **rabeprazole, lansoprazole,** and **pantoprazole** (Fig. 45-6).

All of the proton pump inhibitors are prodrugs that require activation in the acidic environment of the parietal cell canaliculus. Oral formulations of these drugs are enteric-coated to prevent premature activation. The prodrug is converted to its active **sulfenamide** form in the acidic canalicular environment, and the sulfenamide reacts with a cysteine residue on the H^+/K^+-ATPase to form a covalent disulfide bond

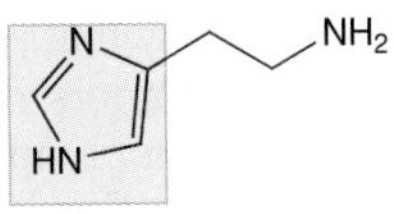

Histamine
(imidazole ring)

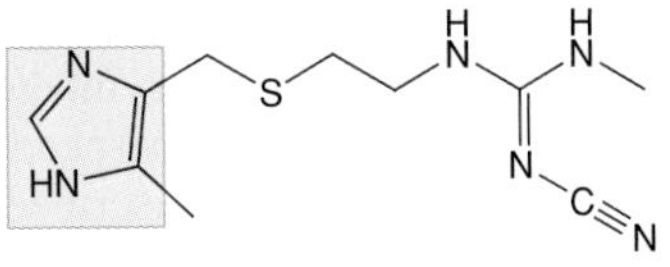

Cimetidine
(imidazole ring)

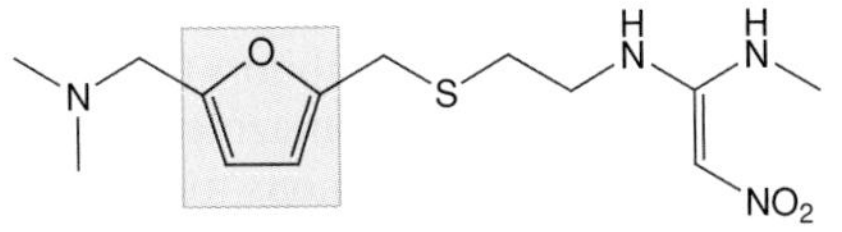

Ranitidine
(furan ring)

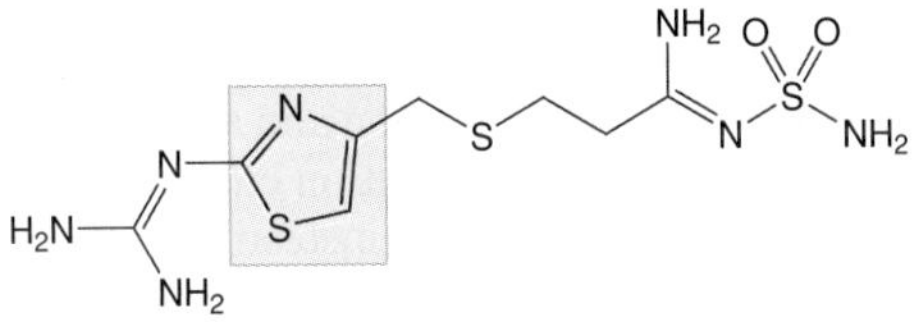

Famotidine
(thiazole ring)

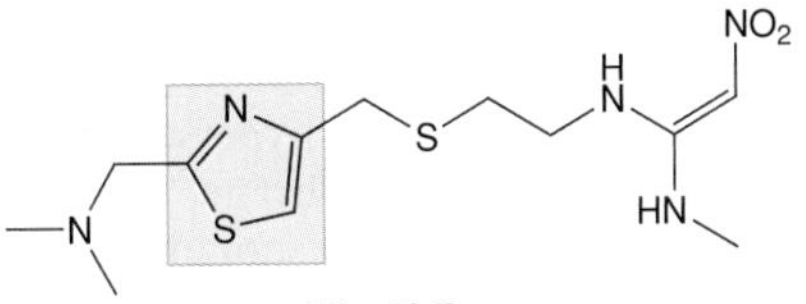

Nizatidine
(thiazole ring)

Figure 45-5. Histamine H2 receptor antagonists. H2 receptor antagonists share moieties related to histamine, providing a structural rationale for inhibition of the H2 receptor. For a more detailed description of the structure of these agents, see the legend to Figure 42-5.

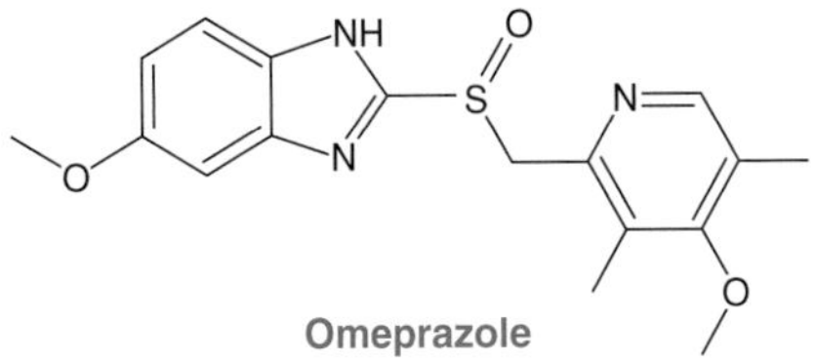

Omeprazole

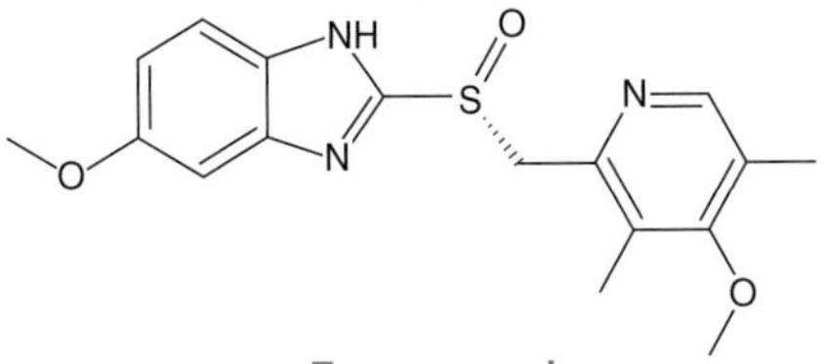

Esomeprazole

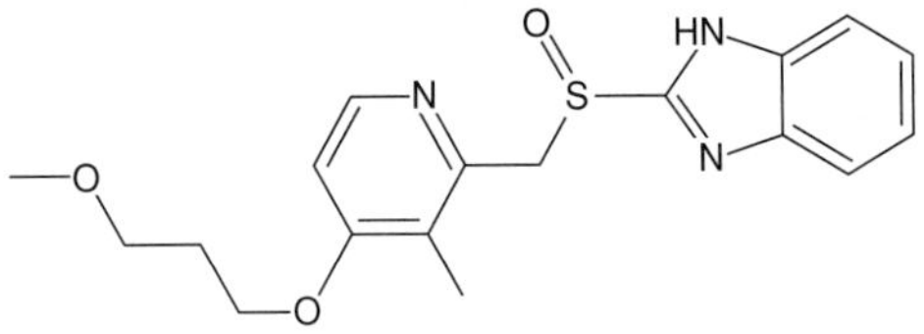

Rabeprazole

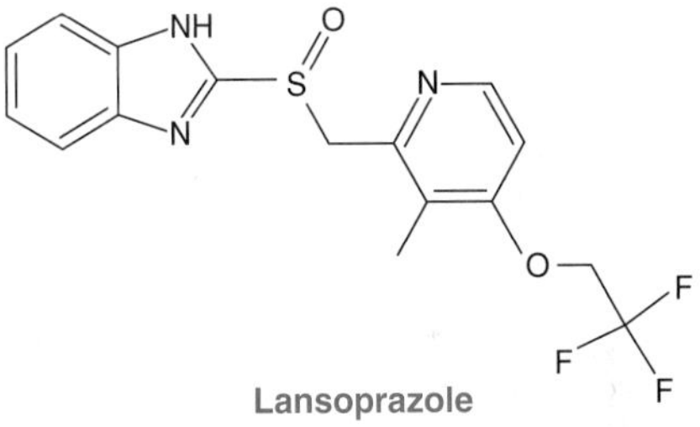

Lansoprazole

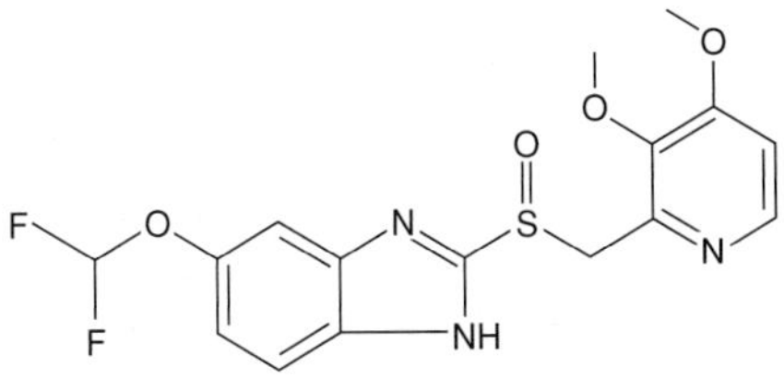

Pantoprazole

Figure 45-6. Proton pump inhibitors. The proton pump inhibitors are a family of structurally related prodrugs that are all activated by the mechanism shown in Figure 45-7. Note that esomeprazole is the (*S*)-enantiomer of omeprazole, which is formulated as a racemic mixture of (*R*)- and (*S*)-enantiomers.

(Fig. 45-7). Covalent binding of the drug inhibits the activity of the proton pump irreversibly, leading to prolonged and nearly complete suppression of acid secretion. In order for acid secretion to resume, the parietal cell must synthesize new H^+/K^+-ATPase molecules, a process that requires approximately 18 hours.

The five available proton pump inhibitors have similar rates of absorption and oral bioavailability. Rabeprazole and lansoprazole appear to have a significantly faster onset of action than omeprazole and pantoprazole. Comparisons of effectiveness suggest that esomeprazole inhibits acid secretion more effectively than other proton pump inhibitors at therapeutic doses.

Clinical Indications

Proton pump inhibitors are used to treat *H. pylori*-associated ulcers and hemorrhagic ulcers and to allow continued use of NSAIDs in a patient with a known peptic ulcer.

Proton pump inhibitors are preferred for the treatment of peptic ulcer disease when there is an accompanying *H. pylori* infection because they contribute to eradication of the infection by inhibiting the growth of *H. pylori.*

Proton pump inhibitors are also effective in preventing recurrent hemorrhagic ulcers. Clot formation involves processes that are impaired in acidic environments, and the profound suppression of gastric acid secretion by proton pump inhibitors helps maintain clot integrity in the ulcer bed. For example, an intravenous infusion of omeprazole is able to

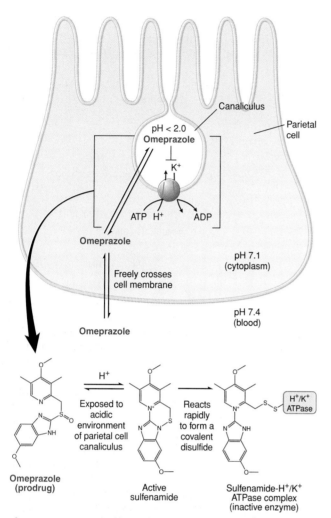

Figure 45-7. Mechanism of action of omeprazole, a proton pump inhibitor. Omeprazole freely enters the cytoplasm of the parietal cell (pH 7.1) in uncharged form. In the acidic environment of the parietal cell canalicular system (pH <2.0), omeprazole is converted to its active sulfenamide form. The sulfenamide reacts with a cysteine residue on the H^+/K^+-ATPase to form a covalent disulfide bond. Covalent modification of the H^+/K^+-ATPase inhibits the activity of the proton pump and thereby prevents acid secretion.

maintain the intragastric pH above 6.0, thereby supporting platelet aggregation and clot stability (see below).

Proton pump inhibitors are superior to H2 receptor antagonists (ranitidine) for healing of NSAID-associated gastric and duodenal ulcers when the patient continues NSAID use, most likely because proton pump inhibitors are better able to sustain a constant increase in gastric pH.

Several considerations may favor the use of H2 receptor antagonists over proton pump inhibitors. H2 receptor antagonists have been in use longer than proton pump inhibitors, and their adverse effects are better studied. This may be an especially important consideration for pregnant women because H2 receptor antagonists (with the exception of cimetidine) have proven to be safe in pregnancy, whereas the safety of proton pump inhibitors in pregnancy is less certain. Use of proton pump inhibitors is therefore discouraged during pregnancy unless absolutely necessary. In addition, H2 receptor antagonists are generally less expensive than proton

pump inhibitors. The possibility that proton pump inhibitors may cause gastric carcinoid tumors is sometimes raised as a concern for long-term proton pump inhibitor therapy, although this association has not been observed in humans.

In the introductory case, Tom was first given a proton pump inhibitor because he was found to have an associated *H. pylori* infection. He was given an H2 receptor antagonist for the second episode because there was no associated *H. pylori* infection and the H2 receptor antagonist was more affordable. After realizing that Tom needed to continue using aspirin, however, Dr. Smith prescribed a proton pump inhibitor to allow for the concomitant use of the NSAID.

Formulations

Four of the five proton pump inhibitors (omeprazole, esomeprazole, lansoprazole, and pantoprazole) are available in intravenous dosage forms. Intravenous formulations of proton pump inhibitors are useful clinically because this delivery route bypasses the harsh acidic environment of the stomach and upper duodenum. Intravenous delivery allows more of the drug to reach its site of action in the parietal cell canaliculus without degradation. For example, esomeprazole has a twofold higher peak concentration and a 66% to 83% greater area under the plasma concentration curve (AUC) when the dose is delivered intravenously instead of orally. The U. S. Food and Drug Administration (FDA) has approved intravenous formulations of lansoprazole (7-day limit), esomeprazole (10-day limit), and pantoprazole (10-day limit) for treatment of erosive esophagitis in patients unable to take oral medications. Intravenous pantoprazole is also approved for treatment of the gastrin-induced hypersecretory state associated with Zollinger-Ellison syndrome.

The intravenous formulation should be reserved for patients who require profound acid suppression or who are unable to take oral medications. Patients with erosive esophagitis and patients with compromised gastrointestinal absorption are also candidates for therapy with intravenous proton pump inhibitors. One good indication for an intravenous proton pump inhibitor would be upper gastrointestinal hemorrhage with endoscopic evidence of a visible blood vessel, because gastric acid impairs clot formation (see above). Because of the short half-life of the proton pump inhibitors (approximately 1 hour), it may be necessary to use a loading dose of medication followed by a continuous intravenous infusion. An oral formulation should be substituted for the intravenous infusion once the bleeding has stopped, because there is no significant difference between the oral and intravenous dosage forms in terms of acid suppression.

Metabolism and Excretion

The five available proton pump inhibitors have similar rates of metabolism. Four of these drugs are metabolized by cytochrome P450 enzymes in the liver (specifically, by CYP2C19 and CYP3A4). Rabeprazole is largely metabolized through a nonenzymatic reduction pathway. Box 45-1 describes the effect of pharmacogenetic differences on the P450-mediated metabolism of omeprazole, lansoprazole, esomeprazole, and pantoprazole.

After metabolism by the liver, proton pump inhibitor me-

An individual's response to treatment with a proton pump inhibitor (PPI) may vary from a marked decrease in acid secretion to little change in acid secretion. The pharmacogenetics of drug metabolism is the major factor responsible for this variation. Omeprazole, lansoprazole, esomeprazole, and pantoprazole are extensively metabolized in the liver to less active or inactive metabolites; of these four PPIs, omeprazole is the most extensively metabolized and pantoprazole is the least extensively metabolized. Metabolism of the PPIs involves two cytochrome P450 isoenzymes, CYP2C19 and CYP3A4 (also called P450 2C19 and P450 3A4, respectively). CYP2C19 is responsible for the major metabolism of PPIs, while CYP3A4 functions as an ancillary metabolic pathway when the main pathway through CYP2C19 is saturated. Studies have shown that individuals have different rates of metabolism and clearance of these drugs because of genetic polymorphisms in their CYP2C19 isoenzymes.

Two polymorphisms of CYP2C19 (CYP2C19m1 and CYP2C19m2) are associated with decreased enzyme activity. Carriers of two copies of the polymorphisms are "poor metabolizers" of PPIs. Carriers of one copy of the polymorphisms are "intermediate to extensive metabolizers;" their rate of CYP2C19-mediated drug metabolism is reduced but not to the extent of individuals with two copies of the polymorphisms. These polymorphisms exist most commonly in Asian populations: 20% of some Asian populations are poor metabolizers, whereas only 2% to 6% of Caucasian populations are poor metabolizers.

Compared to normal individuals ("extensive metabolizers") taking the same dose of omeprazole, lansoprazole, esomeprazole, or pantoprazole, poor metabolizers exhibit decreased clearance of the PPI, leading to higher serum concentrations of the drug as well as greater degrees of acid inhibition. Fortunately, the standard recommended doses of PPIs take into account these differences, and most patients reach a sufficient degree of acid inhibition regardless of the variability in metabolism of these drugs. Pharmacogenetic differences in PPI metabolism can lead to potentially significant drug–drug interactions, however. To date, only omeprazole has been found to interact with other drugs metabolized by CYP2C19. Although clinically significant interactions generally do not occur, awareness should be high if patients are taking omeprazole concomitantly with warfarin, phenytoin, diazepam, or carbamazepine. In the future, screening for the presence of CYP2C19 polymorphisms could allow physicians to determine which PPI is most appropriate for each patient and what dosage should most effectively favor acid inhibition while avoiding drug-drug interactions.

tabolites are excreted via the kidney. Patients with chronic kidney disease generally do not require adjustment of the standard dose. However, patients with liver failure should be treated with lower doses of these drugs. Elderly patients do not generally require dose reduction even though plasma clearance is reduced, because the plasma half-life is short and accumulation does not typically occur. Elderly patients with concomitant renal and liver dysfunction should receive lower doses to avoid an increased risk of adverse effects.

Proton pump inhibitors cross the human placental barrier. Given the absence of animal data demonstrating the safety of these drugs, their use is discouraged during pregnancy. A recent meta-analysis of human studies did not indicate an increased rate of malformations in children born to women who took proton pump inhibitors during the first trimester of pregnancy.

Adverse Effects

Proton pump inhibitors are generally well tolerated. Adverse effects may include headache, nausea, disturbed bowel function, and abdominal pain. On occasion, proton pump inhibitors cause such a large decrease in acid secretion that enteric infections (such as *Salmonella*) occur because the ingested bacteria are not killed by stomach acid. Another potential concern is the large increase in plasma gastrin associated with proton pump inhibitor use. Because gastric acid is a physiologic regulator of gastrin secretion by G cells in the gastric antrum, the decreased acid secretion caused by proton pump inhibitor therapy leads to increased gastrin release. The trophic effects of gastrin can induce hyperplasia of ECL cells and parietal cells in the gastric mucosa. Although rats treated for long durations with omeprazole developed gastric carcinoid tumors, these tumors have not been observed in humans. Patients with Zollinger-Ellison syndrome usually develop ECL and parietal cell hyperplasia and some develop carcinoid tumors, but no increase in carcinoid tumors has been found in Zollinger-Ellison patients taking proton pump inhibitors. Hypergastrinemia can also result in rebound hypersecretion of acid upon discontinuation of the proton pump inhibitor.

Anticholinergic Agents

Anticholinergic agents such as **dicyclomine** antagonize muscarinic ACh receptors on parietal cells and thereby decrease gastric acid secretion. However, anticholinergic agents are seldom used in the treatment of peptic ulcer disease because they are not as effective as H2 receptor antagonists or proton pump inhibitors. These agents also have many adverse effects, including dry mouth, blurred vision, cardiac arrhythmia, and urinary retention.

AGENTS THAT NEUTRALIZE ACID

Antacids are used on an as-needed basis for symptomatic relief of dyspepsia. These agents neutralize hydrochloric acid by reacting with the acid to form water and salts. The most widely used antacids are mixtures of **aluminum hydroxide** and **magnesium hydroxide**. The hydroxide ion reacts with hydrogen ions in the stomach to form water, while the magnesium and aluminum react with bicarbonate in pancreatic secretions and with phosphates in the diet to form salts. Common adverse effects associated with these antacids include diarrhea (magnesium) and constipation (aluminum). When antacids containing aluminum and magnesium are taken together, constipation and diarrhea may be avoided. Antacids containing aluminum can bind phosphate; the resulting hypophosphatemia can cause weakness, malaise, and anorexia. Patients with chronic kidney disease should avoid magnesium-containing antacids because they can lead to hypermagnesemia.

Sodium bicarbonate reacts rapidly with HCl to form water, carbon dioxide, and salt. Antacids containing sodium bicarbonate have high amounts of sodium; in patients with hypertension or fluid overload, sodium-containing antacids can result in significant sodium retention.

Calcium carbonate is less soluble than sodium bicarbonate; it reacts with gastric acid to produce calcium chloride and carbon dioxide. Calcium carbonate is not only useful as an antacid, but can also serve as a calcium supplement for prevention of osteoporosis. The high calcium content of this antacid formulation may cause constipation.

AGENTS THAT PROMOTE MUCOSAL DEFENSE

Agents that promote mucosal defense are used in the symptomatic relief of peptic ulcer disease. These drugs include coating agents and prostaglandins.

Coating Agents

Sucralfate, a complex salt of sucrose sulfate and aluminum hydroxide, is a coating agent used to alleviate the symptoms of peptic ulcer disease. Sucralfate has little ability to alter gastric pH. Instead, in the acidic environment of the stomach, this complex forms a viscous gel that binds to positively charged proteins and thereby adheres to gastric epithelial cells (including areas of ulceration). The gel protects the luminal surface of the stomach from degradation by acid and pepsin. Because sucralfate is poorly soluble, there is little systemic absorption and no systemic toxicity. Constipation is one of the few adverse effects. In addition, sucralfate may bind to drugs such as quinolone antibiotics, phenytoin, and warfarin and limit their absorption.

Colloidal bismuth is a second coating agent used in peptic ulcer disease. Bismuth salts combine with mucus glycoproteins to form a barrier that protects an ulcer from further damage by acid and pepsin. Bismuth agents may stimulate mucosal bicarbonate and prostaglandin E_2 secretion and thereby also protect the mucosa from acid and pepsin degradation. Colloidal bismuth has been found to impede the growth of *H. pylori* and is frequently used as part of a multidrug regimen for the eradication of *H. pylori*-associated peptic ulcers (see below).

Prostaglandins

Prostaglandins can be used in the treatment of peptic ulcer disease (see Chapter 40), specifically in the treatment of NSAID-induced ulcers. NSAIDs are ulcerogenic because they inhibit prostaglandin synthesis and thereby interrupt the "gastroprotective" functions of PGE_2, which include reduced gastric acid secretion and enhanced bicarbonate secretion, mucus production, and blood flow.

Misoprostol is a prostaglandin analogue used to prevent NSAID-induced peptic ulcers. Its most frequent adverse effects are abdominal discomfort and diarrhea. In clinical practice, these adverse effects often interfere with patient compliance. Misoprostol is contraindicated in women who are (or may be) pregnant because of the possibility of generating uterine contractions that could result in abortion (see Chapter 28, Pharmacology of Reproduction).

AGENTS THAT MODIFY RISK FACTORS

Diet, Tobacco, and Alcohol

As in the introductory case, diet therapy typically involves recommendations to avoid caffeine-containing products because of their ability to increase acid secretion. Avoidance of alcohol and cigarette smoking is also advised. Excessive alcohol intake is directly toxic to the mucosa, and is associated with erosive gastritis and an increased incidence of peptic ulcers. Cigarette smoking is thought to decrease the production of duodenal bicarbonate and diminish mucosal blood flow, leading to a delay in ulcer healing.

Treatment of *H. pylori* Infection

Elimination of *H. pylori* can lead to cure of *H. pylori*-associated peptic ulcers. Treatment for *H. pylori* infection uses broad-spectrum antibiotics, such as **amoxicillin** or **tetracycline** combined with **metronidazole** or **clarithromycin,** together with bismuth citrate and a proton pump inhibitor or ranitidine. Common regimens involve **triple therapy** with amoxicillin, clarithromycin, and a proton pump inhibitor, or **quadruple therapy** with tetracycline, metronidazole, a proton pump inhibitor, and bismuth.

H. pylori may develop resistance to antibiotic therapy. Metronidazole resistance has been reported in the United States in patients with *H. pylori* infections. Resistance to clarithromycin is less common. Three-point mutations in the clarithromycin-binding site on *H. pylori* 23S rRNA (A2143G, A2142G, and A2142C) appear to be responsible for clarithromycin resistance, and the A2143G mutation has been associated with a very low bacterial eradication rate. In the introductory case, Tom was given clarithromycin instead of metronidazole because the former drug is less commonly associated with drug resistance.

The adverse effects of therapy for *H. pylori* infection include hypersensitivity reactions to penicillin analogues, nausea, headache, and antibiotic-induced diarrhea caused by superinfection with *Clostridium difficile*. These effects, along with the complicated dosing schedules associated with triple therapy and quadruple therapy, can lead to noncompliance. Resistance to *H. pylori* is a growing concern, and antibiotic regimens will need to evolve in order to meet the challenge.

◾ *Conclusion and Future Directions*

Peptic ulcer disease is responsible for significant morbidity and mortality in the United States. Because more than one pathophysiologic mechanism is often involved in the disease, multiple pharmacologic agents may be required for its prophylaxis and treatment (Fig. 45-4). Pharmacologic agents active against peptic ulcer disease decrease acid secretion, promote mucosal defense, and modify risk factors. Use of intravenous proton pump inhibitors and screening for cytochrome P450 polymorphisms may allow enhancement and customization of pharmacologic therapy for patients at risk. Improved treatment of *H. pylori* infection has the potential to decrease the overall incidence of peptic ulcer disease. COX-2 inhibitors have fallen short of expectations because of adverse cardiovascular effects. It remains to be seen whether new NSAIDs can be developed that do not promote peptic ulcer formation and have an acceptable cardiovascular effect profile.

Many new antisecretory agents are under development. **Tenatoprazole** is a proton pump inhibitor with a much longer plasma half-life (5 to 7 hours) than the 1 to 2 hours characteristic of the classic proton pump inhibitors. The longer half-life may translate into better control of acid secretion over a prolonged period. **Potassium-competitive acid blockers** are an investigational class of drugs that act by competitively inhibiting potassium entry into the parietal cell; these drugs bind ionically to the proton pump at or near the potassium binding site in a K^+-competitive manner. **CCK$_2$ receptor antagonists** may be useful for decreasing gastrin-mediated acid secretion; these agents are under investigation. Finally, an anti-gastrin vaccine designed to neutralize the gastrin-17 hormone is under development.

Suggested Reading

Baker DE. Intravenous proton pump inhibitors. *Rev Gastroenterol Disord* 2006;6:22–34. (*Discusses similarities and differences among intravenous proton pump inhibitors.*)

de Argila CM. Safety of potent gastric acid inhibition. *Drugs* 2005; 65(Suppl 1):97–104. (*Reviews proton pump inhibitor metabolism and drug-drug interactions.*)

De Francesco V, Margiotta M, Zullo A, et al. Clarithromycin-resistant genotypes and eradication of *Helicobacter pylori*. *Ann Intern Med* 2006;144:94–100. (*Discusses clarithromycin-resistant genotypes in* H. pylori.*)

Esplugues JV. A pharmacological approach to gastric acid inhibition. *Drugs* 2005;65(Suppl 1):7–12. (*Discusses pharmacology and adverse effects of individual proton pump inhibitors.*)

Spechler SJ. Peptic ulcer disease and its complications. In: Feldman M, Friedman LS, Sleisenger MH, eds. *Sleisenger and Fordtran's gastrointestinal and liver disease.* 7th ed. Philadelphia: WB Saunders; 2002:747–782. (*Reviews the pharmacology of peptic ulcer disease.*)

Suerbaum S, Michetti P. *Helicobacter pylori* infection. *N Engl J Med* 2002;347:1175–1186. (*Reviews the epidemiology, pathogenesis, and treatment of* H. pylori *infection.*)

Vakil N. New pharmacological agents for the treatment of gastro-oesophageal reflux disease. *Aliment Pharmacol Ther* 2004;19: 1041–1049. (*Summarizes data on new antisecretory agents.*)

Drug Summary Table | Chapter 45 Integrative Inflammation Pharmacology: Peptic Ulcer Disease

Drug	Clinical Applications	Serious and Common Adverse Effects	Contraindications	Therapeutic Considerations
H2 RECEPTOR ANTAGONISTS *Mechanism—Decrease acid secretion by inhibiting histamine binding to H2 receptors on parietal cells*				
Cimetidine	Peptic ulcer disease Gastroesophageal reflux disease (GERD) Erosive esophagitis Gastric acid hypersecretion	*Necrotizing enterocolitis in fetus or newborn, agranulocytosis, psychotic disorder* Headache, dizziness, arthralgia, myalgia, constipation, diarrhea, gynecomastia, galactorrhea, loss of libido	Hypersensitivity to cimetidine	Cimetidine reduces the cytochrome P450-mediated metabolism of certain drugs, including theophylline, warfarin, phenytoin, lidocaine, and quinidine, delaying the clearance and increasing the plasma levels of these drugs
Ranitidine Famotidine Nizatidine	Peptic ulcer disease Gastroesophageal reflux disease (GERD) Erosive esophagitis Gastric acid hypersecretion	*Necrotizing enterocolitis in fetus or newborn, pancreatitis* Headache, dizziness, arthralgia, myalgia, constipation, diarrhea	Hypersensitivity to ranitidine, famotidine, or nizatidine	Ranitidine can be given IV to treat hypersecretory conditions or to treat patients who are not able to tolerate the oral formulation Bioavailability of nizatidine is higher than that of other H2 receptor antagonists
PROTON PUMP INHIBITORS *Mechanism—Decrease acid secretion by blocking H+/K+-ATPase on parietal cells*				
Omeprazole Esomeprazole Lansoprazole Pantoprazole Rabeprazole	Peptic ulcer disease Gastroesophageal reflux disease (GERD) Erosive esophagitis Gastric acid hypersecretion *H. pylori* gastrointestinal tract infection	*Pancreatitis, hepatotoxicity, interstitial nephritis* Headache, diarrhea, rash, gastrointestinal discomfort, anorexia, asthenia, back pain	Hypersensitivity to omeprazole, esomeprazole, lansoprazole, pantoprazole, or rabeprazole	Proton pump inhibitors are metabolized in the liver by CYP2C19 and CYP3A4 Pantoprazole can be given IV as an alternative therapy in patients who are not able to tolerate oral pantoprazole Drug interaction with ketoconazole or itraconazole due to the acid environment required for absorption of these azole drugs
ANTACIDS *Mechanism—Neutralize gastric acid*				
Aluminum hydroxide	Symptomatic relief of dyspepsia associated with peptic ulcer disease, gastritis, GERD, or hiatal hernia	*Phosphate depletion (severe weakness, malaise, and anorexia)* Constipation, osteomalacia in patients with renal failure	Hypersensitivity to aluminum hydroxide	All antacids can potentially increase or decrease the rate or extent of absorption of concurrently administered oral drugs by changing transit time or by binding the drug
Magnesium hydroxide	Symptomatic relief of dyspepsia associated with peptic ulcer disease, gastritis, GERD, or hiatal hernia	Diarrhea, hypermagnesemia (in patients with renal failure)	Hypersensitivity to magnesium hydroxide	Same as for aluminum hydroxide
Sodium bicarbonate	Symptomatic relief of dyspepsia Metabolic acidosis Urinary alkalinization Uric acid renal stones Diarrhea	Abdominal cramps, flatulence, alkalosis, vomiting	Respiratory alkalosis Hypocalcemia Hypochloremia	Same as for aluminum hydroxide In addition, significant sodium retention in patients with hypertension or fluid overload
Calcium carbonate	Symptomatic relief of dyspepsia Osteoporosis	Hypercalcemia, nausea, vomiting, anorexia	Severe renal insufficiency	Same as for aluminum hydroxide In addition, hypercalcemia can occur in patients with impaired renal function

COATING AGENTS

Mechanism—Coat gastric mucosa with a protective layer

Drug	Clinical Applications	Serious and Common Adverse Effects	Contraindications	Therapeutic Considerations
Sucralfate	Peptic ulcer disease Gastric ulcer disease GERD	*Aluminum accumulation and toxicity (especially in patients with renal impairment)* Constipation	Hypersensitivity to sucralfate	Decreased effectiveness of quinolones (e.g., ciprofloxacin) because of chelation and decreased absorption
Colloidal bismuth	Peptic ulcer disease Gastric ulcer disease GERD Diarrhea with associated abdominal cramps	Darkening of the tongue and/or stool, nausea, vomiting	Known allergy to aspirin or other nonaspirin salicylates	Frequently used as a component of a multidrug regimen for eradication of *H. pylori* because bismuth impedes growth of the organism Reduces absorption of tetracyclines, likely through chelation or by reducing solubility as a result of increasing gastric pH Acute bismuth intoxication is manifested by gastrointestinal disturbance, stomatitis, discoloration of mucous membranes, and potential for kidney and liver damage

PROSTAGLANDINS

Mechanism—Reduce basal and stimulated gastric acid secretion; enhance bicarbonate secretion, mucus production and blood flow

Drug				
Misoprostol	See Drug Summary Table: Chapter 41 Pharmacology of Eicosanoids			

ANTICHOLINERGIC AGENTS

Mechanism—Decrease acid secretion by inhibiting acetylcholine binding to muscarinic ACh receptors on parietal cells

Drug	Clinical Applications	Serious and Common Adverse Effects	Contraindications	Therapeutic Considerations
Dicyclomine	Irritable bowel syndrome Peptic ulcer disease	Dry mouth, blurred vision, tachycardia, urinary retention, constipation	Age less than 6 months Breastfeeding Gastrointestinal obstruction Glaucoma Myasthenia gravis Obstructive uropathy Reflux esophagitis Severe ulcerative colitis or toxic megacolon	Not as effective as H2 receptor antagonists or proton pump inhibitors for the treatment of peptic ulcer disease

46

Integrative Inflammation Pharmacology: Asthma

Joshua M. Galanter and Stephen Lazarus

INTRODUCTION

Asthma is a chronic disease of the airways, marked by intermittent exacerbations of acute disease (asthma attacks). The symptoms of asthma include dyspnea and wheezing as well as mucus production and cough. Asthma is both an obstructive lung disease and an inflammatory disease; the obstructive component is characterized by bronchoconstriction, whereas the inflammatory component is marked by airway edema, goblet-cell hyperplasia, mucus secretion, and infiltration by a wide variety of immune and inflammatory cells that release a number of associated cytokines. Although in most cases the airway obstruction is reversible, over time, asthma may cause airway remodeling and permanent deterioration in pulmonary function.

Medications used to treat asthma act in one of two ways: by relaxing bronchial smooth muscle or by preventing and treating inflammation. This chapter approaches asthma as both a bronchoconstrictive and an inflammatory disease. After discussing the physiologic control of bronchial tone and the function of immune pathways in the airways, the

chapter turns to the pathophysiology of asthma. Current therapies are then discussed, including the pharmacology of both bronchodilators and anti-inflammatory agents.

 Case

Ahmad, a 14-year-old student in the sixth grade, has a long history of allergic rhinitis. He was first diagnosed with asthma at age 6. Ahmad plays soccer during recess but often has to quit early because of difficulty breathing. He has struggled in school because he frequently misses class due to exacerbations of his asthma. When Ahmad was first diagnosed with asthma, his doctor prescribed theophylline, one tablet to be taken twice daily. He has continued on this medicine ever since. Sometimes he also self-administers an inhaled medication containing epinephrine, although afterward he has trouble concentrating because he feels "too nervous."

At home, Ahmad frequently awakens with coughing and chest tightness. He develops symptoms when exposed to cats or cigarette smoke. One night he experiences a severe asthma attack that he cannot control with his aerosolized epinephrine spray. Ahmad is taken to the emergency department of the local hospital. He describes the sensation of a large man sitting on his chest while he is trying to breathe through a narrow straw. He has an incessant cough with thick, clear sputum. His chest examination is notable for bilateral expiratory wheezes and a prolonged expiratory phase. Laboratory tests show that his total white blood cell count is normal (8,200 cells/μL), but there is an excess of eosinophils (9%).

The emergency medicine physician gives Ahmad albuterol, a bronchodilator, administered as a nebulized aerosol. Ahmad's wheezing improves, although he also experiences tremulousness and a rapid pounding of his heart. The physician then administers an intravenous infusion of hydrocortisone, a glucocorticoid, to treat Ahmad's airway inflammation. Every 2 hours, Ahmad receives additional albuterol treatments by nebulizer.

By the end of the night, Ahmad feels he can breathe comfortably again. On his discharge from the emergency department, his mother is given a prescription for an inhaled steroid medication, fluticasone. Ahmad is instructed to use the fluticasone inhaler twice daily, as well as an albuterol inhaler to replace his epinephrine spray. With his new medications, Ahmad has fewer attacks of asthma, although he continues to awaken several nights a week with asthmatic symptoms. He uses the albuterol inhaler several times a day to relieve his cough and wheezing. Ahmad finds that the steroid spray irritates his throat, and he is not as faithful in using it as he knows he should be.

At a checkup later in the year, Ahmad's new doctor recommends that he stop taking the theophylline tablets and instead prescribes a combination inhaler containing fluticasone and salmeterol, a long-acting bronchodilator. He also advises Ahmad to use the albuterol inhaler as needed. With this new regimen, Ahmad finally feels that he is in control of his asthma, and he is able to play soccer and do better in school.

QUESTIONS

■ **1.** Why did Ahmad develop asthma?

■ **2.** Why did epinephrine cause anxiety? Why did albuterol cause fewer adverse effects?

■ **3.** How does theophylline act, and why did Ahmad's new physician discontinue it?

■ **4.** Why did fluticasone cause local throat irritation, and what could Ahmad do to prevent this undesirable effect?

■ **5.** Why are most asthma medications given by the pulmonary route rather than as pills?

PHYSIOLOGY OF AIRWAY SMOOTH MUSCLE TONE AND IMMUNE FUNCTION

Because asthma involves dysfunction in the pathways that regulate both smooth muscle tone and immune function in the airways, it is important to review the normal physiology

of these systems before discussing the pathophysiology of asthma.

PHYSIOLOGY OF AIRWAY SMOOTH MUSCLE CONTRACTION

As discussed in Chapter 7, Principles of Nervous System Physiology and Pharmacology, involuntary responses of smooth muscle are regulated by the autonomic nervous system. In the airways, **sympathetic** (adrenergic) tone causes bronchodilation and **parasympathetic** (cholinergic) tone causes bronchoconstriction. Bronchial smooth muscle tone is also regulated by **nonadrenergic, noncholinergic (NANC)** fibers that innervate the respiratory tree.

Adrenergic receptors mediate sympathetic innervation of the lungs. Airway smooth muscle cells express β_2-**adrenergic receptors** (and, to a lesser extent, β_1-adrenergic receptors). β_2-Adrenergic receptors are activated by **epinephrine**, which is secreted by the adrenal medulla and causes bronchodilation. Exogenous epinephrine was one of the first pharmacotherapies for asthma, and is still available in an over-the-counter formulation that was used by Ahmad. Newer, β_2-selective adrenergic agonists, such as the **albuterol** later prescribed for Ahmad, are now considered the first-line bronchodilators for treatment of acute asthmatic symptoms.

The vagus nerve provides parasympathetic innervation to the lungs. Airway smooth muscle cells express **muscarinic receptors**, especially the excitatory M_3 subtype of muscarinic receptors. Upon stimulation by acetylcholine released by parasympathetic postganglionic neurons, these receptors induce bronchoconstriction. Parasympathetic neurons are dominant in maintaining smooth muscle tone, and **anticholinergic agents** can cause bronchorelaxation. These agents are used primarily in the treatment of chronic obstructive pulmonary disease (see Box 46-1), but can also be used in acute asthma attacks or when β_2-selective adrenergic agonists are contraindicated.

The NANC fibers are primarily under parasympathetic control but release neither norepinephrine nor acetylcholine. Moreover, NANC fibers can be either stimulatory (causing bronchoconstriction) or inhibitory (causing bronchodilation). NANC fibers release neuropeptides, including **neurokinin A**, **calcitonin gene-related peptide**, **substance P**, **bradykinin**, **tachykinin**, and **neuropeptide Y**, all of which are bronchoconstrictors, and **nitric oxide (NO)** and **vasoactive intestinal polypeptide (VIP)**, which cause bronchorelaxation. Although no pharmacologic agents have yet been developed to take advantage of the NANC system, nitric oxide is a marker of the intensity of airway inflammation, and NO measurements have been used to assess the severity of asthma and titrate therapy accordingly.

IMMUNE FUNCTION IN THE AIRWAY

As described in Chapter 40, Principles of Inflammation and the Immune System, **T lymphocytes** play a key role in controlling the immune response. T lymphocytes are divided into CD8$^+$ **T_C (cytotoxic) cells**, which are mediators of cellular adaptive immunity, and CD4$^+$ **T_H (helper) cells**, which regulate adaptive immune responses. T_H cells are further divided into **T_H1** and **T_H2** cells based on the cytokines

Pharmacology of Chronic Obstructive Pulmonary Disease

Chronic obstructive pulmonary disease (COPD) describes a spectrum of disorders that results in obstructive lung disease. Unlike asthma, COPD is generally not reversible. COPD is caused by an abnormal inflammatory response to an inhaled environmental insult. In 90% of cases, this insult to the lungs is tobacco smoke. Clinically, COPD is divided into two frequently overlapping diseases: **emphysema** and **chronic bronchitis.** Pulmonary emphysema refers to alveolar enlargement caused by destruction of alveolar walls, whereas chronic bronchitis is a clinical diagnosis made on the basis of a chronic cough, for 3 or more months during 2 consecutive years, that cannot be attributed to another cause.

COPD is caused by an abnormal response to inhalation of tobacco smoke or other toxic agents. In contrast to asthma, where CD4$^+$ T lymphocytes, B lymphocytes, mast cells, and eosinophils are the primary inflammatory cells, the inflammatory response to tobacco smoke is primarily neutrophilic and monocytic. Tobacco smoke stimulates resident alveolar macrophages to produce chemokines that attract neutrophils. These neutrophils and resident macrophages release proteinases, particularly **matrix metalloproteinases.** The proteinases degrade elastin, which provides elastic recoil to the alveoli, as well as other proteins that compose the matrix supporting the lung parenchyma. Cell death follows, due to impaired attachment to the degraded matrix and to the toxic actions of inflammatory cells. The result is that alveoli degrade and coalesce, forming the characteristic enlargement of air spaces typical of emphysema. There is also enhanced mucus production and fibrosis, although the mechanisms underlying these pathologic phenomena have not been well characterized.

Although it is tempting to think that inflammation in COPD could be held in check by inhaled corticosteroids, steroids are unfortunately of limited benefit in this disease. The lack of steroid efficacy likely results from the fact that the inflammatory cells responsible for COPD

are macrophages and neutrophils, which are less responsive than lymphocytes and eosinophils to the actions of corticosteroids. Moreover, the activity of histone deacetylase is impaired in COPD, so the inhibition of proinflammatory transcription factors is limited. A number of studies have examined the effects of inhaled corticosteroids on lung function in COPD, but none have found a statistically significant benefit. However, inhaled corticosteroids have been found to reduce the frequency and severity of acute exacerbations of COPD. Therefore, while corticosteroids are not routinely recommended for the treatment of COPD, they may be indicated in patients who develop frequent, severe exacerbations.

Because cysteinyl leukotrienes, mast cells, and IgE have no role in the pathophysiology of COPD, specific treatments for asthma that target these pathways are not useful in COPD. Interestingly, **leukotriene B4** is a potent chemotactic factor for neutrophils and, though therapy targeted at this mediator could logically be expected to have a role in COPD, clinical studies of LTB$_4$ antagonism have not shown a benefit to date.

Bronchodilators produce only a modest improvement in airflow in patients with COPD. However, even a small improvement in airflow can significantly improve symptoms in patients with COPD, especially those whose lungs have become hyperinflated. Asthma is punctuated by acute attacks, while most patients with COPD have chronic breathlessness that is worsened with exertion. Therefore, short-acting ''reliever'' medications are less beneficial than long-acting drugs in COPD. Both β-adrenergic agonists and inhaled anticholinergic agents cause bronchodilation in COPD. However, many patients with COPD have concomitant coronary artery disease, so anticholinergic agents may be preferred in this subset of patients. There is evidence that the bronchodilatory effects of β agonists and anticholinergic agents (and theophylline) are additive; therefore, patients with severe COPD may benefit from combination therapy, such as albuterol and ipratropium.

they produce. T$_H$1 cells, which produce **interferon-γ, IL-2,** and **TNF-α,** guide the immune response toward a cellular response involving both T$_H$ and T$_C$ cells. T$_H$2 cells, which produce **IL-4, IL-5, IL-6, IL-9,** and **IL-13,** guide the immune response toward a humoral response based on antibody production by B cells. Because cytokines produced by T$_H$1 and T$_H$2 cells are mutually inhibitory, any given immune stimulus elicits predominantly one or the other response (Fig. 46-1).

All individuals continually inhale environmental allergens such as cat dander, pollen, dust mites, and a host of other antigens. These allergens are phagocytosed by antigen-presenting cells lining the airways. In general, the antigens are ignored by T$_H$ cells and generate only a low level of IgG antibodies and a moderate T$_H$1 response mediated by interferon-γ. In contrast, an exaggerated T$_H$2 response often predominates in asthma, generating the characteristic in-

flammation and bronchial hyperresponsiveness characteristic of the disease (Fig. 46-1).

PATHOPHYSIOLOGY OF ASTHMA

Asthma is a complex disease characterized by airway inflammation, which leads to airway hyperresponsiveness, which causes symptomatic bronchoconstriction. The most prominent clinical feature of asthma is bronchoconstriction, and a simplistic approach to understanding the disease focuses on airway smooth muscle contraction. At its most fundamental level, however, asthma is an inflammatory disease of the airways. As detailed below, the treatment of asthma employs both bronchodilators and anti-inflammatory agents.

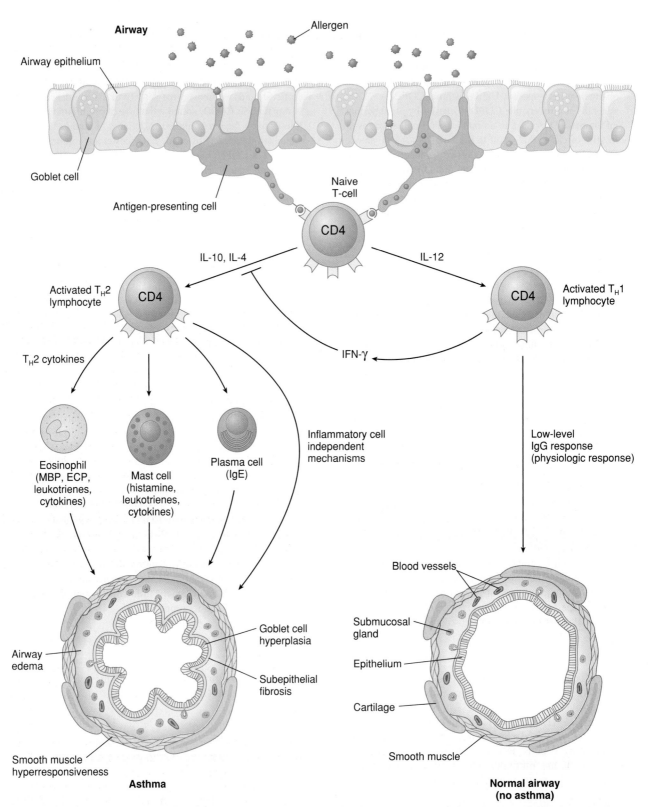

Figure 46-1. Origins of the asthmatic immune response. In nonatopic individuals, antigens derived from allergens are presented by antigen-presenting dendritic cells to engender a T_H1 response that produces only a low-level, physiologic, IgG-predominant response. This response does not cause airway inflammation or bronchoconstriction **(right side).** Interferon-γ, produced by T_H1 lymphocytes, inhibits a T_H2 response. In individuals susceptible to asthma, allergen-derived antigens that are presented to immature CD4+ T cells cause these cells to differentiate into activated T_H2 lymphocytes. The T_H2 lymphocytes release cytokines that recruit to the airway other inflammatory cells, including eosinophils, mast cells, and IgE-producing B cells, which produce an inflammatory response. T cells also induce an asthmatic response directly. The net result—airway hyperresponsiveness, mucus production by goblet cells, airway edema, subepithelial fibrosis, and bronchoconstriction—constitute the asthmatic response **(left side).**

ASTHMA AS A BRONCHOCONSTRICTIVE DISEASE

The propensity of asthmatic airways to constrict in response to a wide variety of stimuli, including allergens, environmental irritants, exercise, cold air, and infections, is termed **hyperresponsiveness**. Two features of airway hyperresponsiveness separate the asthmatic response to stimuli from the nonasthmatic response: **hypersensitivity** and **hyperreactivity**. Hypersensitivity describes a normal response at abnormally low levels of stimuli; i.e., the airways of asthmatics constrict too readily. Hyperreactivity describes an exaggerated response at normal to high levels of stimuli; i.e., the airways respond too vigorously. In Figure 46-2, hypersensitivity describes a shift of the stimulus-response curve to the left, while hyperreactivity describes an upward shift.

The causes of airway hyperresponsiveness in asthma have not been completely elucidated. The hyperreactive response may be explained by the hyperplasia and hypertrophy of the airway smooth muscle that develops as part of the inflammatory response. The hypersensitivity response may be related to an observation that the amount and activity of **myosin light chain kinase** is increased in the bronchial smooth muscle of patients with asthma.

ASTHMA AS AN INFLAMMATORY DISEASE

Although the primary symptoms of most asthmatic patients are due to bronchoconstriction, the underlying cause of asthma is an allergic inflammation of the airways. The inflammatory process is visible histologically as airway edema, goblet cell hyperplasia, subepithelial fibrosis, increased mucus secretion, and infiltration by a variety of inflammatory cells, including T_H2 lymphocytes, antigen-presenting cells, plasma cells, mast cells, neutrophils, and eosinophils (Fig. 46-1). Many inflammatory mediators and cytokines govern the interplay among these inflammatory cells. Anti-inflammatory medications, particularly corticosteroids, are mainstays in the pharmacologic treatment of asthma. As the complex pathophysiology of asthma is further elucidated, more targeted therapies will be developed.

T_H2 Cells and the Origin of Asthma

One theory suggests that asthma (and other allergic diseases) is caused by a cellular imbalance favoring T_H2 lymphocytes over T_H1 lymphocytes and a humoral response involving strong IgE-mediated reactions rather than low-level IgG responses. T_H2 lymphocytes contribute to asthma through three mechanisms. First, in patients with a hereditary predisposition to **atopy** (from the Greek meaning ''out of place''), an allergen can trigger a **type I hypersensitivity** response. In normal (nonatopic) individuals, an allergen is phagocytosed by antigen-presenting cells, stimulating a low-level T_H1 response that includes the production of appropriate amounts of IgG antibodies directed against the allergen. In atopic individuals, however, the same allergen induces a strong T_H2 response that includes the production of IL-4, which induces B cells to produce exaggerated amounts of IgE antibodies directed against the allergen (Fig. 46-1). The IgE antibodies bind to high-affinity IgE receptors on mast cells, and crosslinking of the IgE receptors upon re-exposure to the allergen causes mast-cell degranulation (Fig. 46-2, and see below). Second, T_H2 cells can directly induce a **type IV hypersensitivity** reaction through the production of IL-13 (and, to a lesser degree, IL-4). In the airway, IL-13 causes goblet cell hyperplasia, increased mucus production, and smooth muscle hyperresponsiveness (Fig. 46-1). Third, T_H2 lymphocytes recruit eosinophils by producing IL-5 as well as GM-CSF and IL-4. These cytokines induce eosinophil proliferation and release from the bone marrow and promote eosinophil survival in the circulation and tissues. As in many patients with asthma, Ahmad had a high level of circulating eosinophils.

What causes the imbalance between T_H1 and T_H2 lymphocytes in patients with asthma? The exact reasons are unknown but likely involve environmental effects on genetically susceptible individuals. It is known through epidemiologic studies that exposures to tuberculosis, viruses such as measles and hepatitis A, older siblings, and other children through attendance at a day-care facility, particularly in the first 6 months of life, are associated with a decreased incidence of asthma. One leading theory suggests that a ''Western lifestyle,'' including decreased exposure early in life to microbes that engender T_H1-lymphocyte responses, contributes to the development of asthma and other allergic diseases in susceptible individuals. Although this ''hygiene hypothesis'' is probably too simplistic to explain the origins of a complex disease such as asthma, it forms a useful model for thinking about the disease as well as a possible explanation for the dramatic rise in the incidence of asthma in the Western hemisphere. It is impossible to know exactly what caused Ahmed's asthma; however, the fact that he had allergic rhinitis suggests that he had an atopic predisposition triggered by cat dander and possibly other antigens.

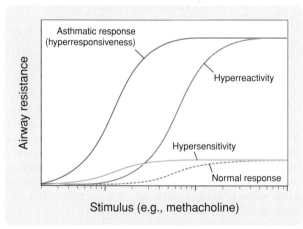

Figure 46-2. Airway hyperresponsiveness in asthma. Nonasthmatics have a low-level response to a stimulus that produces mild, if any, bronchoconstriction at normal to high doses (normal response). An asthmatic patient has hyperresponsive airways that demonstrate exaggerated bronchoconstriction at low doses of the stimulus (hyperresponsiveness). The two components of hyperresponsiveness are hypersensitivity (a normal response to abnormally low doses of a stimulus) and hyperreactivity (an exaggerated response to normal to high doses of a stimulus).

Plasma Cells, IgE, Mast Cells, and Leukotrienes

As noted above, IgE-mediated type I hypersensitivity responses are one mechanism by which allergens cause the pathologic and clinical manifestations of asthma (Fig. 46-3). The allergic response is initiated when a dendritic cell phagocytoses an inhaled allergen. The dendritic cell presents the processed allergen to T_H2 cells and activates them. The activated T_H2 cells bind and activate B cells via CD40 on the B-cell surface. Activated T_H2 cells also generate IL-4 and IL-13, which induce B-cell transformation into IgE-producing plasma cells.

IgE circulates briefly in the bloodstream before binding to high-affinity IgE receptors (**FcϵRI**) on mast cells. Upon re-exposure, the allergen binds to mast cell-bound IgE and crosslinks the FcϵRI receptors, thereby activating the mast cell. The activated mast cell degranulates, releasing its preformed inflammatory mediators. These molecules include **histamine**, proteolytic enzymes, and certain cytokines (such as **platelet-activating factor**). The activated mast cell also releases **arachidonic acid** from its plasma membrane and produces **leukotrienes** and **prostaglandin D$_2$** (Fig. 46-4).

Acutely, mast-cell degranulation produces bronchoconstriction and airway inflammation. Histamine released by the mast cells promotes capillary leakage, leading to airway edema. Mast cells also release **leukotriene C$_4$** (LTC$_4$), which is subsequently converted into **LTD$_4$** and **LTE$_4$** (see Chapter 41, Pharmacology of Eicosanoids). These three leukotrienes, called **cysteinyl leukotrienes**, are central to the pathophysiology of asthma because they induce marked bronchoconstriction. *Leukotriene D$_4$ is 1,000 times more potent than histamine in producing bronchoconstriction.* Leukotrienes also cause mucus hypersecretion, capillary leakage, and vasogenic edema, and recruit additional inflammatory cells. The effect of the leukotrienes, though slower in onset, is more powerful and sustained than that of the preformed mediators. The leukotrienes were called **slow-reacting substance of anaphylaxis** (**SRS-A**) before their actual structures were identified.

Mast cells recruit other inflammatory cells via the release of chemokines and cytokines. This produces a delayed reaction that develops 4 to 6 hours after exposure to allergen (Fig. 46-3). Mast cells also release **tryptase**, a protease that activates receptors on epithelial and endothelial cells, inducing the expression of adhesion molecules that attract eosinophils and basophils. Tryptase is also a smooth muscle mitogen, causing hyperplasia of airway smooth muscle cells and contributing to airway hyperresponsiveness. The production of IL-1, IL-2, IL-3, IL-4, IL-5, GM-CSF, interferon-γ, and TNF-α by mast cells contributes to chronic inflammation and the chronic asthmatic reaction. Finally, mast cells release proteases and proteoglycans that act on supporting airway structures to produce chronic changes in the airway (also called **airway remodeling**). Unlike the reversible component of bronchoconstriction that characterizes the acute asthmatic reaction, the airway remodeling induced by chronic inflammation may be irreversible.

Eosinophils

The major physiologic role of eosinophils is to defend against parasitic infections. Eosinophils originate in the bone marrow and are stimulated by IL-3, IL-5, and GM-CSF pro-duced by T_H2 lymphocytes and mast cells. Eosinophils migrate from the bloodstream to the airway by binding to specific adhesion molecules, particularly VCAM-1, and by traveling along chemokine gradients to sites of inflammation. Once recruited to the airway, eosinophils have a complex, multifunctional role in asthma. Activated eosinophils secrete cytotoxic granules that cause local tissue damage and induce airway remodeling. Eosinophils also release cytokines and chemokines that recruit other inflammatory cells. Finally, these cells release lipid mediators and neuromodulators that affect airway tone.

The toxic granules of eosinophils contain a number of cationic proteins—including **major basic protein** (MBP), **eosinophilic cationic protein** (ECP), **eosinophil peroxidase**, and **eosinophil-derived neurotoxin**—that are directly damaging to the bronchial epithelium. For example, ECP can breach the integrity of target cell membranes by forming ion-selective, voltage-insensitive pores, and eosinophil peroxidase catalyzes the production of highly reactive oxygen species that oxidize target cell proteins and induce apoptosis. Eosinophils also produce **matrix metalloproteinases** that contribute to airway remodeling.

Eosinophils contribute both directly and indirectly to airway hyperresponsiveness. MBP and ECP affect smooth muscle tone and induce hyperresponsiveness. These proteins also damage inhibitory M2 muscarinic receptors, increasing vagal tone. Eosinophil-derived cysteinyl leukotrienes and neuropeptides (such as substance P) increase vasodilation, vascular permeability, mucus hypersecretion, and airway smooth muscle contraction.

Finally, eosinophils are immunomodulatory cells that can amplify the immune response in asthma. Eosinophils upregulate endothelial adhesion molecules and thereby recruit other inflammatory cells. Eosinophils are also antigen-presenting cells capable of activating T lymphocytes.

PHARMACOLOGIC CLASSES AND AGENTS

The pharmacologic agents used to treat asthma are divided into two broad categories: **relievers** and **controllers** (also called **preventers**). This distinction emphasizes the clinical uses of these agents and helps patients understand and comply with the prescribed regimen. This classification scheme also relates to the mechanisms of action of antiasthma drugs. *In general, bronchodilators, which alleviate smooth muscle bronchoconstriction, are used as relievers, and anti-inflammatory medications, which decrease airway inflammation, are used as controllers.* There is also evidence that some medications—**methylxanthines**, for example—have both bronchodilatory and anti-inflammatory effects. In the introductory case, Ahmad was given a combination of an anti-inflammatory agent (fluticasone) and a long-acting bronchodilator (salmeterol, a long-acting β_2-agonist) as controllers, with albuterol (a short-acting β_2-agonist) as a reliever.

BRONCHODILATORS

Bronchodilators affect airway smooth muscle tone by acting on autonomic nervous system receptors and signaling path-

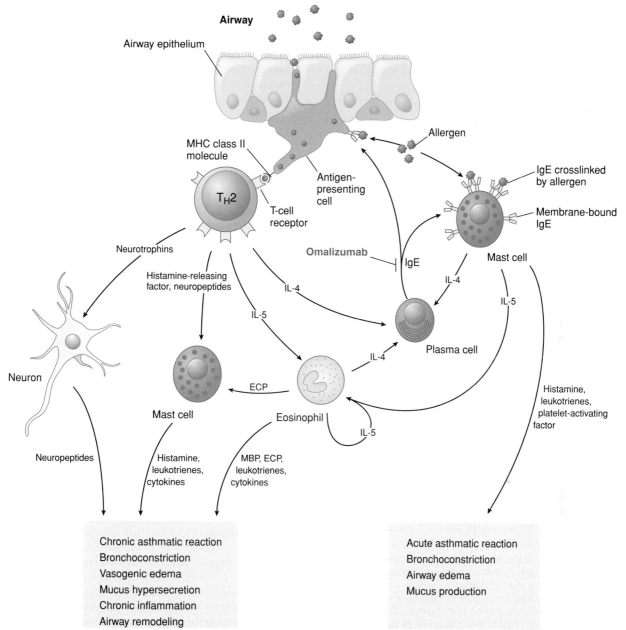

Figure 46-3. The allergic response in asthma. Asthma produces acute and chronic inflammatory responses in the airways. Antigen-presenting cells phagocytose and process allergens, presenting the antigens to CD4$^+$ T cells. These cells differentiate into cytokine-producing T_H2 lymphocytes. The T_H2 cells release IL-4 and IL-5, which recruit B cells and eosinophils, respectively. The B cells differentiate into IgE-producing plasma cells, and the IgE binds to the FcϵRI receptors on mast cells and antigen-presenting cells. Upon re-exposure to the allergen, the FcϵRI-bound IgE is crosslinked, inducing the mast cell to degranulate and release preformed and newly generated inflammatory mediators—including histamine, the cysteinyl leukotrienes, platelet-activating factor, and other cytokines—which cause the acute asthmatic reaction. Chronically, T_H2 cells and mast cells produce circulating IL-5 that recruits eosinophils, and T_H2 cells release products that stimulate local mast cells and neurons. Together, the inflammatory mediators and catabolic enzymes produced by eosinophils, mast cells, and neurons cause a chronic asthmatic reaction characterized by bronchoconstriction, airway edema, mucus hypersecretion, chronic inflammation, and airway remodeling.

Omalizumab is a humanized monoclonal antibody against the FcϵRI-binding domain on IgE. By preventing IgE from binding to the IgE receptor (FcϵRI) on mast cells, omalizumab inhibits mast cell degranulation upon re-exposure to allergen and thereby modulates the acute allergic response. Omalizumab also down-regulates FcϵRI on antigen-presenting cells, diminishing antigen processing and presentation to CD4$^+$ lymphocytes. Because fewer immature T cells are induced by allergen to differentiate into T_H2 lymphocytes, the chronic asthmatic reaction is also blunted.

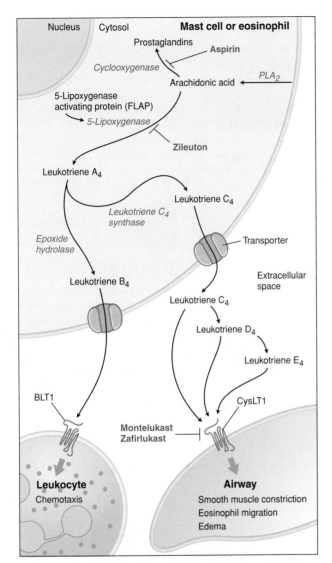

Figure 46-4. The leukotriene pathway in asthma. Leukotrienes are some of the most potent bronchoconstrictors known and are important mediators of inflammation in the airway. Drugs that inhibit leukotriene production or receptor binding have a role in asthma therapy. Leukotrienes are formed when arachidonic acid is released from the inner leaflet of the plasma membrane by the action of phospholipase A_2 (PLA$_2$), and converted to leukotriene A_4 by the action of 5-lipoxygenase upon activation of the latter enzyme by 5-lipoxygenase activating protein (FLAP). Leukotriene A_4 is converted to leukotriene C_4 by the action of leukotriene C_4 synthase, and leukotriene C_4 is transported out of the cell. Leukotriene C_4 is converted to leukotriene D_4 and then to leukotriene E_4; all three of these cysteinyl leukotrienes bind to CysLT1 receptors expressed on airway smooth muscle cells, leading to bronchoconstriction and airway edema. Leukotriene A_4 is converted to leukotriene B_4 by epoxide hydrolase in mast cells and eosinophils. Leukotriene B_4 is transported out of the cell and binds to BLT1 receptors expressed on leukocytes, leading to leukocyte chemotaxis and recruitment. The leukotriene pathway can be inhibited by the 5-lipoxygenase inhibitor zileuton or by the CysLT1 receptor antagonists montelukast and zafirlukast.

ways. Sympathetic activation (mediated primarily by β_2-adrenergic receptors) results in bronchodilation, while parasympathetic stimulation (mediated by muscarinic acetylcholine receptors) results in bronchoconstriction. Because sympathomimetics cause rapid relaxation of airway smooth muscle, β_2-adrenergic agonists are particularly effective in the treatment of acute asthma exacerbations.

Anticholinergics

Anticholinergic agents were the first medications used to treat asthma in Western medicine. As early as 1896, Stedman's *Twentieth Century Practice of Modern Medical Science* suggested that asthma attacks could be treated by smoking "asthma cigarettes" containing **stramonium** extracted from the plant *Datura stramonium*. The active ingredients in stramonium were the anticholinergic belladonna alkaloids. To this day, asthma exacerbations that are not responsive to inhaled β_2-adrenergic agonists, or where inhaled beta agonists are contraindicated (such as in patients with cardiac ischemia or arrhythmia), can be treated with inhaled **ipratropium bromide**.

Ipratropium bromide is a quaternary ammonium salt derived from **atropine**. Because inhaled atropine is highly absorbed across the respiratory epithelium, it causes many systemic anticholinergic effects, including tachycardia, nausea, dry mouth, constipation, and urinary retention. Unlike atropine, ipratropium is not significantly absorbed, and these adverse systemic effects are minimized. Nonetheless, inhaled ipratropium can cause dry mouth and gastrointestinal upset through its deposition in the mouth and inadvertent oral absorption.

Tiotropium, a long-acting anticholinergic agent, has recently been approved by the U. S. Food and Drug Administration (FDA) for the treatment of **chronic obstructive pulmonary disease** (COPD; Box 46-1). Like ipratropium, tiotropium is a quaternary ammonium salt that produces few systemic effects because it is not systemically absorbed upon inhalation.

Atropine, ipratropium, and tiotropium are competitive antagonists at muscarinic acetylcholine receptors. Of the four muscarinic receptor subtypes expressed by the lung (M_1, M_2, M_3, and M_4), the excitatory M_3 receptor is the most important in mediating smooth muscle contraction and mucus gland secretion in the airway. Ipratropium and tiotropium antagonize the effect of endogenous acetylcholine at M_3 receptors, leading to bronchorelaxation and decreased mucus secretion. Tiotropium has a long duration of action largely because of its slow dissociation from M_1 and M_3 receptors.

Ipratropium and tiotropium are used mainly to treat COPD, where the major reversible bronchoconstrictive component is mediated by cholinergic neural tone. In chronic asthma, cholinergic stimulation has only a secondary role in causing bronchoconstriction, although increased vagal stimulation at night may be an important contributor to nighttime symptoms. Ipratropium is not formally approved by the FDA for asthma, but studies have suggested therapeutic uses for the drug in the treatment of acute asthma exacerbations and as rescue therapy in the subset of patients who cannot tolerate β-adrenergic agonists.

Beta-Adrenergic Agonists

Because β_2-adrenergic stimulation of airway smooth muscle leads to relaxation, it follows that systemic or aerosolized administration of agents that stimulate β_2-adrenergic receptors would be effective as a therapy for asthma. One early treatment for asthma involved the subcutaneous administration of **adrenaline (epinephrine)**. By the middle of the 20th century, epinephrine was made into an inhaled formulation that is still available today. Traditional Chinese practitioners have for centuries made use of the nonselective adrenergic agonist **ephedrine (Ma-Huang)** as a remedy for asthma.

Epinephrine is a nonselective adrenergic agonist that binds to α-, β_1-, and β_2-adrenergic receptors (see Chapter 9, Adrenergic Pharmacology). Epinephrine causes cardiac stimulation via β_1 receptors, leading to tachycardia, palpitations, and potentially arrhythmias, and peripheral vasoconstriction via α receptors, leading to hypertension. These systemic effects explain Ahmad's nervousness and difficulty concentrating after using inhaled epinephrine.

A selective β-adrenergic agonist, **isoproterenol**, was later developed as an alternative to epinephrine. Isoproterenol stimulates both β_1 and β_2 receptors and therefore causes both bronchodilation and cardiac stimulation. Isoproterenol has been used in inhaled form to treat asthma, although systemic absorption of drug can lead to tachycardia and arrhythmias. An epidemic of asthma deaths in Britain in the mid-1950s was associated with the use of high-dose isoproterenol, prompting a search for agents that were more selective for β_2 receptors.

The first agents to offer relative β_2 selectivity were **isoetharine** and **metaproterenol**, although both drugs had moderate β_1 effects. The newer drugs **terbutaline, albuterol, pirbuterol,** and **bitolterol** (in order of discovery) bind to β_2-adrenergic receptors 200 to 400 times more strongly than to β_1 receptors and cause significantly fewer cardiac effects than the less selective adrenergic agonists. Albuterol was the first of the strongly β_2-selective agents to be available in inhaled form, further reducing systemic effects. Modern inhaled β_2-selective agonists were the first drugs to allow regular treatment of asthma with an acceptable adverse-effect profile. Nonetheless, at high doses, especially if taken orally, even these drugs can cause cardiac stimulation. In addition, since β_2-adrenergic receptors are expressed in peripheral skeletal muscle, activation of these receptors can result in a tremor.

Albuterol is a racemic mixture of two stereoisomers, R-albuterol (or **levalbuterol**) and S-albuterol. Levalbuterol, which is now available as a pure enantiomer, has tighter binding to β_2 receptors and is more β_2-selective, while S-albuterol is more active at β_1 receptors. The S isomer also induces airway hyperresponsiveness, at least in animal models, although in clinical practice this has not been significant. Nonetheless, there appears to be a subset of patients who are more sensitive to the β_1 effects of S-albuterol and who report decreased tachycardia and palpitations when taking levalbuterol.

Beta-adrenergic receptors are coupled to the stimulatory G protein G_s (see Chapter 9). The α subunit of G_s activates adenylyl cyclase, which catalyzes the production of cyclic adenosine monophosphate (cAMP). In the lung, cAMP

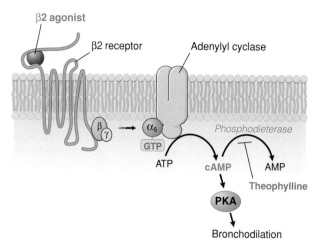

Figure 46-5. Mechanism of the β_2 agonists and theophylline. In airway smooth muscle cells, the activation of protein kinase A by cAMP leads to phosphorylation of a number of intracellular proteins and thus to smooth muscle relaxation and bronchodilation. Any therapy that increases the level of intracellular cAMP can be expected to lead to bronchodilation. In practice, this can be accomplished in one of two ways: by increasing the production of cAMP or by inhibiting the breakdown of cAMP. cAMP production is stimulated by β_2-agonist mediated activation of β_2-adrenergic receptors, which are G protein-coupled receptors. cAMP breakdown is inhibited by theophylline-mediated inhibition of phosphodiesterase.

causes a decrease in the intracellular calcium concentration and, via activation of protein kinase A, both inactivates myosin light chain kinase and activates myosin light chain phosphorylase (Fig. 46-5). In addition, the β_2 agonists open large-conductance calcium-activated potassium channels (K_{Ca}) and thereby tend to hyperpolarize airway smooth muscle cells. The combination of decreased intracellular calcium, increased membrane potassium conductance, and decreased myosin light chain kinase activity leads to smooth muscle relaxation and bronchodilation.

There appears to be variability in clinical response among patients using β_2 agonists. Researchers studying the effect of **single nucleotide polymorphisms (SNPs)** in the β_2 receptor gene have compared patients homozygous for the most common genotype to patients homozygous for the second most common genotype. While most studies have found that the magnitude of the bronchodilator response is no different between patients with the two genotypes, lung function appears to deteriorate faster over time among patients with the less common genotype.

Most β_2-adrenergic agonists have a rapid onset of action (15 to 30 minutes), a peak effect at 30 to 60 minutes, and a duration of action of approximately 4 to 6 hours. This time course of drug action makes the β_2 agonists good candidates for use as asthma relievers (or rescue inhalers) during acute attacks. However, this profile also makes the β_2 agonists poor candidates for control of nocturnal asthma and for prevention of attacks, unless they are used prophylactically before a known trigger such as exercise. Two newer agents, **formoterol** and **salmeterol**, are known as **long-acting beta agonists (LABAs)**. The LABAs were engineered with lipophilic side chains that resist degradation. As such, these agents have a 12- to 24-hour duration of action, making them good candidates for prevention of bronchoconstriction. Although formoterol and salmeterol are reasonable asthma controllers, these agents do not treat the underlying inflammation and, as such, can be dangerous if used as monotherapy. Because salmeterol has a slower onset of action than albuterol, it should not be used for acute asthma flares. Formoterol does have a rapid onset of action and can be used as a rescue inhaler, although it is not yet approved for this indication in the United States. It should be noted that clinical studies have shown higher mortality among asthma patients taking long-acting beta agonists. It is not yet known whether the association can be attributed to the LABAs, but the controversy has spurred caution in the use of these drugs.

Methylxanthines

Two methylxanthines, **theophylline** and **aminophylline**, are used in asthma treatment. The mechanism of action of these drugs is complex, but their primary bronchodilatory effect appears to be due to nonspecific inhibition of phosphodiesterase isoenzymes. Inhibition of phosphodiesterase types III and IV prevents cAMP degradation in airway smooth muscle cells, leading to smooth muscle relaxation by the cellular and molecular mechanisms detailed above (i.e., decreased intracellular calcium, increased membrane potassium conductance, and decreased myosin light chain kinase activity). As shown in Figure 46-5, the bronchodilatory effect of the methylxanthines results from perturbation of the same pathway that is initiated by β agonists, although the methylxanthines act downstream of β-receptor stimulation.

The methylxanthines also inhibit phosphodiesterase isoenzymes in inflammatory cells. Inhibition of phosphodiesterase type IV in T lymphocytes and eosinophils has an immunomodulatory and anti-inflammatory effect. By this mechanism, theophylline can control chronic asthma more effectively than would be expected on the basis of its bronchodilatory effect alone. Some of the adverse effects of the methylxanthines, including cardiac arrhythmias, nausea, and vomiting, are also mediated by phosphodiesterase inhibition, although the responsible isoenzymes remain to be elucidated.

Theophylline is a structural relative of **caffeine**, differing only by a single methyl group, and caffeine is an adenosine receptor antagonist. Adenosine receptors are expressed on airway smooth muscle cells and mast cells, and antagonism of these receptors could play a role in preventing both bronchoconstriction and inflammation. In fact, coffee has been used as a medication for asthma. However, experiments with specific adenosine receptor antagonists that do not inhibit phosphodiesterase have shown little bronchodilation, suggesting that phosphodiesterase inhibition is the major mechanism of action of the methylxanthines. Nonetheless, adenosine receptor antagonism is responsible for many of the secondary effects of theophylline, including increased ventilation during hypoxia, improved endurance of diaphragmatic muscles, and decreased adenosine-stimulated mediator release from mast cells. In addition, some of the adverse effects of theophylline are mediated through adenosine receptor antagonism, including tachycardia, psychomotor agitation, gastric acid secretion, and diuresis.

Because the methylxanthines are nonselective and have multiple mechanisms of action, they cause multiple adverse effects and have a relatively narrow therapeutic index. Moreover, there is significant interindividual variation in the metabolism of theophylline by the P450 isoenzyme CYP3A, and theophylline use is susceptible to drug-drug interactions with P450 inhibitors such as cimetidine and the azole antifungals. At supratherapeutic levels, theophylline produces nausea, diarrhea, vomiting, headache, irritability, and insomnia. At even higher doses, seizures, toxic encephalopathy, hyperthermia, brain damage, hyperglycemia, hypokalemia, hypotension, cardiac arrhythmias, and death can occur. For this reason, the role of theophylline in the treatment of chronic asthma has diminished. Theophylline is still used occasionally with routine monitoring of plasma drug levels when β-adrenergic agonists and corticosteroids are ineffective or contraindicated. Ahmad was prescribed theophylline when he was young, but he was later switched to the fluticasone/salmeterol combination because these agents have fewer adverse effects and are more effective than theophylline.

ANTI-INFLAMMATORY AGENTS

As detailed above, allergic inflammation provides the pathophysiologic basis for asthma. To control persistent asthma and prevent exacerbations of acute asthma, treatment should generally include anti-inflammatory agents, known as asthma controllers. Corticosteroids have long been mainstays of asthma treatment, although the profound adverse effects of systemically administered corticosteroids remained problematic until the development of inhaled formulations. Three additional classes of drugs with anti-inflammatory mechanisms of action are the cromolyns, the leukotriene-pathway modifiers, and a humanized monoclonal anti-IgE antibody.

Corticosteroids

Inhaled corticosteroids are the major preventive treatments for patients with all but the mildest forms of asthma. Corticosteroids have been used in asthma since the 1950s, but the adverse effects of systemic corticosteroids prevented their widespread adoption except for patients with the most serious cases. Because inhaled corticosteroids produce higher local drug concentrations in the airway than an equivalent dose of systemically administered corticosteroids, a lower overall dose can be administered, reducing the likelihood of significant systemic effects.

Corticosteroids alter the transcription of many genes. In general, corticosteroids increase the transcription of genes coding for the β_2-adrenergic receptor and a number of anti-inflammatory proteins such as IL-10, IL-12, and IL-1 receptor antagonist (IL-1ra). Corticosteroids decrease the transcription of genes coding for many pro-inflammatory (and other) proteins; examples include IL-2, IL-3, IL-4, IL-5, IL-6, IL-11, IL-13, IL-15, TNF-α, GM-CSF, SCF, endothelial adhesion molecules, chemokines, inducible nitric oxide synthase (iNOS), cyclooxygenase (COX), phospholipase A_2, endothelin-1, and NK_1-2 receptor. IL-4 is important in inducing B-cell production of IgE, while IL-5 is an important recruiter of eosinophils (Fig. 46-3). *Therefore, inhibition of IL-4 and IL-5 markedly reduces the inflammatory response in asthma.* Moreover, corticosteroids induce apoptosis in a number of inflammatory cells, particularly eosinophils and T_H2 lymphocytes. Corticosteroids do not directly affect mast cells, probably because most of the mast cell mediators are preformed; however, mast cells are indirectly inhibited over time as the entire inflammatory response is muted.

Corticosteroids reduce the number of inflammatory cells in the airways and the damage to airway epithelium. Vascular permeability is also reduced, leading to resolution of airway edema. In addition, although steroids do not directly affect the contractile function of airway smooth muscle, over time the reduced inflammation leads to a reduction in airway hyperresponsiveness. The net result is that corticosteroids reverse many of the features of asthma. Unfortunately, steroids are merely suppressive and do not cure asthma. In addition, steroids cannot reverse airway remodeling caused by long-standing, poorly controlled asthma. Nonetheless, because the effects of these agents are so far-reaching, inhaled corticosteroids are the most important drug class in most cases of asthma.

Most systemic effects can be mitigated, if not eliminated, by delivering corticosteroids directly to the airway, i.e., by inhalation. Although all corticosteroids are active in asthma when given systemically, substitution at the 17α position increases topical absorption and allows them to be active when given by inhalation (see Fig. 27-7). Such steroids include **beclomethasone**, **triamcinolone**, **fluticasone**, **budesonide**, **flunisolide**, **mometasone**, and **ciclesonide**. Even though only 10% to 20% of the administered dose is delivered to the airways by inhalation (the rest is deposited in the oropharynx and swallowed, unless the mouth is rinsed after using the inhaler), this produces a much higher airway concentration of drug than would occur with a similar dose administered systemically. Inhaled delivery allows dosing in the hundreds-of-micrograms range, as compared to the tens-of-milligrams that must be given systemically to achieve a similar anti-inflammatory effect. In addition, the newer steroids (all but beclomethasone and triamcinolone) are subject to first-pass metabolism in the liver, such that much of the inadvertently swallowed dose does not reach the systemic circulation.

The combination of lower dose and first-pass metabolism in the liver limits the incidence of adverse effects of inhaled corticosteroids. At sufficiently high doses, however, enough drug is absorbed through the gastrointestinal tract and pulmonary epithelium to cause systemic effects with prolonged use, including osteopenia or osteoporosis in adults and a delay in growth in children (although the children do eventually catch up). In addition, inhaled steroids can cause local adverse effects, including oropharyngeal candidiasis due to oropharyngeal deposition and hoarseness due to laryngeal deposition. These effects can be prevented by using a large-volume spacer to capture large droplets of steroid that would be deposited in the oropharynx and by rinsing the mouth after use. In the introductory case, Ahmad found the local adverse effects of fluticasone troubling until he was told how to minimize these effects by using a spacer and rinsing his mouth.

Cromolyns

Roger Altounyan was a physician with a predictable asthmatic response to guinea pig dander. In the 1960s, Dr. Altounyan tested a series of synthetic compounds based on a traditional Egyptian folk remedy for their ability to decrease his response to guinea pig dander extracts. These tests resulted in his discovery of a novel class of compounds, of which two—**cromolyn** (also known as **disodium cromoglycate**) and **nedocromil**—have since entered clinical practice.

Studies showed that cromolyn inhibits the immediate allergic response to an antigen challenge but does not relieve an allergic response once it has been initiated. Further studies found that cromolyn decreases the activity of mast cells, preventing release of their inflammatory mediators upon antigen challenge. For this reason, cromolyn is commonly viewed as a "mast-cell stabilizing agent." This view is somewhat simplistic, however, as the release of inflammatory mediators from eosinophils, neutrophils, monocytes, macrophages, and lymphocytes is also inhibited. The underlying molecular mechanism of action has not been elucidated but may involve inhibition of chloride ion transport, which in turn affects calcium gating to prevent mediator release from intracellular granules.

Because it prevents the acute allergic response in susceptible patients, cromolyn has found a role as a prophylactic therapy in patients with allergic asthma associated with specific triggers. It has also been useful in patients with exercise-induced asthma, as it can be taken immediately prior to exercise. Clinical experience has shown that cromolyn is more effective in children and young adults than in older patients.

Cromolyn has a better safety profile than any other asthma medication, largely due to its low systemic absorption. Cromolyn is administered by inhalation; less than 10% of the drug that reaches the lower airway is systemically absorbed, and less than 1% of the drug that reaches the gastrointestinal tract is absorbed. Cromolyn is generally less effective than inhaled corticosteroids, particularly in cases of moderate and severe asthma. Moreover, it must be taken four times daily.

Leukotriene Pathway-Modifying Agents

The central role of leukotrienes in the pathogenesis of asthma suggests that one therapeutic strategy could be to inhibit steps in the leukotriene pathway. This strategy has been employed in two ways to date, and a third is under development. The leukotriene pathway is initiated when arachidonic acid is converted to leukotriene A_4 by the enzyme 5-lipoxygenase. Inhibition of 5-lipoxygenase by the drug **zileuton** reduces the biosynthesis of LTA_4 and its active derivatives, the cysteinyl leukotrienes (Fig. 46-4). A second strategy involves inhibition of the cysteinyl leukotriene receptor CysLT1, which is stimulated endogenously by LTC_4, LTD_4, and LTE_4. **Montelukast**, **zafirlukast**, and **pranlukast** (the latter approved in Japan) are CysLT1 receptor antagonists (Fig. 46-4). A third strategy involving inhibition of the protein that activates 5-lipoxygenase (**5-lipoxygenase-activating**

protein or **FLAP**) is being actively explored, although no approved agents work by this mechanism.

The leukotriene pathway inhibitors have two major clinical effects. In patients with moderate or severe asthma who have pulmonary function impairment at baseline, zileuton, montelukast, and zafirlukast produce an immediate, albeit small, improvement in lung function. This effect is likely due to antagonism of the abnormally constricted bronchial tone that is thought to result from cysteinyl leukotriene stimulation of CysLT1 receptors at baseline. With chronic administration, the leukotriene-modifying agents reduce the frequency of exacerbations and improve control of asthma—as evidenced by fewer symptoms and less-frequent use of inhaled β agonists—even in patients who have mild asthma and only episodic symptoms. Nonetheless, compared to the effect of inhaled corticosteroids, the effect of leukotriene pathway modifiers on lung function and symptom control is limited. Because the leukotriene pathway is just one of several processes responsible for the inflammatory response in asthma, it is not surprising that leukotriene pathway modifiers are less effective than inhaled corticosteroids, which have much broader anti-inflammatory effects.

Unlike most of the other drugs used in the treatment of asthma, the leukotriene-modifying agents are all available as oral tablets rather than inhaled formulations. One advantage of an oral dosage form is that many patients, particularly children, find it easier to take a pill than use an inhaler, so compliance is frequently better. Moreover, because inhalers are often used improperly, there is a higher likelihood with pills that the intended dose is delivered. In addition, because orally delivered drugs are absorbed systemically, the drugs can be used to treat other coexisting allergic diseases such as allergic rhinitis. On the other hand, there is also a higher probability of systemic adverse effects.

All three leukotriene-modifying agents are well tolerated and have few extra-pulmonary effects, particularly compared to oral corticosteroids. Zileuton has a 4% incidence of hepatotoxicity, so periodic liver function testing is required. The leukotriene receptor antagonists are considered generally safe but have been associated with Churg-Strauss syndrome on rare occasions. Churg-Strauss syndrome is a serious granulomatous vasculitis affecting the small arteries and veins of the lungs, heart, kidneys, pancreas, spleen, and skin. Because Churg-Strauss syndrome is independently associated with asthma and eosinophilia, it is not clear whether the reported reactions represent a distinct effect of the drug or an unmasking of the pre-existing syndrome due to the reduction in corticosteroid use allowed by the addition of a leukotriene receptor antagonist to the therapeutic regimen.

Anti-IgE Antibodies

Given the prominence of IgE-mediated allergic responses in asthma, it follows that removal of IgE antibodies from the circulation could mitigate the acute response to an inhaled allergen. **Omalizumab** is a humanized mouse monoclonal antibody that binds to the high-affinity IgE-receptor (FcεRI)-binding domain on human IgE. Omalizumab both decreases the quantity of circulating IgE and prevents the remaining IgE from binding to mast-cell FcεRI (Fig. 46-3). Because it does not crosslink FcεRI-bound IgE, omalizumab does not typically induce anaphylaxis. Furthermore, omalizumab af-

fects both the early- and late-phase asthmatic responses to challenge by an inhaled allergen. In response to the lower levels of circulating IgE, the FcεRI receptor on mast cells, basophils, and dendritic cells is down-regulated. Receptor down-regulation reduces stimulation of T$_H$2 lymphocytes and decreases the late-phase asthmatic response beyond the decrease that could be expected from removal of the circulating IgE alone.

Because it is an antibody, omalizumab must be administered parenterally. In practice, it is given subcutaneously every 2 to 4 weeks. Although its high cost and the inconvenience of parenteral administration have limited the use of omalizumab to severe cases of asthma, it also reduces the dose of steroids needed for disease control as well as the number of exacerbations in moderate asthma. Despite the fact that it is a humanized antibody in which 95% of the original mouse amino acid sequence has been replaced by the corresponding human sequence, on rare occasions omalizumab is recognized as an antigen and triggers an immune response.

DRUG DELIVERY

Many of the adverse effects of drugs used to treat asthma, especially the corticosteroids and β agonists, can be minimized by delivery of the drug directly to the airway. There are three principal delivery systems for inhaled drugs: **metered-dose inhalers**, **dry-powder inhalers**, and **nebulizers**. In a metered-dose inhaler, a compressed gas such as Freon®, or a more environmentally friendly hydroalkane, propels a fixed dose of drug out of the device upon activation of the canister. Although the canisters are easy to use, they do require coordination between inhalation and actuation of the device. This is not the case for a dry-powder inhaler, where the act of inspiration creates turbulent flow within the device that aerosolizes and scatters a dry powder. Some patients find dry-powder inhalers easier to use than metered-dose inhalers, but others find the powder irritating or find they cannot generate a sufficient inspiratory force to activate the device. Nebulizers pass a compressed gas such as oxygen through a liquid formulation of the medication to convert it into a mist that is then inhaled. Although nebulizers are not as portable as the other delivery devices, they can be used in a hospital or home setting for treatment of acute asthmatic exacerbations.

CLINICAL MANAGEMENT OF ASTHMA

Treatment of asthma should be based on the severity of disease. A general guideline stipulates that the smallest dose of medication needed for adequate control of symptoms should be used. As a practical matter, this means adjusting the dose of medication to achieve adequate control, and then reducing it to the lowest effective dose. A step-care approach has been advocated to facilitate the ambulatory treatment of asthma. This approach classifies patients into one of four clinical categories (Table 46-1). For example, in patients with mild intermittent asthma who have no impairment in lung function, and who have symptoms occurring no more than twice a week and nocturnal awakenings due to asthma no more than twice a month, disease can be controlled with inhaled β agonists as needed before exposure to known

TABLE 46-1	Clinical Management of Asthma		
SEVERITY OF ASTHMA	**CLINICAL CHARACTERISTICS**	**SHORT-TERM RELIEF**	**LONG-TERM CONTROL**
Mild intermittent (Step 1)	Symptoms ≤2 times/week Nocturnal awakenings ≤2 times/month Exacerbations brief Lung function normal between exacerbations Limited peak flow variability	Short-acting β-agonist as needed for symptoms or prior to expected exposures	No medications necessary
Mild persistent (Step 2)	Symptoms >2 times/week Nocturnal awakenings >2 times/month Exacerbations brief and may affect activity Lung function normal when asymptomatic Peak flow decreased 20%–30% when symptomatic	Short-acting β-agonist as needed for symptoms	Preferred: inhaled low-dose corticosteroid Alternative: leukotriene-pathway modifier, mast-cell stabilizer, or theophylline
Moderate persistent (Step 3)	Daily symptoms Nocturnal awakenings >1 time/week Frequent exacerbations lasting days, affecting activity Lung function 60%–80% of predicted Peak flow variability >30%	Short-acting β-agonist as needed for symptoms	Preferred: Low- to medium-dose inhaled steroid and long-acting inhaled β-agonist Alternatives: Medium-dose inhaled steroid alone; or low- to medium-dose inhaled steroid plus sustained-release theophylline; or low- to medium-dose inhaled steroid plus leukotriene-pathway modifier
Severe persistent (Step 4)	Continual symptoms Limited activity Frequent nocturnal awakenings Frequent, severe exacerbations Lung function <60% of predicted Peak flow variability >30%	Short-acting β-agonist as needed for symptoms	Preferred: High-dose inhaled corticosteroid and long-acting inhaled β-agonist Oral corticosteroids if needed Addition of more controllers has not been studied adequately

asthma triggers, and for relief of symptoms once they have occurred. Patients with more frequent or severe symptoms, or with impairment in lung function, should be treated with regular preventive therapy such as inhaled corticosteroids at escalating doses, depending on severity of symptoms. Other medications, such as long-acting β agonists or leukotriene-modifying agents, may be added to facilitate improved control. Combination agents that include an inhaled corticosteroid and a long-acting inhaled β agonist (such as the fluticasone/salmeterol formulation ultimately given to Ahmad and the budesonide/formoterol combination that has been approved by the FDA and is scheduled to become available in 2007) can improve compliance by reducing the number of inhalers needed.

As in Ahmad's case, asthma management also involves avoiding environmental exposures known to provoke airway inflammation. For example, eliminating environmental tobacco smoke has been shown to reduce symptoms and the frequency of asthma attacks in children whose parents or caregivers are cigarette smokers.

Conclusion and Future Directions

Although the increasing incidence of asthma entails a significant burden of disability, economic cost, and death, research has uncovered key features of asthma pathophysiology that are useful for pharmacologic management of the disease. At its core, asthma is a disease caused by an aberrant inflammatory response in the airways that leads to airway hyperresponsiveness and bronchoconstriction. There is no cure for asthma, but a therapeutic approach that treats both aspects of asthma by using anti-inflammatory medications and bronchodilators, along with the avoidance of known triggers, can be successful in achieving long-term clinical control and enabling successful management of the disease in most patients.

As our understanding of the pathophysiology of asthma has improved, new targets for therapeutic intervention have become available. In general, research has focused on three areas: improving existing therapies by altering the ratio of benefit to adverse effect, devising new targeted therapies, and attempting to prevent or reverse permanent airway remodeling in long-standing asthma. One example of the first approach is the development of novel inhaled corticosteroids with reduced systemic effects. For example, one novel corticosteroid is an inactive ester that is activated in airway epithelium, reducing systemic absorption of active drug. There is also an ongoing search for glucocorticoid receptor modulators that retain anti-inflammatory activity while minimizing the risk of adverse effects.

A number of inflammatory cytokine inhibitors are under development as potential new therapeutics. However, the complex nature of asthma means that inhibition of a single pathway may not significantly affect the disease. For example, an anti-IL-5 antibody failed in clinical trials, despite successfully reducing the number of circulating and airway eosinophils. Nonetheless, studies are ongoing with inhibitors of IL-13 and IL-9 and with the inhibitory cytokine IL-10. Studies are also ongoing with cell-adhesion inhibitors and chemokine inhibitors, which may prevent the recruitment and transit of inflammatory cells to the airway.

Two phosphodiesterase type IV (PDE IV) inhibitors, **roflumilast** and **cilomilast**, are in advanced clinical trials for asthma. Phosphodiesterase type IV hydrolyzes cAMP in airway smooth muscle cells, and a compound that inhibits PDE IV is expected to lead to airway smooth muscle relaxation and relief of bronchoconstriction. Both compounds are also being evaluated for the treatment of COPD.

Suggested Reading

Barnes PJ. New drugs for asthma. *Nat Rev Drug Discov* 2004;3: 831–844. (*Discusses novel therapeutics in the treatment of asthma and future targets for new drugs.*)

Chu EK, Drazen JM. Asthma: one hundred years of treatment and onward. *Am J Respir Crit Care Med* 2005;171:1203–1208. (*Historic view of the evolution of asthma therapy over the last 100 years.*)

Drazen JM. Treatment of asthma with drugs modifying the leukotriene pathway. *N Engl J Med* 1999;340:197–206. (*Discusses the mechanism of action of the leukotriene pathway-modifying agents.*)

http://www.nyc.gov/html/doh/html/asthma/asthma.shtml. (*Contains an overview of a public health department's approach to reducing asthma morbidity in children.*)

Peachell P. Targeting the mast cell in asthma. *Curr Opin Pharmacol* 2005;5:251–256. (*Discusses the role of the mast cell in the pathogenesis of asthma and examines existing treatments for asthma that target the mast cell as well as targets for future intervention.*)

Rhen T, Cidlowski JA. Anti-inflammatory action of glucocorticoids—new mechanisms for old drugs. *N Engl J Med* 2005; 353:1711–1723. (*Discusses the molecular mechanisms by which glucocorticoids act and efforts to develop novel glucocorticoids with improved adverse-effect profiles.*)

Strunk RC, Bloomberg GR. Omalizumab for asthma. *N Engl J Med* 2006;354:2689–2695. (*Discusses the use of omalizumab for asthma, including its mechanism, clinical studies, clinical use, and potential adverse events, together with recommendations for its use.*)

Drug Summary Table   Chapter 46 Integrative Inflammation Pharmacology: Asthma

Drug	Clinical Applications	Serious and Common Adverse Effects	Contraindications	Therapeutic Considerations
ANTICHOLINERGICS				
Mechanism—Antagonists at muscarinic receptors on airway smooth muscle and glands, leading to decreased bronchoconstriction and mucus secretion				
Ipratropium Tiotropium	Asthma COPD Rhinitis	*Paralytic ileus, angioedema, bronchospasm* Abnormal taste, dry mouth, dry nasal mucus, constipation, tachycardia, urinary retention	Hypersensitivity to ipratropium or tiotropium Hypersensitivity to soya lecithin or related food products (inhalation aerosol)	Tiotropium has a long duration of action because of slow dissociation kinetics from M1 and M3 receptors
BETA-ADRENERGIC AGONISTS				
Mechanism—Agonists at beta-adrenergic receptors on airway smooth muscle; act through a stimulatory G protein (Gs) to cause smooth muscle relaxation and bronchodilation				
Epinephrine	Asthma Anaphylaxis Cardiac arrest Open-angle glaucoma	*Cardiac arrhythmias, hypertensive crisis, pulmonary edema* Tachycardia, palpitations, sweating, nausea, vomiting, tremor, nervousness, dyspnea	Narrow-angle glaucoma (ophthalmic form) Within 2 weeks use of MAOI (inhalation form)	Epinephrine is a non-selective adrenergic agonist that binds to α, β1, and β2 adrenergic receptors Causes cardiac stimulation via β1 receptors and hypertension via α receptors
Isoproterenol	Asthma Cardiac arrest Decreased vascular flow Heart block Shock Stokes-Adams syndrome	*Tachyarrhythmia, palpitations, dizziness,* headache, tremor, restlessness	Tachyarrhythmias Angina pectoris Digitalis-induced tachycardia or heart block	Stimulates both β1 and β2 receptors and therefore causes both bronchodilation and cardiac stimulation
Isoetharine Metaproterenol Terbutaline Albuterol Levalbuterol Pirbuterol Bitolterol	Asthma COPD	Similar to isoproterenol, except with significantly fewer cardiac effects due to β2 receptor selectivity	Hypersensitivity to isoetharine, metaproterenol, terbutaline, albuterol, levalbuterol, pirbuterol, or bitolterol	These agents are selective agonists at β2 receptors The newer agents terbutaline, albuterol, pirbuterol, and bitolterol bind to β2 adrenergic receptors 200 to 400 times more strongly than to β1 receptors, and cause fewer cardiac effects than the less selective adrenergic agonists Levalbuterol has a stronger β2 binding affinity and is more β2 selective than racemic albuterol
Formoterol Salmeterol	Asthma COPD	Similar to isoproterenol, except with significantly fewer cardiac effects due to β2 receptor selectivity	Hypersensitivity to formoterol or salmeterol	Due to their lipophilic side chains that resist degradation, formoterol and salmeterol are long-acting β2 agonists (LABAs) with a duration of action lasting 12 to 24 hours Salmeterol should not be used for acute asthma flares due to its slow onset of action
METHYLXANTHINES				
Mechanism—Nonselective phosphodiesterase inhibitors that prevent the degradation of cAMP; also act as adenosine receptor antagonists. The combined effect is smooth muscle relaxation and bronchodilation.				
Theophylline Aminophylline	Asthma COPD	*Ventricular arrhythmia, seizure* Tachyarrhythmias, vomiting, insomnia, tremor, restlessness	Hypersensitivity to theophylline or aminophylline	Nonspecific inhibitors of phosphodiesterases that inhibit phosphodiesterase in both airway smooth muscle and inflammatory cells While inhibition of phosphodiesterase type III and IV in smooth muscle results in bronchodilation, inhibition of phosphodiesterase type IV in T cells and eosinophils causes an immunodulatory and anti-inflammatory effect

(Continued)

Drug Summary Table   Chapter 46 Integrative Inflammation Pharmacology: Asthma (*Continued*)

Drug	Clinical Applications	*Serious* and Common Adverse Effects	Contraindications	Therapeutic Considerations
				Plasma levels must be monitored to prevent toxic levels of these agents Avoid coadministration with fluvoxamine, enoxacin, mexiletine, propranolol, and troleandomycin due to increased risk of theophylline toxicity Avoid coadministration with zafirlukast because theophylline can decrease plasma concentration of zafirlukast

INHALED CORTICOSTEROIDS
Mechanism—Inhibit COX-2 action and prostaglandin biosynthesis by inducing lipocortins, activating endogenous anti-inflammatory pathways, and other mechanisms

Drug	Clinical Applications	*Serious* and Common Adverse Effects	Contraindications	Therapeutic Considerations
Beclomethasone Triamcinolone Fluticasone Budesonide Flunisolide Mometasone Ciclesonide	See Drug Summary Table: Chapter 27 Pharmacology of the Adrenal Cortex			

CROMOLYNS
Mechanism—Inhibit chloride ion transport, which in turn affects calcium gating to prevent granule release, possibly decreasing mast cell response to inflammatory stimuli

Drug	Clinical Applications	*Serious* and Common Adverse Effects	Contraindications	Therapeutic Considerations
Cromolyn Nedocromil	Asthma Allergic rhinitis Keratitis Keratoconjunctivitis Mast cell disorder Vernal conjunctivitis	Abnormal taste, burning sensation in eye, cough, throat irritation	Hypersensitivity to cromolyn or nedocromil	Used primarily as prophylactic therapy in patients with allergic asthma associated with specific triggers Useful in patients with exercise-induced asthma; can be taken immediately prior to exercise More effective in children and young adults than in older patients Excellent safety profile, but less efficacious than other asthma medications

LEUKOTRIENE PATHWAY-MODIFYING AGENTS
Mechanism—Zileuton inhibits 5-lipoxygenase, thereby decreasing synthesis of leukotrienes; montelukast and zafirlukast are leukotriene receptor antagonists

Drug	Clinical Applications	*Serious* and Common Adverse Effects	Contraindications	Therapeutic Considerations
Zileuton Montelukast Zafirlukast	See Drug Summary Table: Chapter 41 Pharmacology of Eicosanoids			

ANTI-IMMUNOGLOBULIN E ANTIBODIES
Mechanism—Humanized mouse monoclonal antibody against the high-affinity IgE-receptor (FcεRI)-binding domain on human IgE. Prevents IgE from binding to FcεRI on mast cells and antigen-presenting cells; also, decreases the quantity of circulating IgE. The combined effect is a decrease in the allergic response in asthma.

Drug	Clinical Applications	*Serious* and Common Adverse Effects	Contraindications	Therapeutic Considerations
Omalizumab	Asthma	*Extremely rare anaphylactic reactions* Injection site reaction, rash, headache	Hypersensitivity to omalizumab	Affects both the early- and late-phase asthmatic responses to challenge by an inhaled allergen Administered subcutaneously every 2–4 weeks High cost limits its use to severe cases of asthma

47

Integrative Inflammation Pharmacology: Gout

Ehrin J. Armstrong and Lloyd B. Klickstein

INTRODUCTION

Gout is a uniquely human disease. Most mammals possess uricase, an enzyme that metabolizes purine breakdown products into a freely water-soluble substance, allantoin. Humans, in contrast, excrete most purines as sparingly soluble uric acid. High plasma levels of uric acid can lead to deposition of uric acid crystals in joints, most frequently the first metatarsophalangeal joint (great toe). Acute attacks of gout cause intense pain but typically occur infrequently. A number of rational therapies exist for the treatment of gout, including drugs that suppress the immune response to crystal deposition, agents that limit the extent of inflammation, agents that reduce uric acid synthesis, and agents that increase the renal excretion of uric acid. These pharmacologic interventions provide effective therapy for most cases of gout.

Case

Mr. J, a 52-year-old man, awakens one morning with excruciating pain in his great toe. Even the weight of the bedsheet is enough to make him want to scream; he is unable to put on a sock or shoe. Worried that something terrible has occurred, Mr. J rushes to his doctor. Based on the history and physical findings, the physician diagnoses an acute attack of gout. The physician prescribes ibuprofen, which relieves the pain after 2 days. Mr. J is then well until 5 years later, when the symptoms recur and he treats himself with ibuprofen, successfully. Subsequently, Mr. J learns to anticipate the attacks, which slowly increase in frequency until they occur once weekly. He uses ibuprofen at the first hint of pain.

The morning after one of his attacks begins, Mr. J goes to his doctor because the pain is not relieved with ibuprofen. Focused examination reveals a swollen, red and warm left knee, right midfoot, and right first metatarsophalangeal joint. There are 0.5-cm mobile nodules near the olecranon bilaterally and another at the inferior pole of the right patella. The rest of the exam is unremarkable. The physician aspirates Mr. J's left knee, revealing a cloudy yellow fluid that, on microscopic exam, contains numerous leukocytes. Abundant needle-shaped microscopic crystals are also seen, some of them intracellular. An x-ray of the left knee is normal except for the presence of an effusion; a film of the right foot shows an erosion of the distal first metatarsal.

Mr. J is treated with colchicine for 3 days and naproxen for 2 days. His condition improves rapidly. Three weeks later, he returns to his physician while feeling well. He is given a prescription for allopurinol to take on a long-term basis and one for colchicine to take during the first few months of allopurinol therapy.

QUESTIONS

■ **1.** Why was ibuprofen effective for most of Mr. J's acute attacks of pain?
■ **2.** How do ibuprofen and colchicine reduce the inflammatory response during an acute attack of gout?
■ **3.** How does allopurinol act? Will it alter the frequency of Mr. J's painful attacks?
■ **4.** Why does Mr. J take colchicine during the first few months of treatment with allopurinol?

PHYSIOLOGY OF PURINE METABOLISM

Gout is a disease caused by imbalances in purine metabolism. To understand the cause and treatment of gout, it is necessary to recall the principles of nucleotide biochemistry. Although pyrimidines such as cytosine, thymidine, and uracil are straightforward for the body to metabolize and excrete, it is a challenge to metabolize purines (most notably the nucleotides guanine and adenine). The intermediates of purine metabolism are toxic, necessitating tight regulation of purine synthesis and degradation. Furthermore, the final breakdown product of purine metabolism is uric acid, which is barely soluble in blood or urine. Increased plasma levels of uric acid are the strongest risk factor for gout, although, for poorly understood reasons, not everyone with high plasma uric acid levels develops gout.

Purines are synthesized via two general pathways: **de novo synthesis** and the **salvage pathway** (Fig. 47-1). The first step in the de novo pathway is the reaction of phosphoribosyl pyrophosphate (**PRPP,** a ribose sugar with two pyrophosphates attached) with glutamine. PRPP provides the ribose sugar as one precursor for the nascent nucleotide. Hydrolysis of the pyrophosphate in a later step makes the de novo pathway irreversible. Glutamine is the precursor for inosine monophosphate (IMP), a precursor that is common to adenine and guanine biosynthesis. The reaction of PRPP with glutamine is catalyzed by the enzyme amidophosphoribosyltransferase (**amidoPRT**). AmidoPRT is activated allosterically by high levels of PRPP; PRPP is thus both a substrate and an activator of amidoPRT. In general, *the cellular level of PRPP is the most important determinant of de novo purine synthesis.* High PRPP levels result in enhanced de novo purine synthesis, whereas low PRPP levels decrease the rate of synthesis.

The salvage pathway is the second important mode of purine synthesis. The first step in the salvage pathway is catalyzed by the key regulatory enzyme hypoxanthine-guanine phosphoribosyltransferase (**HGPRT**). HGPRT transfers PRPP to either hypoxanthine or guanine, resulting in the formation of IMP or guanosine monophosphate (GMP), respectively. Nucleotide interconversions can then yield adenosine triphosphate (ATP) and guanosine 5'-triphosphate (GTP).

Increased activity of the salvage pathway has two impor-

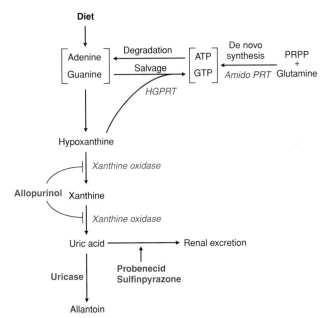

Figure 47-1. Purine metabolism. Purines (adenine and guanine) can be formed via de novo synthesis or dietary salvaging. The de novo pathway utilizes the amino acid glutamine and phosphoribosyl pyrophosphate (PRPP) in a reaction catalyzed by amidophosphoribosyltransferase (amidoPRT). The salvage pathway converts dietary guanine or adenine to nucleotides. Hypoxanthine-guanine phosphoribosyltransferase (HGPRT) phosphorylates and ribosylates dietary adenine and guanine, creating the purine nucleotides used for DNA and RNA synthesis. Degradation converts all purines to xanthine and ultimately uric acid, which is excreted by the kidneys or gastrointestinal tract *(not shown).* Pharmacologic interventions that reduce plasma urate consist of reducing urate synthesis (allopurinol and its metabolite oxypurinol), increasing urate excretion (probenecid and sulfinpyrazone), or converting urate to the more soluble allantoin (uricase).

tant consequences. First, increased scavenging activity depletes cells of PRPP, thus decreasing the rate of de novo purine synthesis. Second, the salvage pathway leads to the generation of more ATP and GTP. Increased levels of these nucleotides inhibit amidoPRT in a feedback manner, also resulting in decreased de novo purine synthesis.

Although purines can be synthesized by these two interrelated pathways, *degradation occurs via a convergent mechanism* (Fig. 47-1). Adenosine monophosphate (AMP) is deaminated, dephosphorylated, and deribosylated, forming hypoxanthine. GMP is also deaminated, dephosphorylated, and deribosylated, forming hypoxanthine. Hypoxanthine, which is moderately soluble, is oxidized to xanthine. Thus, xanthine is the common product of purine metabolism. A further oxidation step converts xanthine to uric acid. The enzyme **xanthine oxidase** catalyzes the oxidation of hypoxanthine to xanthine and xanthine to uric acid.

Cross-talk between the de novo and salvage pathways is important for overall regulation of purine metabolism. The de novo pathway is the most important generator of purine breakdown products. *High de novo pathway activity increases purine turnover, resulting in higher plasma uric acid concentrations.* In contrast, increased salvage pathway activity leads to decreased de novo synthesis and reduced plasma uric acid levels.

The importance of cross-talk in purine metabolism is demonstrated by several inherited enzyme disorders. Certain genetic polymorphisms that increase PRPP synthase activity lead to increased intracellular levels of PRPP; because PRPP activates amidoPRT, high levels of PRPP cause greater de novo purine synthesis, leading to increased turnover and degradation of purines and increased plasma levels of uric acid. Similarly, genetic deficiencies of HGPRT (the critical enzyme in the salvage pathway) lead to decreased salvage pathway activity and increased de novo purine synthesis and degradation, resulting in increased uric acid levels. The inherited absence of HGPRT results in **Lesch-Nyhan syndrome**, a devastating disorder characterized by self-mutilation, mental retardation, and hyperuricemia. Partial defects in HGPRT (e.g., polymorphisms in the HGPRT gene that lead to decreased HGPRT synthesis or activity) are thought to explain some cases of hereditary gout.

Uric acid is eliminated by the kidney (65%) and the gastrointestinal (GI) tract (35%). Uric acid is filtered and secreted by the kidney by the same mechanisms that process other organic anions. Approximately 90% of filtered uric acid is reabsorbed, and only 10% appears in the urine. Renal excretion is important for the maintenance of normal plasma uric acid levels, and renal failure often leads to high plasma urate levels.

PATHOPHYSIOLOGY OF GOUT

The likelihood of developing gout correlates strongly with increased plasma uric acid levels. Uric acid is a weak acid (pKa = 5.6); at physiologic pH, 99% of plasma uric acid is in the ionized, urate form. The normal urate concentration in human plasma is 4 to 6 mg/dL, reflecting a balance of urate synthesis, breakdown, and excretion. Urate is sparingly soluble: the plasma becomes saturated if urate levels exceed 6.8 mg/dL. A plasma level over 7.0 mg/dL for men or 6.0 mg/dL for women is classified clinically as hyperuricemia. The gender difference may be attributable to differences in urate excretion between women and men.

Any variable that decreases the solubility of urate can promote urate crystal deposition. Gout occurs most commonly in peripheral joints. Urate is less soluble at lower temperatures, which may explain the peripheral distribution of urate crystal deposition. Also, joint synovial fluid is more acidic than blood, favoring crystal formation.

The pathogenesis of gout is thought to reflect deposition of urate crystals in the periarticular fibrous tissue of synovial joints after years of hyperuricemia. However, it is also possible to develop gout without hyperuricemia (e.g., due to an immune response to urate or to preferential deposition of urate in synovial fluid).

The natural history of gout has four stages (Table 47-1). First, asymptomatic hyperuricemia develops, either because of increased purine breakdown or decreased excretion of urate. Because most cases of hyperuricemia never develop into gout, there is no indication for treatment of hyperuricemia in the absence of gout. It is, however, important to determine the cause of marked hyperuricemia: such causes can include lymphoma (increased purine turnover) and renal failure (decreased excretion of urate).

For patients with symptomatic gout, the second phase involves an acute attack of arthritis. Typically, this involves the rapid onset of acute pain in a single joint, as occurred in Mr. J. More than 50% of patients with gout have their first attack in the first metatarsophalangeal joint (pain at this site is referred to as **podagra**), and almost all patients with symptomatic gout have podagra at some point. Without treatment, an acute attack of gout may last for hours to days but usually resolves spontaneously. It is not understood what causes the periodic onset of gout attacks, or why these attacks resolve spontaneously.

The end of an attack leads to the third, intercritical phase, characterized by hyperuricemia without acute symptomatic

TABLE 47-1	Natural History of Gout	
STAGE	**FEATURES**	**PHARMACOLOGIC INTERVENTION**
1. Asymptomatic hyperuricemia	Plasma urate >6.0 mg/dL in women, >7.0 mg/dL in men	None
2. Acute gout	Acute arthritis	NSAIDs
	Typically first metatarsophalangeal joint	Colchicine
		Glucocorticoids
	Excruciating pain	
3. Intercritical phase	Asymptomatic hyperuricemia	None
	10% may never have another acute attack	
4. Chronic gout	Hyperuricemia	Allopurinol
	Development of tophi	Probenecid
	Recurrent attacks of acute gout	Sulfinpyrazone

Note that the degree of hyperuricemia correlates with the likelihood of developing gout; however, developing gout without hyperuricemia is possible. No pharmacologic intervention is indicated for asymptomatic hyperuricemia, but the cause should be investigated.

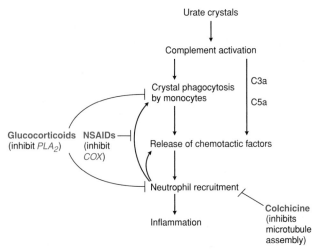

Figure 47-2. Inflammation in a gouty joint. During an acute attack of gout, urate crystals in the synovial fluid and synovial tissue activate complement. Complement activation leads to phagocytosis of opsonized crystals by monocyte/macrophages and release of chemotactic factors such as C3a and C5a. Monocyte-secreted factors and other chemotactic factors stimulate neutrophil recruitment, which leads to a positive feedback loop involving IL-8 and leukotriene B_4 release (not shown). The combination of these factors constitutes the inflammatory response typical of acute gout. Pharmacologic interventions consist of inhibiting the inflammatory response, either by inactivating monocytes and neutrophils (glucocorticoids and colchicine) or by decreasing the levels of inflammatory mediators released (glucocorticoids and NSAIDs).

gout. Some individuals will experience only one acute attack of gout and remain in the intercritical phase for long periods or even for the remainder of their lives. Five years after his initial attack, Mr. J developed chronic, recurrent attacks of gout, the fourth phase. Typically, these attacks become polyarticular and more severe. Chronically high levels of plasma uric acid can also lead to deposition of urate crystals around synovial joints, called **tophi**. Tophi can stimulate an inflammatory response that eventually destroys the synovial lining and cartilage.

A working model has been proposed for the inflammatory reaction in the joint (Fig. 47-2). Central to this model is the phagocyte response to urate crystal deposition in the synovial fluid and synovium. Initially, urate crystals in the synovial fluid cause complement activation and phagocytosis of the crystals by monocytes. In turn, complement activation and monocyte activation release chemotactic factors such as C5a and IL-8, which recruit other inflammatory cells. Neutrophils release lysosomal enzymes and previously phagocytosed urate crystals into the joint, recruiting additional neutrophils. These processes cause the intense pain characteristic of an acute attack of gout, while the chronic inflammatory response to urate crystals can cause cartilage destruction.

PHARMACOLOGIC CLASSES AND AGENTS

There are two main strategies for the treatment of gout: (1) management of acute attacks of gouty arthritis; and (2) long-

term management of chronic gout. Although some of the same drugs are used in treating acute and chronic gout, the aims of therapy differ in the two cases. The goal of acute gout management is to control pain, using drugs that limit joint inflammation. In contrast, therapy of the chronic disease aims to modify purine metabolism to achieve normal concentrations of plasma urate. Thus, pharmacologic agents for the treatment of chronic gout modify either the increased production of urate or the decreased renal clearance of urate.

MANAGEMENT OF ACUTE GOUT: SUPPRESSORS OF LEUKOCYTE RECRUITMENT AND ACTIVATION

Nonsteroidal Anti-Inflammatory Drugs (NSAIDs)

Metabolites of arachidonic acid play an important role in the inflammatory response to urate crystals in the joint. NSAIDs inhibit cyclooxygenase (COX) and thereby inhibit prostaglandin and thromboxane synthesis (see Chapter 41, Pharmacology of Eicosanoids). These drugs were effective for most of Mr. J's acute attacks of gout; his pain responded well to ibuprofen. Clinically, **indomethacin** is one of the NSAIDs used most often to treat acute attacks of gout. The choice of an NSAID or colchicine (see discussion below) for treatment of acute gout is generally based on the adverse-effect profile. The serious adverse effects of NSAIDs include bleeding, salt and water retention, and renal insufficiency. COX-2 selective inhibitors are potentially useful for the management of acute gout attacks because they may decrease the risk of gastrointestinal bleeding, although concerns about adverse cardiovascular effects limit their long-term use.

Colchicine

Colchicine binds to tubulin, inhibiting its polymerization and preventing the formation of microtubules. Colchicine inhibits cell division because microtubules are critical for the alignment and separation of chromosomes during mitosis (see Chapter 37, Pharmacology of Cancer: Genome Synthesis, Stability, and Maintenance). Microtubules are also essential in intracellular trafficking. In an acutely inflamed joint, colchicine limits the inflammatory response by inhibiting neutrophil activation. The mechanisms of neutrophil inhibition include: (1) decreased trafficking of phagocytosed particles to lysosomes; (2) decreased release of chemotactic factor; (3) decreased motility and adhesion of neutrophils; and (4) decreased tyrosine phosphorylation of neutrophil proteins, with a resulting decrease in leukotriene B_4 synthesis. Colchicine can also be administered in low doses as a prophylactic therapy for chronic gout, to inhibit the occurrence of acute attacks. Drugs that alter urate homeostasis are often coadministered initially with colchicine to avoid precipitating an acute attack of gouty arthritis (see discussion below).

Colchicine causes several important adverse effects. Colchicine inhibits the turnover of epithelial cells in the gastrointestinal tract, and diarrhea is a common complication of moderate or high doses of the drug. Colchicine is myelosuppressive, particularly in high doses or in combination with

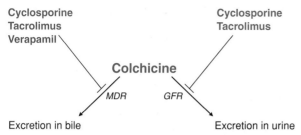

Figure 47-3. Important drug interactions involving colchicine. Cyclosporine and tacrolimus (immunosuppressant drugs frequently prescribed after organ transplantation) and verapamil (a Ca^{2+} channel blocker used to treat hypertension and some cardiac arrhythmias) each inhibit the activity of the multidrug-resistance (MDR) protein responsible for the hepatic excretion of colchicine. Cyclosporine and tacrolimus are also nephrotoxic, acting to reduce the glomerular filtration rate (GFR); this side effect can compromise the renal excretion of colchicine. Therefore, coadministration of colchicine with cyclosporine, tacrolimus, or verapamil can lead to toxic plasma levels of colchicine at otherwise therapeutic doses.

Figure 47-4. Mechanism of allopurinol action. Allopurinol is a structural analogue of hypoxanthine *(similarity is highlighted in blue).* Oxidation of allopurinol yields oxypurinol, a noncompetitive inhibitor of xanthine oxidase. (At low doses, allopurinol is a competitive inhibitor of xanthine oxidase.) Inhibition of xanthine oxidase decreases the production of uric acid by inhibiting two steps in its synthesis. The increased plasma levels of xanthine and hypoxanthine are tolerated because these metabolites are more soluble than uric acid.

other myelosuppressive agents such as ganciclovir or azathioprine. Colchicine undergoes extensive enterohepatic recirculation, and drug secretion into the bile is mediated by the liver multidrug-resistance (MDR) protein. Repeated delivery of colchicine to the GI tract likely explains why diarrhea is a common adverse effect of the drug. Drugs that inhibit the liver MDR protein, such as cyclosporine and verapamil, can significantly increase the fraction of a colchicine dose that is delivered to the systemic circulation (Fig. 47-3). By this mechanism, such drugs can cause systemic colchicine toxicity that may not be accompanied by diarrhea because the GI exposure to colchicine is decreased. Accordingly, the dose of colchicine should be lowered when the drug is administered concurrently with any drug known to inhibit MDR activity.

Glucocorticoids

Glucocorticoids have powerful anti-inflammatory and immunosuppressive effects (see Chapter 27, Pharmacology of the Adrenal Cortex). Glucocorticoids inhibit numerous steps in the inflammatory response during an acute attack of gout. Because they have widespread adverse effects when administered systemically, glucocorticoids are used in the treatment of acute polyarticular gout or when there are contraindications, such as renal insufficiency, to other effective therapies. When an acute attack of gout occurs in a single joint and is unresponsive to NSAIDs or colchicine, depot preparations of prednisolone or another glucocorticoid can be injected directly into the site of inflammation.

MANAGEMENT OF CHRONIC GOUT: AGENTS THAT LOWER PLASMA URATE CONCENTRATION

Agents That Decrease Uric Acid Synthesis

Allopurinol is an example of a drug designed to inhibit a well-understood biochemical pathway. Allopurinol is a structural analogue of xanthine. By inhibiting xanthine oxidase, allopurinol decreases the concentration of uric acid in

the blood (Fig. 47-4). Because of its close structural similarity to xanthine, allopurinol also acts as a substrate for xanthine oxidase. The oxidized form of allopurinol, known as **oxypurinol,** inhibits xanthine oxidase by preventing molybdenum in the active site of the enzyme from interconverting between the $+4$ and $+6$ oxidation states, essentially "freezing" the enzyme. Recall that xanthine oxidase is important for two sequential steps in purine degradation—oxidation of hypoxanthine to xanthine, and oxidation of xanthine to uric acid. Therefore, inhibiting xanthine oxidase results in increased plasma levels of hypoxanthine and xanthine (see Fig. 47-1). Unlike uric acid, hypoxanthine and xanthine are moderately soluble in blood and can be filtered by the kidney without crystal deposition.

Allopurinol is used in the treatment of chronic gout, especially in cases caused by increased purine degradation. It should not be administered during an acute attack of gout because disruption of urate homeostasis can potentially worsen or precipitate acute attacks of gouty arthritis. Therefore, *an NSAID or colchicine is often coadministered during the first 4 to 6 months of allopurinol therapy to reduce the chance of precipitating an acute attack of gout.* This was the concern that prompted Mr. J's doctor to coadminister colchicine during his first few weeks of allopurinol therapy.

Because allopurinol inhibits purine degradation, caution should be used when a patient is taking other purine analogues. For example, azathioprine and its active form 6-mercaptopurine (see Chapter 37) are anticancer and immunosuppressive drugs that contain a purine backbone, and 6-mercaptopurine is metabolized by xanthine oxidase (Fig. 47-5). Inhibition of xanthine oxidase by allopurinol can result in toxic levels of coadministered mercaptopurine or azathioprine because of decreased degradation of the latter

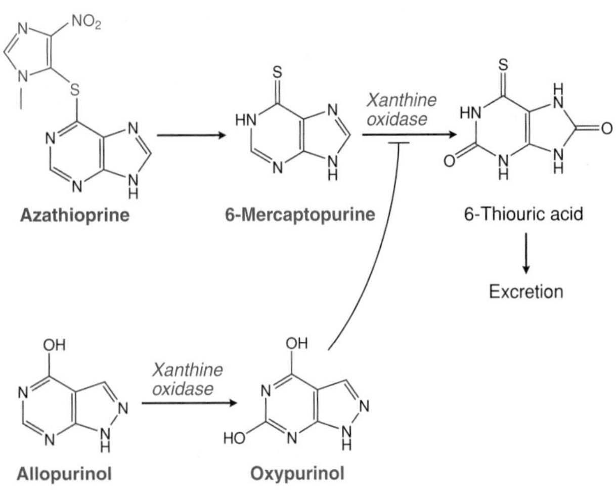

Figure 47-5. Interaction between 6-mercaptopurine and allopurinol. 6-Mercaptopurine and azathioprine (a prodrug) are metabolized and eliminated from the body via the same pathways as other purines. Allopurinol and its metabolite, oxypurinol, inhibit xanthine oxidase, thereby inhibiting the breakdown of 6-mercaptopurine. Decreased degradation causes plasma levels of 6-mercaptopurine to rise. When coadministering 6-mercaptopurine and allopurinol (for example, in cancer chemotherapy), the dose of 6-mercaptopurine should be substantially reduced.

drugs. Therefore, the dose of mercaptopurine or azathioprine should be reduced by approximately 75% when allopurinol is coadministered. In some cases, switching from azathioprine to a nonpurine immunosuppressive drug, such as mycophenolic acid (see Chapter 44, Pharmacology of Immunosuppression), is another option.

Although allopurinol is generally well tolerated, several important adverse effects should be considered when prescribing this agent. A small percentage of patients taking allopurinol may develop a hypersensitivity reaction characterized by a rash that, in rare instances, can progress to Stevens-Johnson syndrome. For this reason, all patients who develop a cutaneous reaction to allopurinol should discontinue the drug. Rarely, allopurinol may also cause leukopenia, eosinophilia, and/or hepatic necrosis.

Febuxostat, a nonpurine small-molecule inhibitor of xanthine oxidase, is also being evaluated for the treatment of chronic gout. In a large clinical trial, febuxostat was as effective as allopurinol in preventing recurrent flares of gout. Unlike allopurinol, febuxostat undergoes extensive hepatic metabolism, and it may not require dose adjustment in renal insufficiency. Further studies will be necessary to define the adverse-effect profile of febuxostat.

Agents That Increase Uric Acid Excretion

Because the kidney reabsorbs a substantial amount of filtered uric acid, a pharmacologic agent that blocks tubular reabsorption increases uric acid excretion. Such drugs are called **uricosuric agents.**

Probenecid was one of the first drugs used to increase urate excretion. It is an inhibitor of the basolateral anion exchanger of the proximal tubule. This exchanger acts to enhance the secretion of many anions, including drugs. However, studies also indicate that the proximal tubule anion exchanger mediates urate *reabsorption.* The mechanism is not known; urate reabsorption may be coupled to the secretion of other anions. Therefore, although inhibiting the anion exchanger increases the plasma concentration of many organic anions and drugs, such as penicillin, such inhibition *decreases* the plasma concentration of urate by decreasing urate reabsorption.

In patients with gout, probenecid is useful for the treatment of chronic hyperuricemia. Probenecid shifts the balance between renal excretion and endogenous formation of urate, thereby lowering plasma urate, dissolving urate crystals, and reversing the crystal deposition in synovial joints. However, increasing renal urate excretion can predispose to formation of urate stones in the kidney or ureter. This complication can be prevented by making the urine less acidic, commonly by coadministration of oral calcium citrate or sodium bicarbonate: uric acid has a pKa of 5.6, and it remains predominantly in the more soluble neutral form if the urine pH is above 6.0. Because probenecid inhibits the secretion of most anions, the dose of other drugs excreted by this pathway should be reduced when probenecid is coadministered. Low-dose aspirin may antagonize probenecid action; the mechanism of this antagonism is unknown.

Sulfinpyrazone is a uricosuric agent that acts by the same mechanism as probenecid. It is more potent than probenecid, and it is effective in mild-to-moderate renal insufficiency. In addition to acting as a uricosuric, sulfinpyrazone has antiplatelet effects; it should therefore be used with caution in patients taking other antiplatelet agents or anticoagulants. A significant percentage of patients taking sulfinpyrazone develop hematologic toxicity—this adverse effect has limited widespread use of the drug.

Benzbromarone is a uricosuric agent with a mechanism of action similar to that of probenecid and sulfinpyrazone. Benzbromarone may have greater uricosuric efficacy than probenecid and sulfinpyrazone, particularly in patients with impaired renal function. However, the frequent incidence of hepatotoxicity has limited widespread use of the drug. Benzbromarone is not approved for use in the United States but it is available in Europe.

Losartan is an angiotensin II receptor antagonist (see Chapter 21, Pharmacology of Vascular Tone) that has a modest uricosuric effect. Losartan may be a logical therapeutic choice in patients with concomitant hypertension and gout, although no controlled studies have been performed to prove that losartan reduces the incidence of acute gouty attacks.

Agents That Enhance Uric Acid Metabolism

Most mammals other than humans express the enzyme uricase. This enzyme oxidizes uric acid to allantoin, a compound that is easily excreted by the kidney. In cancer chemotherapy, the rapid lysis of tumor cells can liberate free nucleotides and greatly increase plasma urate levels. By this mechanism, **tumor lysis syndrome** can lead to massive renal injury. Exogenous **uricase** can be coadministered with cancer chemotherapy to reduce plasma urate levels rapidly, and thereby to prevent renal damage. Allopurinol can also be used to prevent this component of tumor lysis syndrome.

Currently, uricase is available in Europe as a protein purified from the fungus *Aspergillus flavus*. A recombinant version of the *Aspergillus* uricase, **rasburicase,** is available in the United States. A small percentage of patients have allergic reactions to the foreign protein. Pegylated formulations of uricase, which have a longer plasma half-life, are also under investigation.

Conclusion and Future Directions

Gout can be thought of as a disorder of purine metabolism and excretion. An imbalance between urate synthesis and excretion leads to hyperuricemia; in some individuals, hyperuricemia progresses to gout. Acute therapeutic interventions are aimed at symptomatic treatment of gouty attacks; these treatments interrupt inflammatory pathways by inhibiting neutrophil and monocyte activation. Treatments for chronic gout lower plasma urate levels by re-establishing the balance between urate synthesis and excretion. Allopurinol inhibits urate synthesis; probenecid increases renal urate ex-

cretion. New therapies are under development; for example, febuxostat is being studied as a potential alternative to allopurinol in chronic gout. Recombinant uricase rapidly decreases plasma urate levels by converting uric acid to allantoin, thereby preventing the adverse renal consequences of tumor lysis syndrome.

Suggested Reading

Becker MA, Schumacher HR, Wortmann RL, et al. Febuxostat compared with allopurinol in patients with hyperuricemia and gout. *N Engl J Med* 2005;353:2450–2461. *(Phase III trial comparing febuxostat with allopurinol.)*

Bomalaski JS, Clark MA. Serum uric acid-lowering therapies. *Curr Rheumatol Rep* 2004;6:240–247. *(Reviews development of and indications for uricase and pegylated uricase.)*

Schlesinger N. Management of acute and chronic gouty arthritis. *Drugs* 2004;64:2399–2416. *(Clinical management of acute and chronic gout.)*

Drug Summary Table **Chapter 47 Integrative Inflammation Pharmacology: Gout**

Drug	Clinical Applications	Serious and Common Adverse Effects	Contraindications	Therapeutic Considerations
SUPPRESSORS OF LEUKOCYTE RECRUITMENT AND ACTIVATION				
Mechanism—Interrupt inflammatory pathways that cause inflammation in a gouty joint; see specific drug				
Colchicine	Acute gout Prevention of recurrent gout attacks	*Myelosuppression, neuromyopathy* Diarrhea, nausea, abdominal pain	Severe cardiac, gastrointestinal, or renal disease Hepatic failure Blood dyscrasias	Colchicine inhibits microtubule formation by binding to tubulin heterodimers; inhibition of microtubule assembly interrupts cellular motility and other processes necessary for neutrophil-mediated inflammatory reaction Concomitant administration of cyclosporine, tacrolimus, or verapamil may increase plasma levels of colchicine
Ibuprofen Indomethacin	See Drug Summary Table: Chapter 41 Pharmacology of Eicosanoids			
Prednisone Methylprednisolone	See Drug Summary Table: Chapter 27 Pharmacology of the Adrenal Cortex			Methylprednisolone may be injected into an inflamed joint for treatment of acute gout
INHIBITORS OF URIC ACID SYNTHESIS				
Mechanism—Inhibit xanthine oxidase, the enzyme that converts hypoxanthine and xanthine to uric acid; decreased uric acid levels lead to less urate crystal formation				
Allopurinol Oxypurinol	Prevention of recurrent gout attacks Cancer-related hyperuricemia Calcium and uric acid renal calculus	*Agranulocytosis, aplastic anemia, renal failure, hepatic necrosis, Stevens-Johnson syndrome, toxic epidermal necrolysis* Pruritus, rash, gastrointestinal disturbance	Idiopathic hemochromatosis	Allopurinol is an inhibitor and substrate for xanthine oxidase; the product of allopurinol oxidation (oxypurinol) also inhibits xanthine oxidase Oxypurinol is available on a compassionate use basis Both drugs increase levels of azathioprine, 6-MP Amoxicillin, ampicillin, and thiazide diuretics may increase risk of severe rash
Febuxostat	Investigational			Non-purine small-molecule inhibitor of xanthine oxidase
AGENTS THAT INCREASE URIC ACID EXCRETION				
Mechanism—See specific drug				
Sulfinpyrazone Probenecid	Prevention of recurrent gout attacks	*Leukopenia, thrombocytopenia, bronchoconstriction in patients with asthma, aplastic anemia (probenecid), hepatic necrosis (probenecid), anaphylaxis (probenecid)* Gastrointestinal disturbance	Acute gout attack Blood dyscrasias Children under 2 years of age Coadministration of salicylates Uric acid kidney stones	Sulfinpyrazone and probenecid inhibit renal tubule basolateral anion exchanger, leading to increased excretion of uric acid Sulfinpyrazone and probenecid increase levels of penicillin and other anionic compounds; may also increase levels of nitrofurantoin Benzbromarone is a more potent uricosuric available in Europe Probenecid increases the serum level of methotrexate
Losartan	Hypertension Prevention of recurrent gout attacks	*Angioedema, rhabdomyolysis, thrombocytopenia* Anemia, fatigue, back pain, hypoglycemia	Pregnancy	Losartan is an angiotensin II receptor antagonist with a modest uricosuric effect
AGENTS THAT ENHANCE URIC ACID METABOLISM				
Mechanism—Enzyme that converts sparingly soluble urate to the more soluble allantoin				
Rasburicase	Tumor lysis syndrome	*Hemolysis, methemoglobinemia, neutropenia, respiratory distress, sepsis* Rash, gastrointestinal disturbance, fever	Glucose-6-phosphate dehydrogenase (G6PD) deficiency Known *Aspergillus* sensitivity	Rasburicase is a recombinant form of *Aspergillus* uricase that converts sparingly soluble urate to the more soluble allantoin Pegylated formulations with a longer half-life are under investigation

VII

Fundamentals of Drug Development and Regulation

48

Drug Discovery and Preclinical Development

John L. Vahle and Armen H. Tashjian, Jr.

INTRODUCTION

Over the past decade, the U. S. Food and Drug Administration (FDA) has approved approximately 200 new drugs and biologics. These "new drugs" include approximately 125 "new molecular entities," which are active substances that have never before been approved for therapeutic use. Many such drugs have enabled treatments for diseases that were previously untreatable. Others have yielded expanded treatment options because they are more efficacious and/or less toxic than previously available treatments. In the fight against infectious diseases, for example, pharmaceutical and biotechnology companies, university laboratories, and others continue to develop new agents to fight diseases that have become resistant to existing treatments. With new technologies, genetic knockout animal models, and information from the human genome project, it is anticipated that important new classes of drugs will continue to be discovered in the coming decades.

The development of a new drug is difficult and costly. Very few molecules that reach the development stage are ultimately approved as drugs: of 10,000 compounds considered promising from the results of initial screening assays, fewer than 10 make it to clinical trials, and only 2 are eventually approved. Furthermore, the costs associated with discovering and developing a new drug can range from 0.8 to 1.7 billion dollars. Although the development of new drugs is a risky venture, successful drugs can be quite profitable for those willing to take such risks. The most commercially successful drugs, such as **atorvastatin**, have annual sales of more than 12 billion dollars.

Increased attention has recently been focused on the inability of the biomedical research community to produce innovative new therapies. The challenges involved in drug discovery and development were highlighted (along with potential solutions) in the 2004 report of the FDA Critical Path Initiatives (see Suggested Reading). This report noted that both the National Institutes of Health (NIH) budget and pharmaceutical company research and development spending approximately doubled over a 10-year period beginning in 1993. The added investment did not increase the rate of development of new medicines, however, as evidenced by a decline in major drug and biological product submissions to the FDA. While several potential solutions have been offered to address this issue, it is important to note that a joint report by the FDA and the Association of American Medical Colleges highlighted the critical role of physician-scientists in improving the effectiveness of drug discovery and development.

This chapter describes the phases of drug discovery and development and the scientific disciplines that are involved in these phases. **Drug discovery** spans the period from the identification of a potential therapeutic target to the selection of a single molecule for testing in humans. **Drug development** is generally defined as the period from the preclinical studies that support initial clinical trials through approval of the drug by regulatory authorities. The process of drug discovery and development is complex, requiring contributions from many otherwise disparate scientific disciplines.

■ Case

In 1987, researchers at Abbott Laboratories decided to target human immunodeficiency virus (HIV) protease in their search for a novel antiviral therapeutic. Abbott chose the protease because it is essential to HIV's replication and because it has an unusual substrate specificity (see Chapter 36, Pharmacology of Viral Infections). Because the natural substrate for the enzyme contains a phenylalanine-proline bond, a rare cleavage site for mammalian proteases, researchers reasoned that a drug that inhibits HIV protease would have relatively few adverse effects.

In 1989, crystallographers at Merck announced that they had elucidated the crystal structure of HIV protease. Based on the newly solved structure, researchers now knew that the viral protease was a symmetric dimer of two identical subunits (Fig. 48-1; see also Fig. 36-9 and Box 36-3). Using a molecular model, researchers at Abbott designed an analogue of the enzyme's natural substrate by replacing the proline in the natural sequence with a phenylalanine—this analogue was a symmetric molecule containing identical amino acids on each end of the structure. They also replaced the peptide bond in the center of the molecule with a functional group that mimicked the transition state of the

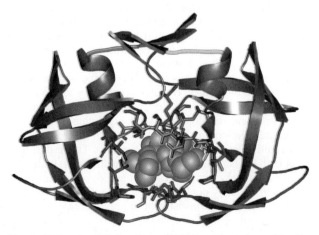

Figure 48-1. Crystal structure of HIV-1 protease bound to ritonavir. The structure of HIV protease is shown as a ribbon, with ritonavir *(blue space-filling model)* occupying the active site. The rotational axis of symmetry of the enzyme is evident; this was the basis for the design of the drug. Using the crystal structure of HIV protease, researchers were able to fine-tune the structure of the inhibitor to achieve a K_i of less than 5 nM (also, see Fig. 36-9).

enzymatic reaction but was resistant to cleavage by the protease. Although this first molecule was a weak inhibitor of viral protease, the researchers used knowledge about the enzyme's structure to add additional functional groups to the molecule that would likely increase its potency. The result was a drug candidate that bound the enzyme with 10,000-fold higher affinity than the first structure; however, this candidate displayed poor pharmacokinetics.

Chemists continued to alter functional groups on the candidate drug until **ritonavir,** a highly potent molecule with acceptable pharmacokinetic properties, was created. Incidentally, studies of ritonavir in tissue culture showed that it inhibited a cytochrome P450 enzyme involved in the metabolism of other candidate protease inhibitors.

In 1996, about 9 years after the initial research began, the FDA approved ritonavir for marketing. In 2000, based on pharmacokinetic and clinical studies showing that ritonavir increases the bioavailability of a second protease inhibitor, **lopinavir**, the FDA approved the marketing of a combination drug that contains both ritonavir and lopinavir.

QUESTIONS

■ **1.** What methods can researchers use to "discover" new drugs such as ritonavir?
■ **2.** How can structural information about a molecular target help in the drug discovery process?
■ **3.** How do researchers evaluate drug candidates?
■ **4.** How do drug development investigations help to elucidate likely therapeutic features of a drug candidate, such as its pharmacokinetics and toxicity?

THE DRUG DISCOVERY PROCESS

The term **drug discovery** refers to the process by which pharmaceutical, biotechnology, academic, and government laboratories identify or screen compounds to find potentially active therapeutic agents. Screening consists of testing many compounds in assays relevant to the disease in question: a compound that passes such a screen is called a **hit.** If the compound or its structural derivatives continue to show promise after further biological and chemical characterization, it becomes a **lead.** Drug discovery should ideally be cost-effective, producing hits that have a high likelihood of conversion to leads and eventually to successful drugs (Fig. 48-2).

Two basic strategies are used to identify hits. In a **compound-centered** approach, a compound is identified by one of several methods (described below), and its biological profile is explored. If the compound displays desirable pharmacologic activity, it is refined and developed further. In a **target-centered** approach, which is now the more common mode, the putative drug target is identified first. The potential target could be a receptor thought to be involved in a disease process, a critical enzyme, or another biologically important molecule in the disease pathway. Once the target is identified, researchers search for compounds that interact with the target as agonists, antagonists, or modulators. The search may be systematic, using information about the struc-

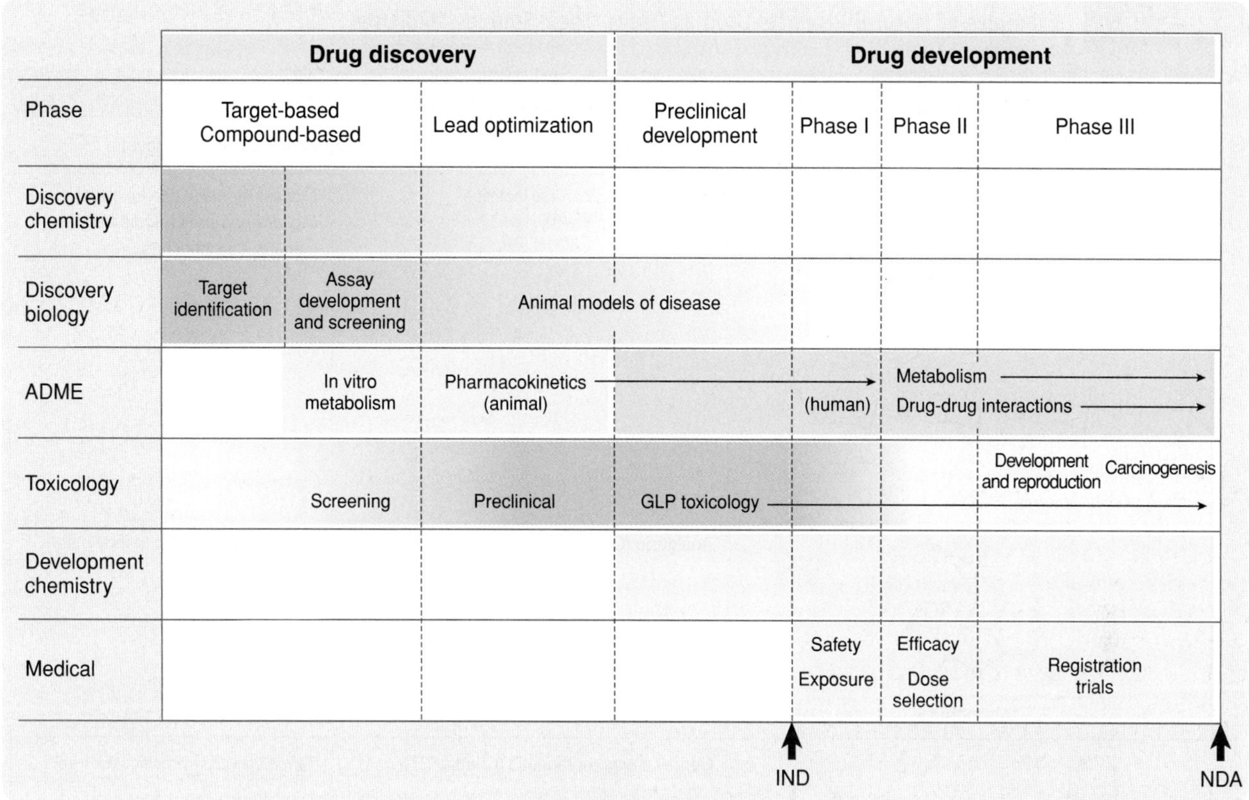

	Drug discovery			Drug development		
Phase	Target-based Compound-based	Lead optimization	Preclinical development	Phase I	Phase II	Phase III
Discovery chemistry						
Discovery biology	Target identification / Assay development and screening	Animal models of disease				
ADME	In vitro metabolism	Pharmacokinetics (animal)	⟶ (human)		Metabolism ⟶ / Drug-drug interactions ⟶	
Toxicology	Screening	Preclinical	GLP toxicology ⟶			Development and reproduction / Carcinogenesis ⟶
Development chemistry						
Medical				Safety / Exposure	Efficacy / Dose selection	Registration trials

↑ IND   ↑ NDA

Figure 48-2. Sequence of phases of drug discovery and development. The important points to note are the general sequence of activities and the considerable overlap of functions with time. The process is highly interactive among several disciplines in an attempt to obtain the molecule with the greatest efficacy, fewest adverse effects, and greatest safety. The clinical trials and regulatory approval phases are described in Chapter 49. The entire process from hit to drug approval can take 8 to 12 years and cost more than $1 billion. IND, investigational new drug application; NDA, new drug application; ADME, absorption, distribution, metabolism, excretion; GLP, good laboratory practices.

ture of the target as a starting point, or it may take a **shotgun approach,** whereby all the compounds in a large library of substances, synthesized via **combinatorial chemistry,** are tested in a high-speed automated assay. After any of these approaches identifies a hit, the hit is then often modified with the aid of specific knowledge about its target. For example, such knowledge can be used to design a high-throughput screen that will test the biological activity of compounds generated by chemical modifications of the original hit.

COMPOUND-CENTERED DRUG DESIGN

Natural and Synthetic Compounds

Traditionally, drugs were discovered using a compound-centered approach. Many of the earliest drugs discovered were **natural products** isolated from plants, molds, or other organisms. Often, the discoveries were made serendipitously. For example, **penicillin** (see Chapter 33, Pharmacology of Bacterial Infections: Cell Wall Synthesis) was discovered when Alexander Fleming observed that spores of the contaminant mold *Penicillium notatum* inhibited bacterial growth in a petri dish. Other natural products that have been transformed into successful drugs include **paclitaxel,** a chemotherapeutic derived from the Pacific yew tree, **morphine,** an opioid analgesic obtained from the opium poppy, **streptokinase,** a thrombolytic agent obtained from strepto-

coccal bacteria, and **cyclosporine,** an immunosuppressive agent obtained from a fungus. Table 48-1 lists a number of drugs obtained from natural products.

There are several advantages to examining natural products as a source for potential drugs. First, natural products have a reasonable likelihood of biologic activity. Second, it may be easier to isolate a compound from its natural source than to synthesize a compound de novo, especially if the structure of the compound is complex or requires difficult synthetic manipulations. **Paclitaxel,** for example, has a complex structure that contains four fused rings, one of which contains eight carbons. A chemical synthesis of the compound took over 50 steps to complete and had a total yield of less than 1%. Third, it may be feasible to use the natural compound as a starting point for synthetic fine-tuning, i.e., to form a **semisynthetic** product. Of course, natural products also have disadvantages: it often takes significant effort to isolate a natural product, without a guarantee of success. Although natural products are more likely than many synthetic compounds to have biological activity, it may be difficult to predict which assay system would be optimal for testing the function of these molecules. Even if it is found to be pharmacologically active, a natural product can be expensive to isolate and modify.

Synthetic compounds are now frequently used to search for new drugs. Researchers can construct a library consisting of thousands of compounds with differing structural charac-

TABLE 48-1	Examples of Natural Products Used as Drugs, Their Sources, and Uses	

DRUG	CLINICAL USE AND CHAPTER REFERENCE	SOURCE
Cyclosporine	Immunosuppressant (Chapter 44)	*Beauveria nivea* (fungus)
Digoxin	Antiarrhythmic, cardiac inotrope (Chapters 18, 19, 24)	*Digitalis lanata* (white foxglove), *Digitalis purpurea* (purple foxglove), numerous other plants
Morphine	Analgesic (Chapter 16)	*Papaver somniferum* (poppy plant)
Paclitaxel	Cancer chemotherapeutic (Chapter 37)	*Taxus brevifolia* (Pacific yew tree)
Penicillin G	Antibacterial (Chapter 33)	*Penicillium chrysogenum* (mold)
Reserpine	Antihypertensive (Chapter 24)	*Rauwolfia serpentina* (plant)
Streptokinase	Thrombolytic (Chapter 22)	Beta-hemolytic streptococci (bacteria)

The structures of streptokinase and cyclosporine are too complex to include in this table.

teristics, tailored for a particular type of investigation: a library could, for example, consist of numerous compounds that have a phenylalanine-proline bond or that are likely agonists or antagonists of a particular class of receptors.

Analogues of Natural Ligands

An alternative compound-centered approach uses the natural ligand (often an agonist) of a receptor as the starting point for drug development. For example, because lack of **dopamine** is associated with Parkinson's disease (see Chapter 12, Pharmacology of Dopaminergic Neurotransmission), one of the first effective treatments involved administering the drug **levodopa** (L-DOPA), a metabolic precursor of dopamine. **Insulin** was developed in much the same way; once it was discovered that the signs and symptoms of diabetes were caused by low insulin levels, insulin was administered exogenously as an effective treatment.

The natural agonist for a receptor can also serve as a skeleton on which chemical modifications can be made. These changes can alter the compound's binding affinity, physiologic effect (such as converting an agonist into an antagonist; see Chapter 1, Drug-Receptor Interactions), distribution, metabolism, or pharmacokinetics. This approach was employed in the development of **cimetidine** (see Chapter 42, Histamine Pharmacology), an H2 receptor antagonist. Starting with histamine, researchers made successive modifications in the structural skeleton to synthesize an antagonist with high affinity for the receptor and decreased toxicity. Similarly, modified insulins with different pharmacokinetic properties are now used to treat patients with diabetes.

Modifying a small-molecule agonist has a relatively high likelihood of success. Because the natural agonist is biologically active, chemical derivatives of that compound are also likely to be biologically active. Of course, problems may also arise. Dopamine formed from exogenous L-DOPA can bind to receptors in undesirable areas of the brain and cause hallucinations. Moreover, many disease processes are not mediated by the interaction of a small-molecule agonist and its receptor. Many targets for drug molecules are ion channels or proteins that interact with other proteins, and hence are not amenable to this agonist analogue approach.

TARGET-CENTERED DRUG DESIGN

In a target-centered approach to drug discovery, researchers use a validated biochemical or molecular target to search for hits. This approach has several advantages. First, if the target has been associated with a disease process, a hit that successfully interacts with the target has a relatively high likelihood of useful pharmacologic activity. Second, because the target is known, it may be easier to devise assays capable of isolating the effect of an agent on the target. This is especially true for disease processes too complex to observe in cell or tissue preparations. For example, although a potential drug's effect on the process of atherosclerosis may be difficult to measure rapidly, it is relatively easy to measure whether the drug inhibits an enzyme shown to be involved in the pathogenesis of atherosclerosis, such as HMG-CoA reductase (see Chapter 23, Pharmacology of Cholesterol and Lipoprotein Metabolism). As knowledge of the pathophysi-

ology of disease processes has increased, target-centered approaches to drug discovery have become increasingly successful, and many new drugs have been discovered using target-centered methods. HIV protease inhibitors, such as **ritonavir**, are notable examples of a drug class discovered using a target-centered approach. In an alternative approach, dissection of the underlying biological pathway has allowed the development of macromolecules, including antibodies, as novel pharmaceuticals to interrupt the pathway (Box 48-1).

BOX 48-1. **Macromolecular Biologics and Therapeutics**

Increasingly, pharmaceutical and biotechnology companies are turning toward large molecules such as **peptides, peptidomimetics, proteins, antisense oligonucleotides,** and **monoclonal antibodies.** The pharmacologic properties and clinical utility of these therapies are described in Chapter 53, Protein-Based Therapies.

The approach to the discovery and development of these molecules can differ significantly from that for small molecules. Consider, for example, the development of agents for the treatment of diseases related to an insufficiency or lack of an endogenous compound, such as **insulin** for diabetes, **erythropoietin** for anemia, or a coagulation factor (**factor VIII** or **factor IX**) for an inherited coagulopathy. In these situations, referred to as *replacement therapy,* it is not necessary to perform extensive screening of a large number of molecules to determine whether the endogenous molecule needs to be modified. Therefore, these agents may rapidly move into development and human testing.

Natural or modified macromolecules are increasingly used not only to replace but also to modulate physiologic processes, and engineered macromolecules such as antibodies are being used in the treatment of disease (Table 48-2). In the case of antibodies, the drug discovery and development process may involve modifications that increase the affinity or specificity of the antibody for the desired molecular target or that ''humanize'' the antibody in order to minimize its immunogenic potential. Because these types of molecules must typically be administered parenterally, the need to screen for acceptable pharmacokinetic properties is lessened. Furthermore, the required discovery biology and animal toxicity testing may not be as extensive, because there is often less risk of ''off-target'' toxicity with biologic agents. Manufacturing a biologic product may be more challenging, however: the major challenges are to develop a system capable of producing the desired macromolecule in a bacterium, yeast, or a mammalian cell, and then to isolate the compound in pure form from the large mixture of metabolic products that often result from the synthesis. Faithfully reproducing the complex procedures involved in macromolecule synthesis and purification makes the preparation of generic biologic drugs a substantial challenge.

TABLE 48-2	Examples of Macromolecular Therapies		
NAME	**INDICATION**	**MOLECULAR CATEGORY**	**ORIGIN**
Antivenin	Snake bite	Antibody	Equine or cell culture
Erythropoietin	Anemia	Growth factor	Bacteria (recombinant human)
Heparin	Anticoagulant	Glycosaminoglycan	Porcine or bovine
Human growth hormone	Growth retardation	Hormone	Bacteria (recombinant human)
Insulin	Diabetes	Hormone	Bacteria (recombinant human)
Parathyroid hormone	Osteoporosis	Hormone	Bacteria (recombinant human)
Streptokinase	Thrombolytic	Protein	Streptococcus
Trastuzumab	Cancer	Antibody	Chinese hamster ovary cell culture (humanized monoclonal antibody)

High-Throughput Screening

The simplest target-centered approach involves rapidly screening many molecules using an assay based on the drug target. **High-throughput screening** uses a target-based assay and robotic automation to test thousands of compounds in a few days.

Two aspects are critical in this approach. First, a large library of compounds must be available for screening. Second, a robust assay that leads to rapid identification of true hits must be developed. The assay may be as simple as determining the binding affinity of drug candidates for a receptor (see Chapter 2, Pharmacodynamics), or it may be more sophisticated, involving complicated biochemical or cell-based manipulations. The library is then "run through" the assay, and any hits giving a positive signal are examined more closely. An assay performed in a 96- or 384-well plate allows researchers to screen many compounds simultaneously. In addition, once a library of compounds has been established, the same library can be run through many different assays. The quality of the results is dependent on the quality of the assay and the compounds in the library, so a poorly designed assay or a limited library may result in false hits or miss viable candidates. In practice, because high-throughput screening places a premium on rapid assays, false positives and false negatives are not uncommon. Even when a true hit is found, it will most likely need to be refined to increase its binding affinity or to change its pharmacologic properties (specificity, solubility, stability, kinetics, etc.); this process is called "**hit-to-lead development.**"

Combinatorial Chemistry

One important refinement in the process of high-throughput screening has been the introduction of **combinatorial chemistry.** In a strategy analogous to that used by nature to construct a wide variety of proteins from a relatively small number (approximately 20) of amino acids, combinatorial chemistry uses a relatively small number of precursor molecules to generate a large number of compounds. Researchers are not limited to natural substances; instead, they generally use a group of precursors with common functional groups and divergent side chains. For example, a researcher starting with three sets of 30 precursor building blocks can create 27,000 (30 × 30 × 30) different compounds in two syn-

thetic steps (Fig. 48-3). One could theoretically create each compound individually in its own reaction well, but in practice it is easier to synthesize the molecules on a solid support such as a polystyrene bead. In a **parallel synthesis,** the beads are split so that thousands are reacted at once and then successively recombined and split to undergo successive reactions. This strategy drastically reduces the number of reactions in the synthesis (30 at a time instead of 27,000 at a time, in the previous example). However, the challenge then becomes sorting the beads in order to know which compound

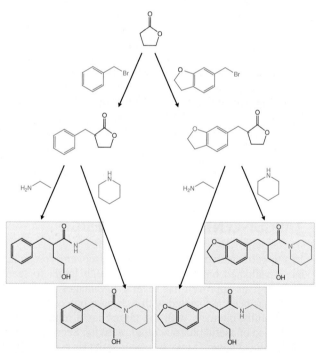

Figure 48-3. Diversity through combinatorial chemistry. Combinatorial chemistry uses simple building blocks to produce a complex library of compounds. In this example, the functionalized skeleton (black) has multiple sites of attachment. Two building blocks (blue) combine with the functionalized skeleton to produce a wide variety of products. In this example, two different side groups for each of the two building blocks results in four (2^2) possible products. Combinatorial chemistry libraries use several building blocks, each with up to 20 or more different side groups, and can produce thousands of complex molecules using the same basic chemistry.

has been synthesized on each bead. Researchers have solved this problem by **tagging** each bead with a unique chemical code, such as a ribonucleotide sequence, during each reaction. To identify a bead that bears a successful hit compound, the tag is cleaved, amplified by standard methods, and sequenced. The code then reveals to which reactions the bead has been exposed and consequently the identity of the successful compound. Large chemical libraries can be synthesized in this manner and then screened in high-throughput assays for activity, sometimes with the compounds still attached to the beads. The use of combinatorial chemistry and high-throughput screening is termed a **shotgun approach,** because researchers test a wide range of compounds blindly against a single target. This approach can also be modified to search for a particular result by using "**biased libraries**" for different types of targets. For example, researchers have synthesized large libraries of compounds that are more likely to interact with G protein-coupled receptors, proteolytic enzymes, kinases, or ion channels, based on the structural characteristics of each target class.

Structure-Based Drug Design

Another target-centered approach is termed **structure-based drug design** or **rational drug design**. In this approach, a drug candidate is discovered using the three-dimensional structure of the target obtained through **nuclear magnetic resonance** (NMR) or **x-ray crystallography**. In theory, researchers could identify the active site within the structure of the target, use modeling algorithms to study the shape of the active site, and design a candidate drug molecule to fit into the active site. More commonly, though, the target is cocrystallized with a substrate analogue or receptor ligand (agonist or antagonist) in order to identify the structure of the active site. The structure of the analogue is then modified to increase the molecule's affinity, as was done in the case of ritonavir (see the case that opens this chapter). Alternatively, researchers can refine the structure of a new compound that binds to the target in a screening assay. By iteratively improving the fit of the prototypic molecule in the active site of the target, the binding affinity is increased (Fig. 48-1).

There are several advantages to a structure-based drug design approach. The refined hit (also called *lead*) compounds are often extremely potent, with binding affinities in the nanomolar range. Moreover, only a limited number of candidates need to be tested because there is a high likelihood that one or more of the designed compounds will bind the target. In addition, iterative modification of the compound is relatively straightforward because it is known which parts of the molecule are critical for binding to the active site of the target. Thus, in comparison to a structure-blind approach, fewer analogues are prepared in a structure-based approach, but each analogue has a higher likelihood of activity. One disadvantage to this approach is that the modified compounds are often more difficult to synthesize because the molecular design demands specific functionalities in specific locations of the molecule. Another disadvantage is that obtaining a crystal structure of the target can be difficult, especially for membrane-bound proteins. Often, other methods of drug design yield hits long before the target can be crystallized. However, even if the initial hit com-

pound results from another method, that hit can often be refined into a lead using a structure-based design approach.

As illustrated in the introductory case, rational drug design has been critical for the development of HIV protease inhibitors such as ritonavir. Structure-based methods have also been used to develop a second class of antiviral drugs, the neuraminidase inhibitors (see Chapter 36). As structure-based drug design gains feasibility, more drugs will be produced using structural information about the target even if the initial hits are discovered through other methods.

LEAD OPTIMIZATION

The early drug discovery process will typically identify a promising group of lead molecules that appear to interact with the target in a desirable way. For these promising molecules, however, many of the physical, chemical, biological, and pharmacologic properties that are important attributes of an effective drug remain unknown. **Lead optimization** is the stage of drug discovery where these properties are characterized and refined, with the ultimate goal of selecting a single molecule to enter into clinical testing and formal drug development.

In practice, most lead compounds have one or more characteristics (e.g., low solubility, low oral bioavailability, complex metabolism, high toxicity) that make them poor candidates for clinical use. Using the data generated in lead optimization, it is often possible to modify the structure of the molecule to overcome these deficiencies. As exemplified in the introductory case, precursors of ritonavir went through several modifications before a final compound was chosen to enter clinical trials.

A variety of factors may cause a molecule to be terminated at the lead optimization stage. These include:

- Failure to demonstrate efficacy in a rigorous animal model of human disease
- Failure to attain adequate systemic exposures following oral administration (low bioavailability)
- Extensive or complex metabolism within the body, resulting in the generation of potentially dangerous reactive metabolites
- Extremely low solubility that prevents preparing a suitable formulation for dosing
- Toxic effects in preliminary animal toxicology studies
- In vitro evidence that the molecule may damage DNA (genotoxicity)
- Extremely difficult chemical synthesis that cannot be "scaled up" in a cost-effective manner

PHASES OF DRUG DEVELOPMENT

The outcome of the lead optimization process is the selection of a molecule suitable for testing in humans. At this point, the molecule moves from drug discovery to drug development. Early drug development consists of preclinical activities designed to support clinical trials and clinical drug development. The initial preclinical phase of drug development includes the following activities:

- Manufacture, formulation, and packaging of a sufficient amount of high-quality drug material for both definitive animal safety testing and clinical trial use
- Animal toxicology and pharmacokinetic studies to support the safety of initial drug administration in humans
- Preparation of regulatory documents and submissions to regulatory authorities; these activities are described in more detail in Chapter 49, Clinical Drug Evaluation and Regulatory Approval

Initial planning for clinical drug development proceeds concurrently with preclinical drug development. Key initial activities include defining outcome objectives for the clinical trial, selection of clinical trial investigators, and development of clinical trial protocols. The initial regulatory filings must include detailed protocols to allow regulators to assess the safety of the proposed clinical investigation.

The clinical development of the drug candidate refers to a wide range of studies conducted in humans. As described in more detail in Chapter 49, these studies are divided into three phases, with the goal of providing a rigorous test of the safety and efficacy of the molecule. Clinical studies may be conducted in various patient populations and disease states. The number, duration, and complexity of the required clinical trials depend on the nature of the proposed disease indication for the drug. For example, an assessment of the ability of a drug to lower blood pressure in hypertensive patients may require only a few weeks of dosing, whereas the ability of a molecule to reduce the risk of fracture in a patient with osteoporosis may require 2 years of drug administration.

Although evaluating the effects of the molecule in humans is the primary focus of the drug development phase, extensive activities must also be completed by various scientific disciplines to support both these clinical trials and the ultimate regulatory approval of the drug. These activities are described in the following section, and they must be carefully coordinated in order for drug development to proceed as effectively as possible.

KEY DISCIPLINES IN DRUG DISCOVERY AND DEVELOPMENT

Having discussed the overall process of drug discovery and development, we now turn to the fundamental tools—from basic chemistry and biology to manufacturing and formulation—that are crucial in the discovery and development of new therapeutic agents.

DISCOVERY CHEMISTRY

Chemistry and biology work hand-in-hand in the early phases of drug discovery. In compound-centered drug design, medicinal chemists begin the discovery process by preparing the molecules to be tested in biological and pharmacologic assays. In target-centered design, the process begins with the identification of potential drug targets against which chemists then design and prepare the molecules for testing. Thus, in both approaches there is close interaction and collaboration between chemists and biologists.

Initially, the amount of a drug candidate needed to run a simple screening assay is small—typically less than 1 mg. This is important, because synthesizing or isolating even small amounts of a compound can be expensive, at least until the synthesis can be refined. Once a lead is identified, gram quantities are needed to carry out biological, toxicity, and chemical characterization studies. Kilogram quantities are required when a drug enters clinical trials and, if a drug is approved, plants need to manufacture material on a scale sufficient to meet expected use. Quality and documentation of the specifications of the manufacturing process must be maintained throughout the scale-up (see Chapter 49).

Chemical characterization refers to the chemical properties of the drug candidate, including physical characteristics such as melting point, crystal form, and solubility, as well as purity and stability. The physical and chemical characteristics of a drug candidate are critical for determining how the drug could best be administered and stored (Table 48-3). The compound's chemical structure is commonly elucidated using a range of techniques, including mass spectrometry, which gives the compound's molecular weight; elemental analysis, which determines its atomic composition; NMR, which elucidates the types and patterns of chemical bonds present; and x-ray crystallography, which determines its three-dimensional structure. It is also important to distinguish among various isomers of the same compound, because biological activity is often isomer-selective. For exam-

TABLE 48-3	Information Obtained in Chemical Characterization Studies	
TYPE OF ASSAY	**EXPERIMENTAL TECHNIQUE**	**CLINICAL IMPLICATIONS**
Characterization, structure	NMR, IR spectroscopy; mass spectrometry, x-ray crystallography	Isomeric purity, active compound
Impurities	HPLC, GC, mass spectrometry	Possible adverse reactions from impurities, toxicology
Partition coefficient	Octanol/water partition	Pharmacokinetics, including absorption, distribution, metabolism, and excretion; tissue distribution
Solubility	Solubility in various solvents	Pharmacokinetics, including absorption, distribution, metabolism, and excretion; formulations
Stability	Stability measurements under different conditions (heat, cold, humidity, light)	Shelf life, degradation products

ple, propranolol (see Chapter 24, Integrative Cardiovascular Pharmacology: Hypertension, Ischemic Heart Disease, and Heart Failure) is a mixture of l and d isomers, but only the l isomer acts as a β-adrenoceptor antagonist.

Chemists also characterize physical properties of the molecule, such as the pK_a of an acidic or basic drug, which are used in developing the formulation (see below). In addition, the drug's solubility is measured in a variety of solvents, especially water, to provide information on the molecule's likely oral bioavailability and possible hepatic metabolism. The partition coefficient describes how the molecule distributes between an aqueous solvent, analogous to blood, and a hydrophobic solvent, analogous to the plasma membrane. Finally, the compound's stability and impurity profiles must be determined.

DISCOVERY BIOLOGY: BIOCHEMICAL ASSAYS, CELLULAR ASSAYS, AND ANIMAL MODELS

The goal of discovery biology is to determine whether a molecule is likely to be efficacious in a particular disease state. Effectiveness may be assessed at the biochemical, cell, tissue, organ, and organism levels. If undesirable biological properties are found, it may be possible to modify the structure so as to improve its pharmacologic profile. In general, biochemical and cell-based assays are used early in the drug discovery process, while more complex organ and whole-animal studies are used in the lead optimization phase to characterize the pharmacologic properties of the molecule.

Biochemical assays evaluate the mechanism of action of the drug candidate at a molecular level. **Receptor binding assays** measure both the binding affinity and selectivity of the molecule for the target receptor. **Enzyme activity assays** measure the ability of the drug to inhibit the activity of a target enzyme. Selectivity for the desired target is critically important in the design and testing of lead molecules.

In **cellular assays,** researchers aim to determine whether the lead molecule(s) acts appropriately in an environment that more closely approximates its in vivo use. For example, if the drug is designed to act in the cytoplasm, then it is essential to determine whether the drug can cross the plasma membrane. Early assessment of potential toxicity may be measured by incubating the lead molecule with a variety of tissues or cells, such as liver cells or cell extracts, to investigate its metabolic products, as well as how the molecule affects liver enzymes or interacts with other drugs. The ability of ritonavir to inhibit cytochrome P450 enzymes was found in such an assay. Drug-induced changes in complex patterns of gene expression can be assessed using gene array chips capable of measuring mRNA levels for thousands of genes simultaneously.

Finally, at the highest level of complexity, the effects of the drug candidate on whole organisms are established. Ideally, **animal models** are used that mirror the critical aspects of human pathophysiology for the target disease. For example, cancer chemotherapeutic agents can be tested in nude (T-cell–deficient) mice that have been injected with human tumor cells. Similarly, drugs for the treatment of postmenopausal osteoporosis can be tested in rats that have been ovariectomized to mimic the postmenopausal state. Table 48-4 describes just a few of the many animal models used by pharmaceutical researchers.

ABSORPTION, DISTRIBUTION, METABOLISM, AND EXCRETION (ADME)

Studies characterizing the fate of a molecule following its administration are critical in understanding the potential effectiveness as well as the safety of that molecule. Such studies collectively describe the ADME profile of the molecule. The basic principles investigated in the course of these studies are described in Chapters 3 and 4. These studies are initially conducted on animals, and complementary information is obtained during clinical drug development.

The systemic exposure of a drug candidate is typically determined in pharmacokinetic studies, in which the concentration of drug in the systemic circulation is measured at

TABLE 48-4 Examples of Efficacy Models Used in Drug Discovery

DISEASE	ANIMAL MODEL	DRUG EXAMPLE
Cancer	Tumor xenografts in nude mice	Cisplatin
Diabetes	Genetically predisposed rodents (Zucker Diabetic Fatty Rat)	Insulin
		Metformin
		Thiazolidinediones
Hypercholesterolemia	Genetically hypercholesterolemic rats/mice	Statins
	Diet-induced hypercholesterolemia	
Obesity	db/db and ob/ob rats	Orlistat
		Rimonabant
		Sibutramine
Postmenopausal osteoporosis	Ovariectomized rats	Bisphosphonates
		SERMs (raloxifene)
		Teriparatide
Rheumatoid arthritis	Collagen-induced arthritis	Anti-TNF antibodies

various time points after administration. Important parameters include the maximal (''peak'') level of systemic exposure, the time after drug administration at which the maximal systemic exposure occurs, the overall systemic exposure during a treatment interval, and the length of time for which the drug remains in the circulation. These parameters are measured for different administered dose levels and are also evaluated for acute (single-dose) and chronic (repeat-dose) administrations. The tissues to which the drug distributes and the routes of excretion of the drug are typically measured by administering radiolabeled drug and then measuring the radioactivity levels in the different organs and body fluids.

As described in Chapter 4, metabolism or biotransformation refers to the processes by which biochemical reactions alter drugs within the body. As drug discovery and development progresses, there is a continual accrual of data to understand these processes for a candidate drug. Initial studies are often conducted in vitro, using animal and human microsomes or hepatocytes as the source of the drug-metabolizing enzymes. Measured parameters include the metabolic stability of the drug and its ability to inhibit or induce important drug-metabolizing enzymes. The latter studies help to assess the potential of the molecule to cause metabolic drug-drug interactions. As drug development progresses, studies are conducted to characterize the metabolic fate of the candidate drug in both animals and humans. In addition, formal drug-drug interaction studies are performed to determine whether the candidate drug is likely to affect the metabolism of other drugs that are already in clinical use for the target disease state.

TOXICOLOGY

Animal toxicity studies are conducted to determine whether it is safe to initiate clinical trials with the drug candidate and ultimately to market the drug. Studies of increasing duration and complexity are completed as the molecule proceeds through clinical drug development. The animal toxicity testing program is customized based on the desired therapeutic goal. For example, a drug designed to be used acutely in a critical care setting would require only short-term animal studies, whereas an agent intended for chronic use would require studies encompassing nearly the lifetime of the animal. Because these animal toxicity studies are critical to an accurate assessment of the potential risks to clinical trial subjects from administration of the drug candidate, they are proscribed by a complex set of regulations. To ensure the quality of the study data, pivotal toxicology studies that directly support a clinical trial must be conducted under a set of rules called the Good Laboratory Practices (GLP).

Many drug discovery organizations will perform an initial assessment of the molecule's toxicity during lead optimization. At this stage, the toxicity assays may involve the potential of the molecule to alter DNA (genotoxicity testing), its potential to affect the cardiovascular system (cardiovascular pharmacology testing), and its toxicity in short-term animal studies. These studies may provide insights into the mechanisms of potential toxic effects of the molecule. They can also ascertain whether acceptable margins of safety are likely to be found in later phases of drug development. Significant

target organ toxicity (functional and/or histopathological) is a frequent source of molecule termination at this phase of drug development.

As the molecule proceeds into the testing required for clinical trial authorizations, a more comprehensive set of toxicity studies is conducted. Some of the most important safety data derive from **repeat-dose toxicity studies**. In general, these studies are conducted in both a rodent (e.g., rat or mouse) and a nonrodent (e.g., dog or monkey) species. Animals in these studies are administered various dose levels of the molecule for periods of time (e.g., 2 weeks to 1 year) that depend on the duration of the proposed clinical trial. Repeat-dose toxicity studies evaluate body weight, clinical signs, and clinical laboratory parameters (hematology, clinical chemistry, and urinalysis). A histologic evaluation of all organ systems is also performed. Safety pharmacology studies are used to assess potential undesirable drug effects on the central nervous, cardiovascular, and respiratory systems. Genotoxicity is thoroughly assessed; animal studies are performed to characterize effects on fertility, reproduction, and development; and the ability of the drug to induce tumors in animal models is measured. In sum, the results of these comprehensive animal studies identify the potential toxicities that might occur upon administration of the drug to humans, and assess the systemic exposures and durations of treatment that would likely produce these adverse effects.

DEVELOPMENT CHEMISTRY: CHEMICAL SYNTHESIS, SCALE-UP, AND MANUFACTURING

An effective chemical synthesis must satisfy several requirements. Ideally, it should require few synthetic steps. Each additional step in a synthesis increases the possibility of impurities, decreases the yield (the amount of material obtained at the end of the synthesis), and increases the cost. If multiple isomers of a compound are possible products of the synthesis, then a synthesis that produces only the target isomer is preferable. Finally, the synthesis should be amenable to scale-up.

Two techniques, **retrosynthetic analysis** and **convergent synthesis,** aid in the establishment of a good synthetic scheme. In a retrosynthetic analysis, key steps are developed by examining important structural elements in the final product and figuring out how specific reactions could lead to the product (Fig. 48-4). This procedure is performed iteratively so that a complex final molecule is reduced to simpler intermediates. The advantage of such an approach is that it greatly simplifies planning the synthesis of a complex product and readily leads to a convergent synthesis. In a convergent synthesis, individual parts of a molecule are synthesized separately, and the parts are assembled only near the end of the synthesis (Fig. 48-5). This increases the overall yield of the synthesis by reducing the number of linear steps required and allows each key component of the final product to be optimized individually. These two methods are complementary and are often employed together in planning the chemical synthesis of a compound.

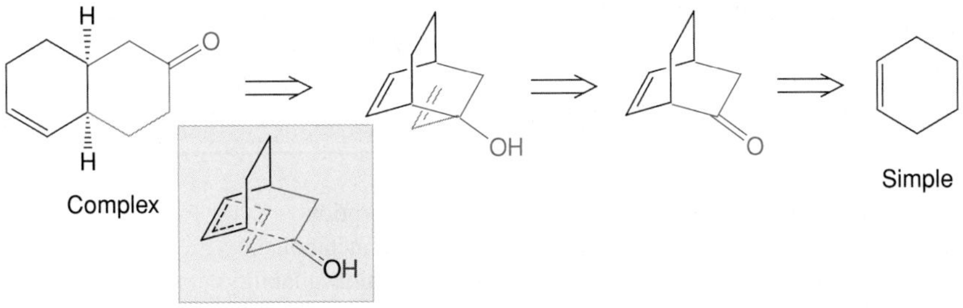

Figure 48-4. Retrosynthetic analysis of a complex molecule. A retrosynthetic analysis of a complex molecule, such as the illustrated bicyclic compound, allows the identification of simple starting materials such as cyclohexadiene. Analysis of the structural element *(blue)* demonstrates the creative process required to envision how a complex structure could be deconstructed into its component parts. The structure in a blue box illustrates the thinking required when deconstructing a molecule. These simple starting materials can then be combined in a series of steps to create the complex molecule. For simplicity, the synthetic details are not shown.

For early drug development, the goal of development chemistry is to generate enough product to meet the demands of chemical and biological characterization, particularly for animal toxicology and formulation studies. As the scale of the need increases, the synthesis strategy must evolve. For example, a chemical synthesis often starts out using available raw materials, which may include expensive specialty chemicals. However, as the scale of the synthesis increases, these reagents must be replaced with cheaper (and/or safer) alternatives. Furthermore, in an early synthetic scheme each intermediate is isolated, purified, and characterized to ensure that each sequential step of the synthesis is effective. However, as chemists gain more experience with the synthesis, multiple steps may be combined without isolating intermediates or purifying the products of each reaction, in a so-called **one-pot synthesis.**

Once the synthesis strategy of a drug candidate has been fully developed, process chemists must then adapt the synthesis for large-scale commercial manufacturing. This process must be initiated before a drug is approved, because the approval process requires that several batches of the drug be successfully manufactured, formulated (see below), and rigorously tested for quality and stability. A pharmaceutical company must also be prepared to meet market demands immediately after approval, which means that a manufacturing process must be established before the commercial launch of the drug.

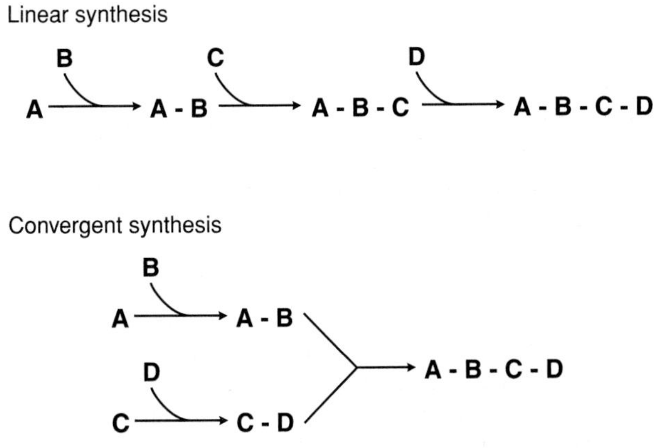

The process chemist must ensure that the synthesis is safe and meets environmental regulations for emissions and disposal of water. This may preclude the use of certain solvents that are commonly used by synthetic chemists in small-scale syntheses.

FORMULATION

Drugs must be in a form that can be administered to humans in a measured dose. The type of formulation depends on the intended route of administration (Table 48-5). **Enteral formulations,** which include oral, sublingual, and rectal dosage forms, are designed to be absorbed across portions of the digestive tract. **Parenteral formulations** include intravenous, intramuscular, and subcutaneous injections, inhalants, topical formulations, and transdermal patches. The preferred route of administration is determined by many variables, including the drug's stability and its pharmacokinetic properties of absorption, distribution, metabolism (including first-pass metabolism), and excretion. Oral dosage forms are favored for drugs that are relatively stable in the digestive tract, are not rapidly metabolized in the liver, have high oral bioavailability, and do not require an immediate action. Parenteral dosage forms are preferred for drugs that must be fast-acting and are more reliably absorbed by nonenteral than by enteral routes. Macromolecules, which generally have little or no oral bioavailability, are typically administered via injection (see Chapter 53, Protein-Based Therapies).

Most drugs are administered orally in either tablet or capsule form. In addition to the measured dose of the drug, most tablets contain **binders,** which keep the components together, and **stabilizers,** which enhance the drug's shelf life. For acid-sensitive drugs, it is often possible to coat the tablet with an **enteric coating** that is acid-resistant but dissolves in the intestine. Formulation chemists can also manipulate the rate at which the tablet or capsule dissolves, thus enabling ''sustained-release'' formulations, whereby the drug is released slowly over the course of hours (see Chapter 54, Drug Delivery Modalities).

The absorption profile and first-pass metabolism are typi-

Figure 48-5. Convergent versus linear synthesis. In a linear synthesis, each component is added sequentially. In a convergent synthesis, each component is assembled separately and then combined in the last step. The convergent synthesis approach generally results in higher yields. The *arrows* indicate sequential synthetic reactions.

TABLE 48-5	Advantages and Disadvantages of Common Formulations

FORMULATION	ADVANTAGES	DISADVANTAGES	EXAMPLES
Enteral			
Oral	Ease of administration	Slow absorption	Acetaminophen
		First-pass metabolism	Oxycodone
		Reduced bioavailability	Pravastatin
Sublingual	Rapid action	Few drugs are absorbed by this	Nitroglycerin
	No first-pass metabolism	route	
Rectal	Rapid action	Uncomfortable	Morphine
	No first-pass metabolism		
Parenteral			
Intravenous	Rapid action	Risk of infection	Lidocaine
	High bioavailability	Uncomfortable	Morphine
	Can control dose easily	Must be administered by trained	tPA
		personnel	
Intramuscular	Sustained release possible	Uncomfortable	Demerol
		Adverse reaction possible	Growth hormone
Subcutaneous	Slow action	Poor compliance	Insulin
Transdermal	Sustained release	Poor absorption	Estrogen
	No first-pass metabolism	Slow action	Nicotine (patch)
Inhalation	Large surface area for absorption	Inconvenience (device)	Albuterol
	Convenience (no injection)		Glucocorticoids (asthma)
			Insulin

cally not issues for drugs delivered intravenously. However, the drug must be dissolved in a vehicle, usually water. Moreover, the solution must be made isotonic with plasma by adding osmotically active compounds such as saline, dextrose, or mannitol, so that the solution does not cause hemolysis. The solution must also be sterile for intravenous injection. Finally, a drug is often less stable in solution than as a solid, so formulation chemists must test its stability in solution. If the drug is unstable, it may be prepared as a **lyophilized powder** that can be dissolved in water or buffer immediately before administration.

Conclusion and Future Directions

The discovery and development of new drugs is a complex process that often requires 10 or more years and hundreds of millions of dollars. Researchers start by searching for a biologically active compound. This may involve a drug-centered approach or a target-centered approach. New pharmacologic targets are currently being identified by gene sequencing, by analysis of genetic factors that predispose to disease, by gene knockout experiments in laboratory animals, and by other techniques. For example, it is now possible to target proteins that enable the expression of genes rather than the gene products themselves. In addition, information about genetic polymorphisms may enable the products of specific, mutant genes to be the targets of new drugs (see Chapter 52, Pharmacogenomics). Finally, new methods to discover compounds that interact with these targets are also becoming available.

Suggested Reading

Burke MD, Schreiber S. A planning strategy for diversity-oriented synthesis. *Angew Chem Int Ed* 2004;43:46–58. *(Tools used by synthetic organic chemists to synthesize a specific target molecule or a large library.)*

Drews J. Drug discovery: a historical perspective. *Science* 2000; 287:1960–1964. *(Historic description of the major methods of drug discovery.)*

Levine RR. *Pharmacology, Drug Actions and Reaction.* 6th ed. New York: Parthenon Publishing; 2000. *(Explains how new drugs are discovered and describes the drug development process through clinical development.)*

Pritchard JF, Jurima-Romet M, Reimer ML, et al. Making better drugs: decision gates in nonclinical drug development. *Nat Rev Drug Discov* 2003;2:542–553. *(Explores the key scientific questions that are addressed during drug discovery and preclinical development.)*

Rademann J, Günther J. Integrating combinatorial synthesis and bioassays. *Science* 2000;287:1947–1948. *(Novel techniques for screening large libraries of compounds.)*

Sams-Dodd F. Strategies to optimize the validity of disease models in the drug discovery process. *Drug Discov Today* 2006;11: 355–363. *(Discusses how to optimize animal models of human disease to allow selection of better drug candidates.)*

United States Food and Drug Administration, United States Department of Health and Human Services. *Innovation or stagnation: challenge and opportunity on the critical path to new medical products.* 03/16/04. Available at http://www.fda.gov/oc/initiatives/criticalpath/whitepaper.pdf. *(Discusses current challenges and opportunities in the development of new drugs, biologic products, and medical devices.)*

49

Clinical Drug Evaluation and Regulatory Approval

John L. Vahle and Armen H. Tashjian, Jr.

INTRODUCTION

Controlled clinical trials provide the scientific and legal basis by which regulatory authorities around the world evaluate new prescription drugs and approve them for sale. In the United States, the regulatory review of drugs is the responsibility of the **U. S. Food and Drug Administration (FDA)**. Over the past 50 years, improved methods for large-scale clinical studies have precipitated a shift toward evidence-based medicine and helped to accelerate the pace of drug development. A total of 119 New Drug Applications (NDA) and 6 Biologic License Applications (BLA) were approved by the FDA in 2004. Of these approvals, 31 drugs and 5 biologic agents were new and innovative medicines that had not been previously approved. As shown in Figure 49-1, the annual number of approved new drugs has varied from 17 to 53 over the past 10 years, with considerable year-to-year variation.

Drug discovery and development remains a lengthy, high-risk, and complex process. According to the Pharmaceutical Research and Manufacturers of America, of every 5,000 to 10,000 chemically synthesized molecules that are screened

as potential drugs, only 1 becomes an approved drug. The previous chapter (Chapter 48, Drug Discovery and Preclinical Development) outlines the early preclinical phase of drug development from target identification to candidate selection. This chapter describes the process by which new candidate drug molecules are evaluated and approved for marketing and sale in the United States.

Case

Throughout the 1980s, Pfizer invested in research and development of a drug intended for the treatment of hypertension and angina. During clinical trials, the hoped-for efficacy was minimal; however, investigators (and subjects) observed that impotent men receiving the treatment were able to achieve erections. Pfizer subsequently patented this molecule for the treatment of erectile dysfunction (ED) and proceeded with its development. Between July 1993 and January 1997, 21 studies involving 3,000 subjects ages 19 to 87 were undertaken. In March 1998, Pfizer received approval from the FDA to market sildenafil citrate as an oral

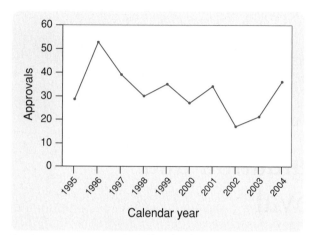

Figure 49-1. Drug review and approval. The FDA has approved an average of 31 new drugs and biologics each year over the past 10 years.

therapy for ED. The drug was approved under the trade name Viagra.

Sildenafil proved to be successful in treating ED. The drug also offered patients greater convenience over existing treatments, which included an alprostadil pellet inserted into the urethra; an alprostadil injection administered directly into the base of the penis; and a constriction loop designed to slow venous outflow from the penis. Despite its widespread adoption, however, sildenafil was linked to a small number of deaths. In the 6 months following approval, a period during which more than 6 million prescriptions were dispensed, the FDA received reports of 130 deaths. Of these deaths, 77 were the result of cardiovascular events such as myocardial infarction, cardiac arrest, and

coronary artery disease. Subsequent testing revealed conditions, situations, or drug interactions (such as concomitant use of nitrates) that represent contraindications to the use of sildenafil. As a result, the FDA ordered Pfizer to amend its label to include expanded warnings of potential cardiovascular adverse effects and drug interactions. In July 2005 the FDA reported in an alert that a small number of men lost sight in one eye some time after taking sildenafil. This type of vision loss is called nonarteritic anterior ischemic optic neuropathy (NAION). The alert was followed by an additional update of the sildenafil label (and the labels for other drugs of the same class, vardenafil and tadalafil); the new labels gave a narrower description of the type of patients for whom sildenafil and other type V phosphodiesterase inhibitors are believed to be safe and appropriate.

QUESTIONS

■ **1.** What ethical standards govern the relationship between physicians and patients in clinical research?
■ **2.** What testing must a drug undergo in order to gain approval for marketing?
■ **3.** What are the differences among phases I, II, and III clinical trials of a drug candidate?

HISTORY OF THE U. S. FOOD AND DRUG LAW

Drug development, testing, and approval is a lengthy process, the major milestones of which are shown in Figure 49-2. Achievement of each of these milestones requires the

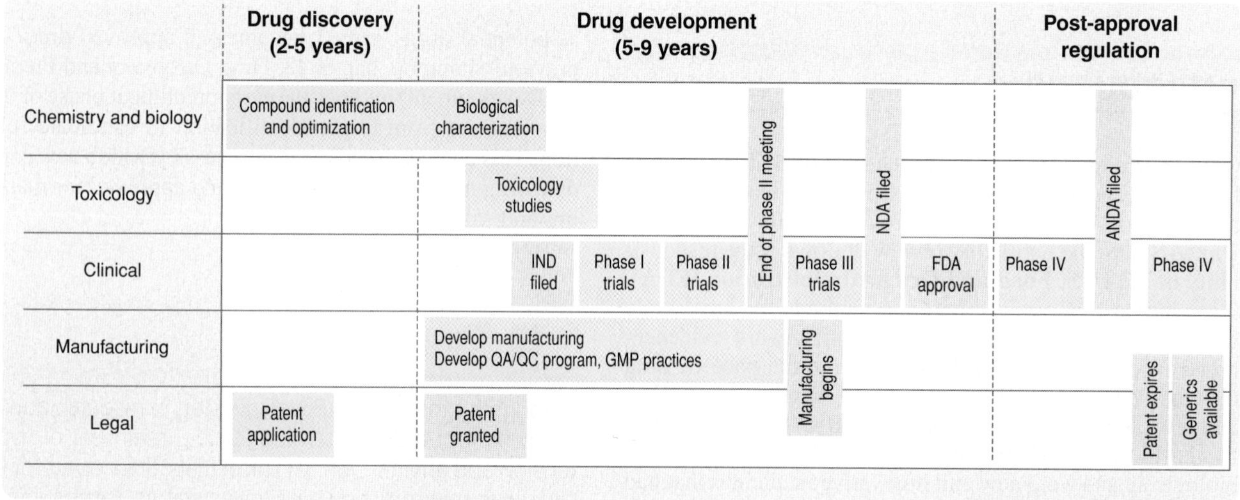

	Drug discovery (2-5 years)	Drug development (5-9 years)								Post-approval regulation	
Chemistry and biology	Compound identification and optimization	Biological characterization									
Toxicology			Toxicology studies								
Clinical				IND filed	Phase I trials	Phase II trials	End of phase II meeting	Phase III trials	NDA filed	FDA approval	Phase IV	ANDA filed	Phase IV
Manufacturing		Develop manufacturing Develop QA/QC program, GMP practices						Manufacturing begins			
Legal	Patent application	Patent granted									Patent expires	Generics available

Figure 49-2. Life cycle of drug approval. The life cycle of approval for a new drug is complex, requiring an average of 11 years for completion. Drug discovery, discussed in Chapter 48, produces a new drug molecule. The first patents are usually filed at this stage and are granted several years later. The drug development process requires that biological characterization and toxicology studies in animals are conducted before an Investigational New Drug (IND) Application can be filed. In turn, an IND is required for the start of clinical trials. At the conclusion of successful clinical trials, a drug company files a New Drug Application (NDA), which is reviewed by the FDA. Once a drug is approved, it must be monitored for safety for the remainder of its lifespan (so-called phase IV). The first of the drug's patents expire 20 years after its application. Abbreviated New Drug Applications (ANDAs) can be filed before the original patent expires. Once a patent expires, generic versions of that drug can become available.

cooperation of researchers, clinicians, patients, pharmaceutical or biotechnology companies, and government regulators.

Regulation of drugs in the United States has evolved considerably during the last century. At and before the start of the 20th century, tampering with and mislabeling of food and drugs were common. By 1906, public outcry over the unsanitary and unsafe conditions of the meatpacking industry—described in Upton Sinclair's *The Jungle*—prompted Congress to pass the **Pure Food and Drugs Act.** The Act charged the Bureau of Chemistry in the U. S. Department of Agriculture with overseeing these new requirements of the law:

- Drugs must meet published standards of purity and quality.
- Manufacturers must provide correct and truthful labeling for all drugs.
- Interstate and foreign commerce in adulterated and misbranded food and drugs is prohibited.
- Also prohibited are the adulteration of food by the removal of valuable constituents, the substitution of ingredients so as to reduce quality, the addition of deleterious ingredients, and the use of spoiled animal and vegetable products.

The need to create a separate regulatory agency was eventually recognized, and the Food, Drug, and Insecticide Agency was created in 1927. This Agency was subsequently reorganized and renamed the U. S. Food and Drug Administration in 1930.

In 1937, more than 100 Americans — many of them children—died after consuming "Strep-Elixir," an untested product containing a sulfonamide and a chemical analogue of antifreeze, diethyleneglycol. In response, Congress passed the 1938 Food, Drug, and Cosmetic Act, which mandated that manufacturers must obtain premarket approval of new drugs from the FDA, and that this approval must be contingent on demonstrated safety and purity of the product. The Durham-Humphrey Amendment of 1951 clarified the types of drugs that require medical supervision for their use and restricted sales of those drugs to patients with a prescription from a licensed health care professional.

Another key event in the history of drug regulation was the discovery that thalidomide, used to treat morning sickness, caused birth defects in large numbers of babies born in Europe. This issue created widespread support for stronger drug regulation and led to passage of the Kefauver-Harris Amendments in 1962. Several important features of these amendments substantially changed the drug development and approval process in the United States. The amendments included the following new requirements (among others):

- Proof of both efficacy and safety prior to approval
- Compliance with Good Manufacturing Practices (GMP)
- Mandatory reporting of adverse events
- Assurance of informed consent from clinical trial subjects
- Complete public information on the drug (which led to the development of modern drug labeling)

Table 49-1 provides a chronology of major legislation affecting the scope and direction of the FDA's oversight of drug evaluation and approval.

ETHICS IN CLINICAL DRUG INVESTIGATION

Regulatory agencies around the world have codified standards of ethical behavior for all parties involved in clinical research, including clinicians, pharmaceutical companies, and medical institutions. The ethical relationship is governed by the notion that clinical trial research represents a partnership between investigator (physician) and subject (patient). Four major ethical principles, established by the **International Conference on Harmonization** and the **Declaration**

TABLE 49-1	Major Legislation Affecting FDA Regulation

LEGISLATION	OUTCOME
Pure Food and Drugs Act of 1906	Requires truthful labeling for all drugs
1912 Amendment to the Pure Food and Drugs Act	Prohibits fraudulent advertising claims
Food, Drug and Cosmetic Act of 1938	Requires proof of a drug's safety and purity
Durham-Humphrey Amendment of 1951	Grants FDA authority to determine which drugs may be sold without a prescription
1962 Kefauver-Harris Amendments to the Food, Drug and Cosmetic Act	Requires proof of efficacy as well as safety for new drugs and drugs approved since 1938; also establishes guidelines for adverse event reporting, clinical testing, and advertising
Orphan Drug Amendments of 1983	Provides incentives to manufacturers of drugs that treat orphan diseases
Drug Price Competition and Patent Restoration Act (Hatch-Waxman Act) of 1984	Abbreviates and modifies New Drug Applications (NDAs) for generic drugs; creates patent life extensions for delay caused by FDA review; extensions are limited to 5 extra years or 14 years post-NDA approval
Expedited Drug Approval Act of 1992	Allows accelerated FDA approval for drugs of significant medical need but requires detailed postmarketing surveillance

of Helsinki, support this partnership. These principles are as follows:

- The trial must minimize the risks for participants.
- Provisions must be made for the overall care of the patient.
- The investigator is responsible for terminating the trial when the risks become incompatible with the goals of the trial.
- Adverse events must be reported immediately to an ethics or safety committee.

Furthermore, investigators must ensure the fair and equitable selection of subjects by limiting enrollment in the study to patients with conditions that may benefit from the drug in question. This requirement balances the potential risks, many of which are unknown, with the potential benefits, the type and extent of which are also unknown.

In addition, investigators must obtain subjects' **informed consent**. Informed consent is not just a signed document, but rather a process in which patients (1) are made aware of the potential risks and benefits of the trial and (2) must make an informed decision to participate voluntarily in a clinical study. For patients with poor prognoses, informed consent encompasses the understanding that the research likely will not benefit them, but may benefit future patients.

At the institutional level, the FDA relies on independent **Institutional Review Boards** (IRBs) or **Independent Ethics Committees** (IECs) to ensure the rights and welfare of those participating in clinical trials. FDA regulations mandate that clinical study protocols be reviewed for legal and ethical issues by an IRB/IEC. These regulations give IRBs/IECs the authority to approve, require modification of, or disapprove research in human subjects. Specifically, the IRB/IEC must determine whether the proposed research:

- Minimizes potential risk to human subjects
- Poses risks that are reasonable relative to the anticipated benefit and potential scientific gain of the research
- Includes equitable selection of subjects
- Provides for an effective informed consent process
- Contains safeguards for vulnerable populations, such as children and the mentally disabled

IRB/IEC oversight and approval begins before the commencement of human trials and continues for the duration of clinical trials. The membership of an IRB/IEC consists of five or more experts and laypersons from various backgrounds. Federal regulations stipulate that IRB membership must include at least one member whose primary expertise is in a scientific area, one member whose primary expertise is in a nonscientific area, and one member who is not affiliated with the institution overseeing the clinical research protocol. In addition, the other members' qualifications must be such that the IRB is able to evaluate research proposals in terms of institutional requirements, applicable law, standards of professional practice, and community attitudes. Thus, many IRBs include clergy, social workers, and attorneys as well as physicians, scientists, and other health care professionals.

DRUG EVALUATION AND CLINICAL DEVELOPMENT

The investigation of a new drug candidate comprises several phases, beginning with preclinical evaluation and proceed-

ing through phase III clinical studies. At the conclusion of this process, the FDA may consider the molecule for approval as a new drug.

AUTHORIZATIONS TO INITIATE CLINICAL TRIALS

Preclinical research establishes the potential efficacy and safety of a compound for use in human trials. During this stage of testing, described in Chapter 48, a compound is studied to determine its biological actions, chemical properties, and metabolism, and a process is developed for its synthesis and purification.

The International Conference on Harmonization (ICH) has established requirements for the animal studies used to support different types of clinical trials. The primary studies used to support clinical drug development are animal toxicity studies and investigations on the absorption, distribution, metabolism, and excretion of the compound. As described in Chapter 48, the duration of animal studies is determined by the length of the clinical trials being undertaken. Short-term testing (2 to 4 weeks) is often used to support initial clinical trials, while studies of up to 9 to 12 months may be required to support large phase III trials in which patients may receive the investigational drug for a number of months. Many potential drug candidates either do not proceed to human trials or are removed from clinical testing due to potential adverse safety findings in the animal studies.

The mechanism for seeking approval to initiate clinical trials in the United States is the submission of an **Investigational New Drug** application (IND) to the FDA. The IND contains data from the preclinical studies, data from prior clinical investigations (if available), the proposed protocol for human trials, and other background information. The IND also contains a document referred to as the **Clinical Investigator's Brochure** (CIB). The CIB is provided to regulators, clinical investigators, and IRBs/IECs; it represents a summary of all available information on the investigational drug and may be several hundred pages in length. The IND must also contain information on the composition and stability of the drug and evidence that the drug can be manufactured in consistent batches for clinical trials. The IND does not grant a manufacturer permission to market a drug. Rather, it grants an exemption from a federal law that prohibits unapproved drugs from being shipped in interstate commerce; this exemption is a necessary part of multicenter clinical investigation. Commercial INDs are submitted by sponsors with the ultimate goal of obtaining approval for marketing and sale of a new drug product. Noncommercial filings, such as **Investigator, Emergency Use,** and **Treatment INDs,** are used for different purposes, as described below.

The FDA must review the IND within 30 days and decide whether human trials may begin. Figure 49-3 is a flowchart representing the process used by the FDA to review an IND. The areas of review include a **chemistry review,** a **pharmacology/toxicology review,** and a **medical review**. The chemistry review evaluates the stability of the drug and the reproducibility of its synthesis and purification. In particular, evaluators review any chemistry or manufacturing differences between the material being proposed for clinical use and the material used in animal toxicology trials. The

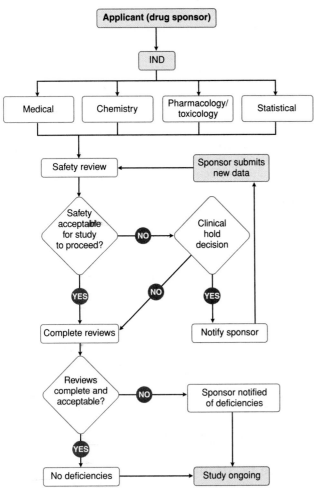

Figure 49-3. Process of investigational new drug review. When an IND is filed, the FDA has 30 days to review the application. This flow diagram shows the process of internal review that is undertaken by the FDA. The drug sponsor provides medical, chemical, pharmacology/toxicology, and statistical data for the compound; these data are reviewed by separate committees within the FDA. If the safety of the compound is deemed acceptable, an IND is approved once the application is complete. If the safety of the compound is deemed unacceptable for clinical trials or more data are needed, the sponsor is given the opportunity to submit new results from further testing. In some cases, a study is allowed to proceed while the sponsor is answering any deficiencies *(not shown)*. *Blue boxes* correspond to actions by the drug sponsor; *white boxes* correspond to actions by the FDA.

pharmacology/toxicology review evaluates animal pharmacology and toxicology data; this review provides an integrated summary of potential safety concerns. The medical review evaluates all of the data relevant to the proposed clinical trial protocol to ensure that participants will not be exposed to undue risk. Medical reviewers may also determine whether the proposed clinical studies are likely to yield results sufficiently robust to support subsequent clinical trials.

If the IND review does not identify any safety concerns, the IND is considered open or active after the 30-day wait period. If the review reveals the potential for unreasonable risk to participants, the FDA contacts the sponsor, and a **clinical hold** is issued, preventing initiation of human studies. The sponsor must address any issues in question before the clinical hold is lifted. A clinical hold may be issued at any time during clinical drug development; such a hold can be based on new findings from animal studies, clinical data indicating an unacceptable risk profile, or a finding that a sponsor did not accurately disclose the risk of the study to investigators or subjects.

Throughout the process of drug development, the sponsors of the program have the opportunity to consult with the regulatory agencies through formal meetings. The meetings may be conducted to gain input on a variety of topics, such as the acceptability of a manufacturing process, the design of preclinical studies or clinical trials, or the choice of appropriate endpoints to support the eventual approval of the drug.

CLINICAL TRIALS

Once the IND is active and an IRB approves a study protocol, clinical studies proceed in three phases (see Table 49-2). Trial protocols must be structured to provide reliable answers to specific questions, and must consider the following:

- Which prospectively defined outcome variables are feasible to measure and are scientifically valid
- Whether a control group is possible and what treatments, if any, need to be used in control group subjects
- The ease with which subjects and investigators may be blinded
- The definition and scope of disease
- The numbers of participating trial sites and subjects

Study investigators must assess chance, bias, and confounding factors affecting the trial and incorporate measures to address these issues. **Subject bias** can often be countered by providing a placebo, an inert substance with the same appearance as the drug under investigation. **Observer bias**

TABLE 49-2	Clinical Drug Testing in Humans		
	NUMBER OF SUBJECTS	**LENGTH OF PHASE**	**PURPOSE**
Phase I	20–100	Several months	Mainly safety
Phase II	Up to several hundred	Several months to 2 years	Effectiveness and short-term safety
Phase III	Several hundred to several thousand	1–4 years	Safety, dosage, effectiveness

can be countered by blinding, usually by coding the drug and placebo so that their identities are masked and the investigators cannot ''see'' which subjects are being administered which treatment. When the identity of the intervention is unknown to both subject and observer, the study is a **double-blind** study.

The natural fluctuation and spontaneous remission of many diseases also confound clinical trials. A **crossover design,** in which each study group is given the test drug alternately with placebo, can protect against the misinterpretation of results due to natural variation in the disease process. The presence of comorbid diseases and their treatment or risk factors, known or unknown, represents a third major confounder of clinical trials. Careful medical histories and **randomization of subjects** can counter some of the effects of these risk factors. In addition to the strategies mentioned above—use of placebos, blinded studies, crossover design, and randomization—a large sample size helps to minimize the effect of these factors. Phase III trials, the key studies that form the primary basis for regulatory approval, are often referred to as **pivotal trials** and are *randomized, placebo-controlled, double-blind studies.*

Table 49-2 summarizes the representative number of subjects, length of time required, and purpose of each phase of clinical trials.

Phase I Studies

Phase I studies generally involve between 20 and 100 healthy normal subjects and are intended to establish the safety and tolerability of a drug. If high levels of toxicity are expected, such as with many cancer drugs, patients with the target condition may be used in place of healthy volunteers. The focus of phase I investigation is the drug's overall effect and kinetics in the body, including **maximum tolerated dose,** absorption, distribution, metabolism, and excretion. To determine the effect of varying doses, subjects are started on a dose anticipated to have little effect, and receive increasing doses thereafter.

The primary goal of phase I studies is to establish safety, toxicity, kinetics, and major adverse effects. Phase I studies may involve **nonblinded trials,** in which subject and investigator are both aware of what is being administered. Phase I studies must yield sufficient information about a drug's pharmacokinetics to inform the design of scientifically valid phase II studies. For example, knowing the drug's volume of distribution and clearance enables study designers to determine an appropriate maintenance dose and dosing frequency for phase II and III trials.

Although phase I trials focus on safety and tolerability, **biomarkers** of the desired pharmacologic effect are increasingly being used to provide data early in drug development on the potential effectiveness of the molecule. One example of a simple marker would be the phenotyping of lymphocytes in the peripheral blood, for agents designed to inhibit B cells; more generally, cell-based or biochemical assays are used to detect whether the drug has effectively regulated the targeted enzyme or tissue.

A relatively new concept in clinical development is the use of ''prephase I'' studies that are conducted under an **exploratory IND**. This approach allows a clinical investigator to perform very limited clinical investigations based on a reduced amount of chemistry and animal toxicology data. These early clinical investigations are limited to low doses and very short durations of treatment (at most, a few days). It is anticipated that these investigations will facilitate efficient drug development by allowing investigators to test specific hypotheses in human subjects more efficiently.

Phase II Studies

Phase II studies may involve up to several hundred subjects with the medical condition of interest. Phase II clinical trials have multiple objectives, including the acquisition of preliminary data regarding the effectiveness of the drug for treatment of a particular condition. Like phase I trials, phase II trials continue to monitor safety. Because phase II studies enroll more patients, they are capable of detecting less common adverse events. Phase II studies also evaluate **dose-response** and dosing regimens, which are critically important in establishing the optimum dose or doses and frequency of administration of the drug.

A typical phase II design may involve either **single-blind** or **double-blind** trials in which the drug of interest is evaluated against placebo and/or an existing therapy. The trial usually compares several dosing regimens to obtain optimum dose range and toxicity information. The results of phase II studies are critically important in establishing a specific protocol for phase III studies. Phase II results can also be used to pinpoint additional data that must be collected in phase III trials, such as monitoring of liver function tests if phase II data suggest possible hepatotoxicity.

Phase III Studies

Phase III studies involve several hundred to several thousand patients and are conducted at multiple sites and in settings similar to those in which the drug would ultimately be used. Phase III studies are based on specific **clinical endpoints** (also known as **primary endpoints**) or **surrogate endpoints** (also known as **secondary endpoints**). Examples of primary endpoints include survival, improvement in patient functional status, or improvement in how patients feel. Examples of surrogate endpoints include markers for decreased disease burden, such as a reduction in the plasma levels of biochemical markers (e.g., glucose and LDL cholesterol), an increase in cardiac output, or a reduction in size of a tumor. *Although surrogate endpoints are usually easier to measure, a drug's approval usually depends on demonstrating effectiveness in improving primary endpoints.*

To distill true effects from placebo effects and from natural fluctuations in the course of disease, phase III studies typically employ randomized, controlled, double-blind trials with multiple study arms. Because of the large number of patients under study, phase III trials typically provide an adequate basis for extrapolating the results to the general population.

Before the start of phase III trials, the sponsor and the FDA conduct an **''End of Phase II'' meeting.** The purpose of this meeting is to establish the safety of proceeding with phase III studies and to cement study objectives and designs. Before the ''End of Phase II'' meeting, the FDA encourages sponsors to submit preclinical data supporting the clinical indication for the drug, chemistry data, animal data, results of phase I and II studies, statistical methods and protocols for phase III studies, and proposed labeling for the drug.

The FDA requires satisfactory compliance with specified endpoints that are often determined by the FDA or in conjunction with the drug's sponsor. If the results of phase I and II studies do not satisfy these requirements, the FDA can mandate additional studies or issue a clinical hold before allowing phase III investigation to begin.

DRUG APPROVAL PROCESS

FDA REVIEW

Approval of new drugs in the United States is based on the NDA. The NDA must contain all relevant data that a sponsor has collected during research and development of the proposed new drug. As such, the data gathered for the IND are integrated into the NDA. The FDA mandates that every NDA must contain the following sections: index, summary, chemistry, manufacturing and quality control, samples, methods validation, package and labeling, nonclinical pharmacology and toxicology, human pharmacokinetics, metabolism and bioavailability, microbiology, clinical data, safety update report (typically submitted 120 days after NDA submission), statistical information, case report tabulations, case report forms, patent information, patent certification, and other information. The typical length of an NDA submission is more than 1,000 pages. To facilitate the submission of these data to regulatory agencies in a variety of countries, the data are presented in a format referred to as the **Common Technical Document (CTD).**

Upon receipt by the FDA, an NDA is routed to a specific review division based on the proposed indication for the drug. A review team initially determines whether the NDA will receive a priority or standard review. A priority review is granted based on the existence of unmet medical need and the absence of prior marketed therapies that have similar therapeutic qualities. The FDA strives to complete all priority reviews within 6 months and all standard reviews within 10 months. The NDA also undergoes a preliminary review to assess the completeness of the information submitted.

The FDA organizes this review into several categories, which may include the following: **medical review, biopharmaceutical review, statistical review, pharmacology review, chemistry review,** and **microbiology review.** Within each of these groups, FDA experts review the data package submitted to the agency and provide an assessment of the safety and efficacy of the proposed new drug. Figure 49-4 is a flowchart representing the process used by the FDA to evaluate an NDA.

In addition to reviews internal to the Agency, the FDA may also call on **external advisory committees** for input on NDAs. These committees provide non-FDA input and allow for consultation with outside experts in a particular field. Although the FDA usually incorporates advisory committee recommendations into its decisions, these external opinions are not binding.

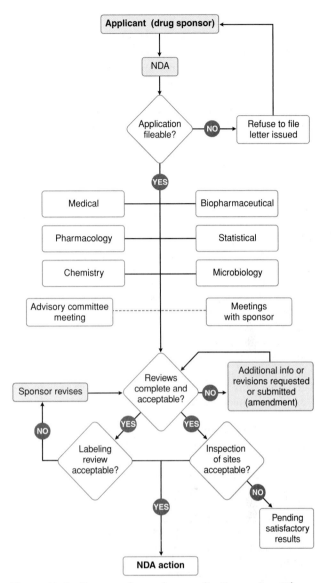

Figure 49-4. Process of new drug application review. When a new drug application (NDA) is filed, the drug sponsor provides data regarding the drug's medical, pharmacologic, chemical, biopharmaceutical, statistical, and microbiologic characteristics; these data are reviewed by separate committees at the FDA. The FDA or an FDA Advisory Committee (optional) may meet with the sponsor. If the review is complete and acceptable, then the drug application is reviewed for acceptable labeling (official instructions for use). The manufacturing sites and sites where significant clinical trials are performed also undergo review. *Blue boxes* correspond to actions by the drug sponsor; *white boxes* correspond to actions by the FDA.

During the review process, the FDA maintains ongoing communication with the sponsor regarding scientific or other issues that arise during review. Meetings are held between the sponsor and the agency, particularly if additional data are needed. The FDA frequently asks the sponsor questions in writing, and the sponsor may submit additional data or a new analysis of previously available data to assist in addressing these questions. Substantial amounts of new information are considered an amendment of the NDA, and can prolong the time to approval.

FDA APPROVAL

The FDA may take three possible actions on an NDA—an NDA may be **approved, not approved,** or ruled **"approvable."** If the Agency deems an NDA not approved or approvable, it must list the deficiencies in the application and provide suggested changes. Often the FDA meets with the sponsor to discuss what steps must be taken to secure approval. "Not approved" applications may require significant new studies to be undertaken, and such applications are frequently abandoned. "Approvable" applications usually need relatively minor modifications to the NDA but may also require new analyses or additional supporting data.

In general, of every 100 INDs submitted, 70 complete phase I trials and proceed to phase II; approximately 33 of the original 100 complete phase II and proceed to phase III; 25 to 30 of the original 100 complete phase III; and 20 of the original 100 are ultimately approved for marketing.

APPROVAL IN OTHER COUNTRIES

Before drugs may be sold in countries outside the United States, they must first be evaluated and approved by the appropriate regulatory authorities in that country. In some countries, this may include a comprehensive review of all the data, similar to the NDA review. In other countries, a more limited review may occur if the drug has already been approved in one of the major foreign markets (United States, Europe, Japan). During these reviews, a regulatory authority may require additional types of studies that were not required for U. S. approval. In addition, worldwide regulatory agencies may have different approaches to the type and amount of data required in product labeling. In Europe, many drugs are first evaluated by the **European Medicines Evaluation Agency** and then approved by the **European Union.** In Canada, **Health Canada** administers the regulations embodied in the **Canadian Food and Drugs Act.** In Japan, approval of new drugs is granted by the **Ministry of Health and Welfare.**

SPECIAL SITUATIONS

Accelerated development and approval status, or **"fast track"** status, may be given to products that demonstrate the potential to fulfill an unmet medical need for a serious or life-threatening disease. For a drug with this status, approval may be granted based on the evaluation of surrogate endpoints. An accelerated review period for such an NDA may be only 6 months, as compared to the standard review time of 10 to 12 months. As a condition of expedited review and approval, the FDA may require the sponsor to conduct post-approval (phase IV) studies to define more extensively the clinical benefit and safety of the drug. If clinical benefit or safety is not confirmed in such studies, the FDA may withdraw the approval without the process it would follow for drugs that had received standard approval.

The FDA has specific regulations for the development and approval of drugs for **orphan diseases**, defined as diseases that affect fewer than 200,000 individuals in the United States. Absent additional incentives, pharmaceutical companies would typically be disinterested in developing products for such small markets. In an attempt to encourage development of drugs for rare diseases, Congress passed the **Orphan Drug Act** in 1983. The legislation offers financial incentives to companies that develop orphan drugs. In addition, an orphan drug enjoys exclusive approval for the orphan indication for 7 years following approval. Since 1983, the FDA has approved more than 180 such products. Examples are

- Infliximab—for Crohn's disease
- Thalidomide—for an inflammatory symptom in Hansen's disease (leprosy)
- Denileukin diftitox—for cutaneous T-cell lymphoma following failure of other treatments
- Atovaquone—for *Pneumocystis carinii* pneumonia.

The FDA has created **compassionate use protocols**, also known as treatment investigational new drug applications (**treatment INDs**), to expand access to investigational drugs. These protocols permit promising investigational therapies to be used, before general approval, for extremely sick patients who are not eligible for an ongoing clinical trial. Three conditions must be satisfied in order for an investigational drug to be eligible for a compassionate use protocol: (1) the drug must show preliminary evidence of efficacy; (2) patients must be likely to die or suffer rapid disease progression within several months, or to die prematurely without treatment; and (3) there must be no comparable approved therapy to treat the disease at that stage.

DRUG LABELING

Each country's regulatory bodies establish a standard format and organization for labeling an approved drug in that country. A **drug label** must include the drug's proprietary and chemical name, formula and ingredients, clinical pharmacology, indications and usage, contraindications, warnings, precautions, adverse reactions, drug abuse/dependence potential, overdosage, dosage, and rate and route of administration, and how the drug is supplied. In the United States, this information is also known as the drug's **package insert.** When a new drug approaches approval, the FDA reviews and negotiates the final package insert with the sponsor to ensure that the labeling is justified by the data submitted in the NDA. To provide more accessible and informative drug information, the FDA has instituted structured product labeling, which provides key information important to prescribers in a standardized format. Figure 49-5 displays a sample package insert.

Regulatory agencies may use additional methods to ensure that the important attributes of the drug are clearly communicated. For example, in the United States, package inserts for drugs that have certain safety risks include a **"black box" warning**, in which key safety information is prominently displayed. In addition, the FDA may require sponsors to create **Medication Guides** for mandatory distribution to patients; these guides communicate critical safety information in language that is readily understandable.

DRUG NAMING

Another facet of drug approval involves the determination of a drug's name. A drug is known by two principal names,

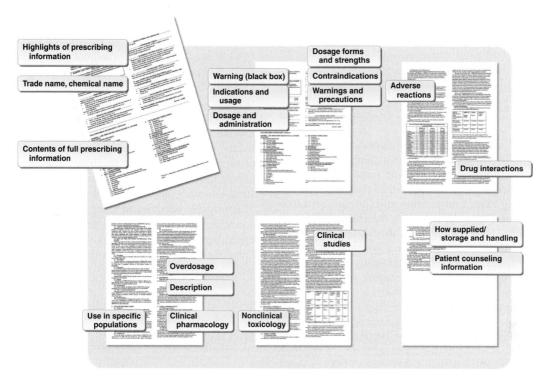

Figure 49-5. Sample package insert. The package insert contains several mandated sections, as highlighted. These sections include the trade and chemical names of the drug, highlights of prescribing information, "black-box" warnings, indications and usage, dosage and administration, dosage forms and strengths, contraindications, warnings and precautions, adverse reactions, drug interactions, use in specific populations, overdosage, drug abuse/dependence *(not shown for this drug),* description (which frequently contains the molecular structure), clinical pharmacology, nonclinical toxicology, clinical studies, how the drug is supplied (e.g., tablet, liquid) and handling, and patient counseling information.

the **generic name** and the **brand-name** (or **trade name**). A drug's generic name is based on its chemical name and is unprotected by a trademark. However, the generic name must be approved and registered with the **U. S. Patent and Trademark Office** (PTO). For example, sildenafil citrate is the generic name by which Viagra is known. In contrast, a drug's brand-name refers to the exclusive name of a substance or drug product owned by a company under trademark law, regardless of whether the name has been registered with the PTO. Viagra is the trade name for sildenafil citrate.

ADDITIONAL INDICATIONS

Once a drug is approved, physicians and certain other health care professionals are permitted to prescribe the drug in various doses or dosage regimens. Providers may also prescribe the drug for additional clinical indications, known as **"off-label" use.** Physicians are also permitted to conduct investigational studies with the drug, provided that they follow the rules of informed consent and have obtained IRB approval for the studies. Although health care providers are permitted to use a drug off-label, such use may nonetheless subject them to medical malpractice liability just as any other treatment decision could. Pharmaceutical companies, however, may not market the drug for any indications other than those for which it has been approved by the FDA. Current regulations prohibit pharmaceutical companies from providing any marketing materials, including scientific articles, on the off-

label use of a drug, unless such materials are requested by a physician. In order to market a drug for a new indication, a pharmaceutical company must conduct an additional program of development to prove that the drug is safe and efficacious for that new indication. These data are then submitted to regulatory authorities and subjected to additional review prior to the granting of approval for the new indication.

REGULATORY ASPECTS OF DRUG PRODUCTION AND QUALITY CONTROL

In addition to demonstrating a drug's safety and efficacy, manufacturers must also comply with FDA regulations for manufacturing as a requirement for drug approval. The **"Good Manufacturing Practice"** (GMP) guidelines govern quality management and control for all aspects of drug manufacturing, and the FDA makes unannounced inspections of manufacturing facilities to determine compliance. FDA regulations specify impurity tolerance levels, quality control procedures, and testing of sample batches.

A company must obtain prior FDA approval before implementing any manufacturing change that is determined by FDA to have substantial potential to affect the safety or effectiveness of a drug through alterations in its identity, strength, quality, purity, or potency. Other changes may be implemented either with or without submission of a supplemental NDA. Changes not requiring a supplement may be noted in the report filed annually with the FDA or on another date determined by the agency.

GENERIC DRUGS

The FDA also oversees approval of **generic drugs**, which the agency defines as drugs that are comparable to innovator drugs in dosage form, safety, strength, route of administration, quality, performance characteristics, and intended use. Under the **Drug Price Competition and Patent Term Restoration Act of 1984,** also known as the **Hatch–Waxman Act,** a company may submit an **Abbreviated New Drug Application** (ANDA) before the patent governing the brand-name drug expires. However, the company must wait for the original drug's patent to expire before it can market a generic version. The first company to file an ANDA has the exclusive right to market the generic drug for 180 days.

ANDAs for generic drugs are not required to provide data establishing safety and efficacy, because this has been established in the NDA for the innovator drug. To establish **bioequivalence**, which is required in the ANDA, sponsors may submit a formulation comparison, comparative dissolution testing (where there is a known correlation between in vitro and in vivo effects), in vivo bioequivalence testing (comparing the rate and extent of absorption of the generic with that of the reference product), and, for nonclassically absorbed products, a head-to-head evaluation of comparative effectiveness based on clinical endpoints.

In addition, an ANDA sponsor must provide evidence that its manufacturing processes and facilities, as well as any outside testing or packaging facilities, are in compliance with federal **GMP** regulations.

NONPRESCRIPTION DRUGS AND SUPPLEMENTS

The 1951 **Durham-Humphrey Amendment** to the Food, Drug and Cosmetic Act defined prescription drugs as drugs that are unsafe for use except under professional supervision. In determining which drugs do not require a prescription, the FDA examines a drug's toxicity and the facility with which a condition may be self-diagnosed. Because over-the-counter (OTC) drugs are sold in lower doses than their prescription counterparts, and are used primarily to treat symptoms of disease, the FDA requires their labels to contain the following:
• Intended uses of the product, as well as the product's effects
• Adequate directions for use
• Warnings against unsafe use
• Adverse effects
Although OTC products present a potential danger of misuse or misdiagnosis in the absence of physician oversight, the increased availability of these products has provided many

U. S. citizens with access to effective and relatively inexpensive treatments.

The **Dietary Supplement Health and Education Act** of 1994 defines a **dietary supplement** as any product intended for ingestion as a supplement to the diet, including vitamins, minerals, herbs, botanicals, other plant-derived substances, amino acids, concentrates, metabolites, and constituents and extracts of these substances. The FDA oversees the safety, manufacturing, and health claims made by dietary supplements. The FDA does not, however, evaluate the efficacy of supplements as it does for drugs. The FDA may restrict or halt the sale of unsafe supplements, but it must demonstrate that such supplements are unsafe before taking action. This recently occurred in December 2003, when the FDA announced a rule banning dietary supplements containing ephedrine alkaloids (**ephedra**), after reviewing the substantial number of adverse events (including deaths) associated with these products.

DRUG PATENTS

A patent may confer legal protection on a drug's composition of matter, its use, or the process by which it is manufactured. **Composition of matter patents** grant exclusive rights to an individual chemical compound or a range of compounds and may hint at synthesis or potential uses. **Use patents** grant exclusive rights for a type of compound in a particular therapeutic area. **Process patents** grant exclusive rights to the complete process by which a compound is synthesized.

U. S. law grants a patent to a technology that is novel, useful, and not obvious to someone with appropriate expertise. This technology may not be publicly disclosed for more than a year, even by those applying for the patent. Application for a patent requires the applicant to disclose all work previously undertaken in that field by anyone, as well as the anticipated use for the technology at the time. Patents in the United States are valid for a period of 17 years from the issue date, if filed before June 1995, and for a period of 20 years from the filing date, if filed after June 1995.

◼Conclusion and Future Directions

Specific laws and regulations have been put in place to provide for the development of new drugs, while at the same time assuring privacy and safety for the individuals participating in clinical trials. Regulatory approval of new drugs follows a lengthy process of preclinical and clinical studies. Each phase of development provides critical information that defines the study protocol for subsequent investigations. However, no amount of animal and clinical data can guarantee complete safety for all future patients. Thus, the FDA and drug manufacturers continue to monitor the adverse effects, manufacturing processes, and overall safety of a drug for its lifetime (see Chapter 50, Systematic Detection of Adverse Events in Marketed Drugs). In the future, there will be an increased focus on evaluating the safety of new medicines, both during clinical trials and after the drug is approved and introduced into larger, more diverse patient populations.

 Suggested Reading

Center for Drug Evaluation and Research, Food and Drug Administration, United States Department of Health and Human Services. The CDER Handbook. Revised 03/16/98. Available at http://www.fda.gov/cder/handbook/. *(Describes the processes by which the FDA evaluates and regulates drugs, including new drug evaluation and postmarketing monitoring of drug safety and effectiveness.)*

Goldstein I, Lue TF, Padma-Nathan H, et al. Oral sildenafil in the treatment of erectile dysfunction. *N Engl J Med* 1998;338: 1397–1404. *(Randomized, controlled, double-blind phase III study of the efficacy and safety of sildenafil in the treatment of erectile dysfunction.)*

Nightingale SL. Viagra approval information on the Internet [from the Food and Drug Administration]. *JAMA* 1998;279:1684. *(Summarizes the basis for FDA approval of sildenafil, with link to Internet address containing FDA's review of the drug, approval letter, professional labeling, and information for consumers.)*

Salonia A, Rigatti P, Montorsi F. Sildenafil in erectile dysfunction: a critical review. *Curr Med Res Opin* 2003;19:241–262. *(Reviews the clinical literature on sildenafil, focusing on the results of long-term postmarketing studies of drug effectiveness and safety.)*

50

Systematic Detection of Adverse Events in Marketed Drugs

Jerry Avorn

INTRODUCTION

Medications act by interfering with one or more aspects of molecular and cellular function. It is rarely if ever possible to do so without also creating an unintended effect caused by that perturbation or by another, perhaps unexpected drug action. Because all drugs have risks, the goal of pharmacotherapy cannot be to prescribe a risk-free regimen. Instead, it is to ensure that the risks of drug therapy are as low as possible and commensurate with a medication's clinical benefit.

Some adverse effects of a drug are apparent during its early development and often result from the same on-target mechanism responsible for its therapeutic effect (e.g., cytotoxic cancer chemotherapy). Even in such situations, however, it is necessary to know how those expected adverse effects will be manifested when the drug is in widespread use—in terms of both their frequency and their severity. After a drug has been approved for clinical use, the goal then becomes detecting and quantifying the risks as quickly and rigorously as possible.

Serious or even life-threatening adverse effects have led to recent withdrawals of widely used drugs. These withdrawals have heightened the sensitivity of clinicians and patients to the emerging field of pharmacoepidemiology—the measurement of drug effects in large "real-world" populations of patients. Advances in informatics and analytic techniques in this field hold promise for enhancing our understanding of often inevitable drug risks so that they can be better understood and then employed to put a drug's benefits into a proper context and guide clinical decision-making and regulatory action.

Case

Edna C is a 42-year-old woman with severe type II diabetes. She has had difficulty complying with her insulin regimen, and on recent office visits her hemoglobin A1c levels have been unacceptably high. Her physician has heard about an advance in the management of diabetes, a novel class of medications known as thiazolidinediones (TZDs). These drugs do not influence insulin secretion but instead enhance its action at target tissues. Eager to try and manage Ms. C's condition with this approach, her doctor prescribes the first drug in this class to be approved for clinical use, troglitazone (Rezulin). Soon, Ms. C's blood sugars and hemoglobin A1c levels decrease to normal values, and she experiences less polyuria and fatigue.

Three months after beginning troglitazone, Ms. C complains of flu-like symptoms, nausea, and loss of appetite. Shortly thereafter, her husband notes that her complexion has become "sallow." Five days later she is lethargic and her skin is frankly jaundiced. Her total bilirubin level is 10.7 mg/dL (normal, 0.0 to 1.0 mg/dL), and her serum transaminase levels are 30 times the upper limit of normal. Within a week she is comatose, and her physicians make a diagnosis of fulminant acute hepatic necrosis, probably caused by troglitazone. An acceptable donor match is found, and Ms. C undergoes a successful liver transplant.

Within weeks, similar case reports cause manufacturers or regulatory authorities in most nations to suspend the use of troglitazone. The drug remains available in the U.S. market, where proponents argue that the public health benefits of potentially better diabetes control outweigh the relatively rare cases of hepatotoxicity that the new medication may cause. During this time, dozens of additional cases of troglitazone-induced liver failure are reported; 2 years later, it is withdrawn from the U. S. market as well.

Newer agents in the same class (pioglitazone, rosiglitazone) were introduced into practice following the withdrawal of troglitazone. While similar to the older drug in their structure and mechanism of action, they do not appear to present the same risk of liver damage and continue in widespread use. Ms. C is doing well with her transplanted liver but requires chronic use of immunosuppressive drugs. Her diabetes is in excellent control on insulin and metformin.

QUESTIONS

■ **1.** How are drug risks ascertained before FDA approval, and what are the strengths and weaknesses of that process?

■ **2.** How do physicians and patients learn about the frequency and severity of adverse drug effects after approval?

■ **3.** How is the risk-benefit profile of a drug monitored after it is in widespread clinical use?

■ **4.** Given that all medications have some adverse effects, how safe is "safe enough" in relation to a drug's benefits?

CHALLENGES IN THE ASCERTAINMENT OF DRUG SAFETY

The randomized controlled clinical trial (RCT) is the gold standard for determining the efficacy of a drug, and is the sole criterion used by regulatory agencies, such as the U. S. Food and Drug Administration (FDA), in deciding whether to approve a new medication for use. But this valuable tool

also has limits, and it is important to understand those limits when assessing the benefits and risks of a given agent.

STUDY SIZE AND GENERALIZATION

Compared to the number of patients who eventually use a drug, the number of subjects in clinical trials supporting the approval of that drug is relatively modest. Approval decisions are generally made on the basis of trials that include 2,000 to 4,000 participants, or fewer for rare conditions. If a particular adverse event occurs just once in every 1,000 patients, it may not occur at all during clinical trials. When that event does occur, it is difficult or impossible to determine whether its rate of occurrence is meaningfully greater among study subjects vs. controls. One in 1,000 may seem like a rare event, but if 10 million people take a drug each year, that rate would result in 10,000 occurrences of the adverse event annually. For a life-threatening adverse effect such as fulminant hepatotoxicity, this could have important clinical and public health consequences.

Subjects in clinical trials of new drugs are nearly always volunteers—individuals who have come forward to participate in medical research and have given their informed consent to take part in the study. There is ample evidence demonstrating that such individuals tend to be different from the more typical patients who will receive the drug when it is in routine use; study subjects tend to be younger, healthier, better educated, and of higher socioeconomic status. Sometimes this is because of the nature of who volunteers for medical research, but often it is because of the exclusion criteria of study protocols. Some protocols prohibit participation of patients over a given age cutoff (such as 65 or 70), even if the drug is expected to be used disproportionately by the elderly. Entry criteria often exclude patients who have important comorbidities other than the disease being studied (thereby excluding those who are take multiple other medications). While this may be the ''cleanest'' way to test the efficacy of a new agent, there is growing concern that the data thus generated have limited generalizability to the populations who ultimately use these products. Others are excluded for unassailable ethical reasons, such as not allowing pregnant women or children into most preapproval drug trials. However, when such patients then take these drugs in routine care, there is little information to guide their use.

By definition, clinical trials are conducted by physicians and support staff with experience in clinical research and in settings accustomed to such activities. Their actions are guided by study protocols that require monitoring for adverse effects as well as efficacy, and ensuring that patients are taking the prescribed product as directed. This, too, is far different from routine care in typical settings, where compliance is generally much lower, and surveillance for early detection of adverse events is far less.

SURROGATE OUTCOMES AND COMPARATORS

It would be difficult to delay the approval of every new antihypertensive drug until it had been shown to reduce stroke rates, or not to allow a new lipid-lowering drug on the market until it had been shown to prevent myocardial infarctions. Such a requirement could delay the availability of potentially useful new therapies, as well as further increase their cost. As a consequence, new products may be approved on the basis of their effect on "surrogate outcomes," such as blood pressure for antihypertensives, serum LDL levels for statins, intraocular pressure for drugs used to treat glaucoma, or biomarkers of tumor growth for drugs used in oncology. *While such a metric can be useful in making drug approval quicker and more efficient, it is reliant on the association between the surrogate marker and the clinical outcome of concern.* These may correlate well, but not always. For example, the antiarrhythmics **encanide** and **flecanide** reduced the surrogate outcome of ventricular ectopy following myocardial infarction. However, a larger study (the CAST trial) demonstrated that they actually increased mortality in such patients, despite their success in "treating" the surrogate marker.

Whenever feasible, placebos are the comparison treatment most preferred by manufacturers and the FDA. If it is ethically or pragmatically impossible to conduct placebo-controlled trials (e.g., with a new AIDS drug or for long-term management of pain), then an active comparator is used. Comparisons between drug and placebo provide the clearest contrasts and the most straightforward statistical analysis, and there is no possibility of confusion resulting from therapeutic or adverse events caused by an active agent used in the control group. Placebo controls also make it possible to approve new products whose efficacy is similar to that of existing drugs; performing "equivalency" or "noninferiority" studies against active therapies requires larger numbers of patients and is more demanding statistically.

However, while the "better than placebo" comparison may be sufficient for a manufacturer to meet FDA's legal requirements for drug approval, the data it yields often fall short of what the clinician, patient, or payor would want to know about a new drug's safety or comparative effectiveness. A new drug may work better than placebo, but is it better than an existing treatment a physician may choose instead? Or is it even as good? The new drug may produce more adverse effects (e.g., rhabdomyolysis with a statin), but is the rate higher than that seen with older therapies? And even if it is, does the new drug also provide better prevention from ischemic cardiac events? If so, the trade-off might be acceptable; if not, it would not be. But if no such comparative data exist, the question cannot even be considered.

DURATION AND POST-APPROVAL STUDIES

The duration of efficacy trials for certain new drugs can be as short as 8 to 16 weeks. Although surrogate endpoints or outcome data may be sufficient for meeting a legal definition of efficacy, such short-term trials may yield little useful information about benefits and risks that occur beyond this time frame. In addition, the FDA requires a minimum of 6 months of safety testing for a new drug that is designed for chronic use (where chronic is defined as any period longer than 6 months). Even this duration of safety testing may be relatively short, however, for a chronically administered medication that may be taken for a number of years.

On occasion, in approving a new drug for widespread use, the FDA will ask the manufacturer to conduct additional postmarketing studies (sometimes called *phase IV studies*) to address questions that were not resolved by the evidence submitted prior to approval. Sometimes, useful new data about a drug's benefits and risks are obtained in this way. But the agency has little authority to oblige a drug's sponsor to complete these studies, since its main regulatory power, once a drug has been approved, is confined to the "nuclear option" of threatening to take it off the market—an action that is often not possible in the absence of additional data. Each year, the agency reports how well such "postmarketing commitments" are being met by manufacturers. A recent report by the Government Accountability Office noted that up to half of the "mandated" postmarketing safety studies requested by the agency had not been initiated, even years after the drug had entered widespread use.

PHARMACOEPIDEMIOLOGY

Pharmacoepidemiology is the study of drug outcomes in large populations of patients. To understand this approach, it is necessary to think about drug effects in ways that are different from those of conventional pharmacology (Table 50-1). This perspective considers the *population* as the experimental system being studied. Medications are introduced into the system much as they might be studied in tissue culture, in a patient, or in an isolated single-cell preparation. The differences are that, in populations, randomization generally does not occur, outcomes are measured in terms of probabilities (or rates) of events, the intervening decision-making and behavior of doctors and patients can alter the

TABLE 50-1	Conventional Pharmacology versus Pharmacoepidemiology
CONVENTIONAL PHARMACOLOGY	**PHARMACOEPIDEMIOLOGY**
Modest number of patients studied	Populations of patients studied
Direct dose-response relationships	Define probabilities of benefit and risk
Focus on biology	Focus on behavior of prescribers and patients
Outcomes over short time frame	Longer time frame of study
Rare events difficult to study	Able to identify rare events

drug's effect, and the scales used in the analysis are much larger than those of conventional pharmacology, ranging to millions of patients and years of exposure.

The importance of pharmacoepidemiology is highlighted by a number of prominent drug withdrawals in recent years. Each of these withdrawals was preceded by severe or even fatal adverse effects that had been unrecognized or underappreciated at the time of approval (Table 50-2). Using the tools of pharmacoepidemiology, it is possible to identify adverse effects that may be overlooked in randomized trials because those adverse effects are uncommon, represent an increase in risk from an already high baseline (e.g., doubling of the risk of myocardial infarction or stroke in older patients), occur primarily in patient groups underrepresented in clinical trials (e.g., the elderly, children, pregnant women), require many months or years to develop, occur primarily with coadministration of specific other drugs, and/or occur primarily in patients with a specific comorbidity or genotype.

SOURCES OF PHARMACOEPIDEMIOLOGIC DATA

Once a drug is in routine use, information about its adverse effects can come from a variety of sources. These include (1) spontaneous reports submitted to the FDA or manufacturer by physicians, other health professionals, or patients; (2) analysis of large data sets assembled by HMOs, government programs, or private insurers in the course of paying for prescriptions and clinical services; (3) ongoing registries of patients given a specific medication; and (4) individual ad-hoc studies designed to answer a specific question. Each approach has its own strengths and weaknesses, which must be considered in assessing the quality of the evidence derived from a particular source.

Spontaneous Reports

By default, spontaneous reports are one of the most heavily relied-upon sources of information used by the FDA in tracking the adverse effects of marketed drugs. Such reports are sent in by practitioners or patients to drug makers or to the FDA, describing an adverse outcome in a patient that may have been drug-related. A strength of spontaneous reports is that they are often the first signal of an effect that was not previously suspected (e.g., cardiac valvulopathy in patients taking fenfluramine-type diet aids).

While such reports can be useful to generate new hypotheses, they have important limitations. First, the majority (90% to 99%) of drug-induced illness is never reported; this is true even for previously unknown, serious adverse effects. The rate of reporting is influenced heavily by the newness of a drug, by reports in the medical literature and lay media, and by other factors. Because such reports originate in undefined populations of users, it is difficult to learn much from their frequency—an important issue in trying to compare the rates of a particular known adverse effect between one drug and other members of the same class. Limited availability of clinical data about the reported case can also hamper efforts to assess confounders (see discussion below) that may distort the drug-outcome relationship.

Automated Databases

Automated health care utilization databases have become increasingly important for defining associations among medications and adverse effects. Increasingly, prescriptions filled by patients are recorded in a computerized database, often for billing purposes. Likewise, individual clinical encounters (e.g., physician visits, hospitalizations, procedures, diagnostic tests) are also recorded for the same reason, usually with one or more associated diagnoses. Even when these services are delivered in an uncoordinated manner (as for most Medicare or Medicaid patients), the data trail produced makes it possible to measure the frequency of use of a given drug in a defined population of patients, as well as the frequency of specific outcomes (desired or undesired) in users of such drugs. If a population is relatively well defined and stable (as may be the case in a health maintenance organization, at least for a subset of patients), it is possible to evaluate exposures and outcomes in a relatively closed and well characterized population. If clinical information is available in such claims data (e.g., diagnoses, number and lengths of hospitalizations for specific reasons), one can conduct rigorous studies of specific drug-outcome relationships, as described below. An important limitation of such utilization-based databases has been the limited and often unvalidated nature of diagnostic information, particularly in the outpatient setting. As the quantity and quality of such information increase, however, this limitation will diminish.

TABLE 50-2	Important Withdrawals of Widely Used Drugs	
TRADE NAME	**GENERIC NAME**	**REASON FOR WITHDRAWAL**
Duract	Bromfenac	Hepatotoxicity
Posicor	Mibefradil	Hypotension, bradycardia
Fen-phen	Fenfluramine/phentermine	Pulmonary hypertension, cardiac valvulopathy
Rezulin	Troglitazone	Hepatotoxicity
Baycol	Cerivastatin	Rhabdomyolysis
PPA	Phenylpropanolamine	Intracerebral hemorrhage
Vioxx	Rofecoxib	Myocardial infarction, stroke
Bextra	Valdecoxib	Stevens-Johnson syndrome, myocardial infarction

Patient Registries

For some drugs, the manufacturer is asked by the FDA to keep track of all patients (or a well-defined sample of all patients) who use the drug. This request may be made both to define and prevent specific dangerous adverse effects (e.g., the agranulocytosis that can result from the antipsychotic medication clozapine).

Ad Hoc Studies

Many important questions in pharmacoepidemiology cannot be addressed by these methods, but must instead be answered by collecting data de novo on particular groups of patients with a given disease, or patients taking a particular class of medications. One example is the definition of sudden uncontrollable somnolence (sometimes called "sleep attacks") in patients taking dopamine agonists for Parkinson's disease (PD). Such events were not systematically documented in most large clinical trials of these drugs, are not likely to be recorded as a new diagnosis in an office visit, and, to determine whether some drugs cause this problem more than others, would require interviewing a large sample of PD patients who are using different classes of medications.

STUDY STRATEGIES

Once a source of pharmacoepidemiologic data has been identified, statistical methods are used to evaluate those data and reach conclusions about the associations between a drug and possible adverse effects. Most of the data collected for this purpose are observational, and the two most common types of analyses used to evaluate these data are cohort studies and case-control studies. Such studies are designed to evaluate statistically the risk associated with exposure to a particular drug or with a particular adverse outcome.

Cohort and Case-Control Studies

In cohort studies, one identifies a group of patients exposed to a given drug (e.g., patients with arthritis treated with a particular NSAID), and another group of patients who are as similar as possible to the exposed group, but did not take the drug of interest (e.g., patients with arthritis of comparable severity who were treated with another NSAID). Both groups are then followed over time to determine how many in each group develop an adverse effect of interest (e.g., myocardial infarction; Fig. 50-1). While this can be done on a real-time basis, it is more often the case that exposure (or nonexposure) several years previously is defined from an existing database, so that subsequent events can be analyzed retrospectively, without requiring the passage of time for follow-up. Cohort studies are preferred if one wants to measure actual incidence rates (i.e., the likelihood of a given outcome following use of a particular drug).

In case-control studies, one specifies the case-defining outcome event (e.g., myocardial infarction) and identifies a group of patients in a population who have experienced that event. These are the cases. The controls are patients in the same population who are as similar as possible to the cases but have not had the outcome of interest (e.g., patients of

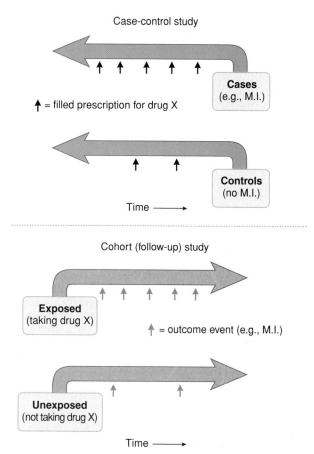

Figure 50-1. Schematic design of case-control and cohort studies. Top. In a case-control study, cases are identified as a group of patients in a population who have experienced the case-defining outcome event (e.g., myocardial infarction), and controls are patients in the same population who are as similar as possible to the cases but have not had the outcome of interest. All medications taken by cases and controls are reviewed retrospectively to determine whether drug use was higher among cases than among controls. **Bottom.** In a cohort study, two groups of patients are identified—one group who are exposed to a given drug and another group who are as similar as possible to the exposed group but do not take the drug of interest. Both groups are followed over time to determine how many in each group develop a specified outcome event of interest (e.g., myocardial infarction).

similar age and gender, and with similar cardiac risk factors, who have not had a myocardial infarction). One then looks back in time to review all the medications that were taken by cases and by controls, to determine whether drug use was higher among cases than among controls (Fig. 50-1). It is more difficult to measure incidence rates in a case-control study than in a cohort study. However, the case-control design is more efficient if the outcome of interest is rare and one has to interview all study participants, because it is possible to focus on a selected group of patients already known to have had the outcome of interest.

Evaluation of Risk

At the most basic level, cohort and case-control studies yield data that comprise a 2 × 2 table defined by the presence or absence of exposure to the drug of interest as well as the

	Adverse outcome	No adverse outcome
Drug exposure	A **Exposure +** **Outcome +**	B **Exposure +** **Outcome –**
No drug exposure	C **Exposure –** **Outcome +**	D Exposure – Outcome –

Figure 50-2. Basic analysis of data from case-control and cohort studies. The 2 × 2 table is defined by the presence or absence of exposure to the drug of interest as well as the presence or absence of the outcome of concern. Cells *A* to *D* include, respectively, patients who took the drug of interest and had the outcome *(A)*, patients who took the drug but did not have the outcome *(B)*, patients who did not take the drug but had the outcome anyway *(C)*, and patients who did not take the drug and did not have the outcome *(D)*. In simple terms, the product *A* × *D* divided by the product *B* × *C* reflects the strength of the drug-outcome association. For case-control studies (provided that the case outcome is not common), this ratio is termed the *odds ratio;* for cohort studies, this ratio is termed the *relative risk.*

presence or absence of the adverse outcome. The data can be arranged in four cells, as shown in Figure 50-2: patients who took the drug of interest and had the outcome *(A)*; patients who took the drug but did not have the outcome *(B)*; patients who did not take the drug but had the outcome anyway *(C)*; and patients who did not take the drug and did not have the outcome of interest *(D)*.

Cells *A* and *D* are concordant for the drug-outcome relationship, and cells *B* and *C* are discordant for this association. In simple terms, the product *A* × *D* divided by the product *B* × *C* reflects the strength of such an association. For cohort studies, this is referred to as the **relative risk**; for case-control studies (as long as the case outcome is not common), this is known as the **odds ratio.** A relative risk (or odds ratio) of 2 means that patients using the drug are twice as likely to have the outcome as patients not using that drug; a relative risk or odds ratio of 0.5 means that drug users are half as likely as non-users to experience that outcome (i.e., the drug has a protective effect for that outcome).

ISSUES IN STUDY DESIGN AND INTERPRETATION

Epidemiologists and statisticians have developed several strategies to correct for the problems inherent in observational studies. To address most forms of confounding, researchers attempt to learn as much as possible about the characteristics of patients who use each drug regimen under study. Were the patients who were prescribed one drug older than patients given a comparator drug? Or sicker? Or more likely to be taking (or not taking) other medications that could influence the likelihood of a given outcome? For example, in a study comparing rates of myocardial infarction in patients taking **rofecoxib** (Vioxx) with those taking **celecoxib** (Celebrex), **ibuprofen** (Motrin), or no NSAID, one would want to know as much as possible about the patients' history of cardiovascular disease as well as their cardiac risk factors. If these characteristics are evenly balanced across the ''groups'' of users of different drugs, there is not likely to be a problem. However, if not (for example, if users of rofecoxib were more likely to be smokers than users of celecoxib, or less likely to take prophylactic doses of aspirin), this would have to be adjusted for in the analysis.

Ascertaining Drug Exposures and Outcomes

In a clinical trial, it is clear which drug a patient takes, because that drug is part of a protocol. In an observational study, however, drug use must be ascertained by other means. One of the most powerful means of verifying drug usage is by scanning the electronic records that are created when a patient fills a prescription. For patients with drug insurance, such as Medicaid, health maintenance organization coverage, or potentially Medicare, these records can then be aggregated to provide a complete and reliable record of all the prescriptions a patient actually filled.

Computer-based health care utilization files can also be used to measure outcomes, such as hip fracture, myocardial infarction, or pulmonary embolus. Such measurements can be performed with considerable power, as these diagnoses are likewise recorded routinely in the course of administering and paying for services in the health care system. A great deal of care must be exercised in evaluating this diagnostic information. Whereas a filled prescription for a 30-day supply of simvastatin 30 mg is specified unambiguously in a pharmacy data file, the presence (or absence) of a code for depression or drug allergy or heart failure may represent a much wider variety of actual diagnoses. Some diagnoses can be made with certainty from computer-based claims data, such as a hip fracture repaired surgically or a hospitalization for myocardial infarction. Others may require validation of a computer-based diagnosis by reviewing the primary medical record. This problem will diminish as more clinical information is recorded electronically and direct access to the ''primary medical record'' is possible on the computer. These issues also present less of a problem for pharmacoepidemiologic studies that are based primarily on review of the medical record.

Confounding by Indication

In a randomized trial, subjects are assigned arbitrarily to one treatment versus another. If the study is large enough and the randomization works well, it is likely that differences in outcomes between subjects in the different study arms must be the result of the different treatments they received, because they were (by definition) similar in all other respects. By contrast, in an observational study, the researcher is obliged to study outcomes in patients for whom a physician has already chosen to prescribe Drug A versus Drug B versus no drug. It is therefore necessary to move beyond the simple 2 × 2 formulation described previously in order to adjust the observed relationships so as to control for these differences—differences that may have existed before the patients took the drugs under study.

For example, a group of individuals who take antihypertensive medications are likely to have more cardiovascular disease than a group of age- and sex-matched individuals in the same community who do not take antihypertensive medications. Of course, this is not because blood pressure medicines cause heart disease. It is well established that antihypertensive medications reduce the risk of cardiovascular disease (including heart failure, myocardial infarction, and stroke) in patients with high blood pressure. These medications reduce the risk of heart disease, but they do not reduce it to zero. Furthermore, many patients with hypertension start therapy later in life, or do not comply adequately with their prescribed regimens. As a result, antihypertensive medication users overall have a *higher* rate of heart disease than demographically identical individuals who do not take blood pressure medication. This problem is known as "*confounding by indication.*"

Selection Bias

A second problem is produced by the fact that, in epidemiological studies, patients' drug use is determined by their physicians and not by the observer. For example, when **fluoxetine** (Prozac) first introduced the selective serotonin reuptake inhibitor (SSRI) class of antidepressants in the late 1980s, reports emerged that patients given the new drug were more likely to commit suicide than patients taking older antidepressants such as the tricyclic antidepressants (**amitriptyline**, **nortriptyline**, **desipramine**). Indeed, concern persists (based on placebo-controlled randomized trials) that SSRIs may precipitate suicidal thoughts or attempts in some patients, especially adolescents and children. However, the early reports of increased risk make it clear that selection bias could provide an alternative explanation for suicide in fluoxetine users. Patients who were doing well on the older antidepressants would have been less likely to be switched to the newer drug when it was first marketed. Trial of a new medication would have occurred disproportionately more in depressed patients who were not doing well—perhaps those who were continuing to threaten suicide. Moreover, the LD_{50} for the older drugs is low because of their cardiovascular toxicity, whereas it is much harder to ingest enough of an SSRI for a fatal overdose. Thus, a physician would prefer a potentially suicidal patient to have a supply of fluoxetine at home rather than a supply of tricyclic antidepressants. Whatever the underlying risk of suicide caused by either drug, these factors alone would combine to create a profile of higher suicide rates among fluoxetine users compared to tricyclic antidepressant users in an observational assessment.

The "Healthy User" Effect

Several epidemiological studies of drug use and outcomes have defined relationships that have not been borne out in randomized controlled trials (e.g., reduced rates of cardiac disease, incontinence, and depression in women taking postmenopausal estrogen; reduced rates of cancer and Alzheimer's disease in patients taking statins). Such studies often seem to be flawed by what can be called the "healthy user effect." Patients who are regular users of any preventive

medication appear to be different from those who do not exhibit this behavior: they are more likely to visit their doctor seeking preventive therapy, or are at least open to receiving it, and their physicians are frequently also sufficiently prevention-oriented to write such a prescription. Perhaps most importantly, patients who repeatedly refill their prescriptions in a regular and long-lasting way are clearly in a minority. They are probably also more likely to engage in other health-promoting behaviors, such as tobacco avoidance, weight control, exercise, and adherence to their other prescribed drug regimens.

Several large randomized trials have proven a similar point: patients randomized to placebo who comply with their study regimen have fewer cardiac events than patients in the placebo group who do not comply. Because the content of the placebo could not have produced this effect, these findings provide clear evidence that patients who consistently behave in a health-promoting manner are more likely to have better clinical outcomes, apart from the therapeutic effect of a specific drug in their regimen. To address this issue in observational studies, some research groups have begun to use only "active controls" as comparator groups—comparing patients adherent to statin regimens with patients adherent to regimens of other preventive drugs—rather than simply comparing such patients with patients who are not statin users.

Interpreting Statistical Significance

In evaluating the results of both observational studies and randomized trials, it is conventional to use a *p*-value of 0.05 as a threshold or benchmark for statistical significance. This criterion is often mistakenly interpreted to mean that a finding is "real" if the between-group difference is below that value and "not real" if it is above. However, more sophisticated readers of the literature understand that such a cutpoint is largely arbitrary (compared to, for example, a *p*-value of 0.03 or 0.07), and that attention must also be paid to the magnitude of the difference. For example, a $p < 0.05$ difference between a new drug and placebo may be clinically meaningless if there is only a 2% difference in effect size. It may be necessary for regulatory purposes (such as the FDA approval of a new drug) to have a widely agreed-upon benchmark level of significance in comparing efficacy endpoints, but the limits of this approach must be understood.

The situation is even more critical in assessing the statistical significance of data about adverse events, whether from a randomized trial or from an observational analysis. It is useful to recall that the *p*-value is determined by both sample size and the magnitude of an observed difference. Most clinical trials are powered to be large enough to detect a difference between a study drug and its comparator in producing a clinical outcome that is relatively common (e.g., reduction in blood pressure or LDL level). As a result, however, such studies are not likely to have adequate statistical power to find a "significant" difference between groups for outcomes that are much more rare (e.g., reduction in renal function). Adherence to a "$p < 0.05$" standard for uncommon adverse effects can lead to dismissal of important risks that a study may not have been powered to detect.

The solution is not to embrace all differences in adverse effect rates regardless of their statistical properties. Instead, it is to consider such rate differences thoughtfully and to seek additional evidence to clarify worrisome relationships even if they are not "significant" in *p*-value terms. For example, when the FDA was evaluating the risk of suicidal thoughts and actions in adolescents and children taking SSRI antidepressants in placebo-controlled trials, the rates of these relatively rare outcomes were generally higher in the treated patients than in those randomized to placebo. Each individual study did not find a $p < 0.05$ level of significance for these differences. However, when the FDA aggregated the data from all such trials (in some cases, years after the studies were completed), it became clear that the difference across all studies was clear and consistent (and also met the conventional $p < 0.05$ level).

The opposite problem arises when considering the statistical significance of data from large population-based epidemiological studies. Here, sample size (power) is not a limitation, especially when studies employ data on several hundred thousand patients through use of an automated claims database. A 4% or 5% difference in rates of a given effect (either therapeutic or adverse) may achieve a *p*-value of 0.001, simply because of the huge size of the population studied. But here, even if the finding appears to have statistical significance, a difference of such small magnitude may have little or no clinical importance.

ADVERSE DRUG EFFECTS AND THE HEALTH CARE SYSTEM

The series of withdrawals of commonly used drugs in the 1990s and early 2000s led to renewed interest in developing ways to prevent such problems, or at least to limit the number of patients exposed to risk by identifying adverse effects earlier. As a result, the concept of "risk management" has become an important theme in drug development and regulation.

BALANCING BENEFITS AND RISKS

As noted above, new products are typically not compared with existing alternatives when they are evaluated for approval, and such studies are not commonly performed after approval either. For drugs with known risks, it is therefore difficult to know whether an adverse effect occurs more commonly with a new drug than with another drug in the same class (e.g., gastrointestinal hemorrhage with NSAIDs, or rhabdomyolysis with statins). A higher rate of a given adverse event might be acceptable for a particular drug if it were accompanied by substantially greater efficacy. In this case, however, the absence of head-to-head clinical trials makes it difficult to make such an evaluation. Thus, in most instances, the individual clinician is left to make therapeutic decisions without the data needed to make such choices rigorously.

The 30 billion dollars spent annually by the pharmaceutical industry to market its products is often heavily "front-end loaded," with vast sums spent soon after a drug is launched in order to maximize sales for as many years as possible while its patent is still in effect. Ironically, this means that the heaviest promotion of a drug occurs during the period in which there is least experience with its use and effects in the population as a whole. At the time of approval, there may not be much (or even any) information in the peer-reviewed literature about a drug's efficacy and safety, so promotional sources of information are often the primary means by which physicians learn about new products. Industry critics have argued that these materials often emphasize therapeutic benefits more persuasively than they communicate risk.

ROLE OF THE FDA

After 5 years on the market and use by an estimated 20 million patients, rofecoxib (Vioxx) was withdrawn in 2004 when it was found to double the risk of myocardial infarction and stroke. This event captured the attention of the public like no drug crisis since the discovery in 1961 that thalidomide caused major fetal malformations. The thalidomide tragedy had helped spark a wave of drug regulatory reforms that gave the FDA new authority to demand proof of efficacy before a drug was approved. (This requirement was not in place previously.) The withdrawal of Vioxx also prompted calls for regulatory reform, particularly in the way adverse events are detected and followed up, but the political response was far more muted. One area of vigorous debate was the FDA's lack of clear authority to require postmarketing studies of drug risks. While the agency holds considerable sway over manufacturers during the initial drug approval process, it has very few powers to compel further study of a drug once it is on the market. Governmental reviews have demonstrated that, even when postmarketing safety studies are mandated at the time of approval, they are often not completed or even initiated. This helps explain the tardiness with which important adverse effects are detected and acted on. Rationalizing the national response to this problem remains a key goal for public policy.

LEGAL AND ETHICAL ISSUES

The adverse event situations of recent years have caused many in the medical profession, the government, and the public to ask how responsibility should be apportioned for discovering and acting on important adverse effect data. For the most part, industry and FDA officials have argued that present laws are satisfactory, and that it is adequate for a company to adhere to the requirements for submitting spontaneous adverse event reports to the agency. However, the failure of this system to provide early warning concerning the risks of the now-withdrawn drugs listed in Table 50-2 has caused others to call for a more demanding standard. They have suggested that a company must serve as "steward of its molecule," responsible for proactive research into possible harms beyond the minimum required by law. Juries and courts have agreed with this notion; legal settlements exceeded 1 billion dollars for **cerivastatin** (Baycol) and 21 billion dollars for **fenfluramine** and **dexfenfluramine** (Redux), even in the absence of criminal convictions.

■Conclusion and Future Directions

To answer the questions raised in this chapter, one necessary ingredient is the availability of rigorous and comprehensive data about risks and benefits in large populations of typical patients. Such data are needed to allow decisions—made both at the bedside and at policy levels—to be based on science rather than hunches, fear, or hype. Several directions have been proposed to address the "data gap" concerning the adverse effects of drugs. These advances can be divided into three distinct domains: biology, epidemiology, and policy.

From a biologic perspective, the systematic detection of adverse effects will benefit from the development of biomedical research tools to predict the toxicities of new compounds more accurately and to flag them for intensive surveillance once a drug is marketed. Pharmacogenomics (see Chapter 52) is addressing many of these questions from the perspective of inherited differences in drug metabolism (pharmacokinetics) and drug responses (pharmacodynamics).

Within the discipline of epidemiology, large-scale studies will be facilitated by the increased availability of large automated databases of drug use and clinical records, such as those housed in health maintenance organizations or government insurance programs. These data will be made even more useful by the growing sophistication of advanced methodological tools, such as propensity scores and instrumental variables to improve control for confounding in observational studies.

Ultimately, changes in policy will be necessary to ensure vigilance in detection of adverse events. Proposed changes include a "safety fee" of a few cents per prescription to support publicly funded studies of the risks of marketed drugs; a new governmental entity to fund drug safety research and comparative trials of similar products; an analogue of the National Transportation Safety Board (NTSB) to study "drug crashes" much as the NTSB studies plane or train crashes—like the NTSB, this analogue would be independent of the federal agency and companies involved in the routine workings of that sector; new regulatory powers for the FDA that would enable it to require manufacturers to complete needed safety studies; and mandatory reassessment of all new drugs after 2 or 3 years of widespread use, to measure their true rate of adverse effects in routine practice.

Suggested Reading

Avorn J. *Powerful Medicines: the Benefits, Risks, and Costs of Prescription Drugs.* New York: Knopf; 2005. *(An examination of the interrelationships among pharmaceutical companies, the FDA, and drug prescribing practices.)*

Ray WA, Stein CM. Reform of drug regulation—beyond an independent drug safety board. *N Engl J Med* 2006;354:194–201. *(Proposal for a regulatory authority that includes centers for new drug approval, postmarketing studies, and drug information.)*

Schneeweiss S, Avorn J. A review of uses of health care utilization databases for epidemiologic research on therapeutics. *J Clin Epidemiol* 2005;58:323–337. *(Reviews strengths, limitations, and applications of health care use databases.)*

Strom B. *Pharmacoepidemiology.* New York: John Wiley & Sons; 2005. *(A comprehensive textbook on pharmacoepidemiology.)*

U. S. Government Accountability Office. Drug safety: improvement needed in FDA's postmarket decision-making and oversight process. March 2006. *(Highlights recent policy debate over postmarketing surveillance.)*

Wood AJ. A proposal for radical changes in the drug-approval process. *N Engl J Med* 2006;355:618–623. *(Proposes economic incentives for improving long-term safety data, postmarketing surveillance, use of surrogate endpoints, and development of drugs with high commercial risk.)*

VIII

Poisoning by Drugs and Environmental Toxins

51

Poisoning by Drugs and Environmental Toxins

Sarah R. Armstrong, Joshua M. Galanter, Laura C. Green, and Armen H. Tashjian, Jr.

INTRODUCTION

Toxicology is the study of deleterious effects of physical, chemical, or biological substances. The systematic study of toxicology predates that of pharmacology, and the discovery of most pharmacologically active agents before the 20th century derived from the study of these substances as poisons. Today, toxicology also includes many public health elements, such as **occupational safety** and **environmental toxicology,** which seek to limit environmental exposures to acceptable levels; **analytic toxicology,** the qualitative or quantitative evaluation of the presence of toxic substances; and **forensic toxicology,** the use of toxicology for legal purposes.

This chapter describes the acute and chronic effects of important **xenobiotic** toxins, meaning agents not taken for beneficial effect. Because the human body does not differentiate between a xenobiotic taken for therapeutic purpose and

a ''poison,'' the distinction between drug and toxin is somewhat artificial. Thus, the principles of pharmacology discussed earlier in this text are also pertinent to the study of toxicology and are not repeated here. This chapter includes the treatment of some commonly overdosed therapeutics, although the mechanisms of toxicity of these agents may be discussed elsewhere in this book.

Case

The W family is out of money. Times are difficult, with few opportunities in the sheet metal industry. After a few months of trying to make ends meet, Mr. W decides to stop paying the electricity bill. Instead, he borrows a propane generator from a friend who works in the air conditioning business. Mr. and Mrs. W and their teenage son set up the generator in the garage attached to the house, so no one will be able to see that they are using it as a source of electricity. That night, they gather together in the living room to watch television.

The next morning, a neighbor knocks on the front door, but there is no response. He looks in the living room window, and, to his horror, sees three people lying motionless on the couch. He calls the police, who break down the door and confirm that all the family members have died, including the two dogs and a cat.

QUESTIONS

■ **1.** Which toxin(s) could have caused the deaths of all the family members and their pets?

■ **2.** Why weren't the family members alarmed by any symptoms of the toxin(s)?

■ **3.** Which routine laboratory test(s) could confirm the likely cause of death?

■ **4.** What might have been the source of the toxin(s)?

ACUTE XENOBIOTIC TOXICITY

Numerous substances can cause serious acute illness, including death. This section describes some of the more frequent nonpharmaceutical causes of acute poisoning and their toxic mechanisms.

CARBON MONOXIDE

The combustion (burning) of any organic material produces **carbon monoxide (CO)** gas and other products of incomplete combustion. Improperly operating combustion devices, such as home-heating furnaces, may release significant concentrations of CO, and even properly operating devices, if not adequately ventilated, may permit accumulation of CO to toxic and even lethal levels. People have also been poisoned by CO in exhaust from powerboats, mines, liquefied petroleum gas (LPG)- or propane-burning forklifts and ice resurfacers, automobiles, buildings, and many other sources. Many fatalities due to fire are caused primarily by inhalation of CO. In addition, methylene chloride, a chemical found in paint strippers, is metabolized to CO after inhalation. Because CO is colorless and odorless, and its acute effects are nonspecific, many jurisdictions require CO monitors and alarms in dwellings.

CO causes tissue hypoxia by binding more strongly (more than 200-fold) to the heme iron in hemoglobin than does O_2, thereby reducing the transport of oxygen in the blood (Fig. 51-1). In addition, **carboxyhemoglobin (COHb)** shifts the dissociation curve for oxyhemoglobin (OHb) to the left, impeding the dissociation of O_2. CO also binds to cytochromes and to myoglobin in heart and skeletal muscle; this bound CO can serve as an internal reservoir of CO as COHb concentrations in the blood decrease. The degree to which binding to hemoglobin versus cytochromes is responsible for toxicity is unclear.

Because initial symptoms of CO poisoning are nonspecific, including headache, dizziness, nausea, and shortness of breath, both an accurate diagnosis and removal from expo-

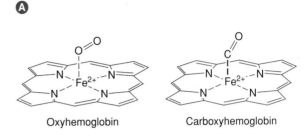

Oxyhemoglobin   Carboxyhemoglobin

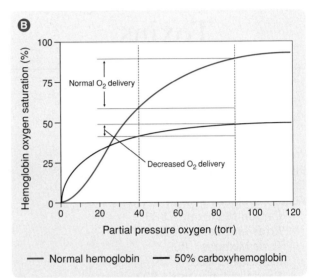

Figure 51-1. Mechanism of carbon monoxide poisoning. A. The oxygen binding site of hemoglobin is a ferrous heme that can reversibly bind oxygen. Carbon monoxide prevents oxygen binding by forming a bond to ferrous heme that is significantly stronger than the heme-oxygen bond *(shorter bold line)*. **B.** Carbon monoxide interferes strongly with oxygen transport not only because it prevents oxygen binding, but also because it increases the affinity of heme for oxygen. Under normal conditions *(blue line)*, hemoglobin is 85% saturated with oxygen in the alveoli (where the partial pressure of oxygen is approximately 90 torr). At tissue partial pressures (40 torr), normal hemoglobin is 60% saturated with O_2. Thus, under normal conditions, 25% of the hemoglobin sites deliver their oxygen to the tissues. When 50% of oxygen binding sites are occupied by carbon monoxide *(black line)*, hemoglobin oxygen saturation can be no more than 50% at a partial pressure of 90 torr. At tissue partial pressures (40 torr), the hemoglobin oxygen saturation is still over 35%, indicating that less than 15% of the heme sites have delivered their oxygen to the tissues.

sure can be delayed. Measurement of COHb is straightforward, however, and concentrations higher than about 2% in nonsmokers or 5% to 10% in smokers indicate an unusual exposure. (Note that pO_2 is likely normal in a CO-poisoned patient.) Signs and symptoms of acute poisoning track fairly well with COHb concentrations, with severe headache, vomiting, and visual disturbances at 30% to 40% COHb and collapse and convulsions at 50% to 60% COHb. Death is likely at 70% COHb or more and possible at lower concentrations. Survivors of CO poisoning with severe cerebral hypoxia are at risk of permanent brain damage. Because the COHb concentration depends on the atmospheric CO level, activity level, duration of exposure, and other factors, no single threshold of toxicity exists. However, current CO alarms for use in homes must sound at concentrations of 70 ppm or greater, depending on how long that concentration has been present.

The half-life of COHb is approximately 5 hours in room air but decreases to about 90 minutes in a 100% O_2 environment at normal pressure. Hyperbaric oxygen therapy (3 atmospheres, 100% O_2) can reduce the half-life to about 20 minutes.

In the introductory case, carbon monoxide produced by the portable propane generator was the toxin that led to the deaths in the W family. Placement of the generator in the garage resulted in circulation of carbon monoxide throughout the house, rather than as exhaust to the environment. The W family did not react to the presence of carbon monoxide because it lacks an odor; this is why the family died while watching television, without any apparent alarm. If they had had a carbon monoxide detector in the house, their deaths might have been prevented.

ACIDS AND BASES

Strong acids, alkalis (caustic agents), oxidants, and reducing agents damage tissue by altering the structure of proteins, lipids, carbohydrates, and nucleic acids so severely that cellular integrity is lost. These substances, such as **potassium hydroxide** in drain cleaners and **sulfuric acid** in car batteries, produce **chemical burns** by hydrolyzing, oxidizing, or reducing biological macromolecules or by denaturing proteins. High concentrations of **detergents** can also cause nonspecific tissue damage by disrupting and dissolving the plasma membrane of cells.

Although some of these agents may target particular macromolecules, direct tissue-damaging agents tend to be relatively nonspecific. Thus, the systems most commonly affected are those most exposed to the environment. Skin and eyes are frequently affected by splashes or spills. The respiratory system is affected when toxic gases or vapors are inhaled, whereas the digestive system is affected by accidental or deliberate ingestion.

Many agents can cause damage to deep tissues after breaking through the barrier formed by the skin. Other agents are able to pass through the skin causing relatively little local damage, but destroy deeper tissues such as muscle or bone. For example, **hydrofluoric acid** (HF; found in, among other products, grout cleaner) causes milder skin burns than an equivalent amount of **hydrochloric acid** (HCl). However, once HF reaches deeper tissue, it destroys the calcified matrix of bone. In addition to the direct effects of the acid, the release of calcium stored in bone can cause life-threatening cardiac arrhythmias. For this reason, HF can be more dangerous than an equivalent amount of HCl.

Three characteristics determine the extent of tissue damage: the compound's identity, its concentration/strength, and its **buffering capacity,** or its ability to resist change in pH or redox potential. As mentioned above, HF is more injurious than an equivalent amount of HCl. In general, a stronger acid or base (measured by pH) or oxidant or reductant (measured by redox potential) will cause more damage than an equivalent compound at a more physiologic pH or redox potential. A solution of 10^{-2} M sodium hydroxide in water has a pH of 12 but has a low capacity to cause tissue damage, because it has a small buffering capacity and is rapidly neutralized by body tissue. In contrast, a buffered solution of pH 12, such as that found in wet ready-set concrete [made with buffered $Ca(OH)_2$], can cause more serious alkali burns because tissues cannot readily neutralize the material's extreme pH.

TOXIC MIXTURES

Poisonings by some materials are unusual because the important "mechanism" occurs before exposure. For example, acute upper and lower respiratory symptoms may occur after inhalation of vapors evolved when household bleach (aqueous sodium hypochlorite) is mixed, either knowingly or unknowingly, either with aqueous ammonia or with acids such as phosphoric acid-based floor or ceramic cleaners. In each case, the materials react to form a variety of toxic products such as monochloramine and dichloramine, ammonia gas, chlorine gas, hydrochloric acid, and hydrochlorous acid. Severe exposure can cause pulmonary edema and damage. Note that the relevant cleaning agents do not always carry the appropriate warnings against mixing.

PESTICIDES

Pesticides include insecticides, herbicides, rodenticides, and other compounds designed to kill unwanted organisms in the environment. By their nature, pesticides—of which there are hundreds (both natural and synthetic)—are biologically active; however, the degree of their specificity toward target organisms varies, and thus many of these compounds cause toxicity in humans. In addition, commercial pesticides typically contain "inactive" ingredients (inactive with respect to the desired activity) that may contribute to human toxicity, and some contain synergists to increase the lethality of the active ingredient toward the target. Some of the more common acute poisonings involve organophosphate and pyrethroid insecticides and rodenticides.

Organophosphate insecticides, derived from phosphoric or thiophosphoric acid, include **parathion, malathion, diazinon, fenthion, chlorpyrifos**, and many other chemicals. These widely used compounds are acetylcholinesterase (AChE) inhibitors due to their ability to phosphorylate AChE at its esteratic active site (Fig. 51-2). Inhibition of AChE, and consequent accumulation of acetylcholine at cholinergic junctions in nerve tissue and effector organs, produces acute muscarinic, nicotinic, and central nervous system (CNS) effects such as bronchoconstriction, increased bronchial secretions, salivation, lacrimation, sweating, nausea, vomiting, diarrhea, and miosis (muscarinic signs), as well as twitching, fasciculations, muscle weakness, cyanosis, and elevated blood pressure (nicotinic signs). CNS effects can include anxiety, restlessness, confusion, and headache. Symptoms usually occur within minutes or hours of exposure and resolve within a few days in nonlethal poisonings.

Toxic exposures may occur by inhalation, ingestion, or dermal contact, depending on the product formulation and manner of use or misuse. Toxic secondary exposures have

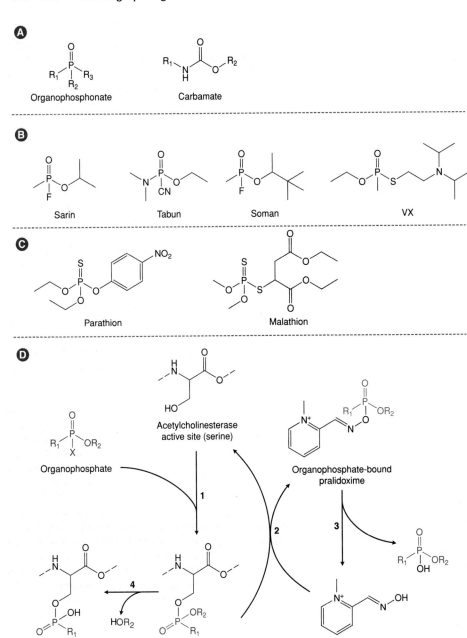

Figure 51-2. Structures and mechanisms of acetylcholinesterase inhibitors. A. Structures of typical acetylcholinesterase inhibitors, an organophosphonate on the left and a carbamate on the right. **B.** Structures of the principal nerve gases sarin, tabun, soman, and VX, which are potent inhibitors of human acetylcholinesterase. **C.** Structures of the organophosphate insecticides parathion and malathion. The thiophosphate bonds between the sulfur and phosphorus are oxidized more efficiently by arthropod oxygenases than by mammalian oxygenases, so the compounds are less toxic to humans than the structurally related nerve gases. **D.** Organophosphates attack the serine active site in acetylcholinesterase, forming a stable phosphorus-oxygen species *(1)*. Pralidoxime abstracts the organophosphate from serine, restoring active acetylcholinesterase *(2)*. Organophosphate-bound pralidoxime is unstable and spontaneously regenerates pralidoxime *(3)*. Organophosphate-bound acetylcholinesterase can lose an alkoxy group, in a process called *aging*. The end product of aging is more stable and cannot be detoxified by pralidoxime.

occasionally occurred in people coming into close contact with the victim of direct exposure; for example, emergency responders and emergency department staff have suffered organophosphate toxicity after contacting—or simply being near—contaminated clothing, skin, secretions, or gastric contents.

Because the common organophosphate insecticides are metabolized and excreted relatively rapidly, the toxins do not accumulate in the body. However, the toxic effect may increase after repeated exposure because recovery of cholinesterase activity, either by dissociation of the phosphorylated AChE or de novo synthesis of the enzyme, is slow in the absence of treatment. Because the organophosphate insecticides are preferentially toxified by arthropod cholinesterases and/or preferentially detoxified by mammalian carboxyes-

terases, these compounds are more toxic to arthropods than to humans, an example of **selective toxicity**—although toxicity to humans exists as well.

Pyrethroid insecticides, such as **permethrin, deltamethrin, cypermethrin,** and **cyfluthrin,** are semisynthetic chemicals that are structurally related to the naturally occurring pyrethrins found in chrysanthemum flowers. The pyrethroids (and pyrethrins) have very high affinity for plasma membrane sodium channels, and, while they do not alter activation of sodium currents by membrane depolarization, they significantly delay termination of the action potential. Pyrethroids are common agricultural pesticides and are also found in some household products, including antilice shampoos.

Two classes of pyrethroids have been defined based on

activity determined largely in laboratory experiments. Type I pyrethroids do not contain a cyano group, produce shorter-duration sodium tail currents and repetitive discharges, and cause a **tremor (T) syndrome** in mammals that can include fine tremor, increased response to stimuli, and hyperthermia. Type II pyrethroids usually contain a cyano group, produce a longer-duration sodium tail current and stimulus-dependent nerve depolarization and block, and cause a **choreoathetosis-with-salivation syndrome (CS)** that may include sinuous writhing (choreoathetosis) and salivation, coarse tremor, clonic seizures, and hypothermia. A few pyrethroids elicit intermediate syndromes. As in laboratory animals, T and CS signs are seen in people with large acute exposures to pyrethroids, as may occur during agricultural use of these insecticides. Pyrethroids are often formulated with a **synergist**, such as piperonyl butoxide, that inhibits insect cytochrome P450 enzymes (and thus metabolism) and increases pyrethroid toxicity.

Pyrethroids are relatively low in toxicity to humans, but a small number of case reports of death in asthmatics exposed to pyrethroid-containing dog shampoos suggests a potential for exacerbation of asthma. Occupational exposure to pyrethroids often involves both inhalation and dermal exposure, since the insecticides are typically sprayed and workers may be caught in the drift. Absorption is rapid across the lung but very slow across the skin. Common symptoms include paresthesias (most frequently facial skin), dizziness, headache, blurred vision, nasal and laryngeal irritation, and shortness of breath. It is not clear to what extent other chemicals in the insecticidal formulation, such as petroleum hydrocarbons, contribute to these symptoms.

FOOD CONTAMINANTS

An estimated one in four Americans experience significant **foodborne illnesses** each year. The mechanisms of food poisoning involve either infection, which typically manifests one to several days after exposure, or intoxication from a preformed microbial or algal toxin, with symptoms occurring within a few hours following exposure. Infectious food poisoning is typically caused by species of *Salmonella, Listeria, Cryptosporidium,* or *Campylobacter.* Less common but quite virulent are poisonings by enteropathogenic *Escherichia coli,* which can cause sometimes fatal hemorrhagic colitis and hemolytic-uremic syndrome (HUS), likely through the uptake of pathologic bacterial proteins by host cells.

Food intoxication is often caused by toxins elaborated by *Staphylococcus aureus* or *Bacillus cereus,* or by marine algal toxins ingested via seafood. *S. aureus* produces a variety of toxins; the staphylococcal enterotoxins (SE) cause emesis by stimulating receptors in the abdominal viscera. Improper food handling after cooking, followed by poor refrigeration, contaminates high-protein foods such as meats, cold cuts, and egg and dairy products.

B. cereus is a common contaminant of cooked rice. It produces several toxins that cause vomiting and diarrhea. Of particular concern is the production of **cerulide**, a small, cyclic peptide that stimulates intestinal 5-HT$_3$ receptors, resulting in emesis. The peptide is heat-stable to 259 °F for

up to 90 minutes, so reheating of contaminated cooked rice will typically not prevent intoxication.

Most algal toxins are neurotoxic and heat-stable, so, again, cooking leaves the toxins intact. Algal toxins such as **saxitoxins** are a group of approximately 20 heterocyclic guanidines that bind with high affinity to the voltage-dependent sodium channel, thus inhibiting neuronal activity and causing tingling and numbness, loss of motor control, drowsiness, incoherence, and, with sufficient doses (greater than about 1 mg), respiratory paralysis.

Many foodborne illnesses appear to be caused by pathogens that are not yet characterized. (It is estimated that more than 90% of the microbial species on earth have yet to be isolated and identified.) Moreover, novel pathogens can emerge because of changing ecologies or technologies, or can arise via transfer of mobile virulence factors such as bacteriophages.

TOXIC PLANTS AND FUNGI

Acute illness can also be caused by mistaken ingestion of nonfood items, such as poisonous mushrooms collected by amateur mycologists or any number of poisonous plants. The highly toxic "death cap" mushroom, for instance, *Amanita phalloides*, produces numerous cyclopeptide toxins that are not destroyed by cooking or drying, have no distinctive taste, and are taken up by hepatocytes. The **amatoxins** bind strongly to RNA polymerase II, greatly slowing RNA and protein synthesis and leading to hepatocyte necrosis. The somewhat less toxic phallotoxins and virotoxins interfere with F- and G-actins in the cytoskeleton. Consumption of *Amanita* species or their relatives can thus cause severe liver dysfunction, even hepatic (and renal) failure and death. Initial symptoms of poisoning, such as abdominal pain, nausea, severe vomiting and diarrhea, fever, and tachycardia, may occur 6 to 24 hours after consumption of the mushrooms. Hepatic and renal function may deteriorate even while the initial symptoms abate, leading to jaundice, hepatic encephalopathy, and fulminant liver failure; death may occur 4 to 9 days after consumption. There is no specific antidote.

An anticholinergic syndrome may be caused by deliberate or accidental ingestion of **jimson weed**, a plant belonging to the *Datura* family. All parts of the plant are toxic, but the seeds and leaves, in particular, contain atropine, scopolamine, and hyoscyamine. These compounds are rapidly absorbed and produce anticholinergic symptoms such as mydriasis, dry, flushed skin, agitation, tachycardia, hyperthermia, and hallucinations. The mnemonic for anticholinergic effects, "blind as a bat, dry as a bone, red as a beet, mad as a hatter, and hot as a hare," is applicable to jimson weed poisoning.

Some plants in the families *Umbelliferae* (such as parsley, parsnip, dill, celery, and giant hogweed), *Rutaceae* (such as limes and lemons), and *Moraceae* (such as figs) contain **psoralen isomers (furocoumarins)** in leaves, stems, or sap that can be absorbed into the skin after contact. Subsequent exposure to UV-A radiation of wavelength >320 nm (generally via sunlight) can excite furocoumarins, which then form DNA-damaging adducts in epidermal tissue. Within 2 days, burning, redness, and blistering are observed in areas of contact with the plant and light; after healing, hyperpigmentation may persist for months. The response is greater with increasing plant contact, humidity, and duration and intensity of radiation exposure. This nonallergic **phytophototoxic** mechanism is the basis of PUVA therapy for eczema and other dermatological disorders.

CHRONIC XENOBIOTIC TOXICITY

Chronic toxicity refers to the often irreversible effects of repeated exposure to a toxin. Chronic toxicities of some of the more prevalent xenobiotics are described below.

TOBACCO

Cigarette smoke is the most commonly encountered and important toxin in the United States. It is responsible for about 30% of all U. S. cancer deaths and for significantly increased risks of pulmonary disease and cardiovascular disease. Tobacco smoke causes not only lung cancer but also cancers of the oral cavity, esophagus, pancreas, and bladder. Passive smoking—that is, the exposure of nonsmokers to cigarette side-stream smoke—is also believed to cause cancer and cardiovascular disease, although the magnitude of these risks is less clear than it is for smokers. The carcinogenicity of cigarette smoke is likely due to the combined actions of many of the dozens of carcinogens, including benzo-(a)pyrene, among the 4,000 chemicals in cigarette smoke (Fig. 51-3). A number of these carcinogens are not limited to the particle phase, or "tar," but are in the gas phase as well. "Low tar" cigarettes are as carcinogenic and cause as much cardiovascular disease as "regular" cigarettes.

ETHANOL

Excessive consumption of **ethyl alcohol** is also a common and complex toxic exposure. Binge drinking occurs in a sizable minority of adolescents; in adults with coronary artery disease, binge drinking can cause myocardial ischemia and angina. Acutely, alcohol is a sedative (see Chapter 11, Pharmacology of GABAergic and Glutamatergic Neurotransmission, and Chapter 17, Pharmacology of Drug Dependence and Addiction) and causes psychomotor retardation. The largest fraction of morbidity and mortality from alcohol intoxication results from injuries suffered (not to mention inflicted) while impaired.

Chronic excess drinking increases the risk of cirrhosis, hepatocellular carcinoma, pancreatitis, hemorrhagic stroke, and heart failure. The pathophysiology of alcoholic cardiomyopathy is complex and appears to involve cell death and pathologic changes in myocyte function. Women tend to be more susceptible than men to alcoholic cardiomyopathy.

The mechanism of alcoholic hepatotoxicity is also multifactorial. First, it is associated with a nutritional deficiency, as chronic alcohol abusers obtain most of their calories from alcohol. This leads to a hypermetabolic state and increased oxygen demand in the liver. In turn, poorly perfused centri-

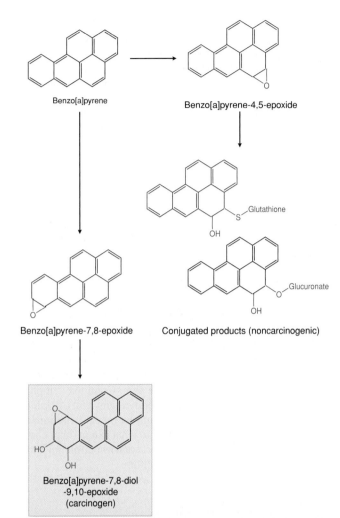

Figure 51-3. Metabolism of benzo[a]pyrene. Benzo[a]pyrene is a precarcinogen that can be metabolized by a variety of pathways. Oxidation at the so-called bay region produces the ultimate carcinogen benzo[a]pyrene-7,8-diol-9,10-epoxide, which can cause double-stranded breaks in DNA. On the other hand, oxidation at the so-called K region produces the 4,5-epoxide of benzo[a]pyrene. Opening of the epoxide and conjugation with glutathione or glucuronate produces noncarcinogenic conjugated products that are hydrophilic and can be excreted.

lobular hepatocytes are threatened. The metabolism of alcohol generates NADH and NADPH, which shift the redox potential of the hepatocyte. The altered redox potential leads to increased production of lactic acid and uric acid and to hypoglycemia. Finally, ethanol metabolism produces harmful reactive species, including acetaldehyde (by the action of alcohol dehydrogenase) and hydroxyl radicals, superoxide anions, and hydrogen peroxide (produced by the action of the enzyme P450 2E1).

Ethanol is believed to cause tumors directly in the oropharynx, larynx, and esophagus, where it may act synergistically with tobacco smoke. Ethanol is also associated with hepatocellular carcinoma, both by inducing chronic regeneration of damaged tissue and by inducing P450 2E1, which can activate carcinogens.

Ethanol is also a teratogen; it causes **fetal alcohol syndrome,** the most common preventable cause of mental retardation. Despite extensive research, the mechanism of fetal alcohol syndrome remains unknown.

Light-to-moderate ingestion of alcohol, on the other hand, appears to protect against heart disease. The mechanisms that mediate this risk reduction may include increased production of high-density lipoprotein cholesterol, plasminogen, and tissue plasminogen activator, coupled with decreased production of fibrinogen and lipoprotein(a), decreased platelet aggregation, and altered endothelial function.

LEAD

Lead is ubiquitous in the environment, both because of its persistence and because of its formerly widespread use in paints, plumbing, solder, and as an additive in gasoline. Lead exposure causes neural toxicity, making exposure a particular concern for fetuses and children up to the age of about 7 years. Young children are also at risk because they are more likely than adults to eat lead-contaminated paint dust or soil. Although the half-life of lead in soft tissues is relatively short, its half-life in bone is more than 20 years; a substantial exposure in early childhood could result in elevated bone lead levels for decades. Despite a fivefold decrease in the exposure to lead in the United States since the 1940s, nearly one million U. S. children are believed to be at risk for lead poisoning. Some impoverished children are at particular risk because of a combination of residence in improperly maintained, formerly lead-painted dwellings, waterborne exposures from old lead plumbing, and/or inadequate dietary intake of calcium and iron.

Lead causes a disruption of the blood-brain barrier, allowing both lead and other potential neurotoxins to reach the CNS. There, lead can block voltage-dependent calcium channels, interfere with neurotransmitter function, and, most importantly, interfere with cell-cell interactions in the brain; the latter effect causes permanent changes in neuronal circuitry. Overt lead encephalopathy, which is fortunately rare in the United States today, results in lethargy, vomiting, irritability, and dizziness and can progress to altered mental status, coma, and death. More important is the risk, in children, of an IQ deficit of approximately two to four points for every 10-μg/dL increase in blood lead concentration.

Lead interferes with the synthesis of hemoglobin at multiple steps, causing a microcytic, hypochromic anemia. Specifically, lead inhibits the action of **delta-aminolevulinic acid dehydratase (ALA-D)**, which catalyzes the synthesis of porphobilinogen, a heme precursor. Lead also inhibits the incorporation of iron into the porphyrin ring.

In the kidney, lead causes both reversible and irreversible toxicity. Lead can interfere reversibly with energy production in proximal tubular cells by interfering with mitochondrial function, resulting in decreased energy-dependent reabsorption of ions, glucose, and amino acids. Chronic exposure to lead results in interstitial nephritis, with the eventual development of fibrosis and chronic kidney disease.

CADMIUM

Cadmium dusts and fumes may be encountered in various occupations. Cadmium is toxic to several organs and may be carcinogenic to the lung and prostate, but it also has particular toxicity to the kidney following inhalation exposure. Abnormal renal function, consisting of proteinuria and decreased glomerular filtration rate (GFR), was first reported in cadmium workers in 1950 and has been confirmed in numerous investigations. The proteinuria consists of low-molecular-weight proteins such as β_2-microglobulin, retinol binding protein, lysozyme, and immunoglobulin light chains; these proteins are normally filtered in the glomerulus and reabsorbed in the proximal tubules. Cadmium-exposed workers also have a higher rate of kidney stone formation, perhaps due to disruption of calcium metabolism as a consequence of renal damage.

There is good evidence that renal tubular dysfunction occurs only after a threshold concentration of cadmium is reached in the renal cortex. The threshold varies among individuals but has been estimated to be approximately 200 μg/g wet weight. Several studies of the prevalence of proteinuria in worker populations suggest that inhalation exposure in excess of about 0.03 mg/m^3 for 30 years is associated with increased risk of tubular dysfunction. Unfortunately, removal from exposure does not necessarily halt disease in workers with cadmium-induced kidney damage, and progressive decreases in GFR and end-stage renal disease may occur. Progression of disease may depend both on the body burden of cadmium and the severity of proteinuria at last exposure. Unless renal damage is significant, urinary cadmium concentration reflects the body burden of the metal.

Although renal damage is clearly due to accumulation of cadmium in the kidney, the molecular mechanism of this damage is unclear. Metallothionein may be involved; this cadmium-binding protein, which is synthesized in the liver and kidney, appears both to facilitate transport of cadmium to the kidney and to promote retention of cadmium in the kidney.

DUSTS

Numerous cases of occupational lung injury are caused by inhalation of dusts of various kinds, such as coal dust, asbestos, crystalline silica, or talc. Various forms of **asbestos**, such as amosite and crocidolite, are carcinogenic to the lung and/or mesothelium after long-term exposure to fibers of respirable size (<10 μm). The widespread use of asbestos-containing products in shipbuilding, construction, textiles, and other industries in past decades has caused a large number of cancer cases; in fact, because of latency, this number is still increasing. Although the use of asbestos has been much curtailed in the United States, older products (such as pipe insulation) are still in use and present opportunities for continued exposure. Excessive exposures due to natural outcroppings of asbestos-containing rocks may also be problematic, especially in certain regions of California, and extensive mining of vermiculite in Libby, Montana, has apparently led to an increased risk of mesothelioma. Asbestos also causes severe nonmalignant respiratory disease, called **asbestosis**, characterized by fibrotic lesions in the lung parenchyma that limit gas exchange. The mechanism(s) by which asbestos fibers damage the lung or pleura are not clear but may involve production of reactive oxygen species by macrophages attempting to destroy the fibers. Fiber characteristics such as composition, length, and diameter also play a role in toxicity. The risk of lung cancer in a person with asbestos exposure is greatly increased by cigarette smoking, by more than the sum of the independent risks due to asbestos and smoking as separate factors—an unfortunate example of **synergism** in carcinogenesis.

Black lung, or **coal worker's pneumoconiosis (CWP)**, is another nonmalignant (but potentially fatal) fibrotic lung disease induced by excessive coal dust exposure. The simple form of CWP may not markedly limit respiration and affect only small areas of the lung, whereas progressive CWP can develop and worsen even in the absence of continued exposure, leading to severe emphysema. Interestingly, coal dust does not appear to increase the risk of lung cancer. Although worker exposures to coal dust have been limited by U. S. regulations in recent decades and underground mining is less common than in the past, thousands of coal miners in other countries, especially China, are at risk for CWP and related illnesses.

TREATMENT FOR ACUTE EXPOSURES

In all toxic exposures, the patient should be removed from the contaminated environment and stabilized with standard life-supportive measures. Once a patient is stabilized acutely, measures should be taken to identify the precise toxic exposure. In some cases, history and physical examination is sufficient, while in other cases, advanced laboratory testing may be required.

Once a poison has been identified, several strategies are used to minimize harm, based on the nature of the inciting toxin. One strategy is to alter the toxicokinetics of a poison so as to minimize exposure by (1) decreasing the absorption of the toxin, (2) preventing toxication of a benign compound, or (3) increasing the metabolism or elimination of the toxin. A second strategy aims to inactivate a toxin by binding a small molecule or antibody to it and thus prevent the toxin from interfering with essential biochemical and cellular processes. A final strategy is to counteract the action of the toxin at the biochemical, cellular, or whole-body level.

Table 51-1 (end of chapter) lists selected major poisons along with their mechanism of toxicity, receptor or target, clinical signs, and antidote (if any).

PRINCIPLES FOR TREATING THE ACUTELY POISONED PATIENT

The initial approach to the treatment of a poisoned patient is to eliminate further exposure. In many cases, this step alone is effective because the body's homeostatic mechanisms can minimize injury by responding adequately to some brief exposures. For example, acute symptoms caused by inhalation of high concentrations of **trichloroethylene** vapor are readily reversed after removal of the patient to fresh air.

Once the patient has been removed from the exposure, supportive measures such as securing the airway, ensuring ventilation and end-organ perfusion, and correcting electrolyte abnormalities are undertaken. For example, overdose of a **beta-adrenergic antagonist** is treated by giving **glucagon** to increase heart rate and blood pressure and parenteral fluids to treat hypotension. Glucagon increases cAMP in cardiac cells by stimulating glucagon receptor-mediated activation of adenylyl cyclase. Glucagon is also locally metabolized to a "mini-glucagon" fragment that increases intracellular Ca^{2+} (and hence contractility) by stimulating phospholipase A_2. If necessary, the heart can be paced using external paddles or a transvenous pacing wire. **Salicylate** poisoning, which causes a metabolic acidosis, is treated with aggressive electrolyte management: **sodium bicarbonate** is administered both to maintain a normal serum pH and to alkalinize the urine. Alkalinizing the urine promotes the renal excretion of salicylate.

The next step is to establish the nature of the poison. Sometimes this is known from the history, such as an occupational exposure, or from evidence gathered at the scene, such as an empty pill bottle. Other times, the patient's symptoms are consistent with a particular **toxidrome.** For example, the symptoms of cholinergic overload (vomiting, diarrhea, peripheral vasodilation, loss of accommodation, and pupillary constriction) in an agricultural setting suggest exposure to a pesticide. Frequently, however, particularly in an obtunded patient, it may be necessary to obtain plasma toxicology data or other specialized information to determine definitively the poison and to tailor treatment accordingly.

TOXICOKINETIC-BASED TREATMENTS

Toxicokinetic approaches aim to minimize the opportunity for the poison to cause end-organ damage by decreasing the quantity of the agent in the body. This can be accomplished by preventing the poison from being absorbed, preventing toxication, enhancing the toxin's metabolism, or enhancing its elimination.

Prevention of Absorption

It is occasionally possible to prevent gastrointestinal absorption of material that has been ingested but not yet absorbed by performing gastric lavage. In very rare instances, emesis may be induced instead of gastric lavage. The most common method of inducing emesis is with **ipecac syrup,** which acts via a dual mechanism within approximately 15 to 30 minutes of administration. Locally, it irritates the gastrointestinal tract, while centrally, it activates the chemoreceptor trigger zone in the area postrema of the brain (see Chapter 13, Pharmacology of Serotonergic and Central Adrenergic Neurotransmission). **Chemical adsorption** of a toxin onto **activated charcoal** is another way to prevent the absorption of ingested toxins. Activated charcoal powder provides a large surface area onto which many small organic molecules can be adsorbed. The charcoal then passes through the gastrointestinal tract and is eliminated in the feces, along with the adsorbed toxin. In general, activated charcoal is more effective for hydrophobic substances and ineffective for most inorganic salts. In some cases, **multiple-dose activated charcoal** can be given to interfere with enterohepatic circulation of drugs that have been absorbed systemically.

Inhibition of Toxication

It is sometimes possible to prevent toxication by inhibiting the enzymes involved in converting the xenobiotic into its toxic product. In practice, few specific metabolic enzymes are targets of therapy because most of the enzymes are part of the cytochrome P450 system. However, one target for such an approach is **alcohol dehydrogenase,** which converts alcohols into their corresponding aldehydes. In many cases, the parent alcohol is not particularly toxic and can be excreted renally, but the aldehyde metabolite or a more downstream metabolite is significantly more toxic. For example, formate is a toxic metabolite of methanol (wood alcohol), and glycolic acid is the toxic metabolite of ethylene glycol (a bifunctional alcohol and a component of antifreeze) that causes dose-dependent CNS depression and elevated anion gap metabolic acidosis. Because **ethanol** is also metabolized by alcohol dehydrogenase, it can function as a competitive inhibitor for both methanol and ethylene glycol. Historically, patients who had ingested methanol or ethylene glycol were kept inebriated with oral or IV ethanol solutions to minimize the formation of the more toxic metabolites. More recently, the competitive alcohol dehydrogenase inhibitor **fomepizole** has been employed. Unlike ethanol, fomepizole is not itself metabolized by alcohol dehydrogenase and does not cause symptoms of inebriation.

Enhancement of Metabolism (Detoxication)

It is theoretically possible to accelerate the metabolism of a toxic substance by inducing the appropriate cytochrome P450 isoenzyme. Unfortunately, because the process of induction takes time, this approach is not suitable for acute intoxications and is not generally used clinically.

In some cases, the metabolic actions of non-P450 enzymes that are dependent on cofactors or cosubstrates may be accelerated by the addition of these cofactors. The most dramatic example is cyanide poisoning, which is treated with a ''kit'' containing **amyl nitrite** or **sodium nitrite** and **sodium thiosulfate** (Fig. 51-4). The nitrites act by oxidizing hemoglobin to methemoglobin to provide a substrate that can compete with cytochrome *c* oxidase for cyanide molecules (see below). The methemoglobin-bound cyanide is then oxidized to the relatively nontoxic thiocyanate by the enzyme **rhodanese** (also known as *transsulfurase*). The addition of thiosulfate provides a ready source of sulfur for the detoxication reaction and enhances cyanide metabolism.

Another example of providing the substrate for a detoxification reaction is the use of N-acetylcysteine in the treatment of **acetaminophen** poisoning. Acetaminophen can be converted into the hepatotoxic metabolite N-acetyl-*p*-benzoquinoneimine (NAPQI) by the action of P450 enzymes in the liver (Fig. 51-5). NAPQI can be detoxified by conjugation with glutathione. However, if the acetaminophen dose is sufficiently large, then glutathione stores are depleted and liver toxicity can result. Glutathione stores can be replenished by administering **N-acetylcysteine** (NAC), a metabolic precursor of glutathione.

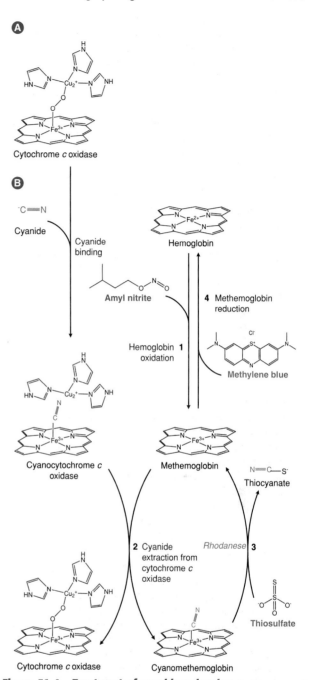

Figure 51-4. Treatment of cyanide poisoning. A. Structure of the copper/heme active site of cytochrome *c* oxidase, the enzyme responsible for the final step of the electron transport chain (the four-electron reduction of oxygen to water). Here, the enzyme is depicted after reducing oxygen to the bridging peroxide form. **B.** Cyanide displaces oxygen because it forms an extremely stable bond with the ferric heme group in cytochrome *c* oxidase. Treatment of cyanide poisoning involves *(1)* oxidation of the ferrous heme in hemoglobin to its ferric form (methemoglobin) by amyl nitrite or sodium nitrite. Methemoglobin competes strongly for cyanide *(2)*, facilitating its removal from the active site of cytochrome *c* oxidase, and acting as a sink for circulating cyanide. Cyanide is converted to thiocyanate via the action of rhodanese, a mitochondrial enzyme *(3)*. The addition of sodium thiosulfate provides the sulfur needed for the conversion of cyanide to thiocyanate. Once cyanide has been detoxified, methemoglobin can be returned to its ferrous form *(4)* by the addition of methylene blue.

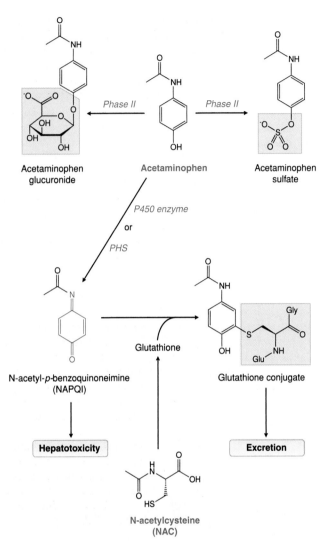

Figure 51-5. Mechanism of acetaminophen poisoning and treatment. Acetaminophen is not toxic by itself but can be converted to toxic metabolites in the liver by the oxidative action of P450 enzyme or prostaglandin H synthase (PHS). Most acetaminophen is conjugated to sulfate or glucuronate via conjugation (phase II) reactions. However, a small amount is oxidized to N-acetyl-*p*-benzoquinoneimine (NAPQI), which can bind to hepatic proteins and cause centrolobular necrosis (hepatotoxicity). NAPQI can be conjugated to glutathione to form the nontoxic glutathione conjugate. In cases of acetaminophen overdose, glutathione is depleted, and NAPQI is free to cause hepatotoxicity. N-acetylcysteine (NAC) can be administered as an antidote. NAC, which is a metabolic precursor for glutathione, repletes hepatocellular glutathione levels and thereby prevents NAPQI-induced hepatotoxicity.

Enhancement of Elimination

Facilitating the elimination of a toxin is a common method of treating an acutely poisoned patient. This can be accomplished either by enhancing renal clearance of the toxin or by artificially clearing the toxin from plasma. The former is accomplished by preventing tubular reabsorption of the toxin (**ion trapping**), while the latter is accomplished by means of **hemodialysis, hemofiltration,** or **hemoperfusion.**

Ion trapping involves alkalinization of the urine to enhance renal clearance of a weakly acidic toxin. In ion trap-

ping, the neutral form of the toxin is filtered through the glomerulus, and this form becomes deprotonated in the alkalinized (basic) urine. The ionized form of the toxin is not reabsorbed and is therefore excreted in the urine. Clinically, ion trapping is accomplished by administering bicarbonate to the patient and titrating to a urine pH of 7.5 to 8.5. This technique has been especially effective in improving the elimination of salicylates and phenobarbital. Although acidification of the urine to enhance clearance of a basic toxin is theoretically possible, the practical dangers of iatrogenic metabolic acidosis preclude this approach.

The techniques of hemodialysis, hemofiltration, and hemoperfusion depend on extracorporeal purification of the blood. For this reason, these techniques only work with substances that have a relatively small volume of distribution, so that removal of the toxic substance from the blood does not leave a large, inaccessible reservoir in the body tissues. Hemodialysis is generally useful for small molecules that have a small volume of distribution, are relatively water soluble, and are not highly bound to plasma proteins (which cannot cross the dialysis membrane).

In hemofiltration, the blood is filtered through a variable-sized porous membrane, which allows plasma with a varying amount of protein to be removed in the ultrafiltrate. Because the plasma is exposed to a filter rather than a semipermeable membrane, larger molecules can be cleared with hemofiltration than with hemodialysis.

In hemoperfusion, blood is passed through a cartridge where it comes in contact with an **ion-exchange resin** or activated charcoal that can adsorb the toxin. Ion-exchange resins bind inorganic salts and exchange them for electrolytes such as sodium or chloride. Because of the direct contact between blood and the adsorbent material, hemoperfusion poses a risk of thrombosis. In addition, the ion-exchange resin is not selective in its ion binding and can deplete plasma of calcium and magnesium.

In extreme circumstances, it may be possible to conduct a **plasma exchange** or an **exchange transfusion,** whereby the patient's plasma or blood is removed and replaced with transfused plasma or whole blood from a donor. This technique is generally reserved for newborns.

INACTIVATION OF POISONS

Inactivation is one approach to reducing the activity of toxins that have entered the circulation and cannot be eliminated readily. An inactivator, such as a chelator or antibody, binds to the toxin and thereby prevents interaction of the toxin with target tissues. The complexes of toxin and inactivator are then cleared from the body. An inactivating substance must have a high affinity for the toxin so that equilibrium strongly favors the inactivated complex, and the complex formed must have low toxicity.

Heavy Metal Chelators

The inactivation and removal of toxic heavy metals such as lead, mercury, or cadmium, and of overdoses of metals such as iron or copper, can be accomplished by binding the metal to a small molecule containing a nucleophilic electron donor such as an amine, hydroxide, carboxylate, or mercaptan to form a **metal-ligand complex.** A **chelator,** which in Greek means ''claw,'' is a multidentate structure with multiple binding sites (Fig. 51-6). Binding the metal at multiple sites shifts the equilibrium constant in favor of metal ligation. High-affinity metal-ligand binding is critical because the chelator must compete with tissue macromolecules for binding. In addition, the chelator should be nontoxic and water-soluble, and the complex should be readily cleared. Finally, an ideal chelator should have a low binding affinity for endogenous ions such as calcium. To prevent the depletion of tissue calcium, many chelators are administered as their calcium complexes. The target metal is then exchanged for calcium, and the body's calcium stores are not depleted.

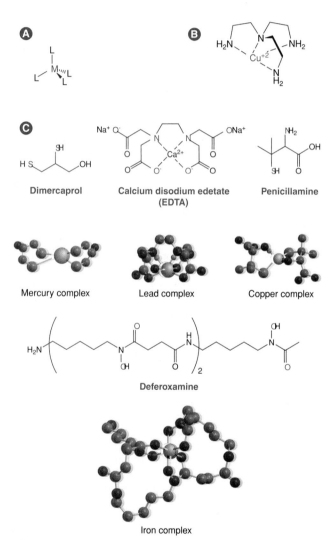

Figure 51-6. Heavy metal chelators. A. A ligand *(L)* is a compound containing a Lewis base (such as amine, thiol, hydroxyl, or carboxylate groups) that can form a complex with a metal *(M).* **B.** A chelator is a multidentate ligand, that is, a ligand that can bind to a metal through multiple atoms, as in this example of a tetra-amino ligand bound to copper *(Cu²⁺)* via its four amine groups. **C.** The structures of dimercaprol, calcium EDTA, penicillamine, and deferoxamine are shown; the groups that form bonds with the metal are identified in *blue.* Three-dimensional structures of the mercury complex of dimercaprol, the lead complex of EDTA, the copper complex of penicillamine, and the iron complex of deferoxamine are also shown. Here, the heavy metal is highlighted in *blue.* For simplicity, hydrogen atoms are not shown.

The most important heavy metal chelators are **edetate disodium** (the calcium, disodium complex of EDTA), which can be used to bind lead; **dimercaprol** (also known as **British anti-Lewisite** or **BAL**), which binds gold, arsenic, lead, and mercury to its two thiol groups; and **succimer** (2,3-dimercaptosuccinic acid), which has supplanted dimercaprol for the removal of lead, cadmium, mercury, and arsenic. **Deferoxamine** is used for the removal of toxic levels of iron, such as would occur in accidental overdoses of iron-containing supplements or in patients with transfusion-dependent anemias. **Deferasirox** is an orally bioavailable iron chelator that has recently been approved by the U. S. Food and Drug Administration (FDA); this agent may supplant deferoxamine for many conditions associated with chronic iron overload. Removal of copper, typically in patients with Wilson's disease, is accomplished with **penicillamine** or, for patients who do not tolerate penicillamine, **trientine.**

Antivenins and Antibody Binding

Antibodies are also used as inactivators because they have high affinity and high specificity for their substrates. **Antivenins** are antibodies against a venom. They are produced by inoculating an animal, usually a horse, with small amounts of the venom to incite a humoral antibody response. Upon injection into a patient who has been exposed to the venom, the purified horse antiserum binds and inactivates the venom.

Another use of an antibody as an inactivator is the binding of digoxin with **digoxin immune Fab.** This treatment is used in cases where the patient is experiencing signs or symptoms due to toxic plasma levels of the drug. As the name implies, the antibody includes only the Fab fragment of the immunoglobulin. Digoxin immune Fab is derived from immunized sheep.

One danger inherent in the use of antibodies as inactivators is the risk of developing serum sickness, a type III hypersensitivity reaction. Both antivenins and digoxin immune Fab can cause serum sickness.

PHARMACOLOGIC TREATMENT

For toxins that act via a specific metabolic pathway, treatment can be rendered by administering a drug with the opposite pharmacologic action, or by bypassing the metabolic pathway that has been inhibited. Four broad categories of pharmacologically mediated treatments are used to counteract poisonings: (1) a receptor antagonist can block the effect of a toxin that acts as an agonist at the receptor or that potentiates the action of the receptor's endogenous ligand; (2) a receptor agonist or a drug that enhances the physiologic action of the endogenous ligand can restore balance at a receptor that has been blocked by a toxin acting as a receptor antagonist; (3) a drug can restore the physiologic function of an enzyme or receptor by removing a toxin from the active site of the protein; (4) it is sometimes possible to bypass the metabolic pathway completely by taking advantage of pharmacologic targets downstream of the inhibited receptor or enzyme.

Pharmacologic Antagonism

Conceptually, the simplest treatment for poisoning is the administration of an antagonist that blocks the action of a toxin that, directly or indirectly, results in supraphysiologic activation of a receptor. For example, an opioid overdose can be treated with **naloxone,** a pharmacologic antagonist of the opioid receptor. Naloxone has a rapid onset of action and is highly potent; indeed, if no improvement is seen within 10 minutes after naloxone doses of up to 10 mg, a different diagnosis or multiple toxic entities should be considered. Naloxone has a relatively short half-life, so it must be given every 1 to 4 hours to provide adequate receptor antagonism while the opioid is being cleared.

Flumazenil is a pharmacologic antagonist at the $GABA_A$ (benzodiazepine) receptor and is used to treat benzodiazepine overdose. Like naloxone, flumazenil has a rapid onset of action and is highly potent; its effects should be seen within 5 minutes at a dose of not more than 3 mg. Flumazenil also has a short half-life (approximately 1 hour) and must be given frequently to provide adequate receptor antagonism while the benzodiazepine is being cleared.

Pharmacologic antagonism can also be used when the toxic agent is not a direct agonist but rather indirectly increases the concentration of the natural ligand for a receptor. AChE inhibitors produce a supraphysiologic concentration of acetylcholine in the synaptic cleft and a characteristic toxidrome of cholinergic excess—bradycardia, miosis, hypersalivation, sweating, diarrhea, vomiting, bronchoconstriction, weakness, respiratory paralysis, and convulsions. Although it is sometimes possible to restore AChE activity (see below), the treatment of AChE inhibition generally depends on administering an anticholinergic agent, such as **atropine.** By antagonizing the muscarinic acetylcholine receptor, atropine restores cholinergic balance and prevents bronchoconstriction, the most common cause of death in patients with exposure to AChE inhibitors. Atropine does not antagonize nicotinic acetylcholine receptors and cannot reverse muscular paralysis.

Pharmacologic Enhancement of Physiologic Function

When the toxin is a competitive receptor antagonist, administering an agonist or a compound that enhances agonist activity can be an effective treatment. For example, ingestion of berries or seeds (such as from jimson weed) containing **belladonna alkaloids** causes an atropine-like anticholinergic effect that can result in delirium, coma, and respiratory collapse. Treatment involves the administration of **physostigmine,** which blocks AChE to increase cholinergic tone. It should be noted that atropine, an anticholinergic agent, is the treatment of choice for organophosphate poisoning of AChE, whereas an AChE inhibitor is the treatment of choice for poisoning with an anticholinergic toxin.

Active Site Restoration

The effects of some toxins that bind covalently to the active site of a receptor or an enzyme can be counteracted by a pharmacologic agent that displaces the toxin and thereby restores enzyme or receptor activity. This strategy is best illustrated by the treatment for toxic agents that bind or oxidize heme groups. The three prototypic toxins that act on heme groups are **carbon monoxide** (which acts on hemoglobin), **cyanide** (which acts on cytochrome c oxidase), and xenobiotics such as **nitrate**, a common water contaminant in rural areas (which is reduced in the body to **nitrite**, which then oxidizes hemoglobin to methemoglobin).

Treatment for carbon monoxide and cyanide poisoning involves displacing the small molecule from its heme target. For carbon monoxide poisoning, high concentrations of oxygen are administered. The oxygen competes with carbon monoxide for hemoglobin, and the free carbon monoxide is exhaled. Higher concentrations of oxygen result in greater displacement and more rapid elimination of carbon monoxide. In cases of severe poisoning, a patient may be placed in a **hyperbaric oxygen chamber** that delivers oxygen at partial pressures above atmospheric pressure.

Cyanide cannot be displaced by oxygen. However, cyanide has a greater affinity for methemoglobin than for cytochrome c oxidase (Fig. 51-4). Thus, by oxidizing hemoglobin to its ferric state (methemoglobin) with amyl nitrite or sodium nitrite, a competitor for cyanide is generated. Cyanide is then converted to thiocyanate with the aid of sodium thiosulfate. Once the danger of cyanide toxicity has passed, the ferric iron in methemoglobin can be reduced to its ferrous state by administration of the active redox agent **methylene blue.** Under normal circumstances, the concentration of methemoglobin is kept low via two reducing pathways, the NADH diaphorase pathway, which accounts for $>95\%$ of methemoglobin reducing activity, and the NADPH diaphorase pathway, which accounts for the remainder. Methylene blue is reduced to leukomethylene blue by NADPH diaphorase; leukomethylene blue then reduces methemoglobin to hemoglobin, thereby restoring its oxygen-carrying capacity.

Acute treatment for organophosphate poisoning involves restoration of the active site of the enzyme. While the administration of anticholinergic agents such as atropine can block the effect of excess acetylcholine at muscarinic receptors, it cannot restore the enzymatic function of AChE. However, **pralidoxime** can enhance the hydrolysis of the serine-phosphate bond between the organophosphate and AChE. Pralidoxime contains a quaternary ammonium group that places an oxime nucleophile in close proximity to the electrophilic phosphate group on the organophosphate (Fig. 51-2). The organophosphate then binds to pralidoxime, releasing AChE. The resulting phosphorylated oxime is unstable in water and degrades. Unfortunately, the phosphorylated AChE can also undergo ''aging'' through hydrolysis of an alkyl side-group, and the aged enzyme is then resistant to the action of pralidoxime. Therefore, pralidoxime should be given as soon as possible after exposure to an organophosphate.

Metabolic Pathway Alternatives

It is sometimes possible to bypass a toxin-inhibited enzymatic reaction entirely, either by supplying the enzymatic product or by enhancing an alternative metabolic pathway. An example of this therapeutic strategy is the administration of **vitamin K** in cases of certain **anticoagulant** poisonings. **Warfarin**, discussed in Chapter 22, Pharmacology of Hemostasis and Thrombosis, and certain anticoagulants used as rodenticides, including **brodifacoum, diphacinone,** and derivatives, inhibit the regeneration of vitamin K from its epoxide form. Vitamin K is needed for the carboxylation of glutamate to form γ-carboxyglutamate, converting precursor coagulation factors into their active forms. Hence, the depletion of reduced vitamin K stores results in the depletion of coagulation factors, thereby inhibiting hemostasis and facilitating bleeding. One treatment for overdose or poisoning with these anticoagulants is the administration of supplementary vitamin K, to enable the liver to generate the active coagulation factors. However, because it takes time for the liver to synthesize coagulation factors, vitamin K therapy generally requires a number of hours to improve coagulation function. Thus, it may be necessary in cases of bleeding, surgery, or trauma to bypass the entire metabolic pathway by administering **fresh frozen plasma** (FFP), which contains the active forms of the coagulation factors.

Conclusion and Future Directions

Much of the treatment for toxic exposures focuses on the acutely poisoned patient. However, most of the morbidity associated with toxic exposures is caused by chronic exposures and may be clinically apparent only years after the initial exposure. In fact, there is generally no specific treatment for injury caused by chronic toxic exposures, and much of the available treatment is symptomatic and supportive.

Thus, the study of toxicology includes not only **mechanistic toxicology,** on which this chapter has focused, but also **descriptive toxicology** and **regulatory toxicology.** Descriptive toxicology is concerned with the determination of which compounds are toxic and what their toxic effects are; regulatory toxicology helps develop public policy that reasonably minimizes exposure to toxic compounds. In the United States, several regulatory agencies are charged with forming such policy. The **FDA** seeks to ensure the safety of the food supply, approve new therapeutic agents, and withdraw approvals of unsafe agents or medical devices (see Chapter 48, Drug Discovery and Preclinical Development, and Chapter 49, Clinical Drug Evaluation and Regulatory Approval). The **Environmental Protection Agency (EPA)** establishes and enforces policy with regard to environmental pollution and its public health consequences. The **Occupational Safety and Health Administration (OSHA)** regulates workplace exposures, while the **Consumer Products Safety Commission (CPSC)** acts to ensure the safety of consumer goods.

The application of a mechanistic understanding of toxicity is expected to improve regulatory toxicology and thus enhance public health, particularly with respect to the health implications of exposure to low levels of pollutants in the wider environment and the prevention of dangerous adverse effects of pharmaceuticals. Significant advances in toxicology, as in pharmacology and medical sciences, may be promoted by progress in genomics, development of "gene chips," and tools of computational biology that identify genetic or other traits responsible for individual responses to drugs and toxins.

Suggested Reading

Bornaya J, Glantz S. Cardiovascular effects of secondhand smoke: nearly as large as smoking. *Circulation* 2005;111:2684–2698. *(Discusses the health risks and toxic mechanisms of second-hand smoke.)*

Klaassen CD, ed. *Casarett & Doull's Toxicology: The Basic Science of Poisons.* 6th ed. New York: McGraw-Hill; 2001. *(A comprehensive textbook of toxicology, this resource provides a solid foundation for the understanding of toxicology. It includes sections on general principles, toxicokinetics, nonspecific toxicity, organ-specific toxicity, toxic agents, environmental toxicology, and applications of toxicology, including a chapter on clinical toxicology.)*

Lang CH, Frost RA, Summer AD, et al. Molecular mechanisms responsible for alcohol-induced myopathy in skeletal muscle and heart. *Int J Biochem Cell Biol* 2005;37:2180–2195. *(Reviews cellular and molecular mechanisms by which alcohol impairs skeletal and cardiac muscle function, with special emphasis on alterations in signaling pathways that regulate protein synthesis.)*

Smilkstein MJ, Knapp GL, Kulig KW, et al. Efficacy of oral N-acetylcysteine in the treatment of acetaminophen overdose. Analysis of the national multicenter study (1976 to 1985). *N Engl J Med* 1988;319:1557–1562. *(Established the clinical benefit of treating acetaminophen toxicity by providing N-acetylcysteine, a source of cysteine for the production of glutathione.)*

Tauxe RV. Emerging foodborne pathogens. *Int J Food Microbiol* 2002;78:31–41. *(Overview of common sources of food poisoning.)*

Toxnet. Available at http://toxnet.nlm.nih.gov/. *(This government resource, sponsored by the National Library of Medicine, contains a vast database of both toxic substances and articles in the field of toxicology.)*

Tzipori S, Sheoran A, Akiyoshi D, et al. Antibody therapy in the management of Shiga toxin-induced hemolytic uremic syndrome. *Clin Microbiol Rev* 2004;17:926–941. *(Reviews the structure and mechanism of action of Shiga toxins, produced by E. coli O157:H7 and other enteropathic bacteria, the manifestations and treatment of hemolytic uremic syndrome, and the potential utility of antibody therapy.)*

Weaver LK, Hopkins RO, Chan KJ, et al. Hyperbaric oxygen for acute carbon monoxide poisoning. *N Engl J Med* 2002;347:1057–1067. *(Although hyperbaric oxygen had been postulated to help treat carbon monoxide poisoning and has been used since 1960, this study established its clinical efficacy in reducing cognitive deficits at 6 weeks and 12 months.)*

TABLE 51-1 **Mechanisms of Toxicity, Targets/Receptors, Clinical Signs, and Antidotes of Selected Poisons**

POISON	MECHANISM OF TOXICITY	TARGET/RECEPTOR (IF APPLICABLE)	CLINICAL SIGNS (ALL REQUIRE SUFFICIENTLY HIGH EXPOSURES/DOSES AND ARE NOT EXPECTED IN ALL SETTINGS)	ANTIDOTE (IF AVAILABLE)
Acetaminophen	Converted to reactive NAPQI in the liver	N/A	Hepatotoxicity	N-acetylcysteine
Acid anhydrides	Strong nucleophiles; cause type II hypersensitivity reactions	N/A	Eye and skin irritants	None
Amyl nitrite	Oxidizes hemoglobin to methemoglobin	Hemoglobin	Cyanosis, nausea, vertigo, vomiting, collapse, tachycardia, tachypnea, coma, convulsions, and death	Methylene blue
Anabolic steroids		Steroid receptors	Lipoprotein disturbances, cardiac disease, hepatoma, psychiatric disturbances, and hypogonadal states	None
Aniline dyes	Oxidize hemoglobin to methemoglobin	Hemoglobin	Cyanosis, nausea, vertigo, vomiting, collapse, tachycardia, tachypnea, coma, convulsions, and death	Methylene blue
Antivenins	Cause type III hypersensitivity reactions	N/A	Serum sickness	None
Arsenic	May replace phosphate in several reactions; binds cysteine residues in proteins; alters DNA methylation; oxidative stress; alters cell proliferation; tumor promoter	N/A	Carcinogen (skin, lung, liver)	Dimercaprol
Asbestos	Inhaled fibers lodged in alveoli. Fibers elicit iron deposition. Fibers also attract macrophages → inflammatory reaction → collagen formation	N/A	Pulmonary fibrosis, lung cancer, mesothelioma, possibly gastrointestinal cancer	None
Atropine	Antagonist at cholinergic receptors	Muscarinic cholinergic receptors	Glaucoma, tachycardia	Physostigmine
Benzene	Converted to reactive phenols and polyphenols in the liver	N/A	CNS depression (acutely) Bone marrow depression, leukemia (chronically)	None
Benzocaine	Oxidizes hemoglobin to methemoglobin	Hemoglobin	Cyanosis, nausea, vertigo, vomiting, collapse, tachycardia, tachypnea, coma, convulsions, and death	Methylene blue
Beryllium	Inhaled particles can elicit granuloma formation	N/A	Chemical pneumonitis; suspected carcinogen; lung hypersensitivity	None
Botulinum toxin	Blocks release of acetylcholine	Synaptobrevin or synapse-associated proteins	Muscular paralysis	None

Brodifacoum	Prevents clotting factor synthesis by inhibiting vitamin K regeneration	Epoxide reductase	Bleeding	Vitamin K Fresh frozen plasma
Cadmium	Inhibits synthesis of alpha-1-antitrypsin; causes proteinuria	N/A	Carcinogenic; vomiting, pulmonary edema (acute); emphysema, renal failure, osteomalacia (chronic)	Succimer
Calcium hydroxide	Caustic (alkali) agent; chemical burns	N/A	Chemical burns	None
Carbon monoxide	Binds to hemoglobin, preventing oxygen transport; shifts oxygen saturation curve to the left, preventing oxygen unloading	Hemoglobin	Headache, cardiac ischemia (in patients with pre-existing heart disease), lactic acidosis; neurologic symptoms including seizures, coma, and death	Hyperbaric oxygen
Carbon tetrachloride	Converted to reactive trichloro radical in the liver	N/A	Hepatotoxicity, renal toxicity	None
Chlorpyrifos	Inhibits acetylcholinesterase	Acetylcholinesterase (directly); acetylcholine receptors (indirectly, by increasing concentration of acetylcholine at the synapse and neuromuscular junction)	Nausea, vomiting, diarrhea, hypersalivation, muscle paralysis, bradycardia	Atropine Pralidoxime
Cigarette smoke	Chemical carcinogenesis, among other mechanisms	N/A	Lung cancer, oropharyngeal cancer, other cancers; emphysema; cardiovascular disease	None
Coal dust	Fine particles irritate the lungs and mucous membranes	N/A	Mucous membrane irritation; pulmonary irritation; pneumoconiosis	None
Copper	Generates free radicals	N/A	Hepatotoxicity; cerebellar dysfunction; hematuria, proteinuria, oliguria, and/or uremia	Penicillamine, trientine
Cyanide	Binds to cytochrome c oxidase, preventing reduction of oxygen to water, halting electron transport chain	Cytochrome c oxidase	Lactic acidosis, irregular respirations; convulsions, coma; death	Amyl nitrite Sodium nitrite Sodium thiosulfate
Diazinon	Inhibits acetylcholinesterase	Acetylcholinesterase (directly); acetylcholine receptors (indirectly, by increasing concentration of acetylcholine at the synapse and neuromuscular junction)	Nausea, vomiting, diarrhea, hypersalivation, muscle paralysis, bradycardia	Atropine Pralidoxime
Digoxin	Increases intracellular Ca^{2+} concentration	Na^+/K^+ ATPase	Ventricular extrasystole, AV block	Digoxin Fab
Diisocyanates	Cause type II hypersensitivity reactions	N/A	Atypical asthma; respiratory irritation	None
Dioxin	Various; induces P450 via Ah receptor	Aryl hydrocarbon receptor	Possible carcinogenesis; porphyria cutanea tarda; chloracne	None

(Continued)

TABLE 51-1 Mechanisms of Toxicity, Targets/Receptors, Clinical Signs, and Antidotes of Selected Poisons (*Continued*)

POISON	MECHANISM OF TOXICITY	TARGET/RECEPTOR (IF APPLICABLE)	CLINICAL SIGNS (ALL REQUIRE SUFFICIENTLY HIGH EXPOSURES/DOSES AND ARE NOT EXPECTED IN ALL SETTINGS)	ANTIDOTE (IF AVAILABLE)
Diphacinone	Prevents clotting factor synthesis by inhibiting vitamin K regeneration	Epoxide reductase	Bleeding	Vitamin K Fresh frozen plasma
Ethanol	Stimulates GABA receptors, inhibits glutamate receptors; nutritional deficiencies; metabolized to toxic intermediates (acetaldehyde)	GABA receptors (enhances effect), glutamate receptors (inhibitor)	CNS depression (acutely); hepatic cirrhosis, cardiomyopathy (chronic); fetal alcohol syndrome	None
Ethylene glycol	Converted to oxalic acid → calcium oxalate crystals in the kidney	N/A	Acute renal failure	Ethanol Fomepizole
Fenthion	Inhibits acetylcholinesterase	Acetylcholinesterase (directly); acetylcholine receptors (indirectly, by increasing concentration of acetylcholine at the synapse and neuromuscular junction)	Nausea, vomiting, diarrhea, hypersalivation, muscle paralysis, bradycardia	Atropine Pralidoxime
Glycol ethers	Direct nephrotoxin	N/A	Kidney and liver damage	None
Halothane	Alters liver proteins to elicit autoimmune reaction	N/A	Autoimmune hepatitis	None
Hay dust	Causes type I, type III hypersensitivity reaction	N/A	Allergic rhinitis; asthmatic bronchoconstriction; hypersensitivity pneumonitis	Antihistamines Glucocorticoids
Hydralazine	Causes autoimmune reaction by inducing autoantibodies against myeloperoxidase	N/A	Lupus-like syndrome	None
Hydrochloric acid	Strong acid; chemical burns	N/A	Chemical burns	None
Hydrofluoric acid	Strong acid; leaches bone → hypercalcemia	N/A	Chemical burns, hypercalcemia	Treatment for hypercalcemia
Iron	Generates free radicals; accumulates in cardiac tissue with hemosiderin → cellular degeneration and fibrosis	N/A	Hepatotoxicity, cardiotoxicity	Deferoxamine
Isoniazid	Causes autoimmune reaction by inducing autoantibodies against myeloperoxidase	N/A	Lupus-like syndrome	None

Lead	Binds to cysteine residues in proteins. Destroys blood-brain barrier; interferes with voltage-dependent calcium channels, neuronal cell-cell signaling, and neurotransmitter function; inhibits hemoglobin synthesis	Multiple: Pyrimidine 5'-nucleotidase; δ-aminolevulinic acid dehydratase (ALA-D)	Hypochromic anemia; developmental delays; encephalopathy; probable human carcinogen; renal toxicity; peripheral neuropathy	Edetate calcium disodium, Dimercaprol, Succimer
Malathion	Inhibits acetylcholinesterase	Acetylcholinesterase (directly); acetylcholine receptors (indirectly, by increasing concentration of acetylcholine at the synapse and neuromuscular junction)	Nausea, vomiting, diarrhea, hypersalivation, muscle paralysis, bradycardia	Atropine, Pralidoxime
Mercury	Alkyl compounds are direct neurotoxins (reactive species); mercuric salts bind cysteine residues in proteins, causing changes in protein structure	N/A	Interstitial pneumonitis, membranous colitis (acute); psychotic reactions, renal failure, muscle tremors, dementia, cerebral palsy, mental retardation (chronic); teratogen	Dimercaprol, Succimer
Methanol	Liver: formaldehyde; Retinal cells: formic acid (neurotoxin)	N/A	Blindness	Ethanol, Fomepizole
Methyldopa	Causes autoimmune reaction	N/A	Hemolytic anemia	None
Metoclopramide	Oxidizes hemoglobin to methemoglobin	Hemoglobin	Cyanosis, nausea, vertigo, vomiting, collapse, tachycardia, tachypnea, coma, convulsions, and death	Methylene blue
Mold spores	Cause type I, type III hypersensitivity reaction	N/A	Allergic rhinitis; asthmatic bronchoconstriction; hypersensitivity pneumonitis	Antihistamines, Glucocorticoids
Morphine	Opioid agonist	Opioid receptors	Respiratory depression, constipation, nausea, vomiting, sedation, euphoria, peripheral vasodilation, urinary retention, miosis, drug dependence	Naloxone
MPTP	Converted to MPT$^+$, a neurotoxin	N/A	Parkinsonian symptoms	None
Nitric acid	Causes type I hypersensitivity reaction	N/A	Asthmatic bronchoconstriction	None
Nitrites	Oxidize hemoglobin to methemoglobin	Hemoglobin	Cyanosis, nausea, vertigo, vomiting, collapse, tachycardia, tachypnea, coma, convulsions, and death	Methylene blue
Nitrogen mustards	Alkylate DNA	N/A	Skin blistering; carcinogenesis	None
Nitroglycerin	Oxidize hemoglobin to methemoglobin	Hemoglobin	Cyanosis, nausea, vertigo, vomiting, collapse, tachycardia, tachypnea, coma, convulsions, and death	Methylene blue
Parathion	Inhibits acetylcholinesterase	Acetylcholinesterase (directly); acetylcholine receptors (indirectly, by increasing concentration of acetylcholine at the synapse and neuromuscular junction)	Nausea, vomiting, diarrhea, hypersalivation, muscle paralysis, bradycardia	Atropine, Pralidoxime

(Continued)

TABLE 51-1   Mechanisms of Toxicity, Targets/Receptors, Clinical Signs, and Antidotes of Selected Poisons *(Continued)*

POISON	MECHANISM OF TOXICITY	TARGET/RECEPTOR (IF APPLICABLE)	CLINICAL SIGNS (ALL REQUIRE SUFFICIENTLY HIGH EXPOSURES/DOSES AND ARE NOT EXPECTED IN ALL SETTINGS)	ANTIDOTE (IF AVAILABLE)
Pentadecacatechol	Causes type IV hypersensitivity reaction	N/A	Contact dermatitis	None
Pet dander	Crosslinks IgE; causes type I hypersensitivity reaction	N/A	Allergic rhinitis; asthma	Antihistamines Glucocorticoids
Platinum chloride	Crosslinks IgE; causes type I hypersensitivity reaction	N/A	Asthmatic bronchoconstriction	None
Primaquine	Oxidizes hemoglobin to methemoglobin	Hemoglobin	Cyanosis, nausea, vertigo, vomiting, collapse, tachycardia, tachypnea, coma, convulsions, and death	Methylene blue
Procainamide	Causes autoimmune reaction by inducing autoantibodies against DNA	N/A	Lupus-like syndrome	None
Sarin	Inhibits acetylcholinesterase	Acetylcholinesterase (directly); acetylcholine receptors (indirectly, by increasing concentration of acetylcholine at the synapse and neuromuscular junction)	Nausea, vomiting, diarrhea, hypersalivation, muscle paralysis, bradycardia	Atropine Pralidoxime
Silica	Inhaled, fine particles of crystalline silica are deposited in the lungs, eliciting an inflammatory reaction	N/A	Pulmonary fibrosis; lung cancer; scleroderma	None
Soman	Inhibits acetylcholinesterase	Acetylcholinesterase (directly); acetylcholine receptors (indirectly, by increasing concentration of acetylcholine at the synapse and neuromuscular junction)	Nausea, vomiting, diarrhea, hypersalivation, muscle paralysis, bradycardia	Atropine Pralidoxime
Sulfonamides	Oxidize hemoglobin to methemoglobin	Hemoglobin	Cyanosis, nausea, vertigo, vomiting, collapse, tachycardia, tachypnea, coma, convulsions, and death	Methylene blue
Sulfur dioxide	Causes type I hypersensitivity reaction	N/A	Asthmatic bronchoconstriction	None
Sulfuric acid	Strong acid	N/A	Chemical burns	None
Tabun	Inhibits acetylcholinesterase	Acetylcholinesterase (directly); acetylcholine receptors (indirectly, by increasing concentration of acetylcholine at the synapse and neuromuscular junction)	Nausea, vomiting, diarrhea, hypersalivation, muscle paralysis, bradycardia	Atropine Pralidoxime

Substance	Mechanism	Site/Target	Effects	Antidote
Talc	Inhaled particulates cause granuloma formation	N/A	Pulmonary fibrosis	None
Tetrachloroethylene (perchloroethylene)	Converted to reactive species via the action of cytochrome P450 enzyme	N/A	CNS depression (acutely); possible carcinogenesis	None
Tricyclic antidepressants	Quinidine-like effect on sodium channel; lengthen QRS interval	Sodium channels	Ventricular arrhythmias, hypotension, heart block, bradyarrhythmias, asystole	Sodium bicarbonate
Trinitrotoluene	Oxidizes hemoglobin to methemoglobin	Hemoglobin	Cyanosis, nausea, vertigo, vomiting, collapse, tachycardia, tachypnea, coma, convulsions, and death	Methylene blue
Urushiol	Causes type IV hypersensitivity reaction	N/A	Contact dermatitis	Glucocorticoids
VX	Inhibits acetylcholinesterase	Acetylcholinesterase (directly); acetylcholine receptors (indirectly, by increasing concentration of acetylcholine at the synapse and neuromuscular junction)	Nausea, vomiting, diarrhea, hypersalivation, muscle paralysis, bradycardia	Atropine Pralidoxime
Warfarin	Prevents clotting factor synthesis by inhibiting vitamin K regeneration	Epoxide reductase	Bleeding; teratogenic, causing facial defects	Vitamin K Fresh frozen plasma

IX

Frontiers in Pharmacology

52

Pharmacogenomics

Liewei Wang and Richard M. Weinshilboum

INTRODUCTION

Previous chapters have described drugs in the context of their molecular targets and their metabolism. Although modern pharmacologic agents can be used successfully to treat or control diseases that range from hypertension to infection with human immunodeficiency virus (HIV), there are large individual variations in response to drug therapy. These variations can range from potentially life-threatening adverse drug reactions to equally serious lack of therapeutic efficacy. Many factors can influence the drug response phenotype, including age, gender, and underlying disease, but genetic variation also plays an important role. Interindividual differences in the genes that encode drug targets, drug transporters, or enzymes that catalyze drug metabolism can affect profoundly the success or failure of pharmacotherapy.

Pharmacogenetics is the study of the role of inheritance in variation in drug response. The convergence of recent advances in genomic science and equally striking advances in molecular pharmacology has resulted in the evolution of pharmacogenetics into pharmacogenomics—terms that are often used interchangeably. The promise of pharmacogenetics-pharmacogenomics is the possibility that knowledge of a patient's DNA sequence could be used to enhance pharmacotherapy, maximizing drug efficacy by targeting drugs only to those patients who are most likely to benefit while, at the same time, reducing the incidence of adverse drug reactions.

This chapter describes the principles of pharmacogenetics and pharmacogenomics as well as recent developments in this discipline. Examples are cited in which knowledge of pharmacogenetics-pharmacogenomics can help individualize drug therapy.

Case

Robert H, a 66-year-old man, is shoveling snow one wintry morning in Minnesota when he slips and falls on a patch of ice. He immediately feels pain in his left hip and is unable to stand. He is brought to the hospital, where x-rays reveal that he has fractured his hip. He undergoes surgery the next day and is discharged to a rehabilitation hospital 3 days later. After less than 24 hours at the rehabilitation hospital, Mr. H develops the sudden onset of pleuritic chest pain. He is brought to the Emergency Department, where a CT scan with intravenous contrast reveals a pulmonary embolus. He is treated with heparin and is anticoagulated with warfarin at a starting dose of 5 mg each day, with a target international normalized ratio (INR) of 2.0–3.0. Mr. H is discharged back to his rehabilitation hospital and referred to his local physician. When the INR is subsequently measured, it is 6.2, a value associated with an increased risk of hemorrhage. He is taking no other medication that might interfere with plasma levels of warfarin. The physician advises Mr. H to stop taking warfarin for 2 days. After multiple attempts at adjusting his dose of warfarin, Mr. H eventually reaches a stable INR of 2.5 when taking 1 mg of warfarin each day.

QUESTIONS

■ **1.** What additional laboratory information could assist in anticoagulating this patient?

■ **2.** Would that information have helped in the selection of Mr. H's initial warfarin dose?

■ **3.** What molecular mechanisms could be responsible for the apparent sensitivity of this patient to warfarin?

PHYSIOLOGY

Three types of interindividual genetic variation can influence pharmacotherapy: variation in proteins involved in drug metabolism or transport (pharmacokinetic variation); variation in drug targets or pathways associated with those targets (pharmacodynamic variation); and genetic variation associated with idiosyncratic drug effects.

GENOMIC VARIATION AND PHARMACOGENOMICS

The human genome contains approximately three billion nucleotides. Current estimates are that the genome contains between 25,000 and 40,000 genes that, through alternative splicing and posttranslational modification, may encode 100,000 or more proteins. Any two people differ on average at about one nucleotide in every 1,000 in their genome, totaling an average interindividual difference of 3 million base pairs throughout the genome. The majority of these differences are so-called **single nucleotide polymorphisms** or **SNPs** (pronounced "snips"), in which one nucleotide is exchanged for another at a given position. SNPs and other differences in DNA sequence can occur anywhere in the genome, in both coding regions and noncoding regions. If a SNP changes the encoded amino acid, it is called a nonsynonymous coding SNP (cSNP). The remaining differences in DNA sequence involve insertions, deletions, duplications, and reshufflings, sometimes of just one or a few nucleotides but occasionally of whole genes or larger DNA segments that include many genes. Functionally significant DNA sequence differences tend to fall within genes, either within their coding sequences or in the promoters, enhancers, splice sites, or other sequences that control gene transcription or mRNA stability. Taken together, these differences constitute each person's genetic individuality. Some of that individuality affects the way in which each person will respond to drug treatment.

PHARMACOLOGY

The concept that inheritance might be an important determinant of individual variation in drug response emerged half

a century ago. It originally grew out of clinical observations of striking differences among patients in their response to "standard" doses of a drug. Those observations, in addition to twin and family studies that showed inherited variations in plasma drug concentrations and other pharmacokinetic parameters, led to the birth of pharmacogenetics. Many of those original examples of pharmacogenetic variation, and many of the most striking examples even today, involve *pharmacokinetics*—factors that influence the concentration of drug reaching its target(s). However, examples of pharmacogenetic variation in the drug target, so-called *pharmacodynamic factors,* are also being reported with increasing frequency.

VARIATION IN ENZYMES OF DRUG METABOLISM: PHARMACOKINETICS

Inherited variation in enzymes that catalyze drug metabolism is the most common factor responsible for pharmacogenetic variation in response to medications. The enzymes involved in drug metabolism are discussed in Chapter 4, Drug Metabolism. There are two broad categories of drug-metabolizing enzymes: those that catalyze phase I reactions (functionalization reactions that typically involve oxidation or reduction) and those that catalyze phase II reactions (typically, conjugation reactions that add groups, such as glucuronic acid, that enhance drug solubility and thus drug excretion). Phase I and phase II reactions do not necessarily occur in that order, and metabolic intermediates resulting from both types of reactions may be pharmacologically active. In fact, some medications are administered as inactive prodrugs that must undergo phase I and/or phase II metabolism before they can exert their pharmacologic effect.

Genetic polymorphisms are common in enzymes that catalyze drug metabolism, and clinically significant polymorphisms have been found in nearly all of the major enzymes involved in both phase I and phase II reactions (Table 52-1). Two "classic" examples are provided by the inherited variations in the enzymatic hydrolysis of the short-acting muscle relaxant succinylcholine by the enzyme butyrylcholinesterase (BChE) and the enzymatic acetylation of drugs such as the antituberculosis drug isoniazid (see Chapter 33, Pharmacology of Bacterial Infections: Cell Wall Synthesis). Patients with variations in BChE have a decreased rate of metabolism of acetylcholine and its analogues, resulting in prolonged paralysis after drug exposure. A genetically polymorphic phase II enzyme, N-acetyltransferase 2 (NAT2), catalyzes the acetylation of isoniazid. Patients treated with isoniazid can be classified as either "slow acetylators" who metabolize isoniazid slowly and have high blood drug levels, or "fast acetylators" who metabolize isoniazid rapidly and have low blood drug levels. Family studies have shown that the rate of isoniazid biotransformation is inherited. The slow-acetylator phenotype is associated with drug toxicities that result from excessive drug accumulation; examples include hydralazine- and procainamide-induced lupus and isoniazid-induced neurotoxicity. Although the antihypertensive agent hydralazine is rarely used today in the treatment of hypertension, this drug has recently re-emerged as one of the two active components in BiDil, a combination drug

TABLE 52-1	Examples of Genetic Polymorphisms and Drug Metabolism

ENZYME	AFFECTED DRUG, CLASS, OR COMPOUND
Phase I (Oxidation/Reduction) Enzyme	
CYP1A2	Acetaminophen, caffeine, propranolol
CYP1B1	Estrogens
CYP2A6	Halothane, nicotine
CYP2B6	Cyclophosphamide
CYP2C8	Paclitaxel, retinoic acid
CYP2C9	Nonsteroidal anti-inflammatory drugs, phenytoin, warfarin
CYP2C19	Omeprazole, phenytoin, propranolol
CYP2D6	Antidepressants, β-adrenergic antagonists, codeine, debrisoquine, dextromethorphan
CYP2E1	Acetaminophen, ethanol
CYP3A5	Calcium channel blockers, cyclosporine, dapsone, etoposide, lidocaine, lovastatin, macrolides, midazolam, quinidine, steroids, tacrolimus, tamoxifen
Phase II (Conjugation) Enzyme	
N-Acetyltransferase 1	Sulfamethoxazole
N-Acetyltransferase 2	Dapsone, hydralazine, isoniazid, procainamide, sulfonamides
Sulfotransferases (SULTs)	Acetaminophen, dopamine, epinephrine, estrogens
Catechol-O-methyltransferase	Catecholamines, levodopa, methyldopa
Histamine N-methyltransferase	Histamine
Thiopurine S-methyltransferase	Azathioprine, mercaptopurine, thioguanine
UDP-glucuronosyltransferases	Androgens, ibuprofen, irinotecan, morphine, naproxen

approved for the treatment of patients with symptomatic heart failure. It is of interest that the U. S. Food and Drug Administration (FDA) has approved BiDil for use only in patients of African ancestry, presumably because of an ethnically dependent genetic difference in response to this drug.

Early examples of pharmacogenetics, such as those represented by BChE and NAT2, served as a stimulus to search for additional examples. Most of the second-generation examples continue to be associated with pharmacokinetics and continue to be recognized from clinical observations—often from adverse drug responses. They have been studied most often either by administering a "probe drug" to a group of subjects and measuring plasma or urinary drug and/or metabolite concentrations, or by directly assaying a drug-metabolizing enzyme in an easily accessible tissue such as the red blood cell (e.g., a series of methyltransferase enzymes). Two prototypic examples that have become pharmacogenetic "icons" are the **cytochrome P450 2D6 (CYP2D6)** and **thiopurine S-methyltransferase (TPMT)** genetic polymorphisms. Because of the clinical implications of these polymorphisms, the FDA in its 2003 "Guidance on Pharmacogenomic Data" cited CYP2D6 and TPMT as examples of valid pharmacogenomic biomarkers.

CYP2D6 is a member of the cytochrome P450 (CYP) family of microsomal, phase I drug-metabolizing enzymes. CYP2D6 contributes to the metabolism of a large number of medications, including antidepressants, antiarrhythmics, and analgesics. The CYP2D6 polymorphism was originally described by two different laboratories studying two different probe drugs, the antihypertensive **debrisoquine** and the oxytotic agent **sparteine**. The frequency distribution of the debrisoquine urinary metabolic ratio, the ratio of the parent drug to its oxidized metabolite, is shown in Figure 52-1A for a Northern European population. Shown at the far right of the figure is a group of "poor metabolizers" of debrisoquine, subjects homozygous for recessive alleles (genes) coding for enzymes with decreased activity; shown in the middle is the large group of "extensive metabolizers," subjects heterozygous or homozygous for the "wild type" allele; and shown at the far left is a small subset of "ultrarapid metabolizers," some of whom have multiple copies of the CYP2D6 gene.

Several molecular genetic mechanisms are responsible for variation in CYP2D6 enzyme activity, including nonsynonymous cSNPs, gene deletion, and gene duplication; some ultrarapid metabolizers can have up to 13 copies of the gene. It has been estimated that 5% to 10% of Caucasians are CYP2D6 poor metabolizers. Among East Asians, in contrast, the poor-metabolizer phenotype is present at a frequency of just 1% to 2%. The ultrarapid metabolizer phenotype, rare in most Caucasian populations, has a frequency of 3% in Spaniards and up to 13% in Ethiopians. These ethnic differences have potentially important medical implications, because CYP2D6 metabolizes many commonly prescribed medications, including the β-adrenergic blocker **metoprolol**, the neuroleptic **haloperidol**, the opioids **codeine** and **dextromethorphan**, and the antidepressants **fluoxetine**, **imipramine**, and **desipramine**, among many others (Table 52-1). Therefore, poor metabolizers for CYP2D6 can potentially experience an adverse drug effect when treated with standard doses of agents such as metoprolol that are inactivated by CYP2D6, whereas codeine is relatively ineffective in poor metabolizers because it requires CYP2D6-catalyzed metabolism to form the more potent opioid morphine. Conversely, ultrarapid metabolizers may require unu-

A   CYP2D6 pharmacogenetics

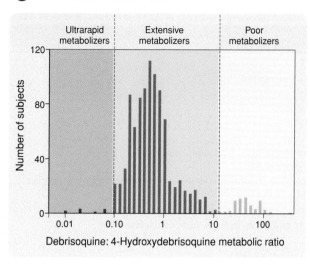

B   AmpliChip CYP450 array

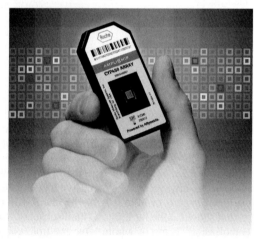

Figure 52-1.   CYP2D6 pharmacogenetics. **A.** Frequency distribution of the metabolic ratio for the cytochrome P450 2D6 (CYP2D6)-catalyzed metabolism of debrisoquine to form its 4-hydroxy metabolite. Data for 1,011 Swedish subjects are plotted as the ratio of metabolites in the urine. Most subjects metabolize debrisoquine extensively, while some subjects metabolize the compound ultrarapidly and others metabolize the compound poorly. **B.** The AmpliChip CYP450 array can be used to determine variant genotypes for cytochrome P450 genes that influence drug metabolism.

sually high doses of drugs that are inactivated by CYP2D6, but those same subjects can be "overdosed" with codeine, suffering respiratory depression or even respiratory arrest in response to "standard" doses. In the past, an individual's genotype for CYP2D6 and many other genes encoding drug-metabolizing enzymes was inferred from phenotype, e.g., the urinary metabolic ratio that can be measured by assaying the urinary excretion of a specific metabolite after the administration of a probe drug (Fig. 52-1A). As discussed below, genotype assignment is now increasingly dependent on DNA-based tests performed with devices such as the "chip" shown in Figure 52-1B.

Thiopurine S-methyltransferase (TPMT) represents another example of an important and clinically relevant genetic polymorphism for drug metabolism. This example has also served as an important pharmacogenetic model system. TPMT catalyzes the S-methylation of thiopurine drugs such as **6-mercaptopurine** and **azathioprine** (Chapter 37, Pharmacology of Cancer: Genome Synthesis, Stability, and Maintenance). Among other indications, these cytotoxic and immunosuppressive agents are used to treat acute lymphoblastic leukemia of childhood and inflammatory bowel disease. Although thiopurines are useful drugs, they have a narrow therapeutic index, i.e., the difference between the toxic and therapeutic dose is small, with occasional patients suffering from life-threatening thiopurine-induced myelosuppression.

In Caucasians, the most common variant allele for TPMT is *TPMT*3A*; the gene frequency is approximately 5%, so 1 in 300 subjects carries two copies of the TPMT*3A allele. TPMT*3A is predominantly responsible for the trimodal frequency distribution of the level of red blood cell TPMT activity shown in Figure 52-2. TPMT*3A has two nonsynonymous cSNPs, one in exon 7 and another in exon 10 (Fig. 52-2). The presence of TPMT*3A results in a striking decrease in tissue levels of TPMT protein. Mechanisms responsible for the observed decrease in TPMT*3A protein level

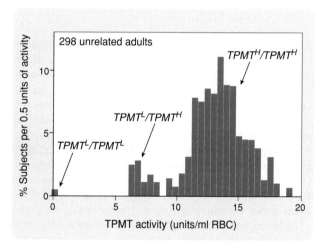

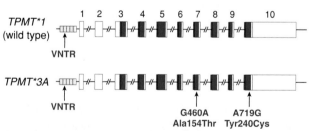

Figure 52-2.   TPMT pharmacogenetics. Frequency distribution of red blood cell (RBC) thiopurine S-methyltransferase (TPMT) activity for 298 unrelated Caucasian subjects. *TPMT^L* indicates an allele or alleles for the trait of low activity, while *TPMT^H* refers to the "wild type" (*TMPT*1*) allele for high activity. The observed trimodal frequency distribution for RBC TPMT activity is due mainly to the effect of *TPMT*3A*, the most common variant allele for low activity in a Caucasian population. *TMPT*1* and *TPMT*3A* differ by two nonsynonymous single nucleotide polymorphisms (SNPs), one in exon 7 and one in exon 10.

include both accelerated TPMT*3A degradation and intracellular TPMT*3A aggregation, probably as a result of protein misfolding. As a result, drugs such as 6-MP are poorly metabolized and may reach toxic levels. *Subjects homozygous for TPMT*3A are at greatly increased risk for life-threatening myelosuppression when treated with standard doses of thiopurine drugs.* These patients have to be treated with approximately one-tenth to one-fifteenth the standard dose. There are striking ethnic differences in the frequency of variant alleles for TPMT. For example, TPMT*3A is rarely observed in East Asian populations, while *TPMT*3C*, which has only the exon 10 SNP, is the most common variant allele in those populations.

Because of its clinical significance, TPMT was the first example selected by the FDA for public hearings on the inclusion of pharmacogenetic information in drug labeling. For the same reason, clinical testing for TPMT genetic polymorphisms is widely available. The phenomenon of marked changes in the level of a protein as a result of the alteration of only one or two amino acids in the protein has been observed repeatedly for many other genes of pharmacogenetic significance and is a common explanation for the functional effects of nonsynonymous cSNPs.

The BChE, NAT2, CYP2D6, and TPMT genetic polymorphisms all behave as monogenic (single-gene) Mendelian traits, as do many other early examples from pharmacogenetics. However, pharmacogenetics-pharmacogenomics has now moved beyond monogenic pharmacokinetic traits, and the focus increasingly involves functionally and clinically significant variation in drug targets as well as drug-metabolizing enzymes. Variation can also involve multiple genes that influence both pharmacokinetics and pharmacodynamics.

VARIATION IN DRUG TARGETS: PHARMACODYNAMICS

Drugs generally exert their effects by interacting with specific target proteins. Therefore, genetic variations in these target proteins, or in signaling pathways downstream from the target proteins, can influence the outcome of pharmacotherapy (Table 52-2). Furthermore, variation in drug targets can occur either as a result of variation in germ-line DNA or, in the case of cancer, through variation in somatic DNA present in the tumor. One example of genetic variation for a drug target in germ-line DNA involves a class of drugs that is used to treat asthma. As noted in Chapter 46, Integrative Inflammation Pharmacology: Asthma, the antiasthma medication **zileuton** decreases airway inflammation by inhibiting the enzyme **5-lipoxygenase,** an enzyme encoded by the gene *ALOX5*. Variations in 5-lipoxygenase illustrate the point that variation in many areas of a gene can affect protein function. The functional significance of nonsynonymous cSNPs—and their ability to alter the amount of protein expressed—was highlighted in the previous section on TPMT pharmacogenetics. In addition, however, polymorphisms in regulatory regions, such as the gene promoter, can influence transcription and thereby alter protein expression. The promoter of the *ALOX5* gene displays variation in the number of tandem repeats of the sequence GGGCGG. These repeat sequences bind the transcription factor complex Sp1, which up-regulates *ALOX5* transcription.

The most common *ALOX5* allele contains five repeats and is present in about 77% of *ALOX5* genes. As a result, approximately 94% of the population has at least one copy of the five-repeat allele. The most common variant alleles contain four and three repeats and are present at frequencies of about 17% and 4%, respectively. Because of increased Sp1 binding, people who carry the five-repeat allele are thought to express more 5-lipoxygenase than those who lack it. Interestingly, there seems to be no relationship between the presence or absence of the five-repeat allele and the severity of asthma in the population; i.e., this *ALOX5* promoter polymorphism does not seem to affect the disease process itself. However, in trials of a 5-lipoxygenase inhibitor related to zileuton, only subjects who had at least one copy of the five-repeat allele responded to the drug. This result suggests that zileuton-like compounds are unlikely to help the 6% of the population who lack the five-repeat allele, and that identifying this subgroup would allow the use of alternative, more effective, medications. *This example also illustrates an important principle, that a polymorphism need not cause a disease to influence the treatment of that disease.*

An example of genetic variation in a drug target in somatic (tumor) DNA involves gain-of-function mutations in the gene encoding the **epidermal growth factor receptor (EGFR)** (also known as *HER1* or *ErbB1*) in patients with nonsmall cell lung cancer (NSCLC). Two groups reported in 2004 that, in patients with NSCLC, response to the EGFR inhibitor **gefitinib** was influenced strongly by these somatic DNA mutations, i.e., subjects with sequence variation in the portion of the gene encoding the ATP binding site of this receptor tyrosine kinase responded more favorably to gefitinib therapy than did patients without such mutations.

TABLE 52-2	Examples of Genetic Polymorphisms and Drug Targets
PROTEIN	**AFFECTED DRUG CLASS (EXAMPLE)**
5-Lipoxygenase	Zileuton
Angiotensin-converting enzyme (ACE)	ACE inhibitors (lisinopril)
Apolipoprotein E	Statins (pravastatin)
β₂-Adrenergic receptor	β-Adrenergic agonists (albuterol)
Epidermal growth factor receptor	Gefitinib
Sulfonylurea receptor	Tolbutamide
Vitamin K epoxide reductase complex 1	Warfarin

EGFR is often overexpressed in these tumors, and several drugs targeting this receptor have been tested clinically. It was already known that NSCLC patients of East Asian origin responded more favorably to gefitinib therapy than Caucasian patients did, and one of the two original studies reported that somatic mutations in *EGFR* occurred in 15 of 58 randomly selected tumors obtained from patients in Japan but in only 1 of 61 from the United States—illustrating, once again, striking ethnic differences in pharmacogenetic effects. The example provided by gefitinib may represent the future of oncology, where both somatic and germ-line mutations/polymorphisms may be considered prior to initiating a therapeutic program. This example and the *ALOX5* example also demonstrate that pharmacodynamic-pharmacogenetic variation (i.e., variation in genes encoding drug targets) can be just as important, if not more important, than the pharmacokinetic-pharmacogenetic variation represented by CYP2D6 and TPMT. Table 52-2 lists several polymorphisms in genes encoding drug target proteins that have been associated with variation in drug response.

PATHWAY-BASED PHARMACOGENETICS-PHARMACOGENOMICS

The preceding examples, *CYP2D6*, *TPMT*, *ALOX5*, and *EGFR*, all involve clinically significant pharmacogenetic variation as a result of sequence variation in a single gene, i.e., monogenic inheritance. Figure 52-3 illustrates this pharmacokinetic-pharmacodynamic pharmacogenomic dichotomy, using the four major examples cited in this chapter. However, it is also possible for multiple genes encoding proteins that influence both pharmacokinetics and pharmacodynamics to alter the drug response phenotype.

One good example is provided by the anticoagulant warfarin. Warfarin (see Chapter 22, Pharmacology of Hemostasis and Thrombosis) is one of the most widely prescribed oral anticoagulants in both North America and Europe. However, in spite of the existence of a laboratory test that is used universally to follow warfarin's effect on coagulation (INR), serious adverse reactions—involving both hemorrhage and undesired thrombosis—continue to complicate warfarin therapy. These complications are illustrated by the case of Mr. H at the beginning of this chapter: after a "standard" dose of warfarin, his INR was elevated to 6.2, a level associated with increased risk for hemorrhage.

Why might that have occurred? First, we need to remember that warfarin is a racemic mixture. S-warfarin is three to five times more potent than R-warfarin, and S-warfarin is metabolized predominantly by the cytochrome P450 isoform **CYP2C9**. CYP2C9 is a highly polymorphic gene, and the variant alleles *CYP2C9*2* (Arg144Cys) and *CYP2C9*3* (Ile358Leu) are associated with only 12% and 5%, respectively, of the level of enzyme activity observed with the wild-type allele (*CYP2C9*1*). Patients who carry these variant alleles require decreased doses of warfarin to achieve an anticoagulant effect, and these same subjects have increased risk for hemorrhage during warfarin therapy. However, this pharmacokinetic-pharmacogenetic variation fails to explain most of the variance in the therapeutic warfarin dose in patients who are anticoagulated with this powerful, but potentially dangerous, drug.

The molecular target for warfarin was not identified until 2004. The gene encoding that target, **vitamin K epoxide reductase complex 1, *VKORC1***, was also cloned that year. When the *VKORC1* gene was sequenced in a number of patients, although no nonsynonymous cSNPs were found, a series of haplotypes (combinations of SNPs on a single chromosome) was observed that were associated with warfarin dose requirement. In one study, patients with *VKOCR1* haplotypes that were associated with a low dose requirement had an average warfarin maintenance dose approximately half of that required by subjects with haplotypes associated with a high dose requirement. Several subsequent studies have confirmed that *VKORC1* haplotype is associated with approximately 25% to 30% of the variance in warfarin maintenance dose, while 5% to 15% can be explained by *CYP2C9* genotype. The roles of CYP2C9 and VKORC1 in warfarin pharmacokinetics and pharmacodynamics are shown schematically in Figure 52-4. Because the genes encoding both of these proteins contribute to variation in drug response, genotyping for *CYP2C9* as well as haplotyping for *VKORC1* could represent a useful strategy for the determination of an initial warfarin dose for Mr. H.

Warfarin provides a striking example of a situation in which pharmacokinetic-pharmacogenetic data proved inadequate for clinical translation because those data explained too little of the variation in therapeutic drug dose. However, when *CYP2C9* polymorphisms and *VKORC1* haplotypes were both determined, it became possible to assess genetic variation both in drug metabolism and in the drug target, and to move beyond the monogenic pharmacogenetics represented by NAT2, CYP2D6, and TPMT. Therefore, warfarin represents, probably in a simplified form, the type of polygenic, pathway-based pharmacogenetic-pharmacogenomic model that may become increasingly common in the future.

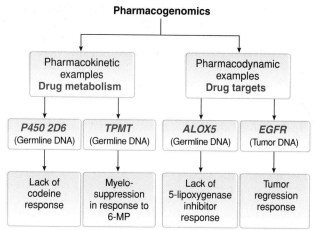

Figure 52-3. Pharmacokinetic and pharmacodynamic pharmacogenomics. The figure depicts the major pharmacokinetic (drug metabolism) and pharmacodynamic (drug target) examples described in this chapter. Shown are the affected gene (in italics), whether germ-line or somatic (e.g., tumor) DNA is involved, and the clinical response observed in the presence of the variant allele(s). *P450 2D6*, cytochrome P450 2D6 gene; *TPMT*, thiopurine S-methyltransferase gene; *ALOX5*, 5-lipoxygenase gene; *EGFR*, epidermal growth factor receptor gene; 6-MP, 6-mercaptopurine.

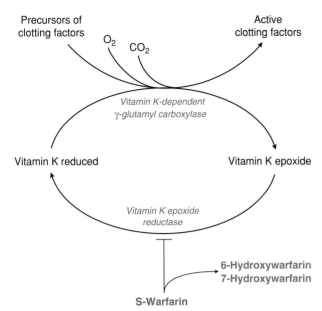

Figure 52-4. Warfarin pharmacokinetics and pharmacodynamics. Vitamin K is a required cofactor for the posttranslational γ-carboxylation of glutamate residues in certain clotting factor precursors (see Chapter 22). Vitamin K is oxidized to the inactive epoxide as a consequence of the carboxylation reaction. The enzyme vitamin K epoxide reductase (VKORC1) converts the inactive epoxide into the active, reduced form of vitamin K. Warfarin acts as an anticoagulant by inhibiting VKORC1 and thereby preventing the regeneration of reduced vitamin K. S-warfarin is metabolized to 6-hydroxywarfarin and 7-hydroxywarfarin by cytochrome P450 2C9.

IDIOSYNCRATIC DRUG REACTIONS

An additional way in which genetic variation might influence pharmacotherapy involves idiosyncratic drug reactions. These effects differ from the other examples described in this chapter in that they are not known to be caused by differences in either drug metabolism or drug targets. Instead, idiosyncratic effects seem to result from interactions between the medication and a unique aspect of the physiology of the individual patient. A "classic" example illustrating this least predictable effect of interindividual genetic variation is represented by idiosyncratic drug reactions associated with functional deficiency of the enzyme **glucose 6-phosphate dehydrogenase** (G6PD; see Chapter 35, Pharmacology of Parasitic Infections). This enzyme is involved in protecting red blood cells from oxidative injury. A number of polymorphisms result in this condition. The most common involves a cSNP that causes an amino acid substitution, resulting in a 90% to 95% reduction of G6PD enzyme function. That allele, A^-, is present in 10% to 20% of Africans and is thought to provide protection against malaria. A different G6PD-inactivating polymorphism is found at lower frequency among subjects of Mediterranean, Middle Eastern, Indian, and Southeast Asian descent, and a third polymorphism is also present in Southeast Asia. A number of medications cause oxidative stress on red blood cells as an effect unrelated to their intended targets or their metabolic clearance. These drugs include sulfonamides, antimalarials, and the analgesic agents acetaminophen and ibuprofen, among others. Individuals with G6PD deficiency who are exposed

to these medications may develop acute and, at times, severe hemolytic anemia.

By definition, idiosyncratic effects are difficult or impossible to predict. However, information emerging from genomic, proteomic, and metabolomic research may prove useful in the future in the development of pharmacogenomic screens for unanticipated drug interactions. At present, unfortunately, idiosyncratic effects cannot be predicted.

MODERN PHARMACOGENETICS-PHARMACOGENOMICS

Completion of the Human Genome Project and the ongoing refinement of the HapMap project point the way to future developments in pharmacogenetics and pharmacogenomics in this "post-genomic" era. Application of modern genomic assay techniques, when combined with an increasing focus on pharmacokinetic pathways—pathways that encompass genes encoding all of the drug-metabolizing enzymes and transporters that could influence the final concentration of drug reaching the target—together with pharmacodynamic pathways that include the drug target and signaling pathways downstream from that target, may represent the future for this aspect of "individualized medicine." To attain the goal of truly personalized drug therapy, and to translate genomic knowledge fully into clinical practice, will require the clinical application of high-throughput genotyping technologies. Numerous platforms for genotyping have been developed and refined, and new ones are being developed. As an example, the CYP450 gene chip shown in Figure 52-1B has already been introduced into clinical practice. To apply genotype information to select responsive patients, and then to treat these patients pharmacologically on the basis of genotype, will require a comprehensive knowledge of genotype-phenotype correlations.

However, to achieve truly individualized drug therapy, we need not only to understand the science underlying pharmacogenetics and pharmacogenomics and to develop state-of-the-art technologies to detect and assay DNA sequence data, but also to translate that knowledge into the clinic. That translation process will require active involvement of the FDA and the pharmaceutical industry, which develops virtually all new drugs. In 2003 the FDA issued a Draft Guidance with regard to pharmacogenomic data, and this draft was approved in 2005. The FDA also initiated a series of public hearings with regard to the incorporation of pharmacogenomic data into drug labeling. These hearings began with thiopurine drugs and TPMT, and were followed by hearings on a genetic polymorphism in *UGT1A1*, a gene encoding a phase II enzyme involved in the biotransformation of the antineoplastic agent irinotecan. Public hearings have recently been held on *CYP2C9*, *VKORC1*, and warfarin.

The attention given to pharmacogenetics-pharmacogenomics by the FDA is having an impact on the pharmaceutical industry, especially within the context of the unfortunate series of events that resulted in the withdrawal of the COX-2 inhibitor rofecoxib (Vioxx) from the market for reasons of safety. It is unclear whether pharmacogenetics played a role in the Vioxx-induced cardiovascular disease that led to the withdrawal of that drug. However, pharmacogenetics almost certainly could contribute to postmarketing surveillance, not only to help avoid adverse reactions, but also to help "rescue" drugs that might be of benefit to groups of patients selected on the basis of genetic variation in drug response. The latter situation was recently highlighted when a polymorphism in the β_1 adrenoceptor was shown to influence response to the β_1-adrenergic antagonist bucindolol—both in vitro and in patients with heart failure. This β-antagonist had initially failed in a clinical trial that did not include genotyping, probably because only patients with the wild type β_1-adrenoceptor genotype had the desired clinical response.

Conclusion and Future Directions

Pharmacogenetics and pharmacogenomics involve the study of ways in which gene sequence variation affects the response of individual patients to medications. The goal of pharmacogenetics and pharmacogenomics is to maximize efficacy and minimize toxicity, based on knowledge of an individual's genetic composition. Although many factors other than inheritance influence differences among patients in their response to drugs, the past half-century has demonstrated that genetics is an important factor responsible for variation in the occurrence of adverse drug reactions or the failure of individual patients to achieve the desired therapeutic response. Pharmacogenetics has evolved during that half-century from classical examples, such as CYP2D6 and TPMT, to include more complex situations such as that represented by warfarin pharmacogenetics, involving both pharmacokinetic and pharmacodynamic pharmacogenetic variation. This area of genomic medical science also presents unique challenges in its translation into the clinic. However,

there can no longer be any doubt that pharmacogenetics will be applied to clinical medicine with increasing breadth and depth, and that, ultimately, it will enhance our ability to individualize drug therapy.

Suggested Reading

Broder S, Venter JC. Sequencing the entire genomes of free-living organisms: the foundation of pharmacology in the new millennium. *Ann Rev Pharmacol Toxicol* 2000;40:97–132. *(Overview of genome sequencing and a primer on the possible implications of genetic diversity for pharmacology.)*

Drazen JM, Yandava CN, Dube L, et al. Pharmacogenetic association between *ALOX5* promoter genotype and the response to anti-asthma treatment. *Nat Med* 1999;22:168–171. *(Original study that showed different pharmacologic responses in people with different polymorphisms of the ALOX5 gene.)*

Evans WE, McLeod HL. Pharmacogenomics—drug disposition, drug targets, and side effects. *N Engl J Med* 2003;348:538–549. *(Review describing the integration of genomics with pharmacogenetics.)*

Rieder MJ, Reiner AP, Gage BF, et al. Effect of *VKORC1* haplotypes on transcriptional regulation and warfarin dose. *N Engl J Med* 2005;352:2285–2293. *(Description of VKORC1 haplotypes, CYP2C9 genotypes, and their relationship to warfarin dose.)*

Wang L, Weinshilboum R. Thiopurine S-methyltransferase pharmacogenetics: insights, challenges and future directions. *Oncogene* 2006;25:1629–1638. *(Overview of the scientific development of a "classic" pharmacogenomic trait, with an emphasis on mechanisms linking genotype to phenotype.)*

Weinshilboum RM, Wang L. Pharmacogenetics and pharmacogenomics: development, science and translation. *Annu Rev Genomics Hum Genet* 2006;7:223–245. *(Review of pharmacokinetic and pharmacodynamic pharmacogenomic variation, as well as challenges to the translation of this science into the clinic.)*

53

Protein-Based Therapies

Benjamin Leader and David E. Golan

INTRODUCTION

More than any other class of macromolecules in the human body, proteins play dynamic and diverse roles. Proteins catalyze biochemical reactions, form receptors and channels in membranes, provide intracellular and extracellular scaffolding support, and transport molecules within a cell or from one organ to another. Over the past 40 years, scientists have not only deciphered the genetic code—the blueprint for protein production—but have also determined the complete genetic sequence for many organisms including humans. It is currently estimated that there are 25,000 to 40,000 different genes in the human genome, and, with alternative splicing of genes and posttranslational modification of proteins (e.g., by cleavage, phosphorylation, acylation, and glycosylation), the number of functionally distinct proteins is likely to be much higher. Viewed from the perspective of disease mechanisms, these estimates pose an immense challenge to modern medicine, as disease may result when any one of these proteins contains mutations or other abnormalities or is present in an abnormally high or low concentration. Viewed from the perspective of therapeutics, however, these estimates represent a tremendous opportunity to harness protein-based therapies to alleviate disease. At present, more than 70 different proteins or peptides are approved for clinical use by the U. S. Food and Drug Administration (FDA), and many more are in development.

Protein-based therapeutics have several advantages over small-molecule drugs (SMDs). First, proteins often serve a highly specific and complex set of functions that cannot be mimicked by chemical compounds. Second, because the action of proteins is highly specific, there is often less potential for protein-based drugs to interfere with normal biological processes and cause adverse effects. Third, because the body naturally produces many of the proteins that are used as therapies, such drugs are often well tolerated and are less likely to elicit immune responses. Fourth, for diseases in which a gene is mutated or deleted, protein-based therapies can provide effective replacement treatment without the need for gene therapy, which is not currently available for most genetic disorders. Fifth, the clinical development and FDA approval time of protein therapies may be faster than that of SMDs; a study published in 2003 showed that the average clinical development and approval time was more than 1 year faster for 33 protein therapies approved between 1980 and 2002 than for 294 SMDs approved during the same time period. Finally, because proteins are unique in form and function, pharmaceutical companies are able to obtain far-reaching patent protection for protein therapeutics. The last two advantages make proteins attractive from a financial perspective compared to chemical compounds, which can frequently be copied with slight modifications that circumvent patent protection and may take longer to obtain regulatory approval.

Modern protein therapeutics are purified from a wide variety of different organisms and increasingly are produced by genetic engineering using recombinant DNA technology.

Nonrecombinant proteins are purified from their native source, such as **pancreatic enzymes** from hog and pig pancreas and **alpha-1-proteinase inhibitor** from pooled human plasma. Production systems for recombinant proteins include bacteria, yeast, insect cells, mammalian cells, and transgenic animals and plants. The system of choice can be dictated by the cost of production or the modifications of the protein (e.g., glycosylation, phosphorylation, or proteolytic cleavage) that are required for biological activity. For example, bacteria do not perform glycosylation reactions, and each of the other biological systems listed previously produces a different type or pattern of glycosylation. Protein glycosylation patterns exert dramatic effects on the activity, half-life, and immunogenicity of the recombinant protein in the body. As one example, the half-life of native erythropoietin, a growth factor important in erythrocyte production (see below), can be lengthened by increasing the glycosylation of the protein. **Darbepoetin** is an erythropoietin analogue engineered to contain two additional amino acids that are substrates for N-linked glycosylation reactions. When expressed in Chinese hamster ovary (CHO) cells, the analogue is synthesized with five rather than three N-linked carbohydrate chains; this modification causes the half-life of darbepoetin to be threefold longer than that of erythropoietin.

Recombinantly produced proteins have all the advantages of nonrecombinant proteins, with the following additional benefits. First, transcription and translation of the exact human gene lead to a higher specific activity of the protein and a decreased chance of immunologic rejection by the patient (see the example below of bovine insulin compared to recombinant human insulin). Second, recombinant proteins are often produced more efficiently and inexpensively and in potentially limitless quantity. One striking example is found in the protein-based therapy for Gaucher's disease, a chronic congenital disorder of lipid metabolism caused by a deficiency of the enzyme beta-glucocerebrosidase. Most patients with this disease have an enlarged liver and spleen, increased skin pigmentation, and painful bone lesions. Although patients can be treated with **beta-glucocerebrosidase** purified from human placenta, this treatment requires purification of protein from 50,000 placentas per patient per year. This requirement obviously places a practical limit on the amount of purified protein available for patients with the disease. A recombinant (although extremely expensive) form of beta-glucocerebrosidase is now available. The recombinant protein is not only available in sufficient quantities to treat many more patients with the disease, but it also eliminates the risk of transmissible (e.g., viral or prion) diseases associated with purifying the protein from human placentas. This illustrates the third benefit of recombinant proteins over nonrecombinant proteins, which is the reduction of exposure to animal or human diseases. A fourth advantage is that recombinant technology allows the modification of a protein to improve function or specificity. Again, recombinant beta-glucocerebrosidase provides an interesting example. When this protein is made recombinantly, a change of amino acid arginine-495 to histidine allows the addition of mannose residues to the protein. The mannose is recognized by endocytic carbohydrate receptors on macrophages and many other cell types, allowing the enzyme to enter these cells more efficiently and to cleave the intracellular lipid that has accumulated in pathologic amounts. This results in an improved therapeutic outcome.

Perhaps the best example of how protein therapies are both produced and used therapeutically is provided by the history of **insulin** in the treatment of diabetes mellitus type I (DM-I) and type II (DM-II). Untreated, DM-I is a disease that leads to severe wasting and death due to lack of the protein hormone, insulin, which signals cells to perform a number of functions related to glucose homeostasis and intermediary metabolism. In 1922, insulin was first purified from bovine and porcine pancreas and used as a lifesaving daily injection in patients with DM-I. At least three challenges prevented widespread use of this protein therapy: (1) increasing the availability of animal pancreas for purification of insulin; (2) reducing the cost of insulin purification from animal pancreas; and (3) overcoming the immunologic reaction of some patients to animal insulin. These problems were addressed by isolating the human insulin gene, "recombining" the gene with bacterial DNA, and engineering *Escherichia coli* using this recombinant DNA technology to express human insulin. By growing vast quantities of these bacteria, large-scale production of human insulin was achieved. The resulting insulin was abundant, inexpensive, of low immunogenicity, and free from other animal pancreatic substances. Recombinant insulin was the first commercially available recombinant protein therapeutic; it was approved by the US FDA in 1982, and has been the major therapy for DM-I (and a major therapy for DM-II) ever since.

The 25 years since the approval of insulin by the FDA have seen a remarkable expansion of proteins in the pharmacologic armamentarium used by physicians to treat disease. As noted previously, more than 70 different proteins (over 40 of which are produced recombinantly) are currently approved by the FDA for clinical use. Protein-based therapies are, and will continue to be, a mainstay in treating human disease.

Case

M. R. is a 55-year-old traveling salesman who presents to the emergency department of a small rural hospital with left chest pain and lightheadedness. The pain started suddenly 1 hour ago when he was carrying a large box. At first M. R. felt as if he was going to pass out, but the pain and lightheadedness improved at rest and eventually resolved after 20 minutes. M. R. denies any other symptoms, and he has no history of medical problems. He takes no medications, he is not a smoker, and his father died unexpectedly in a car accident at age 53. On physical exam, M. R. is afebrile with heart rate 100 beats/min, blood pressure 150/90 mm Hg, and respiratory rate 16 breaths/min. His pulse-oximeter displays 96% on a nasal cannula with oxygen flowing at 2 liters per minute. He appears to be comfortable and the remainder of his physical exam is notable only for an S4 heart sound. There is no evidence of fecal occult blood. His ECG demonstrates sinus tachycardia with no ST segment elevation. His chest x-ray is normal. His STAT chemistry panel shows normal sodium, potassium, chloride, bicarbonate, blood urea nitrogen (BUN), and creatinine levels. Cardiac biomarkers and coagulation studies are pending. M. R. is given aspirin, metoprolol, and sublingual nitroglycerin upon his arrival in the emergency department.

On admission to hospital, M. R.'s troponin T returns at 1.34 ng/mL (normal, 0 to 0.1 ng/mL), and he develops 2-mm ST segment depression in leads V1–V3 when he has chest pain. At this time, he is also given heparin, abciximab, and clopidogrel, and his chest pain resolves. His clinical course is stable overnight.

The next day, however, M. R. develops crushing substernal chest pain and diaphoresis, and his ECG shows 4-mm ST segment elevation in leads V2–V4. Because cardiac catheterization is not available at the regional cardiac center for at least 4 hours, M. R. is given tenecteplase in the coronary care unit, and his aspirin, metoprolol, nitroglycerin, heparin, and clopidogrel are continued. He stabilizes on this regimen.

After an otherwise uneventful 5-day hospitalization, M. R. is transferred to the regional cardiac center for catheterization, with a diagnosis of unstable angina that evolved into an ST elevation myocardial infarction. Outpatient plans include cardiac rehabilitation and treatment with aspirin, metoprolol, enalapril, spironolactone, and sublingual nitroglycerin as needed.

QUESTIONS

- ■ **1.** By what mechanism does abciximab act?
- ■ **2.** How could abciximab augment the function of clopidogrel and aspirin in this case?
- ■ **3.** By what mechanism does tenecteplase act?
- ■ **4.** How does the action of tenecteplase differ from that of heparin?

USES OF PROTEINS IN MEDICINE

Proteins from both recombinant and nonrecombinant sources are employed in a wide variety of medical applications, ranging from alleviating mild digestive ailments to correcting lethal protein deficiencies to diagnosing infectious diseases. *An appreciation of the many therapeutic uses of proteins may be gained by categorizing such therapies according to their mechanism of action* (Table 53-1; see also an expanded version of this table at the end of the chapter). A few of these proteins can be used clinically in more than one application; such proteins may therefore fall into more than one category.

GROUP I: PROTEIN THERAPEUTICS WITH ENZYMATIC OR REGULATORY ACTIVITY

Proteins in this category function via a classic paradigm in which a specific endogenous protein is deficient, and the deficit is then remedied by therapy with exogenous protein. *Group Ia* proteins are used to replace a particular activity in cases of protein deficiency or abnormal protein production. These proteins are used in a range of conditions, from providing **lactase** in patients lacking this gastrointestinal en-

zyme to replacing vital blood clotting factors such as **factor VIII** and **factor IX** in hemophiliacs. A classic example, as mentioned above, is the use of **insulin** for the treatment of diabetes. Another important example is the treatment of cystic fibrosis, the most common lethal genetic disorder. In this disease, defects in the chloride channel encoded by the *cftr* gene lead to abnormally thick secretions, which can (among other effects) block pancreatic enzymes from traveling down the pancreatic duct into the duodenum. This prevents food from being properly digested and results in malnutrition. Patients with cystic fibrosis are often treated with a combination of **pancreatic enzymes** isolated from pigs—including lipases, amylases, and proteases—that allow for digestion of lipids, sugars, and proteins. Patients who have had their pancreas removed or who suffer from chronic pancreatitis can benefit from this therapy as well. Other striking examples include the treatment of Gaucher's disease with **Cerezyme** or **Ceredase**, mucopolysaccharidosis I with **laronidase**, Fabry disease with **agalsidase beta**, congenital alpha-1-antitrypsin deficiency with **alpha-1-proteinase inhibitor**, and severe combined immunodeficiency (SCID) with **adenosine deaminase**. **Pooled immunoglobulins** are used to treat patients with primary immunodeficiencies.

It may sometimes be desirable to augment the activity of a particular plasma protein that is present in normal amounts. *Group Ib* proteins are administered to enhance the magnitude or timing of a particular protein activity. Recombinant proteins in this category have been immensely successful in treating hematopoietic defects. The most prominent example is recombinant **erythropoietin**, a protein hormone secreted by the kidney that stimulates erythrocyte production in the bone marrow. In patients with chemotherapy-induced anemia or myelodysplastic syndrome, recombinant erythropoietin is used to increase erythrocyte production and thereby ameliorate the anemia. In patients with chronic kidney disease, whose levels of endogenous erythropoietin are below normal, recombinant protein is administered to correct this deficiency. **Darbepoetin alfa** is a recombinant variant of erythropoietin with a longer half-life (see Introduction). Neutropenic patients can be treated with **granulocyte** or **granulocyte-monocyte colony stimulating factor (G-CSF or GM-CSF,** respectively), which stimulate an increase in the number of neutrophils produced by the bone marrow to allow these patients to better combat microbial infections. Similarly, thrombocytopenic patients can be treated with **interleukin-11** (IL-11), which increases platelet production and thereby prevents bleeding complications.

In vitro fertilization (IVF) and immunoregulation are two other active areas for the application of *Group Ib* proteins. Increased levels of **follicle stimulating hormone (FSH)** are normally produced by the anterior pituitary gland just prior to ovulation. These high levels of FSH can be augmented by treatment with recombinant FSH, leading to maturation of an increased number of follicles and to an increased number of oocytes available for IVF. Similarly, recombinant **human chorionic gonadotropin (hCG)** is employed in assisted reproductive technology to promote follicle rupture, a process that must occur before the oocytes can be transported into the fallopian tubes for fertilization. A much larger array of protein therapies has been developed and is in active use for purposes of immunoregulation. Chronic hepatitis B

TABLE 53-1 — A Functional Classification of Protein-Based Therapies

Group I: Protein Therapeutics with Enzymatic or Regulatory Activity

Ia: Replacing a protein that is deficient or abnormal

Factor VIII	Beta-glucocerebrosidase	Pancreatic enzymes (lipase, amylase, protease)
Factor IX	Laronidase	
Insulin	Agalsidase beta	Lactase
Insulin analogues (lispro, aspart, glargine)	Alpha-1-proteinase inhibitor	Adenosine deaminase
Growth hormone (GH)		Pooled immunoglobulins

Ib: Augmenting an existing pathway

Erythropoietin	Type I alpha-interferon	Tissue plasminogen activator (tPA), alteplase
Darbepoetin alfa	Interferon alpha-2a (IFNα-2a)	
Granulocyte colony stimulating factor (G-CSF)	Peginterferon alfa-2a	Reteplase (deletion mutein of plasminogen activator (rPA)
Granulocyte-macrophage colony stimulating factor (GM-CSF)	Interferon alfa-2b (IFNα-2b)	Tenecteplase
	Peginterferon alfa-2b	Factor VIIa
Interleukin-11 (IL-11)	Interferon beta-1a (rIFN-β)	Drotrecogin alfa (activated protein C)
Human follicle stimulating hormone (FSH)	Interferon beta-1b (rIFN-β)	Teriparatide (human parathyroid hormone 1-34)
	IFN-gamma	Exenatide
Human chorionic gonadotropin (HCG)	Interleukin-2 (IL-2), epidermal thymocyte activating factor (ETAF), aldesleukin	Platelet-derived growth factor (PDGF)
		Trypsin
		Nesiritide

Ic: Providing a novel function or activity

Papain	L-asparaginase	Lepirudin
Collagenase	PEG-asparaginase	Streptokinase
Dornase alfa, human deoxyribonuclease I		Etanercept

Group II: Protein Therapeutics with Special Targeting Activity

IIa: Interfering with a molecule or organism by binding to it and thereby blocking its function or targeting it for degradation

Rituximab	Alefacept	Omalizumab
Alemtuzumab	Efalizumab	Palivizumab
Cetuximab	Infliximab	Enfuvirtide
Bevacizumab	Anakinra	Abciximab
	Muromonab-CD3	Ovine digoxin immune serum, Fab fragment
	Daclizumab	Pegvisomant
	Basiliximab	

IIb: Stimulating a signaling pathway

Trastuzumab	Tositumomab

IIc: Delivering other compounds or proteins

Gemtuzumab ozogamicin	I-131 tositumomab

Group III: Protein Vaccines

IIIa: Protecting against a deleterious foreign agent

HBsAg	OspA

IIIb: Treating an autoimmune disease

Glatiramer acetate (formerly copolymer-1)
Anti-Rh IgG

IIIc: Treating cancer

Currently in clinical trials

Group IV: Protein Diagnostics

DPPD	Growth hormone releasing hormone (GHRH)	Thyroid stimulating hormone (TSH)
HIV antigens		Glucagon
Hepatitis C antigens	Secretin	

and C, Kaposi's sarcoma, melanoma, and some types of leukemia and lymphoma have been treated with one or more of the following forms of interferon: **consensus interferon (interferon alpha)**, **interferon alpha-2a**, **peginterferon alfa-2a**, **interferon alfa-2b**, and **peginterferon alfa-2b**. "Peginterferon" refers to a modified form of the protein in which the polymer polyethylene glycol (PEG) is added to prolong the absorption, decrease the renal clearance, retard the enzymatic degradation, increase the elimination half-life, and reduce the immunogenicity of interferon. Multiple sclerosis can be treated with **interferon beta-1a** and **interferon beta-1b**. **Interferon gamma** can be used to treat severe osteopetrosis and chronic granulomatous disease (CGD), and metastatic renal cell carcinoma and melanoma can be treated with **interleukin-2**.

Group Ib proteins can also have lifesaving effects on the processes of thrombosis and hemostasis. **Alteplase**, recombinant tissue plasminogen activator (tPA), is used to treat life-threatening blood clots in conditions such as coronary artery occlusion and pulmonary embolism. Endogenous tPA is secreted by the endothelial cells that line blood vessels. The secreted tPA normally cleaves plasminogen to plasmin, which then degrades fibrin and thereby lyses fibrin-based clots. Although endogenous tPA may be present at normal or even increased levels near the site of a blood clot, administration of relatively large amounts of exogenous tPA may be required to disrupt these clots. **Reteplase**, a genetically modified form of recombinant tPA, is also used to treat ST elevation myocardial infarction. **Tenecteplase**, another genetically engineered derivative of tPA, has greater specificity than tPA for binding to plasminogen and therefore causes more efficacious lysis of fibrin in blood clots. Tenecteplase was the tPA derivative used to reopen M. R.'s occluded coronary artery when he sustained an ST elevation myocardial infarction the day after his admission to hospital. Unlike the anticoagulant heparin, which could prevent propagation of the existing clot but could not lyse the existing clot, the thrombolytic agent tenecteplase could disrupt the clot in M. R.'s coronary artery (see Chapter 22, Pharmacology of Hemostasis and Thrombosis, and Chapter 24, Integrative Cardiovascular Pharmacology: Hypertension, Ischemic Heart Disease, and Heart Failure). Supraphysiologic levels of coagulation **factor VIIa** may catalyze thrombosis and thereby stop life-threatening bleeding in patients with hemophilia A or B. Recent studies have suggested that recombinant **activated protein C** can improve immunoregulation and prevent excessive clotting reactions in patients with severe, life-threatening sepsis and organ dysfunction.

A variety of other disease states are also treated with *Group Ib* proteins. Severe osteoporosis is treated with daily injections of **teriparatide (human parathyroid hormone 1-34 (PTH 1-34))**, which stimulates bone formation. Type II diabetes is treated with the recently approved incretin mimetic **exenatide**. Exenatide is a recombinantly produced 39-amino acid peptide whose sequence overlaps partially with that of glucagon-like peptide-1 (GLP-1). Like GLP-1, exenatide reduces glucose levels by a number of mechanisms, including suppression of excess glucagon production, enhancement of the insulin response to a glucose load, slowing of gastric emptying leading to slower glucose absorption, and decreasing appetite. Healing of skin ulcers and other

wounds can be enhanced by the use of **platelet-derived growth factor (PDGF)** or **trypsin**. Decompensated heart failure can be treated with **nesiritide**, recombinant B-type natriuretic peptide, which causes vascular smooth muscle relaxation and thereby allows the heart to pump against lower levels of systemic vascular resistance. As illustrated by the previous examples, modern medicine has not only identified important human proteins and their functions, but can now also modify protein activity levels when the human body is unable to do so optimally.

Occasionally, the activity of a particular protein is desirable even though the body does not normally express that activity. *Group Ic* proteins contain examples of this paradigm, including both foreign proteins with novel functions and endogenous proteins that act at a novel time or place in the body. **Papain**, for example, is a protease purified from the *Carica papaya* fruit. This protein is used therapeutically to degrade proteinaceous debris in wounds. **Collagenase**, obtained from fermentation by *Clostridium histolyticum*, can be used to digest collagen in the necrotic base of wounds. The protease-mediated debridement or removal of necrotic tissue is helpful in the treatment of burns, pressure ulcers, postoperative wounds, carbuncles, and other types of wounds. **Recombinant human deoxyribonuclease I** also has a novel use. Normally found inside human cells, this recombinant enzyme can be used to degrade the DNA left over from dying neutrophils in the respiratory tract of patients with cystic fibrosis. Such DNA could otherwise form mucous plugs that obstruct the respiratory tract and lead to pulmonary fibrosis, bronchiectasis, and recurrent pneumonias. Thus, recombinant protein technology has allowed modern medicine to employ a normally intracellular enzyme in an extracellular environment.

There are many other successful examples of this innovative approach to protein therapy. It has been known for a number of years that certain forms of acute lymphoblastic leukemia (ALL) are unable to synthesize asparagine and therefore require the availability of this amino acid in order to survive. **L-asparaginase**, purified from *E. coli*, can be used to lower serum levels of asparagine in such patients and thereby inhibit cancer cell growth. Studies of the medical leech, *Hirudo medicinalis*, revealed that its salivary gland produces hirudin, a potent thrombin inhibitor. The gene for this protein was then identified, cloned, and used recombinantly to provide a new protein therapy, **lepirudin**, which prevents clot formation in patients with heparin-induced thrombocytopenia (HIT). Physicians and scientists can harness other organisms to produce proteins capable of breaking up clots that have already formed; for example, **streptokinase** is a plasminogen activating protein produced by group C beta-hemolytic streptococci. **Etanercept** is a novel fusion between two human proteins, tumor necrosis factor receptor (TNFr) and the Fc region of the human antibody protein IgG1. The TNFr portion of the molecule binds excess TNF in the plasma, while the Fc portion of the molecule targets the TNF for destruction (see discussion below). By combining these two functions, the drug neutralizes the deleterious effects of TNF (a cytokine that stimulates increased activity of the immune system), and thereby provides an effective therapy for inflammatory arthritis and psoriasis.

GROUP II: PROTEIN THERAPEUTICS WITH SPECIAL TARGETING ACTIVITY

The exquisite binding specificity of **monoclonal antibodies** can be exploited in a variety of ways using recombinant DNA technology. Many *Group IIa* proteins, also known as **immunoadhesins**, use the antigen recognition sites of immunoglobulin molecules to guide the body's immune system to destroy specifically targeted molecules or cells. Other immunoadhesins neutralize molecules by simple physical occupation of a functionally important region of the molecule. Immunoadhesins combine the antigen recognition sites of known immunoglobulins with the Fc region of the same or a related immunoglobulin. The Fc region can *target a soluble molecule for destruction* because cells of the immune system can recognize the Fc region, endocytose the attached molecule, and break down the molecule chemically and enzymatically. When bound to specifically recognized molecules on the surface of a cell, the Fc region can *target the cell for destruction* by the immune system. Cell killing can be mediated by macrophages, by other immune cells, or by complement fixation.

Infliximab is a *Group IIa protein*. Like etanercept (see above), this recombinantly produced monoclonal antibody binds TNF-α and is used to neutralize the action of TNF-α in inflammatory conditions such as rheumatoid arthritis and inflammatory bowel disease. Another example of the use of a *Group IIa* protein is the prevention of severe infection by respiratory syncytial virus (RSV), which is one of the leading causes of hospital admissions for pediatric respiratory illness. High-risk patients are given a recombinantly produced monoclonal antibody, **palivizumab**, which binds to the RSV F protein and thereby directs the immune-mediated clearance of virus from the body. **Enfuvirtide** is a third example of a *Group IIa protein* that is also used to treat an important infectious disease; by binding to gp120/gp41, the HIV envelope protein responsible for fusion of the virus with host cells, this 36-amino acid peptide prevents the conformational change in gp41 required for viral fusion and thereby inhibits viral entry into the cell.

The field of antibody-mediated molecular and cellular inhibition has virtually exploded with new applications to treat human diseases. Recently developed *Group IIa* protein therapeutics are too numerous to describe in detail; a partial listing of targeted diseases and the *Group IIa* proteins used to treat the diseases is as follows: B-cell non-Hodgkin's lymphoma (CD20 targeting protein, **rituximab**); B-cell chronic lymphocytic leukemia (B-CLL) (CD52 targeting protein, **alemtuzumab**); colorectal cancer (epidermal growth factor [EGF] inhibitors, **cetuximab** and **bevacizumab**); psoriasis (CD2 inhibitor, **alefacept**, and CD11a inhibitor, **efalizumab**); rheumatoid arthritis (IL-1 receptor antagonist, **anakinra**); transplanted organ rejection (CD3 inhibitor, **muromonab-CD3** [OKT3]); renal transplant rejection (CD25 inhibitors, **daclizumab** and **basiliximab**); seasonal allergic asthma (mast cell receptor inhibitor, **omalizumab**); cardiac ischemia (platelet glycoprotein IIb/IIIa [gpIIb/IIIa] antagonist, **abciximab**); digoxin toxicity (digoxin inhibitor, Fab portion of **ovine digoxin immune serum**); and acromegaly (growth hormone receptor inhibitor, **pegvisomant**). The number of such treatments in use today is an indication that many more

protein therapeutics utilizing the exquisite specificity of monoclonal antibodies are yet to come. Abciximab was the monoclonal antibody used to augment the antiplatelet effects of aspirin and clopidogrel in treating M. R.'s non-ST elevation myocardial infarction. By preventing the binding of fibrinogen to gpIIb/IIIa on the platelet surface, abciximab effectively inhibits the platelet aggregation step of primary hemostasis (see Chapters 22 and 24).

Many important processes are modulated by cell surface receptors that are activated upon binding of their cognate ligands. By binding to such receptors, *Group IIb* targeting proteins can activate cell signaling pathways and profoundly affect cell function. Outcomes range from cell death (through the induction of apoptosis) to down-regulation of cell division to increased cell proliferation. Although it has been difficult to prove that a particular target-binding protein mediates an in vivo effect through the modulation of a particular signaling pathway, in vitro evidence suggests that this type of modulation is the mechanism of action of certain therapeutic proteins. For example, the treatment of certain breast cancers, in which the malignant cells express the Her2/Neu cell surface receptor, is enhanced by the addition of **trastuzumab** (an anti-Her2/Neu monoclonal antibody) to the therapeutic regimen. Although trastuzumab contains an Fc region, it is unlikely that simple targeting of the immune system to breast cancer cells by trastuzumab is sufficient to mediate cell killing. This is because many other monoclonal antibodies, with similar abilities to target breast cancer cells, have failed to show efficacy in vivo. Rather, because the anti-Her2/Neu antibody has been shown in vitro to induce intracellular signaling events that control the growth of breast cancer cells, it is likely that receptor-mediated signaling accounts for the efficacy of trastuzumab in vivo. Another example can be found in the treatment of CD20-positive follicular non-Hodgkin's lymphoma. **Tositumomab**, a monoclonal antibody directed against CD20, is thought to inhibit this type of lymphoma by signaling the cancer cells to undergo cell death via CD20-mediated apoptosis. Although few *Group IIb* proteins are currently in clinical use, more are in development and will likely be available in the coming years.

One of the great challenges in drug therapy is the selective delivery of SMDs and proteins to the intended therapeutic target. The body normally uses proteins to achieve specialized transport and delivery of molecules. An active area of current research is focused on understanding the principles of protein-based, targeted delivery of molecules, so that these principles can be applied to modern pharmacotherapy. There are currently two examples of *Group IIc* proteins, which enable drug delivery to a specific site. Both examples are in the area of cancer therapeutics. **Gemtuzumab ozogamicin** links the binding region of a monoclonal antibody directed against CD33 with calicheamicin, a small-molecule chemotherapeutic agent. By using this therapy, the toxic compound is selectively delivered to CD33-positive acute myeloid leukemia (AML) cells, resulting in the selective killing of these cells. Similarly, refractory CD20-positive non-Hodgkin's lymphoma cells can be destroyed selectively by **I-131 tositumomab**, a monoclonal antibody directed against CD20 and linked to the radioactive iodine isotope I-131.

In addition to these two current examples, developments

are in progress that illustrate where the field may be headed. For example, herpes simplex virus produces a protein, VP22, that enters human cells. VP22 has been used in vitro to deliver proteins or other compounds to the nucleus. In one application, VP22 was used to convey the tumor suppressor protein p53 to cultured osteosarcoma cells that lacked the p53 gene (and hence the protein). Reintroduction of p53 led to apoptosis of the cells. It is thought that a novel and effective therapy for certain forms of cancer could employ protein-based targeting of the p53 gene.

Another challenging area of research involves the delivery of proteins and other macromolecules to the central nervous system (CNS). With current technology, the blood-brain barrier (BBB) makes such delivery virtually impossible. Animal experiments have demonstrated, however, that fusion proteins combining a therapeutic protein with a protein that naturally has specific access through the BBB can allow successful delivery of the therapeutic protein to the CNS. For example, a fragment of the tetanus toxin protein that naturally crosses the BBB has been shown in animal experiments to deliver the enzyme superoxide dismutase to the CNS. This type of therapeutic could potentially be used to treat neurological disorders such as amyotrophic lateral sclerosis, in which CNS levels of superoxide dismutase are reported to be low. Exciting prospects also exist for the treatment of other disorders of the CNS in which levels of a particular protein are abnormal.

GROUP III: PROTEIN VACCINES

As recombinant DNA technology was being developed, great strides were also being made in understanding the molecular mechanisms that allow the immune system to protect the body against infectious diseases and cancer. Consequently, *Group III* proteins have been successfully applied as prophylactic or therapeutic vaccines. For humans to develop effective immunity against foreign organisms or cancer cells, immune cells such as helper T cells must be activated. Immune cell activation is mediated by antigen-presenting cells, which display on their surface specific oligopeptides that are derived from proteins found in foreign organisms or cancer cells. Vaccination against certain organisms such as polio or measles has most often been achieved by injecting heat-killed or attenuated forms of these pathogens. Unfortunately, these methods have involved a certain amount of unavoidable risk of infection or adverse reaction. By specifically injecting the appropriate immunogenic (but nonpathogenic) protein components of a microorganism, vaccines can hopefully be created that provide immunity in an individual without exposing the individual to the risks of infection or toxic reaction.

Group IIIa proteins are used to generate protection against infectious diseases or toxins. One successful example is the **hepatitis B vaccine**. This vaccine was created by producing recombinant HBsAg protein, a noninfectious protein of the hepatitis B virus. When immunocompetent humans are challenged and rechallenged with this protein, significant immunity results in the large majority of individuals. Similarly, the noninfectious lipoprotein on the outer surface of *Borrelia burgdorferi* has been engineered into a vaccine for Lyme disease **(OspA).**

In addition to generating protection against foreign invaders, recombinant proteins can induce protection against an overactive immune system that attacks its own body or "self." One theory is that administering large amounts of this self-protein causes the body's immune system to develop tolerance to that protein by eliminating or deactivating cells that react against the self-protein. *Group IIIb* proteins are used to treat patients with disorders that arise from this type of autoimmune phenomenon. One example is the use of **glatiramer acetate**, a short peptide of four amino acids. When administered to patients, this protein can improve the symptoms of certain forms of multiple sclerosis, an autoimmune disorder that targets the nervous system. Immunologic acceptance of a fetus during pregnancy represents a special situation with respect to vaccine use. Occasionally, a pregnant woman can reject a fetus after she has been immunized against certain antigens carried by a fetus from a previous pregnancy. Administration of **an anti-Rh(D) immunoglobulin** prevents the sensitization of an Rh-negative mother at the time of delivery of an Rh-positive neonate. Because the woman fails to develop antibodies directed against the fetal Rh antigens, immune reactions and pregnancy loss do not occur in subsequent pregnancies, even when the new fetus carries the Rh antigens.

Group IIIc proteins will likely be used to vaccinate against some cancers. Although there are currently no FDA-approved recombinant anti-cancer vaccines, promising clinical trials employ patient-specific cancer vaccines. For example, a vaccine for B-cell non-Hodgkin's lymphoma makes use of transgenic tobacco plants (*Nicotiana benthamiana*). Each patient with this type of lymphoma has a malignant proliferation of an antibody-producing B-cell that displays a unique antibody on its surface. By subcloning the idiotype region of this tumor-specific antibody and expressing the region recombinantly in tobacco plants, a tumor-specific antigen is produced that can be used to vaccinate a patient. (This is somewhat ironic, in that the immune system is being vaccinated to protect against an antibody-producing cancer.) This process requires only 6 to 8 weeks from biopsy of the lymphoma to a ready-to-use, patient-specific vaccine. As the genomes of infectious organisms and the nature of autoimmune diseases and cancer are more fully elucidated, more recombinant proteins will undoubtedly be developed for use as vaccines.

GROUP IV: PROTEIN DIAGNOSTICS

Although *Group IV* proteins are not used to treat disease, purified and recombinant proteins used for medical diagnostics bear mentioning here because they are invaluable in the decision-making process that precedes the treatment and management of many diseases. A classic example is the **purified protein derivative (PPD)** test, which determines whether an individual has been exposed to antigens from *Mycobacterium tuberculosis*. In this test, a noninfectious protein component of the organism is injected under the skin of an immunocompetent individual. An active immune reaction is interpreted as evidence that the patient has been previously infected by *M. tuberculosis* or exposed to the antigens of this organism. Another important example of protein diagnostics involves the natural and recombinant **human immunodeficiency virus (HIV) antigens** that are essential components of common screening (enzyme immunoassay) and confirmatory (western blot) tests for HIV infection. In these tests, the antigens serve as "bait" for specific antibodies to HIV *gag*, *pol*, and *env* gene products that have been elicited in the course of infection. Oral versions of HIV tests have also become available. Hepatitis C infection is diagnosed by using recombinant **hepatitis C antigens** to detect antibodies directed against this virus in the serum of potentially infected patients.

Another example illustrating the use of proteins for diagnosis is provided by recombinant **growth hormone releasing hormone (GHRH)**. This protein stimulates somatotroph cells of the anterior pituitary gland to secrete growth hormone. Used as a diagnostic, GHRH can help to determine whether pituitary growth hormone secretion is defective in patients with clinical signs of growth hormone deficiency. Similarly, the recombinant human protein **secretin** is used to stimulate pancreatic secretions and gastrin release and thereby to aid in the diagnosis of pancreatic exocrine dysfunction or gastrinoma. In patients with a history of thyroid cancer, recombinant **thyroid stimulating hormone (TSH)** is an important component of the surveillance methods used to detect residual thyroid cancer cells. Before the advent of recombinant TSH, patients with a history of thyroid cancer were required to stop taking replacement thyroid hormone in order to develop a hypothyroid state to which the anterior pituitary gland would respond by releasing endogenous TSH. TSH-stimulated cancer cells could then be detected by radioactive iodine uptake. Unfortunately, this method required patients to experience the adverse consequences of hypothyroidism. The availability of recombinant instead of endogenous TSH not only allowed patients to remain on replacement thyroid hormone but also resulted in improved detection of residual thyroid cancer cells. Finally, recombinant **glucagon** can be used to slow gastric motility, allowing higher resolution radiologic studies of the gastrointestinal tract.

CHALLENGES OF PROTEIN-BASED THERAPEUTICS

Numerous proteins are used therapeutically in clinical medicine. Nonetheless, failed protein therapies have far outnumbered the successes. The production of biologically active proteins can be difficult for a number of reasons. Drug delivery (*pharmacokinetics*) provides one of the greatest challenges to successful protein therapy. Proteins are large molecules with both hydrophilic and hydrophobic properties that can make entry into cells and other compartments in the body difficult. Protein solubility, route of administration, and distribution are all factors that can hinder the successful application of protein therapy. The stability of the protein inside the body is another important pharmacokinetic issue. The half-life of a therapeutic protein can be drastically affected by proteases, protein-modifying chemicals, or other clearance mechanisms.

One special pharmacokinetic issue is that the body may mount an *immune response* against the therapeutic protein.

In some cases, this immune response can neutralize the protein and can even cause a harmful reaction in the patient. Immune responses can be generated against *Group Ia* therapeutic proteins used to replace a factor that has been missing since birth; for example, antifactor VIII antibodies ("inhibitors") can develop in patients with severe hemophilia A who are treated with **recombinant human factor VIII**. More commonly, however, immune responses are generated against proteins of nonhuman origin. Until recently, the widespread clinical application of monoclonal antibodies has been limited by the rapid induction of immune responses against this class of therapeutic proteins. With the advent of methods to develop "humanized" antibodies, in which portions of the antibody that are not critical for antigen-binding specificity are replaced with human immunoglobulin sequences that confer stability and biologic activity on the protein but do not provoke an "antiantibody" response, this limitation has been overcome, at least in some cases.

In order for a protein to be physiologically active, posttranslational modifications such as glycosylation, phosphorylation, and proteolytic cleavage are often required. These requirements may dictate the use of specific cell types that are capable of expressing and modifying the recombinant protein appropriately. In addition, recombinant proteins must be synthesized in a genetically engineered cell type for *large-scale production*. The host system must produce not only biologically active protein but also a sufficient quantity of this protein to meet clinical demand. The system must allow purification and storage of the protein in a therapeutically active form for extended periods of time. The protein's stability, folding, and tendency to aggregate may be very different in large-scale production and storage systems than in the small-scale systems used to produce the protein for animal testing and clinical trials. Some have proposed engineering host systems that coexpress a chaperone or foldase with the therapeutic protein of interest, but these approaches have had limited success. Potential solutions could include the development of systems in which entire cascades of genes involved in protein folding are induced together with the therapeutic protein; the impetus for this work is the observation that plasma cells utilize such gene cascades to produce large quantities of monoclonal antibody. Although bacteria and yeast are generally considered easy to culture, certain mammalian cell types can be more difficult and more costly to culture. Other methods of production, such as genetically engineered animals and plants, could provide a production advantage. Transgenic cows, goats, and sheep have been engineered to secrete protein in their milk, and transgenic chickens that lay eggs filled with recombinant protein are anticipated in the future. Transgenic plants can inexpensively produce vast quantities of protein without waste or bioreactors, and potatoes can be engineered to express recombinant proteins and thereby to make edible vaccines. Lastly, microliter-sized culture systems may be able to predict the success of large-scale culture systems and thereby provide substantial cost savings by focusing investment on systems that are more likely to succeed.

Another important challenge is that the *costs* involved in developing protein therapies can be prohibitive. Because most protein-based therapeutics are produced by companies that must remain financially solvent, cost can often be the most crucial issue. For example, the switch to recombinant methodology from laborious purification of placentally derived protein has allowed the production of sufficient beta-glucocerebrosidase to treat Gaucher's disease in many patients. Even so, the cost of the recombinant protein can be hundreds of thousands of dollars per patient per year, which prevents some patients from receiving the necessary therapy.

The example of Gaucher's disease highlights one final and substantial challenge associated with protein therapeutics: *ethics*. The possibility of expensive treatments for small but severely ill patient populations (such as patients with Gaucher's disease) presents a serious dilemma in health care with respect to allocation of financial resources. Furthermore, the very definition of illness or disease may be challenged now that protein therapies can ''improve upon'' conditions previously viewed as variants of normal. For example, the definition of short stature may begin to change with the possibility of using growth hormone to increase the height of a child.

Conclusion and Future Directions

Modern medicine stands at the edge of an entirely new pharmacology. For the first time in history, physicians seek to manage disease at the level of the genetic and protein information that underlies all biology. Protein-based therapies are playing an increasingly important role in the pharmacologic treatment of disease. The potential for new therapies is virtually endless, given the thousands of proteins produced by the human body and the many thousands of proteins produced by other organisms. The early success of recombinant insulin production in the 1970s created an atmosphere of enthusiasm and hope that was unfortunately followed by an era of disappointment when the vaccine attempts, nonhumanized monoclonal antibodies, and cancer trials in the 1980s were largely unsuccessful. Despite these setbacks, significant progress has recently been made. Exciting new means of production are changing the scale, cost, and even route of administration of recombinant protein therapies, and the large number of protein therapies both in current clinical use and in phase III clinical trials attests to the promise of this technology.

It is likely that novel protein-based therapies will be available shortly for many types of cancer, autoimmune disorders, neurologic diseases, graft rejection, microbial diseases, and vascular and hematologic regulation. In fact, recombinant human proteins now make up the majority of FDA-approved biotechnology medicines, which include monoclonal antibodies, natural interferons, vaccines, hormones, modified natural enzymes, and various cell therapies. It is becoming apparent that recombinant proteins not only provide alternative treatments for particular diseases, but can also be used in combination with small-molecule drugs to provide additive or synergistic benefit. Treatment of EGFR-positive colon cancer is illustrative of this point: combination therapy with the SMD **irinotecan**, which prevents DNA repair by inhibiting DNA topoisomerase, and the recombinant monoclonal antibody **cetuximab**, which binds to and inhibits the extracellular domain of the EGFR, results in increased survival in colorectal cancer patients. The therapeutic synergy between irinotecan and cetuximab may be due to the fact that both drugs inhibit the same EGFR signaling pathway, with one drug (cetuximab) inhibiting the initiation of the pathway and the other drug (irinotecan) inhibiting a target downstream in the pathway. Although the success of any particular protein therapy will depend on its pharmacodynamic, pharmacokinetic, and safety profiles, one can confidently predict that protein therapies will have an expanding role for years to come.

In the first edition of this textbook, this chapter contained an extended discussion of gene therapy, including the rationale for gene therapy, the requirements for safe and effective gene therapy, and the applications and limitations of viral gene therapy vectors. Three years later, however, gene therapy remains an unfulfilled promise. It is an attractive notion that genetically based diseases could be treated directly by transfer of genetic material into diseased cells, tissues, and organs, and many such gene therapy ''warheads'' have been successfully designed. However, significant problems have arisen in the efficient delivery of the genetic material without causing serious adverse effects. For example, several children with a life-threatening form of severe combined X-linked immunodeficiency (SCID-X1) developed acute leukemia as a consequence of gene therapy using a retroviral vector that had integrated in or near a leukemia oncogene, and a healthy volunteer died in a phase I clinical trial designed to test the safety of an engineered recombinant adenovirus vector. There are currently no gene-based therapeutics approved for clinical use, although it is hoped that many such therapeutics will be developed in the future as scientists and physicians work to address the safety issues associated with the currently available gene delivery modalities. Interested readers are referred to Chapter 49, Protein-Based and Gene Therapies, in the *first* edition of this textbook, and to the review article by Verma and Weitzman cited below.

Suggested Reading

Banting FG, Best CH, Collip JB, et al. Pancreatic extracts in the treatment of diabetes mellitus. *Can Med Assoc J* 1922;12: 141–146. (*Describes the treatment of diabetes by an extract from pancreas—later shown to be insulin.*)

Gross ML. Ethics, policy, and rare genetic disorders: the case of Gaucher disease in Israel. *Theor Med Bioeth* 2002;23(2): 151–170. (*Discusses interface of ethics and cost in the use of protein therapeutics for lifesaving treatment of genetic disorders.*)

Hodi FS, Dranoff G. Combinatorial cancer immunotherapy. *Adv Immunol* 2006;90:341–368. (*Reviews current preclinical and clinical research on use of cancer vaccines, monoclonal antibodies, recombinant cytokines, and adoptive cell infusions in combination treatment of cancer.*)

Leader B, Golan DE. Recombinant and non-recombinant protein therapies in medicine. *Nat Rev Drug Discov,* 2007. In press. (*Fully referenced review article from which this chapter is adapted.*)

Mahmood I, Green MD. Pharmacokinetic and pharmacodynamic considerations in the development of therapeutic proteins. *Clin Pharmacokinet* 2005;44:331–347. (*Reviews pharmacokinetic and pharmacodynamic challenges in therapeutic protein development.*)

Verma IM, Weitzman MD. Gene therapy: twenty-first century medicine. *Annu Rev Biochem* 2005;74:711–738. (*Reviews challenges and opportunities for gene therapy.*)

Weiner LM. Fully human therapeutic monoclonal antibodies. *J Immunother* 2006;29:1–9. (*Reviews methods of engineering chimeric and humanized monoclonal antibodies.*)

TABLE 53-1 A Functional Classification of Protein-Based Therapies

Group I: Protein Therapeutics with Enzymatic or Regulatory Activity

Ia: Replacing a protein that is deficient or abnormal

CATEGORY (r, RECOMBINANT; n, NONRECOMBINANT)	PROTEIN	TRADE NAME	FUNCTION	EXAMPLES OF CLINICAL USE
Hemophilia (coagulation factor deficiencies)				
rIa	Factor VIII	Bioclate, Helixate, Kogenate, Recombinate, ReFacto	Coagulation factor	Hemophilia A
rIa	Factor IX	BeneFix	Coagulation factor	Hemophilia B
Endocrine disorders (hormone deficiencies)				
rIa, rIb	Insulin	Humulin, Novolin	Regulates blood glucose, shifts potassium into cells	Diabetes mellitus, diabetic ketoacidosis, hyperkalemia
rIa, rIb	Insulin lispro	Humalog	Insulin analogue with faster onset of action and shorter duration of action	Diabetes mellitus
rIa, rIb	Insulin aspart	NovoLog	Insulin analogue with faster onset of action and shorter duration of action	Diabetes mellitus
rIa, rIb	Insulin glargine	Lantus	Insulin analogue with slower onset of action and longer duration of action	Diabetes mellitus
rIa, rIb	Growth hormone (GH)	Genotropin, Humatrope, NorlVitropin, Nutropin, Protropin, Saizen, Serostim	Anabolic and anticatabolic effector	Growth failure due to GH deficiency or chronic renal insufficiency, Prader-Willi syndrome, Turner syndrome, AIDS wasting or cachexia with antiviral therapy
Lysosomal storage disorders (metabolic enzyme deficiencies)				
rIa	Beta-glucocerebrosidase	Cerezyme	Hydrolyzes glucocerebroside to glucose and ceramide	Gaucher's disease
nIa	Beta-glucocerebrosidase	Ceredase	Hydrolyzes glucocerebroside to glucose and ceramide; purified from pooled human placenta	Gaucher's disease
rIa	Laronidase	Aldurazyme	alpha-L-iduronidase is an enzyme that digests endogenous glycosaminoglycans (GAGs) within lysosomes, and thereby prevents an accumulation of GAGs that can cause cellular, tissue, and organ dysfunction	Hurler and Hurler-Scheie forms of mucopolysaccharidosis I (MPS I)
Pulmonary and gastrointestinal tract disorders				
rIa	Agalsidase beta (human α-galactosidase A)	Fabrazyme	Enzyme that hydrolyzes globotriaosylceramide (GL-3) and other glycosphingolipids, reducing deposition of these lipids in capillary endothelium of the kidney and certain other cell types	Fabry disease; prevents accumulation of lipids that could lead to renal and cardiovascular complications

nla	alpha-1-Proteinase inhibitor	Prolastin, Aralast	Inhibits elastase-mediated destruction of pulmonary tissue; purified from pooled human plasma	Congenital alpha-1-antitrypsin deficiency
nla	Pancreatic enzymes (lipase, amylase, protease)	Arco-Lase, Cotazym, Pancrease, Viokase, Creon, Zymase, Donnazyme	Digests food (protein, fat, and carbohydrate); purified from hogs and pigs	Cystic fibrosis, chronic pancreatitis, pancreatic insufficiency, post-Billroth II gastric bypass surgery, pancreatic duct obstruction, steatorrhea, poor digestion, gas, bloating
nla	Lactase	Lactaid	Digests lactose; purified from fungus *Aspergillus oryzae*	Gas, bloating, cramps, diarrhea due to inability to digest lactose
Immunodeficiencies				
nla	Adenosine deaminase	Adagen (pegademase bovine, PEG-ADA)	Metabolizes adenosine, prevents accumulation of adenosine; purified from cows	Severe combined immunodeficiency disease (SCID) due to adenosine deaminase (ADA) deficiency
nla	Pooled immunoglobulins	Octagam	Intravenous immunoglobulin preparation	Primary immunodeficiencies
Ib: Augmenting an existing pathway				
Hematopoiesis				
rIb	Erythropoietin	Epogen, Procrit	Stimulates erythropoiesis	Anemia of chronic disease, myelodysplasia, anemia due to renal failure or chemotherapy, preoperative preparation
rIb	Darbepoetin alfa	Aranesp	Modified erythropoietin with longer half-life; stimulates red blood cell production in the bone marrow	Treatment of anemia in patients with chronic renal insufficiency and chronic renal failure ($+/-$ dialysis)
rIb	Granulocyte colony stimulating factor (G-CSF)	Filgrastim	Stimulates neutrophil proliferation, differentiation and migration	Neutropenia in AIDS or post-chemotherapy or bone marrow transplantation, severe chronic neutropenia
rIb	Granulocyte-macrophage colony stimulating factor (GM-CSF)	Leukine, Sargramostim	Stimulates proliferation and differentiation of neutrophils, eosinophils and monocytes	Leukopenia, myeloid reconstitution post-bone marrow transplantation, HIV/AIDS
rIb	Interleukin-11 (IL-11)	Neumega Oprelvekin	Stimulates megakaryocytopoiesis and thrombopoiesis	Prevention of severe thrombocytopenia, especially after myelosuppressive chemotherapy
Fertility				
rIb	Human follicle-stimulating hormone (FSH)	Gonal-F/ Follistim	Augments ovulation	Assisted reproductive technology for infertility
rIb	Human chorionic gonadotropin (HCG)	Ovidrel	Stimulates ovarian follicle rupture and ovulation	Assisted reproductive technology for infertility

(Continued)

TABLE 53-1   **A Functional Classification of Protein-Based Therapies** *(Continued)*

CATEGORY (r, RECOMBINANT: n, NONRECOMBINANT)	PROTEIN	TRADE NAME	FUNCTION	EXAMPLES OF CLINICAL USE
Immunoregulation				
rIb	Type I alpha-interferon, interferon alphacon-1, consensus interferon	Infergen	Unknown, immunoregulator	Chronic hepatitis C infection
rIb	Interferon alpha-2a (IFNα-2a)	Roferon-A	Unknown, immunoregulator	Hairy cell leukemia, chronic myelogenous leukemia, Kaposi's sarcoma, chronic hepatitis C infection
rIb	Peginterferon alfa-2a	Pegasys	Unknown, immunoregulator	Adults with chronic hepatitis C who have compensated liver disease and who have not been previously treated with interferon alpha; used alone or in combination with ribavirin (Copegus)
rIb	Interferon alfa-2b (IFNα-2b)	Intron A	Unknown, immunoregulator	Hepatitis B, melanoma, Kaposi's sarcoma, follicular lymphoma, hairy cell leukemia, condylomata acuminata, hepatitis C
rIb	Peginterferon alfa-2b	PEG-Intron	Recombinant interferon alpha-2b conjugated to polyethylene glycol (PEG) in order to increase half-life	Adults with chronic hepatitis C who have compensated liver disease and who have not been treated previously with interferon alpha
rIb	Interferon beta-1a (rIFN-β)	Avonex, Rebif	Unknown, antiviral and immunoregulator	Multiple sclerosis
rIb	Interferon beta-1b (rIFN-β)	Betaseron	Unknown, antiviral and immunoregulator	Multiple sclerosis
rIb	IFN-gamma, interferon-gamma-1b	Actimmune	Increases inflammatory and antimicrobial response	Chronic granulomatous disease (CGD), severe osteopetrosis
rIb	Interleukin-2 (IL-2), epidermal thymocyte activating factor (ETAF), aldesleukin	Proleukin	Stimulates T and B cells, natural killer cells, and lymphokine-activated killer (LAK) cells	Metastatic renal cell cancer, melanoma
Hemostasis and thrombosis				
rIb	Tissue plasminogen activator (tPA), alteplase	Activase	Promotes fibrinolysis by binding fibrin and converting plasminogen to plasmin	Pulmonary embolism, myocardial infarction, occlusion of central venous access devices
rIb	Reteplase (deletion mutein of plasminogen activator (rPA))	Retavase	Contains the non-glycosylated kringle 2 and protease domains of human tPA; functions similarly to tPA	Management of acute myocardial infarction, improvement of ventricular function

rlc, rlb	Tenecteplase	TNKase	Tissue plasminogen activator with greater specificity for plasminogen conversion; has amino acid substitutions of Thr103 to Asp, Asp117 to Gln, and Ala for amino acids 296-299; promotes fibrinolysis by binding fibrin and converting plasminogen to plasmin	Acute myocardial infarction
rlb	Factor VIIa	NovoSeven	Pro-thrombotic (activated factor VII; initiates the coagulation cascade)	Hemorrhage in patients with hemophilia A or B and inhibitors to factor VIII or factor IX
rlb	Drotrecogin alfa (activated protein C)	Xigris	Anti-thrombotic (inhibits coagulation factors Va and VIIIa), anti-inflammatory	Severe sepsis with a high risk of death
Other				
rlb	Teriparatide (human parathyroid hormone 1-34)	Forteo	Markedly enhances bone formation; administered as a once-daily injection	Severe osteoporosis
rlb, rlc	Exenatide	Byetta	Incretin mimetic with actions similar to glucagon-like peptide-1 (GLP-1); increases glucose-dependent insulin secretion, suppresses glucagon secretion, slows gastric emptying, decreases appetite	Type 2 diabetes resistant to treatment with metformin and a sulfonylurea
rlb	Platelet-derived growth factor (PDGF), becaplermin	Regranex	Promotes wound healing by enhancing granulation tissue formation and fibroblast proliferation and differentiation	Debridement adjunct for diabetic ulcers
nlb	Trypsin	Granulex	Proteolysis	Decubitus ulcer, varicose ulcer, debridement of eschar, dehiscent wound, sunburn
rlb	Nesiritide	Natrecor	Recombinant B-type natriuretic peptide	Acute decompensated congestive heart failure
Ic: Providing a novel function or activity				
nlc	Papain	Accuzyme, Panafil	Protease from the *Carica papaya* fruit	Debridement of necrotic tissue or liquefaction of slough in acute and chronic lesions, such as pressure ulcers, varicose and diabetic ulcers, burns, postoperative wounds, pilonidal cyst wounds, carbuncles, and other wounds
nlc	Collagenase	Collagenase, Santyl	Collagenase obtained from fermentation by *Clostridium histolyticum*; digests collagen in necrotic base of wounds	Debridement of chronic dermal ulcers and severely burned areas
rlc	Dornase alfa, human deoxy-ribonuclease I	Pulmozyme	Degrades DNA in purulent pulmonary secretions	Cystic fibrosis; decreases respiratory tract infections in selected patients with FVC greater than 40% of predicted
nlc	L-asparaginase	ELSPAR	Provides exogenous asparaginase activity, removing available asparagine from serum; purified from *E. coli*	Acute lymphocytic leukemia (ALL), which requires exogenous asparagine for proliferation

(Continued)

TABLE 53-1 A Functional Classification of Protein-Based Therapies *(Continued)*

CATEGORY (r, RECOMBINANT; n, NONRECOMBINANT)	PROTEIN	TRADE NAME	FUNCTION	EXAMPLES OF CLINICAL USE
nIc	PEG-asparaginase	Oncaspar	Provides exogenous asparaginase activity, removing available asparagine from serum; purified from *E. coli*	Acute lymphocytic leukemia (ALL), which requires exogenous asparagine for proliferation
rIc	Lepirudin	Refludan	Recombinant hirudin, a thrombin inhibitor from salivary gland of medicinal leech *Hirudo medicinalis*	Heparin-induced thrombocytopenia (HIT)
nIc	Streptokinase	Streptase	Converts plasminogen to plasmin; produced by group C beta-hemolytic streptococci	Acute evolving transmural myocardial infarction, pulmonary embolism, deep vein thrombosis, arterial thrombosis or embolism, occlusion of arteriovenous cannula
rIc	Etanercept	Enbrel	Dimeric fusion protein between recombinant soluble tumor necrosis factor receptor (TNFr) and Fc portion of human IgG1	Moderate to severe active rheumatoid arthritis (RA) after failing other therapies, moderate to severe active polyarticular juvenile RA

Group II: Protein Therapeutics with Special Targeting Activity
IIa: Interfering with a molecule or organism by binding to it and thereby blocking its function or targeting it for degradation

Cancer

rIIa	Rituximab	Rituxan	Chimeric (human/mouse) mAb that binds CD20, a transmembrane protein found on over 90% of B-cell non-Hodgkin's lymphomas	Treatment of relapsed or refractory, low-grade or follicular, CD20-positive B-cell non-Hodgkin's lymphoma
rIIa	Alemtuzumab	Campath	Humanized monoclonal antibody directed against CD52 antigen on T and B cells	B-cell chronic lymphocytic leukemia (B-CLL) in patients who have been treated with alkylating agents and who have failed fludarabine therapy
rIIa	Cetuximab	Erbitux	mAb that binds epidermal growth factor receptor (EGFR)	Colorectal cancer
rIIa	Bevacizumab	Avastin	mAb that binds epidermal growth factor receptor (EGFR)	Colorectal cancer

Immunoregulation

rIIa	Alefacept	Amevive	mAb that binds CD2 on the surface of lymphocytes and inhibits interaction with leukocyte function-associated antigen 3 (LFA-3); this association is important for the activation of T lymphocytes in psoriasis	Adults with moderate to severe chronic plaque psoriasis who are candidates for systemic therapy or phototherapy
rIIa	Efalizumab	Raptiva	Humanized monoclonal antibody directed against CD11a	Adults with chronic moderate to severe plaque psoriasis who are candidates for systemic therapy

	Generic	Trade name	Description	Indication
rIIa	Infliximab	Remicade	Monoclonal antibody that binds and neutralizes TNF-α, preventing induction of pro-inflammatory cytokines, changes in endothelial cell permeability, activation of eosinophils and neutrophils, induction of acute phase reactants, and enzyme elaboration by synoviocytes and/or chondrocytes	Rheumatoid arthritis, Crohn's disease
rIIa	Anakinra	Kineret, Antril, Synergen	Recombinant interleukin-1 receptor antagonist	Moderate to severe active rheumatoid arthritis in adults who have failed one or more disease modifying antirheumatic drug
Transplantation				
rIIa	Muromonab-CD3	Orthoclone/OKT3	Monoclonal antibody that binds CD3 and blocks T cell function	Acute renal allograft rejection or steroid-resistant cardiac or hepatic allograft rejection
rIIa	Daclizumab	Zenapax	Humanized IgG1 mAb that blocks cellular immune response in graft rejection by binding the alpha chain of CD25 (IL-2 receptor) and thereby inhibiting the IL-2 mediated activation of lymphocytes	Prophylaxis against acute allograft rejection in patients receiving renal transplants
rIIa	Basiliximab	Simulect	Chimeric (human/mouse) IgG1 that blocks cellular immune response in graft rejection by binding the alpha chain of CD25 (IL-2 receptor) and thereby inhibiting the IL-2 mediated activation of lymphocytes	Prophylaxis against allograft rejection in renal transplant patients receiving an immunosuppressive regimen including cyclosporine and corticosteroids
Pulmonary disorders				
rIIa	Omalizumab	Xolair	IgG monoclonal antibody that inhibits IgE binding to the high-affinity IgE receptor on mast cells and basophils, decreasing activation of these cells and release of inflammatory mediators	Adults and adolescents (at least 12 years old) with moderate to severe persistent asthma who have a positive skin test or in vitro reactivity to a perennial aeroallergen and whose symptoms are inadequately controlled with inhaled corticosteroids
rIIa	Palivizumab	Synagis	Humanized IgG1 mAb that binds the A antigenic site of the F protein of the respiratory syncytial virus	Prevention of respiratory syncytial virus infection in high-risk pediatric patients
Infectious diseases				
rIIa	Enfuvirtide	Fuzeon	36 amino acid peptide that inhibits HIV entry into host cells by binding to the HIV envelope protein gp120/gp41	Adults and children (at least 6 years old) with advanced HIV infection

(Continued)

TABLE 53-1 A Functional Classification of Protein-Based Therapies (Continued)

CATEGORY (r, RECOMBINANT; n, NONRECOMBINANT) PROTEIN	TRADE NAME	FUNCTION	EXAMPLES OF CLINICAL USE
Cardiovascular disorders			
rIIa Abciximab	ReoPro	Fab fragment of chimeric (human/mouse) mAb 7E3 that inhibits platelet aggregation by binding to the glycoprotein IIb/IIIa integrin receptor	Adjunct to aspirin and heparin for prevention of cardiac ischemia in patients undergoing percutaneous coronary intervention or patients about to undergo percutaneous coronary intervention with unstable angina not responding to medical therapy
nIIa Ovine digoxin immune serum, Fab fragment	DigiFab	Monovalent fragment antigen-binding (Fab) immunoglobulin fragment obtained from sheep immunized with a digoxin derivative	Digoxin toxicity
Endocrine disorders			
rIIa Pegvisomant	Somavert	Recombinant human growth hormone conjugated to PEG; blocks the growth hormone receptor	Acromegaly
IIb: Stimulating a signaling pathway			
rIIb, rIIa Trastuzumab	Herceptin	Monoclonal antibody that binds Her2/Neu cell surface receptor and controls cancer cell growth	Breast cancer
rIIb (rIIc) Tositumomab	Bexxar	Monoclonal antibody that binds CD20 surface antigen and stimulates apoptosis	CD20-positive follicular non-Hodgkin's lymphoma, with and without transformation, in patients whose disease is refractory to rituximab and has relapsed following chemotherapy
IIc: Delivering other compounds or proteins			
rIIc Gemtuzumab ozogamicin	Mylotarg	Humanized anti-CD33 IgG4 kappa monoclonal antibody conjugated to calicheamicin, a small-molecule chemotherapeutic agent	Relapsed CD33-positive acute myeloid leukemia in patients who are more than 60 years old and are not candidates for cytotoxic chemotherapy
rIIc (rIIb) I-131 tositumomab	Bexxar	Monoclonal antibody coupled to radioactive iodine-131; binds CD20 surface antigen and delivers cytotoxic radiation (used after tositumomab without I-131)	CD20-positive follicular non-Hodgkin's lymphoma, with and without transformation, in patients whose disease is refractory to rituximab and has relapsed following chemotherapy

Group III: Protein Vaccines

IIIa: Protecting against a deleterious foreign agent

rIIIa	HBsAg	Engerix, Recombivax HB	Noninfectious protein on surface of hepatitis B virus	Hepatitis B vaccination
rIIIa	OspA	LYMErix	Noninfectious lipoprotein on outer surface of *Borrelia burgdorferi*	Lyme disease vaccination

IIIb: Treating an autoimmune disease

rIIIb	Glatiramer acetate (formerly copolymer-1, consists of acetate with L-Glu, L-Ala, L-Tyr, L-Lys)	Copaxone	Unknown, modifies immune response, may not act by classical vaccine mechanisms	Relapsing-remitting multiple sclerosis
rIIIb	Anti-Rh IgG	Rhophylac	Neutralizes Rh antigens that could otherwise elicit anti-Rh antibodies in an Rh-negative individual	Routine antepartum and postpartum prevention of Rh(D) immunization in Rh(D)-negative women; Rh prophylaxis in case of obstetric complications or invasive procedures during pregnancy; suppression of Rh immunization in Rh(D)-negative individuals transfused with Rh(D)-positive red blood cells

IIIc: Treating cancer
Currently in clinical trials

Group IV: Protein Diagnostics

rIV	DPPD	Recombinant purified protein derivative (DPPD)	Noninfectious protein from *Mycobacterium tuberculosis*	Diagnosis of tuberculosis exposure
rIV	HIV antigens	Enzyme immunoassay (EIA), western blot, OraQuick, Uni-Gold	Detects human antibodies to HIV	Diagnosis of HIV infection
rIV	Hepatitis C antigens	Recombinant immunoblot assay (RIBA)	Detects human antibodies to hepatitis C virus	Diagnosis of hepatitis C exposure
rIV, rIa	Growth hormone releasing hormone (GHRH)	Geref	Recombinant fragment of GHRH that stimulates growth hormone (GH) release by somatotroph cells of the pituitary gland	Diagnosis of defective growth hormone secretion
rIV	Secretin	ChiRhoStim, ChiRhoClin	Stimulation of pancreatic secretions and gastrin	Aid in the diagnosis of pancreatic exocrine dysfunction or gastrinoma; facilitates identification of the ampulla of Vater and accessory papilla during endoscopic retrograde cholangiopancreatography

(Continued)

TABLE 53-1   A Functional Classification of Protein-Based Therapies (*Continued*)

CATEGORY (r, RECOMBINANT; n, NONRECOMBINANT)	PROTEIN	TRADE NAME	FUNCTION	EXAMPLES OF CLINICAL USE
rIV	Thyroid stimulating hormone (TSH), thyrotropin	Thyrogen	Stimulates thyroid epithelial cells or well-differentiated thyroid cancer tissue to take up iodine and produce and secrete thyroglobulin, triiodothyronine, and thyroxine	Adjunctive diagnostic for serum thyroglobulin testing in the follow-up of patients with well-differentiated thyroid cancer
rIV, rIb	Glucagon	GlucaGen	Pancreatic hormone that increases blood glucose by stimulating the liver to convert glycogen to glucose	Diagnostic aid to slow gastrointestinal motility in radiographic studies; reversal of hypoglycemia

54

Drug Delivery Modalities

Joshua D. Moss and Robert S. Langer

INTRODUCTION

Drugs are typically administered in either pill or injection form, with limited control over release-rate and localization. More advanced drug delivery systems have recently been developed, however. The goal of these new technologies is to alter four pharmacokinetic properties: (1) absorption of the drug, including the period of time over which it is released into the systemic circulation or at its final site of action; (2) distribution of the drug, whether it be to the entire body or to a specific tissue or organ system; (3) metabolism of the drug, either to be avoided entirely or used to convert a prodrug to an active form; and (4) elimination of the drug.

This chapter describes several existing and emerging delivery modalities and discusses how these modalities influence one or more of these four properties. The field of drug delivery is large and encompasses many disciplines, and this discussion will highlight approaches that illustrate these properties rather than provide an exhaustive description of all ongoing practice and research. The highlighted modalities include the novel use of existing delivery routes, polymer-based delivery, and liposome-based delivery.

Case

March 1988: Mr. F is 13 years old. His parents begin to notice that he is tired much of the time, despite getting plenty of sleep. He can no longer participate on his school's track team because he becomes exhausted in the middle of races—the same races he had often won less than a year earlier. Also, Mr. F complains of being thirsty constantly and, as a result, consumes large quantities of water. Mr. F goes to his family physician, who measures his blood glucose level at 650 mg/dL (approximately six times normal levels) and makes an initial diagnosis of type I diabetes mellitus. The diagnosis is confirmed in the hospital, where Mr. F's physicians stabilize his blood glucose and develop an insulin therapy regimen. He is taught how to draw a drop of blood from his fingertip to measure his blood glucose and how to give himself subcutaneous injections of insulin. Each day, Mr. F injects recombinant human insulin before breakfast and before dinner.

January 1997: Throughout high school and most of college, Mr. F rarely monitors his glucose levels and purposely keeps them higher than recommended. He wants to be as "normal" as possible, which for him means never allowing his glucose level to fall so low as to require food in the middle of a class or at other unusual times. As Mr. F becomes older, he begins to appreciate that avoiding the long-term consequences of poorly controlled diabetes—atherosclerosis, retinopathy, nephropathy, and peripheral neuropathy, among others—is worth the inconvenience of better control. He switches to a four-injection per day regimen and begins checking his blood glucose four to five times each day. Eventually, he switches from multiple subcutaneous injections (MSI) to continuous subcutaneous insulin infusion (CSII) with an insulin pump. The pump delivers a constant basal level of insulin that can be supplemented with bolus releases before meals, thereby more closely approximating the body's normal control of blood glucose levels.

September 2014: Back in 1997, Mr. F used his insulin pump for only about 3 months, deciding that the small machine he needed to keep constantly attached to his body was not compatible with his active lifestyle or self-image. He resumed MSI therapy for several more years, until he began participating in human trials for a new, implantable insulin delivery system. Now, a 2-year supply of insulin is incorporated into a polymer matrix that can be implanted in the subcutaneous fat of the abdomen. A device in Mr. F's wristwatch constantly measures his glucose levels transdermally, and it transmits instructions to a magnetic oscillator implanted near the polymer delivery system. The dosing advantages of the insulin pump are thus achieved without Mr. F feeling limited or tied to a machine in any way. He simply has the polymer system replaced every 2 years and makes minor daily adjustments to the programmed delivery parameters in his wristwatch device. Mr. F is looking forward to receiving a transplant of pancreatic beta cells, developed from his own stem cells, that will cure his diabetes.

QUESTIONS

■ **1.** Why is oral administration of insulin not practical? What other routes could be tried?

■ **2.** How can polymers be used to optimize and simplify administration of some drugs?

NOVEL USE OF EXISTING DELIVERY ROUTES

ORAL DELIVERY

Oral administration of small molecules is currently the most common method of drug delivery. The main advantages of oral delivery are ease of use and relatively low cost, both of which can improve patient compliance. However, incomplete absorption, metabolism of the drug during absorption, and metabolism of the drug during the first pass through the liver can decrease bioavailability of the drug. The variability of these factors, as well as limitations in dosing frequency, also affect the ability to maintain a therapeutic drug concentration in the blood. In addition, only relatively small molecules can be used in conventional pills: the intestine generally cannot absorb large molecules intact. Intact peptide and protein drugs, such as insulin, are poorly absorbed orally because of proteolysis in the digestive tract. Recent advances

and ongoing research in oral drug delivery are beginning to address these issues.

Sustained or **extended release formulations** can prolong plasma drug concentrations with less frequent doses. In early approaches to sustained release, pill or capsule solubility was modified with one or more inert substances known as **excipients.** By formulating the drug in an emulsion or suspension that is relatively difficult to digest, the period of time over which the drug dissolves and is absorbed can be extended. Similar results have been achieved by coating the drug with substances such as cellulose derivatives or wax. This approach is used in a wide variety of both prescription and over-the-counter medicines. Another successful and more recent approach to sustained release oral formulations involves an osmotic pump capsule (see below).

Techniques are also being researched for delivery of larger molecules, such as proteins and DNA, in oral formulations. Several designs make use of drug-carrying vehicles, including liposomes and microspheres. **Liposomes,** small vesicles with lipid bilayer membranes, are lipophilic and can be taken up by intestinal Peyer's patches when targeted to M-cells (specialized epithelial cells) with appropriate ligands. Certain types of liposomes have been moderately successful in experimental oral vaccine delivery; their use in intravenous delivery systems is discussed below. Polyanhydride **microspheres,** which adhere strongly to the intestinal mucosal surface, have been shown to penetrate intestinal epithelium. After the microspheres are absorbed, presumably because they can stay in contact with the intestinal epithelium for long periods of time, the complex molecules carried within them can be released into the blood.

Another potential approach to delivering proteins orally involves targeting the drug to the colon, which has lower levels of protease activity than the upper gastrointestinal tract. For example, microsphere delivery vehicles can be synthesized from polymers that have enzymatically degradable azoaromatic cross-links. The colon has a relatively high concentration of azoreductases, resulting in degradation of the microspheres and protein release within the colon. Substances that transiently increase the permeability of colonic epithelium, possibly coincorporated in the microspheres, may improve the absorption of proteins delivered to the colon. Another approach involves carrier molecules that may be able to shuttle large molecules across the epithelial lining of the intestine.

PULMONARY DELIVERY

Patients suffering from asthma and other respiratory diseases have long been able to treat their condition by inhaling aerosols of drugs directly into their lungs: β_2-adrenergic agonists, such as albuterol, and glucocorticoid analogues are widely used examples of such locally delivered drugs. In early metered-dose inhaler designs, many of which are still used, the drug is delivered in liquid form using a high velocity chlorofluorocarbon (CFC) propellant. With this technique, very little drug is reproducibly delivered to the lung—often less than 10%. Particles often accumulate in the mouth and throat, and many are immediately exhaled. Components of the immune system and macrophages in the lung can also clear some of the drug before it can act. In addition, many patients use their inhalers incorrectly; common mistakes include not shaking the inhaler well enough, pressing the inhaler too early or too late during inhalation, or using an empty inhaler. Incorrect use further reduces delivery efficiency.

Inhaler design continues to improve. Recent advances include more consistent dosing, greater ease of use via electronic breath actuation, and non-CFC propellants. The aerosol formulations have also been improved by adjusting several properties of the particles themselves. For example, optimized particle chemistry and surface morphology can minimize undesirable particle-particle aggregation. Similarly, particle solubility can be modified to influence the rate of therapeutic release once delivered. Dry-powder aerosol clouds that reach deep into the lungs can be generated by blowing compressed air into a drug powder, breaking the powder into tiny (1 to 5 μm) particles inside the inhaler. Devices that take advantage of these improvements have reduced both dosing frequency and cost for local applications of pulmonary drug delivery in patients with asthma and cystic fibrosis.

The lung also offers several potential advantages for noninvasive, systemic delivery of molecules. The large alveolar surface area, thin tissue lining, and limited numbers of proteolytic enzymes make the lung an ideal location for proteins and peptides to enter the bloodstream. A dry-powder aerosol device has recently been approved for the pulmonary delivery of insulin. In addition to insulin, other biotherapeutics that are currently administered subcutaneously—such as growth hormone, glucagon, and α_1-antitrypsin—are being investigated for inhalation therapy.

One approach to achieving increased delivery efficiency is the design of large, highly porous aerosol particles with very low densities. Such particles tend to aggregate less than smaller, denser particles, resulting in more efficient aerosolization. In addition, these particles have an ''aerodynamic diameter,'' a parameter based on both density and actual particle dimensions, similar to conventional aerosol particles; thus, they can reach the deep parts of the lung through an airstream, despite their relatively large (5 to 20 μm) size. Once deposited, the particles can escape clearance by alveolar macrophages, because phagocytosis of particles by macrophages diminishes with increasing particle size beyond 2 to 3 μm. Thus, drugs can be delivered more efficiently over longer periods of time. In one study, insulin was encapsulated in biodegradable polymer microspheres. Some of the microspheres were small and nonporous, and some were large and porous (low density), but both types had similar aerodynamic diameters. When the microspheres were delivered into the lungs, the relative bioavailability of the large, porous insulin particle was about seven times greater, and the total time of insulin release into the systemic circulation was about 24 times longer, than that of the conventional particle.

TRANSDERMAL DELIVERY

The stratum corneum, composed of lipids and keratinocytes, is the outermost skin layer and the major barrier to transdermal transport. Small, lipophilic drugs have been successfully delivered through the skin into the systemic circulation by passive diffusion at low flux rates, thereby avoiding first-pass metabolism by the liver. Currently, passive transdermal patches are available for hormone replacement and for pharmacologic treatment of motion sickness, angina, nicotine withdrawal, hypertension, pain, and other conditions.

In addition to providing greater bioavailability while remaining noninvasive, transdermal delivery systems are often associated with fewer adverse effects than conventional oral dosage forms. For example, liver damage during first-pass metabolism is avoided when a drug is delivered by the transdermal route. Thus, more sophisticated transdermal systems are under development in an attempt to provide these advantages for drug molecules that are normally unable to penetrate the skin. **Iontophoresis** is one approach to enhancing the transport of charged low molecular mass molecules through the skin. Iontophoresis involves the application of low-voltage electric pulses for long time periods; this technology is already used clinically for local applications, such as therapy for hyperhidrosis (excessive perspiration), and it is under development for systemic delivery of small-molecule analgesic drugs. The use of high-voltage pulses for a short time period—on the order of milliseconds—is also being explored. In human cadaver skin, which is commonly used as a model for skin transport, such high-voltage pulses have been shown to induce temporary pores. This phenomenon, known as **electroporation,** will potentially allow systemic delivery of large, charged molecules, such as heparin and oligonucleotides.

Ultrasound enhancement of drug delivery through the skin, termed **sonophoresis,** is also being explored for molecules such as insulin, interferon, and erythropoietin. Application of ultrasound to the skin results in cavitation, the formation of tiny air-filled spaces in lipid bilayers of the stratum corneum. The net result of cavitation is disordering of the lipid bilayers, enhancing diffusivity of the drug through the skin by up to 1,000 times. Sonophoresis does not damage the skin, which typically regains its normal structure within 2 hours, and no undesirable effects have been observed in early clinical trials.

Sonophoresis can also be used to remove diagnostic samples from the extracellular space under the stratum corneum. Experiments have been devised in which a reservoir was placed between an ultrasound transducer and a rat's skin, and interstitial fluid was extracted. Theophylline, glucose, cholesterol, urea, and calcium could be measured in the sample; the glucose measurements were accurate enough to be used as a surrogate for blood glucose monitoring in diabetics. With a portable ultrasound transducer, this technique could be incorporated in a futuristic device such as the one Mr. F used in 2014.

POLYMER-BASED DELIVERY SYSTEMS

GENERAL MECHANISMS

Polymer-based drug delivery systems gradually release drugs into their surroundings. Polymer delivery mechanisms are widely used in diverse applications such as birth control, chemotherapy, and antiarrhythmic therapy. These systems offer advantages in both controlled release and targeting of drugs and are thus the focus of much research. Drug delivery from a polymer-based system can be achieved via three general mechanisms: (1) diffusion; (2) chemical reaction; and (3) solvent activation (Fig. 54-1).

Diffusion

Diffusion from either a reservoir or a matrix is the most common release mechanism. In a reservoir system, the drug is contained within a polymer membrane through which it diffuses over time (Fig. 54-1A). Norplant, a long-term contraceptive system (no longer marketed in the U.S.), acts by this principle. **Levonorgestrel,** a synthetic progestin, is stored in small silicone tubes implanted in the arm. The drug diffuses slowly through the polymer capsule over the course of 5 years, providing effective long-term contraception. (For a further discussion of progestin action on the menstrual cycle, see Chapter 28, Pharmacology of Reproduction.) However, such reservoir systems are limited by the size of the drug molecules being delivered. Molecules larger than approximately 300 Daltons (Da) are unable to diffuse through the polymer shell.

In one common matrix system design, the drug is contained in a series of interconnecting pores within the polymer, rather than in one large reservoir. This system is less limited by the size of the drug molecules because each pore can accommodate molecules with molecular weights of several million Daltons. The rate of diffusion between the pores—and thus through the matrix and out of the system—is controlled architecturally; tight constrictions and tortuous connections between pores prevent rapid release of the stored drug. One such system is used clinically to administer **gonadotropin releasing hormone (GnRH) analogues.** GnRH analogues are peptide hormones that, when administered continuously, inhibit anterior pituitary gland production of gonadotropins (LH and FSH) and are useful in the treatment of sex-hormone–dependent diseases such as prostate cancer. A major previous limitation of this therapeutic approach was the short in vivo half-life of GnRH analogues following intramuscular injection. When the drug is incorporated into polymer microcapsules, and the capsules are injected intramuscularly, the half-life of GnRH is extended significantly, so that therapeutic concentrations are maintained over a period of 1 to 4 months. Drug delivery by the microcapsule system utilizes two mechanisms: first, the drug diffuses out of the microcapsules; and second, the polymer matrix itself degrades slowly. The second mechanism of polymer-based drug delivery involves a chemical reaction between the polymer and water (see below).

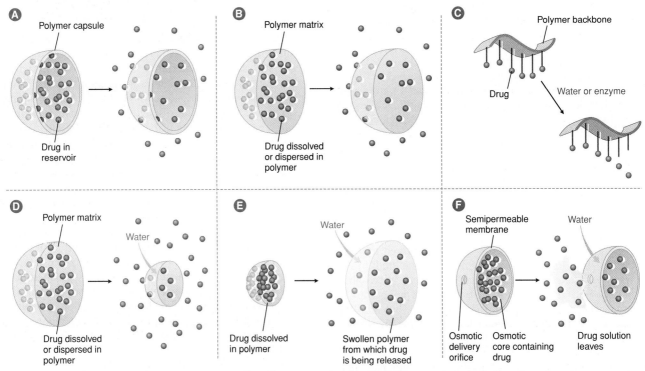

Figure 54-1. Polymer release mechanisms. In all panels except *C,* the simplified diagrams represent polymeric systems in cross section. The most common release mechanism is diffusion, whereby the drug migrates from its initial location in the polymer system to the polymer's outer surface and then to the body. **A,B.** Diffusion can occur from a reservoir, in which a drug core is surrounded by a polymer film, or from a matrix, where the drug is uniformly distributed through the polymeric system. **C,D.** Drugs can also be released by chemical mechanisms such as cleavage of the drug from a polymer backbone or hydrolytic degradation of the polymer. **E.** Exposure to a solvent can also activate drug release. For example, the drug can be retained in place by polymer chains; upon exposure to environmental fluid, the outer polymer regions begin to swell, allowing the drug to diffuse outward. **F.** An osmotic system in the form of a tablet with a laser-drilled hole in the polymer surface can provide constant drug release rates. Water diffuses through the semipermeable membrane into the tablet along its osmotic gradient, swelling the osmotic core inside the tablet and forcing drug solution out through the hole. Combinations of the previously described approaches are possible. Release rates can be controlled by the nature of the polymeric material and the design of the system.

Chemical Reaction

In **chemical reaction-based systems,** part of the system is designed to degrade over time. Degradation can involve either a chemical or enzymatic reaction. In some designs, covalent bonds that connect the drug to a polymer are cleaved in the body by endogenous enzymes (Fig. 54-1C). Such polymer-drug complexes are typically administered intravenously, and the use of water-soluble polymers such as polyethylene glycol (PEG) increases the biological half-life of the drug considerably. For example, PEG-Intron, a pegylated form of **interferon-α2b,** has been approved by the U.S. Food and Drug Administration (FDA) for weekly administration; this treatment for hepatitis C infection previously required injections three times as often. In the case of the intramuscular GnRH microcapsules discussed above, the polymer itself is degraded in a reaction with water (Fig. 54-1D).

Most insoluble polymers considered for these applications exhibit bulk erosion (i.e., the entire matrix dissolves at the same rate), which results in larger pores and a more sponge-like and unstable structure. This pattern of degradation makes constant release rates difficult to achieve and creates the potential risk of undesirable ''dose dumping.'' Novel polymers have been designed to overcome this problem by optimizing degradation for controlled drug delivery (i.e., through surface erosion). For example, a polymer with desirable erosion properties can be engineered by using hydrophobic monomers connected by anhydride bonds. The hydrophobic monomers exclude water from the interior of the polymer matrix, eliminating bulk erosion. In contrast, the anhydride bonds are highly water reactive, allowing surface erosion in the aqueous environment of the body. This design allows the polymer to degrade from the outside only (Fig. 54-2). The rate of degradation can be controlled by using a combination of monomers, one more hydrophobic than the other. The length of time that the polymer persists is specified by the ratio of monomers used, and a drug that is uniformly distributed within such a polymer matrix will be released constantly over time. Based on these principles, Gliadel has become the first controlled-release system for an anticancer drug to receive FDA approval. After surgeons remove glioblastoma multiforme, an aggressive form of brain cancer, they place up to eight small polymer-drug wafers at the tumor site. As the polymer surface erodes over 1 month, the drug **carmustine** (an alkylating agent; see Chapter 37, Pharmacology of Cancer: Genome Synthesis, Stability, and Maintenance) is slowly released. The concentration of carmustine at the tumor site is maintained at a level high enough to kill many of the remaining tumor cells, while adverse effects of systemic delivery are avoided. This treatment significantly prolongs the lives of patients with this cancer.

Solvent Activation

The third mechanism for polymer-based drug delivery is **solvent activation,** in which the solvent does not react with the polymer chemically, but rather initiates drug release via **osmosis** (Fig. 54-1E) or swelling (Fig. 54-1F) of the system. One widely used example of such a system is an extended release oral formulation of **nifedipine,** a calcium channel

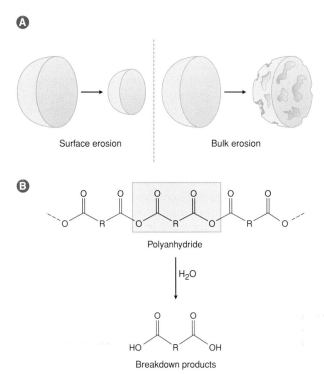

Figure 54-2. Surface erosion using polyanhydride polymers. A. Surface erosion of degradable polymer delivery devices allows for more accurately controlled release rates and is therefore preferable to bulk erosion. **B.** Polyanhydrides are used to promote surface erosion. They have hydrophobic monomers that exclude water from the interior of the polymer matrix and prevent bulk erosion. However, the monomers are linked by water-soluble anhydride bonds, allowing breakdown at exposed surfaces.

blocker (see Chapter 21, Pharmacology of Vascular Tone). The drug is mixed with an osmotically active agent, such as a salt, and coated with a membrane that is permeable to water but not the drug. A small hole is then drilled in the capsule membrane with a laser. After ingestion, the constant osmotic influx of water through the membrane forces the drug out of the pill through the hole, thereby controlling release. This delivery technique, when compared to conventional (immediate release) oral formulations, provides patients greater relief from ischemic events with fewer adverse effects. Concerta, an extended release formulation of **methylphenidate,** uses a similar system to treat children with attention deficit hyperactivity disorder (ADHD).

INTELLIGENT DELIVERY

There are situations in which pulsatile delivery is desirable to mimic the body's natural pattern of producing chemicals. In the case of Mr. F, the insulin pump he wore provided a constant, basal rate of insulin to maintain his blood glucose levels between meals. When Mr. F ate, he could set the pump to provide an additional bolus of insulin and thereby prevent a sudden, excessive rise in blood glucose concentration. Several innovative approaches have been taken to incorporate such versatility in polymer-based drug delivery systems, which have traditionally been designed to deliver drugs at constant or decreasing release rates.

In one early design, magnetic beads were incorporated in the polymer matrix together with a 2-year supply of insulin. The system was then implanted subcutaneously in rats, where the insulin was slowly released by diffusion out of the matrix, as discussed above. When an oscillating magnetic field was applied externally, movement of the magnetic beads within the matrix caused alternating expansion and contraction of the drug-carrying pores. The insulin could thus be effectively squeezed out of the matrix, resulting in higher dose delivery for as long as the oscillating magnetic field was applied. This system significantly lowered blood glucose levels in the treated rats compared to control rats and may eventually become a viable method of insulin delivery. In Mr. F's hypothetical future, the implanted magnetic oscillator allowed him to administer a rapid bolus of insulin simply by selecting the appropriate program on his wristwatch controller, which sent the instructions to the implanted device via a radiofrequency signal.

Other methods of increasing the rate of drug diffusion from a polymer matrix include the application of either ultrasound or electric current. Ultrasound delivered at an appropriate frequency can have an effect similar to that of the magnetic bead system. Ultrasound causes cavitation (the formation of tiny air pockets) in the polymer, disrupting the porous architecture to facilitate faster drug release. Applying an electric current to certain polymers can induce electrolysis of water at the polymer surface, lowering local pH and disrupting hydrogen bonding within the complex. The polymer subsequently degrades at a faster than normal rate, allowing transient release of larger drug doses. Pulsatile delivery can also be achieved via local environmental stimuli. For example, hydrogels (materials composed of polymers and water) can be designed to sense changes in temperature, pH, and even specific molecules by virtue of their structure.

A silicon microchip delivery system that offers even more control over release rates has recently been designed. The microchip contains up to 1,000 tiny drug reservoirs, each covered with a thin gold film. Applying a small external voltage to an individual implanted reservoir dissolves the gold film electrochemically, releasing the drug stored in that reservoir. Because the reservoirs can be loaded and opened individually, almost limitless possibilities exist for both dosing of single drugs and combining multiple drugs.

TARGETING

Accurate targeting allows for larger, more effective doses to reach the tissues of interest without risking the toxic effects of systemic delivery. The first variable that can be controlled is the anatomic placement of the polymer-based drug delivery system; the carmustine wafer delivery system discussed earlier makes use of this basic consideration. Other notable examples include Estring, a vaginal ring that delivers **estradiol** for vaginal dryness; Vitrasert, an eye implant that delivers **ganciclovir** for the treatment of cytomegalovirus retinitis in AIDS patients (see Chapter 36, Pharmacology of Viral Infections); and drug-eluting stents that deliver **sirolimus** or **paclitaxel** for the prevention of in-stent restenosis in coronary angioplasty (see Chapter 44, Pharmacology of Immunosuppression). Many tissues are accessed practically only via the bloodstream, however, making targeted delivery

more difficult. Both passive and active targeting techniques have been developed to direct polymer-based systems to specific tissues following intravenous administration.

Passive targeting exploits vascular differences between the target tissue and other tissues to deliver drugs selectively. For example, high-molecular mass polymer-drug complexes accumulate in some tumor tissues to a greater extent than in normal tissues because the tumor has more permeable capillary beds. Therefore, rather than using lower doses of low-molecular mass anticancer drugs, which rapidly pass through all cell membranes and distribute throughout the body, larger and more effective doses of high-molecular mass polymer-drug conjugates can be used to target tumors. In addition, the polymer-drug conjugates can be constructed in such a way as to allow enzymatic cleavage of the drug after the complex has left the bloodstream and been taken up by tumor cells (Fig. 54-1F). In one example of such a system, the anticancer drug **doxorubicin** (see Chapter 37) is conjugated to a water-soluble, nonimmunogenic polymer through a peptidyl linker. The polymer-drug complex accumulates in mouse melanoma tumors at concentrations up to 70 times greater than in normal tissue because of the relatively leaky microvasculature in the tumor. Once inside the tumor cells, the peptidyl linker is cleaved by lysosomal proteases, releasing the cytotoxic drug. The polymer portions of the complex either degrade or are eliminated by the kidneys.

In **active targeting,** the polymer-drug conjugate is linked to a molecule that is recognized specifically by cell surface receptors in the tissue of interest. For example, a human IgM antibody directed against a tumor-associated antigen can be used to target a polymer-doxorubicin complex to malignant tissues. Linked to the polymer with an acid-labile bond, the doxorubicin is selectively released in the acidic environment of the tumor. In another system, galactose is used to target a polymer-drug complex to the liver via the hepatocyte cell surface asialoglycoprotein receptor.

LIPOSOME-BASED DELIVERY SYSTEMS

Drugs attached to a single polymer chain are stable structures that can remain in the circulation for long periods of time; the drug polymer complexes discussed above in the context of tissue targeting are examples of such systems. However, these polymer chains can accommodate only small amounts of drug, thus limiting the dose per unit volume administered. The potentially high drug-carrying capacity of **liposomes,** small vesicles with lipid bilayer membranes, makes them an attractive option for a circulating drug delivery system.

Important considerations in the design of liposome-based delivery systems include tissue targeting and protection from the immune system. Highly specific antibodies, analogous to those used for active targeting of polymer-drug complexes, can be used to improve tissue targeting. For example, antibodies against the *Her2* proto-oncogene, implicated in the progression of breast cancer and other cancers, are being explored for tumor targeting. Similarly, antibodies against E-selectin, an endothelial-specific surface molecule, can be used to target vascular endothelial cells. Protection of liposomes from the immune system can be accomplished by the addition of water-soluble polymers to the liposomal surface. As discussed above, moieties such as PEG increase the hydrophilicity of the structures to which they are attached; in this case, liposomes are made more hydrophilic in the blood and are therefore less liable to be taken up by the reticuloendothelial system. Because liposomes with the PEG moiety (''stealth liposomes'') have a prolonged circulation time (days), larger doses can be administered without the risk of drug toxicity. These principles have been used to develop liposomes loaded with **daunorubicin** and **doxorubicin** in the treatment of several tumors, including HIV-associated Kaposi's sarcoma. Liposomal **amphotericin B,** used to treat fungal infections, has been approved for clinical application in cancer patients (see Chapter 34, Pharmacology of Fungal Infections). Also, liposomal **cyclosporine** is being studied for targeted immunosuppression following transplant surgery (see Chapter 44).

Conclusion and Future Directions

The delivery modalities described in this chapter represent selected novel approaches to optimizing absorption, distribution, metabolism, and excretion of drugs. There are several advantages of improved drug delivery:

- Drug levels can be continuously maintained in a therapeutically desirable range. Sustained release oral formulations, large particles that can be inhaled, and many polymer-based designs have this desirable property.
- Harmful adverse effects can be reduced by preventing transient high peak blood levels of drug. Designs that alter absorption kinetics, targeted delivery systems (e.g., antibody-labeled polymer-drug complexes), and systems that avoid first-pass liver metabolism (e.g., transdermal delivery of drugs normally taken orally) achieve this goal.
- The total amount of drug required can be reduced, as with advanced inhaler designs. Both a decrease in the number of required dosages and a less invasive administration route contribute to improved patient compliance. Mr. F's case illustrates the influence of lifestyle factors on patient compliance.
- Pharmaceuticals with short half-lives, such as peptides and

proteins, can be successfully delivered using controlled-release polymer-based delivery systems.

Advanced drug delivery technologies also introduce new concerns that must be considered in their design. For example, each material put in the body, as well as its degradation products, must be evaluated for toxic effects; this factor is especially important for synthetic materials such as polymers. Other potential dangers must be avoided, such as unwanted rapid release of the drug from a system intended for sustained release. Discomfort caused by the delivery system or its insertion is another potential disadvantage: Mr. F's insulin pump, while providing better control of his diabetes, was uncomfortable to him. Finally, advanced technology is often accompanied by increased cost, which can be a problem for patients, their insurance companies, and hospitals.

Despite these obstacles, advanced drug delivery technologies play an increasingly valuable role in making the pharmacologic management of disease safer, more effective, and more agreeable to patients.

Suggested Reading

Edwards DA, Ben-Jabria A, Langer R. Recent advances in pulmonary drug delivery using large, porous inhaled particles. *J Appl Physiol* 1998;84:379–385. (*Review of aerodynamic diameter principles and the potential advantages and applications of large, porous inhaled particles.*)

Langer R. Drug delivery and targeting. *Nature* 1998;392:5–10. (*Review of drug delivery techniques, with emphasis on polymer and liposome-based systems as well as novel use of delivery routes.*)

Langer R. Drugs on target. *Science* 2001;293:58–59. (*Short review that addresses some of the challenges of gene therapy delivery systems.*)

Langer R. Where a pill won't reach. *Sci Am* 2003;April:50–57. (*Broad overview of concepts in drug delivery.*)

Leong KW, Brott BC, Langer R. Bioerodible polyanhydrides as drug-carrier matrices: I. Characterization, degradation, and release characteristics. *J Biomed Mater Res* 1985;24:1463–1481. (*Good starting point for learning more about polymer matrix design.*)

Santini JT Jr, Cima MJ, Langer R. A controlled-release microchip. *Nature* 1999;397:335–338. (*More detailed information about intelligent drug delivery using silicon microchips with arrays of drug reservoirs.*)

CREDIT LIST

Figure 1-1: Adapted from an illustration (www.genome.gov/Pages/Hyperion//DIR/VIP/ Glossary/Illustration/protein.shtml) on the National Human Genome Research Institute web site: www.nhgri.nih.gov

Figure 1-2: Data used to render the image in panel A were deposited in the RCSB Protein Data Bank (www.rcsb.org/pdb, PDB ID: 1FPU) by Schindler T, Bornmann W, Pellicena P, et al. Structural mechanism for STI-571 inhibition of Abelson tyrosine kinase. *Science* 2000;289:1938–1942, Figure 1. Panels B and C were adapted with permission from Schindler T, et al (ibid., Figures 1 and 2).

Figure 2-7: Adapted with permission from Stephenson RP. A modification of receptor theory. *Brit J Pharmacol* 1956;11:379–393, Figure 10.

Figure 3-1: Adapted with permission from Hardman JG, Limbird LE, eds. *Goodman & Gilman's The Pharmacological Basis of Therapeutics*, 10th ed. New York: The McGraw-Hill Companies, 2001:3, Figure 1-1.

Figure 3-7: Adapted with permission from Katzung BG, ed. *Basic & Clinical Pharmacology*, 7th ed. New York: Lange Medical Books/The McGraw-Hill Companies, Inc., 1998:38, Figure 3-2.

Figure 4-2A: Adapted with permission from Katzung BG, ed. *Basic & Clinical Pharmacology*, 7th ed. New York: Lange Medical Books/The McGraw-Hill Companies, Inc., 1998:52, Figure 4-3.

Figure 7-14: Adapted with permission from Goldstein GW, Laterra J. Appendix B: Ventricular organization of cerebrospinal fluid: blood-brain barrier, brain edema, and hydrocephalus. In: Kandel ER, Schwartz JH, Jessell TM, eds. *Principles of Neural Science*, 4th ed. New York: The McGraw-Hill Companies, 2000:1291, Figure B-4.

Figure 8-2: Adapted with permission from Changeux JP. Chemical signaling in the brain. *Sci Am* 1993;269:58–62.

Figure 8-4: Adapted with permission from Kandel ER, Schwartz JH, Jessell TM, eds. *Principles of Neural Science*, 4th ed. New York: The McGraw-Hill Companies, 2000:188, Figure 11-1.

Table 8-5: Adapted with permission from Hardman JG, Limbird LE, eds. *Goodman & Gilman's The Pharmacological Basis of Therapeutics*, 10th ed. New York: The McGraw-Hill Companies, 2001:159, Table 7-1.

Table 9-1: Adapted with permission from Hardman JG, Limbird LE, eds. *Goodman & Gilman's The Pharmacological Basis of Therapeutics*, 10th ed. New York: The McGraw-Hill Companies, 2001:137, Table 6-3.

Table 10-1: Adapted with permission from Carpenter RL, Mackey DC. Local anesthetics. In: Barash PG, Cullen BF, Stoelting RK, eds. *Clinical Anesthesia*, 2nd ed. Philadelphia: Lippincott, 1992:509–541.

Figure 11-2B: Adapted with permission from Cooper JR, Bloom FE, Roth RN. *Biochemical Basis of Neuropharmacology*, 7th ed. New York: Oxford University Press, 1996: Figures 6-1 and 6-11.

Figure 11-4: Adapted with permission from Neelands TR, Greenfield J, Zhang J, et al. $GABA_A$ receptor pharmacology and subtype mRNA expression in human neuronal NT2-N cells. *J Neurosci* 1998;18:4993–5007, Figure 1a.

Figure 12-4: Adapted with permission from Hardman JG, Limbird LE, eds. *Goodman & Gilman's The Pharmacological Basis of Therapeutics*, 10th ed. New York: The McGraw-Hill Companies, 2001:554, Figure 22-5.

Figure 12-5: Adapted with permission from Seeman P. Dopamine receptor sequences. Therapeutic levels of neuroleptics occupy D2 receptor, clozapine occupies D4. *Neuropsychopharmacology* 1992;7:261–284, Figure 2.

Figure 12-9: Adapted with permission from Seeman P. Dopamine receptors and the dopamine hypothesis of schizophrenia. *Synapse* 1987;1:133–152.

Figure 14-3: Adapted with permission from Lothman EW. Pathophysiology of seizures and epilepsy in the mature and immature brain: Cells, synapses and circuits. In: Dodson WE, Pellock JM, eds. *Pediatric Epilepsy: Diagnosis and Therapy*. New York: Demos Publications, 1993:1–15.

Figure 14-4: Adapted with permission from Lothman EW. The neurobiology of epileptiform discharges. *Am J EEG Technol* 1993;33:93–112.

Figure 14-5A: Adapted with permission from Kandel ER, Schwartz JH, Jessell TM, eds. *Principles of Neural Science*, 4th ed. New York: The McGraw-Hill Companies, 2000:899, Figure 45-9.

Figure 15-2: Adapted from Miller KW. General anesthetics. In: Wolff ME, ed. *Burger's Medicinal Chemistry and Drug Discovery, Volume 3: Therapeutic Agents*, 5th ed. Hoboken, New Jersey: John Wiley & Sons, 1996: Figure 36-2. This material used by permission of John Wiley & Sons, Inc.

Figure 15-6: Adapted with permission from Eger EI. *Anesthetic Uptake and Action*. Baltimore: Williams & Wilkins, 1974: Figure 4-7.

Figure 15-7: Adapted from Eger EI. Uptake and distribution. In: Miller RD, ed. *Anesthesia*, 5th ed. Philadelphia: Churchill Livingstone, 2000: Figure 4-2. With permission from Elsevier.

Figure 15-9: Adapted with permission from Eger EI. *Anesthetic Uptake and Action*. Baltimore: Williams & Wilkins, 1974: Figures 7-1 and 7-8.

Figure 15-10: Adapted from Eger EI. Uptake and distribution. In: Miller RD, ed. *Anesthesia*, 5th ed. Philadelphia: Churchill Livingstone, 2000: Figure 4-10. With permission from Elsevier.

Figure 15-12: Adapted with permission from Eger EI. *Anesthetic Uptake and Action*. Baltimore: Williams & Wilkins, 1974: Figure 14-8.

Figure 15-13: Adapted with permission from Trevor AJ, Miller RD. General anesthetics. In: Katzung BG, ed. *Basic & Clinical Pharmacology*, 7th ed. New York: Lange Medical Books/The McGraw-Hill Companies, Inc., 1998:421, Figure 25-6.

Figure 17-5: Adapted from Jones RT. The pharmacology of cocaine smoking in humans. In: Chiang CN, Hawks RL, eds. *NIDA Research Monograph 99* (Research Findings on Smoking of Abused Substances), 1990:30–41.

Figure 18-1: Adapted from Ackerman M, Clapham DE. Normal cardiac electrophysiology. In: Chien KR, Breslow JL, Leiden JM, Rosenberg RD, Seidman CE, eds. *Molecular Basis of Cardiovascular Disease: A Companion to Braunwald's Heart Disease*. Philadelphia: WB Saunders, 1999:282, Figure 12-1. With permission from Elsevier.

Figure 18-2: Adapted from Ackerman M, Clapham DE. Normal cardiac electrophysiology. In: Chien KR, Breslow JL, Leiden JM, Rosenberg RD, Seidman CE, eds. *Molecular Basis of Cardiovascular Disease: A Companion to Braunwald's Heart Disease*. Philadelphia: WB Saunders, 1999:284, Figure 12-2. With permission from Elsevier.

Figure 18-3: Adapted from Ackerman M, Clapham DE. Normal cardiac electrophysiology. In: Chien KR, Breslow JL, Leiden JM, Rosenberg RD, Seidman CE, eds. *Molecular Basis of Cardiovascular Disease: A Companion to Braunwald's Heart Disease*. Philadelphia: WB Saunders, 1999:282,284, Figures 12-1 and 12-2. With permission from Elsevier.

Figure 18-5: Adapted with permission from Lilly LS, ed. *Pathophysiology of Heart Disease*, 2nd ed. Baltimore: Williams & Wilkins, 1998:241, Figure 11.7.

Figure 18-6: Adapted with permission from Lilly LS, ed. *Pathophysiology of Heart Disease*, 2nd ed. Baltimore: Williams & Wilkins, 1998:241, Figure 11.8.

Figure 18-7: Adapted with permission from Lilly LS, ed. *Pathophysiology of Heart Disease*, 2nd ed. Baltimore: Williams & Wilkins, 1998:243, Figure 11.9.

Figure 18-9A: Adapted with permission from Lilly LS, ed. *Pathophysiology of Heart Disease*, 2nd ed. Baltimore: Williams & Wilkins, 1998:371, Figure 17.11B.

Figure 18-10: Adapted with permission from Lilly LS, ed. *Pathophysiology of Heart Disease*, 2nd ed. Baltimore: Williams & Wilkins, 1998:371, Figure 17.11A.

Figure 18-11: Adapted with permission from Lilly LS, ed. *Pathophysiology of Heart Disease*, 2nd ed. Baltimore: Williams & Wilkins, 1998:376, Figure 17.12.

Figure 18-12: Adapted with permission from Lilly LS, ed. *Pathophysiology of Heart Disease*, 2nd ed. Baltimore: Williams & Wilkins, 1998:377, Figure 17.13.

Figure 18-13: Adapted with permission from Lilly LS, ed. *Pathophysiology of Heart Disease*, 2nd ed. Baltimore: Williams & Wilkins, 1998:380, Figure 17.14.

Figure 19-1: Adapted with permission from Katz AM. Congestive heart failure: role of altered myocardial cellular control. *N Engl J Med* 1975;293:1184–1191 and Lilly LS, ed. *Pathophysiology of Heart Disease*, 2nd ed. Baltimore: Williams & Wilkins, 1998:11, Figure 1.9.

Figure 19-2: Adapted with permission from Katz AM. *Physiology of the Heart*, 2nd ed. New York: Raven Press, 1992:187, Figure 8.4.

Figure 20-10: Adapted from Skorecki KL, Brenner BM. Body fluid homeostasis in congestive heart failure and cirrhosis with ascites. *Am J Med* 1982;72:323–338, Figure 1. With permission from Elsevier.

Figure 20-11: Adapted with permission from Seldin DW, Giebisch G, eds. *The Kidney: Physiology and Pathophysiology*, 3rd ed. Philadelphia: Lippincott Williams & Wilkins, 2000:1494, Figure 54-8.

Figure 20-12: Adapted with permission from Katzung BG, ed. *Basic & Clinical Pharmacology*, 8th ed. New York: Lange Medical Books/The McGraw-Hill Companies, Inc., 2001:173, Figure 11-6.

Figure 21-1: Adapted with permission from Greineder K, Strichartz GR, Lilly LS. Basic cardiac structure and function. In: Lilly LS, ed. *Pathophysiology of Heart Disease*, 2nd ed. Baltimore: Williams & Wilkins, 1998:9, Figure 1.7. Adapted from Berne RM, Levy MN. Control of cardiac output: coupling of heart and blood vessels. In: *Cardiovascular Physiology*. St. Louis: Mosby Year Book, 1997: Figure 9.2. With permission from Elsevier.

Figure 21-10: Adapted with permission from Benowitz NL. Antihypertensive agents. In: Katzung BG, ed. *Basic & Clinical Pharmacology*, 7th ed. New York: Lange Medical Books/The McGraw-Hill Companies, Inc., 1998:168 and Kalkanis S, Sloane D, Strichartz GR, Lilly LS. Cardiovascular drugs. In: Lilly LS, ed. *Pathophysiology of Heart Disease*, 2nd ed. Baltimore: Williams & Wilkins, 1998:360, Figure 17.7.

Figure 22-1A–D: Adapted from Cotran RS, Kumar V, Collins T, eds. *Robbins Pathologic Basis of Disease*, 6th ed. Philadelphia: WB Saunders Company, 1999: Figure 5-5. With permission from Elsevier.

Figure 22-1E: Courtesy of James G. White.

Figure 22-2: Adapted from Cotran RS, Kumar V, Collins T, eds. *Robbins Pathologic Basis of Disease*, 6th ed. Philadelphia: WB Saunders Company, 1999: Figure 5-7. With permission from Elsevier.

Figure 22-3: Adapted from Cotran RS, Kumar V, Collins T, eds. *Robbins Pathologic Basis of Disease*, 6th ed. Philadelphia: WB Saunders Company, 1999: Figure 5-7. With permission from Elsevier.

Figure 22-11: Adapted from Cotran RS, Kumar V, Collins T, eds. *Robbins Pathologic Basis of Disease*, 6th ed. Philadelphia: WB Saunders Company, 1999: Figure 5-12. With permission from Elsevier.

Figure 23-1: Adapted from Larsen PR, Kronenberg HM, et al., eds. *Williams Textbook of Endocrinology*, 10th ed. Philadelphia: WB Saunders, 2003: Figure 34-5. With permission from Elsevier.

Figure 23-2: Adapted with permission from Scapa Ef, Kanno K, Cohen DE. Lipoprotein metabolism. In: Benhamou JP, Rizzetto M, Reichen J, Rodés J, Blei A, eds. *The Textbook of Hepatology: From Basic Science to Clinical Practice*, 3rd ed. Oxford, UK: Blackwell, 2007: Figure 2.

Figure 23-6B: Adapted with permission from Mahley RW, Ji ZS. Remnant lipoprotein metabolism: Key pathways involving cell-surface heparan sulfate proteoglycans and apolipoprotein E. *J Lipid Res* 1999;40:1–16.

Figure 23-8: Adapted with permission from Quinn MT, Parthsarathy S, Fong LG, Steinberg D. Oxidatively modified low density lipoproteins: a potential role in recruitment and retention of monocyte/macrophages during atherogenesis. *Proc Natl Acad Sci USA* 1987;84:2995–2998, Figure 1.

Figure 23-9B: Adapted with permission from Scapa Ef, Kanno K, Cohen DE. Lipoprotein metabolism. In: Benhamou JP, Rizzetto M, Reichen J, Rodés J, Blei A, eds. *The Textbook of Hepatology: From Basic Science to Clinical Practice*, 3rd ed. Oxford, UK: Blackwell, 2007: Figure 6B.

Figure 23-11: Adapted from Vaughan CJ, Gotto AM Jr, Basson CT. The evolving role of statins in the management of atherosclerosis. *J Am Coll Cardiol* 2000;35:1–10. With permission from Elsevier.

Table 23-1: Adapted from Jonas A. Lipoprotein structure. In: Vance DE, Vance JE, eds. *Biochemistry of Lipids, Lipoproteins and Membranes,* 4th ed. Amsterdam: Elsevier, 2002:483–504. With permission from Elsevier.

Table 23-4: Adapted from Grundy SM, Cleeman JI, Merz CN, et al. Implications of recent clinical trials for the National Cholesterol Education Program Adult Treatment Panel III Guidelines. *J Am Coll Cardiol* 2004;44:720–732. With permission from Elsevier.

Figure 24-1: Adapted with permission from Deshmukh R, Smith A, Lilly LS. Hypertension. In: Lilly LS, ed. *Pathophysiology of Heart Disease*, 2nd ed. Baltimore: Williams & Wilkins, 1998:270, Figure 13.3.

Figure 24-2: Adapted with permission from Deshmukh R, Smith A, Lilly LS. Hypertension. In: Lilly LS, ed. *Pathophysiology of Heart Disease*, 2nd ed. Baltimore: Williams & Wilkins, 1998:286, Figure 13.10.

Figure 24-5: Adapted with permission from Lilly LS, ed. *Pathophysiology of Heart Disease*, 2nd ed. Baltimore: Williams & Wilkins, 1998:141, Figure 6.5.

Figure 24-6: Adapted from Gould KL, Lipscomb K. Effects of coronary stenoses on coronary flow reserve and resistance. *Am J Cardiol* 1974;34:48–55, Figure 2. With permission from Elsevier.

Figure 24-7: Adapted with permission from Libby P. Current concepts of the pathogenesis of acute coronary syndromes. *Circulation* 2001;104:365–372.

Figure 24-8: Adapted with permission from Libby P. Current concepts of the pathogenesis of acute coronary syndromes. *Circulation* 2001;104:365–372.

Figure 24-10: Adapted with permission from Frankel SK, Fifer MA. Heart failure. In: Lilly LS, ed. *Pathophysiology of Heart Disease*, 2nd ed. Baltimore: Williams & Wilkins, 1998:199, Figure 9.5.

Figure 24-11: Adapted with permission from Harvey RA, Champe PC, eds. *Lippincott's Illustrated Reviews: Pharmacology*. Philadelphia: Lippincott Williams & Wilkins, 1992: 157, Figure 16-6.

Table 24-1: Data (available at hin.nhlbi.nih.gov/nhbpep_slds/jnc/jncp2_2.htm) from The Seventh Report of the Joint National Committee on Prevention, Detection, Evaluation, and Treatment of High Blood Pressure, 2003 (available on the National Heart, Lung, and Blood Institute web site at www.nhlbi.nih.gov/guidelines/hypertension/).

Table 24-4: Adapted from Kaplan NM. Systemic hypertension: therapy. In: Zipes DP, Libby P, Bonow RO, Braunwald E, eds. *Braunwald's Heart Disease*, 7th ed. Philadelphia: Elsevier Saunders, 2005: Table 38-4. With permission from Elsevier.

Figure 27-2: Adapted from Cotran RS, Kumar V, Collins T, eds. *Robbins Pathologic Basis of Disease*, 6th ed. Philadelphia: WB Saunders Company, 1999: Figure 26-27. With permission from Elsevier.

Figure 27-8: Adapted from Cotran RS, Kumar V, Collins T, eds. *Robbins Pathologic Basis of Disease*, 6th ed. Philadelphia: WB Saunders Company, 1999: Figure 26-27. With permission from Elsevier.

Figure 28-5: Adapted with permission from Thorneycroft IH, Mishell DR Jr, Stone SC, et al. The relation of serum 17-hydroxyprogesterone and estradiol-17β levels during the human menstrual cycle. *Am J Obstet Gynecol* 1971;111:947–951.

Figure 29-4: Adapted with permission from Braunwald E, Fauci AS, et al, eds. *Harrison's Principles of Internal Medicine*, 15th ed. New York: The McGraw-Hill Companies, 2001: Figure 33-34.

Figure 31-5: Adapted from Haskell CM, ed. *Cancer Treatment*, 3rd ed. Philadelphia: WB Saunders Company, 1990:5, Figure 1.2. With permission from Elsevier.

Figure 32-2C: Data used to render the image were deposited in the RCSB Protein Data Bank (www.rcsb.org/pdb, PDB ID: 1AFZ) by Zegar IS, Stone MP. Solution structure of an oligodeoxynucleotide containing the human N-Ras codon 12 sequence refined from 1H NMR using molecular dynamics restrained by nuclear overhauser effects. *Chem Res Toxicol* 1996;9:114–125.

Figure 32-3: Adapted with permission from Dekker NH, Rybenkov VV, et al. The mechanism of type IA topoisomerases. *Proc Natl Acad Sci USA* 2002;99:12126–12131, Figure 1.

Figure 32-4: Adapted with permission from Berger JM, Gamblin SJ, Harrison SC, Wang JC. Structure and mechanism of DNA topoisomerase II. *Nature* 1996;379:225–232, Figure 5.

Figure 32-7: Adapted with permission from PharmAid. Copyright 2003, Jeffrey T. Joseph and David E. Golan.

Figure 35-1: Adapted with permission from Miller LH, Baruch DI, Marsh K, Doumbo OK. The pathogenic basis of malaria. *Nature* 2002;415:674–679, Figure 2.

Figure 35-4: Adapted from www.cdc.gov/ncidod/emergplan/box23.htm

Figure 35-6: Adapted with permission from Huston CD, Haque R, Petri WA. Molecular-based diagnosis of Entamoeba histolytica infection. *Expert Rev Mol Med* 1999 Mar 22; 1999:1–11, Figure 1.

Figure 36-3: Adapted from an illustration kindly provided by Professor Stephen Harrison, Department of Biological Chemistry and Molecular Pharmacology, Harvard Medical School.

Figure 36-4: Adapted from Hay AJ. The action of adamantanamines against influenza A viruses: inhibition of the M2 ion channel protein. *Sem Virol* 1992;3:21–30, Figure 3. With permission from Elsevier.

Figure 36-10A: Data used to render the image were deposited in the RCSB Protein Data Bank (www.rcsb.org/pdb, PDB ID: 2BAT) by Varghese JN, McKimm-Breschkin JL, Caldwell JB, Kortt AA, Colman PM. The structure of the complex between influenza virus neuraminidase and sialic acid, the viral receptor. *Proteins* 1992;14:327–332.

Figure 36-10C: Adapted with permission from Lave WG, Bischofberger N, Webster RG. Disarming flu viruses. *Sci Amer* 1999;280: 78–87.

Figure 37-8: Adapted with permission from Shiloh Y. ATM and related protein kinases: Safeguarding genome integrity. *Nat Rev Cancer* 2003;3:155–168, Box 2.

Figure 37-9: Adapted with permission from de Lange T. Shelterin: The protein complex that shapes and safeguards human telomerases. *Genes Dev* 2005;19:2100–2110, Figure 2.

Figure 37-11: Adapted with permission from Lodish H, Berk A, et al, eds. *Molecular Cell Biology*, 4th ed. New York: W.H. Freeman and Company/Worth Publishers, 2000:797, Figure 19-2.

Figure 37-12: Adapted with permission from Lodish H, Berk A, et al, eds. *Molecular Cell Biology*, 4th ed. New York: W.H. Freeman and Company/Worth Publishers, 2000:806, Figure 19-15.

Figure 37-21A: Data used to render the image were deposited in the RCSB Protein Data Bank (www.rcsb.org/pdb, PDB ID: 1AO1) by Caceres-Cortes J, Sugiyama H, Ikudome K, et al. Interactions of cobalt(III) pepleomycin (green form) with DNA based on NMR structural studies. *Biochemistry* 1997; 36:9995–10005.

Figure 37-21B: Data used to render the image were deposited in the RCSB Protein Data Bank (www.rcsb.org/pdb, PDB ID: 1AIO) by Takahara PM, Rosenzweig AC, Frederick CA, Lippard SJ. Crystal structure of double-stranded DNA containing the major adduct of the anticancer drug cisplatin. *Nature* 1995;377:649–652.

Figure 37-21C: Data used to render the image were deposited in the RCSB Protein Data Bank (www.rcsb.org/pdb, PDB ID: 1D10) by Frederick CA, Williams LD, Ughetto G, et al. Structural comparison of anticancer drug/DNA complexes adriamycin and daunomycin. *Biochemistry* 1990;29:2538–2549.

Figure 37-22: Adapted with permission from Downing KH. Structural basis for the interaction of tubulin with proteins and drugs that affect microtubule dynamics. *Ann Rev Cell Dev Biol* 2000;16:89–111, Figure 9.

Figure 38-4A: Adapted with permission from Mani A, Gelmann EP. The ubiquitin-proteasome pathway and its role in cancer. *J Clin Oncol* 2005;23:4776–4789, Figure 1.

Figure 40-1: Adapted with permission from Janeway CA, Travers P, Walport M, eds. *Immunobiology: The Immune System in Health and Disease*, 4th ed. New York: Garland Publishing, Inc., 1999:4, Figure 1.3.

Figure 40-4: Adapted from Abbas AK, Lichtman AH, Pober JS. *Cellular and Molecular Immunology*, 4th ed. Philadelphia: WB Saunders, 2000:169, Figure 8-3. With permission from Elsevier.

Figure 40-5: Adapted from Abbas AK, Lichtman AH, Pober JS. *Cellular and Molecular Immunology*, 4th ed. Philadelphia: WB Saunders, 2000:173, Figure 8-5. With permission from Elsevier.

Figure 40-6: Adapted with permission from Janeway CA, Travers P, Walport M, eds. *Immunobiology: The Immune System in Health and Disease*, 4th ed. New York: Garland Publishing, Inc., 1999:378, Figure 10.11.

Table 40-2: Adapted from Cotran RS, Kumar V, Collins T, eds. *Robbins Pathologic Basis of Disease*, 6th ed. Philadelphia: WB Saunders Company, 1999: Table 3-7. With permission from Elsevier.

Figure 41-3: Adapted with permission from Serhan CS. Eicosanoids. In: Kooperman WJ, ed. *Arthritis and Allied Conditions: A Textbook of Rheumatology*, 14th ed. Philadelphia: Lippincott Williams & Wilkins, 1999: 516, Figure 24.2.

Figure 41-5: Adapted with permission from Serhan CS. Eicosanoids. In: Kooperman WJ, ed. *Arthritis and Allied Conditions: A Textbook of Rheumatology*, 14th ed. Philadelphia: Lippincott Williams & Wilkins, 1999: 524, Figure 24.6.

Figure 42-2: Adapted with permission from Janeway CA, Travers P, Walport M, eds. *Immunobiology: The Immune System in Health and Disease*, 4th ed. New York: Garland Publishing, Inc., 1999:474, Figure 12.12.

Figure 42-3: Adapted with permission from Leurs R, Church MK, Taglialatela M. H1-antihistamines: Inverse agonism, anti-inflammatory actions and cardiac effects. *Clin Exp All* 2002;32:489–498, Figure 1.

Figure 43-1: Adapted from Cotran RS, Kumar V, Collins T, eds. *Robbins Pathologic Basis of Disease*, 6th ed. Philadelphia: WB Saunders Company, 1999: Figure 14-1. With permission from Elsevier.

Figure 44-7: Adapted with permission from Fox DA. Cytokine blockade as a new strategy to treat rheumatoid arthritis: inhibition of tumor necrosis factor. *Arch Intern Med* 2000;160:437–444, Figure 1.

Figure 44-8: Adapted with permission from Fox DA. Cytokine blockade as a new strategy to treat rheumatoid arthritis: inhibition of tumor necrosis factor. *Arch Intern Med* 2000;160:437–444, Figure 2.

Figure 46-1: Adapted from Mason RJ, Broaddus VC, Murray JF, Nadel JA, eds. *Murray and Nadel's Textbook of Respiratory Medicine*, 4th ed. Philadelphia: WB Saunders Company, 2005. With permission from Elsevier.

Figure 46-3: Adapted from Mason RJ, Broaddus VC, Murray JF, Nadel JA, eds. *Murray and Nadel's Textbook of Respiratory Medicine*, 4th ed. Philadelphia: WB Saunders Company, 2005. With permission from Elsevier.

Figure 46-4: Adapted with permission from Drazen JM. Treatment of asthma with drugs modifying the leukotriene pathway. *N Engl J Med* 1999;340:197–206, Figure 1.

Figure 48-1: Data used to render the image were deposited in the RCSB Protein Data Bank (www.rcsb.org/pdb, PDB ID: 1HXW) by Kempf DJ, Marsh KC, et al. ABT-538 is a potent inhibitor of human immunodeficiency virus protease and has high oral bioavailability in humans. *Proc Natl Acad Sci USA* 1995;92:2484–2488.

Figure 48-4: Adapted with permission from Schreiber SL. Target-oriented and diversity-oriented organic synthesis in drug discovery. *Science* 2000;287:1964–1969.

Figure 49-1: Data from Center for Drug Evaluation and Research 2005 Report to the Nation: Improving Public Health Through Human Drugs, US Food and Drug Administration, http://wwww.fda.gov/cder/reports/rtn/2005/rtn2005.pdf

Figure 49-3: Reproduced from the CDER handbook, US Food and Drug Administration, http://www.fda.gov/cder/handbook

Figure 49-4: Reproduced from the CDER handbook, US Food and Drug Administration, http//www.fda.gov/cder/handbook

Table 49-1: Adapted with permission from Katzung BG, ed. *Basic & Clinical Pharmacology*, 7th ed. New York: Lange Medical Books/The McGraw-Hill Companies, Inc., 1998:68, Table 5-5.

Table 49-2: Adapted from http://www.fda.gov/fdac/special/newdrug/testtabl.html

Figure 52-1A: Adapted with permission from Bertilsson L, Lou YQ, Du YL, et al. Pronounced differences between native Chinese and Swedish populations in the polymorphic hydroxylations of debrisoquin and S-mephenytoin. *Clin Pharmacol Ther* 1992;51: 388–397. [Erratum, *Clin Pharmacol Ther* 1994;55:648]

Figure 52-1B: Photo of the AmpliChip CYP450 array was provided by Roche Diagnostics.

Figure 52-2: Adapted with permission from Weinshilboum RM, Sladek SL. Mercaptopurine pharmacogenetics: Monogenic inheritance of erythrocyte thiopurine methyltransferase activity. *Am J Human Genet* 1980;32: 651–662 and Weinshilboum R, Wang L. Pharmacogenomics: Bench to bedside. *Nature Rev Drug Discovery* 2004;3:739–748.

INDEX

Note: Page numbers followed by *f* denote figures; those followed by a *t* denote tables; those followed by *b* indicate a box.